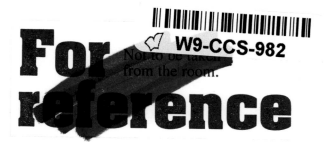

ENCYCLOPEDIA OF

Substance Abuse
Prevention, Treatment,
&Recovery

Editorial Board

ENCYCLOPEDIA OF
Substance Abuse Prevention, Treatment, & Recovery

1

GARY L. FISHER
NANCY A. ROGET

University of Nevada, Reno

Editors

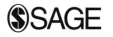

Los Angeles • London • New Delhi • Singapore • Washington DC

A SAGE Reference Publication

For information:

 SAGE Publications, Inc.
2455 Teller Road
Thousand Oaks, California 91320
E-mail: order@sagepub.com

SAGE Publications Ltd.
1 Oliver's Yard
55 City Road
London EC1Y 1SP
United Kingdom

SAGE Publications India Pvt. Ltd.
B 1/I 1 Mohan Cooperative Industrial Area
Mathura Road, New Delhi 110 044
India

SAGE Publications Asia-Pacific Pte. Ltd.
33 Pekin Street #02-01
Far East Square
Singapore 048763

Printed in the United States of America.

Library of Congress Cataloging-in-Publication Data

Encyclopedia of substance abuse prevention, treatment, and recovery / editors, Gary L. Fisher, Nancy A. Roget.
   p. cm.
Includes bibliographical references and index.
ISBN 978-1-4129-5084-8 (cloth : alk. paper)
  1. Substance abuse—Encyclopedias. I. Fisher, Gary L. II. Roget, Nancy A.
  [DNLM: 1. Substance-Related Disorders—Encyclopedias—English. WM 13 E5825 2009]

RC563.4.E53 2009
362.2903—dc22   2008022786

This book is printed on acid-free paper.

08 09 10 11 12 10 9 8 7 6 5 4 3 2 1

Publisher/Acquisitions Editor:	Rolf A. Janke
Acquisitions Editor:	Jim Brace-Thompson
Editorial Assistant:	Michele Thompson
Developmental Editor:	Yvette Pollastrini
Reference Systems Manager:	Leticia Gutierrez
Production Editor:	Tracy Buyan
Copy Editors:	Colleen Brennan, Renee Willers
Typesetter:	C&M Digitals (P) Ltd.
Proofreaders:	Wendy Jo Dymond, Scott Oney
Indexer:	Mary Fran Prottsman
Cover Designer:	Candice Harman
Marketing Manager:	Amberlyn Erzinger

Contents

List of Entries

Reader's Guide

The Reader's Guide is provided to assist readers in locating articles on related topics. It classifies entries into 18 general topical categories: Behavioral Addictions; Classifications of Drugs of Abuse; The Criminal Justice System and Substance Abuse; Engagement and Intervention; Family and Community Issues; Models of Addiction; Neurobiology of Addiction; Prevention Theories, Research, Techniques, Strategies, and Effectiveness; Professional Issues in Addictions; Public Policy Development; Recovery; Relapse Prevention; Research and Evaluation Issues in Substance Abuse Prevention and Treatment; Screening, Assessment, and Diagnosis; Sociocultural and Historical Perspectives on Drug Use; Special Populations: Etiology, Prevention, and Treatment; Substance Abuse Health-Related Issues; Substance Abuse in the Workplace and School; Treatment Theories, Research, Techniques, Strategies, and Effectiveness. Entries may be listed under more than one topic.

Behavioral Addictions

Anorexia Nervosa
Bulimia Nervosa
Cross-Addictions
Gamblers Anonymous
Gambling, Pathological
Gambling, Problem
Internet Addiction
National Council on Problem Gambling
National Gambling Impact Study Commission
Other Addictions
Sex Addiction
Shopping Addiction
Substitute Addictions

Classifications of Drugs of Abuse

Alcohol
Amphetamines
Amyl Nitrite
Anabolic Steroids
Anxiolytic Drugs
Barbiturates
Benzodiazepines
Buprenorphine
Caffeine
Central Nervous System Depressants
Central Nervous System Stimulants
Club Drugs
Cocaine and Crack
Drugs, Classification of
Ecstasy
Fentanyl
Hallucinogens
Heroin
Illicit and Illegal Drugs
Inhalants
Levo-Alpha Acetyl Methadol
Marijuana
Methadone
Methamphetamine
Methods of Drug Administration
Morphine
Naltrexone
Opioids
Over-the-Counter Drugs
OxyContin
Prescription Drugs
Tobacco

The Criminal Justice System and Substance Abuse

Blood Alcohol Concentration
Coercion and Treatment
Court-Mandated Treatment
Crime and Substance Abuse
Criminal Justice Populations

About the Editors

Gary L. Fisher, Ph.D., is the founder and the first director of the Center for the Application of Substance Abuse Technologies at the University of Nevada, Reno. Since 1993, he has received more than $28 million in state and federal grants in the alcohol and other drug field and was the first director of the Mountain West Addiction Technology Transfer Center and the Western Region Center for the Application of Prevention Technologies.

In addition to numerous scholarly articles, Dr. Fisher is the author of six books. His first book, *The Survival Guide for Kids With Learning Differences*, has sold more than 80,000 copies and has been translated into six languages. His textbook, *Substance Abuse: Information for School Counselors, Social Workers and Therapists*, is in its fourth edition. As a result of this textbook, the National Board of Addiction Examiners made Fisher its "Author of the Year" in 1999. Dr. Fisher's most recent book, *Rethinking Our War on Drugs: Candid Talk About Controversial Issues,* was published in 2006.

After receiving a master's degree in 1974, Dr. Fisher began his professional career as a school psychologist in the Seattle area. He received his Ph.D. in applied educational psychology from the University of Washington in 1982 and accepted a teaching position in 1983 at the University of Nevada, Reno. He has a faculty appointment as Professor at that institution and is a licensed psychologist in Nevada.

Nancy A. Roget is the executive director of the Center for the Application of Substance Abuse Technologies at the University of Nevada, Reno, a grant-funded organization involved with training and technical assistance in substance abuse prevention, treatment, and recovery. She is the principal investigator and project director for federal and state grants and has created innovative initiatives, including an online minor in addiction counseling and prevention services. From 1994 to 2001, Ms. Roget taught undergraduate and graduate courses in addiction counseling at the University of Nevada, Reno. Previously, she directed community-based substance abuse treatment programs for adolescents and their family members for 14 years. She holds a master's degree from San Diego State University in Rehabilitation Counseling (1979). Ms. Roget maintains Nevada licenses as a marriage and family therapist and as an alcohol and drug counselor. She has written several training manuals and peer-reviewed journal articles. Ms. Roget has devoted her entire professional career (almost 30 years) to the substance abuse treatment field working as a counselor, treatment coordinator, executive director, trainer, lecturer, project manager, and principal investigator.

Contributors

Ruwida Abdel-Al
University of Nevada, Las Vegas

Eric C. Albers
University of Nevada, Reno

Daniel N. Allen
University of Nevada, Las Vegas

Jane Appleyard Allen
American Legacy Foundation

Susan L. Ames
*Institute for Health Promotion
and Disease Prevention
Research, University of
Southern California*

Ananda B. Amstadyer
*Medical University of South
Carolina*

Shawna M. Andersen
Butler Hospital

Leandro Anit
*University of Nevada School
of Medicine*

Christina M. Armstrong
University of Nevada, Las Vegas

Larry Ashley
University of Nevada, Las Vegas

Stephanie Asteriadis
University of Nevada, Reno

Nathan Azrin
Nova Southeastern University

Daniel M. Bagner
Brown Medical School

Kelly M. Banna
*Medical University of South
Carolina*

Arielle Baskin-Sommers
Brown University

Robinder P. Bedi
University of Victoria

Danielle T. Bello
University of Nevada, Las Vegas

Patricia S. Berry
Prevention First

James Bethea
St. John's University

Arthur W. Blume
*University of North Carolina
at Charlotte*

Ricky N. Bluthenthal
*California State University,
Dominguez Hills*

David Borsos
Chestnut Hill College

Jennifer L. Boulanger
University of Nevada, Reno

Warren G. Bowles III
*Southern Illinois University
Carbondale*

Angela D. Broadus
University of Nevada, Reno

Joanne Brosh
University of Nevada, Reno

Nancy Brown
University of South Carolina

Betty J. Buchan
University of Alaska, Anchorage

Meggan M. Bucossi
Butler Hospital

M. Audrey Burnam
RAND Corporation

Daniel J. Calcagnetti
Fairleigh Dickinson University

Stacy B. Calhoun
*University of California, Los
Angeles*

Barbara Campbell
*Oregon Health & Science
University*

Michael D. Campos
*University of California, Los
Angeles*

Nathan Cardon
*University of Nevada School of
Medicine*

Alan A. Cavaiola
Monmouth University

Sherry Dyche Ceperich
University of Virginia

James G. Chan
Pegasus Consulting, Inc.

Yael Chatav
Brown University

Tony Clark
Hazelden Foundation

Samantha S. Clinkinbeard
University of Nebraska, Omaha

Timothy B. Conley
University of Montana

James J. Costello
Emporia State University

Desirée A. Crèvecoeur
University of California, Los Angeles

Chad L. Cross
University of Nevada, Las Vegas

Alicia L. Danforth
Los Angeles BioMedical Research Institute, Harbor-UCLA Medical Center

Carolyn Davis
Altarum Institute

S. J. Davis
Southern Illinois University Carbondale

Jennifer M. Day
Auburn University

Catherine L. Dempsey
University of Arizona

Jared P. Dempsey
Medical University of South Carolina

Thomas F. Denson
University of Southern California

Caitlin H. Diggles
Brown University

Tiara M. Dillworth
University of Washington

Gail D. Dixon
Florida Certification Board

Bradley C. Donohue
University of Nevada, Las Vegas

D. Gent Dotson
Southern Illinois University

Holly R. Dotson
University of New Orleans

Crissa Draper
University of Nevada, Reno

Carlton T. Duff
University of Alberta

Andrea L. S. Dugan
University of Nevada, Reno

Peggy Dupey
University of Nevada School of Medicine

Thomas G. Durham
The Danya Institute

Denise L. Everett
Quest Counseling and Consulting, Inc.

William Fals-Stewart
University of Rochester

Leah Farrell
Virginia Tech

Sarah W. Feldstein
Brown University Medical School

Ann-Marie Fenner
University of Nevada, Reno

Gary L. Fisher
University of Nevada, Reno

Michael Flaherty
Institute for Research, Education and Training in Addiction

Patrick M. Flynn
Texas Christian University

Katherine W. Follansbee
University of Florida

John Fordham
University of Nevada, Las Vegas

Julie Franks
Harlem Hospital Center

Kevin C. Frissell
Westat

Elizabeth C. Gallon
James Madison University

Michelle D. Garner
University of Washington, Tacoma

Cynthia Jean Gaughf
University of Southern Mississippi

Peter Gaumond
Abt Associates, Inc.

Jason E. Glenn
University of Texas Medical Branch

Abigail A. Goldsmith
University of Cincinnati

Suzanne Gorney
University of Nevada, Las Vegas

Debra L. Gresham
Florida Department of Children & Families

Jean E. Griffin
University of Nevada, Las Vegas

Heather M. Griffiths
Fayetteville State University

Charles S. Grob
Harbor-UCLA Medical Center

Melanie L. Gulmatico-Mullin
University of Nevada, Las Vegas

Glen Hanson
University of Utah

Thomas Harrison
University of Nevada, Reno

Joyce A. Hartje
University of Nevada, Reno

Steven C. Hayes
University of Nevada, Reno

Sarah H. Heil
University of Vermont

Julianne C. Hellmuth
University of Tennessee, Knoxville

Jordana L. Hemberg
University of California, Los Angeles

Christian S. Hendershot
University of Washington

Peter S. Hendricks
University of California, San Francisco

Jennifer E. Hettema
University of California, San Francisco

Stephen T. Higgins
University of Vermont

Heather H. Hill
University of Nevada, Las Vegas

Tom Hill
Altarum Institute

Valerie Hobson
Texas Tech University

David C. Hodgins
University of Calgary

Julie A. Hogan
University of Nevada, Reno

Christina Holman
University of Nevada, Las Vegas

Grace S. Hubel
Medical University of South Carolina

Li-Ching Hung
Mississippi State University

Scott Hunt
Fielding Graduate University

Darryl S. Inaba
Genesis, CNS Productions

Melissa M. Irniger
University of Nevada, Reno

Janita Jerup
University of Nevada, Reno

Rhonda Jeter
Bowie State University

Ann Johnson
Southern Illinois University Carbondale

Mary Beth Johnson
Addiction Technology Transfer Center National Office

Sharon D. Johnson
University of Missouri, St. Louis

Valerie L. Johnson
Rutgers, The State University of New Jersey

David A. Jones
Silom International

Hendree E. Jones
Johns Hopkins University

Nicole A. Kahhan
University of Florida

Jennifer D. Karmely
University of Nevada, Las Vegas

Michelle L. Kelley
Old Dominion University

Scott Kellogg
New York University

Maureen C. Kenny
Florida International University

Jason Kilmer
Evergreen State College

Mora Kim
University of Nevada, Las Vegas

Keith Klostermann
University of Rochester

D. Shane Koch
Southern Illinois University Carbondale

Karen Kopera-Frye
University of Nevada, Reno

Lynn Kunkel
Oregon Health & Science University

Debra Langer
Institute for Research, Education and Training in Addictions

John Waldemar Lazzari
University of Nevada, Reno

Brian D. Leany
University of Nevada, Las Vegas

Ireon Lebeauf
University of Nevada, Reno

David M. Ledgerwood
Wayne State University

Robert F. Leeman
Yale University School of Medicine

Matthew Leone
University of Nevada, Reno

Barry M. Lester
Warren Alpert Medical School of Brown University

Carl G. Leukefeld
University of Kentucky

Michael Levin
University of Nevada, Reno

Therissa A. Libby
The T. A. Libby Group

Jason Lillis
VA Palo Alto Health Care System, Stanford University Medical School

Robert J. Lindsey
National Council on Alcoholism and Drug Dependence

Tanja C. Link
University of Kentucky

Diane E. Logan
University of Washington

Michael D. Loos
University of Wyoming

Sarah A. Lowrey
University of Nevada, Reno

Nora Luna
University of Nevada, Reno

Tory Lynch-Dahmm
Chestnut Health Systems

Terri-Lynn MacKay
University of Calgary

Michael B. Madson
University of Southern Mississippi

Jill M. Manit
University of Nevada, Reno

Peter Mansky
Nevada Health Professionals Assistance Foundation

Patricia A. Markos
University of Wisconsin, La Crosse

Alan Markwood
Chestnut Health Systems, Inc.

G. Alan Marlatt
University of Washington

Steve Martino
Yale University

Jeanne Martino-McAllister
James Madison University

Dennis McCarty
Oregon Health & Science University

Patricia A. McCoy
Community Crisis Services, Inc.

Robert J. Meyers
University of New Mexico

Karen Mooney
Colorado Department of Human Services

Keith Morgen
Monmouth University

Sabina Mutisya
University of Nevada, Reno

Peter L. Myers
Essex County College

Frank Norton
Bowie State University

Joseph Nowinski
University of Connecticut Health Center

Timothy J. O'Farrell
Harvard Medical School at the VA Boston Healthcare System

Emire Olmeztoprak
University of Nevada, Las Vegas

Eileen McCabe O'Mara
Hazelden Foundation

Carrie B. Oser
University of Kentucky

Karen Chan Osilla
RAND Corporation

José Pacheco
Independent Consultant

Robert Packer
Washington State University

Rosalie Liccardo Pacula
RAND Corporation

Penny Booth Page
Rutgers University Center of Alcohol Studies

Matthew Parra
University of Nevada School of Medicine

Candace Peters
University of Iowa

Melissa Piasecki
University of Nevada School of Medicine

Daniel J. Pilowsky
Columbia University & New York State Psychiatric Institute

Nancy A. Piotrowski
California School of Professional Psychology

Amanda Jeffrey Platter
Virginia Consortium Program

Marc N. Potenza
Yale University School of Medicine

Chaithra Prasad
University of Nevada, Reno

Katherine A. Pryde
Swedish Medical Center

Sandra M. Radin
University of Washington

Carol Randall
University of Nevada, Las Vegas

Elke Rechberger
VDT, Inc.

Richard R. Reich
University of South Florida

Judith Resell
*University of California,
Los Angeles*

Patricia Katherine Riggs
*University of California, San
Diego*

Paula Riggs
*University of Colorado, Denver,
School of Medicine*

Rostyslaw W. Robak
Pace University

Nancy A. Roget
University of Nevada, Reno

Laurie J. Rokutani
*Mid-Atlantic Addiction Technology
Transfer Center and Virginia
Commonwealth University*

John M. Roll
Washington State University

Paul M. Roman
University of Georgia

David Rosenbloom
*Boston University School of
Public Health*

Frederick Rotgers
*Philadelphia College of
Osteopathic Medicine*

Emily Rothman
*Boston University School of
Public Health*

Jill Russett
College of William and Mary

Goal Auzeen Saedi
*Oregon Health & Science
University*

Meri Shadley
University of Nevada, Reno

Amy Shanahan
*Northeast Addiction Technology
Transfer Center*

Samantha Sharp
*University of Nevada School
of Medicine*

Stephen J. Sheinkopf
Brown Medical School

Clayton Shorkey
University of Texas at Austin

Yan Shu
University of Nevada, Reno

Stacey C. Sigmon
University of Vermont

Karen Z. Silcott
*University of Nevada,
Las Vegas*

D. Dwayne Simpson
Texas Christian University

Sherry Lynn Skaggs
University of Delaware

Anne Helene Skinstad
*University of Iowa and
Prairielands Addiction
Technology Transfer Center*

Cary Stacy Smith
Mississippi State University

Jane Ellen Smith
University of New Mexico

Joseph L. Smith
*Tompkins Cortland Community
College*

Joshua P. Smith
*Medical University of South
Carolina*

Ira Sommers
*California State University,
Los Angeles*

Susan C. Sonne
*Medical University of South
Carolina*

Kathryn J. Speck
Doane College

Nicolette Stephens
Al-Anon Family Groups, Inc.

Merridy Lynne-Young
Stephenson
University of Nevada, Reno

Stefanie A. Stern
RAND Corporation

Lauren Stevens
University of Nevada, Reno

Patricia L. Stilen
*University of Missouri,
Kansas City*

Maxine Stitzer
*Johns Hopkins University School
of Medicine*

Victor B. Stolberg
Essex County College

William W. Stoops
University of Kentucky

Gregory L. Stuart
*University of Tennessee
at Knoxville*

Barbara Sullivan
University of Utah

An-Pyng Sun
University of Nevada, Las Vegas

Steven Sussman
*University of Southern
California*

Griffin P. Sutton
*University of Nevada,
Las Vegas*

Sumner Jay Sydeman
Northern Arizona University

Ralph Tarter
University of Pittsburgh

Andrew Tatarsky
New York University

Laura A. Taylor
*Southern Connecticut State
University*

Pat Taylor
Faces & Voices of Recovery

Jeff R. Temple
*University of Texas Medical
Branch, Galveston*

Dennis L. Thombs
University of Florida

Rachel D. Thompson
University of Cincinnati

Ellen Tuchman
New York University

Michael Uebel
*Austin Center for Relational
Psychoanalysis and
Psychotherapy*

Roberto Valdez
*University of Nevada,
Las Vegas*

Donna M. Vallone
American Legacy Foundation

Vincent Van Hasselt
Nova Southeastern University

Elizabeth Van Vleck
Emporia State University

Michael Vanyukov
University of Pittsburgh

Amanda Villamar
*University of Nevada,
Las Vegas*

Serena Wadhwa
*Great Lakes Addiction
Technology Transfer
Center*

Margaret L. Walsh
University of Nevada, Reno

Tiffany Walsh
Attorney, Independent Practice

Zach Walsh
Brown University

Judith A. Waters
Fairleigh Dickinson University

Pamela Waters
*Southern Coast Addiction
Technology Transfer Center*

Noreen Watson
*Medical University of South
Carolina*

Megan V. Webster
*University of Nevada,
Las Vegas*

Bryan J. Wedel
James Madison University

Maria Theresa Wessel
James Madison University

J. Lee Westmaas
American Cancer Society

Tara White
Brown University

Keith Whyte
*National Council on Problem
Gambling*

Charles B. Winick
Nova Southeastern University

Katie M. Winters
University of Victoria

Jennifer P. Wisdom
Columbia University

Kristina Wood
*California School of Professional
Psychology*

Briana A. Woods
University of Washington

Li-Tzy Wu
Duke University

Z. Helen Wu
*University of Texas Medical
Branch*

Natalie G. Wuitchik
University of Victoria

Sarah Winsland Yip
*University College
London*

Heidi Zosel
University of Nevada, Reno

Jake P. Zucker
*University of Nevada Medical
School*

William A. Zule
RTI International

Michael Zvolensky
University of Vermont

Introduction

The alcohol and other drug (AOD) field occupies a unique place within the disciplines that are called "health sciences," "human sciences," or "helping professions." These disciplines (e.g., medicine, nursing, social work, psychology, public health, counseling) have long-standing and well-established scientific foundations but rely on the skills of professionals for effective practice. The AOD field also is dependent on the skills of practitioners but does not have the same credibility as the other disciplines because its historical foundation of science is relatively new compared with the other fields. Justifiably or not, the AOD field has been perceived as relying on paraprofessionals for treatment and on tradition, rather than science, for clinical practices. Furthermore, the AOD treatment field has always had, and continues to have, a heavy component of spirituality in the approaches used. This aspect, more than any other, separates the AOD field from other human service professions.

However, in the past 20 years, there has been a tremendous explosion in the knowledge base of all aspects of the AOD field. The recognition of the enormous economic and human costs of alcohol and other drug abuse has stimulated research interest in the biological basis of addiction and effective practices in prevention and treatment. Certification and licensure requirements for prevention and treatment providers have become more rigorous. Formal training programs to prepare professionals have been instituted in colleges and universities. In short, the AOD field has begun to resemble other helping professions: There is a well-established knowledge base, formal training programs to prepare the workforce, and standards of practice established by states.

Although the evolution of the AOD field is positive, the speed of this maturity presents challenges for those who are preparing for careers in the field and those already in practice who wish to be up-to-date. Therefore, this encyclopedia is an effort to compile information on as many relevant topics as possible into one volume. An encyclopedia entry cannot substitute for an in-depth analysis of a complex topic.

However, it can serve to provide a condensed version of a subject, along with guides for further study for those who require additional information.

Terminology

As is the case with many areas in the helping professions, terminology can be confusing. The term *alcohol and other drugs* (*AOD*) has been used in this introduction to clearly indicate that alcohol is a drug and should not be omitted from any discussion about drugs. The phrase "illicit drugs" refers to illegal drugs and legally prescribed drugs used for recreational purposes. "Illegal drugs" are those substances that cannot be used for any medical purpose in the United States (e.g., marijuana, heroin) and drugs that are only allowed to be used for medical purposes in very restrictive situations (e.g., cocaine, methamphetamine). Many other terms can have technical meanings but also are used in general contexts. *Substance abuse* is probably the best example. The *Diagnostic and Statistical Manual of Mental Disorders, Fourth Edition, Text Revision* (*DSM-IV-TR*) contains specific criteria for a diagnosis of a substance abuse disorder. However, the term is frequently used in a general sense, including in the title of this encyclopedia and in the name of federal agencies (e.g., Center for Substance Abuse Treatment, Center for Substance Abuse Prevention), to refer to all aspects of the AOD field. William White, a well-known recovery advocate, has argued that the term *substance abuse* is stigmatizing and inappropriate. *Abuse* has negative connotations (e.g., physical abuse, sexual abuse), and those people who have problems with alcohol and other drugs normally have great love, respect, and admiration for the substances they use. Unfortunately, it is difficult to change habits with regard to the use of the term *substance abuse*. Therefore, there are places in this volume where the term is used in a general sense and other places where *substance abuse* refers to the specific condition as defined in the *DSM-IV-TR*.

The use of terms such as *alcoholic, alcoholism, addict, drug addiction, chemical dependency*, and *substance dependence* can also be problematic. This is not an issue that is unique to the AOD field. Professionals in the mental health field may use the term *neurosis* in a very specific sense or to generally refer to a variety of mental disorders. Similarly, you will find that the various contributors to this encyclopedia may use different terms to describe the same condition. For example, we (your editors) use the term *addiction* or *addict* when referring to any condition or person who is dependent (according to the *DSM-IV-TR*) on alcohol or other mind-altering drugs. Some of the contributors use the term *chemical dependency* to refer to substance dependence. Obviously, *alcoholic* and *alcoholism* refer to dependence on alcohol. For nearly everyone, *drug addiction* is used to describe dependence on illicit drugs. However, some people, when using the term *addicts,* are describing only those individuals who are dependent on illicit drugs. The context of the discussion should help the reader discern the exact meaning of the term used in the entry. Similar to the term *substance abuse, substance dependence* has a technical meaning when used to describe the condition in the *DSM-IV-TR*. However, some authors use the term in a general sense.

The final terminology issue involves the term used to describe groups such as Alcoholics Anonymous. Historically, these groups were called *self-help groups*. However, a more enlightened term is *support groups*. Alcoholics Anonymous and other groups of this type are designed to support recovery from AOD and other addictions. The self-help movement in psychology is completely different than the process of Twelve-Step recovery groups. Thus, we have made every attempt to ensure that the term *support groups*, instead of *self-help groups*, is used throughout the encyclopedia.

Audience

This encyclopedia is intended for use by pre-service and in-service addiction prevention and treatment providers and allied professionals. Allied professionals include those in the following fields: criminal justice, counseling, social work, public health, nursing, medicine, other health care professions, education, and family studies. All of these allied professions encounter individuals with substance use issues or the consequences from substance abuse.

In the past 10 years, colleges and universities have increased the number of formal training programs for addiction prevention and treatment providers. These programs may be undergraduate minors or majors or graduate specializations. The number of courses required, the content of these courses, and the breadth of material varies widely. Therefore, the material in this encyclopedia can serve as a supplement to the courses these students take. With regard to students in allied professions, some are required to take one or more courses in the AOD field, some have elective options, and some have no opportunity for formal course work. Regardless of our feelings about this, the lack of formal training in the AOD field for many pre-service students in allied professions is a reality. Given the prevalence of substance use problems that these potential professionals will encounter, it is essential that they have resources to gain knowledge in this area.

Similarly, the professional already working in the addiction field or in a related profession may have limited time to search for information about specific subjects in the field. This encyclopedia should be a resource for these in-service workers.

Scope and Rationale

In any discipline, it is a challenge to determine what topics to cover in order to provide a comprehensive view of the field. In this encyclopedia, our goal is that readers should be able to find information on almost every contemporary and historical issue in the AOD field that would be of interest to those in prevention, treatment, or recovery studies or practice. In attempting to reach this goal, decisions were made about topics to include and topics to exclude. The rationale for both types of decisions is important.

The process used to select topics is described in the next section. However, as editors, we did organize this process to achieve our goal for this encyclopedia. We were guided by this question: What information in the AOD field do addiction treatment and prevention professionals and allied professionals (social workers, counselors, therapists, psychologists, educators, criminal justice workers, health care professionals) need in their work with clients? We have been involved in pre-service and in-service training of all of these groups for many years, so we used this experience to guide our initial selection of possible categories and topics. Practical, rather than academic, considerations were a priority. Therefore, compared with other compilations of topics in this field, you will find less emphasis on neurobiology and pharmacology. These are important topics. However, we find that practitioners require a basic, rather than in-depth, understanding in these areas. A probation officer needs to know the signs and symptoms of methamphetamine use. He or she does not need to understand the neurobiology of stimulant addiction.

We also decided to have limited coverage of specific programs and specific drugs. With regard to the former, there is a great deal of activity in identifying evidence-based programs and practices in prevention and treatment. We have topics on both of these issues. However, if this encyclopedia is to have any long-lasting value, it does not make sense to have entries on all current evidence-based programs and practices (a rather long list) when new ones are being identified on a regular basis. We have made sure that readers are made aware of resources to find which programs and practices are identified as evidence based. The evidence-based programs and practices that do have entries have been in the field for extended periods of time. In future editions of this encyclopedia, we have no doubt that others will be included.

The coverage of specific drugs was handled in two ways. First, there are entries on broad categories of mind-altering substances. Second, for the most common legal and illicit substances, there are specific entries. There are also entries for those pharmacological agents used in addiction treatment and categories of drugs used in the treatment of other mental disorders. If you are looking for information on an obscure substance, you probably won't find it here. In keeping with our goal for this encyclopedia and the question that guided selection of topics, we could not justify allocating limited space to every possible drug in existence. However, in the Appendix, there is a table listing 58 different drugs and substances with the corresponding relevant entry. For example, if a reader was interested in information on the minor tranquilizer Ativan, he or she would be directed to the entry on benzodiazepines.

The topics in this encyclopedia are not limited to drugs and evidence-based practices in prevention and treatment. For example, for readers who are interested in the topic of co-occurring disorders, there is an entry on this general topic, as well as specific entries on Antisocial Personality Disorder, Anxiety Disorders, Attention Deficit Hyperactivity Disorder, Borderline Personality Disorder, Depression, and Post-Traumatic Stress Disorder. It should be noted that each of these specific entries involves the relationship of the disorder to substance use disorders.

Because the volume is designed to be useful to those who are intending to work, or are already working, in the AOD field, as well as those working in allied professions, there are many topics that will be of interest to criminal justice professionals, school personnel, counselors and therapists, health care professionals, social workers, and others. The categories of topics covered in the encyclopedia are listed in the Reader's Guide. Hopefully, the breadth of these categories demonstrates the commitment to the inclusion of topics that would be relevant to our broad audience.

Selection Criteria and Methodology

The initial compilation of topics was completed by the editors. We used our own textbook, other textbooks, and our experience to develop this list. Each topic was placed in one or more of the categories listed in the Reader's Guide. This initial list was circulated to our editorial board for criticism and suggestions. Their input resulted in the addition of topics, deletion of redundant topics, and terminology changes in the topics and categories. The revised topic and category list was then approved by the editorial board. In some cases, a topic was suggested by a potential contributor. We added several entries as a result of these suggestions.

Contributors were recruited through several different processes. First, we circulated a general invitation to contribute through professional organizations such as the International Coalition for Addiction Studies Education and universities with departments or centers focused on the substance abuse field. This was an effective method of involving numerous faculty members in the United States and Canada in preparing entries, and we have contributions from faculty at well-known research centers such as the University of Washington, Brown University, Yale, and the University of California at Los Angeles. We encouraged contributors to forward the solicitation to colleagues, and this also resulted in recruiting authors from other institutions. Prospective contributors were asked to identify topic areas in their area of expertise, and the available entries in the topic areas were then forwarded to them.

Targeted solicitations were sent to organizations, agencies, and individuals. For example, we asked some private research centers to contribute entries on prevention topics. Representatives from agencies such as Join Together were recruited to write the entries on their organizations. The executive director of Faces and Voices of Recovery submitted several entries on recovery topics. Individuals with expertise in a specific topic were identified by editorial board members, by other contributors, or through our own contacts. While these experts did not always accept our invitation, they would usually recommend someone else with expertise in the topic.

Potential contributors with faculty appointments at colleges and universities were assumed to be qualified to be authors. In some cases, we received inquiries from graduate students or clinicians. Graduate students were required to have a faculty member coauthor the entry or to submit a résumé and writing sample that established their qualifications and ability to write. Similarly, clinicians who wished to contribute were asked to submit résumés and writing samples.

Entries were reviewed by one or both of the editors for accuracy, knowledge of the topic, coverage, and writing proficiency.

How to Use This Encyclopedia

Obviously, if a reader wants information on a specific topic, the index should be used to determine if the topic is covered. Blind entries refer the reader to the title of an entry with a synonymous heading. For example, if a reader wanted to find information on driving while intoxicated, he or she would be referred to the entry Driving Under the Influence. At the end of each entry, there is a section titled *See also*. This section assists the reader in finding related entries of interest. Finally, every entry has a section titled *Further Readings*, which will allow the reader to pursue the topic in more depth.

Rather than searching for a specific topic, readers may wish to pursue a number of different topics within a broad theme. The Reader's Guide contains 18 topic categories with specific entries for each category. Quite often, an entry fits in more than one category. The Reader's Guide will cross-reference a specific entry to each relevant category. For example, a reader who is interested in the category Treatment Theories, Research, Techniques, Strategies, and Effectiveness will find that the entry Support Groups is cross-referenced in the categories of Relapse Prevention and Recovery. This should assist readers in finding all entries of interest.

Acknowledgments

It is always difficult to predict the amount of work involved in any huge project. The senior editor (Gary Fisher) was contacted about his interest in this encyclopedia by Neil Salkind, a literary agent and professor who had previously edited an encyclopedia for Sage Publications. Gary had just finished a book and was applying for a sabbatical leave. So, timing and Neil's salesmanship led to Gary agreeing to be the editor for the project. After seeing the extent of work required, Gary recruited Nancy Roget to coedit the encyclopedia. After going through this process, we are not sure that thanking Neil would be appropriate. However, we do acknowledge his skills of persuasion.

With nearly 350 entries and hundreds of authors, many people contributed to the success of this encyclopedia. First, we appreciate the willingness of the members of our editorial board, all of whom are eminent professionals in the field, to lend their experience and expertise: Tim Condon, Jeanne Obert, Tom McLellan, Peter Nathan, Nancy Petry, and Bill Wendt. Our managing editor, José Pacheco, was a great asset with many of the organizational tasks of the project. We want to thank the very professional and efficient staff from Sage Publications who worked closely with us during all phases of the encyclopedia. Jim Brace-Thompson, acquisitions editor, stayed in contact with us and monitored the progress of the project. He was always encouraging and responsive. The reference systems manager, Leticia Gutierrez, and the reference systems coordinator, Laura Notton, handled all the issues with technology and contracts. Leticia was very patient with us as we fumbled with mastering the organizational technology. In the copyediting stage, we were very fortunate to work with an extremely thorough, efficient, and responsive team: Tracy Buyan, production editor, and Colleen Brennan and Renee Willers, copy editors. We especially want to thank Yvette Pollastrini, our developmental editor. Yvette read all the entries and corresponded with us about numerous issues regarding format, content, and authors. She was consistently professional and efficient and had a major role in the timely completion of this encyclopedia.

Obviously, this encyclopedia could not have been developed without the contributions of all of the scholars and clinicians who wrote entries. We are indebted to all of them. However, we want to especially acknowledge Gregory Stuart, formerly a faculty member at Butler Hospital in the Brown University Department of Psychiatry and Human Behavior and now at the University of Tennessee at Knoxville. Greg became so enthused with the project that he recruited numerous colleagues, former students, and his current students to contribute to the encyclopedia. His efforts were invaluable.

A project such as this is time-consuming and intense. We are blessed with supportive families who enable us to do this kind of work. We want to express our love and appreciation to our spouses Carole (Gary's wife) and Ray (Nancy's husband) and our children: Aaron, Brooke, Colin, and Jacob (Gary's in alphabetical order) and Spencer (Nancy's).

Gary L. Fisher and Nancy A. Roget

A

ABSTINENCE

See SOBRIETY

ABSTINENCE VIOLATION EFFECT

The abstinence violation effect (AVE) includes the cognitive and emotional responses a substance abuser may experience after breaking a rule for abstinence. In 1985, Alan Marlatt and Judith Gordon proposed the AVE as an important ingredient of relapse and a variable needing to be addressed as part of their relapse prevention model. In 2001, George Parks, Britt Anderson, and Alan Marlatt suggested that the AVE included the attributions and cognitive dissonance that develop following a lapse in alcohol or other drug use by a substance user who had previously made an active decision to maintain abstinence. It has been hypothesized that a slip or lapse, the first violation of the abstinence goal, has the potential to turn into a full-blown relapse depending upon the attributions an individual applies to the lapse and the level of cognitive dissonance experienced in relation to the lapse.

Cognitive dissonance is a psychological phenomenon that develops when there is a disagreement between goals or values and behavior. In the case of the AVE, cognitive dissonance occurs when an individual identifies her- or himself as an abstainer, while at the same time experiencing thoughts and urges to use alcohol and other drugs. The abstinence "rule" creates the value that, in order to be successful in recovery, a substance abuser must not act on these urges. If the individual encounters high-risk situations (i.e., any situation that increases the risk of a potential relapse), succumbs to urges, and breaks the abstinence rule, a lapse has occurred.

This cognitive dissonance is further complicated by the attributions ascribed to the lapse. The most extreme of these attributions often seen in AVE are internal, stable, and global. In other words, in extreme cases of negative attributions, individuals will view the lapse as an internal flaw ("I should have controlled this") that is stable across time ("I will never get clean") and is attributed to global causes that disregard the context of the situation ("No matter what, I am a failure"). This can result in feelings of being a failure, of being a bad person, or of disappointing those who are closest. These attributions also cause the individual to have a decreased level of self-efficacy (i.e., confidence in the ability to make a behavior change) because of a perception that urges cannot be controlled. Negative attributions, coupled with these decreased feelings of self-efficacy, may lead to increased amounts of cognitive dissonance. As a result of the increased cognitive dissonance, decreased self-efficacy, and negative attributes, substance abusers may feel out of control and as if it is "too late" to seek help. Further, the person may come to believe that "all is lost" in relation to abstinence and that she or he may as well return to previous substance use behaviors. This is an example of dichotomous thinking associated with substance use and the AVE. Thus, the individual may continue to use alcohol and other drugs because of their dichotomous thinking, fail to seek help, and relapse.

AVE may also be seen in substance abusers who endorse controlled substance use. In this case, AVE is called the rule violation effect. The psychological phenomenon associated with AVE is similar to that of the rule violation effect. Instead of the abstinence rule being violated, it is the self-imposed rule for controlling the substance of choice that is violated.

In 1996, William Miller, Verner Westerberg, Richard Harris, and Scott Tonigan suggested that the AVE was predictive in those who experienced relapse. More specifically, they found that those who view their dependence as a disease and commit to a total abstinence belief (i.e., all-or-nothing thinking) experienced more guilt over a lapse and felt as if they had failed. Therefore, relapse prevention approaches, such as the cognitive behavioral approach proposed by Marlatt and colleagues, usually address AVE and methods to cope with an initial lapse or slip.

In 1985, Marlatt and Gordon outlined several strategies for decreasing the negative emotions caused by the AVE in order to prevent the progression of a lapse into a full-blown relapse. The first step in relapse prevention is intervening in the events that occurred to precipitate the lapse. This process includes identifying high-risk situations and possible methods to manage those situations. Second, substance abusers should be prepared to experience feelings of guilt following a lapse and to understand that these feelings are to be expected. Counselors can facilitate this preparation by discussing lapses with clients before they occur, including the feelings of guilt that usually occur following a lapse. Although these feelings may be powerful, clients can be reminded that, by identifying negative emotions and reminding themselves that such emotions are normal, the guilt can be minimized and does that have to lead to a relapse. The third step involves establishing a renewed commitment to abstinence following a lapse. Specifically, a lapse can be conceptualized as the beginning of a new learning process and as an opportunity to recommit to abstinence. Recommitting to an abstinent state after a lapse can allow for change in the negative attributions (e.g., "I should have controlled this") that lead to decreased self-efficacy for positive behavior change (e.g., remaining abstinent). After this renewed commitment, the client should look back over the events that lead to the lapse. During this review, clients can examine whether there is something that they could learn from the lapse to help them cope with similar situations in the future. Counselors and clients can use this information to develop a new plan for recovery based on what was learned from the lapse. Finally, it is important for the client to understand that they have outlets for support, such as their therapist, Twelve-Step group, and sponsors, and that, when in trouble, it is acceptable to ask for help.

Turning the negative emotions caused by the cognitive dissonance and attributions that cause AVE into a learning experience can allow for growth following a lapse. This growth can be empowering, can increase self-efficacy, and can lead to a situation in which the individual is better prepared for high-risk situations that previously may have led to a lapse.

Cynthia Jean Gaughf and Michael B. Madson

See also Cognitive Behavioral Therapy; High-Risk Situations; Relapse; Relapse Prevention

Further Readings

Marlatt, G. A., & Gordon, J. R. (1985). *Relapse prevention: Maintenance strategies in the treatment of addictive behaviors*. New York: Guilford Press.

Marlatt, G. A., & Witkiewitz, K. (2005). Relapse prevention for alcohol and drug problems. In G. A. Marlatt & D. M. Donovan (Eds.), *Relapse prevention: Maintenance strategies in the treatment of addictive behaviors* (pp. 1–44). New York: Guilford Press.

Miller, W. R., Westerberg, V. S., Harris, R. J., & Tonigan, J. S. (1996). What predicts relapse? Prospective testing of antecedent models. *Addiction, 91,* S155–S172.

Parks, G. A., Marlatt, G. A., & Anderson, B. K. (2003). Cognitive-behavioural alcohol treatment. In N. Heather & T. Stockwell (Eds.), *The essential handbook of treatment and prevention of alcohol problems* (pp. 69–86). New York: Wiley.

ACAMPROSATE

Acamprosate (calcium acetyl homotaurinate) is a drug used in conjunction with psychosocial treatment to facilitate abstinence in alcohol-dependent individuals who have recently stopped drinking. Acamprosate has been prescribed in Europe for nearly 20 years. In 2004, it was approved by the U.S. Food and Drug Administration (FDA), becoming the third drug (along with disulfiram and naltrexone) to receive FDA approval for the treatment of alcohol dependence.

Developed by Merck, acamprosate is marketed under the brand name Campral (delayed-release tablets) and distributed in the United States by Forest Laboratories, Inc.

Acamprosate is structurally similar to the naturally occurring brain amino acid taurine and the neurotransmitter gamma-aminobutyric acid (GABA). Although its precise mechanism of action is unknown, acamprosate is thought to facilitate abstinence by normalizing alcohol-induced neurotransmitter imbalances in the central nervous system. Specifically, chronic alcohol consumption can lead to compensatory upregulation (overactivity) of the excitatory glutamate system and downregulation (underactivity) of the inhibitory GABA system. If the glutamate system becomes overactive to compensate for the presence of alcohol, the removal of alcohol may result in a surge in glutamate activity. This neurotransmitter imbalance has been proposed to contribute to some of the aversive aspects of withdrawal and may therefore heighten the risk of relapse. Acamprosate, a weak inhibitor of glutamate activity and possible instigator of GABA activity, is thought to limit glutamate hyperactivity during and after withdrawal (specifically, by targeting N-methyl-D-aspartate receptors), thereby helping to normalize the balance between glutamate and GABA systems. This proposed mechanism of action is distinct from that of other drugs used for treating alcohol dependence: Acamprosate does not alter the rewarding effects of alcohol (as does naltrexone), nor does it alter acute pharmacological effects of alcohol (as does disulfiram).

A number of double-blind, placebo-controlled trials support the efficacy of acamprosate for reducing the incidence of relapse in patients with alcohol dependence. Most studies were conducted in Europe and included adults (18–65 years old) meeting criteria listed in the *Diagnostic and Statistical Manual of Mental Disorders, Third Edition* or *Third Edition, Text Revision* (*DSM-III* or *DSM-III-TR*) for alcohol dependence. Nearly all participants had attained at least several days abstinence prior to study onset. Typically, participants in acamprosate (2 grams per day (g/day) or 1.3 g/day) and placebo conditions also received psychosocial support, with treatment duration ranging from 3 to 12 months. Results from these studies, summarized in several reviews and meta-analyses, suggest a consistent and significant (although modest) effect of acamprosate for increasing continuous abstinence rates (number of days from treatment initiation until the first drinking day) and cumulative abstinence duration (percentage of nondrinking days during the trial period). Despite some variability in findings across studies, acamprosate generally appeared to increase abstinence rates by a factor of 1.5 to 2. The drug proved effective across a range of patient characteristics, and its benefits were often sustained after treatment ended.

In contrast to findings from European studies, initial findings from large-scale trials in the United States have not been supportive. The COMBINE Study, a randomized, multisite trial that included 1,383 individuals diagnosed with alcohol dependence based on criteria listed in the *DSM-IV-TR* was designed to test the individual and combined effectiveness of acamprosate (3 g/day), naltrexone, and a combined behavioral intervention (CBI). Interventions were delivered during a 16-week outpatient program and participants were assessed for up to 1 year following treatment. Whereas naltrexone and CBI each reduced drinking independently, acamprosate had no effect on primary drinking outcomes and did not enhance the efficacy of naltrexone or CBI. Findings from the COMBINE Study contradicted previous evidence that acamprosate and naltrexone are more effective in combination than alone. However, it has been noted that because these drugs have differing mechanisms of action and are well tolerated together, their combination deserves further consideration. Another randomized, multisite U.S. trial examined acamprosate (2 g/day vs. 3 g/day) versus placebo among 601 participants with *DSM-IV-TR* criteria–based alcohol dependence. Participants also received psychosocial treatment. No significant benefits of acamprosate were found in primary analyses. However, additional analyses showed that acamprosate increased abstinence for a subset of individuals with high initial motivation for abstinence. Although the reasons for discrepancies between European and U.S. studies are not clear, it was noted that most participants in the European studies had undergone recent inpatient detoxification, whereas this practice is relatively uncommon in the United States. Another difference was that the psychosocial treatments were more highly controlled in U.S. trials compared to European studies.

The recommended dosing for acamprosate is 2 g/day (two 333-mg tablets taken 3 times daily).

In some European studies, dosage was reduced to 1.3 g/day for those weighing less than 60 kilograms. Acamprosate has a poor absorption rate (around 10% when taken orally) and acts slowly, taking 5 to 7 days to reach steady-state levels. The drug should be administered soon after abstinence is initiated and should be continued if relapse occurs, as some evidence suggests that relapse severity is reduced among those taking acamprosate. The manufacturer-recommended treatment duration is 1 year. Clinical trials indicate that the drug is safe and well tolerated; it has a relatively mild side effect profile and does not have addictive potential. The most commonly reported side effect is diarrhea; others include headache and nausea. Side effects are usually mild and transient, and drug adherence (i.e., the proportion of prescribed doses taken) is typically high. Acamprosate has no known significant interactions with other medications, including naltrexone and disulfiram, and does not interact with alcohol. Because the drug is eliminated primarily via the kidneys, individuals with liver impairment can use it safely (in contrast to naltrexone). However, it is contraindicated (or dosage should be reduced) in those with renal impairment. Acamprosate is recommended as part of a comprehensive treatment program that includes psychosocial or behavioral approaches.

Christian S. Hendershot

See also COMBINE Study; Naltrexone; Neurobiology of Addiction; Pharmacological Approaches to Treatment; Relapse Prevention

Further Readings

DeWitte, P., Littleton, J., Parot, P., & Koob, G. (2005). Neuroprotective and abstinence-promoting effects of acamprosate: Elucidating the mechanism of action. *CNS Drugs, 19,* 517–537.

Mann, K., Lehert, P., & Morgan, M. (2004). The efficacy of acamprosate in the maintenance of abstinence in alcohol-dependent individuals: Results of a meta-analysis. *Alcoholism: Clinical and Experimental Research, 28,* 51–63.

Mason, B. J. (2005). Rationale for combining acamprosate and naltrexone for treating alcohol dependence. *Journal of Studies on Alcohol, 15*(Suppl.), 148–156.

Scott, L. J., Figgitt, D. P., Keam, S. J., & Waugh, J. (2005). Acamprosate: A review of its use in the maintenance of abstinence in patients with alcohol dependence. *CNS Drugs, 19,* 445–464.

ACCEPTANCE AND COMMITMENT THERAPY

Acceptance and Commitment Therapy (ACT) is a psychological intervention method that applies acceptance and mindfulness processes, and commitment and behavior change processes, to the creation of psychological flexibility. ACT is based on a broad research program in human language and cognition, Relational Frame Theory (RFT). In controlled research, ACT has been shown to be helpful with a wide variety of problems including depression, self-harm, chronic pain, anxiety, psychosis, prejudice, worksite stress, employee burnout, diabetic self-management, adjustment to cancer, obsessive-compulsive disorder, trichotillomania, adjustment to epilepsy, and self-stigma, among others.

In the substance abuse area, ACT is known to be helpful for both clients and therapists. For clients, there are successful controlled studies in the areas of opioid addiction, marijuana abuse, smoking, and group treatment during inpatient drug and alcohol treatment. For therapists, ACT has been shown to reduce burnout among drug and alcohol counselors, to decrease judgmental attitudes toward recipients of care, and to increase openness to learning and adoption of new methods.

The ACT Model of Psychopathology

ACT is an approach that is defined in terms of certain theoretical processes, not a technology per se. From an RFT perspective, the most dominant characteristic of human language and cognition is that it is based on learned, relational, and arbitrarily applicable events. Children can readily be taught to relate events mutually and in combination in distinct ways. For example, children learn to treat events as equivalent, different, opposite, or better than one another. When these "relational frames" are learned, they can be applied to any event and the functions of these events can change as a result.

These abilities are spectacularly useful to humans in domains such as reasoning and problem solving, but they raise challenges. For example, humans can remember events by talking about them because symbols and events are mutually related, but this also means that past painful events can be part of any situation at any time, based only on the minimal cues needed for human thought. Being able to compare events allows relative outcomes to be weighed successfully, but it also allows a person to compare him- or herself to an unrealistic ideal and to be found wanting. Being able to construct temporal sequences allows outcomes to be predicted, but it also allows people to fear the unlikely future or to live in the unresolved past to the extent that the present moment disappears. And because these habits of mind are learned, historical, and useful—even essential—they cannot be stopped, eliminated, or suppressed.

From an ACT point of view, verbal and cognitive processes of this kind are almost too useful in day-to-day problem solving and reasoning; as a result, they often become greatly overextended. Human behavior is often guided by relatively inflexible verbal and cognitive processes rather than by actual experience. This is termed *cognitive fusion,* meaning the domination of verbal regulation over other behavioral processes.

As a result of cognitive fusion, thoughts (e.g., "I'm bad") are treated as one would treat actual referents (i.e., a dangerous object). Emotions become labeled and evaluated, and negative emotions begin to be needlessly tracked and avoided. This centrally important process—experiential avoidance—also becomes overextended, and it persists even when avoidance causes behavioral harm. The goal of life becomes "feeling good" rather than living a valued life. Unfortunately, attempts to avoid uncomfortable private events tend to increase the importance of these very events and sometimes even their magnitude and frequency. Psychological inflexibility is the result of this process, as the long-term desired qualities of life (i.e., values) and committed actions that might lead in that direction take a backseat to more immediate goals of cognitive fusion (e.g., being right), or experiential avoidance (e.g., feeling good at all costs).

Substance abuse often seems to be exacerbated or perhaps even caused by these processes. It is known that substance use often has emotion regulatory functions. Use may be occasioned by difficult feelings, thoughts, or memories. Higher levels of experiential avoidance are correlated with higher levels of substance use. Thus, all of these key processes are targeted in ACT.

Six Core ACT Processes in ACT Interventions

ACT aims to increase psychological flexibility by changing the context in which uncomfortable private events usually occasion experiential avoidance. Psychological flexibility is the ability to contact the present moment more fully as a conscious human being and to change or persist in behavior when doing so serves valued ends. The goal of ACT to get the individual to live a more vital life based on chosen values and direct experiences. Psychological flexibility is established through the following six core ACT processes.

Acceptance

Acceptance is taught as an alternative to experiential avoidance or control strategies. In essence, acceptance occurs when emotions are embraced with awareness and experienced as they are, without attempts to change them in frequency or form. Individuals rarely operate from the perspective that they are a person who is *having an experience* (feeling), which becomes *verbally labeled* (e.g., sad). Rather, emotions are viewed as end states that need to be regulated. For example, when someone feels sad, lonely, or worthless, the focus will generally be less on what that feeling is like than on how to get rid of it. Substance use often provides temporary relief from such feeling states, but the impact is only temporary. When an emotion is avoided, its importance in behavioral regulation is strengthened, not diminished. Acceptance methods teach the client to embrace the feeling as a feeling, without the need to take action to change or get rid of it. The client may learn to note where in his or her body urges appear or to note the rise and fall of sensations. Acceptance flows naturally from a state of cognitive defusion.

Cognitive Defusion

Cognitive defusion techniques attempt to alter the functions of uncomfortable private events by changing the verbal context in which they occur. Said another way, ACT attempts to change the way one *interacts with* or *relates to* thoughts, feelings, and bodily sensations. The main goal is to undermine the excessive literal quality of private events and to relate to them as aspects of ongoing experience. Consider the thought "I can never stop using." ACT would provide a wide variety of contextual altering experiences. For example, the thought could be watched dispassionately, repeated several times out loud until only sounds remains, or treated as an external observation by giving it a shape, size, color, speed, or form. A person could thank his or her mind for such an interesting thought, label the process of thinking ("I am having the thought that I am no good"), or examine the historical thoughts, feelings, and memories that occur while experiencing that thought. All of these procedures attempt to reduce the literal quality of the thought, weakening the likelihood to treat the thought as what it refers to ("I am no good"). The result is usually a decrease in believability of, or attachment to, private events rather than a change in frequency. Disrupting the context of literal language reduces attempts to control or get rid of uncomfortable private events and creates flexibility to behave as one chooses.

Self as Context

Self as context is a transcendent sense of being beyond thoughts, feelings, and bodily sensations. Through experiential exercises, ACT attempts to create a sense of self where one experiences him- or herself to be the arena in which private events occur. From this standpoint, one can be aware of one's own flow of experiences without attachment to them or an investment in what experiences occur. Self as context stands in direct opposition to the traditional sense of self, self as content, where the content of thoughts and feelings are experienced as the essence of one's being. ACT believes that attachment to specific content (e.g., feeling happy, thinking "I am a good, sober, or beautiful person") is unnecessary and often unhelpful. A core ACT exercise has clients experience themselves as a chessboard, on which thoughts and feelings are the pieces fighting a war in which they have no investment. Both the client and the chessboard are in intimate contact with all the pieces and are unthreatened by them. Creating a self as context is used to aid both acceptance and defusion and is an example of both acceptance and defusion processes. The core ACT processes are both overlapping and interrelated.

Being Present

ACT promotes observation and nonjudgmental description of experiences in the present moment.

This is similar to meditation and can also be called mindfulness. The goal is to have clients experience the world more directly, rather than experiencing the world constructed by language, or what ACT calls "the world inside the head." Being present, or mindful awareness, is seen as an overarching meta-skill that can be used to aid in all of the ACT core processes.

Values

In ACT, values are chosen qualities of purposive action. Acceptance, defusion, and being present are not ends themselves; rather, they clear the path for a more vital, successful life. ACT attempts to increase an ability to experience uncomfortable private events if doing so is in the service of value-based life choices. ACT does not suggest one should experience psychological pain for pain's sake. However, if, for example, letting go of substance use contacts historical psychological pain (e.g., negative evaluations of oneself, memories of past failed attempts to keep sober, urges), then ACT provides a space in which one can experience that pain without attachment *in the service of* a valued choice, such as continued sobriety. ACT views values as directions, not outcomes. Life is seen as a process by which valued directions are never attained but rather serve to guide the client through a process of vital living. ACT uses a variety of exercises to help clients choose valued directions in various domains (e.g., family, career, spirituality) while attempting to undermine verbal dominance (e.g., "I should value X" or "A good person would value Y").

Committed Action

Finally, ACT encourages direct changes in behavior that are consistent with chosen value directions. This involves setting short- medium- and long-term behavior change goals while identifying and working through psychological barriers that show up along the way.

Each of the other five ACT core processes plays a role in facilitating behavior change. The six processes can be chunked into two groupings. Mindfulness and acceptance processes involve acceptance, defusion, contact with the present moment, and self as context. Indeed, these four processes provide a workable behavioral definition of mindfulness. Commitment and behavior change processes involve contact with the present moment, self as context, values, and committed action. Contact with the present moment and self as context occur in both groupings because the psychological activity of humans always involves actions in the present by a conscious person.

Conclusion

ACT is part of a larger set of procedures, many of which have been shown to be relevant to substance abuse, including dialectical behavior therapy, functional analytic psychotherapy, mindfulness-based cognitive therapy, and mindfulness-based relapse prevention. No one factor unites these new methods, but all have ventured into areas traditionally reserved for the less empirical wings of clinical intervention and analysis, emphasizing such issues as acceptance, mindfulness, cognitive defusion, dialectics, values, spirituality, and relationship. Their methods are often more experiential than didactic; their underlying philosophies are more contextualistic than mechanistic. Together, they are sometimes labeled "third-generation" behavioral and cognitive therapy.

As the work with ACT shows, these new methods seem to have wide applicability, not just to substance abuse but to a variety of behavioral health problems. In addition, the issues they address are not relevant to a single theoretical wing or camp. Issues of acceptance are as relevant to Twelve-Step programs as to ACT. As such, they seem to have the promise of reducing the barriers that exist between the research and practice base and between the various theoretical and philosophical wings of the field.

Jennifer L. Boulanger, Steven C. Hayes,
and Jason Lillis

See also Behavioral Therapy; Cognitive Behavioral Therapy; Counseling Approaches

Further Readings

Eifert, G., & Forsyth, J. (2005). *Acceptance and commitment therapy for anxiety disorders.* Oakland, CA: New Harbinger.

Hayes, S. C., Follette, V. M., & Linehan, M. (2004). *Mindfulness and acceptance: Expanding the cognitive behavioral tradition.* New York: Guilford Press.

Hayes, S. C., & Smith, S. (2005). *Get out of your mind and into your life.* Oakland, CA: New Harbinger.

Hayes, S. C., & Strosahl, K. D. (2005). *A practical guide to acceptance and commitment therapy.* New York: Springer.

Hayes, S. C., Strosahl, K., & Wilson, K. G. (1999). *Acceptance and commitment therapy: An experiential approach to behavior change.* New York: Guilford Press.

Luoma, J., Hayes, S. C., & Walser, R. (2007). *Learning ACT.* Oakland, CA: New Harbinger.

ACCESS TO RECOVERY

Access to Recovery (ATR) was announced by President George W. Bush in the 2003 State of the Union address as a 3-year, $600-million program intended to expand the array of addiction and recovery services available to individuals with alcohol and other drug problems. The initiative, as originally described by President Bush, was intended to provide 100,000 people annually with access to a comprehensive continuum of treatment and recovery support services. ATR marked the first large-scale federal effort to implement a treatment and recovery support services voucher program. It is notable for the role it has played in supporting the development of recovery support services and in expanding the role of faith-based organizations in treatment and recovery systems. ATR is also notable for including peer-led recovery support services as a key component of service continua.

Through the use of vouchers, ATR has provided an indirect funding mechanism that eliminates many obstacles to reimbursing services provided by faith-based and other small, community-based organizations, many of which might not otherwise have access to government funding. A key goal of ATR has been to expand the array of services made available to individuals seeking help for alcohol and drug problems and thereby to increase choice. Under ATR, recovery support services, that is, nonclinical services that assist individuals in initiating and sustaining recovery, have been emphasized as critical service system components.

ATR required grantees to adopt a standard assessment for services provided under the grant, a system for issuing vouchers that can be redeemed for services at eligible providers, and a mechanism for ensuring that individuals served can choose from among different types of services and provider organizations to meet their needs. Vouchers are intended to support client choice under ATR by making available a broader array of service options than would have been available without the program and by providing a mechanism to ensure that funding follows the individual over time rather than flowing directly to programs through grants or contracts. Vouchers also provide a mechanism for quickly expanding and diversifying a service continuum and, potentially, for allowing service capacity to be more responsive to demand than may be the case under grant or contract-funded addictions treatment systems. A wide variety of recovery support services have been available under ATR programs, ranging from transportation, housing assistance, vocational, employment, educational, and child care services to recovery coaching, peer mentoring, and spiritual support. Faith-based and peer-operated services have played a significant role in ATR. Direct funding of providers by contract, grant, or other mechanism has not been permitted under the program.

In 2004, Congress funded ATR at approximately $100 million per year for 3 years, or half of what President Bush had requested in the 2003 State of the Union Address. ATR was implemented through competitive grants from the Substance Abuse and Mental Health Services Administration (SAMHSA) of the U.S. Department of Health and Human Services to states and tribal organizations. SAMHSA awarded grants of up to $7.6 million annually for 3 years to 14 states and one tribal organization: California, California Rural Indian Health Board, Connecticut, Florida, Idaho, Illinois, Louisiana, Mississippi, New Jersey, New Mexico, Tennessee, Texas, Washington, Wisconsin, and Wyoming.

Under the request for proposals issued by SAMHSA, ATR programs could be implemented directly by the state or tribal authority or through the intermediary of another organization, such as a local government or managed care organization. They could be implemented statewide or in one or more municipalities or counties, regions, networks, or other substate areas.

Among the key challenges grantees faced were identifying the array of recovery support services that would be funded, establishing criteria for enrollment of providers and for ensuring accountability, and engaging faith-based and other community-based organizations that had not previously been part of funded service continua. States and tribal authorities generally specify staff credentialing, facility,

service documentation, and reporting requirements for treatment programs. Whereas some recovery support services, such as childcare, require a license, many do not. When licensing requirements or other standards did not exist, the state or tribal authority had to develop criteria that would protect the safety and interests of those served without making it difficult or impossible for many small organizations to qualify. Establishing provider eligibility and performance criteria and integrating new types of services and organizations with divergent philosophies and approaches into a single continuum of services also sometimes proved difficult.

The development and administration of a voucher system and its operation alongside existing funding systems presented challenges as well. Grantees had to not only design, pilot, and implement a voucher system but also develop mechanisms to ensure accountability across funding systems. In addition to accepting ATR vouchers, participating providers might receive a Substance Abuse Prevention and Treatment Block Grant, general revenue, Medicaid, and other funding from the state or tribe, local government, or other sources. Grantees needed to link existing service tracking and reimbursement systems with the voucher system. ATR grantees had to develop and implement incentive systems to reward provider performance. This required establishing performance criteria and mechanisms to measure and provide feedback on performance in a timely manner. Information systems play a key role, permitting grantees to track vouchers, services, expenditures, fund balances, and performance, and to report to the federal government using required Government Performance and Results Act data.

Under the 2004 ATR grants, initial service targets under the grants were somewhat lower than the 100,000 foreseen in the State of the Union Address. The 15 grantees were expected to serve 75,000 clients (none in the first year, 25,000 in the second year, and 50,000 in the third year). Notably, the service target initially adopted was only 25% lower than the original target, which assumed twice the eventual level of funding. In the months following award, the service target was increased from 75,000 to 125,000, requiring grantees to modify approaches in order to reach the more ambitious targets. As of December 31, 2006, grantees had served a total of 137,579 individuals, exceeding the 3-year target well before the end of the third and final year of the grants.

ATR discharge data through the end of calendar year 2006 appeared promising. Approximately 79% reported no alcohol or other drug use during the 30 days prior to discharge. Among individuals reporting substance use at intake, approximately 69% reported no alcohol or drug use during the month prior to discharge. In addition, at discharge, approximately 21% of individuals not having stable housing at intake reported being in stable housing at discharge, 28% of individuals who were unemployed at intake reported being employed at discharge, and fully 55% of individuals showed improvement on measures of social connectedness from intake to discharge. Among those served, 68% were male.

Through December 31, 2006, 49% of ATR voucher funding was used to purchase recovery support services, and approximately 30% went to faith-based organizations providing treatment or recovery support. Recovery support services were provided to 64% of those served under ATR grants, and nearly 67% received clinical services. Data were not available on the percentage that received both services.

In March 2007, SAMHSA released a second ATR request for proposals (RFP). It made available $96 million to fund up to 18 three-year projects of up to $7 million annually. Notably, the 15 original grantees were eligible to apply under the new RFP, which included about $25 million targeted for treatment and recovery support services addressing methamphetamine dependence. Under the new RFP, SAMHSA sought to serve 135,000 people over the 3 years of the ATR program (25,000 in Year 1, 55,000 in Year 2, and 55,000 in Year 3). Applicants were required to discuss the need for methamphetamine-related services in the communities they proposed to serve and to indicate whether or not they planned to address these needs and, assuming they would address them, how they would do so. The 2007 ATR RFP emphasized cost-effective service mixes that included both treatment and recovery support services. In addition, the RFP stated that treatment and recovery support services might need to be provided concurrently and that, in some cases, recovery support services alone would serve as an appropriate intervention. The 2007 ATR RFP also established a performance incentive system for grantees. In it, SAMHSA informed applicants that the third and final year of each ATR award would be funded at 95% of the level of the prior 2 years. The funding balance achieved through this process would be used to establish a performance award pool.

Grantees that met or exceeded their targets for the number of clients served by 25% or more while meeting or exceeding their targets for 6-month follow-up data and while providing services within approved cost-bands would be eligible to receive a supplemental award of up to 5% of the third year requested amount. Under the incentive plan, third-year awards would range from 95% to 105% of the requested amount. New grantees would be required to show how they would maintain administrative expenses at 15% of the award, the same level as was required for 2004 grantees. Existing grantees who applied for funding under the 2007 RFP would be required to develop a plan for maintaining administrative expenses at 10% of overall costs if they proposed to continue serving the same populations in the same geographic area. Current grantees could negotiate up to 15% administrative expenses if they were expanding the program to new areas or implementing other enhancements that might justify the higher level of administrative expenses.

Overall, Access to Recovery represents an ambitious effort to broaden the options for treatment and recovery support services. There have been, and continue to be, differences of opinion on the types of services that should be funded, the eligibility criteria that should be applied for ATR recovery support providers, and the use of vouchers as a funding mechanism. Although ATR has elicited debate, there is broad consensus in the addictions and recovery field about the need to expand capacity, enhance service continua, and increase the flexibility of treatment and recovery systems. ATR offers an approach for accomplishing all three.

Peter Gaumond

See also Center for Substance Abuse Treatment; Office of National Drug Control Policy; Recovery; Substance Abuse and Mental Health Services Administration; Substance Use Disorders; Treatment of Alcohol and Drug Use Disorders

Further Readings

Substance Abuse and Mental Health Services Administration. (2004). *Access to Recovery (ATR) grants* (TI 04-009) (Initial announcement). Retrieved May 24, 2007, from http://atr.samhsa.gov/2004grant.aspx

Substance Abuse and Mental Health Services Administration. (2007). *Access to Recovery*. Retrieved February 21, 2007, from http://atr.samhsa.gov/index.aspx

Substance Abuse and Mental Health Services Administration. (2007). *ATR: Aggregated data profile.* Retrieved May 24, 2007, from http://atr.samhsa.gov/downloads/Aggregate DataProfileDec06.pdf

Substance Abuse and Mental Health Services Administration. (2007). *Fiscal year 2008: Justification of estimates for appropriations committees.* Retrieved February 21, 2007, from http://www.samhsa.gov/Budget/FY2008/ SAMHSA08CongrJust.pdf

Substance Abuse and Mental Health Services Administration. (2007). *Grant announcement: Access to Recovery* (Initial announcement). Request for applications (RFA) No. TI-07-005. Retrieved June 16, 2008, from http://samhsa .gov/Grants/2007/TI_07_005.aspx

ADDICTION, MODELS OF

Although addictive behaviors have existed for many years, doctors and addictions researchers have been studying them for a relatively short time period. Despite many promising trends, professionals have yet to agree on one model of what causes addictions and how best to treat them. Scientific attempts to explain addictions as some kind of disease or psychological affliction are fairly recent. Until the late 20th century, most of society viewed addictions as a kind of moral failing or character flaw. E. M. Jellenik was one of the first to study alcoholism intensely and scientifically in the 20th century. His research led to the American Medical Association recognizing alcoholism as a disease in 1956. Much work continues on this medical model of addictions, but there are other models as well. The more we understand the etiology of addictions, the better we may be able to help prevent and successfully intervene in their treatment.

The Medical Model

The medical model of addictive behaviors, often called the disease model, proposes that addictions are a disease like any other disease and are not a symptom or manifestation of any other underlying psychological or physical process. The model points out that addictions have many similarities to other diseases. They have a predictable course, which is chronic, progressive, and may lead to death if untreated. There is no cure for the disease, but it can be managed safely much as diabetes and other chronic illnesses are managed. Jellinek outlined four discrete stages in the development of alcoholism: prealcoholic, prodromal, crucial, and chronic.

Given that addiction is a disease, any problems associated with it are a result of the addiction and not a cause of it. These would include issues like depression, anger management, failed relationships, lost jobs, and many other maladaptive effects of chemical dependency. There is a presumed genetic or biological cause for the disease, although the evidence for this is inconclusive as yet. For example, monozygotic twins have the identical genetic code, yet they share the disease of addiction from 40% to 80% of the time depending on the study. However, addictions do seem to run in families. The child of an alcoholic has a probability of developing the disease that is about 10 times as strong as someone with nonalcoholic parents. The uncontrollable urges to use a drink or a drug are often seen as evidence of biological factors. However, some researchers have shown that addicts and alcoholics can control their urges to use through a program of positive reinforcements or rewards.

Recent research into the effects of drugs and alcohol on the brain has shown that there are measurable differences in the parts of the brain that regulate pleasure. This includes the way certain neurotransmitters in the brain, like dopamine, are depleted through excessive substance abuse. Such biological indicators are seen as supporting a medical model of addiction.

The Psychoanalytic Model

Many of the models for addiction parallel the historic and prevailing models that try to explain other psychological disorders. The psychoanalytic tradition and its branches have attempted to explain addictions through analytic concepts and structures. This model avers that addictions are the result of some unconscious psychic conflict or tension. As such, an addiction is the symptom of deeper psychological issues and not a disease unto itself.

For example, a rising urge to express anger, aggression, or another strong emotion could be suppressed or inhibited by the individual's moral code, the Freudian concept of superego, which may be telling the person that it is wrong or forbidden to express such a feeling. The conflict between the need to express the emotion and the opposing demand to suppress the emotion could lead to a conscious or unconscious anxiety around expressing certain feelings. The individual may attempt to avoid this conflicted anxiety through the numbing effects of a drug or alcohol.

Substances can also, then, be used to blunt or avoid other unwelcome or hurtful feelings, thoughts, or memories. This is the concept of self-medication. Rather than try to cope with depression, anxiety or feelings of inferiority, the person uses chemicals to medicate away psychological pain. Again, the drinking or drugging is a symptom of another underlying problem. People who were physically or sexually abused develop addictive behaviors at a rate higher than those who were not abused. This process is also a way of coping with the unbearable pain of the trauma.

The object-relations school of the analytic tradition proposes that psychological problems, including addictions, are the result of deficits in the early relationships or attachment figures in a person's life. Hurtful, abusive, inconsistent, or absent relationships with parents or parenting figures are absorbed or incorporated into a person as a negative view of the self and a negative, even unsafe, view of the world. This model proposes that one way an individual would cope with these harsh or negative internalizations would be to drink or drug them away. The ego psychologists in the Freudian tradition see psychological problems as a result of deficits in the sense of self or the ego. Many people complain of feeling empty inside or having a great void where their core self should be. These individuals are trying to numb that feeling of emptiness by mind-altering substances. These ideas could be interpreted as another perspective on the self-medicating hypothesis.

Critics of these ideas point out that it is impossible to scientifically observe or measure such concepts as a superego or unconscious conflicts. They also question whether these concepts could be applied across cultures, as they are a product of a Western mindset and culture.

Conditioning and Learning Theory Models

Classical conditioning and operant conditioning are other prevailing models used to explain psychological problems that are also used to explain the development of addictions. During his famous experiment in classical conditioning, Ivan Pavlov showed that a dog could be conditioned to salivate at the sound of a bell by pairing the ringing with the appearance of a meat powder. After a while, the dogs would salivate at the sound of the bell independent of any food appearing.

Therefore, a behavior could be developed by associating it with another object or event. The desire to drink or drug, then, could be stimulated by pairing it with something else in a person's life. An individual could begin to associate intoxication with things like fun, sexuality, tension relief, or escape from boredom. Therefore, whenever confronted with these events, a person would feel the urge to drink or drug. A person could also connect urges and cravings to use with the sight of drug paraphernalia, drug-using friends, a corner bar, or beer commercials on television. These stimulating objects, people, or events are often called triggers to use and led to the Alcoholics Anonymous motto of avoiding people, places, and things that are associated with substance use and abuse.

Operant conditioning, developed by B. F. Skinner, states that a person is more likely to repeat a behavior if it is followed by a positive outcome or the removal of a negative one. These outcomes are called positive and negative reinforcements. Therefore, a person is more likely to drink or drug again if the episodes are continually followed by positive or negative reinforcements. A positive reinforcement to drinking or drugging could be a feeling of camaraderie, fun or approval of one's peers. A negative reinforcement could be the removal of a feeling of loneliness, low self-worth, boredom, or even the pain of a hangover or withdrawal symptoms. There are some successful experiments that reward people not to use drugs or alcohol, thereby positively reinforcing abstinence. The concept of enabling could fit into this model because the person doing the enabling is seen as removing the negative consequences of a person's addiction, therefore negatively reinforcing the drinking or drugging. The extra attention from the enabler could also serve as a positive reinforcement to substance abuse.

Albert Bandura is the chief proponent of the social learning model of behavior. This model explains that we learn many behaviors by watching others do them. We are not passive responders to unconscious forces or environmental reinforcements as the psychoanalysts and behaviorists propose. This theory states that we are acted upon by the environment but that we also can act on it through our own power and wishes. The model states not only that we learn by observation but that we also can develop the self-efficacy to control those behaviors or alter the environment.

Therefore, we may learn to drink alcoholically by watching dad or learn to abuse drugs by observing friends. Often, first-time drug users must be taught by their peers how to use the substance and how to recognize and enjoy its effects. The expectations of a user also influence the way the person reacts to a drug or drink. If the individual is told to expect something pleasurable, then that is often what happens. If the individual expects a bad experience, then that is the result. Yet, we can develop the power to decide for ourselves whether or not we will repeat the behaviors that were observed. This is called self-efficacy, the ability to act as an independent individual.

The Biopsychosocial Model

This model of addiction attempts to explain the condition by looking at a combination of causative factors: biological, psychological, and social. It hypothesizes that any addiction may be caused by some combination of these factors but not by one alone. There is assumed to be a genetic or biological predisposition in the physical make-up of a person that sets the stage for an addiction. This could include some combination of genes, changes in brain chemistry, or a deficiency in the ability to metabolize alcohol or other drugs. It is assumed that these biological factors are passed down through the family. Adoption, twin, and half-sibling studies have all shown some support for a tendency for addictions to run in families.

Psychological or personality problems added to the biological predispositions may help trigger addictive behaviors. There have been many attempts over the years to delineate the factors in an addictive personality. At this time there is no consensus on what that might really look like. However, some personality characteristics show up in addicts with some frequency. These factors include high anxiety, depression, emotional lability, impulsivity, low self-image, and a low tolerance for frustration or stress. Addicts often share qualities of poor coping skills, poor interpersonal relationship skills, and an inadequate development and use of good judgment.

One of the criticisms of this list is that it can be difficult to tease out which came first: the personality traits or the addictive behavior leading to the traits. Another criticism is that the list is so broad that it can include almost anyone with any sort of psychological dilemma. Even normally functional people can be depressed, anxious, or impulsive at times.

Social factors are also present to cause and maintain an addiction. This include the covert or overt approval of drinking or drugging in a neighborhood, peer group, or culture. In some low socioeconomic environments, heavy drinking or marijuana use is accepted as a normal part of the daily routine, often because there is little else to do. The peer group of an adolescent often supports drinking or drugging behaviors as a way to prove one's rebelliousness or independence from authority figures. Drinking, especially, is frequently viewed as a rite of passage into adulthood, and the ability to "hold one's liquor" becomes proof of virility. Some cultural groups, like Native Americans, have shown a particular susceptibility to the effects of alcohol. Other cultural groups, like Orthodox Jews and Italian Americans, show lower incidences of alcoholism.

Research has shown that certain cultural factors tend to reduce the incidence of alcohol or drug abuse. Societies that regulate the time, place, and functions of using a mind-altering substance are less prone to addictions. Other factors include a lack of tolerance for inebriation, a strong discouragement of excessive use, and no view of substance use as a social power or rite of passage.

A family system that accepts excessive drinking as a family norm could be a social factor. A spouse who covers for a husband who continually misses work or a husband who makes excuses for a wife who constantly sleeps through her responsibilities is displaying enabling behaviors that are part of the addict's social influences. The lack of legal consequences for alcoholic drinking or drugging could also be a social factor.

The biopsychosocial theory proposes that no one factor can cause an addiction; however, one factor can predispose a person to a problem which can then be triggered by the addition of other factors. Therefore, a biological predisposition can be set off by an accumulation of psychological stresses and supported by factors in the social and family environments. The National Institute on Drug Abuse has estimated that genetics accounts for 30% of the cause of addictions, and other environmental factors account for the other 70%.

The Family Systems Model

Addictions seem to be passed down through families at a higher rate than families without addicted members. Some explain this in terms of genetics or object relations. However, many researchers view the development of addictions from the perspective of the family system as a whole. The family is a complicated interaction of relationships, biology, values, beliefs, actions, and emotions. When there is a dysfunction in the parents or even grandparents, this dysfunctionality ripples through the family system, creating problems that must be accommodated for the family to survive. In a dysfunctional family, the accommodations are usually unhealthy ones. The problems are ignored, denied, seen as normal, unresolved, festering, or acted out in harmful ways among the members of the family.

This is particularly true in a family with one or more parent having an addiction. The problems caused by the addictive behavior ripple through the children, often leading to the development of a substance abuse problem in one or more of them. Children raised in a family with one or more addicted parent have a much stronger chance of developing their own addiction.

One particularly potent method of learning an addiction is by watching it modeled by a parent in the family. When dad is stressed, he drinks. When mom is angry, she pops a pill. Dad blames mom for his drinking, and mom blames the bad grades of the eldest child for her need to take pills. Children learn that coping with problems involves altering the mind in some way rather than resolving the problem. They may also learn that they do not have to take responsibility for their own actions because they can blame others for the drug or alcohol use.

The family systems model proposes that all families seek to have some stability or equilibrium in how they function or exist in daily life. This equilibrium is called homeostasis. It helps family members know what to expect in family roles, emotional expression, communications, and other rules of family life. Although families settle into a homeostasis, it may not always be a healthy one. A family with an addicted parent often develops a dysfunctional homeostasis that accommodates the unpredictability of the disease.

Communications are poor; family members are forbidden to talk about certain topics. The system can stifle legitimate emotional expression or even punish emotions that are taboo. Family rules can be irrational, often meant to deny the problem or to keep the peace despite the problem. The children in the addicted household develop certain predictable and unhealthy roles within the family that help keep the equilibrium. One child may become the "hero" child who carries the accomplishments and pride of the family. Another may be the "mascot" who provides fun or humorous relief. Another child may be the "lost" child who just stays out of the way, and one child usually develops into a "scapegoat" role. The scapegoat is the child who develops obvious problems in school, home, or with substances. The problems of this child serve to take the focus off the addicted parent and the troubles in the marriage.

Abuse of alcohol or drugs is part of the family culture, and the children become acculturated into accepting it as a norm or expected behavior. Denial, avoidance, or minimization of the problem helps it grow and continue in the family and encourages its growth in the next generation. This process also includes enabling, where a spouse covers for the intoxicated effects of the other spouse and may then cover for the child as that person begins to drink or drug. This, then, reinforces the behavior.

So the family system begins to revolve around the effects of the parental drinking or drugging, creating great stress on the health of the family members. Often, the sober parent spends more and more time monitoring and covering for the addicted parent's behavior, leaving less and less time for healthy interactions with the children. The children are then left with fewer positive influences and more psychological distress to handle on their own. This coping often leads to drinking or drugging, the one coping mechanism of choice for the adults in the family.

Conclusion

Attempts to delineate clear models of the causes of addictions have varied over the past 50 years. Some of the models have been proposed from existing models of psychological theory, like psychoanalysis, learning theory, and behaviorism. Others, like the medical model and certain aspects of family systems theory, have been developed specifically in response to studying addictions. All of the models have some elements of truth supported by research. However, the field is moving toward a model that would integrate the best of all of the approaches into a comprehensive one that would explain all the facets of the disease. This would include family and psychodynamic factors as well as behavioral, learning, and biological ones.

David Borsos

See also Biopsychosocial Model of Addiction; Cognitive-Social Learning Model; Disease Concept; Genetic Aspects of Addiction; Moral Model; Psychological Models of Addiction; Sociocultural Models of Addiction

Further Readings

Coombs, R. H. (Ed.). (2005). *Addiction counseling review.* Mahwah, NJ: Lawrence Erlbaum.

Doweiko, H. E. (1999). *Concepts of chemical dependency.* Pacific Grove, CA: Brooks/Cole.

Khantzian, E. J., & Brehm, N. M. (1992). A psychodynamic perspective. In J. Lowinson, P. Ruiz, R. Millman, & J. Langrod (Eds.), *Substance abuse: A comprehensive textbook* (2nd ed., pp. 106–117). Baltimore: Williams & Wilkins.

Lawson, A., & Lawson, G. (1998). *Alcoholism and the family: A guide to treatment and prevention.* Austin, TX: ProEd.

Thombs, D. (1999). *Introduction to addictive behaviors* (2nd ed.). New York: Guilford Press.

ADDICTION SEVERITY INDEX

The Addiction Severity Index (ASI) is probably the most commonly used assessment instrument in the substance abuse treatment field. It is part of most clinical intake assessments in more than 20 states and 50 cities in the United States. The ASI also is included in virtually all clinical trials of patients with substance use disorders. In brief, it is a clinician- or technician-administered, semistructured interview that gathers information on seven functional areas often negatively affected by alcohol and drug abuse: medical status, employment and support, drug use, alcohol use, legal status, family or social status, and psychiatric status. It typically is used upon admission to a treatment program and subsequent follow-up contacts. Clinicians may use the ASI in inpatient and outpatient substance abuse treatment settings to assess problem severity and need for treatment in each of the seven different areas. This information is used to develop treatment plans, monitor patient progress, and measure outcomes over time. Presently, the fifth version of the ASI is in use. Efforts currently are under way to complete a major revision of the ASI (version 6).

The ASI was developed on the premise that individuals with alcohol and drug use disorders often have multiple addiction-related problems that frequently disrupt their lives and impair their capacity to recover from substance abuse. Rather than the substance use itself, these problems often are the major concerns of patients and form the basis of the reasons they seek treatment. In addition, the continued unresolved nature of these problems may often trigger relapse to substance use. The ASI was developed to draw more attention to the specific health and social problems that usually complicate patients' recovery from substance abuse and to promote the inclusion of health and social services as part of the broad array of interventions used to help patients become alcohol and drug free. Recent research has shown that the addition of medical interventions, family or couples therapy, and other health and social services significantly improves the outcomes of standard addiction treatments.

Content of the ASI

The full-length ASI is a 200-item test. It begins with a section on general demographic information and then covers each of the seven problem domains separately, using a common format. Each section includes questions about the frequency, duration, and severity of problems over the patient's lifetime and in the past 30 days. Questions include both objective indicators of problem severity and the patient's subjective assessment of these problems. Item format varies, with yes-no, multiple-choice, and open-ended items in each section. An abbreviated 133-item follow-up version allows for measurement of change and pertains to functioning over the past 30 days. The initial ASI usually takes 45 to 60 minutes to complete; the follow-up version takes about 15 to 20 minutes to complete.

The ASI assesses seven problem domains. The *alcohol* and *drug* domains identify the abuse history, periods of abstinence, history of overdoses and delirium tremens, and lifetime treatments. The *legal status* domain assesses major charges, convictions, current charges, current criminal involvement, and probation or parole status. The *family/social relationships* domain notes the patient's stability and satisfaction with current marital status, living circumstances, free time, and any serious relationship conflicts or lifetime problems with relatives. The *medical* domain assesses lifetime hospitalizations and chronic medical problems. The *employment/support* domain inquires about the patient's education and training background, work skills, longest full-time job, and recent employment patterns. The *psychiatric* domain examines the patient's history of hospitalizations and present and lifetime psychiatric symptoms.

Administration and Scoring

The ASI is designed in an interview format to be used by trained individuals. Successfully trained individuals have included receptionists, college students, police officers, physicians, and research technicians. ASI training typically takes 2 full days to achieve minimally acceptable level of administration skill. Other than face-to-face interviewing, the ASI has been administered successfully over the telephone, although telephone administration is recommended for follow-up evaluations only. A computerized multimedia, self-administered version also is available.

The scoring of the ASI is straightforward. At the end of the assessment of each problem area domain, patients are asked to rate (on a 0–4 scale) two separate questions inquiring about how troubled or bothered they have been by these problems over the past 30 days and the degree to which they feel they need treatment (in addition to any current treatment they may be receiving) for this problem area. Based upon the patient's ratings and the interviewer's interpretation of that information for each functional area, the interviewer also makes severity ratings (0–9) that reflect the degree to which the interviewer believes the patient needs additional treatment. The patient and the interviewer severity ratings are meant to aid initial treatment planning and referral; they are not intended to provide an ongoing measure of improvement with treatment or diagnosis. For this latter purpose, the ASI provides composite scores derived from a defined set of items that reflect current (past 30 day) and potentially alterable functioning within each domain.

Normative data are available for numerous populations, including treated male and female alcohol, opiate, and cocaine abusers. Norms are also given on the basis of the type of treatment episode (inpatient, partial hospitalization, and outpatient substance abuse) and for those with substance abuse problems who are pregnant, out of treatment, incarcerated, psychiatrically ill, coerced, or homeless. Norms are provided for demographic, lifetime ASI items, selected 30-day status items, and composite scores. Tom McLellan and colleagues updated the normative values in 2006 based on the responses on more than 70,000 ASIs administered in more than 300 public and private treatment programs in the United States representing all modalities. These norms provide a means for programs or treatment systems to compare their patient profiles to national data.

The ASI is in the public domain, and there is no charge for its use. The National Institute on Drug Abuse has produced a set of training materials that includes two training videotapes, a training facilitator's manual, a handbook for program administrators, and a resource manual. In addition, a multimedia, interactive CD-ROM self-administered version of the ASI is available. The ASI is available in more than 20 languages, including Dutch, French, German, Japanese, Russian, and Spanish.

Psychometrics and Research

The ASI has been studied extensively. Overall, studies involving the ASI support the consistency (reliability) in which it taps the seven functional areas with each administration, in repeated administrations to the same individuals over time, and between interviewers scoring the same ASI interviews. Computer-administered versions of the ASI also have shown good reliability. The evidence for the ASI's consistency is strongest when it has been studied in primary substance-abusing or substance-dependent patient populations. In general, studies have found that the interviewer severity ratings have been lower than the composite score determinations, leading to the recommendation that only composite scores should be used for monitoring problem severity change over time.

Many efforts have been made to establish that the ASI's scales measure what they have been purported to assess. For example, the ASI seven problem areas have been shown to correspond to scores on other measures assessing similar types of problems (e.g., ASI psychiatric composite scores are positively related to depression inventory scores and symptom checklist scores). Furthermore, several studies have provided support for the ASI's multidimensional scale structure. Two studies have derived the same set of scaled clinical dimensions that corresponded to the seven ASI problem areas in samples of methadone and nonopioid-dependent patients. Other studies have shown that among a mixed sample of substance users, the psychiatric, drug, alcohol, family/social, and legal problem areas seemed most valid, particularly among substance users with concurrent psychiatric disorders.

Based on these studies, the "ASI-Lite" was developed. It contains 111 items, requires about 30 minutes to complete in a semistructured interview, and has become the most popular version of the ASI because of its brevity. Other recent studies have produced new shorter ASI scales (e.g., 74-item and 35-item versions) that preserve the ASI's multidimensionality and permit the assessment of change over time.

Limitations

Limitations of the ASI include the following: (a) Patients are able to easily misrepresent their functioning if they are motivated to conceal their behavior, (b) it is unsuitable for use in a self-report format, (c) the 45- to 60-minute period needed to administer it may be too long for some programs and providers, and (d) it is less reliable in special populations such as with homeless individuals and among those with very severe, chronic mental disorders such as schizophrenia. The suitability of the ASI for adolescent populations also is unclear. A teen-focused version of the ASI shows some initial promise, but the utility of this measure in the field has yet to be established. Another limitation is that each of the specific domains lacks assessment of important information. For example, the medical domain does not ask about current pregnancy status of women or medication adherence. The employment/support domain does not distinguish between problems at work and problems finding work. The alcohol and drug use domains do not assess nicotine use or other commonly abused substances such as ecstasy or steroids. The legal domain does not inquire about whether substance abuse treatment is formally mandated by the legal system. The family/social domain does not adequately assess the degree of interpersonal problems outside the family. The psychiatric domain fails to adequately address the impact of psychological trauma, a problem area frequently co-occurring with substance abuse. Finally, given the somewhat subjective nature of the severity rating determinations, careful training in the consistent administration and scoring of the ASI is required and may demand substantial training resources for clinicians to use the ASI effectively.

Conclusion

The major strength of the ASI is its efficient coverage of the major problem areas for patients with a range of different abused substances, both at the initial evaluation and over the course of treatment. It provides easily comprehensible, rapidly applicable, and clinically relevant data that can be readily used for treatment planning and monitoring, program evaluation, or quality assurance purposes. It also is widely used in the field nationally and internationally and has normative data available from numerous populations. Thus, it can provide a common assessment that may enhance communication between clinicians, agencies, and policy planners. Personnel without advanced clinical training may be trained to use the ASI.

Steve Martino

See also Assessment; Assessment Instruments; Screening; Screening Instruments

Further Readings

Alterman, A. I., McDermott, P. A., Cook, T. G., et al. (1998). New scales to assess change in the Addiction Severity Index for the opioid, cocaine, and alcohol dependent. *Psychology of Addictive Behaviors, 12,* 233–246.

Alterman, A. I., McDermott, P. A., Cook, T. G., Cacciola, J. S., McKay, J. R., McLellan, A. T., et al. (2000). Generalizability of the clinical dimensions of the Addiction Severity Index to nonopioid-dependent patients. *Psychology of Addictive Behaviors, 14,* 287–294.

Butler, S. F., Budman, S. H., Goldman, R. J., Newman, F. L., Beckley, K. E., Trottier, D., et al. (2001). Initial validation of a computer-administered addiction severity index: The ASI-MV. *Psychology of Addictive Behaviors, 15,* 4–15.

Currie, S. R., el-Guebaly, N., & Coulson, R. (2004). Factor validation of the Addiction Severity Index scale structure in persons with concurrent disorders. *Psychological Assessment, 16,* 326–329.

Makela, K. (2004). Studies of the reliability and validity of the Addiction Severity Index. *Addiction, 99,* 398–410.

McDermott, P. A., Alterman, A. I., Brown, L. et al. (1996). Construct refinement and confirmation for the Addiction Severity Index. *Psychological Assessment, 8,* 182–189.

McLellan, A. T., Cacciola, J. S., & Alterman, A. I. (2004). The ASI as a still developing instrument: Response to Makela. *Addiction 99,* 411–412.

McLellan, A. T., Cacciola, J. S., Alterman, A. I., Rikoon, S. H., & Carise, D. (2006). The Addiction Severity Index at 25: Origins, contributions and transitions. *American Journal on Addictions, 15,* 113–124.

McLellan, A. T., Kushner, H., Metzger, D., Peters, R., Smith, I., Grissom, G., et al. (1992). The fifth edition of the Addiction Severity Index. *Journal of Substance Abuse Treatment, 9,* 199–213.

ADDICTION TECHNOLOGY TRANSFER CENTERS

In the early 1990s, managed care began to impact the substance abuse counseling field (e.g., increased clinical documentation requirements, shorter lengths of stay, and justifications for levels of care regarding client placement in treatment). With these and other changes brought on by managed care, the substance abuse treatment workforce came under scrutiny. Prior to this time, most substance abuse counselors were considered "paraprofessionals" with limited formal education and training. Workforce studies that focused on substance abuse counselors revealed that less than half had master's degrees and over two thirds identified themselves as being a person in recovery. Based upon data of this type, the U.S. Congress inquired about the readiness and ability of the substance abuse treatment workforce to function within a managed care environment. After numerous hearings regarding the preparedness of the substance abuse counseling field, a congressional mandate was issued that declared the existence of a shortage of well-trained addiction counselors, especially in the public sector. In response to this congressional mandate in 1992, the Substance Abuse and Mental Health Services Administration (SAMHSA) released a request for proposal to fund addiction training centers across the nation in an effort to improve the training and increase the number of substance abuse counselors.

In 1993, 11 centers across the United States were funded. These centers were located at the following universities and state authority offices: University of California, San Diego; Morehouse; Governor's State; University of Missouri; University of Nevada, Reno; New York; Oregon; Brown University; University of the Caribbean; Texas; and Virginia Commonwealth University. Targeting 24 states and Puerto Rico for services, these 11 centers had three main goals: (1) to increase the number of practitioners (counselors) and other allied health professionals treating individuals with substance use disorders, (2) to formally connect publicly funded substance abuse treatment programs to universities, and (3) to develop addiction counseling curricula and revise existing curricula in universities and colleges. Initially, these centers were called Addiction Training Centers. However, the name was changed to Addiction Technology Transfer Centers (ATTCs) about halfway through the funding period. During this initial

5-year funding period, the ATTCs exceeded the established project goals. Accordingly, thousands of substance abuse counselors and allied health professionals received training, there was an increase in the number of substance abuse counselors earning college degrees or certificates, and numerous university-based addiction counseling curricula were developed.

The most significant achievement of the ATTCs during this first round of funding was the creation of training and curriculum standards for substance abuse counselors and other allied health professionals. A committee of ATTC representatives developed and wrote the publication, *Addiction Counseling Competencies: The Knowledge, Skills, and Attitudes of Professional Practice,* which is considered one of the most popular SAMHSA products. This publication identified transdisciplinary foundations, practice dimensions, and 123 competencies as part of addiction counseling standards. To date, it has been translated and used by 15 different countries, adopted by numerous state certification and licensing boards, and used by colleges and universities to develop curricula.

In 1998, SAMHSA reissued the ATTC request for proposals. Fifteen centers were established (i.e., a national office and 14 regional centers) with the goal to include additional states in the identified service areas. During this 3-year funding period (1998–2001), SAMHSA shifted the focus of the ATTCs from preservice university-based services and programs to professional or continuing education training and technical assistance. Whereas some ATTCs kept their university courses and curricula focus, others shifted to offering more training to substance abuse counselors and other allied health professionals. During this funding period, two ATTC-sponsored activities and products stand out as having a significant impact on the substance abuse counseling field. First, the development and production of the *Change Book* by an ATTC national committee provided a guide to organizations on how to deal with change, with a particular focus on the adoption of evidence-based practices. Second, the ATTC located at Brown University led the ATTC network in the establishment and implementation of online learning opportunities in a continuing education format. Currently, two thirds of the ATTCs regularly offer online education opportunities that increase awareness and build new skills in evidence-based practices for clients with substance use disorders. The ATTCs are considered to be the national innovators and leaders in online learning for substance abuse counselors.

In 2002 the ATTCs were again funded by SAMHSA, with 14 regional centers and 1 national office receiving awards. At this time, all 50 states and associated territories were covered by a designated ATTC, and a regional name was created for each center. The following is a list of the ATTCs and their regions: Caribbean Basin and Hispanic (Puerto Rico and Virgin Islands); Central East (Delaware, Kentucky, Tennessee, Washington, D.C.); Gulf Coast (Louisiana, Mississippi, and Texas); Mid America (Arkansas, Kansas, Missouri, and Oklahoma); Mid Atlantic (Maryland, North Carolina, Virginia, and West Virginia); Mountain West (Colorado, Montana, Nevada, Utah, and Wyoming); New England (Connecticut, Maine, Massachusetts, New Hampshire, Rhode Island, and Vermont); Northeast (New Jersey, New York, and Pennsylvania); Northwest Frontier (Alaska, Idaho, Oregon, Pacific Jurisdictions, and Washington); Pacific Southwest (Arizona, California, and New Mexico); Prairielands (Minnesota, Nebraska, North Dakota, and South Dakota); Southern Coast Region (Alabama and Florida); and Southeast (Georgia and South Carolina). During this funding period, the ATTCs were identified by many in the field as the bridge between researchers and the substance abuse treatment field. Significant achievements during this time included (a) the development and implementation of Leadership Institutes for mid-level managers in substance abuse treatment programs, (b) Web-based learning and training, (c) user-friendly Web sites and databases that help the field (e.g., Academic Addiction Education Programs, Online Addiction Education Learning Opportunities, and Licensing and Certification Regulations by State), and (d) the development of two national products, the *Clinical Supervision Competencies* TAP 21A and revision of the *Addiction Counseling Competences* TAP 21. However, the most noteworthy activity for the ATTCs during this funding period was the development of the Blending Initiative, which was the result of SAMHSA's partnership with the National Institute on Drug Abuse (NIDA). In this initiative, NIDA provided funding to SAMHSA to develop activities and products in order to promote the adoption of substance abuse treatments that have demonstrated efficacy. Specifically, ATTCs were paired with NIDA researchers and community treatment providers to develop products and training activities to help promote the dissemination and use of evidence-based practices. To date, five evidence-based practices (e.g., buprenorphine detoxification, buprenorphine treatment, Addiction Severity Index and treatment planning, motivational interviewing, and motivational incentives) have been disseminated throughout the United States using the resources of the Blending Initiative.

In 2007, the ATTCs were again funded with a similar structure (i.e., 14 regional centers and a national office), with most of the centers remaining unchanged from the previous funding cycle (2001–2006). SAMHSA identified the purpose of the ATTCs to include the following: (a) develop and strengthen the workforce; (b) partner with Single State Authorities, treatment provider associations, addictions counselors, multidisciplinary professionals, faith and recovery community leaders, family members of those in recovery, and other stakeholders; (c) assess the training and development needs of the substance use disorders workforce; and (d) develop and conduct training and technology transfer activities to meet identified needs, with particular emphasis on using evidence-based and promising treatment and recovery practices in recovery-oriented systems of care. Currently, the National ATTC Office Web site (www.nattc.org) provides direct access to all 14 centers and highlights useful products and databases. During the next 5-year funding period (fiscal year 2007–2008 through 2011–2012), the implementation of a national substance abuse workforce study will be one of the most significant activities that will be conducted by the ATTCs. The results of this national survey will provide, for the first time, a national picture of the substance abuse counseling workforce. As such, it will afford the ATTCs and their state and national partners the opportunity to more effectively coordinate their strategies and activities in training and advancing the substance abuse counseling workforce.

Since the early 1990s, the ATTCs have played an instrumental role in helping substance abuse counselors and other allied health professionals improve the quality of services offered to clients and their family members. Today, the ATTCs remain viable, well-established centers with demonstrated expertise in translating research into useful products and practices, providing practitioners with training and technical assistance in multiple formats and venues, and working with a variety of partners and stakeholders to positively impact the substance abuse counseling workforce.

Nancy A. Roget

See also Center for Substance Abuse Treatment; Certification and Licensing; Evidence-Based Prevention and Treatment, Dissemination and Adoption of; Substance Abuse and Mental Health Services Administration

Further Readings

Addiction Technology Transfer Center (ATTC). (n.d.). *About us*. Retrieved November 5, 2007, from http://www.nattc.org/aboutUs.html

Addiction Technology Transfer Center (ATTC). (n.d.). *Timeline*. Retrieved November 5, 2007, from http://www.nattc.org/aboutUs/timeline.html

Addiction Technology Transfer Center (ATTC) Network. (2004). *The change book: A blueprint for technology transfer* (2nd ed.). Kansas City, MO: Addiction Technology Transfer Center (ATTC) National Office. Retrieved November 5, 2007, from http://nattc.org/resPubs/changeBook.html

Center for Substance Abuse Treatment. (2006). *Addiction counseling competencies: The knowledge, skills, and attitudes of professional practice* (Technical Assistance Publication Series 21; DHHS Publication No. SMA 06-4171). Rockville, MD: Substance Abuse and Mental Health Services Administration. Retrieved May 19, 2008, from http://www.nattc.org/resPubs/tap21/accksa.html

Rohrer, S. R., Diesenhaus, H. I., Jaffe, J. H., Morgan, E. T., & Kilpatrick, N. S. (1996). Addiction technology transfer centers (ATTCs). *Substance Abuse, 17*(4), 193–199.

ADOLESCENTS, SUBSTANCE ABUSE AND TREATMENT

Use and abuse of alcohol and illicit drugs by youth is a major public health problem in the United States. Adolescents who use drugs are at higher risk than non-drug-using adolescents for physical and mental health problems and criminal involvement. The social costs of adolescent drug abuse include crime, economic loss, academic disruption, and familial distress. Approximately 7% of adolescents ages 12 to 17 meet criteria for abuse or dependence, but only about 10% of youth with drug abuse problems receive treatment. This entry describes the unique developmental period of adolescence, the epidemiology and nature of adolescent substance abuse, and efforts to prevent and treat alcohol and other substance abuse disorders in adolescents.

Adolescence and Substance Use

The concept of adolescence is a relatively new phenomenon that describes the time between the beginning of puberty and achievement of adulthood. Specific ages in this period vary with a start between 11 and 13 and an end age of 18, 21, or older. The Center for Substance Abuse Treatment defines adolescents as individuals ages 12 to 24.

Adolescent years are characterized by substantial physical, social, and emotional growth, as well as an increasing focus on independence. Conflicts frequently develop between adolescents and their parents or other authority figures due to the presumed vulnerability, impulsivity, rebelliousness, and awkwardness of adolescents. These substantial changes give rise to adolescents' experimentation with different identities and, frequently, with alcohol and other illicit substances. A focus on adolescent drug use as a phenomenon is limited to the relatively recent recognition of adolescence as a period distinct from childhood and adulthood.

As with adult drug use, adolescent drug use is on a continuum of severity from abstinence to dependence. Most information regarding the life course of adolescent drug use is based on experience and research with adults. The view of adult and adolescent drug disorders as fundamentally the same disorder has been questioned in that drug use in adolescence is not necessarily highly predictive of drug use in adulthood. Most drug use peaks in late adolescence. There is controversy regarding whether alcohol and tobacco may be "gateway" drugs that lead to use of illicit drugs, including marijuana. The increased likelihood that an adolescent who uses one illicit drug will use another reflects selective recruitment of people with preexisting traits that may be predisposed to use drugs, peer affiliations with others who use drugs, and socialization into a subculture with favorable attitudes toward the use of drugs.

The diagnostic criteria for drug abuse are similar for all types of substances and across all ages. The *Diagnostic and Statistical Manual of Mental Disorders* defines substance abuse as including a maladaptive pattern of substance use leading to clinically significant impairment or distress, resulting in a failure to fulfill major role obligations, continued use in hazardous situations, and recurrent legal problems or persistent social or interpersonal problems caused or exacerbated by the effects of the substance. Substance dependence diagnoses include increased cognitive, behavioral, and physiological symptoms that indicate decreased control over substance use. Changes from earlier versions of the *Diagnostic and Statistical Manual of Mental Disorders* to the fourth edition increase the diagnostic criteria focus on psychosocial dysfunction and reduce focus on specific behaviors or time periods, which could have the effect of reducing the number of adolescents who meet criteria. The term *abuse,* however, is sometimes used disapprovingly to refer to any use at all, particularly of illicit drugs, or can refer to any non-medical or unsanctioned patterns of use, regardless of consequences. Notably, the International Classification of Diseases and the World Health Organization do not use the term *abuse* and instead address harmful use and hazardous use of drugs.

Epidemiology

The annual National Survey on Drug Use and Health (NSDUH), produced by the U.S. Substance Abuse and Mental Health Services Administration (SAMHSA), is a major source of information on use of illicit drugs, alcohol, and tobacco, in civilian, noninstitutionalized U.S. population, ages 12 and older. According to the NSDUH, current (reported past month) illicit drug use among youth ages 12 to 17 declined from 11.6% in 2002 to 8.3% in 2006. The National Institute on Drug Abuse sponsors the Monitoring the Future study, which surveys 50,000 8th-, 10th-, and 12th-grade students annually about behaviors, values, and attitudes related to drug abuse. The results of this survey are similar to those found in the NSDUH. The Centers for Disease Control and Prevention's Youth Risk Behavior Surveillance System also surveys youth behaviors. The 2004–2006 results indicate 43% of high school students had drunk alcohol, 20% had used marijuana, and 23% had smoked cigarettes during the 30 days preceding the survey.

Alcohol

Alcohol use among adolescents is a concern to those who work in substance abuse because there is a strong relationship between early alcohol use and later problems with dependence and other risk behaviors (dropping out of school, arrests). In 2006, about 10.8 million 12- to 20-year-olds (28.3%) reported drinking alcohol in the past month. Heavy drinking (five or more drinks on the same occasion on 5 or more days in the past month), including binge drinking (five or more drinks within a couple of hours), are significant concerns because of associated health problems. Nearly 7.2 million (18.8%) of 12- to 20-year-olds report binge drinking, and 2.3 million (6.0%) were heavy drinkers. Driving under the influence of alcohol is a considerable public health concern, and the majority of auto crashes involving adolescent drivers also involve the use of alcohol.

Cannabis

Cannabis (including marijuana and hashish) is the most prevalent psychoactive substance (other than alcohol) used by adolescents in the United States. In 2007, the Monitoring the Future survey found that 42% of high school seniors, 31% of 10th graders, and 14% of 8th graders reported lifetime use. Rates of cannabis use are twice that of rates in the early 1990s. According to the NSDUH, current (reported past month) use of marijuana by 12- to 17-year-olds has declined significantly from 8.2% in 2002 to 6.7% in 2006. Young people also compose the majority of marijuana possession arrests, with half of arrestees under age 21. It has been estimated that more than 1 million U.S. teenagers sell marijuana.

Methamphetamine

Methamphetamine is the most prevalent synthetic drug manufactured in the United States, and the use of this powerfully addictive stimulant has significant health effects, including paranoia, hallucinations, and irregular heartbeat. Monitoring the Future reported a drop in annual use among 12th graders from 4.7% in 1999 to 1.7% in 2007, the lowest percentage since the survey started to measure methamphetamine use. The average age of new users dropped from 22.3 years in 1990 to 18.4 years in 2000.

Other Drugs

Rates of adolescent use of other drugs, such as heroin, cocaine, and nonmedical prescription drugs, remain relatively low, with only use of prescription drugs appearing to increase over the past few years. Monitoring the Future reported an increase in the non-medical use of sedatives from 2.8% of high school seniors in 1992 to 6.2% in 2007. There is some evidence that adolescents perceive nonmedical use of prescription drugs to be safer than use of street drugs.

Ethnicity and Gender

There are differences in trends of drug use by ethnicity. According to the NSDUH, among youth ages 12 to 17 in 2006, the rate of current illicit drug use was highest among American Indians and Alaska Natives, about twice the overall rate among youths (18.7% vs. 9.8%, respectively). The rates for other groups were 10.2% among Blacks, 10.0% among Whites, 11.8% among those reporting two or more races, 8.9% among Hispanics, and 6.7% among Asians.

Adolescent males tend to have higher rates of drug use across all drugs than adolescent girls. Adolescent girls' use of drugs is closing the gap, however, with similar rates of use for some drugs, such as nonmedical use of prescription drugs. Males are more likely than females to obtain treatment for drug-related problems. Females are more likely to present with trauma and to be diagnosed with mental health disorders.

Familial Patterns and Co-Occurring Disorders

Adolescents who abuse drugs frequently experience co-occurring medical problems. Medical problems can include problems caused directly by the drug abuse, such as damaged neuronal pathways from methamphetamine use or problems exacerbated by risky behaviors associated with drug use. Adolescents who use drugs intravenously are at particularly high risk for bloodborne pathogens, such as HIV and hepatitis B. Risky behavior and reduced inhibitions during drug use can be associated with unwanted sexual activity, sexually transmitted diseases, physical trauma, and violence. Many female adolescents stop drug use when they discover they are pregnant, but others continue to use during pregnancy, potentially harming both the mother and the fetus.

Developmental research supports the bidirectional impact of drug use and co-occurring psychiatric disorders. Particular temperamental traits, such as being shy, high novelty-seeking, or aggressive, can result in fewer childhood experiences of success or mastery. Adolescents with those childhood experiences who also have family problems, self-regulation difficulties, or poor social skills may associate with a peer group that is supportive of drug use. For example, many adolescents experience dysfunctions in the maintenance of a safe environment, which may include poor adult supervision, poor family communication, poor academic performance, a deviant peer group, and overt conflict or violence. Drug use contributes to further marginalization of adolescents from potentially positive school or family associations and increased involvement with deviant peers. Protective factors include family involvement and warmth, religious involvement, academic achievement, and supervision.

Lifetime psychiatric disorder prevalence among adolescents with substance abuse disorders is around 75%. Half of these adolescents have depressive disorders, and another 25% have disruptive disorders, including conduct disorder and attention deficit disorder. Co-occurring trauma has been identified recently as very common among individuals who use drugs and is a potential barrier to treatment. The consideration of the presence of co-occurring psychiatric disorders has changed assessment and treatment procedures in many drug treatment agencies that serve adolescents to view psychiatric disorders as the norm, not the exception.

The presence of co-occurring disorders also has implications in how adolescents obtain treatment for drug use. Many adolescents enter drug treatment indirectly, following identification of drug problems during arrests or mental health service use. In addition, many youth with drug problems receive services from multiple venues, such as drug treatment, mental health treatment, child welfare, and juvenile justice, in which drug use may not be identified as the primary problem. The extent to which the venue of first service (e.g., juvenile justice) affects long-term recovery from drug abuse is not clear.

Adolescents with co-occurring drug use and psychiatric problems have worse outcomes and are costlier to treat than adolescents with either single disorder. The presence of a co-occurring disorder is also associated with different patterns of treatment. Youth with co-occurring mental health and drug abuse disorders are more likely to get treatment only for their mental health disorders, and individuals with only drug abuse disorders are less likely to get any help compared to youth with only mental health disorders. The specific co-occurring disorder can also affect treatment outcomes. For example, youth with conduct disorders are less likely to be successful in drug treatment.

Prevention

Prevention efforts that address substance use rely on data related to perceived risk, availability, and parental disapproval, which are measured annually by the NSDUH. Among youth ages 12 to 17, there were few changes in the perceived risk of marijuana, cocaine, heroin, or LSD use between 2004 and 2006. About a third of adolescents perceived significant risk in smoking marijuana monthly, and half perceived significant risk in weekly use. In 2006, more than half of youth ages 12 to 17 reported that it would be easy for them to obtain marijuana if they wanted some, with about a quarter reporting it would be easy to get cocaine or crack. Ninety percent of youth reported their parents would strongly disapprove of their trying marijuana or hashish.

Prevention activities are structured in a number of ways and are often administered through school or community milieus. Prevention programs can take many forms. Information and affective education approaches seek to prevent drug use by presenting factual information and improving self-esteem; these approaches have not demonstrated strong effectiveness, however. Social-skills training programs enhance skills related to problem solving, assertiveness, self-control, and coping and have demonstrated success. Comprehensive programs address multiple risk factors and may target individuals, families, schools, and communities; these programs demonstrate success relative to programs that focus on only one risk factor or target group.

Several federal and nonprofit organizations fund and evaluate drug prevention activities. The Community Anti-Drug Coalition of America works with nonprofit organizations and community coalitions nationwide to prevent drug abuse. The Office of National Drug Control Policy funds the National Youth Anti-Drug Media Campaign that distributes antidrug messages via media. An independent evaluation, however, demonstrated it raised exposure to antidrug media messages but failed to influence rates of marijuana use. The U.S. Department of Education runs the Safe and Drug-Free Schools Program, which provides grants to reduce drug use and violence at schools. SAMHSA's Center for Substance Abuse Prevention funds programs that provide education and information about the harmful effects of drugs, as well as many evidence-based prevention programs and strategies. Other programs, such as the nonprofit Partnership for a Drug-Free America, distribute antidrug messages and conduct prevention activities.

More than three quarters of adolescents ages 12 to 17 and enrolled in school reported in 2005 that they had seen or heard drug or alcohol prevention messages at school in the past year. Past-month use of an illicit drug was lower for youth exposed to such messages in school (9.2%) than for youth not reporting such exposure (13.2%).

Clinical Treatment

In addition to having different pathways to treatment, adolescents also have unique treatment issues from adults. Adolescents are more likely to be mandated to treatment rather than going voluntarily, they may have less insight into the effects of their substance use, and they may be bothered only by the consequences of their use and not by the use itself. Higher levels of aggression and impulsivity among adolescents often result in challenges in maintaining a safe, therapeutic milieu.

SAMHSA's 2006 National Survey of Substance Abuse Treatment Services identified 91,873 clients under 18 who were in treatment in 2006, which is 8% of all drug treatment clients nationwide. The majority of these clients (84%) were in treatment facilities with special adolescent programs, despite the fact that only 32% of treatment facilities offer specialized adolescent programs.

Treatment of adolescents with substance use disorders is often determined by the severity of drug use, the context of use, and the presence of supports (such as engaged parents) and other problems (such as co-occurring mental or physical disorders). The focus of clinical attention often determines the treatment setting. For some adolescents, this means that their substance use warrants less attention than primary mental health or other symptoms. Adolescents with multiple needs often have difficulty navigating community treatment systems, which typically have different funding sources and poor integration. One community-level intervention designed to increase treatment access and integrated care, Reclaiming Futures, provided community coaching to increase coordination among courts, police, detention facilities, businesses, schools, faith-based organizations, and families to create a network of support for adolescents with substance abuse problems. The program demonstrated success in increasing adolescent access to services, increasing the use of alcohol and drug assessments in the community, and providing targeted treatment for subpopulations.

Several models of treatment have demonstrated success in helping adolescents achieve reduced use or abstinence. Many treatment programs are based on the *Minnesota Model,* which implements group therapy based on the Twelve Steps of Alcoholics Anonymous or similar support groups. This model includes the use of recovering addicts as counselors, availability of aftercare, and intensive attendance at support group meetings. *Motivational Enhancement Therapy* presumes that adolescents need to resolve ambivalence around whether they have a drug problem and increased motivation to stop using. Motivational techniques during assessments or at the beginning of treatment have demonstrated value in establishing a strong treatment alliance. Motivational techniques are frequently supplemented by *Cognitive Behavioral Therapy,* which teaches skills in drug refusal, establishing positive peer networks, coping with stress, and problem solving. Several models of family involvement, such as the *Family Support Network,* which includes group parent meetings and home visits designed to clarify parent and adolescent roles, provide information about substance abuse and recovery processes, improve family organization and communication, and strengthen motivation and commitment to change. The *Adolescent Community Reinforcement Approach* uses functional analyses to identify antecedents and consequences of behaviors associated with drug use, establishing clear and attainable counseling goals and tracking adolescent satisfaction to inform goal planning and reinforcing prosocial behavior. The *Matrix Model* combines structured information, relapse prevention, contingency management, motivational enhancement, family involvement, Twelve-Step program participation, and an exercise program. *Multidimensional Family Therapy* links adolescent changes to parenting practices and therapy alliance. Strategies in this technique include building alliances with adolescents and parents; addressing adolescent themes including abandonment, hope, and trust; and addressing parent themes such as communication, conflict, and positive interactions.

These treatment approaches address adolescent antisocial or family problems generally, with reduced drug use one of many outcomes. *Multisystemic Therapy* considers youth antisocial behavior as multiply determined and linked with characteristics of the youth and family, peer group, school, and community contexts. The therapy builds protective factors and empowers parents to improve parental discipline, reduce association with negative peers, enhance academic or vocational performance, and improve social support. *Functional Family Therapy* is provided for at-risk or delinquent youth and provides parent- and child-focused cognitive and attribution training to reduce family negativity and increase family communication and supportiveness.

The multiple needs of adolescents in drug treatment must be addressed simultaneously (during drug treatment) or sequentially (following drug treatment). Simultaneous treatment requires costly integration of services or case management, and sequential care results in transitions that can be stressful for adolescents. The role of treatment facilities and providers in ameliorating negative effects of transitions in care or improving the quality of care for adolescent patients around the multiple transitions in care they experience is not clear. Drug Strategies, a nonprofit research institute, evaluated the quality of adolescent substance abuse treatment programs and found that even highly regarded programs often do not adequately address assessment and treatment matching, engagement and retention, gender and cultural competence, and treatment outcomes.

Effectiveness of Adolescent Treatment

Federally funded studies have assessed the effectiveness of adolescent drug treatment. The Drug Abuse Reporting Program in the 1970s and the Treatment Outcome Prospective Study in the 1980s assessed adolescent treatment incidental to the adult treatment process, and participating adolescents often received treatment designed for adults. Both studies reported a reduction in adolescents' use of harder drugs (e.g., opiates) and in drug-related behaviors (such as criminal activity), and no change in marijuana or alcohol use. The Drug Abuse Treatment Outcome Studies for Adolescents (DATOS-A) in the 1990s was a multistate, prospective treatment outcome study that included an evaluation of the role of co-occurring psychiatric disorders on treatment processes, retention, and outcomes. DATOS-A demonstrated that engaging in outpatient, residential, or inpatient drug treatment was effective; adolescents showed reduced use of marijuana and other illicit drugs and decreased heavy drinking and criminal involvement. DATOS-A also found that adolescents with a history of physical or sexual abuse demonstrated greater service needs and greater drug severity, and adolescents with co-occurring psychiatric disorders had more service needs and received more services than adolescents without co-occurring psychiatric disorders.

The Cannabis Youth Treatment (CYT) study is the largest clinical trial of adolescent treatment to date. It compared treatment methods of Motivational Enhancement Therapy, Cognitive Behavioral Therapy, Family Support Network, Adolescent Community Reinforcement Approach, and Multidimensional Family Therapy among 600 adolescent cannabis users. All five CYT interventions demonstrated significant improvements among the adolescents in days of abstinence and percentage in recovery (defined as no use or abuse problems and living in the community).

Conclusion

Adolescent substance abuse disorders have demonstrated health risks to those who abuse alcohol or illicit drugs, social costs including crime and family distress, and challenges to communities in adequately addressing adolescents' treatment needs. As epidemiological research elucidates the nature of adolescent substance abuse disorders, treatment research improves the ability to demonstrate positive outcomes for adolescents who receive treatment. Public and private systems providing these services continue to adapt to changing problems and resources, showing promise in reducing the human and social costs of these disorders.

Jennifer P. Wisdom

See also Co-Occurring Disorders; Family Therapy; Gender Issues; Multidimensional Family Therapy

Further Readings

Goplerud, E. N. (Ed.). (1991). *Preventing adolescent drug use: From theory to practice* (OSAP Prevention Monograph No. 8. DHHS Publication No. 91-1725). Rockville, MD: U.S. Department of Health and Human Services, Office for Substance Abuse Prevention.

Liddle, H. A. & Rowe, C. L. (2006). *Adolescent substance abuse: Research and clinical advance*s. Cambridge, UK: Cambridge University Press.

Regents of the University of Michigan. (2007). *Monitoring the Future: A continuing study of American youth.* Retrieved April 2, 2007, from http://www.monitoringthe future.org

Robertson, E. B., David, S. L., & Rao, S. A. (2003). *Preventing drug abuse among children and adolescents: A research-based guide for parents, educators, and community leaders* (2nd ed., NIH Publication No. 04-4212[A]). Bethesda, MD: National Institute on Drug Abuse. Retrieved April 2, 2007, from http://www .drugabuse.gov/pdf/prevention/RedBook.pdf

Stevens, S. J., & Morral, A. R. (2003). *Adolescent substance abuse treatment in the United States.* Binghamton, NY: Haworth Press.

Substance Abuse and Mental Health Services Administration. (2007). *2005 National Survey on Drug Use and Health (NSDUH) results.* Retrieved March 28, 2007, from http://oas.samhsa.gov/NSDUH/2k5NSDUH/2k5results .htm

Vega, W. A., & Gil, A. G. (1998). *Drug use and ethnicity in early adolescence.* New York: Plenum.

ADULT CHILDREN OF ALCOHOLICS

Alcoholism is a progressive and debilitating condition that not only affects the individual but can also have a substantial negative impact on the entire family system. In fact, alcoholism is typically described as a "family illness" due to the stress on the family members. Recent estimates suggest that as many as 20% of children are raised in a family with at least one alcoholic parent. Adult children of alcoholics (ACOAs) are at risk for alcoholism and other related problems, and a considerable amount of research has been conducted in this area. Quantitative research has focused primarily on risk factors of ACOAs that contribute to the development of a substance use disorder. In addition, qualitative and quantitative research has examined the personality and clinical characteristics of ACOAs.

Risk Factors for Later Substance Abuse Problems

Risk factors of ACOAs are variables that influence the development of subsequent problems and can either moderate or mediate the relationship between having an alcoholic parent and negative outcomes. A moderator can strengthen or reduce the likelihood of an ACOA developing subsequent problems. For example, Theodore Jacob and colleagues found that lower socioeconomic status was associated with increased levels of psychopathology in ACOAs. On the other hand, a mediating variable helps account for or explain the relationship between having an alcoholic parent and negative outcomes. For example, it has been suggested that sensitivity to ethanol accounts for an individual's vulnerability to develop alcoholism. Taken together, an ACOA with ethanol sensitivity may have a higher likelihood of developing alcoholism, but this risk may be reduced if this individual was reared in a family with higher socioeconomic status.

Most research in this area focuses on moderating variables, but there have been several notable methodological problems identifying these variables. These problems include small sample sizes, large heterogeneity among groups, lack of inclusion and exclusion criteria, nonadequate control groups, and differential performances (i.e., when performance on task A is different from performance on task B). The heterogeneity among ACOAs can lead to nonsignificant findings; ACOAs without serious negative outcomes may wash out any differences between ACOAs and other groups. For example, Michelle Menees found no differences in recalled disruptions in family environments among ACOAs and non-ACOAs. However, the types of family disruptions that may be specific to ACOAs (e.g., parental abuse and neglect) were not assessed.

Clinical Characteristics of ACOAs

Clinical characteristics of ACOAs have been identified based on the theory that children internalize parental behavior as a result of dysfunctional family systems. The clinical issues hypothesized to be facing some ACOAs include excessive use of denial, all-or-nothing thinking, exaggerated need for control, avoidance of anger and other feelings, avoidance of self-disclosure, lack of trust, and difficulty with intimate relationships. Others have identified characteristics such as depression, isolation, rage, avoidance of feelings, survival guilt, anxiety reactions, sleep disturbances and nightmares, and intrusive thoughts.

Many studies have investigated the clinical characteristics of ACOAs with mixed results and several notable methodological weaknesses. For example, Robert Ackerman found differences between ACOAs and non-ACOAs in 20 adult problems, such as difficulty having fun, constantly seeking approval and affirmation, and difficulty with intimate relationships. However, the results were only descriptive and no statistical analyses were performed in this study, so the conclusions that can be drawn are limited. Many studies of ACOAs use small to moderate sample sizes, which limits the likelihood of statistically significant effects. Therefore, the findings are often

mixed and the evidence is unclear regarding differences between ACOAs and non-ACOAs.

Choosing an appropriate comparison group is important in the investigation of differences between ACOAs and non-ACOAs. Some suggest using comparison groups of adults raised in dysfunctional families without an alcoholic to tease apart the unique contribution of the effect of the alcoholic parent. The results of studies using this type of comparison group have been mixed. Some research has found evidence of codependency in ACOAs. On the other hand, Gary Fisher and colleagues found that ACOAs are not different from adults raised in dysfunctional families and that codependency is not more prevalent in ACOAs. In addition, it is difficult to compare ACOAs to other groups without understanding the typical progression of problems among ACOAs. Despite early findings that ACOAs have significant problems in adulthood even if they do not become an alcoholic or marry an alcoholic, Livia D'Andrea and colleagues found that almost half of ACOAs demonstrated no significant problems.

Although many empirical examinations of clinical characteristics of ACOAs utilized undergraduate samples, recent studies have included more diverse samples such as African Americans and women. Many studies including undergraduate samples found few differences between ACOAs and non-ACOAS and suggest similar adjustment between groups. However, Stephanie Bush and colleagues found ACOAs to have higher levels of depression and lower self-esteem than non-ACOAs. Interestingly, women in this sample had overall higher levels of depression than men, suggesting that there may be groups within ACOAs that are at more risk for later problems. Further research is needed to examine risk and resiliency among various subgroups within the larger group of ACOAs. These factors may carry important ramifications for prevention and treatment efforts.

Assessment and Treatment Considerations

The assessment of ACOAs can be challenging due to the ambiguity of the definition of an ACOA. For example, there is disagreement regarding whether a parent of the ACOA needs to have been formally diagnosed with an alcohol abuse or dependence diagnosis. Alan Berkowitz and Wesley Perkins differentiated between strict and broad definitions of ACOAs. The strict definition of ACOAs required an actual diagnosis of the parent, whereas the adult child's perception of parental drinking problems was sufficient for a broad definition. Although the broader definition may include a larger number of ACOAs, this may be an imprecise diagnostic indicator because the child's perceptions may be inaccurate.

The Children of Alcoholics Screening Test (CAST) is a 39-item diagnostic instrument that asks questions related to parental problems with alcohol. It is designed to measure the chaotic and inconsistent behaviors and experiences of the alcoholic home, such as emotional instability, inconsistent child care, family conflict, and the lack of close, intimate, and trusting relationships between parents and children. Psychometric properties of the CAST are strong, but there has been evidence that distress among the ACOAs may be due more to the impairment of the family than to parental drinking. Although the CAST reflects the stricter definition of an ACOA, Berkowitz and Perkins suggest that it is possible to identify ACOAs by using a single, objective question focusing on the perception of the parent's drinking, and that this method produces prevalence rates similar to those obtained from more detailed diagnostic instruments like the CAST. Regardless, further research is needed to examine the most effective ways to identify ACOAs so that appropriate services and interventions can be provided to these individuals.

There is limited research on the prevention of alcohol-related problems and the treatment of ACOAs. There are two main goals in providing interventions for ACOAs. The first goal is to identify and address early symptoms of problem drinking, and the second goal is to identify dysfunctional behaviors and coping skills that may be predisposing risk factors for drinking or other adult problems. Support groups for ACOAs, such as Codependents Anonymous and Al-Anon, may be appropriate interventions. Other support groups, such as Sex Addicts Anonymous and Emotions Anonymous, could be used as well, depending upon the identified problem of the individual. In fact, some research suggests that families identified as having problems with alcohol prefer group over individual treatment formats. However, limited research has examined the effectiveness of these types of programs.

The mixed results of empirical studies do not suggest that interventions should be tailored specifically for ACOAs because problems among ACOAs may be more similar to those of non-ACOAs with dysfunctional family backgrounds. Nevertheless, the association with alcohol for many ACOAs has been shown to be problematic. Mental health professionals should help their ACOA clients clarify their thoughts and feelings regarding abstention from, or moderation of, alcohol use. Many clients who were raised in homes with alcohol abuse may not identify themselves as ACOAs, so counselors need to be careful about using jargon that may create client resistance. Mental health professionals who use the label ACOA may leave their clients with the impression that this is a widely accepted clinical syndrome, but such a posture would be misrepresenting the empirical findings about ACOAs.

Conclusion

There are mixed opinions about what constitutes the risk factors and clinical characteristics of ACOAs. Although some research suggests increased problems among this group, there are methodological limitations that warrant further attention in this area. It is unclear whether problems are more prevalent in this group and whether problems are linked to parental alcoholism or family functioning. Additional research on the assessment of difficulties among this group is important to provide more effective assessment and refined treatment planning. Regardless, ACOAs who have problems need appropriate services and may benefit from support groups like Al-Anon. More research is needed in the area of prevention and treatment to help provide evidence-based interventions for ACOAs.

Daniel M. Bagner, Gary L. Fisher,
and Gregory L. Stuart

See also Al-Anon; Children of Alcoholics; Codependency

Further Readings

Ackerman, R. J. (1987). *Children of alcoholics* (2nd ed.). New York: Simon & Schuster.

Berkowitz, A., & Perkins, H. W. (1988). Personality characteristics of children of alcoholics. *Journal of Consulting and Clinical Psychology, 56,* 206–209.

Bush, S. I., Ballard, M. E., & Fremouw, W. (1995). Attributional style, depressive features, and self-esteem: Adult children of alcoholic and nonalcoholic parents. *Journal of Youth and Adolescence, 24,* 177–185.

D'Andrea, L. M., Fisher, G. L., & Harrison, T. C. (1994). Cluster analysis of adult children of alcoholics. *International Journal of the Addictions, 29,* 565–582.

Fisher, G. L., Jenkins, S. J., & Harrison, T. C. (1992). Characteristics of adult children of alcoholics. *Journal of Substance Abuse, 4,* 27–34.

Fisher, G. L., Jenkins, S. J., & Harrison, T. C. (1993). Personality characteristics of adult children of alcoholics, other adults from dysfunctional families, and adults from nondysfunctional families. *International Journal of the Addictions, 28,* 477–485.

Jacob, T., Windle, M., & Seilhamer, R. A. (1999). Adult children of alcoholics: Drinking, psychiatric and psychosocial status. *Psychology of Addictive Behaviors, 13,* 3–21.

Jones, J. (1985). *Children of Alcoholics Screening Test.* Chicago: Camelot Unlimited.

Menees, M. M., & Segrin, C. (2000). The specificity of disrupted processes in families of adult children of alcoholics. *Alcohol and Alcoholism, 35,* 361–367.

AFRICAN AMERICANS, ISSUES IN PREVENTION AND TREATMENT

See RACIAL AND ETHNIC MINORITIES, ISSUES IN PREVENTION; RACIAL AND ETHNIC MINORITIES, ISSUES IN TREATMENT

AFTERCARE

See CONTINUUM OF CARE; RELAPSE PREVENTION

AL-ANON

Al-Anon Family Groups, a recovery program for the friends and families of alcoholics, was founded in May 1951 by Lois W. and Anne B. (in Twelve-Step tradition, last names are not used). They share the commonality that another person's drinking has affected their lives in a variety of ways. Al-Anon offers a safe place where people can share their concerns, feelings, and experiences with others who have had similar experiences. The identities of its members are well protected. Although AA and Al-Anon cooperate with one other in the process of recovery, they are not directly affiliated. Membership in Al-Anon does not require any dues and is voluntary.

Al-Anon is structured by the Three Legacies, which are a set of principles adapted from Alcoholics Anonymous that guide the meetings. The theme that ties the principles together is "pass along understanding" through recovery, unity, and service. The first legacy, Recovery through the Twelve Steps, encourages using the Twelve Steps as a tool in finding solutions to problems, changing attitudes and behaviors, and living productive lives. The second legacy, Unity through the Twelve Traditions, is a framework used to help members solve problems, resolve conflict, and conduct group activities. Members are held together by the common desire to be uninfluenced by outside interests that may distract from the Al-Anon experience. The final legacy, Service though the Twelve Concepts of Service, was adapted and changed significantly to fit the needs of Al-Anon Family Groups. The concepts encourage spreading the Al-Anon message worldwide. Members also tend to use these concepts in their personal and work relationships.

Through the three legacies, members realize that they did not cause the alcoholism, they cannot control it, and they cannot cure it. This is sometimes referred to as the 3 C's. They learn that although they cannot change the alcoholic, they can change themselves.

Generally speaking, the families tend to be as uninformed as the alcoholic about the nature of the disease. Nonalcoholic family members are often confused and feel powerless in the face of a disease that is out of control. Many times, it is the nonalcoholic family member who holds the family together and fights for survival of the family system. Over time, life usually becomes miserable and unmanageable. While they have been victimized by the presence of alcoholism in their homes, they also unknowingly perpetuate the cycle by enabling the alcoholic to continue drinking. They do this by making excuses for the alcoholic and covering up the appearance of alcoholism. Thus, it is important that the whole family be involved in a support program in order to recover from the negative influence of alcohol on their lives and relationships.

Although roughly 30% of Al-Anon members have an alcoholic spouse, father, or both, the only requirement for members to attend group meetings is that someone has affected them with his or her drinking. The drinker does not need to be sober, attending Alcoholics Anonymous, or in another recovery program. Since the second step of Al-Anon is to "believe that a power greater than ourselves can restore us to sanity," an important aspect of recovery is a belief in a higher power. However, the program is compatible with all religions and does not endorse a particular religion or higher power. In most Al-Anon groups, there is diversity in religious orientation.

On average, Al-Anon members attend seven meetings a month. The average length of membership is 11.3 years. Females constitute approximately 85% of Al-Anon members, and 25% of the members hold employment in a professional, managerial, or executive position. Fourteen percent of Al-Anon members are dual members of Al-Anon and Alcoholics Anonymous.

An Al-Anon meeting has an average of 12 members gathering together on a weekly basis to share their experiences for the purpose of mutual support. The format of a meeting varies from group to group. Meetings may focus on a specific topic, have a guest speaker, or be a beginner's/newcomer's meeting. Most meetings are "open" meetings, but some are "closed" meetings. A closed meeting welcomes any person who is affected by an alcoholic. Open meetings encourage students, professionals, and the public to sit in on the meeting to listen to members share their stories. Regardless of the meeting topic, most meetings begin with an introduction, which may include announcements or a reading of the Twelve Steps and Twelve Traditions of Al-Anon. Members then have an opportunity to share their experiences and stories with one another if they so choose. Members always have the right to decline. The meetings are generally closed with the Serenity Prayer, or another type of prayer, for members who wish to pray.

Officers are elected by the members to guide the meetings, but they hold no governing authority over the group. Officers are rotated such that many members have the chance to serve the group in different fashions. A group representative is elected to attend district meetings, which are held periodically throughout a region to vote on matters pertaining to the future of Al-Anon.

There are no set rules to abide by at Al-Anon meetings. However, members are discouraged from giving direct advice to each other, questioning or interrupting a member who is speaking, or telling another member what to say, do, or think. Meetings are confidential, and the only personally identifying information is a first name, if it is given. Al-Anon is not a therapy group run by professional counselors. In therapy groups,

clients are treated together for a specific problem, and there is a focus on group process and dynamics. Al-Anon is a support group, which occurs in a nonprofessional environment and is organized and run by its members. In Al-Anon, members relate personal experiences, listen to each other, provide sympathy, and establish social networks.

One important factor in the social supportive relationships of Al-Anon is service. Members take pride in lending themselves to others for help in the same way they were lent help when they first began with the group. This is typically described as mutuality, being able to give back and express gratitude because members want to instill the same hope in others that they have been given. Al-Anon fosters reciprocity and mutuality through service work and sponsorship. Service work is part of the community building that occurs in Al-Anon, and volunteering often helps the member in his or her own recovery. There are different kinds of service. While some people may serve by cleaning up after meetings, others serve as group representatives, on the Board of Trustees, or as sponsors. Sponsoring a member is an effective way to help another member with personal recovery. This relationship is offered on a one-to-one basis, which encourages further sharing of emotions and experiences.

Al-Anon is a chosen community in which members have shared interests and identify with one another on a number of issues. The purpose is not to find a way to make the alcoholic sober; rather, it is for members to focus on themselves and be supported by others who are also affected by someone who drinks. Members learn how to disentangle themselves from the disease of alcoholism, how to set boundaries and limits for themselves, and how to focus on their own emotional health, rather than on the alcoholic. Families of alcoholics experience loneliness and lack familial connection and support, and the common identity of members of Al-Anon is the depletion of resources necessary for coping with living with an alcoholic. Al-Anon supports members during their time of distress by fulfilling needs associated with validation of feelings, thoughts, and emotions. The social support available at Al-Anon has the ability to restore and enhance physical, emotional, and mental health by working through one's experiences in a safe environment.

Al-Anon group meeting information may be obtained by contacting Al-Anon Family Groups listed in a local telephone directory, calling the Al-Anon

Family Group Headquarters, Inc.'s 1-888-4Al-ANON toll-free meeting information line (available Monday–Friday 8 a.m. to 6 p.m. ET), or visiting the Al-Anon Family Group Headquarters, Inc.'s Web site.

Heidi Zosel, Sabina Mutisya,
and Thomas Harrison

See also Adult Children of Alcoholics; Alateen; Alcoholics Anonymous; Codependency; Twelve Steps

Further Readings

Al-Anon/Alateen: http://www.al-anon.alateen.org

Read, E. M. (1995). Posttreatment supervision challenges: Introducing Al-Anon, Nar-Anon, and Oxford House, Inc. *Federal Probation, 59*(4), 18–27.

Southeastern Institute of Research. (2004). *Al-Anon membership survey.* Retrieved May 20, 2008, from http://www.al-anon.org/pdf/survey/survey14.pdf

Zajdow, G. (2002). *Al-Anon narratives: Women, self-stories, and mutual aid.* Westport, CT: Greenwood Press.

ALATEEN

Alateen groups provide a place where young people who are troubled by another person's drinking can share their stories, their strength, and their hope. In the early days of Alcoholics Anonymous (AA) and Al-Anon Family Groups, children and teenagers often attended meetings with their parents. Alateen began with a 17-year-old boy who knew he needed an outlet for sharing his experiences with other young people. His father was a member of AA and mother was a member of Al-Anon Family Groups. At first, he used the Twelve Steps and slogans of AA, but that was not enough. With encouragement from his parents, he asked five teenagers he knew who had parents with a drinking problem to form a group. The purpose of the group was to help teens recover from the effects of someone else's drinking. He wrote to the Al-Anon Clearing House in New York, as did many other teens looking for support, and in 1957 Alateen was established as a part of Al-Anon Family Groups.

Both Al-Anon and Alateen groups have one primary purpose: to help the families and friends of alcoholics. The Al-Anon/Alateen Twelve Steps are adapted from those of AA. Although a separate organization, Al-Anon/Alateen enjoys a cooperative relationship with AA. Each organization often invites the other to participate in special events like conventions and roundups and may work together on community education about the two support programs.

Nearly 1,800 Alateen groups hold weekly meetings throughout the United States, Canada, and worldwide. Many Alateen groups meet at the same location and time as Al-Anon groups for adults. This provides the opportunity for both young people and parents to attend meetings without parents having to arrange rides for the children at a separate time or place. Alateen members report being thankful to have their own meeting to attend while parents go to their meetings.

Every Alateen group has adult Alateen group sponsors who are certified by the state or provincial Al-Anon service structure in accordance with state or provincial laws. The certification includes a minimum age of 21, minimum 2-year membership in Al-Anon Family Groups, and no felony convictions. The Alateen group sponsors do not facilitate the meetings nor do they serve as counselors. Their function is to provide guidance to help the Alateens keep their meetings focused on Al-Anon/Alateen recovery.

Each Alateen meeting is facilitated by an Alateen member who volunteers to present a subject for group discussion. In meetings, Alateens provide each other with mutual support by exchanging their individual experiences about how they apply Alateen's principles to their daily lives. Examples of topics are taking care of myself, attitudes, responsibilities, Step, slogan, or alcoholism as an illness that affects the well-being of all family members. As a result, Alateen members are able to learn from each other about the various choices they have in various situations and the benefits of using Alateen for their recovery.

The membership survey is able to provide some insight as to who are the current members of Alateen. While each Alateen has his or her own individual story, 55% have an alcoholic parent and 23% have an alcoholic grandparent. Nineteen percent of Alateens have a friend who is alcoholic. One Alateen said this about life before Alateen: "My parents would fight basically every day when I was little. I would be afraid of my dad because he drank. I never knew what my dad would do to my mom. I'd get the feeling that he might hit her or worse, kill her. I was young, so I had no clue what was wrong with him."

By attending Alateen meetings, members find that they are not alone in their struggles. Many young people are unaware that their friends have similar experiences. "When I showed up for my first meeting, I was surprised to see so many familiar faces. People I went to school with and some who had even made fun of me. I saw that we had a lot in common. Our family members drank, were violent to us and we were at the end of our rope because we couldn't manage or change our loved ones."

However, Alateens do experience recovery from the effects of another person's drinking on their health. More that 60% of Alateen members reported that their daily functioning at home, school, and work is much improved. Over 75% of the Alateen members reported that Alateen at least somewhat improved their mental health and well-being. This was also the area reported to be the most affected by someone else's drinking, as expressed by one Alateen member: "Before Alateen I was a lonely person with only two friends. I was very pessimistic about myself. I didn't know who I was, what I was doing, or where I was going. I didn't care about anything. In Alateen, I have learned to express myself more, I am more talkative now. I am more optimistic. I am more open-minded and have a lot more self-esteem. Alateen is amazing and I will continue working the program."

Alateen group meeting information is available by contacting Al-Anon Family Groups through a local telephone directory, calling the Al-Anon Family Group Headquarters, Inc.'s 1-888-4AL-ANON toll-free meeting information line (available Monday–Friday, 8 a.m.–6 p.m. ET), or visiting the Al-Anon Family Group Headquarters, Inc.'s Web site. If an Alateen meeting is not available in a local community, please contact the Al-Anon Family Group Headquarters, Inc. for further information at wso@al-anon.org or call 757-563-1600.

Nicolette Stephens

See also Al-Anon; Alcoholics Anonymous; Twelve Steps

Further Readings

Al-Anon Family Group Headquarters, Inc.: http://www.al-anon.alateen.org

Al-Anon Family Groups Headquarters, Inc. (1996). *Courage to be me—Living with alcoholism.* Virginia Beach, VA: Author.

Al-Anon Family Groups Headquarters, Inc. (2001). *Living today in Alateen.* Virginia Beach, VA: Author.

Al-Anon Family Groups Headquarters, Inc. (2003). *Alateen—Hope for children of alcoholics* (Rev. ed.). Virginia Beach, VA: Author.

ALCOHOL

Alcohol is one of the oldest and most widely used psychoactive substances. Alcohol differs from most other psychoactive substances because its use is generally accepted and it is considered a legal recreational substance in most parts of the world. Despite its current acceptance, alcohol is not without its problems. Historically, societal responses to alcohol have ranged from prohibition to unrestricted drinking. Millions of Americans currently suffer from drinking problems, including abuse and dependence. In addition, alcohol use is correlated with a variety of social and health problems, including polysubstance use, fetal alcohol syndrome, aggression and violence, and driving-related accidents.

Alcohol is the popular name for beverages containing the psychoactive ingredient ethanol or ethyl alcohol. For purposes of human consumption, alcohol is produced either through the process of fermentation or through the additional process of distillation. In the presence of yeast, fruits ferment into wine and grains ferment into beer. Wines, excluding fortified wines, typically contain 12% to 14% alcohol by volume. Beers can contain anywhere from 1.5% alcohol by volume in the case of low-alcohol beers to over 10% alcohol by volume for high-gravity beers. To attain concentrations of alcohol above 15%, fermented alcohol must be distilled. Distillation involves the removal of water from a fermented alcohol in order to increase the concentration of alcohol. Distilled alcohol concentrations in the United States are measured in two ways: first, as alcohol by volume (ABV) and, second, as "proof," which corresponds to twice the ABV (e.g., 80 proof = 40% ABV). Common distillation process cannot produce ethanol above 191 proof (approximately 95.5% ABV). Concentrations of ethanol at this level are referred to as grain alcohol and are not intended for human consumption.

Because alcohol concentrations vary by the type of beverage, a standard drink of alcohol in the United States contains 14 grams or one-half ounce of pure alcohol (other countries measure a standard drink as containing 10 grams of pure alcohol). The following beverages contain the same amount of pure alcohol (14 grams) and are equal to a standard drink:

- 12 ounces beer
- 10 ounces microbrew
- 8 ounces malt liquor
- 4 ounces of wine
- 1.25 ounces of 80-proof liquor
- 1 ounce of 100-proof liquor

Pharmacology

Alcohol is a central nervous system depressant, meaning that it depresses, or slows down, the functions of the central nervous system. Although the exact mechanism of neurological action is not clear, the current understanding is that alcohol interacts with a number of neurotransmitters in the central nervous system. Alcohol is believed to have its primary effect on gamma-aminobutyric acid (GABA). GABA is the major inhibitory neurotransmitter in the central nervous system and increases in the presence of alcohol. An increase in GABA is thought to underlie the sedative-hypnotic or depressant qualities of alcohol. Additionally, alcohol inhibits the function of glutamate, which is the brain's major excitatory neurotransmitter. Interference with glutamate appears to affect multiple brain functions, including memory. Alcohol stimulates the release of endorphins, a neurotransmitter similar in structure to opioids, which accounts for the "high" that is attributed to alcohol intoxication, and increases the concentration of dopamine in the reward/pleasure center of the brain. Finally, alcohol is thought to alter serotonin transmission, which is heavily involved with food and water intake, sexual response, and aggression.

Absorption, Metabolism, and Excretion

Approximately 20% of alcohol that is consumed is absorbed into blood vessels lining the stomach. The remainder of consumed alcohol passes from the stomach into the small intestine where it is rapidly absorbed into the bloodstream. Peak levels of blood alcohol occur 30 to 90 minutes after alcohol is consumed. A rapid rate of alcohol absorption into the body and rapid transport across the blood–brain barrier are, in part, responsible for the subjective feeling of intoxication.

The measure of the concentration of alcohol in the bloodstream is *blood alcohol level,* a term commonly associated with laws around drinking and driving. Blood alcohol level is reported as a percentage, given that it represents the percentage of alcohol present in the bloodstream.

The rate at which alcohol is absorbed into the body is determined primarily by the rate of drinking, the amount of alcohol in the beverage consumed, and by the presence of food in the stomach. A person's weight and gender also affect blood alcohol levels. When weight and number of drinks are equal, women absorb approximately 30% more alcohol into the bloodstream than men and feel the effects of alcohol more quickly and with greater intensity than men. A number of factors are responsible for this difference. Women typically have a lower percentage of water in their body, so alcohol is less diluted. Women, also, have less of the enzyme alcohol dehydrogenase in their stomach so less alcohol is metabolized before entering the bloodstream. Finally, hormone levels during menstruation affect the rate of alcohol absorption. Other factors that influence the rate of alcohol absorption include drinking carbonated beverages or drinking warm alcohol (e.g., warm brandy, hot toddies).

The body begins to eliminate alcohol as soon as it is ingested. A small amount of alcohol (up to 10%) is excreted through the lungs and urine without being metabolized by the liver. The majority of alcohol that is ingested is metabolized by oxidation in the liver and then excreted via the kidneys.

While the rate of alcohol absorption is affected by many factors, it is metabolized in the liver at a fairly constant rate. Alcohol dehydrogenase (ADH) transforms alcohol into acetaldehyde, a substance that is highly toxic to the body and liver. Acetaldehyde is then converted by acetaldehyde dehydrogenase (ALDH) into acetic acid, which in turn is oxidized into water and carbon dioxide. Both ADH and ALDH vary in their availability and efficiency, in part, as a result of heredity. Approximately 1 ounce of pure alcohol is eliminated from the body every 3 hours.

Tolerance and Withdrawal

Tolerance reflects the brain's effort to protect itself from the effects of alcohol. When alcohol is consumed over a period of time, the body attempts to become more efficient at metabolizing alcohol. The liver creates more enzymes to process alcohol and the toxic metabolite, acetaldehyde. Therefore, alcohol is eliminated more quickly from the body. Unfortunately, the increase in liver enzymes may also accelerate the elimination of prescription drugs, which ultimately lessens their effectiveness. The brain also responds to the regular use of alcohol. Neurons in the brain become more resistant to alcohol by increasing the number of receptor sites necessary to create an effect. With continued use, GABA receptors become less sensitive to alcohol and to GABA itself. Because the GABA receptor complex interacts with a number of medications, they also become less effective. Finally, drinkers may learn to adapt their behavior to an intoxicated state so that others won't notice. This form of behavioral tolerance is selective, meaning that some behaviors may adapt to the presence of alcohol but others may not. A person may learn to walk steadily under the influence but may not be able to perform behaviors requiring fine motor skills. Tolerance continues to increase until chronic alcohol use begins to damage the liver. The liver eventually becomes less efficient at metabolizing alcohol, which leads to a process of reverse tolerance.

Some research is also examining the role of the environment in the development of tolerance. If one drinks in the presence of distinct cues associated with the presentation of alcohol to the body, there is evidence that the body prepares to receive the drug by increasing central nervous system functions that are normally decreased by alcohol's depressant qualities (i.e., the body makes a conditioned compensatory response).

Although some who drink see having tolerance as a "good" thing (e.g., believing that they can "hold their liquor"), tolerance can result in an increase in negative health risks and, as discussed later in this entry, is one of the criteria for dependence. Just as the body must adapt to heavy chronic alcohol use, it also must respond to the absence of alcohol. As already noted, alcohol changes the brain's balance of several neurotransmitters. Withdrawal is the body's reaction to the disruption of this balance. For instance, alcohol increases the inhibitory neurotransmitter GABA, and the brain responds by increasing excitatory neurotransmitters in addition to decreasing the number of GABA receptors. When a person stops drinking, high levels of excitatory neurotransmitters remain while GABA levels suddenly and rapidly decrease. This rebound effect leads to a state of hyperarousal. The brain's ability to regulate this new imbalance determines in part the intensity of withdrawal symptoms.

Approximately 85% to 95% of those experiencing withdrawal have some form of minor withdrawal. Minor withdrawal symptoms include rapid pulse, insomnia, sweating, increased body temperature, anxiety and/or depression, and nausea or vomiting. If the brain has difficulty regulating the imbalance of neurotransmitters, the person may experience major symptoms of withdrawal. These can include tachycardia (irregular heartbeat), hallucinations, psychomotor agitation, delirium tremens, seizures, and death. Long-term heavy drinkers that have repeated periods of drinking and withdrawal actually increase the intensity of subsequent withdrawal symptoms and are at particular risk for seizures or death.

Withdrawal is often treated by detoxification, or detox. Detox can involve the monitoring of withdrawal symptoms or medication interventions that slow the withdrawal process by the use of GABA-augmenting medications to slow the rebound effect.

Levels of Use

The effects of alcohol are dependent on the amount consumed, the frequency of use, and the duration of use. Light to moderate use is defined as up to 1 drink a day for women and 2 drinks per day for men. Binge drinking involves consuming 5 or more drinks over 2 hours for a male (4 drinks over 2 hours for females). Heavy drinking is conceptualized as 5 or more drinks in one sitting at least 5 times a month.

Acute Effects

It is alcohol's action in the brain that leads to the range of acute effects. Even at low doses, reaction time can be impacted because of alcohol's depressant effects (hence, regardless of the legal limit, driving after drinking any amount of alcohol could be dangerous). Initially, a person who has consumed alcohol may feel relaxed and, in time, feel a "buzz" from alcohol's effects (often described as feeling warm or, paradoxically, feeling energized). This relaxation deepens as blood alcohol level rises. A "point of diminishing returns" occurs between a blood alcohol level of .05% and .06% such that, once exceeded, the positive feelings associated with drinking seem less positive and the negative feelings associated with drinking seem more pronounced. Many people who drink note that efforts to "get their buzz back" once this point is exceeded are unsuccessful; instead, they observe that they feel more tired, sick, and symptoms typically associated with being "drunk."

Over time, the depressant effects are more clearly seen as interfering with the brain's ability to function. Judgment can be impaired at a blood alcohol level of .06% such that decision making, the ability to appraise risks, and the ability to consider consequences are impacted (deficits in these domains can be more pronounced as the blood alcohol level rises). At .08%, the limit associated with being legally intoxicated, nausea can appear and signs of impaired motor coordination are evident. As blood alcohol level increases above .10%, judgment and motor coordination clearly deteriorate.

At much higher doses, it is evident that brain functions are being disrupted. From blood alcohol levels of .15% to .25%, a person is at risk for a "blackout." During a blackout, judgment and risk appraisal are severely affected, and there is evidence that the normal functioning of the hippocampus (a part of the brain affecting a range of cognitive processes, including attention, concentration, and memory) is being interrupted. Following a blackout, a person may report problems in memory ranging from an unclear sense of recent history being recalled when a person is prompted about a detail to entire gaps during the period while intoxicated.

From blood alcohol levels of .25% to .35%, a person is at risk for passing out or losing consciousness. Although lethal accidents can happen across a range of blood alcohol levels, a risk of death becomes a concern with blood alcohol levels over .30%. Blood alcohol levels from .40% to .45% are typically associated with a lethal dose.

Chronic Effects

Because alcohol is readily transported to all the organs of the body, the chronic use of alcohol affects most physiological systems. The liver experiences the greatest impact. Chronic use can lead to a fatty liver, alcoholic hepatitis, and cirrhosis of the liver, which is often fatal. Since alcohol enters the body via the digestive tract, chronic drinking can cause damage to the mouth, esophagus, stomach, and intestinal tract. Effects include gastritis, ulcers, pancreatitis, internal bleeding, and malnutrition. Alcohol can cause a deficiency of vitamin B_1, leading to brain damage and dementia. Chronic drinking can also decrease the

body's ability to manage blood sugar. While small amounts of alcohol are beneficial to the cardiovascular system, chronic heavy drinking can enlarge the heart, increase blood pressure, and increase the risk for intracranial bleeding and strokes. Because alcohol is toxic to cells, neurons in the brain may be killed. Chronic alcohol use can decrease sexual desire and orgasms for women. In men, chronic use can lead to decreases in the male hormone testosterone. Moderate to heavy drinking also increases the risk of cancer, including breast cancer for women, and mouth, throat, esophageal, and rectal cancers for both men and women. Emotional problems and mental illness, particularly depression and anxiety, increase with chronic alcohol use. Finally, heavy drinking is thought to diminish a person's life expectancy by 15 years.

Epidemiology

The natural course of alcohol use and alcohol-related problems looks different depending on the population studied and the research methodology utilized. Far from following a pattern in which use and problems progress to a point in which treatment is essential, research has shown that the majority of people with alcohol problems improve without formal intervention or treatment. Further, this "spontaneous recovery" does not seem to follow or fit a single model or trajectory.

Factors that seem to impact alcohol problems include the co-occurrence of other mental health issues, early initiation of alcohol consumption, and family history (with the acknowledgement, however, that genetics are not a person's destiny). Among adolescents, it seems that conduct problems are the strongest and most consistent predictor of later problems with alcohol. There is great diversity among adults, with stability of drinking patterns and problems varying across age groups. Because many consequences or problems related to alcohol use are commonly reported across a range of drinking patterns, the presence of any one symptom or cluster of symptoms does not suggest or imply that a more significant problem is emerging.

Alcohol Dependence and Alcohol Abuse

The *Diagnostic and Statistical Manual of Mental Disorders, Fourth Edition, Text Revision* outlines criteria for alcohol dependence and alcohol abuse.

Alcohol dependence is characterized by alcohol use leading to clinically significant impairment or distress as indicated by three (or more) of seven criteria occurring within the same 12-month period. These criteria are (1) tolerance; (2) withdrawal; (3) often using alcohol in larger amounts or over a longer period than was intended; (4) having a persistent desire or unsuccessful efforts to cut down or control one's use; (5) taking a great deal of time to obtain, use, or recover from the effects of alcohol; (6) giving up or reducing important social, occupational, or recreational activities because of drinking; or (7) continuing alcohol use despite knowing that one has a persistent or recurrent physical or psychological problem caused or made worse by alcohol. When making a diagnosis, the provider must designate if the individual meets criteria for dependence with physiological dependence (which occurs when tolerance or withdrawal is present) or dependence without physiological dependence (which occurs when three or more criteria, excluding tolerance and withdrawal, are met).

A diagnosis of alcohol abuse involves a pattern of alcohol use leading to impairment or distress as evidenced by endorsement of one or more criteria occurring within a 12-month period. If the individual has ever met criteria for alcohol dependence, a diagnosis of abuse is not made. Criteria for abuse are (1) recurrent alcohol use resulting in a failure to fulfill major role obligations at work, school, or home; (2) recurrent alcohol use in physically hazardous situation; (3) recurrent alcohol-related legal problems; or (4) continued alcohol use despite knowing that one has a persistent or recurrent social or interpersonal problem caused or made worse by alcohol.

Conclusion

In this entry on alcohol, pharmacology, patterns of use, acute effects, chronic effects, epidemiology, and diagnostic issues have been reviewed. It is important to keep in mind that a person's alcohol use should not be interpreted in a vacuum; instead, the context of a person's use should be considered. Alcohol use could be in response to a variety of stressors in a person's life, but use could also be exacerbating or even causing these difficulties. Emphasizing the behavior and the impact of the behavior could be as important as considering the chemical itself.

Scott Hunt and Jason Kilmer

See also Alcohol-Induced Disorders; Alcoholism; Alcohol-Related Birth Defects; Blood Alcohol Concentration; Central Nervous System Depressants; Substance-Induced Withdrawal Delirium; Substance Use Disorders; Underage Drinking

Further Readings

American Psychiatric Association. (2000). *Diagnostic and statistical manual of mental disorders* (4th ed., text rev.). Washington, DC: Author.

Diaz, J. (1997). *How drugs influence behavior: A neurobehavioral approach*. Upper Saddle River, NJ: Prentice Hall.

Inaba, D. S., & Cohen, W. E. (2004). *Uppers, downers, all arounders: Physical and mental effects of psychoactive drugs* (5th ed.). Ashland, OR: CNS Publications.

Larimer, M. E., & Kilmer, J. R. (2000). Natural history. In G. Zernig, A. Savia, M. Kurz, & S. O'Malley (Eds.), *Handbook of alcoholism* (pp. 13–28). Boca Raton, FL: CRC Press.

ALCOHOLIC PERSONALITY

Alcoholism as a label has little specificity. Alcohol abuse and dependence are more specific, behaviorally defined constructs with criteria based on the level of alcohol involvement and the impact of alcohol use on judgment, risk-taking behavior, physical and mental health, and social and occupational functioning. Personality can be thought of as a set of stable, enduring traits that impact social relations, cognition, behavior, and interaction with the environment. Efforts have been made to identify an alcoholic personality; however, current and past research does not support the existence of a single, specific personality structure for individuals with alcohol abuse or dependence. Rather, evidence suggests that broadband personality traits such as those from Hans Eysenck's Big Three model of personality are related to the risk for the development of alcohol abuse or dependence.

The big three traits can be described as extraversion (e.g., sensation seeking, assertiveness, sociability, dominance, venturesomeness), neuroticism (e.g., anxiousness, depressiveness, guilt, low self-esteem), and psychoticism (e.g., aggressiveness, impulsivity, tough-mindedness, creativity, antisociality). Although extraversion, neuroticism, and psychoticism may represent independent risk factors for alcohol abuse or dependence, they may co-occur and increase the risk for the development of alcohol-related problems. The discussion that follows details these traits and their relationship to alcohol abuse and dependence and identifies some parallels, but not complete overlap, between the big three factors and factors employed in one method of subtyping individuals with alcohol problems proposed by C. Robert Cloninger and associates. Although Cloninger's is not the only method for subtyping individuals with alcohol abuse or dependence, it serves as an example of one relatively successful effort to subtype individuals with alcohol problems in a way that meaningfully relates to onset, course, and symptoms based on a three-factor conception of personality.

Extraversion has been shown to be predictive of alcohol abuse or dependence symptoms, with higher levels of extraversion associated with increased alcohol abuse or dependence symptoms. It is not clear to what extent this trait reflects general disinhibition of behavior that may result in difficulties in discontinuing drinking once started, or whether the use of alcohol satisfies the sensation-seeking aspects of this dimension. It may be that individuals high in extraversion use alcohol for its euphoric and social enhancement effects and that alcohol use is sustained through positive reinforcement effects for individuals high in extraversion.

A second broadband personality trait that has been shown to predict alcohol abuse or dependence symptoms is neuroticism or negative emotionality. People who have high levels of negative mood states may use alcohol to relieve these states. Research suggests that negative-emotionality drinking may be more frequent among women relative to men. Individuals high in neuroticism may be more predisposed to physiological dependence on alcohol than those who are not characterized by high neuroticism. The traits of negative emotionality may stabilize or be reduced with a period of abstinence. It may be that the relief of negative mood states reinforces alcohol use negatively, thus sustaining alcohol use.

Psychoticism has been shown to be related to alcohol abuse and dependence and to the risk for later development of frank psychotic processes. Included in this broad trait is impulsivity. Impulsivity, which can be defined as the failure to plan ahead, acting on the spur of the moment without regard for long-term consequences, or the tendency to respond to immediate

rewards strongly without regard for long-term outcomes, has been shown to be related to risk for alcohol disorders. It may be that the immediate effects of alcohol (e.g., euphoria, disinhibition) are rewarding to individuals who are impulsive and outweigh the longer-term negative effects (e.g., health impacts, relationship problems, difficulties in functioning) that result from excessive alcohol use. Antisociality is another component of psychoticism that has been shown to be related to alcohol disorders in that antisocial individuals tend to have earlier age of onset, experience a greater severity of alcohol-related problems, and may respond more poorly to treatment.

A second, three-factor conceptualization of personality that has been found to be related to onset, course, and nature of alcohol-related symptoms is that of Cloninger and colleagues. Cloninger identified three personality components importantly related to two subtypes of alcoholism (Types 1 and 2) identified in twin studies using data from Swedish social services registries. Type 1 alcoholism is a less severe condition that is common among both males and females, generally has a later onset than Type 2, and is not necessarily associated with criminal behavior. Type 2 is a more severe condition that is more common among males, has an age of onset typically during adolescence, and is associated with criminal activity. The traits associated with Cloninger's subtyping are harm avoidance, novelty seeking, and reward dependence. Individuals who are high in harm avoidance tend to be cautious and more inhibited, whereas individuals who are low in harm avoidance are less anxious, more positive, and uninhibited. People high in novelty-seeking traits are impulsive, easily distracted, and open to experience, whereas people low in novelty-seeking traits tend to be more contemplative, less flexible, and detail oriented. High reward dependence describes the tendency to be helpful to others, emotionally attached, and socially sensitive. Low reward dependence reflects a tendency to be socially and emotionally unattached, utilitarian, and less responsive to social cues. Type 1 alcoholism is associated with high harm avoidance, low novelty seeking, and high reward dependence. Type 2 alcoholism exhibits the reverse profile, with low harm avoidance, high novelty seeking, and low reward dependence.

Personality patterns or unique clusters of traits that are maladaptive and cause significant distress or impairment are referred to as personality disorders. Perhaps the two most common personality disorder diagnoses seen among individuals with alcohol abuse or dependence are antisocial personality disorder (ASPD) and borderline personality disorder (BPD). ASPD is a personality disorder that begins early in adolescence and is characterized by the blatant disregard for the emotional and physical rights and safety of others and continued failure to adhere to social norms with regard to behavior, often in the form of criminality. ASPD is more common among men and is associated with an earlier age of onset of alcohol problems, a more severe symptom profile, and poorer prognosis for treatment outcomes. BPD disorder is more common among females and is characterized by frequent, intense mood swings; idealization and devaluation of others; impulsivity; and, possibly, self-injurious behavior. Impulsivity is a common component to both of these disorders; however, negative emotionality may be more predominant in BPD than in ASPD. In fact, ASPD may be characterized by a lack of negative emotionality with significant reward-based impulsivity. Whereas these two disorders may be the most frequently co-occurring personality disorders, personality disorders in general tend to be more frequent among individuals with alcohol abuse or dependence diagnoses relative to the rates seen in the general public.

One issue in the diagnosis of personality disorders in conjunction with alcohol abuse or dependence is to correctly attribute the symptoms related to substance use and the symptoms related to personality pathology. Excluding symptoms that may be substance related significantly lowers the prevalence of personality disorders among those with alcohol abuse or dependence. This is particularly true in the case of the frequently co-occurring ASPD. In fact a number of behaviors meeting criteria for ASPD, including lying, impulsivity and failure to plan ahead, deceitfulness, and reckless behavior, may reflect substance-induced behavior, and may remit upon a period of sobriety. On the other hand, it is possible that one of the manifestations of ASPD and other personality disorders may include problematic substance use (e.g., Cloninger's Type 2 classification).

In summary, although research does not support the existence of a single alcoholic personality, broad-band personality traits are related to an increased risk for alcohol abuse or dependence. These are extraversion, neuroticism, and psychoticism. These traits are independent of each other, can co-occur, and are somewhat similar, but not overlapping, with the traits

identified as components of Cloninger's Type 1 and 2 subgrouping of individuals with alcohol problems. Among individuals with alcohol abuse or dependence, there is an increased prevalence of personality disorders relative to rates observed in the general population. Although other personality disorders can co-occur with alcohol abuse or dependence, the two most commonly found are ASPD and BPD.

Michael D. Campos

See also Alcoholism; Antisocial Personality Disorder; Borderline Personality Disorder; *Diagnostic and Statistical Manual of Mental Disorders*; Genetic Aspects of Addiction

Further Readings

Cloninger, C. R., Sigvardsson, S., & Bohman, M. (1996). Type I and Type II alcoholism: An update. *Alcohol Health & Research World, 20*(1), 18–23.

Grekin, E. R., Sher, K. J., & Wood, P. K. (2006). Personality and substance dependence symptoms: Modeling substance-specific traits. *Psychology of Addictive Behaviors, 20*(4), 415–424.

Kwapil, T. R. (1996). A longitudinal study of drug and alcohol use by psychosis-prone and impulsive-nonconforming individuals. *Journal of Abnormal Psychology, 105*(1), 114–123.

Sher, K. J., & Trull, T. J. (1994). Personality and disinhibitory psychopathology: Alcoholism and antisocial personality disorder. *Journal of Abnormal Psychology, 103*(1), 92–102.

Sher, K. J., Trull, T. J., Bartholow, B. D., & Vieth, A. (1999). Personality and alcoholism: Issues, methods, and etiological process. In H. Blane & E. Leonard (Eds.), *Psychological theories of drinking and alcoholism* (pp. 54–105). New York: Plenum.

ALCOHOLICS ANONYMOUS

Alcoholics Anonymous, most commonly referred to as AA, is a support group for individuals seeking to recover from alcoholism. AA was cofounded in Akron, Ohio, in 1935, through a chance encounter between Dr. Bob (Bob Smith, M.D.) and Bill W. (Bill Wilson), both self-labeled alcoholics who had made many previously unsuccessful attempts to stop drinking. Unbeknownst to them at the time, a friendship began that would lead to the creation of the largest support group for alcoholics. The symbol for AA, which was presented at the International Convention in 1955, is a circle enclosing a triangle. The circle stands for the whole of AA, while the three arms of the triangle stand for AA's three legacies: recovery, unity, and service.

Structure and Membership in AA

AA is often referred to as a fellowship. There are no "rules" or "shoulds"; rather, there are Twelve Steps (suggestions for recovery that help each member's sobriety) and Twelve Traditions (guaranteeing AA's unity covering a guide to better ways of working and living). Because there is no formal membership, no one can be expelled from the group or punished. Members have the ability to interpret the *program,* as it is commonly called, as they like. Most alcoholics will not reach out to AA until they have hit "rock bottom" (had significant losses in their lives).

There is an estimated 1.7 million AA members in 150 countries. Membership is based solely on a desire to stop drinking. One need not be referred to AA, there is no formal registration process, no dues or fee to be paid, and no treatment plan developed. Participation is voluntary, not compulsory, although the criminal justice system may require AA attendance as a condition of probation or parole. The primary components of the AA model are to accept the label of being an "alcoholic," admit loss of control of use of alcohol, express a desire to quit drinking, and to become or remain abstinent from all forms of alcohol and mood-altering drugs. AA functions primarily as a support group for people with a common problem; there is no professional facilitator or group leader. According to AA, groups, which consist of at least two members, are the primary vehicles through which recovery takes place. There are an estimated 100,000 groups worldwide.

The group provides a sense of hope for individuals and has been written about extensively in the group literature. It also allows for a shared sense of purpose, a feeling of progress, and a sense of optimism as individuals recover and see their own change as well as that in others. AA gives many people a sense of faith, which guides them through recovery. Due to the perceived popularity and success of AA, group counseling has become the most popular method of treatment for alcoholism.

Meetings

Meetings, as the groups are referred to, are generally classified as open. Open meetings are available to anyone who wishes to attend, including longtime members and newcomers, alcoholic and nonalcoholic. Closed meetings are limited to individuals who identify themselves as members of the AA fellowship. Typically, closed meetings have a set of discussion topics (steps, the Big Book), and only AA members may attend. These meetings tend to be personal in nature or include an interpretation of the steps and traditions. Groups are available to meet many needs: newcomer groups for AA beginners; Big Book meetings, which center on the reading and interpretation of *Alcoholic Anonymous;* as well as groups that have been established to serve diverse populations, including women's groups, gay and lesbian groups, business-men groups, Hispanic groups, and many others. Meeting times and places are published in newspapers, or a local contact phone number can be obtained through the yellow pages or the AA Web site. Most meetings are held in donated spaces, thus allowing the meeting to take place for free.

For AA, as the name implies, the concept of anonymity is central. This means that individuals use only first names in meetings and are cautioned against disclosing personal identification. It serves three basic purposes for the organization and the membership: It focuses the attention of the new members on the recovery process and away from prestige or grandiosity; through anonymous participation in AA, members can give up their ego-driven struggles; and it provides a safe haven from the stigma attached to alcoholism. AA members are called upon to take responsibility for their actions (past and present), and they can do so in an anonymous setting. Finally, anonymity allows for the inclusive nature of AA, allowing anyone to be a member and reducing self-aggrandizing, favoring instead a new humble self-image for recovering alcoholics. The idea of anonymity has been reduced to some degree over the years, as many members are not afraid to admit they are alcoholics. Generally, though, identities to the press are not revealed, and AA does not seek publicity.

A central tenet of AA is that recovery is a lifelong process, for which there is no treatment but rather a remission of the process through abstinence. Thus, AA members refer to themselves as *recovering,* not recovered, alcoholics. As social relationships are believed to contribute to relapse, AA calls for individuals in recovery to seek new "playmates," implying that individuals must change their interests from consuming alcohol to other things. Those in recovery are urged to be aware of social relationships and activities that can assist in preventing relapse.

The Big Book

The primary philosophy of AA is outlined in what is commonly referred to as the "Big Book," or *Alcoholics Anonymous,* first written by Bill Wilson in 1967. The book consisted mainly of the Twelve Steps, which each AA member is encouraged to complete sequentially. The first step, "We admitted we were powerless over alcohol—that our lives had become unmanageable," is essentially the foundation of AA philosophy; recovery cannot begin until the person admits that he or she is powerless. The steps that follow the first step reinforce the notion that alcohol consumption is insane, is egocentric, and leads to a pattern of self-destruction and harm to others. There is no time frame or particular pattern for step completion; however, most members end up reviewing steps periodically as a way of maintaining their recovery. The concept of completing the Twelve Steps appears overwhelming to many alcoholics; however, the goal is not to complete each one in perfection but rather to grow spiritually. The steps serve as a guide to progress for the alcoholic and are believed to be open to interpretation rather than absolutes.

The Twelve Steps

1. We admitted we were powerless over alcohol—that our lives had become unmanageable.

2. Came to believe that a Power greater than ourselves could restore us to sanity.

3. Made a decision to turn our will and our lives over to the care of God *as we understood Him.*

4. Made a searching and fearless moral inventory of ourselves.

5. Admitted to God, to ourselves, and to another human being the exact nature of our wrongs.

6. Were entirely ready to have God remove all these defects of character.

7. Humbly asked Him to remove our shortcomings.

8. Made a list of all persons we had harmed, and became willing to make amends to them all.

9. Made a direct amends to such people wherever possible, except when to do so would injure them or others.

10. Continued to take personal inventory and when we were wrong promptly admitted it.

11. Sought through prayer and meditation to improve our conscious contact with God *as we understood Him,* praying only for knowledge of His will for us and the power to carry that out.

12. Having had a spiritual awakening as the result of these steps, we tried to carry this message to alcoholics, and to practice these principles in all our affairs.

The Twelve Steps are reprinted with permission of Alcoholics Anonymous World Services, Inc.

An AA guiding principle is that no one can beat alcohol alone. The alcoholic must submit to a Higher Power (most often God) that he or she needs assistance. This reference to a Higher Power in the Twelve Steps is sometimes criticized as including religion. Although the cofounders did not intend for AA to have any religious roots, they believed spirituality played a large role in recovery. The spiritual experience is deemed to give the person new motivation, providing a fresh rebirth and a new opportunity. It is believed that a spiritual awakening can banish the desire to drink. A belief in God is not essential for AA members. However, the belief in a "Higher Power, Power greater than" is essential, as is living by spiritual principles.

AA believes that the self-appraisal portion of the steps is not enough, as people are prone to rationalizations and wishful thinking. Thus, the use of a sponsor is recommended, that is, talking to another person who will provide direct comment and counsel about one's situation. Sponsors are members who are identified as having a relatively long period of sobriety and can act as resource persons to new members, or "pigeons." The sponsor gives advice and direction. The sponsor is supposed to be able to see through resistances and share his or her experience with the new member as a form of ongoing support. The sponsor can assist the member with avoiding relapse, attending meetings, and working the steps of AA. As with much of AA, there is no formal training for sponsors; rather, they rely on their own experience and recovery to assist others.

The Twelve Traditions

In addition to the Twelve Steps, there are the Twelve Traditions of AA. During its first decade, the AA fellowship had accumulated enough experience to assist in establishing a set of group attitudes and principles that were deemed necessary to maintain the survival of the informal structure of the fellowship. In 1946, the cofounders and early members published these as the Twelve Traditions of Alcoholics Anonymous. They were accepted and endorsed by the membership as a whole at the International Convention of AA in Cleveland, Ohio, in 1950. The Twelve Traditions emphasize AA unity, the importance of a higher power, lack of membership requirements, avoiding endorsements, refusal of outside contributions, the necessity of peer support over professional intervention, avoidance of taking a position on outside issues, and the importance of personal autonomy.

Although the Twelve Traditions are not specifically binding on any group, an overwhelming majority of members have adopted them. The Twelve Traditions are neither rules nor regulations nor laws. Members adhere to the Twelve Traditions because they ought to and want to. In an effort to keep AA neutral and focused on its mission, contributions by outside sources are not accepted and from individual AA members are limited to $1,000 a year. AA does not lend its name or logo to any treatment facility organization.

Conclusion

The influence of AA and its Twelve Steps is currently observed in treatments for many other problems, including overeating, gambling, and codependency. There has been tremendous social and political pressure to apply the Twelve Step concept and disease–abstinence model to all psychoactive substances. Approaches based on the AA Twelve-Step model dominate the substance abuse treatment field and are likely to remain influential and popular for years to come.

Maureen C. Kenny and Charles B. Winick

See also Big Book The; Bill W.; Recovery; Support Groups; Twelve Steps

Further Readings

Alcoholics Anonymous World Services, Inc. (2001). *Alcoholics anonymous: The story of how many thousands of men and women have recovered from alcoholism.* New York: Author.

Alcoholics Anonymous World Services, Inc. (2002). *Twelve steps and twelve traditions.* New York: Author.

Alcoholics Anonymous World Services, Inc. (2006). *Alcoholics anonymous big book* (4th ed.). New York: Author.

Hamilton, B. (1995). *Getting started in AA.* Center City, MN: Hazelden.

Lemanski, M. (2001). *A history of addiction and recovery in the United States.* Tucson, AZ: See Sharp Press.

Robertson, N. (1988). *Getting better inside Alcoholics Anonymous.* New York: Morrow.

Wekesser, C. (Ed.). (1994). *Alcoholism.* San Diego, CA: Greenhaven Press.

ALCOHOL-INDUCED DISORDERS

Alcohol is the most commonly used central nervous system (CNS) depressant in the world. A 2006 survey conducted by the Substance Abuse and Mental Health Services Administration found that, in the past month, 50.9% of individuals in the United States used alcohol, 23.0% had engaged in binge drinking (five or more drinks on one occasion), and 6.9% were considered heavy drinkers (five or more episodes of binge drinking in 1 month). Individuals 21 to 25 years of age were the heaviest users, with 68.6% reporting use in the past month, 50% reporting at least one episode of binge drinking, and 16.7% classified as heavy alcohol users. As would be expected based on the high rates of use, mental and physical disorders resulting from the excessive use of alcohol are also highly prevalent. More specifically, approximately 40% of the U.S. population will experience at least one alcohol-related accident during their lifetime; as much as 55% of all driving-related fatalities are associated with alcohol use; and more than 50% of all homicides are alcohol related, with either the perpetrator or the victim intoxicated at the time of the murder. Males have higher rates of problems resulting from alcohol use (60% vs. 30% for females), and males are more often diagnosed with alcohol-related disorders.

The *Diagnostic and Statistical Manual of Mental Disorders, Fourth Edition, Text Revision (DSM-IV-TR)*

includes alcohol-related disorders in its section on substance-related disorders, which includes 10 categories of substances in addition to alcohol, such as opioids, amphetamines, and hallucinogens. Disorders resulting from alcohol use are broken down into two general types of disorders—namely, alcohol use disorders and alcohol-induced disorders. Alcohol use disorders include two diagnoses—alcohol abuse and alcohol dependence; alcohol-induced disorders include alcohol intoxication and alcohol withdrawal, as well as eight different alcohol-induced mental disorders (i.e., alcohol-induced persisting dementia, alcohol-induced persisting amnestic disorder, alcohol-induced delirium, alcohol-induced psychotic disorder, alcohol-induced mood disorder, alcohol-induced anxiety disorder, alcohol-induced sexual dysfunction, and alcohol-induced sleep disorder).

The alcohol-induced mental disorders are diagnosed in lieu of alcohol intoxication or alcohol withdrawal and share symptoms of primary mental disorders described elsewhere in the *DSM-IV-TR* (e.g., the symptoms experienced in alcohol-induced mood disorder with depressive features resemble those of major depressive disorder). Unlike the primary disorders, however, the symptoms are due to the effects of alcohol. The symptoms of alcohol-induced persisting dementia and alcohol-induced persisting amnestic disorder continue long after intoxication or withdrawal has resolved and may be permanent. The symptoms experienced in the other disorders are transient in nature, with onset during either intoxication or withdrawal. Diagnoses are made when the psychological symptoms present are more severe than what typically occurs during intoxication or withdrawal. Thus, whereas some symptoms of anxiety are common during alcohol withdrawal, excessive symptoms of anxiety would warrant a diagnosis of alcohol-induced anxiety disorder. If symptoms persist for more than 4 weeks after acute intoxication or withdrawal has resolved, a formal diagnosis of a primary mental disorder is warranted. Finally, the symptoms in alcohol-induced disorders must cause significant subjective distress or impaired functioning to warrant a diagnosis.

When diagnosing alcohol-induced disorders, the substance thought to be causing the disorder (in this case, alcohol) and the disorder itself are always specified (e.g., alcohol withdrawal or alcohol intoxication). Predominant symptoms and the context in which the symptoms began (i.e., during intoxication or withdrawal) may also be specified. For example,

the diagnosis of alcohol-induced mood disorder with depressed features with onset during withdrawal would be given when depressed symptoms are present that are thought to be associated with alcohol use and which begin during alcohol withdrawal. The link between the symptoms and the alcohol use must be clearly established to allow for a diagnosis. For example, a history of a preexisting mental disorder such as major depressive disorder may preclude the diagnosis of an alcohol-induced mood disorder with depressed features because the symptoms of depression may be indicative of the primary major depressive disorder, whose symptoms may have simply been exacerbated by heavy alcohol use. In these instances, a detailed history must be gained in order to clearly document the onset and offset of alcohol use in relation to onset of psychological symptoms.

Assessment

Because a critical aspect of diagnosing alcohol-induced disorders is to establish the link between alcohol use and onset of psychological symptoms, careful assessment is required, which often involves an extensive psychosocial history. Psychologists, psychiatrists, physicians, licensed or certified addiction counselors, and licensed clinical social workers may all be involved in gathering information, although the specific qualifications required to make diagnoses may vary by state. For some alcohol-induced disorders, such as persisting dementia and persisting amnestic disorder, more specialized training is required to make the diagnosis, which is based not only on the psychosocial interview but also may require a physical and neurological examination (i.e., to include brain imaging procedures), neuropsychological testing to document deficits in memory and other cognitive abilities, and an assessment of functional outcomes. Thus, for some of the alcohol-induced disorders, a diagnosis is made following an extensive evaluation by an interdisciplinary team of professionals, each of whom is specialized to evaluate a specific aspect of the disorder in question.

The assessment of individuals with alcohol-induced disorders can also be complicated by a number of factors unique to those who have substance use disorders. For example, it can often be difficult to assess individuals with substance-induced disorders because there may be strong incentives for these persons to underreport or deny substance use because of possible negative consequences resulting from the admission of use. It may also be the case that individuals with long histories of use may be unable to accurately remember the details of prior use, mainly because some substances can cause deficits in cognitive abilities such as memory. Therefore, individuals with long histories of use may simply be unable to accurately remember the details of prior use. Alcohol-induced dementia and amnestic disorder are extreme examples, where cognitive deficits (the presence of which are required in order to make these diagnoses) interfere with the ability to accurately report a history of alcohol use. However, it is also the case that more subtle deficits in learning and memory, which are more common than amnestic disorder or dementia, may also render a patient unable to accurately recall alcohol use history. As a result, in many cases, an initial suspicion of substance use will require supplemental information in addition to the client's self-reported use. In this regard, it is helpful to obtain collateral reports from significant others, perform drug screening, and review available medical records, with special attention given to patterns of medical problems that are consistent with substance use and whether the client has been prescribed any medications that have a high potential for abuse and dependence (e.g., benzodiazepines).

Specialized psychological and laboratory tests may be helpful when evaluating the quantity and frequency of alcohol use, symptom severity, and the presence of comorbid psychological disorders commonly associated with alcohol use. The Time-Line Follow Back assessment procedure is useful for documenting alcohol use over the prior 4 months. The Substance Abuse Subtle Screening Inventory-3 assists in identifying individuals at risk for alcohol use disorders. The Addiction Severity Index assesses the impact that alcohol use has on medical status, employment status, family and social relationships, legal status, and psychiatric/psychological status. Neuropsychological measures of memory, attention, problem solving, motor speed, and visuospatial abilities are useful in detecting transient and enduring neurocognitive deficits that result from the effects of alcohol on the brain. Useful laboratory tests include gamma-glutamyltransferase and carbohydrate deficient transferrin, which are sensitive state indicators of heavy drinking. Liver function tests such as albumin, total bilirubin, alanine aminotransferase, aspartate aminotransferase, and alkaline phosphatase are useful for

documenting liver damage resulting from heavy alcohol use. Recent alcohol use can be identified through blood alcohol levels, which are determined through blood or urine specimens or by using a breathalyzer.

Alcohol Intoxication and Withdrawal

Alcohol intoxication and alcohol withdrawal are characterized by behavioral, cognitive, and physiological symptoms. Symptoms of alcohol intoxication develop soon after consumption and include slurred speech, impaired coordination and balance, memory and attention problems, poor judgment, and, in severe cases, stupor or coma. Blackouts are sometimes experienced during intoxication and are characterized by amnesia for the period of intoxication. Blackouts are thought to occur when intoxication occurs rapidly, and amnesia resolves as intoxication abates.

Symptoms of alcohol withdrawal typically develop 4 to 12 hours after cessation of alcohol use during which time levels of alcohol in the blood drop quickly. Withdrawal symptoms may include sweating, increased heart rate, insomnia, anxiety, nausea, vomiting, shaky hands, restlessness, and irritability. In rare cases, severe symptoms such as grand mal seizures, hallucinations, and delirium can develop. For the more severe symptoms, medical treatment is necessary during detoxification to avoid serious and sometimes life-threatening medical complications. Withdrawal symptoms can be alleviated by the consumption of alcohol or the administration of another central nervous system depressant, including a benzodiazepine, such as Valium or Klonopin. If left untreated, the milder symptoms will be at their worst around the second day following cessation of drinking and will typically improve by the fifth day. If hallucinations are present during intoxication or withdrawal and are recognized by the individual to be associated with alcohol use, they would be diagnosed by including the specifier "with perceptual disturbances."

Alcohol-Induced Delirium

Delirium is defined as a fluctuating change in consciousness and cognition. Alcohol-induced delirium can occur during intoxication or withdrawal and is characterized by an inability to maintain focused attention, memory impairment, confusion regarding place and time, disturbed language abilities, hallucinations, psychomotor agitation or retardation, emotional disturbances (i.e., depression, anxiety, euphoria, irritability), and alterations in the sleep–wake cycle. Symptoms develop quickly (several hours to several days) and fluctuate over the course of a day. In cases of delirium during intoxication, symptoms develop while the individual is intoxicated and tend to remit within a few hours or a few days following cessation of alcohol use. Symptoms may take longer to resolve in individuals who are older, who have brain damage, or who engage in polysubstance use. Also, intoxication delirium may develop more quickly in those who have a comorbid medical condition (e.g., liver or kidney disease) that causes substances to build up more quickly in the blood.

Delirium during withdrawal is the most severe of the alcohol withdrawal symptoms and is often referred to as delirium tremens, or "DTs." Symptoms generally develop between 3 and 5 hours after cessation of alcohol use, and though they typically last no longer than 5 days, they can last much longer in some cases. Specific symptoms include anxiety, tremors, agitation, hyperactivity of the autonomic nervous system (as evidenced by fever, increased heart rate, increased blood pressure), disturbed sleep, disorientation, delusions, and hallucinations. Following symptom remission, the individual will often fall into a deep and heavy sleep and have little or no memory of the experience upon awakening. Individuals who have sustained head injuries, have other medical illnesses, have a history of alcohol withdrawal or seizure, or who are malnourished are more prone to alcohol-withdrawal delirium. Medical treatment is necessary to avoid serious medical complications.

Alcohol-Induced Persisting Dementia

Dementia is characterized by deficits in memory and in other areas, such as language, executive functions, attention, and visuospatial abilities. Memory deficits include disturbances in the ability to learn new information and difficulties in recalling previously learned information. Other cognitive deficits often include apraxia, or the inability to perform skilled movements, and agnosia, which is the inability to recognize familiar objects, including people. Executive functioning impairments include difficulties in problem solving, planning, initiating appropriate actions, and inhibiting inappropriate behaviors. Alcohol-induced dementia has an insidious onset, often taking many years to develop. Its symptoms are permanent,

persisting long after alcohol consumption has ceased. Some controversy exists regarding the diagnosis, as it is not known whether alcohol-induced dementia can be due to the neurotoxic effects of alcohol on the brain, damage to the brain through other conditions that commonly occur along with alcoholism (e.g., traumatic brain injury, malnutrition), some other brain disorder (Alzheimer's disease), or some combination of these factors.

Alcohol-Induced Persisting Amnestic Disorder

In contrast to dementia, an amnestic disorder affects only the memory, with a relative sparing of other cognitive abilities. Following the onset of an amnestic disorder, there is a marked inability to learn and remember new information, with some impairment in the ability to remember information learned prior to the onset of the disorder. These deficits in learning and memory lead to the severe impairment of social, familial, and vocational functioning.

Individuals who develop alcohol-induced amnestic disorder have usually been extremely heavy users over a period of many years. The biological basis for alcohol-induced amnestic disorder is not the alcohol itself, but rather a deficiency in the B vitamin thiamine. Because thiamine is not stored in the body, but rather maintained through an adequate diet, thiamine can become depleted in individuals who consume extremely large amounts of alcohol over prolonged periods and at the same time neglect eating. With the depletion of thiamine, hemorrhages to structures in the middle of the brain occur, causing a characteristic pattern of symptoms, which include an unsteady gait, nystagmus (involuntary eye movements), ophthalmoplegia (partial or full paralysis of the eyes), and confusion. This acute phase of the disorder is referred to as Wernicke's encephalopathy and, if left untreated, will eventually result in coma and death. Symptoms of Wernicke's encephalopathy typically resolve in 4 weeks with the administration of large doses of thiamine. Most patients then go on to develop an amnestic disorder referred to as Wernicke-Korsakoff's syndrome. As with all amnestic disorders, a severe impairment of memory is present; impairment in other areas of cognitive functioning, such as problem solving and executive functions, may also be present. General intellectual functioning and memory for events prior to the onset of the disorder are typically preserved. Given the severity of this disorder, treatment providers should always consider the patient's nutritional status and administer thiamine prophylactically to prevent the onset of Wernicke's encephalopathy.

Alcohol-Induced Psychotic Disorders

The primary characteristics of an alcohol-induced psychotic disorder are the presence of hallucinations, delusions, or both, which are the direct effects of alcohol use. This disorder is diagnosed only when the hallucinations or delusions are more severe than those that would be "normally" experienced during either intoxication or withdrawal, and only if the individual is unable to recognize that the hallucinations or delusions are due to the effects of alcohol. Alcohol-induced psychotic disorders are diagnosed based on whether symptoms begin during intoxication or withdrawal. If the symptoms begin during alcohol intoxication, they can continue as long as the alcohol is being consumed. If they begin during alcohol withdrawal, the symptoms can last up to several weeks after the end of the withdrawal. Additionally, the diagnosis may also include a subtype to indicate whether hallucinations or delusions are prominent. An alcohol-induced psychotic disorder is not diagnosed if psychotic symptoms only occur during the course of alcohol-induced delirium.

Differentiating alcohol-induced psychotic disorders from primary psychotic disorders can be challenging because substance use may precede or closely coincide with the onset of primary psychotic disorder. In fact, the co-occurrence of substance use disorders in individuals diagnosed with primary psychotic disorders such as schizophrenia is approximately 50%. Thus, clinical factors such as age of onset of psychotic symptoms, chronicity of alcohol use, and duration of symptoms should be considered when making this diagnosis. For example, since the onset of schizophrenia tends to be in the late teens and early twenties, the possibility of alcohol-induced psychotic disorder should be considered for individuals who are experiencing delusions or hallucinations for the first time and are past the typical age of onset for schizophrenia. Because alcohol-induced psychotic disorder is generally only seen in individuals who have a long history of alcohol dependence, the diagnosis becomes even more likely if the individual is, in fact, found to have a long history of alcohol use. Finally, because the

symptoms of alcohol-induced psychotic disorder do not persist past 4 weeks of withdrawal or intoxication, symptoms that persist for longer than this time period should be considered indicative of a primary psychotic disorder.

Alcohol-Induced Mood Disorders

Alcohol-induced mood disorders are characterized by a disturbance in mood that is more severe than what typically occurs during intoxication or withdrawal. These mood symptoms must develop within 1 month of intoxication or withdrawal and persist beyond what is typically expected or observed. While alcohol-induced mood disorders may resemble any of the *DSM-IV-TR* mood episodes, including major depressive, manic, mixed, or hypomanic episodes, it is not necessary that the full criteria for these mood episodes be met in order to diagnose an alcohol-induced mood disorder. The diagnosis includes a specification of the phase during which mood symptoms developed (i.e., during intoxication or withdrawal), as well as a subtype that characterizes the predominant mood symptoms (i.e., depressed, manic, or mixed). A diagnosis of a primary mood disorder should be considered if the mood symptoms either precede use or extend significantly past the cessation of the intoxication or withdrawal period. Similar to alcohol-induced psychotic disorders, the symptoms of an alcohol-induced mood disorder resolve within 4 weeks.

Alcohol-Induced Anxiety Disorders

Alcohol-induced anxiety disorders can occur during either intoxication or withdrawal. Symptoms resemble those experienced in primary (i.e., non-alcohol-induced) anxiety disorders. Alcohol-induced anxiety disorders are diagnosed only when the symptoms experienced are unusually prolonged or intense compared to "normal" anxiety symptoms experienced during alcohol intoxication or alcohol withdrawal. In addition to specifying whether symptoms begin during intoxication or withdrawal, subtype specification is made based on the predominant symptoms, including either generalized anxiety disorder (i.e., excessive worrying in all or multiple areas of life), panic attacks (i.e., the presence of random and unexpected panic attacks), obsessive-compulsive symptoms (i.e., the presence of obtrusive and repeated thoughts accompanied by an inability to get rid of such thoughts, or the need to perform rituals or actions repeatedly in response to a stimulus or to obsessive thoughts, or both), or phobic symptoms (i.e., disorders characterized by the excessive and unreasonable fear of an object, person, or situation).

Alcohol-Induced Sexual Dysfunctions

In contrast to several of the disorders previously mentioned, alcohol-induced sexual dysfunctions occur only during alcohol intoxication. The symptoms experienced must be beyond those which are normally experienced during intoxication. As an example, a sharply decreased sexual libido and difficulty attaining an erection are common occurrences during alcohol intoxication and would thus not be considered symptoms of an alcohol-induced sexual dysfunction. An alcohol-induced sexual dysfunction can occur at the desire, excitement, and orgasm phases of the human sexual response cycle; subtype specifiers are thus included in the diagnosis and are based on during which phase the predominant symptoms occur: desire, arousal, or orgasm. An additional subtype is provided for sexual pain disorder. Alcohol-induced sexual dysfunction appears to be generalized in that it is not limited to a particular partner or situation. Any significant disturbance in normal sexual functioning that occurs either prior to or following alcohol intoxication is more likely a primary sexual disorder rather than one that is alcohol induced.

Alcohol-Induced Sleep Disorders

Alcohol-induced sleep disorders can occur either during alcohol intoxication or alcohol withdrawal and can be further subtyped as insomnia type, hypersomnia type, parasomnia type, or mixed type. The insomnia type is the most common and is characterized by difficulties in falling asleep or maintaining sleep throughout the night. When symptoms appear during alcohol intoxication, they are characterized by an initial period of increased sleepiness followed by a period of both difficulties falling asleep and restless sleep characterized by anxiety-provoking dreams. Alcohol-induced sleep disorders that occur during alcohol withdrawal are characterized by disruption in the normal pattern of sleep with an increase in the intensity and vividness of dreams, as well as difficulty in remaining asleep. Vivid dreams are often anxiety-provoking whether they occur during intoxication or withdrawal. For individuals who have used alcohol heavily and for many years, sleep may continue to be slightly disturbed for years following the cessation of drinking.

Conclusion

Alcohol-induced disorders are a heterogeneous collection of disorders that are grouped together because they are all associated with alcohol use. In some cases, a diagnosis may be relatively straightforward (e.g., alcohol intoxication or alcohol withdrawal), while in others the diagnosis is complicated and requires the expertise of interdisciplinary teams using specialized assessment procedures (e.g., alcohol-induced persisting dementia). Because these disorders cause significant distress and impairment in psychosocial functioning that are above and beyond the effects of alcohol abuse or dependence, it is important for treatment providers to be aware of their diagnostic criteria and to provide the appropriate adjunctive treatment in order to diminish the debilitating effects of these disorders and minimize their negative impact on adjustment following the cessation of substance use.

Griffin P. Sutton and Daniel N. Allen

See also Alcohol; Alcoholism; Central Nervous System Depressants; Substance-Induced Disorders; Substance-Induced Withdrawal Delirium

Further Readings

American Psychiatric Association. (2000). *Diagnostic and statistical manual of mental disorders* (4th ed., text rev.). Washington, DC: Author.

Zernig, G., Saria, A., Kurz, M., & O'Malley, S. S. (Eds.). (2000). *Handbook of alcoholism*. Boca Raton, FL: CRC Press.

ALCOHOLISM

The term *alcoholism* was once the official term for alcohol addiction included in the *Diagnostic and Statistical Manual of Mental Disorders* (*DSM*), published by the American Psychiatric Association. *Alcoholism* has since lost its official status, replaced by the term *alcohol dependence* in both the *DSM* and in the *International Classification of Diseases* (*ICD*), published by the World Health Organization.

Nonetheless, the term *alcoholism* is still typically used by lay persons as well as by researchers and clinicians in the field.

There have been many definitions of alcoholism used over the years. The differences among these definitions are perhaps a testament to the heterogeneous nature of the condition. The current diagnostic criteria used by clinicians and researchers also reflect the many ways in which alcoholism can manifest itself. For example, any given pair of patients, both of whom could be labeled as "alcoholic," will probably share a number of characteristics, but they will likely differ in many ways as well. These differences could include the exact symptoms of their condition, the degree to which their condition includes or does not include a physiological component, and the magnitude and type of negative consequences they have experienced as a result of their drinking.

Definitions

Alcoholism has been defined in many different ways over the years. Authors such as John Saunders have reviewed shifting trends in the prominence of these various definitions. For instance, during the 19th century, it was widely accepted that alcoholism represented a moral failing. A contrasting view is the disease model of alcoholism, in which the condition is viewed as biologically determined and having a predictable progression of symptoms over time. E. M. Jellinek is perhaps the best-known proponent of the disease model, which gained its highest levels of prominence in the 1940s and 1950s but fell out of favor in the 1960s and 1970s.

In 1976, Griffith Edwards and Milton Gross described the seminal concept of the alcohol dependence syndrome (ADS). In contrast with prior approaches, Edwards and Gross's goal was description, rather than taking a firm stance as to how the syndrome develops. Impairment of control over drinking is a central symptom of ADS, which is characterized by both physiological (e.g., tolerance and withdrawal) and psychological aspects (e.g., awareness of compulsive drinking behavior). In Edwards and Gross's view, ADS is one type of alcohol problem with the other type comprising alcohol-related consequences such as injuries or legal trouble. These two types of alcohol problems were viewed as distinct but related, co-occurring in some but not all heavy drinkers. The concept of the ADS was highly

influential and had a great impact on the formation of later editions of the two most widely utilized classification schemes for alcohol use disorders: the *DSM* and the *ICD* manuals.

The *DSM* and *ICD* each contain a list of criteria, some of which need to be met in order for a diagnosis of an alcohol use disorder to be made. The goal of these and other classification systems was to attempt to create a common language among clinicians and researchers, to increase the reliability and validity with which patients are diagnosed, and to obtain accurate statistics as to the prevalence of problem drinking. Although the institution of the *DSM* and *ICD* has led to progress with respect to these goals, debate continues as to which characteristics of problem drinking should be emphasized and de-emphasized.

Diagnostic and Statistical Manual of Mental Disorders (DSM)

The first *DSM* was published by the American Psychiatric Association in 1952. In this first version, substance use disorders were categorized as a subset of personality disorders. Taking their cue from Jellinek, the term *alcoholism* was used, defined as an established alcohol addiction not identifiable as having been caused by another disorder. No specific criteria were provided. In the second edition (*DSM-II*), published in 1968, alcoholism continued to be classified along with the personality disorders. As with *DSM-I*, no specific criteria were offered, although it was advised that withdrawal symptoms were the best evidence for the existence of alcoholism. The first two editions of the *DSM* were based on clinical consensus, as scientific research was limited at the time.

The third edition (*DSM-III*) was published in 1980 and was the first edition to include diagnostic criteria for addiction and was also the first to be based upon research findings. Alcohol use disorders were no longer grouped with personality disorders but were instead a part of a new subset of disorders titled *substance use disorders*. The term *alcoholism* was no longer used. In its place, two types of alcohol use disorders were identified: abuse and dependence. There were three criteria for abuse. For a dependence diagnosis to be made, there had to be evidence of a physiological component, either tolerance or withdrawal. The *DSM-III* was revised, and the *DSM-III-R* was published in 1987. The abuse criteria were reduced from three to two in the *DSM-III-R*, and the dependence diagnosis underwent a significant expansion to nine criteria, of which three had to be met. These changes made in *DSM-III* and *DSM-III-R* were largely based on Edwards and Gross's alcohol dependence syndrome. Like Edwards and Gross's work, the *DSM* took a descriptive approach, avoiding the issue of how addiction develops. The separation of abuse from dependence beginning with *DSM-III* was based on Edwards and Gross's conceptualization of a condition separate from dependence that is typified by alcohol-related consequences. The expanded criteria for dependence in the *DSM-III-R* included both physiological and psychological elements, in accordance with Edwards and Gross's description of dependence as having physiological and psychological aspects.

The *DSM-III-R* was replaced by the *DSM-IV* in 1994. The distinction between alcohol abuse and dependence was retained, and a hierarchical approach to diagnosis was added. With this hierarchical approach, abuse is considered to be a less severe diagnosis that serves as a marker for risk of subsequent development of the more severe condition of dependence. A diagnosis of dependence supersedes an abuse diagnosis in *DSM-IV*, meaning that an individual cannot be diagnosed with both abuse and dependence. There were other changes made in the *DSM-IV* as well. In the *DSM-III-R*, abuse was characterized by social and medical consequences, whereas in the *DSM-IV*, abuse concerns negative legal and social consequences. In the *DSM-IV*, the number of dependence criteria was reduced from nine to seven. Notably, unlike *DSM-III-R*, the *DSM-IV* does not require a physiological component (i.e., tolerance or withdrawal symptoms) in order for a patient to be diagnosed as alcohol dependent. The number of symptoms required to be present for a dependence diagnosis remained three, but the symptoms all now had to occur within a 1-year period.

Diagnostic Criteria for Abuse and Dependence

There are four criteria for alcohol abuse in the *DSM-IV*, of which individuals must demonstrate only one in order to be diagnosed:

1. Problems in fulfilling roles at work, school, or at home resulting from drinking or from being hung over

2. Having repeatedly been in situations in which it was unsafe to drink, referring to situations in which one could have been hurt or in which someone else could have been hurt, with the most frequently cited example being driving while intoxicated

3. Recurrent legal problems resulting from drinking

4. Drinking despite the knowledge that it is causing problems with family or friends

In most clinical or research contexts, if there is evidence of one or more of the four criteria, the assessment would continue in order to assess whether criteria for a diagnosis of dependence is satisfied. In most contexts, if there is no evidence for any of the abuse criteria, then the assessment typically ends.

There are seven criteria for a diagnosis of dependence. Three of these criteria must be met within the past year in order to justify a diagnosis of alcohol dependence. The seven criteria constitute physiological elements of dependence (i.e., tolerance and withdrawal), impairment of control over alcohol use, and other behaviors indicative of a problem with alcohol. Although a physiological component is not required for a diagnosis of alcohol dependence in *DSM-IV*, it has been repeatedly established by Marc Schuckit and colleagues in reports published from 1998 through 2001 that a dependence diagnosis that includes physiological features is associated with poorer subsequent outcomes than a dependence diagnosis without these features. The dependence criteria are as follows:

1. Tolerance, which is a need to consume a considerably greater quantity of alcohol in order to attain similar effects as when one first began drinking, or for individuals who have not increased the quantity of alcohol they typically consume, the consumption of the same level of alcohol as before is associated with substantially weaker effects

2. Withdrawal, or the experience of at least two of the following symptoms during a period of not drinking: autonomic hyperactivity (e.g., sweating or heart racing), increased hand tremor, insomnia, nausea or vomiting, psychomotor agitation, anxiety, seizures or hallucinations, or drinking to relieve or avoid these types of symptoms

3. Frequent consumption of alcohol either more often or in larger amounts than one intended

4. Repeated unsuccessful attempts to quit drinking or to cut back the amount one drinks

5. Spending a lot of time in the process of drinking, including obtaining alcohol, consumption itself, and recovery from alcohol consumption

6. Forfeiting other activities that are enjoyable or important in favor of drinking

7. Continuing to drink with the knowledge that it may be causing physical or psychological harm

A 2004 report from the National Epidemiological Survey of Alcohol and Related Conditions (NESARC) places the prevalence of current (12-month) alcohol abuse at 4.7% (6.9% for males, 2.6% for females) and alcohol dependence at 3.8% (5.4% for males, 2.3% for females). Based on findings from the 2005 National Comorbidity Survey Replication, the lifetime prevalence for abuse was 13.2% and was 5.4% for dependence.

Reliability and Validity of Diagnoses

The reliability and validity of the alcohol dependence diagnosis has been empirically confirmed by several research groups, including Schuckit and colleagues in 2001 and 2002 and Deborah Hasin and colleagues in 2003. The chronic and severe nature of alcohol dependence was demonstrated in a 2001 study by Schuckit and colleagues in which approximately two thirds of subjects diagnosed with alcohol dependence at baseline remained alcohol dependent 5 years later. A report by Schuckit and others from the Collaborative Study of the Genetics of Alcoholism concluded that, with the exception of the third diagnostic criterion relating to the use of alcohol in larger quantities and for longer periods than intended, the criteria for dependence all had similar associations with drinking outcomes 5 years later.

The abuse diagnosis has been found to have lower interrater reliability than that of dependence. Criticisms of the diagnosis of alcohol abuse include questions as to whether alcohol abuse reflects risky behavior more so than a psychiatric disorder. Accordingly, the comorbidity of alcohol abuse with other disorders identified in the *DSM* is not considerable. Although the abuse diagnosis was developed with the thinking that it would act as a marker of high risk for subsequent onset of alcohol dependence, empirical findings from Hasin and colleagues in 1997 and Schuckit and colleagues in 2001 have demonstrated that fewer than 10% of those diagnosed with

abuse at a given time will eventually develop dependence. However, it should be noted that these figures, although low, are higher than the likelihood of alcohol dependence in the general population.

With respect to the division between alcohol dependence and abuse, it seems clear that drinkers meeting criteria for alcohol dependence tend toward worse outcomes than those diagnosed with abuse. In a 1999 report from the National Longitudinal Alcohol Epidemiologic Survey, those with current alcohol dependence consumed significantly more alcohol, were more likely to seek help for their drinking, and had more suicidal ideation or attempts and more blackouts than those diagnosed with abuse. It should also be noted that those diagnosed with abuse scored higher than those with no alcohol-related diagnosis for all of these outcomes except for suicidal ideation or attempts. In this study, a similar pattern emerged for associations between lifetime abuse or dependence and a family history of alcohol dependence. Those with lifetime dependence were more likely than those with lifetime abuse to have this history, and those with lifetime abuse were at greater risk than those without an alcohol-related diagnosis. However, this does not mean that all seven dependence criteria are more severe in nature than all four abuse criteria. Recent findings from the NESARC suggest that the 11 criteria that make up the two diagnoses can be ordered on a continuum. Their findings reaffirmed the severity of tolerance and withdrawal; however, they also found that abuse criterion number four—drinking despite knowledge of social or interpersonal problems—was in the most serious tier. The criterion for dependence related to consumption of larger amounts of alcohol or for a longer time than intended was found to be the least serious. Although the distinction between abuse and dependence might be valid with respect to severity, empirical evidence has challenged abuse and dependence as being two mutually exclusive diagnoses. Based on 1994 findings from the NLAES, a considerable minority of drinkers diagnosed with current alcohol dependence would not have been diagnosed with abuse. Similarly, in the more recent 2004 NESARC data, 33.7% of participants meeting criteria for current alcohol dependence did not meet criteria for abuse (29% in males, 46.1% in females). With respect to lifetime diagnoses, 13.9% of those diagnosed with a history of dependence did not meet criteria for lifetime abuse (10.1% in males, 22.1% in females). These findings strongly challenge the practice of assessing dependence only in patients for whom an abuse criterion has already been met.

An additional question regarding the validity of the abuse and dependence diagnoses concerns their applicability to adolescents. A number of the criteria for a diagnosis of alcohol dependence, such as withdrawal and continued consumption despite physical or psychological harm, are rarely reported by adolescents and thus may be less relevant to them than they are to adults. It has also been suggested that the tolerance criterion may be difficult to apply to adolescents because of wide individual differences in the quantities of alcohol required for adolescents to achieve particular effects. The "more often/larger quantities than intended" criterion might not readily apply to adolescents, as they are less likely to set predetermined limits on their levels of consumption.

In summary, it seems clear from the empirical evidence that alcohol dependence is a reliable and valid diagnosis and that dependence is a chronic and severe condition. Alcohol abuse is a less chronic and less severe condition, as it was intended to be. Further evidence for the validity of the abuse diagnosis can be found in studies showing that those with an abuse diagnosis are at greater risk for negative alcohol-related outcomes than those without such a diagnosis. With respect to challenges to validity, there is evidence for overlap in the severity of individual abuse and dependence criteria in that the seven individual dependence criteria are not more severe in nature than all four abuse criteria. Also, empirical findings have challenged the common practice in which diagnosis for dependence takes place only when at least one criterion for abuse has already been met. There are also questions as to the extent to which the abuse and dependence diagnoses apply to adolescent drinkers.

The fifth edition of the *DSM* is scheduled to be published in 2011. Researchers and clinicians have put forth a number of suggested changes for the diagnoses of substance use disorders. Some have suggested that neurobiological criteria be included. Others have pointed to the role of cultural, ethnic, and religious background in shaping what constitutes safe versus unsafe substance use and that attempts should be made to account for these differences. In response to research identifying differences in the manifestation of abuse and dependence criteria by drinkers at varying age levels, the suggestion has been made to offer separate criteria based on the age group of the patient.

International Classification of Diseases (ICD)

The eighth revision of the *ICD*, published in 1967, included substance-related disorders for the first time. In the *ICD-8*, substance use disorders were classified as a subtype of personality disorders. Alcohol use disorders were referred to as "alcoholism." In the ninth revision of the *ICD*, published in 1978, the World Health Organization made a monumental shift and categorized substance use disorders as their own entity. The term *alcoholism* was dropped and replaced with two categories: dependence and harmful use. The *ICD-10* was published in 1992, making it the most current version of the *ICD*. The dependence/harmful use distinction remained in the *ICD-10*.

There is only one criterion for the diagnosis of harmful use, namely, evidence that substance use has caused the user actual psychological or physical harm. The *ICD-10*'s diagnosis of alcohol dependence diagnosis requires three of the following six criteria:

1. Either a strong desire or compulsion to use a substance

2. Evidence of impaired ability to control substance use, which could relate to problems with avoiding initial use, with terminating use, or with controlling levels of use

3. Experience of withdrawal symptoms or use of a substance to avoid or relieve these symptoms, along with awareness of the deleterious effects of the alcohol use

4. Tolerance to the effects of a substance

5. Progressive neglect of alternative activities or interests, instead taking part in substance use

6. Continuing with substance use despite clear evidence of adverse consequences

The harmful use and dependence diagnoses are used in a hierarchical fashion with harmful use preceding alcohol dependence, although the diagnosis of dependence does not require a previous diagnosis of abuse.

Comparison of the *DSM* and *ICD*

Although earlier versions of the *DSM* and *ICD* were criticized for being too dissimilar, the current *DSM* and *ICD* criteria for alcohol-related disorders have a great deal in common. In both manuals, substance use disorders have been placed in their own category, and two hierarchical diagnoses for problem use are included as well. The *ICD-10* and *DSM-IV* both have a dependence category and a category for an alternative diagnosis, which is deemed less severe. The *DSM-IV* labels this less-severe alternative category as "abuse," whereas the *ICD-10* calls it "harmful use."

The current criteria for substance dependence in both manuals are based on the alcohol dependence syndrome, articulated by Edwards and Gross. Both manuals require the presence of three criteria for a diagnosis to be made; however, the *ICD-10* includes six possible dependence criteria and the *DSM* has seven. The main difference in the criteria for substance dependence in the two manuals is that the *ICD-10* includes a criterion pertaining to compulsion or craving and the *DSM-IV* does not. The concept of impaired control over substance use is covered in two separate criteria in the *DSM-IV*. One concerns substance use in greater quantities or for a longer period than intended, and the other pertains to repeated and unsuccessful attempts to limit substance use. In contrast, the *ICD-10* includes only one impaired control criterion. Also, the *DSM-IV* includes a criterion concerning time spent obtaining, using, and recovering from substance use, whereas the *ICD-10* does not.

There are greater differences between the less-severe diagnoses of alcohol abuse in the *DSM-IV* and harmful use in the *ICD-10*. The *ICD-10* harmful use diagnosis is made up of only one criterion, whereas the *DSM-IV* abuse diagnosis includes four criteria, although only one needs to be met for an abuse diagnosis to be made. The harmful use diagnosis focuses on psychological or medical harm resulting from substance use. It does not include legal or social problems or difficulties in fulfilling one's obligations. It is likely that these difficulties would cause psychological distress, but the *ICD-10* makes no direct reference to these consequences; in contrast, the abuse diagnosis in the *DSM-IV* directly references them.

Alcoholism Subtypes

Given the heterogeneity of alcoholism, a number of research groups have attempted to formulate subtypes of alcoholism. The main objectives of subtyping efforts have been to identify reliable distinctions in the progression of alcoholism and to attempt to

facilitate the matching of individual patients to the most appropriate types of treatment. Arguably, the subtyping schemes that have drawn the most research attention are Robert Cloninger's Type 1/Type 2 distinction, Thomas Babor and colleagues' Type A/B distinction, and the four typologies of Otto Lesch. In Cloninger's taxonomy, Type 1 alcoholics have a later onset of symptoms and display fewer risky behaviors as children, such as engaging in the destruction of property, running away from home, and demonstrating a lack of remorse for their actions, whereas Type 2 alcoholics have an earlier onset, greater frequency of risky childhood behaviors, and high familial risk of alcoholism. There is some degree of overlap between Cloninger's subtypes and Babor's Type A/B distinction. Babor's Type A alcoholics have a later onset of symptoms, fewer childhood risk factors in general, a weak family history of alcohol problems, and overall, less-severe patterns of alcohol consumption. In contrast, Babor's Type B alcoholics are characterized by an early symptom onset, more childhood risk factors, a strong family history of alcohol problems, comorbid psychopathology, and a pattern of heavy drinking. The four Lesch typologies, Types I through IV, entail a number of distinctions. Type I patients tend to drink to avoid withdrawal. Type II patients tend to use alcohol for coping and reduction of anxiety. Type III patients use alcohol primarily to self-medicate, and Type IV patients typically suffer from cognitive impairments that predate their alcohol dependence. Although these various subtyping approaches have had some utility, Babor recently concluded that research on alcoholism subtypes has been inconclusive, and as a result, they do not recommend the incorporation of subtypes into the major psychiatric classification systems at this time.

Robert F. Leeman and Laura A. Taylor

See also *Diagnostic and Statistical Manual of Mental Disorders*; Substance Abuse; Substance Dependence; Substance Use Disorders; Tolerance; Withdrawal

Further Readings

American Psychiatric Association. (1994). *Diagnostic and Statistical Manual of Mental Disorders* (4th ed.). Washington, DC: Author.
Caetano, R., & Tam, T. W. (1995). Prevalence and correlates of *DSM IV* and *ICD-10* alcohol dependence: 1990 US

National Alcohol Survey. *Alcohol & Alcoholism, 30,* 177–186.

Edwards, G., & Gross, M. (1976). Alcohol dependence: Provision description of a clinical syndrome. *British Medical Journal, 1,* 1058–1061.

Hasin, D. S., & Grant, B. F. (2004). The co-occurrence of *DSM-IV* alcohol abuse in *DSM-IV* alcohol dependence: Results of the National Epidemiologic Survey on Alcohol and Related Conditions on heterogeneity that differ by population subgroup. *Archives of General Psychiatry, 61,* 891–896.

Hasin, D., & Paykin, A. (1999). Alcohol dependence and abuse diagnoses: Concurrent validity in a nationally representative sample. *Alcoholism: Clinical and Experimental Research, 23,* 144–150.

Hesselbrock, V. M., & Hesselbrock, M. H. (2006). Are there empirically supported and clinically useful subtypes of alcohol dependence? *Addiction, 101*(Suppl. 1), 97–103.

Rounsaville, B. J., Bryant, K., Babor, T., Kranzler, H., & Kadden, R. (1993). Cross system agreement for substance use disorders: *DSM-III-R, DSM-IV & ICD-10. Addiction, 88,* 337–348.

Saunders, J. B. (2006). Substance dependence and nondependence in the *Diagnostic and Statistical Manual of Mental Disorders* (*DSM*) and the *International Classification of Diseases* (*ICD*): Can an identical conceptualization be achieved? *Addiction, 101*(Suppl. 1), 48–58.

Schuckit, M. A., Danko, G. P., Smith, T. L., & Buckman, K. R. (2002). The five-year predictive validity of each of the seven *DSM-IV* items for alcohol dependence among alcoholics. *Alcoholism: Clinical and Experimental Research, 26,* 980–987.

Schuckit, M. A., Smith, T. L., Danko, G. P., Bucholz, K. K., Reich, T., & Beirut, L. (2001). Five-year clinical course associated with *DSM-IV* alcohol abuse or dependence in a large group of men and women. *American Journal of Psychiatry, 158,* 1084–1090.

World Health Organization. (1992). *The ICD-10 Classification of Mental and Behavioural Disorders.* Geneva: Author.

ALCOHOL MARKETING

Every day young people are inundated with images of alcohol-related products and messages depicting drinking as acceptable behavior. It is commonplace for alcohol advertising to be seen among popular teenage television shows, highlighted in movies, depicted within the pages of magazines, and posted on billboards, as well as heard on local radio stations frequently listened to by minors. Advertising of alcoholic beverages and its influence on both individual consumption and the potential for abuse is understood by professionals in the field of substance abuse considerably differently from the way it is understood by large alcohol-producing corporations. The alcohol industry argues advertising does not promote drinking but rather is a vehicle for producers to increase their share of the market and drive down competition. Those in the substance abuse community counter that alcohol advertising promotes a permissive attitude toward underage drinking and the marketing of such needs to be regulated and reduced.

Although some research supports the notion that alcohol advertising alone does not *cause* greater alcohol consumption, there is considerable evidence suggesting high levels of *correlation* between alcohol advertising and its potential to lead to abuse among youth. Research on alcohol advertising indicates that adolescents' attitude toward drinking alcohol, intention to drink, and underage drinking behavior are influenced by their exposure to alcohol-related media. Knowing that underage consumption of alcohol by minors is significantly associated with alcohol-related motor vehicle crashes, violence, crime, school dropout, and other social and familial problems, it is imperative that alcohol-related advertising does not also contribute to these outcomes. As such, limiting youth exposure to alcohol marketing has become a major public health goal as one means of preventing underage drinking.

Challengers and Proponents

Underage drinkers are exposed to a substantial proportion of alcohol advertising presented in an appealing style to young people. An example of marketing appeal dates back to the use of "Joe Camel" in advertising cigarettes in which a sporty-looking cartoon camel wearing sunglasses is seen smoking a cigarette. Today, youth continue to be flooded with images of alcohol presented in an attractive manner toward this age group. Many young people are familiar with the Budweiser Clydesdales and Bud frogs, Coors Light twins, Absolut Vodka bottles, and other similar alcohol cartoon icons or figures, in part due to the sheer amount of exposure to such content.

Research indicates that images of alcoholic products far outnumber preventative messages. For example, it is estimated there are as many as 226 advertisements for alcoholic products for every one message of "responsible advertising," or that youth ages 12 to 20 are 96 times more likely to see an advertisement for alcohol than about the risks of underage drinking. Studies have established that the exposure of young persons to these messages influences both their beliefs and intentions to drink alcohol. Evidence also shows advertising may have a direct impact on youth drinking practices and associated problems; specifically, the more advertisements youth see, the more they drink. Additionally, communities with more alcohol ads have higher levels of youth drinking.

Each year the alcohol industry spends more than $4.5 billion marketing its products. As part of an incredibly lucrative industry, producers of alcohol products are not always amenable to changing their marketing campaigns. Often one of the greatest contested issues of requiring changes in alcohol advertising is the right to free speech. Enforcing regulations on alcohol advertising comes in direct conflict with the violation of First Amendment rights. The field of substance abuse prevention recognizes the constitutional constraints of attempting to impose restrictions on direct advertising and therefore suggests the most beneficial response is to facilitate public awareness of advertising practices.

Marketing

While not all alcohol advertising is negative, irresponsible marketing specifically targets such populations as underage drinkers, individuals of low socioeconomic status, minority groups, and others that may be particularly vulnerable to its influence. Alcohol advertising falls into two broad categories, both of which need to be addressed concurrently in order to minimize the negative implications of these ads. The first, "measured media," consists of traditional advertising such as electronic media (radio and television), outdoor billboards and signs, and print media (magazines and newspapers). A second form of media, "unmeasured media," includes the nontraditional venues such as sporting and concert events, consumer contests and giveaways, the Internet, and alcohol placement in television and movies. This form of media is associated with "branding," in which alcohol producers attempt to establish a link between a given audience and their loyalty to a particular brand through an emotional connection.

The regulation of alcohol advertising is addressed on multiple levels. Foremost is altering the content and placement of messages. The content of many alcohol advertisements has been found to have images and statements that are attractive and popular among youth. Advertising with particular appeal to youth, such as the popular Super Bowl commercials, should be minimized. Likewise, youth exposure to alcohol-related images should be reduced. This includes limiting advertising to venues such as sporting events or concerts, where there is a potential for a high concentration of youth. Another venue is convenience stores, where a significant proportion of youth are exposed to a high intensity point-of-sale advertisements.

Recommendations for Alcohol Manufacturers

There is little question that images of alcohol are pervasive and likely contribute to the permissive attitudes and values of underage drinking. Rather than the unrealistic solution of eliminating alcohol advertising altogether, research institutes offer recommendations for reducing the impact of alcohol-related marketing specific to youth. At the forefront of this research is the Center of Alcohol Marketing and Youth (CAMY) at Georgetown University. One of their goals is to monitor the marketing practices of the alcohol industry and focus attention and action on industry practices that jeopardize the health and safety of American youth. Through research, CAMY has identified 12 categories of best practices to assist states in regulating the content and placement of alcohol-related advertising

1. Prohibit false or misleading alcohol advertising.

2. Prohibit alcohol advertising that targets minors by excluding the terms *child* and *children* and omitting images or references to characters that may be particularly appealing to young persons, such as "Santa Claus" or the "Easter Bunny."

3. Prohibit images of children in alcohol advertisements.

4. Prohibit images or statements that associate alcohol with athletic achievement or use at sporting events.

5. Prohibit images or statements that portray or encourage intoxication.

6. Establish explicit jurisdiction over in-state electronic media (television and radio), and clearly distinguish between state and federal regulations of such.

7. Restrict outdoor advertising, such as billboards, posters, and banners, in locations where children are likely to be present, most notably in residential areas.

8. Prohibit outdoor alcohol advertising near schools, public playgrounds, churches, and other youth venues by specifying a minimum distance threshold of 500 feet from the location.

9. Restrict alcohol advertising on alcohol retail outlet windows and outside areas by limiting both the amount of space available to advertise as well as the content.

10. Prohibit alcohol advertising on college campuses, such as student newspapers and flyers promoting drink specials.

11. Restrict sponsorship of civic events such as fairs, music events, sporting activities, and the like by excluding giveaways, rebates, and consumer products (e.g., T-shirts) with alcohol logos.

12. Limit giveaways (contests, raffles, etc.) and restrict advertising promotions of prizes.

The Federal Trade Commission regulates most forms of product advertising and works alongside the Bureau of Alcohol, Tobacco, and Firearms, which has the primary responsibility of enforcing associated regulations. In 1999, the FTC completed an investigation of the alcohol industry marketing practices and developed recommended voluntary standards of conduct for manufacturers of alcohol, the retail outlets, and wholesalers. Through these recommendations, efforts have been made to promote self-regulation in the alcohol industry and to reduce the impact of advertising on minors. The FTC emphasizes the responsibility the alcohol industry has in its marketing strategies, specifically related to underage youth. They suggest products, advertising design, and placement of ads meet the following criteria:

- Messages about alcohol do not portray use as a rite of passage from childhood to adulthood or as a necessary element in becoming popular, related to social status, or fulfilling life.
- Alcohol advertising does not disproportionately expose youth to messages about alcohol.

- Advertisements should not be disproportionately appealing to youth or imply, in any manner, that alcohol is acceptable for youth consumption.
- Web site and Internet alcohol advertising is not specifically designed to attract or appeal to youth.

In 2003, the National Academy of Sciences Institute of Medicine released a report to Congress examining the industry's marketing practices and state of America's underage drinking problem. The report outlines three specific recommendations related to alcohol advertising:

- Alcohol companies and advertising media should refrain from marketing practices (to include product design, advertising, and promotions) that have substantial underage appeal and should take reasonable precautions in the time, place, and manner of placement and promotion to reduce youth exposure to alcohol advertising and marketing.
- The alcohol industry should strengthen their advertising codes to preclude placement of commercial messages in venues where a significant proportion of the audience is underage, prohibit messages that have strong underage appeal, and establish independent external review boards to investigate complaints and enforce such codes.
- Congress should appropriate necessary funding to the U.S. Department of Health and Human Services to monitor underage exposure to alcohol advertising and to make these reports available to the public. The report should include information on the estimated number of youth exposed to print and broadcast alcohol advertising to include television and radio broadcasting.

Prevention Strategy Recommendations

Substance abuse professionals support the use and efficacy of a comprehensive approach to prevention. Influencing alcohol marketing is no different, requiring support from multiple sources. In addition to directly addressing the alcohol industry, prevention strategies need to engage multiple stakeholders, such as lawmakers, retail businesses, the entertainment industry, parents, and other adults in the community. For example, specific recommendations for the entertainment industry include reducing advertisements in music and other youth entertainment that depict products or ads that glorify drinking. Other recommendations for alcohol advertising suggest that if the average audience comprises more than 15% of youth (ages 12–20), then that advertising should be prohibited. Finally, monitoring, research, and evaluation of such efforts need to be ongoing.

Conclusion

The alcohol industry is a powerful business that undoubtedly has significant influence on the choices today's youth make about drinking. Despite recommendations to alter advertising and marketing strategies, there is little incentive for the big alcohol businesses to carry them out. Although there has been increased awareness and some changes by the producers of alcohol, the need remains for further steps to be taken to reduce the impact of marketing on underage drinking. Just as it took decades for American to recognize the health risks associated with cigarette smoking and to influence the marketing of nicotine, it will likely take time to influence the marketing of alcohol to underage drinkers. As with any effective prevention strategy, multiple stakeholders need to be involved. Federal, state, and local leaders need to coordinate their efforts to ensure the alcohol industry is being regulated and laws are consistently being enforced. On the other end of the spectrum, adults, youth, and schools should be engaged in evidenced-based prevention programming and increased awareness of the impact of advertising campaigns. Throughout the continuum, the alcohol industry, as well as the entertainment industry which promotes the marketing of products, needs to be invested in reducing the exposure of youth to alcohol advertising. Lastly, efforts must be continually monitored, and research and evaluation must remain a priority.

Jill Russett

See also Environmental Approaches; National Media Campaign; Prevention Strategies; Public Policy, Prevention; Social Norms Marketing; Tobacco Marketing and Countermarketing

Further Readings

Center on Alcohol Marketing and Youth (CAMY). (2003). *State alcohol advertising laws: Current status and model policies*. Washington, DC: Author.

FACE: Resource, Training & Action on Alcohol Issues: http://www.faceproject.org/

Grube, J. W. (2002). Television alcohol portrayals, alcohol advertising and alcohol expectancies among children and adolescents. In S. E. Martin & P. Mail (Eds.), *Effects of the mass media on the use and abuse of alcohol* (pp. 105–121). Bethesda, MD: National Institute on Alcohol Abuse and Alcoholism.

National Academy of Sciences Institute of Medicine. (2003). *Reducing underage drinking: A collective responsibility*. Washington, DC: National Academies Press.

ALCOHOL-RELATED BIRTH DEFECTS

Alcohol use during pregnancy is one of the leading preventable causes of birth defects in the United States. Despite the commonly known risk factors, 14% to 22% of women continue to consume alcohol during pregnancy. Various motivations for continued use have been identified, as well as specific demographic factors linked to continued use; these factors include pregnancy at an early age, low socioeconomic status, ethnicity, and genetic predisposition. The unfortunate consequence of continued alcohol use is fetal alcohol syndrome (FAS), the most frequently occurring alcohol-related birth defect. However, the consequence of maternal drinking is not limited to FAS. Children exposed to alcohol in utero can experience other non-FAS alcohol-related birth defects, such as skeletal and organ abnormalities. These non-FAS abnormalities are often referred to as alcohol-related birth defects (ARBDs). These ARBDs can manifest through cognitive, motor, neurological, physical, speech, mental health, and psychosocial defects. To a large extent, the particular ARBD experienced is determined by the timing, or critical period, of in utero alcohol exposure.

Critical Periods for Prenatal Alcohol Exposure

Studies have shown that the number of women who drink during pregnancy far outnumber the number of children born with an ARBD, indicating that not all children are affected by in utero alcohol exposure. Additionally, children who are affected by maternal alcohol use do not show uniform deficits. There are, however, some factors that have been shown to increase the likelihood of an ARBD occurring, such as the mother's particular metabolism, the pattern of drinking that occurred during pregnancy, and genetic differences. As for the particular type of ARBD that occurs, the most important factor is believed to be the timing of the alcohol exposure during pregnancy, or critical period. For example, early exposure to alcohol causes more craniofacial damage in comparison to exposure later on in the development of the fetus. One particularly significant critical period for fetal development is during the first two months of gestation, which is called the embryonic period. During this time the fetus is undergoing organogenesis, a period in which the majority of organs are forming. Exposure to alcohol during organogenesis can cause severe physical defects characteristic of children born with FAS. Alcohol exposure can also affect the development of sex organs if exposure occurs around the 10th week of gestation, the time in which sex organ differentiation occurs.

Binge Drinking in Pregnant Mothers

A major area of concern for the development of an ARBD is binge drinking among pregnant mothers. Binge drinking is defined as consuming four or more drinks on one occasion for women and five or more drinks on one occasion for men. Although research on this topic is controversial, it has shown that binge drinking tends to be more harmful than other patterns of drinking because it causes significant damage to the brain of the developing fetus. In comparison to more common patterns of drinking, binge drinking episodes cause more prolonged exposure of alcohol to the fetus. This damage can cause global impairment in behavior. For example, binge drinking during pregnancy has been linked to more disinhibited behaviors in the children, when compared to those children who had mothers who did not binge drink. Further, there is strong evidence to suggest that binge drinking may result in lower verbal IQs, more delinquent behaviors, and a greater chance of developing psychological disorders.

Neurological and Developmental Defects

Alcohol can damage many areas of a child's development. However, the most pervasive area of damage to the child is neurological. Although deficits are seen

for specific aspects of the brain, the end result can be a global deficit. General intellectual functioning, academic skills, and social functioning deficits are potential consequences of neurological impairment from in utero alcohol exposure. Furthermore, the neurological damage can result in sleep difficulties tied to abnormal daily physiological rhythms for children with ARBD. In addition to the brain, other areas in the central nervous system can be damaged, such as the spinal cord. Some of the significant defects seen in children born with ARBD include the failure of certain brain structures (such as the corpus callosum) to form, inability of both gray and white brain matter to form, failure of cells to migrate appropriately to the brain during the embryonic stage, and certain brain tissues dying off (e.g., corpus callosum).

Research has suggested that most of the neurological deficits incurred by alcohol consumption are concentrated in the cerebellum and the basal ganglia. The cerebellum is located in the back of the brain and is involved in movement and cognitive processes such as attention. Children that have been exposed to alcohol during fetal development tend to have smaller cerebellums, caused by the decay of cells within this particular structure. As for the basal ganglia, this brain region is located in the white matter of the cerebrum, which controls voluntary movements and cognitive functioning (such as perception, memory, and thinking). Children with ARBDs tend to have smaller basal ganglia in comparison to children without alcohol-related defects. Given that the damage is commonly found in these two particular areas, neurological deficits as a result of ARBD are considered by many researchers to be localized rather than global.

Cognitive and Motor Defects

As a result of ARBD neurological deficits, many children experience decreased cognitive and motor performance. A deficit in intellectual functioning (lower IQ) has long been recognized as a common consequence of maternal drinking. More specifically, children with ARBD tend to have problems remembering information when it is verbally presented to them. Despite this, they do not differ from children without ARBD in retaining learned information. That is, acquiring the information is difficult for children with ARBD, but once the information is retained, the children are able to recall the information at a normal level. Children with ARBD also experience impairment in other facets of cognitive ability, such as visual–spatial functioning (the ability to recall spatial relationships and visual details), and executive functioning (higher-order processing, planning, organizing, abstract thinking), as well as in their ability to be independent. Children with ARBD also have problems with mathematics and problem solving. Other deficits seen are in information processing, including difficulty completing tasks or chores and trouble determining what to do in a given situation. This is often misconstrued as the child being oppositional rather than the child having a deficit in cognitive ability.

Another common deficit for children with ARBD is in attention. Approximately 60% of all children with FAS or ARBD have a problem maintaining attention for an extended of time. These cognitive deficits have also been identified in children who have only been exposed to low levels of alcohol in utero. This is another area that is often misconstrued, in that these attentional difficulties are often thought to be the result of an attention deficit disorder. However, attentional deficits resulting from ARBD, in comparison to those resulting from attention deficit disorder, have a distinct presentation. This differential presentation may help explain and aid in the diagnosis of attention problems in children with alcohol-related birth defects.

In addition to mental functioning deficits resulting from ARBD, these neurological impairments also have a detrimental effect on motor performance. Children with ARBD tend to have problems with their balance and have problems sensing where their bodies are in space, often resulting in the children being perceived as clumsy. These neurological impairments also result in the presentation of other, rather idiosyncratic impairments, such as being more easily upset by sensory input (e.g., bright lights, certain textures of food, and tags in clothing).

Mental Health and Psychosocial Behavior Defects

Individuals with ARBD also experience deficits in mental health, relationships, and interactions with others (e.g., parents, siblings, and friends). Such difficulties are nearly ubiquitous, with 94% of children with FAS having mental health difficulties, the most prevalent being attention deficits. Adults who were born with ARBD also tend to report higher levels of depression. Despite the mixed evidence, researchers have found that children who have been exposed to alcohol during prenatal development tend to show signs that are similar in characteristic to autism. Some of these similarities include impairments in social functioning and language development. Studies have also found that children who have been exposed to alcohol tend to have more psychological problems such as depression, anxiety, and attention problems. In addition to this, there are also deficits in social functioning, such as difficulty making new friends and knowledge of socially acceptable manners. It is important to note, however, that these skills are within the range of ability for children with FAS and ARBD, but they manifest more slowly in comparison to children without ARBDs.

Speech and Language Defects

Children with ARBD tend to exhibit a variety of speech and language deficits, such as delays in speech acquisition, impaired receptive and expressive speech, and impairments in general ability to produce speech. Although ARBD children tend to have average syntax and vocabulary, they often lack the ability to communicate effectively in social situations. This inability may explain why children with ARBD have difficulty forming social relationships and interacting with peers and family.

Physical Deficits

Many cognitive, alcohol-related birth defects cannot be immediately be perceived, aside from physical defects. Children with ARBD often have stunted growth (including decreased height and weight), especially if their mother consumed alcohol during the later stages of in utero development. Mothers, however, who discontinue alcohol usage earlier in the gestational period, tend to have ARBD children who do not exhibit growth abnormalities.

One of the critical diagnostic criteria for diagnosing FAS in a child is noticeable facial deformities. These deformities include small head circumference, skin folds at the corner of the eyes, small eye openings, short noses, thin upper lips, and small midfaces. In addition to this, these children may also have deformities that are found in their nasal structures, which may cause breathing difficulties. Children with ARBD also tend to have smooth philtrums (the groove above the upper lip). However, facial deformities are not present in all children that are exposed to alcohol during prenatal development. Most children with ARBD tend to exhibit neurological and behavioral defects, whereas facial defects are commonly characteristic of FAS. Other physical defects include organ deformities in the heart and in the kidneys.

Secondary Deficiencies of ARBD

As detailed earlier, many children with alcohol-related birth defects often present with problems that are related to primary defects in mental health status, cognition, and physical development. However, these primary deficits also lead to secondary difficulties (problems resulting from the primary deficit). For example, these secondary deficits can include disrupted school experiences. Children with ARBD have a higher risk of not completing their education (in both high school and college). Research has also indicated that children born with ARBD go on to have increased legal and unemployment problems. More atypical secondary problems have also been noted, such as displaying inappropriate sexual behavior. In addition, these children may be more easily pressured by their peers, may repeatedly break rules, and may have difficulties learning from their past mistakes. Given this, health care providers and parents of children with ARBD may benefit from taking these primary and secondary deficits into consideration when dealing with the difficulties arising from ARBD.

Valerie Hobson

See also Binge Drinking; Children of Alcoholics; Fetal Alcohol Syndrome; Fetal Effects of Alcohol and Other Drugs; Maternal Drug Use

Further Readings

Anderson, J., Ebrahim, S., Floyd, L., & Atrash, H. (2006). Prevalence of risk factors for adverse pregnancy outcomes during pregnancy and the preconception period. *Maternal & Child Health Journal, 10,* S101–S106.

Coles, C. (1994). Critical periods for prenatal alcohol exposure. *Alcohol Health & Research World, 18,* 22–30.

King, D. (2006). Alcohol consumption during pregnancy. *International Journal of Childbirth Education, 21,* 25–26.

Maier, S., & West, J. (2001). Drinking patterns and alcohol-related birth defects. *Alcohol Research & Health, 25,* 168–175.

Streissguth, A. (2007). Offspring effects of prenatal alcohol exposure from birth to 25 years: The Seattle Prospective Longitudinal Study. *Journal of Clinical Psychology in Medical Settings, 14,* 81–101.

Warren, K., & Foudin, L. (2001). Alcohol-related birth defects—The past, present, and future. *Alcohol Research & Health, 25,* 153–159.

Welch-Carre, E. (2005). The neurodevelopmental consequences of prenatal alcohol exposure. *Advances in Neonatal Care, 5,* 217–229.

ALCOHOL TESTING

Alcohol testing is used to determine whether an individual is currently using alcohol or has used alcohol in the past. It is utilized in a variety of settings and for a number of different purposes. In treatment settings, alcohol testing is used to monitor patients to ensure that they are abstaining from alcohol while in treatment and that they maintain sobriety once treatment is completed. Alcohol testing is also used in forensic settings, most commonly to determine sobriety for those suspected of operating a motor vehicle while under the influence of alcohol. In this case, alcohol testing may be used for screening in roadside sobriety checks to identify those who are suspected of driving while intoxicated and may be entered as evidence in criminal prosecutions for those found to be intoxicated while driving. Follow-up alcohol testing may be routinely conducted to ensure that those who have been convicted of driving while intoxicated or other offenses are abstaining from alcohol use during probation or parole.

Employers use alcohol testing for pre-employment screening of job applicants, for randomly checking current employees for alcohol use or intoxication on the job, and when there is a suspicion of alcohol use on the job. Less commonly, testing is conducted following an on-the-job accident to determine if alcohol was a causative factor in the accident and to protect the employer from possible liability stemming from the injury. For employees identified as using alcohol, testing may occur as a follow-up to rehabilitation or to certify that the employee is ready to return to work. Private corporations and federal and local government agencies (e.g., police, fire, military, transportation, medical) have relied on alcohol testing for these purposes, particularly when employees perform safety-sensitive activities as part of their routine duties, such as operating motor vehicles.

Schools and parents may also use alcohol testing to confirm suspected use or to ensure abstinence in those who have been identified as using alcohol. In these situations, testing may be performed at the school or in the home with home testing kits. Home testing kits are also available for nursing mothers; this allows the detection of alcohol in breast milk so that the mother can be sure that alcohol has dissipated from her breast milk prior to nursing her infant. Research studies often use alcohol testing as a way to screen out individuals who are currently using or, alternatively, to monitor alcohol use as a study progresses. Insurance companies use alcohol and drug testing to make decisions whether to provide coverage and to establish premiums. Oftentimes, these companies will employ a series of tests to confirm suspicious results that are apparent on routine laboratory testing.

Finally, alcohol testing is used in preventative efforts made possible by the wide availability of breath alcohol tests often referred to as breathalyzers. Some breathalyzers are marketed for personal use so that individuals can monitor their blood alcohol concentration (BAC) when drinking; some breathalyzers are even available at establishments where alcohol is served. Thus, individuals are able to judge their level of intoxication based on their BAC and can use this information to moderate their alcohol intake and avoid driving when they are over the legal BAC limit. Another interesting application of breathalyzer technology is the development of ignition interlock devices. Ignition interlock devices are connected to the car's ignition and the driver must provide a breath sample to start the vehicle. The vehicle will not start until the driver passes the breathalyzer test. These devices can be installed at the driver's discretion to limit other drivers from operating the vehicle while intoxicated (e.g., teenage drivers), but the courts are increasingly mandating them for individuals who are convicted of multiple DUIs (driving while under the influence [of alcohol]). They can be programmed to require multiple breath samples while the vehicle is being operated, as well as to ensure that others cannot provide breath samples on the driver's behalf.

Methods of Testing

Alcohol testing can be accomplished using a variety of techniques using different types of biological samples such as blood, breath, saliva, sweat, urine, or hair. The most common alcohol testing techniques attempt to determine the concentration of alcohol in the blood, and there are various ways of defining blood alcohol concentration (BAC). In the United States, BAC is defined as the weight (or mass) of alcohol measured in grams per volume of blood measured in milliliters (ml). Thus, a BAC of .05% means that there is 0.05 grams of alcohol for every 100 ml of blood.

These testing methods rely on a basic understanding of how alcohol is absorbed, distributed, and disposed of from the body's blood and tissue. During the absorption phase, when alcohol is ingested, a small portion is absorbed into the blood through the mouth. However, the majority is absorbed directly into the blood through the stomach, which absorbs about 20%, and the small intestine, which absorbs the rest. Additionally, some of the alcohol that enters the stomach is not absorbed because it is broken down prior to entering the bloodstream by an enzyme called alcohol dehydrogenase. The rate at which alcohol is absorbed into the blood and the amount that is absorbed is influenced by a number of factors. For example, because women naturally produce less alcohol dehydrogenase, they become intoxicated with less alcohol than men. Presence of food in the stomach, weight, body composition, nutrition and diet, age, type of alcoholic beverage, and rate of alcohol consumption also influence the amount and rate of alcohol absorption into the blood.

After alcohol enters the bloodstream, it is distributed throughout the body to all of its organs in about 90 seconds; the greater the amount of alcohol consumed, the higher the BAC will be. Concentration of alcohol in the blood will reach its highest level (peak), approximately 30 to 60 minutes after alcohol is ingested. Because there is a strong relationship between level of intoxication and BAC, a predictable increase in symptoms of intoxication occurs with rising levels of alcohol in the blood. At BAC levels ranging from .01 to .02, few noticeable symptoms are present although subtle changes can be detected with specialized testing. BAC levels from .03 to .05 are associated with feelings of euphoria, decreased inhibition, and some impairment of judgment and motor coordination. Deterioration in driving skills begins to occur at the .05 level. Feelings of euphoria and disinhibition continue as BAC increases to the .06 to .10 levels, and motor incoordination, impaired judgment, and sexual dysfunction also increase. In all states, the legal limit for operating a motor vehicle is less than .08 for individuals 21 and older, with lower levels for those less than 21 years of age. As BAC increases from .11 to .20, severe intoxication occurs. Stupor and unconsciousness are present for many individuals who have BAC levels of .21 to .30. Marked central nervous system depression occurs at levels above .30, including decreased respiration and heart rate sometimes resulting in death. BAC levels of .40 to .50 are considered the median lethal dose, that is, the concentration that would cause death in half of all adults.

The body disposes of alcohol in the blood a number of ways. A small portion of blood alcohol will evaporate through breath (1%–5%), and some will be excreted through urine (1%–3%) or sweat (.5%), but the liver will dispose of the majority. The liver disposes alcohol in the blood using enzymes (alcohol dehydrogenase, aldehyde dehydrogenase) to break it down into other chemicals (acetaldehyde, acetate), which are then metabolized into water and carbon dioxide. While some variation is present from one individual to the next, the capacity of the liver to dispose of alcohol is typically limited to a rate of approximately one half an ounce of pure alcohol every hour. Put another way, each hour the liver is able to reduce the concentration of alcohol in the blood from between .015 to .018%. In addition to metabolism with alcohol dehydrogenase and aldehyde dehydrogenase, a small portion of the alcohol in the blood is also broken down into chemicals that remain in the blood much longer than that alcohol itself and so can be used to detect alcohol consumption even after BAC levels have reached 0.0.

If more alcohol is consumed than the liver is able to process, the concentration of alcohol in the blood begins to rise and results in increasing symptoms of intoxication. Because individual differences affect the rate of alcohol absorption and disposal, the BAC is preferred over the amount of alcohol consumed in order to judge intoxication, because it is the amount of alcohol in the blood that is responsible for producing alcohol's intoxication effects. However, even with highly accurate estimates of BAC, levels of intoxication can vary among individuals with the same BAC. Tolerance to the effects of alcohol that results from repeated and prolonged use is one major cause of individual differences, although genetic influences and interactions with other medications may also cause variation in intoxication effects.

In addition to tests designed to estimate BAC, a number of additional procedures are available that rely on the measurement of the effects of alcohol on

the body itself (indirect methods) or examine the metabolites of alcohol rather than alcohol itself (direct methods). In the following sections, the most common forms of indirect and direct methods of alcohol testing are discussed, including those that rely on samples of blood, breath, urine, saliva, and hair. Advantages and disadvantages of each method are also discussed.

Blood

The most accurate alcohol tests available to determine BAC rely on analysis of the blood itself. Blood alcohol testing is accomplished by drawing a small sample of blood from the individual. This blood sample is then subjected to a laboratory technique called gas chromatography. Gas chromatography works by separating mixtures of substances back into their original components so that the amount of each component in the mixture can be determined. For alcohol testing, gas chromatography separates the alcohol from the blood. Certain factors that are not related to drinking alcohol may raise the BAC, such as the use of rubbing alcohol may raise the BAC, to clean the site where the blood is drawn and elevated blood ketones in those with diabetes. Medicines and other products that contain alcohol (e.g., mouthwash) will also increase alcohol levels. And, although the alcohol testing is used primarily to detect the levels of drinking alcohol in the blood (ethanol or ethyl alcohol), ingestion of other alcohols such as isopropyl alcohol or methanol may affect the accuracy of the results. Even though blood alcohol testing is the most accurate, it is an invasive and expensive test, so other forms of testing are often used, most notably tests that rely on breath samples. Also, while very accurate in determining the amount of alcohol present in the blood at the time of testing, blood alcohol testing is only sensitive to the presence of alcohol that has been consumed within 3 to 10 hours of testing, depending on the amount of alcohol consumed, and so it provides little information about long-term use, including quantity and frequency of use.

In addition to identifying alcohol in the blood, tests can be conducted that will detect the metabolites of alcohol, which are used to infer recent alcohol use. Examples include tests designed to detect ethyl glucuronide and fatty acid ethyl esters. Ethyl glucuronide results from the breakdown of alcohol and peaks in its blood concentration almost 3 hours after alcohol concentration peaks. Because ethyl glucuronide takes much longer to eliminate from the body than alcohol itself, it can indicate recent alcohol use even after there is no alcohol left in the blood. Fatty acid ethyl esters are also a metabolite that results when alcohol is disposed of by the body. Fatty acid ethyl esters will remain in the blood for up to 24 hours after drinking has ceased. Because fatty acids are not particularly stable in blood samples, they are more commonly examined in other biological samples, such as hair or adipose (fat) tissue. Variation in the levels of some fatty acids may also help clinicians distinguish between individuals who binge drink and those who have more prolonged and chronic consumption.

Finally, laboratory tests that reflect the influence of alcohol on other organ systems have also proved useful in identifying individuals who are heavy alcohol users. For example, tests sensitive to liver damage, such as gamma-glutamyltransferase (GGT), albumin, total bilirubin, alanine aminotransferase, aspartate aminotransferase, and alkaline phosphatase, are sometimes used because heavy drinking often causes liver damage. Because results of these tests are elevated in other medical conditions, they have been criticized for overdetecting or underdetecting individuals with heavy alcohol use. However, a number of newer approaches show promise in this area, including tests of carbohydrate-deficient transferrin (CDT) and the early detection of alcohol consumption test.

CDT is a sensitive state indicator of heavy drinking and one of the most widely used tests of its type. Ten or more days of heavy drinking disrupts the body's normal synthesis of carbohydrates, which is reflected by elevated CDT. This disruption can last up to 3 weeks following cessation of alcohol use. Thus, CDT is particularly useful for detecting heavy chronic alcohol use, although it is not as good for identifying binge drinking. Although CDT and gamma-glutamyltransferase are about equally sensitive, CDT has the advantage of being insensitive to other forms of illness (diabetes, asthma, hypertension) and the effects of many prescribed drugs. Another technique used to identify those who are heavy alcohol consumers does not rely on a single test but rather on a series of routine laboratory tests of, for example, magnesium, cholesterol, iron, white blood cells, platelets, and sodium, among others. This technique, known as early detection of alcohol consumption (EDAC), uses statistical analyses of these laboratory test results to identify patterns that are commonly that found in those known to be heavy drinkers. As the correspondence between the patterns of results increase, the likelihood of heavy alcohol use also increases. Evidence also suggests that the EDAC is able to distinguish between individuals who binge drink and those with a steadier, daily consumption of alcohol.

Breath

Because a small amount of alcohol in the blood passes to the lungs, a breath sample can be used to estimate the concentration of alcohol in a person's blood, referred to as the breath alcohol content (BrAC). In this process, alcohol passes from the blood to the alveoli of the lungs, which are small air sacks where some gases in the blood such as carbon dioxide pass out of the blood and other gases such as oxygen pass into the blood. The amount of alcohol in the blood and the amount that passes from the blood to the alveoli reach a balance, or steady state, so that when breath is exhaled from the lungs, the amount of alcohol in the breath can used to estimate the concentration of alcohol in the blood. On average, the ratio between alcohol in the blood to that in the breath is 2,100:1, a ratio that is often referred to as the blood/breath ratio (BBR). This BBR indicates that there are 2,100 ml of alcohol in the blood for every 1 ml in the breath. Although breathalyzers used in law enforcement are calibrated using this 2,100:1 ratio, the ratio may in fact vary substantially between individuals, which can cause overestimation or underestimation of the actual BAC when using breath samples.

Development of the technology to measure BrAC is attributed to Indiana State Police Captain Robert Borkenstein, who invented a device called a Breathalyzer in 1959. While the first measurement of BrAC occurred much earlier, Borkenstein's Breathalyzer had a number of advantages, including that it was portable. The term *Breathalyzer* was originally the brand name of a series of models made by one manufacturer; today, the term is used in a generic sense to refer to any device that uses breath samples to estimate BAC. Other commercially marketed alcohol breath tests are sold under the brand names of Intoxilyzer, Intoximeter, AlcoHAWK, Alcotest, Alcosensor, and Datamaster. The invention of the breathalyzer was important for a number of reasons, not the least of which was that it provided law enforcement with a non-invasive, low-cost test that provided immediate results that could identify individuals who were driving while intoxicated. Since that time, breathalyzers have become widely available and, as previously mentioned, have been used for prevention purposes by allowing people to monitor their own BACs so they can make an informed decision about continuing to drink and whether or not they are able to safely operate a motor vehicle. Although the technology varies from one device to another, all breathalyzers require individuals to exhale into a tube so that their breath travels across an alcohol-sensing device.

Manual devices used by law enforcement were constructed of chemically sensitive crystals that would turn from yellow to green depending on the amount of alcohol in the breath. These crystals were organized into bands so that the number of crystal bands that turn from yellow to green can determine the BrAC. For these manual devices, BrAC is typically estimated based on ranges, such as .00 to .05, .05 to .10, and so forth. More advanced technology employs infrared spectrophotometers, electrochemical fuel cells, and tin-oxide semiconductors to detect alcohol in the breath. Of these, infrared spectrophotometers provide the most accurate estimation of BAC, and their results can be used as evidence in criminal proceedings. Electrochemical fuel cells sensors are most commonly employed in the handheld devices used by police officers in field sobriety checks and, in many states, are considered to provide only preliminary findings, although these findings can be used to make arrests. Breathalyzers that are designed for personal use employ tin-oxide semiconductors, which are less accurate and much less expensive than the infrared spectrophotometers and electrochemical fuel cells. Despite the fact that they are prone to false positive identifications, these personal breathalyzers provide valuable information regarding BAC to their users, and all are approved by the U.S. Food and Drug Administration. For all of these newer devices, digital readings of BAC are displayed.

Although quite popular, breathalyzers have some limitations, including being susceptible to a number of factors that could artificially increase or decrease their estimates of BAC. Probably the most common source of error is associated with residual alcohol in the mouth that has not been fully absorbed. Residual alcohol can be caused by a recent drinking episode or regurgitating alcohol, or it may be present because of the use of mouthwash or similar products that contain alcohol. Residual alcohol in the mouth will increase the BrAC and thus cause an overestimation of the BAC. Low hematocrit (low volume of cells in the blood), acetone in the breath (sometimes present in those with diabetes), and increased body temperature may also cause overestimates of BAC, whereas hyperventilation, physical activity, and changes in the water content of expired air can cause underestimates of BAC. Because of these factors, it is standard for an observation period of 15 to 20 minutes to precede breathalyzer tests, during which time the test subjects are closely observed to ensure that they do not eat, drink, or vomit. Other limitations include that the breathalyzer can test only for alcohol and not for any other substances, and the breath sample cannot be preserved for future analysis. Despite these limitations, breathalyzers have become increasingly popular over the years because they are a fast, convenient, noninvasive, and inexpensive way to test BAC.

Saliva

Because a small amount of alcohol is excreted through saliva, blood alcohol concentration can also be tested using a saliva sample to determine the saliva alcohol concentration. The testing procedure is straightforward and requires test subjects to provide a saliva sample that is placed on the saliva test strip. Alcohol present in the saliva causes the test strip to change color. The color on the strip is then compared to a standard chart of colors to estimate the amount of alcohol in the blood. Saliva alcohol concentration estimations of blood alcohol are made possible because there is a relatively constant ratio between alcohol contained in the saliva and that contained in the blood (although this ratio is not nearly as well understood as the BrAC ratio of 1,200:1). The color change on the test strip is caused by a reaction between an enzyme that coats the strip and the alcohol in the saliva sample.

Some saliva tests are approved for on the job screening by the U.S. Department of Transportation for safety-sensitive transportation employees involved in, for example, the trucking, railroad, aviation, and mass transit industries. Advantages of this type of test are that, like the breathalyzer, it is a fast, efficient, and cost-effective way to screen for alcohol use. Also, the test results can be copied using a photocopy machine, thus establishing a permanent record of the result. However, there are also certain limitations depending on the type of saliva test used. Some are only sensitive to alcohol above the .02 BAC level, and most have an upper limit of testing (e.g., .145 BAC). Also, there remains some controversy as to how accurately saliva alcohol concentration estimates BAC, although there are some data to suggest that the two are highly correlated. A final consideration is that the enzyme that coats the test strips is sensitive to fluctuations in temperature so that hot temperatures tend to cause overestimation of BAC and cold temperatures cause underestimation of BAC. Ambient air or exposure to temperatures over 80 degrees Fahrenheit can degrade the enzyme so that the test no longer works. Finally, saliva tests typically have a shelf life of up to 1 year (sometimes less), and the test does not provide an indication when a false reading may have occurred or when the saliva sample has been contaminated.

Perspiration

Methods have also been developed to detect alcohol use from perspiration samples as a small amount of blood alcohol is excreted in perspiration. The term *sweat* is used to describe the moisture on the skin that results from perspiration, while the term *insensible perspiration* describes perspiration that evaporates before it is noticed as sweat. The alcohol in both types of perspiration has been referred to as transdermal alcohol and the measurement of it as the transdermal alcohol content (TAC). The ratio between the amount of alcohol present in perspiration and that contained in the blood is not as well understood as it is for breath or saliva samples. Also, it takes some time for alcohol in the blood to diffuse through the skin, which is a complicated process that is determined by a number of factors that may render TAC readings from insensible perspiration unusable to estimate BAC.

One testing approach is to use what has been commonly referred to as a "sweat-patch," which resembles a large Band-Aid that is placed on the skin for as long as 2 weeks during which time it absorbs perspiration. The patch is then removed, and gas chromatography or the fuel cell–based technology used in the breathalyzer test is used to determine the presence of alcohol in the patch. This method of testing does not provide an indication of BAC at specific points in time while the patch was being worn, but it is highly accurate in differentiating between those who use alcohol while wearing the patch and those who do not.

More recently, wearable devices have been developed that that use fuel cell technology similar to that used in a breathalyzer to measure TAC at set time intervals, every 20 minutes for example. These devices can be worn on the wrist or ankle for a month if necessary

and possibly longer. Some also are able to electronically transmit their TAC readings to a modem in the test subject's home; this information is then uploaded to a secure Web site where it is accessible over the Internet to authorized individuals. Because this is a relatively new technology, it has not been nearly as extensively studied as procedures that rely on blood or breath. However, recent research indicates that these monitoring systems are able to distinguish between drinkers and nondrinkers with a high degree of accuracy and between low and high levels of alcohol consumption, but the measurements obtained using these devices are not reliable in estimating BrAC levels. Thus, limitations of these devices are that they can only estimate BAC and provide general time frames during which alcohol was consumed (for fuel cell devices) and so are not particularly useful in situations where BAC is a required test result, such as roadside sobriety checks. There are also concerns that, because readings are taken above the skin and the fuel cell technology is sensitive to other types of alcohol in addition to drinking alcohol, vapors from common household products (e.g., rubbing alcohol, cleaning products) might cause false-positive readings. However, a distinct and substantive advantage to these methods is that they are able to provide monitoring of alcohol use over many days without requiring the test subject to undergo multiple testings (e.g., daily breathalyzer testing, frequent blood draws). Because of this capability, these monitoring devices have had their widest application in the criminal justice system, where monitoring of alcohol use is a requirement of probation or parole.

Urine

Because some alcohol makes its way into the urine, BAC can also be estimated from urine samples. Alcohol begins entering the urine approximately 1 hour after alcohol is consumed and will normally be totally eliminated within 24 hours of drinking. This 24-hour time frame can vary markedly depending on such factors as the amount of alcohol consumed, sex, weight, and age. The ratio of alcohol in the urine to that in the blood is typically assumed to be 1.3:1, although this ratio can vary substantially among individuals. However, the amount of urine in the blood does not correspond to the BAC at the time the urine specimen was collected because alcohol enters the blood much more quickly than it does urine. As a result, it can be difficult to obtain accurate BAC estimates based on the urine specimen.

In addition to directly measuring alcohol content in the urine, some urine tests are designed to identify chemicals that result from the breakdown of alcohol but remain in the body long after alcohol has been metabolized. As previously mentioned, ethyl glucuronide (EtG) is one such chemical that is present in blood, but it is often examined in urine testing because it remains in the urine for as long as 80 hours after drinking has ceased. Some caution should be used when interpreting positive EtG test results, because the test is so sensitive that it may show positive as a result of the use of alcohol-based hand sanitizers or ingestion of medicines or foods that contain small amounts of alcohol. On the other hand, a negative EtG test appears to provide definitive evidence that alcohol has not been consumed.

Hair

Hair samples have also been used to detect alcohol use even though alcohol itself is not stored in the hair. Rather, as hair grows, it absorbs some of the metabolite of alcohol, most notably fatty acid ethyl esters (FAEEs) and EtG. These metabolites will remain in the hair indefinitely. When present in the hair, they suggest that the individual has used alcohol at some point in the past. The more FAEEs and EtG that are present, the more alcohol has been used. Because FAEEs are unstable in the blood, hair analysis is a particularly useful approach because it can identify FAEEs even after several months. The test requires that a hair sample (90 strands of hair) be collected in which hair is cut close to the scalp. The hair is then cleaned and subjected to a chemical process that breaks down the hair and allows EtG or FAEE to be isolated. Because hair grows about one half of an inch each month, a 3-month history could be obtained from a one-and-a-half-inch piece of hair. Of course, it cannot be used with individuals who have shaved their heads (although hair sampled from anywhere on the body can be used). As with the perspiration monitoring devices, the long-term time frame of this test is important advantage. However, it is more expensive than other forms of testing (breath, urine, or saliva) and cannot detect alcohol that was consumed 3 to 9 days before testing.

Conclusion

Many methods can be used to test for alcohol use, and new methods continue to be developed as technology progresses. The best-established and commonly used methods rely on samples of blood, breath, or urine to detect the presence of alcohol at the time of testing or alternatively, in the case of blood and urine, other chemicals that are elevated as a result of the direct or indirect effects of alcohol. Each of the methods has distinct advantages and disadvantages, and the most effective monitoring may result from a combination of these tests. For example, during inpatient treatment, a questionnaire may be used on intake to establish the quantity and frequency of use over the months prior to treatment and identify times during the month when the patient is at greatest risk to use. They may also help quantify the severity of use. Biological tests that provide a longer time frame for detection, such as urine EtG or hair analysis, may also be helpful at intake if there is suspicion regarding underreporting. During treatment, random urine or saliva screening can help ensure abstinence until treatment is completed. Following treatment methods that allow for continuous monitoring (sweat patches, transdermal monitoring) or providing longer time frames for detection may assist in identifying relapse or confirm abstinence. The purpose and goals of the testing program must be identified so that the appropriate tests, or combination of tests, are selected.

Daniel N. Allen and Christina Holman

See also Blood Alcohol Concentration; Driving Under the Influence; Drug Testing; Timeline Followback; Urine Toxicology Testing

Further Readings

Center for Substance Abuse Treatment. (2006, September). The role of biomarkers in the treatment of alcohol use disorders. *Substance Abuse Treatment Advisory, 5*(4), 1–7.

Jenkins, A. J., & Goldberger, B. A. (Eds.). (2002). *On-site drug testing.* Totowa, NJ: Humana Press.

Karch, S. B. (Ed.). (2007). *Forensic issues in alcohol testing.* Boca Raton, FL: CRC Press.

ALCOHOL USE DISORDERS IDENTIFICATION TEST

In the late 1980s, the World Health Organization sponsored the development of the Alcohol Use Disorders Identification Test (AUDIT), a screening test for excessive alcohol consumption that has international applicability to countries with varying economic wealth and standards of living. The AUDIT was the outgrowth of a six, non-Asian country project, and its development and standardization involved approximately 2,000 primary care patients in Australia, Bulgaria, Kenya, Mexico, Norway, and the United States. As a result, the AUDIT became the first widely available screening instrument designed specifically for international use and developed through large-scale cross-cultural research.

The AUDIT is administered orally in an interview setting or as a self-report questionnaire (completed electronically or on paper). Both formats take an average individual approximately 2 minutes to complete, and the test can be hand-scored in about 3 minutes. Although originally developed for use in primary health care settings, the AUDIT has now been used in a variety of situations and has proved to be a versatile screening instrument. The most recent version of the AUDIT manual (*The Alcohol Use Disorders Identification Test: Guidelines for Use in Primary Care, Second Edition*) lists many settings in which the AUDIT has been effectively administered (e.g., emergency room, outpatient clinic, psychiatric hospital, prison), the diverse target groups with which it has been used (e.g., medical patients, psychiatric patients, individuals with impaired social or occupational functioning), and the various professionals who have used it (e.g., nurses, social workers, counselors, human service workers, physicians).

Although there is relatively little research on the use of the AUDIT with women, the manual reports that the AUDIT is equally appropriate for both men and women. In addition, although originally developed for adults, recent research indicates that the AUDIT might also be useful for screening adolescents. However, a growing body of literature is questioning the appropriateness of the AUDIT for elderly individuals based on the relatively poorer performance of the AUDIT in screening individuals of this age group.

The AUDIT consists of 10 questions addressing three separate domains: hazardous alcohol usage (based on drinking frequency, typical quantity, and frequency of heavy drinking), dependence symptoms (based on impaired control over drinking, social role impairment, and morning drinking), and harmful alcohol use (based on guilt after drinking, blackouts, alcohol-related injuries, and level of

concern by others). With the exception of the last two questions (which speak to lifetime usage), the AUDIT items refer to present alcohol use and use within the previous year. The first eight questions offer the respondent five options (which correspond to different levels of either frequency or quantity), while the last two items offer three response options that reflect the occurrence of alcohol-related problems within one's lifetime and how recently these problems have occurred.

The total score on the AUDIT is obtained by summing the scores for each of the 10 items on a 0 (zero) to 4 scale. Consequently, total scores range from 0 to 40, with a score of 8 generally accepted as the cutoff for identifying a potential alcohol use problem. Higher scores are associated with increased likelihood of hazardous or harmful drinking or alcohol dependence and imply that a higher degree of intervention is needed. Nevertheless, some researchers have recommended lowering the cutoff score for certain groups who may be more susceptible to the effects of alcohol (e.g., women, individuals over the age of 65, adolescents).

The AUDIT continues to be used and researched in many countries across the world and has won acclaim for its generalizability across many English-speaking countries. Regardless, some researchers argue that additional international investigation is still required to fully support the currently recommended cutoff scores across nations and cultures. The AUDIT has also been translated into approximately 20 languages. However, because there has been relatively little research on these foreign language versions, their psychometric strength has not yet been well established.

The AUDIT has inspired a widespread and far-reaching body of research, and the performance of the English-language version has been evaluated for about 20 years. According to a review by J. P. Allen and colleagues, the AUDIT is fourth among self-report alcohol-related screening measures in terms of research generated, surpassed only by the CAGE questionnaire (CAGE), the Michigan Alcoholism Screening Test (MAST), and the MacAndrew Alcoholism Scale (MAS). Consistent findings across several academic reviews of the AUDIT (conducted by Allen and colleagues in 1997, D. F. Reinart and Allen in 2002, and again by Reinart and Allen in 2007) have concluded that the AUDIT fares quite well compared to similar screening tests, such as the

CAGE, MAST, and MAS, with respect to reliability, validity, sensitivity, specificity, and predictive validity.

Aside from the fact that the AUDIT is available free of charge, can be administered quickly, is psychometrically sound, and has proven its usefulness across countries, settings, groups, and screening professionals, the AUDIT has several other distinct advantages. Among these advantages are the following: (a) Its large-scale cross-national standardization supports it as the most widely used, if not only, screening instrument designed specifically for international use; (b) it is capable of identifying alcohol-related problems along a wide continuum of varying severity; and (c) it is consistent with alcohol use disorders found in the World Health Organization's *International Classification of Diseases, Tenth Revision (ICD-10)*. Another significant advantage of the AUDIT is that its accompanying manual provides an overarching framework for recommended interventions, based on the individual's score. Scores of 0 to 7 should be followed by alcohol education, 8 to 15 require advice to limit or cut down one's drinking, 16 to 19 suggests the need for brief counseling and continued monitoring in addition to advice, and scores of 20 or higher indicate the need for referral to a specialist for a full diagnostic evaluation and formal treatment.

One key limitation of the AUDIT is that, unlike some tests, it does not include a means of assessing whether an individual's responses are likely to be an accurate reflection of the situation (e.g., due to dishonesty, fatigue, defensiveness, comprehension difficulties, or inattention). As such, the legitimacy of a score produced by the AUDIT is based on the assumption that the individual has the current ability and willingness to provide correct answers.

Since the AUDIT was first introduced, researchers have, for various reasons, developed several alternate forms of the English-language AUDIT (e.g., AUDIT-C, AUDIT-PC, AUDIT-3, and AUDIT-4). Although none of these alternate forms has been studied extensively, the AUDIT-C appears is the most supported by research. Only the original AUDIT and its manual are available free of charge from the World Health Organization Web site.

Robinder P. Bedi and Katie M. Winters

See also CAGE Screening Instrument; Michigan Alcohol Screening Test; Screening; Screening Instruments

Further Readings

Allen, J. P., Litten, R. Z., Fertig, J. B., & Babor, T. (1997). A review of research on the Alcohol Use Disorders Identification Test (AUDIT). *Alcoholism: Clinical and Experimental Research, 21,* 613–619.

Babor, T. F., Higgins-Biddle, J. C., Saunders, J. B., & Monteiro, M. G. (2001). *The Alcohol Use Disorders Identification Test: Guidelines for use in primary care* (2nd ed.). Geneva: World Health Organization.

Reinert, D. F., & Allen, J. P. (2002). The Alcohol Use Disorders Identification Test (AUDIT): A review of recent research. *Alcoholism: Clinical and Experimental Research, 26,* 272–279.

Reinert, D. F., & Allen, J. P. (2007). The Alcohol Use Disorders Identification Test: An update of research findings. *Alcoholism: Clinical and Experimental Research, 31,* 185–199.

World Health Organization: http://www.who.int

ALTERNATIVE ACTIVITIES

Alternative activities provide targeted populations with opportunities to participate in a range of selected substance-free environments. Many alternative approaches consist of activities intended to challenge individuals in safe but novel situations. There was a proliferation of alternative activities in prevention programs following the spread of the concept of natural highs along with the diffusion of the New Games movement in the late 1970s. Alternative activities, as a prevention strategy, should be part of a broader comprehensive prevention program that includes other strategies with demonstrated effectiveness. When functioning as part of an integrated prevention plan, alternative activities help stimulate individual motivation and can help generate increased public and media attention on substance abuse issues, as well as on the critical importance of having ongoing prevention efforts.

Theoretical justification for implementing alternative activities as a prevention strategy has been based on varied prevention assumptions. Many alternative activities are simply offered in the well-intended belief that they provide attractive options that individuals can elect to participate in which might be at least as, or perhaps even more, appealing than engaging in substance use and abuse activities. Afterschool sports activities, such as Midnight Basketball, are examples of such popular alternative activities. In fact, most recreational activities, such as various sports, games, dances, arts and crafts, and other leisure pastimes, can readily be incorporated as alternative activities for use in substance abuse prevention programs. Other alternative activities are selected because it is felt that they can provide participants with useful future life skills, as well as providing for the acquisition of essential knowledge and responsible attitudes necessary for resisting the initiation of drug use. Just Say No organizations were founded on this premise. Skill building has been an integral component of many youth development programs, such as the Boy Scouts and Girl Scouts, 4-H Clubs, YMCA and YWCA, Boys Clubs and Girls Clubs, and Camp Fire Girls. Skill-building alternative activities have also been used with individuals who have already used alcohol, tobacco, or other drugs. A wide array of skills can be the targeted in these alternative activities, such as responsible decision making, the ability to resist peer pressure, and the ability to delay gratification. There are also alternative activities chosen because it is believed that they will offer challenging experiences that, when successfully completed, can boost self-concept, self-esteem, and self-efficacy, as well as promote effective team building. All of these outcomes are hypothesized to aid in resisting drug initiation and subsequent substance use and abuse. Outward Bound and similarly modeled experiences represent this type of alternative activity. Tutoring programs, including cross-age tutoring, are another type of alternative activity designed to develop academic competence, as well as to indirectly enhance interpersonal skills. There are numerous other alternative activities designed to fulfill the various needs that are thought to underlie drug use and abuse. For example, to meet the biological need to relax, individuals might be instructed in specific meditation techniques and yoga postures or be provided biofeedback on meditative brainwave states. Learning to appreciate listening to music might be selected as a strategy to increase sensory awareness. Encounter groups might be conducted to satisfy socialization and acceptance by peer needs.

Environmental approaches that are intended to reduce the desire for and availability of alcohol, tobacco, and other drugs can be combined effectively with alternative activities. For instance, several institutions of higher education have implemented social norms marketing and environmental management programs designed to reduce high-risk drinking and associated negative consequences among college students. Campus-based media campaigns and other alternative strategies have been used in conjunction with environmental strategies in an attempt to correct student misperceptions about the actual alcohol use of other students and to make the campuses less conducive to excessive alcohol use. The sponsoring of alcohol-free events, such as mock-tail (nonalcoholic drinks) parties, is an alternative activity implemented frequently on college campuses.

Community service, which includes service learning, is another broad type of alternative activity for substance abuse prevention. Community service activities might consist of visiting residents in a nursing home or serving food at a homeless shelter. It is felt that participation in meaningful community service activities helps promote the development of social responsibility and personal well-being, as well as closer bonds with the broader community. Mentoring programs, such as that conducted by Big Brothers Big Sisters of America, is another category of alternative activities that are sometimes integrated with community service programs.

Alternative activities have also been targeted at individuals in groups at high risk for substance abuse, such as juvenile delinquents and children of alcoholics or other substance abusers. This has been the case particularly with alternative activities that are, relative to other prevention approaches, more expensive to conduct. For example, wilderness experiences, rock climbing, ropes courses, whitewater rafting, and similar experiences have been used to provide alternative activities to substance abuse for high-risk individuals.

A common critique of the use of alternative activities as a prevention strategy has been the difficulty with measuring their effectiveness at actually preventing alcohol, tobacco, and other drug initiation, use, and abuse. However, meta-analysis of alternative programs has suggested that these activities have the potential to be effective interventions for preventing substance abuse when incorporated into a comprehensive substance abuse prevention program. Alternative activities can, and frequently do, serve as a useful adjunct to comprehensive alcohol, tobacco, and other drug abuse prevention programs.

Victor B. Stolberg

See also Evidence-Based Prevention; Mentoring; National Registry of Evidence-based Programs and Practices; Prevention Evaluation; Prevention Strategies; Refusal Skills

Further Readings

Center for Substance Abuse Prevention's Northeast Center for the Application of Prevention Technologies. (2003). *Alternatives: A strategy for prevention practitioners.* Retrieved May 8, 2007, from http://hhd.org/docs/alternatives_final1.pdf

Kumpfer, K., Morehouse, E., Ross, B., Fleming, C., Emshoff, J., & DeMarco, L. (1988). *Prevention of substance abuse in COSA programs.* Rockville, MD: ADAMHA/OSAP.

National Center for the Advancement of Prevention. (1996). *A review of alternative activities and alternative programs in youth-oriented prevention* (CSAP Technical Rep. No. 13). Washington, DC: Department of Health and Human Services.

Tobler, N. S. (1992). Drug prevention programs can work: Research findings. *Journal of Addictive Diseases, 11,* 1–28.

AMERICAN SOCIETY OF ADDICTION MEDICINE

The mission of the American Society of Addiction Medicine (ASAM) is to increase access to, and improve the quality of, addiction treatment; to educate physicians, including medical and osteopathic students, other health care providers, and the public; to support research and prevention as well as to promote the appropriate role of the physician in the care of patients with addiction; and to establish addiction medicine as a primary specialty recognized by professional organizations, governments, physicians, purchasers and consumers of health care services, and the general public.

Ruth Fox (1895–1989) was the founder of the ASAM. In the early 1950s at the New York Academy of Medicine, Fox established regular meetings with other physicians interested in alcoholism and its treatment. In 1954, these physicians established the New York City Medical Society on Alcoholism with Fox as its first president. As the organization grew, it was subsequently named the American Medical Society on Alcoholism (AMSA).

In 1982, the American Academy of Addictionology was incorporated into the AMSA and began efforts to achieve recognition for this new medical specialty. In June 1988, AMSA was admitted to the American Medical Association (AMA) House of Delegates as a voting member, and in June 1990, the AMA added addiction medicine to its list of designated specialties. In 1989, the organization was renamed the American Society of Addiction Medicine (ASAM) to reflect the AMSA's concern with addictive drugs and its interest in establishing addiction medicine as part of mainstream medicine.

ASAM members are physicians from all medical specialties and subspecialties. They are engaged in private practice, serve as corporate medical directors, and work in group practice or other clinical settings. Some are also involved in research and medical education. To aid these medical professionals, ASAM has created practice guidelines to assist in making clinical decisions. According to ASAM, the physician must make the ultimate decision regarding any specific treatment with consideration of scientific and patient information and in light of the diagnostic and treatment options available.

To further the goal of providing quality care from health care professionals, the ASAM has a code of ethics for its members. The Public Policy Statement on Principles of Medical Ethics was adopted by the ASAM board of directors on October 3, 1992.

The policy states that the ASAM supports a body of ethical statements developed primarily for the benefit of the patient. It states that as members of the medical profession, physicians must recognize their responsibility not only to patients but also to society, to other health professionals, and to themselves.

The ASAM is also prominent in writing publications including the *Principles of Addiction Medicine,* the *Patient Placement Criteria*, and the *Journal of Addiction Medicine.* The *Principles of Addiction Medicine* is currently in its third edition (2007) and provides a comprehensive overview of the diagnosis and treatment of addictive disorders, as well as the management of co-occurring medical and psychiatric conditions. The *Patient Placement Criteria* is currently in its second edition (2007) and is the most widely used and comprehensive national guidelines for placement, continued stay, and discharge of patients with alcohol and other drug problems. Finally, the *Journal of Addiction Medicine* is published quarterly and is free to ASAM members. The journal is a professional forum for new topics, as well as advancements in addiction medicine.

A large component of the ASAM is its advocacy. ASAM's advocacy events and briefings are intended to educate lawmakers about the concept that addiction is a treatable disease. Additionally, these events allow members the opportunity to bring addiction-related issues to the attention of their legislative representatives.

As ASAM looks toward the future, the organization is taking action to ensure that the field of addictions does not become stagnant. In an attempt to allow for easier access and greater exposure, ASAM has a Web site that contains information for professionals and laypersons alike. On the 35th anniversary of the founding of ASAM, the Ruth Fox Memorial Endowment Fund was established. The endowment enables ASAM to move forward with activities that will assist in achieving its mission.

In addition, ASAM has provided medical residents the opportunity to learn about the diagnosis and treatment of alcoholism and other drug dependencies through their mentoring program. To do this, ASAM provides scholarships for physicians-in-training to attend the ASAM annual conference. ASAM also provides rewards to professionals who exemplify the ASAM standards. Each year, ASAM offers five awards in addition to scholarships: the John P. McGovern Award, the R. Brinkley Smithers Distinguished Scientist Award, the ASAM Medical-Scientific Program Committee Award, the Young Investigator Award, and the Annual Awards Recipient.

Since its official inception in 1954, ASAM has developed tremendously. It has incorporated other organizations, grown in awareness and popularity, and become a crucial society for medical professionals dealing with addictions.

Ann-Marie Fenner, Sabina Mutisya,
and Thomas Harrison

See also NAADAC, the Association for Addiction Professionals; National Council on Alcoholism and Drug Dependence; Network for the Improvement of Addiction Treatment; Patient Placement Criteria

Further Readings

American Society of Addiction Medicine: http://www.asam.org/

American Society of Addiction Medicine. (1992). *Code of ethics.* Retrieved March 13, 2007, from http://www.ama-assn.org/ama/pub/category/13352.html

David, M. L. (2001). *ASAM patient placement criteria for the treatment of substance-related disorders.* Chevy Chase, MD: American Society of Addiction Medicine.

Wryobeck, J. M., Chermack, S. T., Closser, M. H., & Blow, F. C. (2006). Using the Addiction Severity Index to predict mental and medical health service utilization. *Journal of Addictive Diseases, 25,* 1–14.

Amotivational Syndrome

Clinical observations of marijuana use in the 1960s led to the development of a label for a constellation of symptoms called "amotivational syndrome," which was thought to be a long-term effect of heavy marijuana use. Symptoms include apathy, decreased productivity, decreased energy levels, depression, inability to concentrate, loss of motivation, and decreased goal-directed behavior. Amotivational syndrome does not refer to the acute intoxication of marijuana but rather the general characteristics of heavy marijuana users even when they are not high from the drug. Many studies in the 1960s and 1970s sought to empirically validate the existence of the syndrome, yet all of the studies had methodological flaws that made it difficult to draw definitive conclusions. As the literature on marijuana use accumulated, research was conducted in controlled laboratory settings, yet only one study involving rhesus monkeys was able to demonstrate the existence of amotivational syndrome. Although the syndrome has not been empirically validated in research on humans, marijuana use has been shown to affect memory and attention, both of which are capacities that could be directly related to motivation levels in an individual.

In the late 1960s, David Smith named the cluster of symptoms associated with motivation levels in marijuana users "amotivational syndrome" as he had observed in adolescents a decreased desire to work or compete. Smith provided two case studies in which the symptoms stopped after a period of abstinence from marijuana. However, in 1982, Smith stated that the impairment in functioning that constituted the syndrome occurred only in a small percentage of users.

Harold Kolansky and William Moore conducted several studies in the early 1970s that provided evidence supporting the existence of an amotivational syndrome among heavy marijuana users. Participants had smoked marijuana 3 to 10 times per week for periods ranging from 16 months to 6 years. The authors reported that all participants demonstrated adverse psychological symptoms such as apathy, flattened affect, confusion, difficulty with short-term memory, and "sluggishness" in mental and physical responses to stimuli. These symptoms emerged when marijuana use was initiated and ceased when drug use stopped. The researchers also asserted that the observed symptoms were associated with longer durations and higher frequencies of marijuana use. The hypothesis that marijuana use led to a cluster of symptoms known as amotivational syndrome was supported by the correlation of severity of symptoms and the length of marijuana use, in addition to the fact that participants' symptoms lessened or stopped after marijuana use ceased. Kolansky and Moore also observed the presence of the syndrome in a sample of 38 adolescents in which they argued that the negative effects of marijuana use were particularly accentuated due to the developmental stage of the participants.

A study examining chronic marijuana exposure in the rhesus monkey provided further evidence for the existence of amotivational syndrome. Monkeys were exposed to marijuana daily for 1 year and pressed a lever for food pellets on a progressive ratio schedule (i.e., every time a pellet was received, more presses of the lever were required to receive another pellet). The researchers found that when exposed to marijuana, breaking points were significantly lower than they were for controls, but they returned to normal when exposure to marijuana was discontinued. Thus, the researchers posited that the result was equivalent to the amotivational syndrome hypothesized to exist in humans.

Research arguing against the existence of amotivational syndrome identifies major methodological flaws in the study designs that make it impossible to draw the conclusion that amotivational syndrome exists. Motivation, a hypothetical construct, is difficult to measure as it cannot be observed directly and can only be operationally defined from some other behavior; thus, there is inherent ambiguity in the construct. Systematic diagnostic criteria for the syndrome were never developed or agreed upon. In the studies conducted in the 1960s and 1970s, there was no way to control for the potency of the marijuana given to participants, rendering it impossible to examine dose–effect relationships. Furthermore, none of the studies supporting the existence of the syndrome used control groups, and many of them derived behavioral data from subjective accounts, rather than using independent and objective measures of behavior.

The numerous studies conducted since the 1960s consistently demonstrate a lack of empirical evidence to support the existence of amotivational syndrome.

Controlled laboratory studies with humans have sought to correct for the methodological flaws in early marijuana research and have not found any significant evidence of an amotivational syndrome. In 1976, Jack Mendelson and colleagues used volunteers to show that amotivational syndrome does not exist. Participants were categorized into "heavy" and "casual" marijuana users based on frequency of reported smoking and were asked to work on simple operant tasks on a fixed interval schedule of reinforcement in a controlled inpatient environment. The reward consisted of earned points based on operant performance, which they could cash in for money or use toward purchasing marijuana cigarettes. Participants served as their own controls during a 5-day baseline period when operant tasks were performed but marijuana was not used. The baseline period was followed by 21 days of marijuana smoking and concluded with a 5-day period of nonsmoking. Results showed that marijuana smoking did not significantly influence the work completed by casual or heavy smokers and produced no changes in operant work. Both groups remained motivated throughout the marijuana-smoking period to earn money in addition to the work they completed to purchase marijuana cigarettes.

A study conducted in Costa Rica also addressed previous methodological flaws by using a holistic perspective of drug abuse. This study used operationally defined testing procedures and accounted for other factors that may explain the presence of amotivational symptoms in addition to marijuana use. Forty-one marijuana users were compared to 41 nonusers. Results showed that 18 users experienced symptoms characteristic of an amotivational syndrome, yet sociocultural factors indicated that marijuana use was not the cause of an unstable lifestyle, and in fact, the participants who endorsed amotivational-like symptoms had experienced major personal and familial problems earlier in their lives. Various other comparisons including intelligence and memory revealed no significant differences between users and nonusers.

The evidence for an amotivational syndrome among chronic marijuana users is equivocal; support for its existence lies mostly in clinical observations, case histories, and research studies that have major methodological flaws, making it difficult to draw conclusions about cause and effect. Furthermore, after conducting a literature review on marijuana and amotivational syndrome, Wayne Hall and colleagues concluded that there is no clear empirical support for such a syndrome and that if it does exist, it occurs in a small percentage of heavy, chronic marijuana users.

Meggan M. Bucossi and Gregory L. Stuart

See also Cannabis Youth Treatment Study; Marijuana

Further Readings

Hall, W., Solowij, N., & Lemon, J. (1994). *The health and psychological consequences of cannabis use* (National Drug Strategy, Monograph Series No. 25). Canberra: Australian Government Publishing Service.

Kolansky, H., & Moore, W. T. (1972). Toxic effects of chronic marihuana use. *Journal of the American Medical Association, 222,* 35–41.

Mendelson, J. H., Kuehnle, J. C., Greenberg, I., & Mello, N. K. (1976). Operant acquisition of marihuana in man. *Journal of Pharmacology and Experimental Therapeutics, 198*(1), 42–53.

Page, B. J. (1983). The amotivational syndrome hypothesis and the Costa Rica study: Relationships between methods and results. *Journal of Psychoactive Drugs, 15*(4), 261–267.

Smith, D. E. (1968). The acute and chronic toxicity of marijuana. *Journal of Psychedelic Drugs, 2*(1), 37–48.

AMPHETAMINES

Amphetamines, including methamphetamine and dextroamphetamine, are psychomotor stimulants that affect the serotonin, epinephrine, norepinephrine, and dopamine levels in the brain. Amphetamines are prescribed to treat various disorders, but they are also illegally manufactured for recreational use. Pharmacotherapies and cognitive behavioral therapies are used to treat amphetamine addictions, and to date, the only empirically validated treatment is the Matrix Model.

Amphetamines closely resemble adrenaline, a naturally produced hormone in the body. Amphetamines cause vasodilation and bronchodilation, as well as an increase in heart rate and blood pressure. Physiological effects of amphetamines vary depending on the dose and method of administration, but include decreased appetite, muscular weakness, respiratory depression, chest pain, hyperactivity, nausea, increased sex drive, dry mouth, headaches, sweating, dizziness, and punding (the repeated performance of some pointless act for an extended time). Psychological effects of amphetamines include euphoria, insomnia, increased concentration and alertness, anxiety, increased sociability or talkativeness, aggression, and antisocial behavior. High doses or continued use of amphetamines can cause a syndrome known as "amphetamine psychosis," characterized by psychotic behavior including paranoia, delusions, and auditory and visual hallucinations. Routes of administration for amphetamines include oral ingestion, smoking (methamphetamine), intranasal, and intravenous (methamphetamine). Khat, the only organically derived amphetamine, is made from the leaves of the Qat tree in East Africa. The leaves are chewed and produce similar feelings of euphoria, as well as having anesthetic effects.

Amphetamines are commonly used to treat attention deficit hyperactivity disorder and are used to treat narcolepsy and other sleeping disorders. However, because amphetamines are so widely prescribed, they are readily, available for recreational use, and recently, public awareness has increased regarding the potential for amphetamines abuse. In addition to amphetamines that are medically prescribed, illegally manufactured amphetamines (e.g., methamphetamine) are commonly abused as well. The National Institute on Drug Abuse estimated that 4.3% of the U.S. population age 12 and older have used methamphetamines at some point in their lives. The prevalence of amphetamine abuse on college campuses in the United States is approximately 10% given that stimulants are often used to stay awake in order to study for extended periods.

Tolerance to amphetamines develops quickly with habitual use; thus, the dose needs to be continually increased to achieve the desired effects. Withdrawal symptoms from amphetamines include intense cravings for the drug, dysphoria, vivid and unpleasant dreams, depression, increased anxiety, decreased energy levels, increased appetite, irritability, and an inability to reach REM (rapid eye movement) sleep cycles. Withdrawal from amphetamines is not medically dangerous and does not usually require inpatient detoxification. However, observation of depressive symptoms and for suicidality is recommended, as the severity of depression is associated with the length of abuse.

According to the U.S. Department of Health and Human Services, the rate of treatment admissions for primary methamphetamine or amphetamine abuse from 1993 to 2003 increased from 13 to 56 admissions per 100,000 patients age 12 or older. In addition, the proportion of primary methamphetamine or amphetamine admissions referred to treatment by the criminal justice system increased from 36% in 1993 to 51% in 2003.

Antidepressant drugs, which affect serotonin levels, are used to treat the depression that occurs when stopping amphetamine use. Sedatives are occasionally used on a short-term basis to treat the anxiety and sleep problems that may occur. An antipsychotic drug may be used to relieve psychotic symptoms such as delusions, paranoia, and hallucinations and also helps to balance dopamine levels.

The Matrix Model, an empirically validated outpatient treatment for stimulant abuse, was developed in the 1980s and has been used in the treatment of more than 1,000 methamphetamine users. The therapist develops a positive relationship with the patient, promoting self-esteem, dignity, and self-worth. Therapists are nonconfrontational, yet realistic and direct in their interactions with patients. The Matrix Model draws from several other empirically validated treatment approaches for drug addictions; thus, it includes information on relapse prevention, family and group involvement, drug education, and information regarding support groups. A treatment manual has been developed, and several studies funded by the National Institute on Drug Abuse have found treatment to be associated with significant reductions in stimulant use.

Numerous drugs have been investigated for the treatment of amphetamine use, including fluoxetine, amlodipine, imipramine, desipramine, and dexamphetamine (used as a substitution treatment), yet none has demonstrated significant levels of efficacy in treating amphetamine abuse. Recently, opioid antagonists (e.g., naltrexone), used for the treatment of opioid dependence, have been investigated for treating amphetamine dependence. Naltrexone blocks the rewarding effects of amphetamines by affecting dopamine levels in the brain. Several studies have reported that naltrexone decreased patients' reports of cravings, consumption, and the feeling of being "high." Opioid blockers have been shown to attenuate specific effects of amphetamines in animal studies and have recently proved effective in decreasing several

subjective effects of amphetamines in studies with healthy, human volunteers. One study, which measured the feasibility of using naltrexone as a pharmacotherapy in amphetamine-dependent participants, found that compliance with treatment (naltrexone plus relapse prevention therapy) was 69%. In this study, naltrexone led to a reduction in the quantity of use and a reduction in the subjective feeling of being "high."

Psychosocial treatments for amphetamine dependence, such as cognitive behavioral therapy (CBT) are currently being utilized, though CBT is not a universally agreed upon treatment for amphetamine dependence. CBT for amphetamine use consists of training in coping skills, self-efficacy and refusal skills, problem-solving skills, self-monitoring, coping with cravings, modeling, planning for relapse prevention, role playing, and behavioral reversal. One study used CBT in combination with motivational interviewing, which is known to be effective in addiction treatment. Results indicated that CBT significantly increased amphetamine refusal self-efficacy ratings posttreatment and was associated with improvements in general health and psychological domains, such as somatic symptoms, anxiety, social dysfunction, and depression. Another study combining CBT with motivational interviewing examined whether there were differences between two sessions and four sessions of CBT in reducing amphetamine use in regular users. Results showed that there was a significant, overall reduction of amphetamine use in both groups, but there was no significant difference in effectiveness between the two- and four-session interventions.

Interpersonal Psychotherapy (IPT), originally used in the treatment of depression, was modified for interventions with cocaine- and stimulant-dependant people in a study conducted with alcohol- and/or stimulant-dependant participants. IPT was used to identify the role of interpersonal relationships in the development and maintenance of stimulant dependence and how these factors could increase or decrease abstinence. Results indicated that IPT did not significantly decrease stimulant use. However, more intense treatment was associated with a better outcome, regardless of the substance that was targeted in the IPT.

Meggan M. Bucossi and Gregory L. Stuart

See also Central Nervous System Stimulants; Illicit and Illegal Drugs; Methamphetamine

Further Readings

Baker, A., Boggs, T. G., & Lewin, T. J. (2001). Randomized controlled trial of brief cognitive-behavioral interventions among regular users of amphetamine. *Addiction, 96,* 1279–1287.

Feeney, G. F. X., Connor, J. P., Young, R. M., Tucker, J., & McPherson, A. (2006). Improvement in measures of psychological distress amongst amphetamine misusers treated with brief cognitive-behavioral therapy (CBT). *Addictive Behaviors, 31,* 1833–1843.

Jayaram-Lindstrom, N., Wennberg, P., Beck, O., & Franck, J. (2005). An open clinical trial of naltrexone for amphetamine dependence: Compliance and tolerability. *Nordic Journal of Psychiatry, 59,* 167–171.

U.S. Department of Health and Human Services. (2006). Trends in methamphetamine/amphetamine admissions to treatment: 1993–2003. *The DASIS Report,* Issue 9. Retrieved May 20, 2008, from http://www.drugabusestatistics.samhsa.gov/2k6/methTx/meth TX.htm

AMYL NITRITE

Amyl nitrite is an inhalant that has recognized medical uses, as well as a history of illicit recreational use. Street names for amyl nitrite include *aimes, ames, amys, pearls,* and *poppers.* Amyl nitrite is usually supplied in thin, glass-covered capsules or ampules that can be easily broken between the fingers. Although intended for medicinal use, these capsules are used as inhalants and are often called *poppers* because of the sound of crushing the capsule and for its rapid euphoric "rush." Amyl nitrite and related substances like isobutyl nitrite are used in several over-the-counter products, such as room deodorizers, polish removers, liquid incense, and video head cleaners. Brand names for some of these products include Locker Room, Rush, Liquid Gold, Bullet, Crypt, TNT, Stag, Ram, Thrust, Rock Hard, Rave, Kix, Hi-Tech, and Snappers. These products are generally sold in clubs, boutiques, gay bars, and sex shops. The recreational use of amyl nitrite and similar substances is largely due to their purported value as aphrodisiacs.

Amyl nitrite is a highly volatile fluid that evaporates at room temperature. It is also highly inflammable and explosive. Amyl nitrite is an organic nitrite, which is a clear, oily, yellowish liquid in appearance, with a fruity odor. It is produced by mixing nitric acid and amylic alcohol.

Amyl nitrite is an effective vasodilator and smooth muscle relaxant. Amyl nitrite is fast acting (5–30 seconds) and has a short duration of action (3–5 minutes). Amyl nitrite is used medically chiefly for the prophylaxis and treatment of angina pectoris. It has also been used to treat cyanide poisoning and renal and biliary colic. However, current Food and Drug Administration regulations prohibit labeling amyl nitrite for any use other than treating angina pectoris (21 CFR 250.102). Amyl nitrite has been used as an aphrodisiac, purported to intensify an orgasm, and is particularly popular by those interested in anal sexual activity, such as homosexual males.

In 1867, Thomas Lauder Brunton, a Scottish medical student, discovered that amyl nitrite relieved the pain of angina pectoris by increasing blood flow to the heart. There was an upsurge in recreational use of amyl nitrite beginning in the early 1960s when the Food and Drug Administration removed the need for a prescription. Amyl nitrite then became very popular in the gay community. It was also used by American soldiers fighting in Vietnam. The ban on the use of amyl nitrite without a prescription was reinstated by the Food and Drug Administration in 1969. To get around this regulatory ban, manufacturers began producing slightly altered formulas that produced similar effects. Butyl nitrite and isobutyl nitrite are examples of some of these slightly modified formulas. In 1988, when the U.S. Consumer Products Safety Commission placed a ban on the sale of butyl nitrite, manufacturers continued to produce slightly adjusted products, such as cyclohexyl nitrite. In street parlance, all of these analogues are typically referred to as amyl nitrite, as well as its other associated street names, such as *poppers.* These products are often used along with other so-called club or rave drugs, like ecstasy (MDMA), ketamine, and gamma-hydroxybutyrate (GHB).

Amyl nitrite relaxes vascular muscle, including that of cardiac muscles, which causes the veins in the heart to dilate, leading to a drop in blood pressure. Pulse rate increases in response to the drop in blood pressure. Dilation of blood vessels in the brain seems to produce an increase of pressure in the brain, which produces the effect usually referred to as a "rush" or "head rush." Headaches are frequently associated with this reaction. Dilation of veins also produces a warm, flush response as blood collects near the skin surface. This also produces a drop in core body temperature.

The body converts amyl nitrite into nitrosamines, which are known carcinogens. In fact, the abuse of amyl nitrite has been associated with Kaposi's sarcoma, a type of skin cancer that increased in prevalence among people with AIDS during the early phases of the pandemic. The use of amyl nitrite also impairs the functioning of the immune system of the body.

Amyl nitrite can produce dizziness, disorientation, drowsiness, and a decreased perception of time. Thus, it should not be used when operating a motor vehicle or other heavy equipment. As it causes intraocular and intracranial pressure, amyl nitrite is also contraindicated for those with glaucoma and recent head injury. It should also not be used by pregnant women, as it can harm the fetus. The possible effects of amyl nitrite use include euphoria, slurred speech, fainting, vasodilatation, nausea, stupor, clammy skin, accelerated heart rate, lowered blood pressure, loss of bladder control, headache, and hallucinations. Amyl nitrite reacts with hemoglobin to form methemoglobin, and at excessive levels of use, this can cause death. Signs of excessive methemoglobin include blue skin, vomiting, shock, and coma. However, methemoglobin bonds with cyanide ions to form cyanmethemoglobin, which has relatively low toxicity and is why amyl nitrite is an effective treatment for cyanide poisoning. Tolerance may develop to amyl nitrite with repeated use over a prolonged period. Withdrawal symptoms include runny nose, loss of appetite, irritability, depression, headache, nausea, cramping, and tremors. There are also concerns over possible liver damage and lung damage from chronic use. Other hazards associated with the nonmedical use of amyl nitrite and similar substances include skin irritation, tracheobronchial irritation, burns, and hypokinetic anoxia, as well as blood disorders and disorders of blood-forming organs. Unconsciousness and even fatalities have been reported from swallowing large quantities of these substances.

Victor B. Stolberg

See also Club Drugs; Drugs, Classification of; Gay, Lesbian, Bisexual, and Transgender Issues; HIV/AIDS; Inhalants

Further Readings

Goode, E., & Troiden, R. R. (1979). Amyl nitrite use among homosexual men. *American Journal of Psychiatry 136,* 1067–1069.

Haverkos, H. W., Kopstein, A. N., Wilson, H., & Drotman, P. (1994). Nitrite inhalants: History, epidemiology, and possible links to AIDS. *Environmental Health Perspectives, 102,* 858–861.

Monroe, J. (2002). *Inhalant drug abusers.* Berkeley Heights, NJ: Enslow.

Young, I. (1999). *The stonewall experiment: A gay psychohistory.* New York: Cassell.

ANABOLIC STEROIDS

Anabolic-androgenic steroids, more commonly known as anabolic steroids, are synthetic structural derivatives of the male sex hormone testosterone. The administration of these substances produces anabolic (i.e., increases in skeletal muscle and lean body mass) and androgenic changes (i.e., masculinization) in men and women. Common routes of administration include oral (e.g., Anadrol, Oxandrin, Dianabol, Winstrol) and intramuscular injection (e.g., Deca-Durabolin, Durabolin, Depo-Testosterone, Equipoise, Tetrahydrogestrinone). Anabolic steroids were developed in the 1930s as a medical treatment for diseases associated with low testosterone, particularly hypogonadism, which can lead to abnormal growth, erectile dysfunction, and infertility. These drugs have demonstrated therapeutic effects for other medical conditions, such as reversing weight and muscle loss (i.e., body wasting) among HIV patients; ameliorating some of the side effects of hysterectomies, such as impaired sexual functioning; and improving the outcomes of burn and other critically injured patients.

Although anabolic steroids can be therapeutic at low doses, the amount administered among recreational users is generally 10 to 100 times what is medically indicated. In contrast, supratherapeutic amounts of anabolic steroids are associated with a wide range of adverse and sometimes irreversible side effects including physical (e.g., hypogonadism, heart disease) and psychological (e.g., depression, aggression, mania) problems. According to the National Institute on Drug Abuse's (NIDA) Monitoring the Future survey conducted in 2007, which questions middle and high school students about drug use behaviors and beliefs, the prevalence of past-year anabolic steroid use among 8th, 10th, and 12th graders was 0.8%, 1.1%, and 1.4%, respectively. Among adult athletes, the prevalence of anabolic steroid use is estimated by NIDA to be between 1% and 6%.

Anabolic steroids are legal in the United States only as a prescription drug. Recreational use of anabolic steroids has been prohibited since 1990 when Congress officially categorized anabolic steroids as a Schedule III controlled substance through the Anabolic Steroid Control Act. By definition, Schedule III drugs have less potential for abuse than Schedules I and II, have a currently accepted medical use in the United States, and have the potential for low to moderate physical dependence or high psychological dependence. Steroid precursors such as androstenedione ("Andro") and dehydroepiandrosterone (DHEA) were not included in the original bill but are metabolized into testosterone and, in high doses, may mimic the effects of anabolic steroids. These and similar substances were marketed as dietary supplements and used as a legal alternative to anabolic steroids until an amendment to the Anabolic Steroid Control Act in 2004 reclassified many of these as controlled substances.

Physiology

In men, the hypothalamus, pituitary gland, and testes are components of a feedback loop that regulates the level of circulating testosterone. The hypothalamus monitors the level of testosterone in circulation and initiates the process of increasing or decreasing testosterone production. If the hypothalamus detects abnormally high levels of exogenous testosterone (as when anabolic steroids are administered), it reduces secretion of gonadotropin-releasing factor; in turn, the pituitary gland decreases the production of follicle-stimulating hormone and luteinizing hormone, which signal the testes to stop producing endogenous testosterone and spermatogenesis. In other words, the exogenous testosterone supplants the endogenous testosterone. The consequent inhibition of testicular function leads to gonadal dysfunction, testicular atrophy, impotence, and infertility.

The hallmark physical changes produced by anabolic steroids, namely, the increase in skeletal muscle and lean body mass, are achieved through dual processes: anabolic and anticatabolic. Anabolic effects refer to the thickening of muscle tissue following the stimulated increase of protein synthesis in muscle cells. The anticatabolic effects are when the anabolic steroids inhibit natural cortisone from breaking down protein into amino acids, which normally releases energy stores during periods of exertion. In combination, these mechanisms make available an unnatural excess of protein in muscle cells, which catalyzes the radical muscle growth.

Methods of Use

Anabolic steroids are often administered recreationally by using stacking, pyramiding, and cycling techniques. Stacking is the administration of two or more anabolic steroids in combination, such as taking an oral anabolic steroid while also receiving intramuscular injections. Pyramiding describes the pattern of varying the amount of drug being administered over a specific time frame, during which the dosage increases until reaching a mid-cycle peak and then tapers off. Cycling refers to the pattern of alternating periods of use with periods of abstinence, usually in 6- or 12-week cycles, ostensibly allowing the body to recover during periods of nonuse. Each of these techniques is designed to optimize the desired effects of anabolic steroids while minimizing the adverse effects; however, empirical investigations have largely failed to validate either of these assumptions.

Reasons for Use

Users of anabolic steroids cite various reasons for their drug consumption, including athletic, cosmetic, and psychological motivations. Notably, anabolic steroids do not induce a sense of euphoria, which is a common motivating factor for using other illicit substances. Rather, the largest consumers of anabolic steroids are athletes who use these drugs for their performance-enhancing effects. Anabolic steroids lead to dramatic muscle growth and increases in lean body mass, strength, competitiveness, and aggression, all of which may provide a competitive edge. Other athletes and nonathletes report a cosmetic desire to alter their physical appearance, specifically to decrease body fat and increase musculature. A subset of these men and women suffer from a psychological condition called muscle dysmorphia. People with this condition have a distorted perception of their bodies and believe themselves to look unfit and weak even if they are, in fact, quite muscular. There is also some evidence to suggest that a minority of people use steroids to cope with histories of physical and sexual abuse. Among these men and women, there may be a belief that an increase in physical size and strength will help to thwart future attacks.

Adverse Effects

Anabolic steroids are known to have serious and sometimes irreversible adverse effects on multiple body systems, some of which can be fatal. In men, elevated levels of testosterone can cause testicular atrophy, infertility, erectile dysfunction, male-pattern baldness, and gynecomastia (breast development); the latter is a result of the anabolic steroids being converted into estradiol, a female sex hormone. In women, high doses of testosterone cause masculinization, including a deepened voice, increased body hair, smaller breasts, coarser skin, balding, and enlargement of the clitoris. Furthermore, anabolic steroids lead to a simultaneous increase in levels of low-density lipo-protein (LDL) or "bad" cholesterol and a decrease in levels of high-density lipo-protein (HDL) or "good" cholesterol, which raises the risk of experiencing a range of cardiovascular problems. Indeed, high doses of anabolic steroids have been related to blood clots, high blood pressure, heart attacks, strokes, and death, even among young, otherwise healthy individuals. Among adolescents, sex hormones including testosterone play a role in regulating skeletal growth during puberty. Excessively high levels of testosterone can permanently stunt growth by prematurely signaling a halt to bone growth. As with all intravenous drug use, there is a risk of contracting an infection such as HIV or hepatitis through needle sharing or by using unsterilized needles or contaminated drugs. Anabolic steroids are also associated with liver disease, including cancer, tumors, cysts, and jaundice. Other physical side effects include severe face and body acne and oily skin. Clearly, supratherapeutic doses of anabolic steroids are highly destructive to the body.

Beyond the physical consequences, the use of anabolic steroids is also associated with adverse psychological effects, including irritability and aggression. In addition, there have been many anecdotal reports of violent episodes of "roid rage," during which one is seemingly unable to control explosions of anger. Withdrawal from anabolic steroids is related to depression, delusions, mood swings, mania, loss of appetite, insomnia, decreased libido, fatigue, psychosis, restlessness, and drug cravings. Moreover,

steroid-induced depression has been implicated in suicide attempts and completions. Notably, the few well-controlled, prospective research studies that have explored the psychological impact of anabolic steroid use and withdrawal suggest that severe psychological side effects may be idiosyncratic and not directly dose dependent and may affect only a minority of users. However, the limitations of these studies prevent the generalization of their findings. Specifically, research in this area has tended to exclude individuals with pre-existing psychiatric conditions, but it is reasonable to assume that underlying mental illness may make one particularly vulnerable to experiencing more severe psychological side effects. In addition, the dose and type of anabolic steroids given to study participants, as well as the method of administration, may not be representative of real-world usage and therefore may limit the applicability of the results.

Treatment

At present, there are no specific guidelines for treating anabolic steroid abuse and dependence. Instead, treatment should be tailored to the individual and can be inpatient or outpatient and include a combination of pharmacological, behavioral, and psychological interventions. Decisions regarding the type and level of care should be guided by the duration and severity of anabolic steroid abuse, symptomatology, and comorbid psychiatric diagnoses. In general, short-term care should be focused on stabilization, for instance, on managing uncomfortable withdrawal symptoms (e.g., joint pain, headaches) and treating acute behavioral and psychological issues, such as agitation, depression, and suicidality. In some cases, this may be accomplished by informing the patient about possible withdrawal symptoms that he or she may experience and by providing support. When indicated, the administration of antidepressants (e.g., selective serotonin reuptake inhibitors), antipsychotics (e.g., Haloperidol), or analgesics (e.g., Tylenol) may be helpful in alleviating specific withdrawal symptoms. In some cases, a tapered regimen of steroids may be prescribed to ease the process of withdrawal; this should be done only under the close supervision of a medical professional. Alternatively, human chorionic gonadotrophin has been used to abate symptoms associated with hypogonadism and to stimulate the production of endogenous testosterone. In turn, the goal of long-term care should be to promote and maintain abstinence.

This may be achieved through ongoing pharmacotherapy (e.g., antidepressants for persistent depression) and psychotherapy to address underlying emotional and behavioral issues that may contribute to anabolic steroid use (e.g., muscle dysmorphia, history of trauma, low self-esteem).

Prevention

As stated earlier, anabolic steroid use has been reported among middle and high school students. In response, two promising group prevention programs targeting adolescent athletes have been developed with the aim of decreasing anabolic steroid use and other risky behaviors. The Adolescents Training and Learning to Avoid Steroids (ATLAS) for males and the Athletes Targeting Healthy Exercise and Nutrition Alternatives (ATHENA) for females are similar programs that educate adolescents about the risks of anabolic steroids and other substances and provide healthy alternatives for achieving the desired physical and motivational effects through nutrition and exercise. Compared to students not receiving the prevention curricula, participating students reported a decrease in current anabolic steroid use and other risky behaviors, such as amphetamine and marijuana use, and an increase in desire to abstain from future steroid use.

Katherine W. Follansbee, Meggan M. Bucossi, and Gregory L. Stuart

See also Athletes and Drug Use; Injection Drug Use; Illicit Drugs and Illegal Drugs; Medical Consequences; Prescription Drugs

Further Readings

Cafri, G., van den Berg, P., & Thompson, J. K. (2006). Pursuit of muscularity in adolescent boys: Relations among biopsychosocial variable and clinical outcomes. *Journal of Clinical Child and Adolescent Psychology, 35,* 283–291.

Goldberg, L., Elliot, D., & Clarke, G. N. (1996). Effects of a multidimensional anabolic steroid prevention intervention: The Adolescents Training and Learning to Avoid Steroids (ATLAS) program. *Journal of the American Medical Association, 276,* 1555–1562.

National Institute on Drug Abuse. (2006). *Anabolic steroid abuse* (NIH Publication No. 00-3721). Retrieved July 12, 2007, from http://www.nida.nih.gov/ResearchReports/Steroids/AnabolicSteroids.html

National Institute on Drug Abuse, anabolic steroid abuse: http://www.steroidabuse.gov

Pope, H. G., Jr., Kouri, E. M., & Hudson, J. I. (2000). Effects of supraphysiologic doses of testosterone on mood and aggression in normal men: A randomized control trial. *Archives of General Psychiatry, 57,* 133–140.

Trenton, A. J., & Currier, G. W. (2005). Behavioural manifestations of anabolic steroid use. *CNS Drugs, 19,* 571–595.

ANOREXIA NERVOSA

Anorexia nervosa is a multifaceted condition of emotional, physical, and behavioral changes associated with an individual's reluctance to maintain a minimally normal body weight (body weight below 15% of what is expected for current age and height); it affects roughly 0.1% of the adult population of the United States. Typically, the individual displays an extreme fear of weight gain and exhibits a distorted perception of his or her size and body shape. Significant weight loss is generally achieved by eating fewer calories than is needed to sustain the body's metabolic requirement. Although anorexia nervosa is primarily diagnosed in adolescent females (accounting for approximately 90% of diagnosed population) around the time of pubertal change, the number of identified males with the disorder is increasing. Males, unlike females, face the stigma of having a gender-inconsistent disorder. Therefore, males may be predisposed to being underdiagnosed.

There are two categories of anorexia nervosa: (1) restrictive and (2) binge-eating or purging type. The restrictive anorexic abstains from habitual characteristics of binge-eating or purging behaviors such as self-induced vomiting or the misuse of enemas, diuretics, or laxatives. The binge-eating or purging anorexic has habitual characteristics of binge-eating or purging behaviors such as self-induced vomiting or the misuse of enemas, diuretics, or laxatives associated with long periods of starvation. Distinct from bulimia nervosa, an individual personifying the binge-eating or purging anorexic type is characterized as significantly underweight.

The following sections discuss the addictive tendencies, preliminary warning signs, symptoms, causes, treatment, and recovery for anorexia nervosa.

Addiction

Strong arguments suggest that anorexia nervosa is a form of addiction. Those afflicted with anorexia are commonly characterized as perfectionists and over-achievers who appear to be in control. This delusion of self-mastery, perfection, and control associated with anxiety and depression are common personality traits that predispose an individual to developing addictive behaviors.

Clinically, supportive arguments affirming that anorexia is an addiction suggest that anorexia and substance abuse behaviors share similar pathology. Both forms of addiction have the potential to progressively become compulsive behaviors. To further demonstrate this point, consider the situation of an anorexic that began a diet to just lose a few pounds and an alcoholic who began using alcohol for recreational purposes only. Both individuals were engaged in what could be considered healthy or harmless activities that eventually developed into destructive, compulsive, and obsessive life-threatening behaviors. Biologically, the victims of anorexia and alcohol need continual and increasing stimuli to achieve the same effect they experienced when they first began their behavior. Therefore, a tolerance is formed: The anorexic must restrict more food and increase exercise to produce the sensations of accomplishment or control just as the alcoholic must consume higher amounts of alcohol to receive the same euphoric effect. Also, behaviors of the alcoholic and anorexic mutually show a strong compulsion to continue the behavior despite the developing destructive medical condition.

The relationship between anorexia and other addictions also share the habitual nature of the attitudes and behaviors, such as frequent episodes, repeated unsuccessful efforts to stop, change of lifestyle, an increase in the severity of symptoms over time, inability to adjust to normative social changes as a result of symptoms associated with the disorder, relapse following treatment, and an increased urge to continue the addiction over time. Addictive psychological and behavioral coping patterns may leave the individual vulnerable to developing other addictions.

Generally, anorexia nervosa is an addictive behavior generally driven by two factors: self-medicating to relieve emotional distress or self-medicating for elated sensation. Once a person begins to starve himself or herself, brain chemistry can be altered; chemicals are produced that provide feelings of peace and ecstasy, thus bringing a temporary release from stress, anxiety, or depression. Starvation and excessive exercise become the positive rewarding behaviors that self-medicate the individual's emotional disturbances.

Warning Signs

Anorexia has an ambiguous etiology. No one victim of anorexia will display every characteristic related to the disorder. Victims may exhibit one or more of the following warning signs.

Eating Behaviors

- Is secretive in eating habits
- Skips meals frequently
- Refuses to eat in front of other people
- Limits or excludes food with high fat or caloric content
- Maintains a restrictive diet
- Avoids red meat
- Chews gum as a substitute for food
- Prepares elaborate meals for family, while refusing to eat the meal
- Obsessively reads food labels for nutritional content

Physiological and Affective Behavior

- Excessive use of laxatives, diuretics, diet pills, street drugs, or natural products to promote weight loss
- Socially withdrawn from friends and family
- Obsessive-compulsive behaviors
- Excessive and compulsive physical activity
- Frequent irritable moods
- Increased isolation over time
- Irrational ideas and denial of disorder
- Feelings of loneliness, depression, anxiety, inadequacy, guilt, or hopelessness

Self-Harm/Self-Injury

- Cuts or burns flesh
- Excessively hits head
- Swallows foreign objects

Symptoms

The most severe symptoms associated with anorexia nervosa resemble those of starvation. There are some similarities in how the individual personifies the associated symptoms, but those suffering from anorexia only look like starving individuals when starvation is well advanced. The body's natural reaction to starvation, induced by anorexia, may include one or more of the following:

- Extremely thin body
- Decreased metabolic rate
- Decreased ability to concentrate
- Dry, nonpliant skin
- Yellow-orange hue to skin tone (due to elevated levels of carotene)
- Brittle nails
- Dramatic loss of scalp hair
- Amenorrhea (loss of menstrual cycle for 3 or more months)
- Insomnia (sleep deprivation)
- Constipation as well as occasional diarrhea
- Lanugo (fine, downlike hair grows all over body)
- Lack of tolerance to cold temperatures
- Tooth loss and bleeding gums
- Electrolyte imbalance
- Diminished reflexes
- Dehydration
- Infertility
- Anemia (low iron in blood)
- Abdominal pain and bloating

Causes

A large proportion of people living in the United States and other Westernized or developed countries are concerned about weight gain or weight loss. Westernized cultures are characterized by their competitive, unrealistic demands for thinness. Today's society is flooded by media images of a happy successful person personified by an actor or model who is young, thin, and toned. An average U.S. child views more than 30,000 television commercials each year or at least 21 hours of television each week filled with media images equating thinness to happiness and success. The response from the viewers is to link self-esteem to weight. Although this does not cause anorexia, the extreme focus on body image in modern culture helps create conditions in which anorexia is more likely to occur.

No single cause of anorexia nervosa has been identified. Each person affected by anorexia nervosa has unique life experiences, exclusive biology, and an individual personality. Therefore, the three influential factors studied by most scientists are biological, psychological, and social. The influence of each factor weighs differently on each person.

There are strong arguments against the idea that biological vulnerability is necessary for an individual to develop anorexia nervosa, but certain psychological characteristics and environmental experiences can reinforce the biological vulnerabilities. It is suggested that dieting during an adolescent's pubertal change (biological), having excessive concern for weight gain (psychological), and focusing on extreme thinness (social) is one way in which the three factors can interact.

Biological

Research suggests that genetic factors account for approximately half of the risk of developing anorexia. Personality characteristics that have a high probability to be genetically transmitted and that are related to anorexia include obsessive-compulsive thoughts or behaviors, anxiety, and perfectionism. The biological study of anorexia nervosa is constantly changing. Therefore, investigating current studies on biological factors is important to understanding the evolution of this disorder.

Psychological

Most individuals suffering from anorexia can be characterized as perfectionists. In other words, these individuals place unrealistic expectations on themselves and others. Regardless of their many achievements, inadequacy and imperfection consume their thoughts. Their reality is often experienced in the extremes, such as either feeling good or bad, successful or unsuccessful, or being thin or fat.

This stressful attitude may be used to avoid sexuality or to attempt to obtain control over their lives. Anorexics often seek to be in control and in charge. Yet, they are often destabilized by their feelings of weakness and powerlessness. By lacking a sense of identity, they attempt to define who they are through an excessive need for social approval and admiration of their exterior.

Social

An individual's social environment may include coworkers, intimate partners, school cliques, or athletic teams. Whatever the social environment, all facets have the potential to generate pressures that invoke anorexia nervosa. In general, individuals vulnerable to anorexia are experiencing loneliness or relationship problems. The person is often unable to construct intimate relationships. This means that the person lacks a confidant with whom fears, insecurities, hopes, dreams, or other personal feelings can be shared.

Treatment and Recovery

Although the early stages of anorexia are difficult to define, the sooner the warning signs are detected and the individual is treated, the easier it is for the individual to recover. Consequently, if warning signs and symptoms are not detected until the individual becomes submerged in addictive behaviors, the individual may struggle with harmful behaviors for an extended period before he or she can begin to recover.

Denial is the defense mechanism used by most individuals during the early stages of anorexia. Individuals often resist treatment because of a false hope that, if they become thin enough, life will become euphoric. Recovery is possible when the illusion that "thinness will bring happiness" dissipates (usually after years of struggling to reach their unattainable goal). At this point, the individual begins to reflect upon the destructive behavior and prepares to take action to live a healthier life.

Recovery is possible, but it is neither quick nor easy. Recovery is a difficult process that can take several years. Four major requirements have been identified for successful recovery in most situations: (1) Seek medical treatment, (2) stay in treatment, (3) make necessary commitments, and (4) resolve core psychological and emotional issues.

With multiple factors influencing anorexia and the unique characteristics for each individual desiring treatment, it is essential that each treatment plan be designed to meet the needs of the client. After an evaluation by a physician or counselor, the following are general possibilities: (a) hospitalization to prevent death, suicide, or medical crisis; (b) a weight restoration program to improve health; (c) medication to relieve depression and anxiety; (d) individual counseling; (e) group counseling; (f) family counseling; and (g) nutrition counseling.

Because anorexia is considered a trait-related disorder, victims are prone to relapses, slips, or partial remission. To prevent feelings of discouragement caused by relapse, it is paramount to include multiple interventions in the treatment plan, thus promoting momentous and enduring personal progress.

Conclusion

A fundamental point to recognize when assisting an individual suffering from anorexia nervosa is an appreciation for the person's need to control everything: life, schedules, family, friends, food, and especially his or her own body. Concerned family members and friends are advised to express unconditional love for the person with anorexia and are encouraged to seek professional help to find the best way to approach and handle their crisis.

Merridy Lynne-Young Stephenson, Sabina Mutisya, and Thomas Harrison

See also Bulimia Nervosa; Co-Occurring Disorders; Cross-Addictions; Gender Issues; Other Addictions

Further Readings

American Psychiatric Association. (2000) Eating disorders. In *Diagnostic and Statistical Manual* (4th ed., text rev., pp. 583–595). Washington, DC: Author.

ANRED: Anorexia Nervosa and Related Eating Disorders, Inc.: http://www.anred.com

Bulik, M. C., Sullivan, F. P., Tozzi, F., Furberg, H., Lichtenstein, P., & Pedersen, L. N. (2006). Prevalence, heritability, and prospective risk factors for anorexia nervosa. *Archives of General Psychiatry, 63,* 305–312.

Davis, C. (2001, February). Addiction and the eating disorders. *Psychiatric Times, 18*(2). Retrieved June 13, 2008, from http://www.psychiatrictimes.com/display/article/10168/54311

Lucas, R. A. (2004). *Demystifying anorexia nervosa: An optimistic guide to understanding and healing.* New York: Oxford University Press.

Maisel, R., Epston, D., & Borden, A. (2004). *Biting the hand that starves you: Inspiring resistance to anorexia/bulimia.* New York: Norton.

Miller W. R., & Heather, N. (1998) *Treating addictive behaviors* (2nd ed., pp. 231–239). New York: Plenum.

ANTABUSE (DISULFIRAM)

Antabuse (trade name) or disulfiram (chemical name) is a small, white tablet that is prescribed to individuals suffering from severe alcoholism. After ingestion, an acute sensitivity to alcohol results, and if any form of alcohol is consumed, the individual experiences a wide variety of sensations—all making him or her nauseated and sick. Disulfiram was not originally created for treating alcoholics. Rather, it was intended as a medication to fight parasites, but individuals charged with checking the drug's efficacy found that if alcohol was consumed after taking the drug, severe symptoms resulted.

When an individual drinks under normal circumstances, the liver breaks the alcohol down from alcohol dehydrogenase to acetaldehyde, and after that, the acetaldehyde is altered to acetaldehyde dehydrogenase, a relatively harmless acetic acid. Disulfiram halts this process by stopping acetaldehyde dehydrogenase. Someone who consumes alcohol after taking disulfiram would have a much higher content of acetaldehyde in his or her blood, with rates as high as 5 to 10 times more than that found in individuals that drank only alcohol. This is called the disulfiram-ethanol reaction. Acetaldehyde is the primary cause of hangovers. Thus, if a person swallows disulfiram before drinking, his or her hangover symptoms usually occur within a 5- to 10-minute period after the first drink. Common reactions include tachycardia (rapid heartbeat), light headiness, nausea, vomiting, skin turning red, pounding in the head and neck, an intensely painful headache, troubled breathing, increased perspiration, dry mouth, and heart palpitations. In addition, people may experience heightened or lowered blood pressure, a general wariness for no apparent reason, an increased inability to move, dizziness, blurred vision, and an overall sense of confusion. These episodes last anywhere from a half an hour up to several hours, depending upon the amount of alcohol consumed.

With even small amounts of disulfiram and alcohol, severe consequences might occur, including complete cessation of breathing, heart attacks, unconsciousness, seizures, or even death. However, these are rare occurrences. On average, a person will feel nauseated and have to vomit, which usually lasts from 1 to 3 hours. After experiencing the consequences of mixing alcohol and disulfiram, one episode of drinking is usually enough.

Patients receive disulfiram in tablets of either 250 milligrams (mg) or 500 mg. The first dosage is often 500 mg for 7 to 14 days, after which one receives a maintenance dosage of 250 mg (range 125–500 mg) per day. At no time should the daily dose exceed 500 mg.

Unlike other medications, tolerance to the drug does not increase over time. On the contrary, the longer an individual takes it, the more powerful the effects are. Disulfiram is assimilated through the stomach and is eradicated gradually. Hence, after first ingesting disulfiram, a person would experience hangover symptoms up to 14 days, if alcohol is consumed. To prevent medical malpractice, the physician must explain in detail the alcohol–disulfiram reaction, as well the length of time the substance stays in the body.

In essence, disulfiram is used in the treatment of alcoholism. It is not an antidote that cures a person of addiction. Although the medication causes severe hangover symptoms, the harmful effects are seldom enough to eradicate the drinking habits of unremitting alcoholics. This is primarily the reason why disulfiram is never prescribed solely by itself. It is usually prescribed to individuals in treatment who plan on maintaining a regimen of complete sobriety.

One common side effect of disulfiram is hepatitis, either cholestatic or fulminant. In addition, it is not uncommon to experience a skin rash, though it is easily controlled by antihistamines. In some patients, drowsiness, erectile dysfunction, acne, frequent headaches, excessive tiredness, and bad breath are experienced during the first 14 days of therapy. However, the symptoms usually disappear with the prolongation of therapy or with decreasing doses. In some cases, when an individual took higher doses, psychotic symptoms appeared; some individuals with masked psychoses had their illness erupt into the open after initially taking the drug.

Contraindications include the following:

1. Pregnant women—The few long-term studies conducted with pregnant women ingesting disulfiram have indicated the presence of birth defects. A

woman who is pregnant, or who might become so, needs to tell her physician.

2. Other medications—Before taking disulfiram, a physician should be told if a patient is taking specific medications such as

   a. Heparin (blood thinner)
   b. Dilantin (anticonvulsant)
   c. Flagyl (antibiotic)
   d. Wellbutrin (bupropion)
   e. Adderall (amphetamine)
   f. Ritalin (methylphenidate)

3. The patient should tell the physician if he or she has any of the following:

   a. Respiratory problems
   b. Diabetes
   c. Seizures
   d. Depression
   e. Cardiovascular disease
   f. Renal disease
   g. Hepatic disease
   h. Skin lesions or skin allergies

4. The patient should tell the physician whether he or she is taking over-the-counter medications that contain alcohol, including cough syrups (Formula 44, Nyquil, Benadryl Elixir), mouthwash (Listerine, Scope).

5. Disulfiram should never be prescribed to individuals taking stimulant drugs such as Ritalin, Concerta, or Focalin or tricyclic antidepressants such as amitriptyline or metronidazole. Disulfiram blocks the enzyme dopamine-beta-hydroxylase from working, which blocks the transfer of the neurotransmitter dopamine becoming norepinephrine. If this is united with the dopamine agonist or grossly affects the reuptake effect of stimulants, an individual could experience psychotic delusions.

How efficacious is disulfiram? The answer is dependent on several factors: (a) client acceptance and compliance, (b) support of the client's loved one(s), and (c) utilization in a comprehensive treatment protocol that includes evidence-based strategies and approaches. If these three conditions are met, the probability of success is greatly enhanced. On the other hand, if used solely by itself, then it is doubtful that disulfiram will have any significant impact on an inveterate alcoholic.

Cary Stacy Smith and Li-Ching Hung

See also Acamprosate; Alcohol; Alcoholism; Naltrexone

Further Readings

Brewer, C. (1987). Disulfiram treatment of alcoholism [Letter]. *Journal of the American Medical Association, 257,* 926.

Hardman, J. G., & Limbird, L. E. (Eds.). (1996). *Goodman and Gilman's the pharmacological basis of therapeutics* (9th ed.). New York: McGraw-Hill.

Hughes, J. C., & Cook, C. C. (1997). The efficacy of disulfiram: A review of outcome studies. *Addiction, 92*(4), 381–395.

Wilson, B. A., Shannon, M. T., & Stang, C. L. (Eds.). (1995). *Nurses drug guide* (3rd ed.). Norwalk, CT: Appleton & Lange.

ANTIANXIETY AGENTS

See ANXIOLYTIC DRUGS

ANTIDEPRESSANT DRUGS

Antidepressants are among the most frequently prescribed agents in medicine. They are a highly effective, relatively safe, and nonaddictive class of therapeutic agents. Antidepressants do not elevate mood in nondepressed people and have no abuse potential. Their primary use is in the treatment of major depressive disorder, although many antidepressants have other established uses such as in the treatment of anxiety and eating disorders.

Our understanding of antidepressants mechanism of action relates to the monoamine hypothesis of depression. This hypothesis suggests that depression follows a dysfunction of one or more of the monoamine neurotransmitters including norepinephrine (NE), serotonin (5-HT), and dopamine (DA). It follows, therefore, that antidepressants work by increasing monoamine-mediated neurotransmission in one or more ways. The three most established hypotheses for mechanism of antidepressant action are (1) reuptake inhibition (i.e., block the reuptake of NE, 5-HT, DA, or all three, into nerve terminals thereby increasing the amount of the monoamine in the synapse); (2) interaction with the 5-HT, NE, or DA receptors to mimic the effects of these natural monoamines; and (3) block inhibition (i.e., block the metabolic degradation of NE, 5-HT, or DA at the nerve terminals to increase the amount in the synapse).

Antidepressants are not general mood elevators and selectively alleviate symptoms of depression, including extreme sadness, loss of interest, decreased energy, inability to concentrate, sleep disturbance, and appetite changes. Because all antidepressants essentially target the same underlying substrate (monoamine neurotransmitters), no antidepressant is superior to others in the treatment of major depressive disorder. Selection of an antidepressant, therefore, depends on a patient's unique symptoms and the different medication side effect and drug interaction profiles.

In general, treatment with antidepressant medications requires 3 to 6 weeks of continuous therapy at therapeutic doses before symptoms of depression improve. Moreover, not every patient given an antidepressant will have improvement in *all* symptoms and some patients will be resistant to treatment and will not respond to one or more medications. Antidepressant use in children, adolescents, and young adults is currently under scrutiny due to a possible increased risk of suicide in these age groups.

Antidepressants in Substance Use Disorders

Depression and anxiety symptoms are prevalent in patients with substance use disorders. Longitudinal studies indicate that depression and anxiety disorders increase the risk for the development of substance use disorders. Marc Schuckit noted substance abuse along with a mood disorder indicates a worse prognosis than the presence of a mood disorder or a substance use disorder alone.

While treatment of depression may improve the outcome of substance abuse treatment, there is still much to be understood about the relationship between mood disorders and substance use. For example, Sandra Brown and Schuckit found that patients with alcohol dependence often reported significantly high levels of anxiety and depression at the time of admission to an inpatient treatment program. Over a period of 4 weeks, the anxiety and mood symptoms normalized for all but a small minority of the patients. Currently, antidepressants are indicated in substance use disorders only when a coexisting

mood or anxiety disorder is established as an independent diagnosis (as opposed to secondary to the substance use disorder). Some authors suggest waiting until 4 weeks of abstinence prior to initiating antidepressant medication. Others support treatment of mood symptoms during early abstinence if the potential benefits of antidepressant medication outweigh the potential risks and costs.

There is little evidence that antidepressants alone are effective in the treatment substance use disorders. One exception is the use of selective serotonin reuptake inhibitors (SSRIs), which may decrease alcohol craving or intake in moderately dependent alcoholics. Patients with co-occurring depression and substance use disorders require multimodal treatment approaches such as antidepressant medication in conjunction with cognitive behavioral therapy or intensive Twelve-Step Facilitation.

Although most antidepressants have no risk of abuse or dependence, published case reports suggest that adolescents crush and insufflate bupropion tablets for a perceived high.

Specific Antidepressants

In this section, the major classes of antidepressants are presented, along with the representative drugs, their side effects, overdose potential, and role in substance use disorders.

Selective Serotonin Reuptake Inhibitors (SSRIs)

Representative Drugs

Fluoxetine (Prozac)

Sertraline (Zoloft)

Paroxetine (Paxil)

Citalopram (Celexa)

Escitalopram (Lexapro)

Fluvoxamine (formerly Luvox)

SSRIs are the most frequently prescribed class of antidepressants due to their reasonably benign side effect profile and lack of potential for abuse. Most of the older SSRIs are now available as generics and are included on insurance formularies.

Side Effects

Most SSRIs carry the risk of significant sexual dysfunction (lack of sexual interest, decreased arousal, delayed or absent orgasm), which occurs in about 50% of patients. Central nervous system activation (restlessness, insomnia, agitation) is common during the initial phase of treatment. Fluoxetine may be more activating than other SSRIs. There is a slight increase in risk of seizures as well. A subgroup of patients report prominent gastrointestinal disturbances (nausea, diarrhea, cramping, heartburn), especially in the first few weeks of treatment. Weight loss is possible during early treatment, with progression to weight gain with long-term use. In adults over 50 years of age, daily SSRI use increases the risk of clinical fragility fractures. SSRIs can prolong bleeding time, which may be a significant consideration in patients with coagulation abnormalities or with a history of gastrointestinal bleeds.

In cases where treatment with an SSRI is abruptly stopped after long-term use, a discontinuation syndrome of nausea, dizziness, anxiety, tremor, and palpitations has been described. This is distinct from "addiction" because there is no compulsive use of the medication or loss of control over use.

Drug Interactions

Serotonin syndrome is a medical emergency that results from using more than one serotonergic medication. Excess serotonin at nerve terminals leads to muscle tremor and rigidity, hyperthermia, restlessness, hallucinations, sweating, nausea, diarrhea, headache, and delirium. Serotonin syndrome can progress to coma and death. Although serotonin syndrome is rare in *pure* SSRI overdoses, it is most commonly seen when SSRIs are combined with, or are prescribed soon after the discontinuation of, another serotonergic agent, such as monoamine oxidase inhibitors. Serotonin syndrome requires emergency hospital evaluation and can be treated with cyproheptadine (Periactin), a drug that blocks the 5-HT receptor from binding to serotonin; management of agitation and elevated vital signs with benzodiazepines can also be helpful.

SSRIs can affect the cytochrome P450 system, which is an enzyme system in the liver responsible for metabolism of many drugs, including various antibiotics, antifungals, and antiseizure medications. A table that details these potential drug interactions can be found at the American Academy of Family Physicians Web site.

Because the SSRIs can decrease the normal clearance of other drugs, plasma drug levels should be monitored in patients taking SSRIs and certain medications to make sure the drug levels do not enter the toxic range. SSRIs can also displace other medications (warfarin, digoxin) from proteins they bind to in the bloodstream and thereby increase blood levels in this manner as well. Clinically significant drug–drug interactions are more common when an SSRI is added to a previously stable medication regimen.

Overdose

SSRIs have a very high therapeutic-to-toxic ratio and are unlikely to be fatal in overdose as a single agent. Many overdose patients use multiple medications and substances, and SSRIs may increase the toxicity of other agents through inhibition of metabolism.

Role in Substance Use Disorders

Research with SSRIs has focused on curbing alcohol and psychostimulant cravings. Because psychostimulants, such as cocaine and methamphetamine, act through altered monoamine levels in the brain, several studies on mice and humans have examined whether SSRIs can decrease drug-seeking behavior and self-administration of stimulants. In mice, blockage of DA and 5-HT receptors has led to behavioral changes consistent with decreased effect of psychostimulants. There is no human research data to suggest that SSRIs have an effect in treating stimulant use disorders.

Atypical Antidepressants

Representative Drugs

Venlafaxine (Effexor, in multiple-release formulations)

Bupropion (Wellbutrin, in multiple-release formulations)

Duloxetine (Cymbalta)

Mirtazapine (Remeron)

Trazodone (Desyrel)

Nefazodone (Serzone)

Side Effects

The side effect profile of atypical antidepressants is varied. Bupropion, in particular, can precipitate psychotic episodes and seizures in susceptible patients due to its effect on increasing DA. Because stimulant use, alcohol withdrawal, and sedative withdrawal can all decrease seizure threshold, bupropion is contraindicated in patients using stimulants, alcohol, or sedatives. Venlafaxine (Effexor) may require blood pressure monitoring in certain patients, as it carries the risk of a rise in blood pressure. This medication can also have significant discontinuation effects. Trazodone carries a rare but significant risk of priapism (abnormal and painful erection), and nefazodone carries a black box warning for liver failure.

Overdose

Atypical antidepressants have a lower therapeutic-to-toxic ratio than the SSRIs. These medications can be dangerous at 10 to 15 times the normal dose. Overdose can result in hallucinations, respiratory failure, cardiovascular abnormalities, convulsions, coma, and death.

Role in Substance Use Disorders

Bupropion has well-known effects in smoking cessation. Numerous studies have found bupropion to enhance one-year smoking abstinence rates in various clinical groups, including smokers with schizophrenia, depression, chronic obstructive pulmonary disease, cardiovascular disease, and healthy smokers. Bupropion may be a helpful adjunct in the treatment of stimulant drug dependence, such as cocaine or methamphetamine dependence. There have been fewer investigations of the use of other atypical antidepressants in substance use disorders.

Tricyclic Antidepressants (TCAs)

Representative Drugs

Nortriptyline (Aventyl, Pamelor)

Imipramine (Tofranil)

Amitriptyline (Elavil)

Desipramine (Norpramin)

Clomipramine (Anafranil)

Indications

TCAs were among the first medications to be used for treatment of depression. Their applications have expanded to include anxiety disorders and off-label use in chronic pain, enuresis, and migraine prophylaxis.

Side Effects

These medications have a wide range of side effects related to their blockage of cholinergic receptors. The side effects include sedation, cognitive impairment, confusion, delirium, dry mouth, blurred vision, constipation, tachycardia, urinary retention, and orthostatic hypotension. TCAs also carry the potential of sexual dysfunction, weight gain, and lowering of the seizure threshold. Patients with prolonged cardiac conduction intervals should not take TCAs because of the potential for abnormal cardiac conduction and precipitation of a cardiac event. TCA use in children has been associated with sudden death.

Overdose

TCAs are highly toxic drugs, and TCA overdose accounts for a large percentage of deaths from antidepressant overdose. Data from the American Association of Poison Control Center's Toxic Exposure Surveillance System show that TCAs were the most common cause of overdose-related death until the 1990s, when analgesics surpassed them as a class. Accidental TCA exposure is seen in toddlers, whereas adolescents and adults tend to present with intentional overdoses. Unlike the relatively benign symptoms of SSRI overdose, TCA overdose can be life threatening, with hyperthermia, hypertension, and cardiotoxicity with arrhythmias. When a TCA overdose is suspected, the emergency medical team will order a TCA level and an electrocardiogram to look for prolongation of the QT interval (measure of the time between the start of the Q wave and the end of the T wave in the heart's electrical cycle). The combination of TCAs with monoamine oxidase inhibitors produces an extremely high risk of serotonin syndrome.

Role in Substance Use Disorders

Although TCA side effects and toxicity have led to their relatively rare use in depression, there is mixed evidence that TCAs, in particular desipramine, can benefit patients with cocaine dependence.

Monoamine Oxidase Inhibitors (MAOIs)

Representative Drugs

Phenelzine (Nardil)

Tranylcypromine (Parnate)

Selegiline (Eldepryl)

Selegiline patch (Emsam)

Side Effects

MAOIs usually rank low among the options for treating depression due to the high risk for hypertensive crisis. This is a condition that can result from MAOI use and ingestion of foods containing tyramine (e.g., beer, wine, cheese, processed meats) or use with other drugs that stimulate the sympathetic nervous system (i.e., over-the-counter cold remedies). A hypertensive crisis can lead to bleeds in the brain and can be fatal. Patients must adhere to a "MAOI diet" and avoid foods that might trigger a crisis. MAOIs are often prescribed with nifedipine (Procardia) to keep on hand in order to counteract a hypertensive crisis if one should occur. MAOIs can also result in serotonin syndrome when combined with SSRIs, atypical antidepressants, TCAs, or when ingested alone in overdose. There is a required 4- to 6-week washout period after the use of an MAOI and the start of another antidepressant. Additional side effects of MAOIs include sexual dysfunction, restlessness, sleep disturbances, and weight gain.

Overdose

Like the TCAs, the MAOIs are also dangerous in overdose with a risk of significant mortality and morbidity at 7 to 10 times the normal dose. The early symptoms of overdose include irritability, anxiety, flushing, sweating, and tachycardia. With severe overdose, patients can develop hyperthermia, hypertonia, seizures, marked hypertension, arrhythmias, cardiovascular collapse, and death.

Role in Substance Use Disorders

Despite the decline in the use of MAOIs for depression, their use in substance use disorders is under active scrutiny. All the MAOIs work by inhibiting monoamine oxidase, the enzyme that breaks down extracellular monoamines such as NE and DA. Selegiline is unique in that it inhibits only the MAO-B isoform of the enzyme and has recently been released in a patch form. This MAOI can prevent the decrease in DA secretion associated with opioid withdrawal and therefore has been used for that purpose. Researchers have identified additional pharmacological effects when used in doses higher than those required for MAO inhibition; it can have psychostimulant effects and neuroprotective effects resulting in behavioral changes in opioid-dependent rats. Whether such high doses can be tolerated in humans and whether the risk-to-benefit ratio is low enough for human use is unknown.

Conclusion

Antidepressants are a unique and versatile group of drugs with many potential benefits. In most cases, animal studies have shown potential benefits in substance use disorders, but clinical trials have not yet shown definitive results. Clinicians will need more evidence before they can confidently prescribe antidepressants to treat substance use disorders. In the meantime, treatment of depression and anxiety that is comorbid with substance use (and that does not resolve with a few weeks of abstinence) includes an antidepressant and/or psychotherapy, along with current interventions for substance use disorders such as Twelve-Step programs, education, psychotherapy, and family involvement.

Chaithra Prasad and Melissa Piasecki

See also Antipsychotic Drugs; Anxiety Disorders; Co-Occurring Disorders; Depression; Pharmacological Approaches to Treatment

Further Readings

American Academy of Family Physicians: http://www.aafp.org/afp/980101ap/cupp.html

Beers, M., Porter, R., Jones, T., Kaplan, J., & Berkwits, M. (Eds.). (2006). *The Merck manual of diagnosis and therapy* (18th ed.). Whitehouse Station, NJ: Merck Research Laboratories.

Brown, S., Irwin, M., & Schuckit, M. (1991). Changes in anxiety among abstinent male alcoholics. *Journal of Studies on Alcohol, 52*(1), 55–61.

Brown, S., & Schuckit, M. (1988). Changes in depression among abstinent male alcoholics. *Journal of Studies on Alcohol, 49*(5), 412–417.

Elkashef, A. M., Rawson, R. A., Anderson, A. L., Li, S. H., Holmes, T., Smith, E. V., et al. (2008). Bupropion for the treatment of methamphetamine dependence. *Neuropsychopharmacology, 33*(5), 1162–1170.

Gabbard, G. (Ed.). (2001). *Treatment of psychiatric disorders* (3rd ed.). Washington, DC: American Psychiatric Press.

Khurshid, K. A., & Decker, D. H. (2004). Bupropion insufflation in a teenager. *Journal of Child and Adolescent Psychopharmacology, 14*(1), 157–158.

Levin, F., & Lehman, A. (1991). Meta-analysis of desipramine as an adjunct in the treatment of cocaine addiction. *Journal of Clinical Psychopharmacology, 11*(6), 374–378.

McEvoy, G. (Ed.). (2007). *AHFS drug information 2007.* Bethesda, MD: American Society of Health-System Pharmacists.

Naranjo, C., Poulos, C., Bremner, K., & Lanctot, K. (1994). Fluoxetine attenuates alcohol intake and desire to drink. *International Clinical Psychopharmacology, 9*(3), 163–172.

Potter, W. A., & Hollister, L. E. (2006). Antidepressant drugs. In B. Katzung (Ed.), *Basic and clinical pharmacology* (10th ed., pp. 475–486). New York: McGraw-Hill.

Schatzberg, A. F., Cole, J. O., & Debattista, C. (2007). *Manual of clinical psychopharmacology* (6th ed.). Washington, DC: American Psychiatric Publishing.

Schuckit, M. (2006). Comorbidity between substance use disorders and psychiatric conditions. *Addiction, 101*(Suppl. 1), 76–88.

Spina, E., Scordo, M., & D'Arrigo, C. (2003) Metabolic drug interactions with the new psychotropic agents. *Fundamental & Clinical Pharmacology, 17*(5), 517–538.

Welsh, C. J., & Doyon, S. (2002) Seizure induced by insufflation of bupropion. *New England Journal of Medicine, 347*(12), 951.

ANTIPSYCHOTIC DRUGS

Antipsychotics are medications that target psychotic symptoms such as delusions and hallucinations. These medications, also known as neuroleptics or major tranquilizers, are also commonly used as mood stabilizers and for nonspecific sedation. The array of antipsychotics is expanding, as new agents are developed with wider applications than those of the older medications. Many substances can produce psychosis, which is often treated with antipsychotic drugs. With one notable exception, antipsychotic drugs have little abuse potential.

Psychosis is defined by *Stedman's Medical Dictionary* as "a mental and behavioral disorder causing gross distortion or disorganization of a person's mental capacity, affective response, and capacity to recognize reality, communicate, and relate to others." All antipsychotics treat psychosis by blocking postsynaptic dopamine (D_2) receptors in the brain. Antipsychotic efficacy appears to occur in a window of 60% to 80% D_2 receptors blockade. Antagonism below 60% confers less antipsychotic effect, whereas blockade of more than 80% of the receptors produces extrapyramidal symptoms.

There are two categories of antipsychotics, typical and atypical, which differ by their receptor activities. These categories are also known as first generation and second generation antipsychotics. In addition to D_2 blockade, atypical antipsychotics are active at serotonin receptors ($5\text{-}HT_2$) and other dopamine receptor subtypes. Atypical agents are thought to bind less tightly to D_2 receptors and occupy these receptors more intermittently than do typical antipsychotics. These variations explain the differences in therapeutic effects and side effects, which may be more benign in the atypical drugs. Other important distinguishing factors between these two classes include cost and Food and Drug Administration (FDA)–approved indications. The atypical agents are newer and much more expensive than the typical agents. The atypical agents have FDA indications as mood stabilizers and are used to treat acute mania and depression and to provide maintenance in bipolar disorder.

Representative Antipsychotics
Typical Antipsychotics

Chlorpromazine (Thorazine)

Haloperidol (Haldol and Haldol decanoate)

Fluphenazine (Prolixin and Prolixin decanoate)

Perphenazine (Trilafon)

Thioridazine (Mellaril)

Thiothixene (Navane)

Pimozide (Orap)

Atypical

Clozapine (Clozaril)

Risperidone (Risperdal)

Olanzapine (Zyprexa)

Quetiapine (Seroquel)

Ziprasidone (Geodon)

Aripiprazole (Abilify)

Side Effects

Antipsychotic medications can produce side effects that range from uncomfortable to life threatening. Some side effects are specific to a single drug. Other side effects are class effects that can occur from any drug in the class. A 2006 study by the National Institute of Mental Health compared the effectiveness and tolerability of the older typical antipsychotics and the newer atypical medications. Many were surprised by the outcome: Three quarters of study patients discontinued the use of a prescribed antipsychotic because of side effects or perceived lack of efficacy. In addition, the older medication, perphenazine, appeared to offer benefits and tolerability comparable to the newer medications. Clozapine stands out among all of the antipsychotics as having more efficacy, especially in treating people with schizophrenia that have not responded to other medications. Clozapine also carries unique risks that require close monitoring.

Generic Side Effects

Extrapyramidal side effects result from the dopamine receptor blockade in brain areas that influence muscle movement and tone. These side effects can present as an acute dystonic reaction, muscle stiffness, tremor, shuffling gait, and flattened facial expression. Acute dystonic reactions are sustained muscle contractions that can be painful and frightening but are very treatable. Extrapyramidal side effects are most common in typical antipsychotics, especially the more potent medications such as haloperidol. Often extrapyramidal symptoms improve with medications such as benztropine (Cogentin). Tardive dyskinesia is a potentially disabling tic disorder that results from exposure to antipsychotics, especially older medications.

Sedation is another side effect common to all antipsychotics. Some antipsychotics such as chlorpromazine are much more sedating and sometimes are used to sedate acutely agitated people. Quetiapine's sedative properties have led to its use in treating anxiety and sleep problems. The multitude of potential side effects with antipsychotic medications suggests that other classes of medications can offer a better risk–benefit profile to treat anxiety or insomnia.

Most typical and atypical antipsychotics are known to cause weight gain and metabolic changes. Ziprasidone and aripiprazole may be the exceptions among atypical antipsychotics, with a benign impact on these factors, and olanzapine may pose the greatest risks. The combination of significant weight gain and changes in metabolism of glucose has resulted in new onset diabetes in some patients treated with some of the atypical antipsychotics. Practice guidelines for the atypical antipsychotics include checking weight and waist circumference during outpatient follow-up visits. A related problem is an alteration of blood lipids. Physicians now routinely monitor lipid panels and glucose levels and may switch medication if a patient's weight or lab values suggest that antipsychotic side effects place general health at risk.

Dopamine blockade by antipsychotics has an unintended side effect of increasing prolactin secretion in the brain. Elevated prolactin levels stimulate breast development and can trigger lactation in some patients. Decreased sexual functioning may result as well. Prolactin elevations are more common in the typical antipsychotics and risperidone.

Some antipsychotics may slow conduction of electrical impulses in the heart. This results in prolongation of the QT interval (measure of the time between the start of the Q wave and the end of the T wave in the heart's electrical cycle) on electrocardiograms. This concern has led to a black box warning for thioridazine and electrocardiogram monitoring for patients who have a preexisting cardiac conduction problem or who are on other drugs that can also prolong the QT interval.

All antipsychotics carry the potential to decrease the seizure threshold and increase the risk of a seizure. Clozapine carries the highest seizure risk. Antipsychotics must be used judiciously in patients who are already at risk for a seizure, such as patients abusing stimulants or undergoing alcohol withdrawal.

Catastrophic side effects are life-threatening problems that may arise from antipsychotic use.

Neuroleptic malignant syndrome (NMS) is a potentially fatal syndrome most associated with typical antipsychotics. Symptoms of NMS are rapidly developing confusion, muscle stiffness, and unstable vital signs. Stimulant use may place people at higher risk of NMS. Agranulocytosis is another catastrophic side effect. It is a loss of white blood cell production leading to elevated risk of infection. Clozapine is the only antipsychotic with a known risk of agranulocytosis, and patients treated with this medication must have frequent blood tests to monitor cell counts.

Antipsychotics in Substance Use Disorders

Illicit drug use can lead to a wide range of psychiatric symptoms, including hallucinations, delusions, and mood disturbances. Psychosis in most cases is transient but sometimes persists long after cessation of substance use. Antipsychotics are used to treat both acute and chronic psychosis resulting from substances.

Substance-Induced Psychotic Disorder

The *Diagnostic and Statistical Manual of Mental Disorders, Fourth Edition, Text Revision (DSM-IV-TR)* defines substance-induced psychotic disorder as a symptom presentation with prominent hallucinations or delusions that developed during substance intoxication or withdrawal and is not better accounted for by another psychotic disorder or by delirium.

A variety of substances from different classes have the potential for inducing psychosis. These include alcohol, amphetamines, cannabis, cocaine, heroin, and hallucinogens. Carol Caton compared patients with substance-induced psychotic disorders with those with a primary psychotic disorder and found the patients with substance-induced psychosis had a significantly later age of onset of psychosis, greater conjugal ties, greater antisocial personality disorder comorbidity, more frequent homelessness, poorer family support, and more likelihood of having a parent with a substance abuse problem. A key factor distinguishing substance-induced psychotic disorders from primary psychosis is the prominence of visual hallucinations in substance-induced psychotic disorders.

The focus of treatment in substance-induced psychosis is symptom management. Patients with psychosis secondary to drug use may need different medications or medication courses than patients with primary psychosis. Antipsychotic medications may be more likely to give adverse effects, such as extrapyramidal symptoms or NMS, in substance-using patients.

Hallucinogen Persisting Perceptual Disorder

Hallucinogenic drugs are the class of substances that can produce a hallucinogenic effect. Drugs in this class are lysergic acid diethylamide (LSD), phencyclidine (PCP, angel dust), tetrahydrocannabinol (THC, which is a constituent of marijuana), amphetamine-like drugs (particularly MDA and MDMA [ecstasy]), psilocybin (mushrooms), and mescaline. Dextromethorphan in over-the-counter cough and cold remedies produces hallucinations when abused at high doses.

Hallucinogens can induce persistent psychosis following the intoxication and withdrawal phases. The *DSM-IV-TR* describes this symptom state as hallucinogen persisting perception disorder (HPPD), which is characterized by the re-experience of the visual symptoms that occurred during intoxication with the hallucinogen. Examples of visual symptoms are geometric hallucinations, false perceptions of movement in the peripheral visual fields, flashes of color, intensified colors, "tracers" (trails of images of moving objects), halos around objects, and size distortions.

According to Espiard, HPPD may persist for as long as 5 years or more. Although there have been no randomized controlled trials or standardized treatment protocols addressing the treatment of HPPD, case reports and case series by Halpem and others have outline various treatment strategies using antipsychotics, anticonvulsants, benzodiazepines, and clonidine.

Stimulant-Induced Psychotic Disorder

Amphetamines have long been used to create an animal model of schizophrenia. It follows that that human abuse of amphetamines will predictably produce psychotic symptoms. These symptoms are typically paranoid delusions, auditory hallucinations, and visual hallucinations. The abuse of stimulant medications prescribed for attention deficit disorder and increases in methamphetamine abuse have contributed to an increased prevalence of stimulant-induced psychosis. Cocaine also can induce psychosis. Methamphetamine, perhaps due to its unique neurotoxicity or to the patterns of prolonged binge use, can cause persistent psychosis, which may last for years after discontinuation of the drug. Studies in Japan by Kunio Yui and colleagues reveal a persistent vulnerability to relapse into a psychotic state when former methamphetamine users are exposed to psychological stressors.

Although antipsychotics are routinely used in patients with stimulant-induced psychosis, a 2007 review revealed no controlled trials of antipsychotics in either short- or long-term treatment of amphetamine psychosis. The only systematic studies of antipsychotics in amphetamine users targeted agitation, not psychosis.

Treatment of Comorbid Substance Use Disorders

People who suffer from schizophrenia and other chronic disorders often have comorbid substance use disorders. Bipolar disorder also carries a high risk for substance use problems. Antipsychotic medications are the first-line treatment for both schizophrenia and bipolar disorder, and there is some evidence that select antipsychotics may be helpful in treating both problems. The first line of evidence comes from studies of the atypical antipsychotic clozapine. In early studies, this drug had the unexpected effect of decreasing cigarette smoking in patients with schizophrenia. Additional research suggests that clozapine may decrease other substance use as well. Olanzapine also shows some promise of helping with comorbid substance use disorders in patients with schizophrenia. These preliminary reports point to a need for systematic research in the efficacy and safety of the atypical antipsychotics for substance use disorders in patients with and without comorbid psychiatric diagnoses.

Abuse Potential of Antipsychotics

Most antipsychotics have unpleasant side effects such as sedation, increased muscle tone, and tremor and do not have any known abuse risk. An exception is quetiapine, an atypical antipsychotic that appears to have reinforcing effects that lead to abuse. The first reports of quetiapine abuse came from reports from correctional settings where the drug was noted to be in circulation as a commodity and abused by intravenous and intranasal administration. In the community, quetiapine has earned the status of attaining street drug names, such as *Quell* and *Susie-Q*. This antipsychotic is sometimes injected with cocaine, known as a *Q-ball*. According to Brian Waters, the sedative and anxiolytic effect of quetiapine in the Q-ball decreases the "crash" associated with cocaine withdrawal and possibly provides a hallucinogenic effect.

Conclusion

Antipsychotic medications have the potential to be tremendously helpful in treating schizophrenia and bipolar disorders. The same medications have the potential for significant side effects, and the atypical antipsychotics have much more serious side effects than originally believed. Although psychotic symptoms are common sequelae of substance abuse, particularly with amphetamines, there is only a very limited database to draw upon for treatment of these symptoms. The emergence of quetiapine as a drug of abuse suggests that antipsychotic medications should be judiciously used and closely monitored.

Melissa Piasecki and Leandro Anit

See also Antidepressant Drugs; Anxiety Disorders; Co-Occurring Disorders; Depression; Pharmacological Approaches to Treatment

Further Readings

Caton, C. L., Drake, R. E., Hasin, D. S., Dominguez, B., Shrout, P. E., Samet, S., et al. (2005). Differences between early-phase primary psychotic disorders with concurrent substance use and substance-induced psychoses. *Archives of General Psychiatry, 62,* 137–145.

Espiard, M. L., Lecardeur, L., Abadie, P., Halbecq, I., & Dollfus, S. (2005) Hallucinogen persisting perception disorder after psilocybin consumption: A case study. *European Psychiatry, 20*(5–6), 458–460.

Green, A. (2005). Schizophrenia and comorbid substance use disorder: Effects of antipsychotics. *Journal of Clinical Psychiatry, 66*(Suppl. 6), 21–26.

Halpern, J. H., & Pope, H. G., Jr. (2003). Hallucinogen persisting perception disorder: What do we know after 50 years? *Drug and Alcohol Dependence, 69*(2), 109–119.

Lieberman, J. A., Stroup, T. S., McEvoy, J. P., Swartz, M. S., Rosenheck, R. A., Perkins, D. O., et al. (2005). Effectiveness of antipsychotic drugs in patients with chronic schizophrenia. *New England Journal of Medicine, 353*(12), 1209–1223.

Marder, S. R., Essock, S. M., Miller, A. L., Buchanan, R. W., Casey, D. E., Davis, J. M., et al. (2007). Quetiapine addiction? (Letter). *American Journal of Psychiatry, 164*(1), 174–175.

Shon, S. (2004). Physical health monitoring of patients with schizophrenia. *American Journal of Psychiatry, 161*(8), 1334–1349.

Srisurapanont, M., Kittiratanapaiboon, P., & Jarusuraisin, N. (2001). Treatment for amphetamine psychosis (Review). *Cochrane Database of Systematic Reviews,* Issue 4, Art. No. CD003026, DOI 10.1002/14651858.CD003026.

Stedman's medical dictionary (28th ed.). (2005). Philadelphia: Lippincott, Williams & Wilkins.

Waters, B. M., & Joshi, K. G. (2007). Intravenous quetiapine-cocaine use (Q-ball). *American Journal of Psychiatry, 164*(1), 173–174.

Yui, K., Ishiguro, T., Goto, K., & Ikemoto, S. (1998). Factors affecting the development of spontaneous recurrence of methamphetamine psychosis. *Acta psychiatrica Scandinavica, 97*(3), 220–227.

ANTISEIZURE DRUGS

Antiseizure medications, also known as anticonvulsants and antiepileptics, treat seizure disorders by decreasing abnormally high levels of brain activity. Various types of seizures exist. The most easily recognized are tonic-clonic seizures, also known as grand mal seizures, with significant muscle activity, loss of consciousness, and often loss of bowel and bladder control. A second type of seizure is absence seizures, which lead to temporary, sometimes brief losses of consciousness and postural tone. Myoclonic seizures are characterized by muscle jerks. These three types are known as generalized seizures because of their widespread effect in the brain. The other category of seizures is called partial, because they involve only one portion of the brain. Partial seizures are further divided into either complex, if they cause loss of consciousness, or simple, if they do not. Temporal lobe seizures, which are commonly complex partial seizures, include a variety of psychological and sensory symptoms such as feelings of unreality and smelling burning rubber. Status epilepticus is a state of continual or closely spaced seizures that can lead to brain damage and death. All of these conditions can be effectively treated with antiseizure medications.

The majority of antiseizure medications are believed to work through one of two mechanisms. One mechanism (for medications like carbamazepine, phenytoin, lamotrigine, oxcarbazepine, valproic acid, and topiramate) is through blocking the channels that regulate sodium flow in brain neurons, and the other mechanism (for phenobarbital, tiagabine, valproic acid, gabapentin, topiramate, and clonazepam) increases the activity of gamma-aminobutyric acid (GABA) neurons in the brain. GABA is the main inhibitory chemical transmitter in the brain, and increasing GABA receptor activity decreases the amount of brain electrical activity and raises the threshold for an epileptic seizure. Other antiseizure drugs decrease calcium channel flow (valproic acid and ethosuximide) or block glutamate transmission (topiramate). These diverse actions all effectively decrease abnormal levels of activation in brain neurons.

Although the drugs in this class were designed to treat seizure disorders, they are also useful in treating other disorders. For patients with bipolar disorder, for example, antiseizure medications have become first-line treatment. Valproic acid, carbamazepine, and lamotrigine are effective treatment of manic episodes. Valproic acid is also effective as a maintenance medication for bipolar disorder and may be a particularly effective treatment for the rapid cycling subtype of bipolar disorder, characterized by four or more mood phases in 1 year. Other clinical uses for antiseizure medications include carbamazepine for trigeminal neuralgia, gabapentin for postherpetic neuralgia (as well as other neurological pain), and phenytoin for migraine headaches. Clonazepam is a benzodiazepine, and its sedating effect led to its use as an adjunct in the treatment of anxiety disorders, such as panic disorder and as a sleep aid.

Valproic acid and carbamazepine have ranges for therapeutic blood levels. Therapeutic use (for seizure disorders or bipolar disorder) requires titration to these ranges. After therapeutic levels are achieved, routine monitoring follows blood levels on a regular basis.

Most antiseizure drugs have low abuse potential because they do not generate euphoric or other reinforcing effects. Significant exceptions are phenobarbital (a barbiturate) and clonazepam, which have sedating and reinforcing effects that can lead to abuse and dependence. In addition, there have been case reports describing gabapentin abuse and withdrawal in patients with preexisting cocaine or alcohol abuse.

Representative Antiseizure Drugs

Older Antiepileptics

Carbamazepine (Tegretol)

Phenytoin (Dilantin)

Phenobarbital (Luminal)

Valproic acid (Depakene, Depakote, and Depakote ER)

Ethosuximide (Zarontin)

Clonazepam (Klonopin)

Newer Antiepileptics

Lamotrigine (Lamictal)

Gabapentin (Neurontin)

Topiramate (Topamax)

Oxcarbazepine (Trileptal)

Antiepileptic Medication Use in Substance Use Disorders

When people with alcohol dependence abruptly decrease or discontinue alcohol use, they are at risk for a variety of problems, including nausea, vomiting, tremor, sleeplessness, and hallucinations. In addition, medically serious and potentially fatal withdrawal symptoms, such as seizures and delirium tremens, can develop. Alcohol withdrawal seizures are usually tonic-clonic seizures and can progress to status epilepticus. Delirium tremens is a related withdrawal syndrome with autonomic hyperactivity (increased blood pressure and heart rate), confusion (delirium), fever, and a high risk of seizures. Abrupt discontinuation of benzodiazepines can lead to a similar withdrawal state, including withdrawal seizures.

Antiseizure drugs are commonly used to treat alcohol withdrawal seizures, usually as an adjunct to benzodiazepines such as lorazepam and diazepam. Barbiturates such as phenobarbital have been used to assess tolerance and to treat withdrawal in patients with elevated seizure risk. Delirium tremens has become a clinical target for antiseizure medications, also as an adjunct to benzodiazepines. A number of research studies suggest gabapentin is useful in the treatment of delirium tremens, likely because of its effects on GABA neurons, the same neurotransmitter affected by alcohol, benzodiazepines, and barbiturates.

There is emerging evidence that topiramate can reduce drinking in people with alcohol dependence. Studies of topiramate in alcohol-dependent patients reveal decreased alcohol use and cravings. The effect size of topiramate in these studies was significant. This antiseizure medication will likely be studied as a treatment for alcohol dependence, both as a solo agent and in conjunction with medication and psychosocial treatments. Topiramate has also been used to treat the withdrawal symptoms of benzodiazepines, including one trial of rapid withdrawal.

The current standard treatment for opioid detoxification is clonidine, a drug that moderates the over-activity of the sympathetic nervous system during withdrawal. Sometimes methadone or buprenorphine are used to withdraw patients from opioids or as a maintenance treatment. Ongoing studies are investigating outcomes of opioid detoxification with antiseizure drugs, such as valproic acid, used in combination with buprenorphine.

When substance abuse is comorbid with other mental illnesses, it complicates the treatment for both disorders. Substance use is particularly common with bipolar disorder: As many as 40% to 70% of bipolar disorder patients have one or more comorbid substance use disorders. There is therapeutic optimism that some patients with bipolar disorder who also have substance use disorders may receive benefits for two clinical problems with a single agent. Valproic acid, lamotrigine, and topiramate appear to have the greatest promise.

Side Effects of Antiseizure Medications

- Children born to pregnant mothers taking antiseizure medications early in pregnancy have an increased risk for abnormalities including neural tube defects (such as spina bifida), facial malformations, and other defects.
- Liver toxicity occurs in a number of these drugs and physicians routinely monitor liver enzymes in patients taking valproic acid or carbamazepine. Pancreatitis is a rare but potentially fatal side effect of valproic acid.
- A severe rash known as Steven Johnson syndrome has been seen in ethosuximide and lamotrigine use.

The rash typically begins around the mouth, nose, and other mucus membranes. Slow upward tapering of the dose may decrease the risk of the rash.

- Gabapentin, topiramate, clonazepam, and phenobarbital are sedating and can cause some ataxia, especially clonazepam and phenobarbital. Patients on these medications should not operate motor vehicles until they know the sedation effects of these medications. Often, tolerance develops to the sedation.
- Clonazepam and phenobarbital carry significant risks of abuse and dependence.
- Valproic acid can lead to hair changes (change in texture, hair loss), weight gain, and tremor. Valproic acid has also been associated with polycystic ovary syndrome.
- Blood problems can occur with commonly used antiseizure drugs. Megaloblastic anemia can occur with phenytoin. Aplastic anemia can be seen in carbamazepine and rarely with valproic acid and phenobarbital. The drop in white blood cells can be life threatening, and patients taking carbamazepine should have regular blood tests to monitor blood counts.
- For patients with seizure disorders, abrupt discontinuation of antiseizure medications can lead to increased numbers of seizures.

Drug Interactions

Antiseizure medications can have complicated drug interactions. Carbamazepine can increase the activity of liver enzymes that metabolize other drugs and decrease their blood levels. It can even induce its own metabolism and thus requires careful monitoring and adjustment to achieve therapeutic blood levels. Phenytoin and phenobarbital also increase the activity of liver enzymes and decrease blood levels of certain medications. In some cases, antiseizure medications lead to a level of increased metabolic clearance that lowers the blood level of other medications, such as birth control pills, to subtherapeutic levels. Interactions with other prescribed medications can raise the blood levels of antiseizure medications. Phenytoin is bound to specific proteins when traveling in the blood and other medications (such as SSRI antidepressants) can displace phenytoin from the proteins. The phenytoin release from bound proteins can then result in toxic blood levels.

Overdose

The antiseizure medications are central nervous system (CNS) depressants, and some can be lethal in an overdose. Like other CNS depressants, the most prominent threat during an overdose is decreased respiratory drive. However, the blood level of many antiseizure medications needs to be very high before it is considered toxic and life threatening. Phenobarbital is an exception to this and, like all barbiturates, carries a high risk of lethality with overdose. Life-threatening overdose with other antiseizure medications is most likely to occur in combination with other CNS depressants, such as alcohol and opioids.

Melissa Piasecki and Matthew Parra

See also Antidepressant Drugs; Antipsychotic Drugs; Co-Occurring Disorders; Pharmacological Approaches to Treatment

Further Readings

Alcohol withdrawal syndrome: How to predict, prevent, diagnose and treat it. (2007, February). *Prescrire International, 16*(87), 24–31.

Beers, M. (2006). Neurological disorders. In R. Porter & T. Jones (Eds.), *The Merck manual of diagnosis and therapy* (18th ed., pp. 1476–1495). Whitehouse Station, NJ: Merck Research Laboratories.

Cheseaux, M., Monnat, M., & Sullino, D. F. (2003). Topiramate in benzodiazepine withdrawal. *Human Psychopharmacology, 18*(5), 375–377.

Nguyen, S. A., Malcom, R., & Middaugh, L. D. (2007). Topiramate reduces ethanol consumption by C57BL/6 mice. *Synapse, 61*(3), 150–156.

Pittenger, C., & Desan, P. H. (2007). Gabapentin abuse, and delirium tremens upon gabapentin withdrawal. *Journal of Clinical Psychiatry, 68*(3), 483–484.

Porter, R. J., & Meldrum, B. S. (2006). Antiseizure drugs. In B. Katzung (Ed.), *Basic and clinical pharmacology* (10th ed., pp. 374–394). New York: McGraw-Hill.

Schatzberg, A. F., Cole, J. O., & Debattista, C. (2007). *Manual of clinical psychopharmacology* (6th ed.) Washington, DC: American Psychiatric Publishing.

Rustembogovic, A., Sofic, E., Tahirovic, I., & Kundurovic, Z. (2004). A study of gabapentin in the treatment of tonic-clonic seizures of alcohol withdrawal syndrome. *Medicinski Arhiv, 58*(1), 5–6.

Voris, J., Smith, N. L., Rao, S. M., Thorne, D. L., & Flowers, Q. J. (2003). Gabapentin for treatment of ethanol withdrawal. *Substance Abuse, 24*(2), 129–132.

ANTISOCIAL PERSONALITY DISORDER

High rates of personality disorder are consistently identified among populations diagnosed with substance use disorders (SUDs). Rates of co-occurrence with SUD are particularly high for personality disorders within the dramatic–erratic (Cluster B) subcategory of the *Diagnostic and Statistical Manual of Mental Disorders, Fourth Edition, Text Revision (DSM-IV-TR)* Axis II. Of the personality disorders, antisocial personality disorder (ASPD) exhibits the highest rates of co-occurrence with SUD. Large-scale epidemiological studies have identified rates of co-occurrence between ASPD and SUD that dramatically exceed rates observed between other forms of psychopathology, and although these rates vary considerably across populations and studies, the prevalence of ASPD among SUD populations is many times higher than the 2% to 3% observed in the general population. Indeed, according to some estimates, individuals with SUD exhibit rates of ASPD of 14% to 55%, and among individuals with ASPD, rates of SUD have been estimated to be as high as 80%. Examination of the nature of the relationships that underlie the co-occurrence of SUD and ASPD may provide important clues to the etiology and maintenance of both disorders and may also have important implications for treatment.

The category of SUD encompasses several disorders, and individual differences have been identified among users of different substances. These differences include different rates of psychiatric comorbidity, and rates of ASPD appear to differ across SUD. Specifically, higher rates of ASPD have been identified among users of illicit drugs relative to those whose substance use is restricted to alcohol. Approximately 15% of individuals with alcohol use disorders display co-occurring ASPD, whereas rates of ASPD as high as 70% have been identified among illicit drug users. This is not surprising, given the centrality of criminality to the ASPD diagnosis. The extent to which these differences are artifacts of the general criminality versus meaningful correlates of core features of ASPD remains unclear.

Diagnostic Criteria

The diagnosis of ASPD requires the presence of conduct disorder (i.e., a behavior pattern of aggression, destruction of property, lying, or all three characteristic) prior to the age of 15 and three of five additional diagnostic criteria. Field trials indicate that interrater agreement for the diagnosis of ASPD is relatively high, particularly compared to other Axis II diagnoses. This reliability is due largely to the emphasis on readily observable behaviors. However, this behaviorally based approach has been widely criticized for sacrificing validity, and it has been argued that the diagnosis lacks specificity, particularly among the correctional populations where the construct is most commonly applied. The behavioral emphasis also complicates the elucidation of the relationship between SUD and ASPD. There is substantial overlap between the *DSM-IV-TR* diagnostic criteria for ASPD and behavior that is characteristic of individuals with SUD, and it is likely that this overlap results in inflated estimates of the meaningful co-occurrence of SUD and prodigious antisociality.

Criteria for ASPD that relate most directly to SUD include the repeated commission of criminal acts, consistent irresponsibility, and disregard for the safety of others. In light of the criminalization of many substances, the presence of SUD might in and of itself warrant a positive score on the ASPD criterion involving criminality. Also, given the high rate of injury, vehicular and otherwise, related to intoxication, many SUD individuals might also meet the criterion of disregard for the safety of others. Finally, given the pervasive sociolegal and professional sanctions related to substance use, the presence of SUD might contribute substantially to a positive score for the irresponsibility criterion. Given this considerable overlap between ASPD diagnostic criteria and SUD related behaviors, the co-occurrence of SUD and APSD may represent, in part, an artifact related to the criminalization of substance use, rather than meaningful covariation in psychopathology.

Psychopathy

In light of the limitations of the ASPD construct, a great deal of research related to individual differences in persistent and prodigious antisociality has focused instead on the construct of psychopathy. The psychopathic personality is characterized by a constellation of traits including impulsivity, callousness, manipulative behavior, and irresponsibility. As conceptualized in the Psychopathy Checklist-Revised (PCL-R), which is the standard measure of psychopathic personality, psychopathy is the best validated and most widely studied clinical construct related to antisocial behavior. One strength of the psychopathy construct is greater specificity relative to ASPD. Base rates of psychopathy in correctional samples generally range from 15% to 25%, whereas rates of ASPD are generally above 50%. Furthermore, the vast majority of psychopathic individuals meet criteria for ASPD, whereas fewer than half of individuals who meet ASPD criteria also meet clinically accepted cutoffs for psychopathy. Another advantage of the psychopathy construct, relative to ASPD, is the inclusion of the affective and interpersonal traits that are central to many clinical conceptions of the pathologically antisocial individual.

Given the lower base rates for psychopathy relative to ASPD, it follows that rates of psychopathy in SUD populations are substantially lower than those observed for ASPD. Because psychopathy is not included among the *DSM-IV-TR* or the *International Classification of Diseases* diagnostic categories, it has not been routinely included in large-scale epidemiological studies, and therefore estimated rates of co-occurrence between psychopathy and SUD in the general population are not available. However, research with SUD samples suggests that approximately 12% of SUD individuals also meet criteria for psychopathy. Estimated rates of SUD among psychopaths in correctional studies show considerable variation across studies. However, these rates are consistently higher than in the general correctional population and, in some instances, even higher than in APSD samples; as many as 93% of psychopathic males have been identified as meeting criteria for alcohol use disorders and 74% for drug use disorders. As is the case for ASPD, differences in rates of co-occurring SUD between psychopathic and nonpsychopathic offenders are greater for use of illicit drugs compared to alcohol use.

An examination at the level of the subcomponents that underlie psychopathy provides further insight into the nature of the relationships among SUD, ASPD, and psychopathy. At least two correlated dimensions underlie PCL-R measured psychopathy: Factor 1 measures callous and unemotional and interpersonal features, and Factor 2 measures a generally antisocial and impulsive lifestyle. Further decomposition indicates that Factor 1 comprises arrogant and manipulative

interpersonal style and deficient affective experience, and Factor 2 comprises impulsive and irresponsible lifestyle and persistent criminality and antisocial behavior. The relationship between psychopathy and ASPD is reliant primarily on the antisocial and deviant behavior captured by Factor 2, with relatively modest relationships observed between ASPD and the core affective and interpersonal traits of psychopathy.

The relationship between psychopathy and SUD displays a pattern that is similar to that observed between psychopathy and ASPD, that is, moderate correlations between SUD and PCL-R total and Factor 2 scores and small or no relationships with Factor 1 scores. In light of this similarity, it has been proposed that the relationship between SUD and psychopathy does not reflect traits specific to psychopathy but is due instead to overlap with ASPD, or with the generally criminal behavior that is common to both disorders. However, there is evidence that the relationship between psychopathy and SUD is not an artifact of general social deviance and that core elements of psychopathy relate to SUD. After accounting for symptoms of ASPD, small to moderate positive relationships have been identified between *DSM–IV-TR* substance dependence symptoms and PCL-R total and Factor 2 scores, and these relationships appear to be consistent across substances. Moreover, these relationships were found to rely primarily on impulsive and irresponsible traits rather than on general antisociality, which suggests that the relationship between SUD and psychopathy may not involve antisociality, per se, but may instead reflect overlap with the impulsive and irresponsible lifestyle common to those who engage in antisocial behavior.

Externalizing

There is substantial evidence for meaningful heterogeneity within SUD populations, and research that has examined this heterogeneity has identified antisociality as an important factor for parsing SUD into meaningful subtypes. One influential SUD typology describes two distinct subgroups that are characterized by distinct precursors, courses, and outcomes. According to this two-cluster model, *Type A* or *Type 1* individuals are characterized by later onset, less comorbidity, better response to treatment, and, importantly, relatively low incidences of antisocial behavior. In contrast, *Type B* or *Type II* individuals are characterized by early onset, poor prognosis for treatment, and high levels of antisocial behavior. Subsequent typologies have added detail to the understanding of heterogeneity in SUD, but antisociality remains central to most classification strategies.

Research examining Type II individuals has consistently identified family history as an important component of this cluster. This apparent heritability suggests a biological component, and developments in behavioral genetics suggest that the shared variance among the features described by Type II may be understood to reflect a latent factor. Specifically, it has been proposed that a common heritable factor, labeled "externalizing," underlies the co-occurrence of disorders characterized by substance use, antisociality, and general disinhibition. The externalizing factor has also been found to correlate highly with Factor 2 of the PCL-R. Twin studies provide powerful evidence for the value of the externalizing construct in understanding the relationship between SUD and ASPD; as much as 80% of the variability in the latent externalizing factor can be accounted for by heritability. In general, externalizing represents a promising focus for future research on these disorders by providing a single locus of examination.

Negative Affect

Externalizing is the most powerful single explanatory factor for understanding the co-occurrence of antisocial behavior and SUD. However, negative affectivity (NA) may also help explain high rates of co-occurrence. NA is related to both SUD and ASPD but is not considered to be part of the externalizing dimension and generally has been found to be unrelated, or inversely related, to core personality features of psychopathy. Indeed, NA is more commonly related to internalizing disorders such as depression and anxiety. Therefore, the relationship among SUD, ASPD, and NA appears to be distinct of the behavioral disinhibition that relates SUD to ASPD via externalizing and psychopathy.

Robust relationships have been identified between NA and SUD, and these relationships are proposed to reflect the self-administration of drugs to relieve unpleasant affective states. There are at least two models that broadly describe the relationship among NA, ASPD, and SUD. In the first model, the antisocial lifestyle associated with ASPD brings about negative life events, which lead to negative affect and to attendant attempts at self-medication. These attempts at self-medication involve substance misuse and the development of SUD. According to the second model, endogenous NA leads to the development of SUD via self-medication. Consequences of SUD, such as vocational failure and the development of antisocial peer relationships, are criminogenic factors that represent risk factors for ASPD. Models of the co-occurrence of SUD and ASPD that posit a mediating role for NA are theoretically appealing, and there is substantial evidence that NA co-occurs with both ASPD and SUD. However, further longitudinal research is necessary to better determine the directionality of the proposed relationships.

Treatment

The co-occurrence of SUD and ASPD may have substantial treatment implications for both disorders. There is evidence that antisociality in general, and psychopathy in particular, may complicate treatment for SUD. Studies involving SUD treatment populations report that ASPD and psychopathy are related to poor compliance with treatment and more rapid relapse. Also, the attenuated concern for the feelings of others and irresponsible attitude toward work that typifies ASPD and psychopathy may reduce the motivational enhancement associated with meeting work and family obligations. Indeed, psychopathy is generally considered to be ego-syntonic (i.e., the individual does not view his or her behavior as problematic), and as such, psychopaths may evince little or no motivation for meaningful compliance with therapeutic recommendations. However, ASPD or psychopathic features should not be considered contraindicative for therapy. Rather, the complications that such factors may present should be considered when setting goals and selecting intervention strategies.

The implications of comorbid SUD in the treatment of ASPD and psychopathy have not received detailed examination. Indeed, comprehensive treatments for these disorders have not been developed. Nonetheless, research on treatments for behaviors that may be related to antisociality, such as intimate partner violence, has emphasized the importance of maintaining a concurrent therapeutic focus on SUD-related issues. Indeed, given the high levels of co-occurrence between SUD and antisociality, treatment for either disorder is likely to benefit from an approach that is sensitive to the implications of comorbidity.

Conclusion

A substantial proportion of individuals who meet criteria for SUD also meet criteria for ASPD, and this high rate of co-occurrence has implications for etiology and treatment of both disorders. This co-occurrence may be attributed, in part, to conceptual overlap in the diagnostic criteria for the two disorders and to the influence of third factors, such as general criminality. However, there is evidence that the co-occurrence also reflects shared risk factors at the trait level. A subset of ASPD individuals meet diagnostic criteria for the more specific construct of psychopathy, and research examining the relationship between psychopathy and SUD can inform our understanding of the relationship between SUD and ASPD. Specifically, research on psychopathy and SUD suggests that the co-occurrence of ASPD and SUD involves personality traits related to behavioral disinhibition. Furthermore, developments in behavioral genetics indicate that the shared variance among disorders characterized by substance use, antisociality, and disinhibition reflects a heritable externalizing factor. Further research aimed at determining factors that moderate the expression of this externalizing disposition may assist in the development of treatments for individuals who suffer from the unfortunate combination of ASPD and SUD.

Zach Walsh and Gregory L. Stuart

See also Coercion and Treatment; Co-Occurring Disorders; Court-Mandated Treatment; Criminal Justice Populations; Treatment in Jails and Prisons; Violence, Intimate Partner and Substance Abuse Treatment

Further Readings

Kreuger, R. F., Hicks, B. M., Patrick, C. J., Carlson, S. R., Iacono, W. G., & McGue, M. (2002). Etiologic connections among substance dependence, antisocial behavior, and personality: Modeling the externalizing spectrum. *Journal of Abnormal Psychology, 111,* 411–424.

Robins, L. N. (1998). The intimate connection between antisocial personality and substance abuse. *Social Psychiatry and Psychiatric Epidemiology, 33,* 393–399.

Taylor, J., & Lang, A. R. (2005). Psychopathy and substance use disorders. In C. J. Patrick (Ed.), *Handbook of psychopathy* (pp. 495–511). New York: Guilford Press.

Trull, T. J., Waudby, C. J., & Sher, K. J. (2004). Alcohol, tobacco, and drug use disorders and personality disorder symptoms. *Experimental Clinical Psychopharmacology, 12,* 65–75.

Walsh, Z., Allen, L. C., & Kosson, D. S. (2007). Beyond social deviance: Substance use disorders and the dimensions of psychopathy. *Journal of Personality Disorders, 21,* 273–288.

ANXIETY DISORDERS

This entry discusses anxiety disorders as co-occurring disorders. Co-occurring disorders are often referred to as being "comorbid" with one another. In mental health treatment and research, comorbidity is quite common; recent epidemiological data suggest that over 40% of individuals with a mental health disorder have one or more additional psychiatric disorders. This is particularly relevant to treatment as patients will often present seeking remedy for one specific problem, while neglecting to mention the difficulties related to the other. Consideration of comorbidity can be the difference between successful and unsuccessful treatment, as one disorder may be caused, in large part, by another disorder. Indeed, comorbidity is frequently linked to poorer prognosis in treatment outcome studies. Comorbidity can also have a substantial fiscal impact; research indicates that treatment cost for one disorder is significantly increased if another disorder is present. Among substance use disorders, consideration of comorbid anxiety disorders is particularly important, as it is seen in nearly 18% of all individuals diagnosed with a substance use disorder.

Types of Anxiety Disorders

Anxiety disorders are the most prevalent category of mental disorders, affecting an estimated 40 million U.S. adults (about 18% of the population) in a given year. The five main anxiety disorders are generalized anxiety disorder, post-traumatic stress disorder, panic disorder, social anxiety disorder, and obsessive-compulsive disorder. Although anxiety disorders are a diverse set of phenotypes, they are alike in that they all involve excessive negative affect typically in the form of fear and anxiety. Anxiety is a state of diffuse arousal following the perception of a real or imagined threat.

This fundamentally experiential, future-oriented, self-focusing emotion can at times be adaptive, as anticipatory problem-solving thoughts are triggered. Yet, anxiety can become excessive, consuming attentional resources and leading to a disabling condition. Anxiety disorders, even when occurring in isolation, are associated with increased morbidity, mortality, and engagement in health risk behaviors. One such health risk behavior is substance misuse, when the anxious individual begins to use substances in a self-medicating fashion. This behavior may negatively reinforce the substance use by alleviating the aversive anxiety state. The negative reinforcement can also lead to an additive effect of the already pharmacologically addictive properties of a substance. The culmination of pharmacological dependence risk, enhanced by negative reinforcement, can contribute to higher risk for abuse and dependence. In fact, anxiety disorders often co-occur with substance use disorders; however, the temporal onset of disorders may also be reversed.

Comorbid Anxiety and Substance Use Disorders

Accurate estimates of the prevalence of this form of comorbidity was lacking until recently, when large-scale projects used criteria from the *Diagnostic and Statistical Manual of Mental Disorders, Fourth Edition* (*DSM-IV*). The two main psychiatric epidemiological studies of the U.S. population (Epidemiologic Catchment Area Survey and the National Comorbidity Survey) used the *DSM-III* criteria. The *DSM-III* did not provide clear guidelines for differentiating between a substance-induced anxiety disorder versus an independent anxiety disorder that is co-occurring with a substance use disorder. The *DSM-IV* added sophistication to make the distinction between an independent disorder versus a substance-induced disorder. For an independent anxiety disorder to be diagnosed, (a) the patient must meet full criteria for the anxiety disorder prior to the commencement of their substance use, or if temporal occurrence cannot be established; and (b) the full anxiety symptoms must persist for at least 1 month following discontinuation of the substance. Conversely, if the anxiety symptoms are ameliorated following cessation and detoxification, then a diagnosis of substance-induced anxiety disorder is warranted. The first epidemiological study to use the *DSM-IV* guidelines for assigning independent

and substance-induced anxiety disorders was the National Epidemiologic Survey on Alcohol and Related Conditions (NESARC).

Data from the NESARC revealed that among individuals with a current substance use disorder, 17.71% also had an independent anxiety disorder. In real population numbers, this prevalence represents 3,435,740 million U.S. adults. Similarly, among those with a current anxiety disorder, 14.96% also met criteria for a current substance use disorder, an estimated 3,440,800 million U.S. adults. Among respondents, less than 1% received a diagnosis of a substance-induced anxiety disorder. The percentage of individuals with a substance-induced anxiety disorder was less than previous estimates, suggesting that use of the old diagnostic criteria yielded an overestimation of prevalence. Another key finding from the NESARC relating to comorbidity was that compared to individuals with a co-occurring substance use disorder and mood disorder, those with comorbid substance use disorders and anxiety disorders were less likely to present for treatment.

Etiology and Temporal Occurrence

Extant research suggests that the relationship between these two classes of disorders is complex and bidirectional. It was commonly believed that anxiety disorders always precede substance use disorders; however, temporality may occur one of three ways: (1) the anxiety disorder precedes the substance use disorder, (2) the substance use disorder precedes the anxiety disorder, or (3) the two disorders have a shared onset. Notably, once the disorders are occurring simultaneously, they may maintain each other. Previous research on the temporal occurrence of anxiety and substance use disorders has focused primarily on alcohol use disorders. Although many of the subsequently mentioned research strategies apply to substance use disorders in general, more research is necessary before conclusions can be drawn regarding the relationship between anxiety disorders and other substances such as cocaine, marijuana, or hallucinogens.

Well-conducted epidemiological studies reveal that the average age of onset of anxiety disorders and substance use disorders is 20.0 and 23.5 years, respectively. It is believed that anxiety disorders have the potential to result in later substance use disorders. Self-medication is a common explanation for this finding. People suffering from anxiety disorders report turning to substances in hopes of alleviating some of their symptoms of anxiety—most often substances that are known to be central nervous system depressants (e.g., alcohol, sedatives, opioids). The relationship between anxiety and alcohol has been tested in a variety of laboratory-based studies. Although the complexity of this relationship leads to limitations in generalizability, some evidence suggests that alcohol can temporarily relieve anxiety; this provides credence to the notion that alcohol has some anxiolytic properties. For example, alcohol has been found to significantly reduce performance anxiety during a public speaking task in persons with social phobia, relative to placebo and control conditions. If anxiety promotes alcohol use, it would be expected that in clinical studies involving successful treatment of anxiety, alcohol use among comorbid individuals would also be reduced or eliminated and that in alcoholism treatment studies, anxiety would predict relapse. In anxiety disorder treatment outcome studies involving persons with generalized anxiety disorder and obsessive-compulsive disorder, symptom reduction has been found to be associated with subsequent decreases in alcohol use; however, treatment studies of comorbid social anxiety disorder and alcohol use disorder do not find that successful treatment of social anxiety symptoms are associated with decreased consumption of alcohol. The presence of an anxiety disorder has been shown to predict a greater likelihood of relapse in treated alcoholics, and persons with high levels of anxiety have been found to be more likely to attribute the cause of their relapse to aversive emotional symptoms.

Although data from prospective studies suggests that a small minority of anxiety disorders (agoraphobia and social anxiety disorder) begin prior to substance use disorders in comorbid individuals, there have also been numerous cases when substance use disorders are prevalent before the onset of (or around the same time as) an anxiety disorder (panic disorder and generalized anxiety disorder). This is often seen in cases involving central nervous system agitators, such as amphetamines. Use of such substances can cause users to experience many symptoms of anxiety—hence, an anxiety disorder following a substance use disorder. Stressors such as job loss, marriage disruption, automobile accidents, and injuries are more likely to be experienced by substance abusers than other individuals, and these stressors may put one at risk for the development of an anxiety disorder.

Chronic substance use may also cause biological changes that generate anxiety. Deficits in the neurotransmitter gamma-aminobutyric (GABA) are known to induce anxiety, and lower levels of GABA as well as increased postmortem GABA receptors in the brain have been found in chronic alcohol abusers. Laboratory studies provide preliminary evidence that long periods of drinking, as well as high doses of alcohol, may lead to increases in anxiety.

Anxiety disorders and substance use disorders may also share a temporal onset. In response to a stressful or traumatic life event, a person may experience symptoms of anxiety and may, at the same time, turn to substances to cope with the distress caused by this event. In such cases, a cyclical process may emerge where substance use is employed as a means of medication for symptoms of anxiety; then, substance use becomes a habit, and habitual use begins to perpetuate anxiety symptoms. For example, after experiencing a traumatic event such as witnessing violence, persons will often learn to fear previously neutral objects and situations that become paired with the traumatic event via conditioning processes. Fear and distress are common following trauma, and these responses typically extinguish once stimuli that have come to produce them are repeatedly experienced in the absence of trauma and new associations can be learned between them and other neutral or positive stimuli. However, persons who successfully escape or avoid the stimuli that have come to produce fear and distress have no opportunity to learn new associations, and, therefore, this escape or avoidance behavior can lead to the development of post-traumatic stress disorder. Alcohol and other substances are known to impair fear extinction processes. Therefore, persons who use substances following trauma may first do so to cope with normal fear and distress reactions; however, their substance use may make them less likely to experience a decrease in these reactions via extinction. Such persons are therefore likely to be at greater risk for post-traumatic stress disorder, and a cycle emerges in which substances are used to ameliorate anxiety symptoms while at the same time perpetuating their existence.

Diagnostic Implications

When a patient presents for treatment of a substance use disorder, identification of a comorbid anxiety disorder may be difficult. The substance of misuse may be masking or "treating" the anxiety to the point that the patient does not consider it a particularly relevant treatment goal. Indeed, the patient may not even mention difficulties with anxiety. Thus, a thorough diagnostic intake, including chronology of onset of all psychiatric symptoms, is imperative in substance use disorder treatment.

Further complicating diagnosis of comorbid anxiety disorders, several symptoms of intoxication and withdrawal can mirror symptoms of anxiety. For example, psychomotor agitation, hypervigilance, and nervousness are quite common among individuals detoxing from alcohol and other depressants. To accurately diagnose an individual with a comorbid anxiety disorder, a period of extended abstinence from the substance used is warranted. The exact length of time should be based on the type and amount of substance being misused. Consideration of half-life of the substance should also be given. For example, a longer period of abstinence is indicated with long-acting substances, such as methadone, whereas for short-acting substances (with a short half-life), such as oxycodone, a shorter period of abstinence would be required.

Brief psychometrically sound screeners are available for both substance use disorders (e.g., Alcohol Use Identification Test, Drug Abuse Screening Test) and anxiety disorders (e.g., Beck Anxiety Disorder Inventory, Posttraumatic Stress Disorder Symptom Checklist, General Health Questionnaire). More detailed clinical interviews, such as the Structured Clinical Interview for DSM-IV may be warranted if patients endorse symptoms on screeners. Emphasis should be given during clinical interviews to ascertain the chronology of symptom of disorder onset.

Treatment Implications

The high rate of comorbidity underscores the need for psychiatric screening at substance use treatment centers and, conversely, for substance use screening at psychiatric treatment centers. Expert consensus has moved from a viewpoint that each disorder should be treated separately to a stance that encourages and supports the use of integrated treatment approaches. Thus, instead of treating anxiety disorders and substance use disorders as independent conditions, unified and integrated treatment of both conditions is encouraged. Attention to comorbidity in the past decade has instigated the development of treatment

manuals to address specific combinations of co-occurring disorders. Furthermore, many of these treatment protocols are gathering empirical support. For example, Seeking Safety, a treatment for comorbid post-traumatic stress disorder and substance use disorders, has been found effective in 12 completed clinical trials.

Despite recent attention to comorbidity, the majority of pharmacotherapy trials for anxiety disorders specifically exclude patients with a co-occurring substance use disorder. Therefore, little is known about the safety and efficacy of agents to treat individuals with both disorders. Pharmacotherapy needs to be given extreme care, as many potential complications can arise when prescribing medications for an individual with comorbid substance use and anxiety disorders. For example, potentially toxic interactions can occur between the drug being used to treat and the drug being misused.

In sum, although research has been rapidly accumulating on these comorbid conditions, much is left to be learned, and discovery of such information is prudent, as the personal and societal costs of these disorders are quite high.

Ananda B. Amstadter, Jared P. Dempsey,
Noreen Watson, and Grace S. Hubel

See also Anxiolytic Drugs; Co-Occurring Disorders; Diagnosis; Post-Traumatic Stress Disorder

Further Readings

Goeders, N. E. (2003). The impact of stress on addiction. *European Neuropsychopharmacology, 13*(6), 435–441.

Goldenberg, I. M., Mueller, T., Fierman, E. J., Gordon, A., Pratt, L., Cox, K., et al. (1995). Specificity of substance use in anxiety-disordered subjects. *Comprehensive Psychiatry, 36*(5), 319–328.

Grant, B. F., Harford, T. C., Muthén, B. O., Yi, H. Y., Hasin, D. S., & Stinson, F. S. (2007). DSM-IV alcohol dependence and abuse: Further evidence of validity in the general population. *Drug and Alcohol Dependence, 86*(2–3), 154–166.

Hung, C. (2001). Meperidine addiction or treatment frustration? *General Hospital Psychiatry, 23*(1), 31–35.

Merikangas, K. R. (1998). Comorbidity of substance use disorders with mood and anxiety disorders: Results of the international consortium in psychiatric epidemiology. *Addictive Behaviors, 23*(6), 893–907.

Nevo, I., & Hamon, M. (1995). Neurotransmitter and neuromodulatory mechanisms involved in alcohol abuse and alcoholism. *Neurochemistry International, 26*(4), 305–336.

Norman, S. B., Tate, S. R., Anderson, K. G., & Brown, S. A. (2007). Do trauma history and PTSD symptoms influence addiction relapse context? *Drug and Alcohol Dependence, 90*(1), 89–96.

ANXIOLYTIC DRUGS

Anxiolytic medications reduce symptoms of anxiety. Hypnotic drugs induce sleep. Both medications can function in either role and are sometimes known as "minor tranquilizers" (to distinguish them from the "major tranquilizers," barbiturates and antipsychotics). Anxiolytics and hypnotics are among the most frequently prescribed medications and have a wide application, including long-term treatment of anxiety disorders, relaxation and sedation before procedures, treatment of acute agitation, and medically managed withdrawal from substances. Despite valid and effective applications in medical practice, almost every drug in this class has significant potential for abuse and dependence with long-term use. This entry reviews the different classes of medications used to treat anxiety and insomnia with an emphasis on the benzodiazepines (BZDs).

Anxiolytics offer predictable, short-term relief from anxiety symptoms related to situational anxiety or a psychiatric disorder. Anxiety is an uncomfortable state of brain overactivity with both emotional symptoms (worry, dread) and physical symptoms (increased muscle tone, increased heart rate, difficulty falling asleep). Normal life events such as public speaking, examinations, or a turbulent flight can cause anxiety. Some people develop anxiety disorders, with abnormally elevated or persistent anxiety that affects their daily functioning. The most common anxiety disorders are phobias, panic disorder, generalized anxiety disorder, post-traumatic stress disorder, and obsessive-compulsive disorder. Anxiety symptoms can also be present as part of another psychiatric disorder, such as major depression or psychosis.

Anxiolytics work by decreasing brain excitability. The primary inhibitory neurotransmitter in the brain is gamma-aminobutyric acid (GABA), which acts on chloride channels on brain cell membranes. BZDs effectively enhance GABA activity at the receptor level by increasing the frequency of chloride channel openings, decreasing the resting tone and subsequent activity level of brain cells. A mild decrease in brain resting tone can induce a state of relaxation. Larger decreases lead to sleep induction.

Newer anxiolytics target different receptors. Buspirone, for example, acts upon serotonin receptors and, in contrast to the fast-acting BZDs, can take 4 to 6 weeks for full effect. The major classes of anxiolytics are presented in this entry, along with the representative drugs, their side effects, overdose potential, and role in substance use disorders. Selective serotonin reuptake inhibitors, monoamine oxidase inhibitors, and other antidepressants treat anxiety disorders over longer periods but have a different mechanism of action and are not classified primarily as anxiolytics.

Benzodiazepines

Representative Drugs

Diazepam (Valium)

Lorazepam (Ativan)

Triazolam (Halcion)

Alprazolam (Xanax)

Oxazepam (Serax)

Midazolam (Versed)

Clonazepam (Klonopin)

Temazepam (Restoril)

Flunitrazepam (Rohypnol, no longer available in United States)

Chlordiazepoxide (Librium)

Flurazepam (Dalmane)

Estazolam (Prosom)

Effects

All BZDs have an identical mechanism of action but differ in their onset and duration of action. The speed with which each of the BZDs affects anxiety depends on its properties and on the mode of administration. Some of the BZDs are highly lipophilic and can act within seconds to minutes because they rapidly pass into brain cells. Other BZDs have an onset of action requiring many minutes. Intravenous and intramuscular administration of BZDs results in faster onset of action (and more potent effect) than oral administration. Midazolam has the most rapid onset of action (seconds), which makes it very useful for medicating patients before they undergo uncomfortable procedures. Clonazepam has the longest half-life of the BZDs, which makes it useful for tapering patients off other BZDs.

The drugs in this class also differ in potency. Clonazepam is the most potent. One milligram (mg) of clonazepam is equivalent to 2 mg of alprazolam or 4 mg of lorazepam (see conversion table Web site of American Academy of Family Physicians at http://www.aafp.org/afp/20000501/2763.html).

Benzodiazepines are very effective for short-term treatment of anxiety (such as a flying phobia). The potential for abuse and dependence increases with exposure. None of the BZDs carries an indication for long-term use. The U.S. Drug Enforcement Agency assigns BZDs to the Schedule IV to reflect these risks. Elderly patients have additional risks with BZD side effects, such as poor balance, poor memory, and confusion. Physicians typically use short-acting benzodiazepines and lower starting doses with elderly patients. Rarely, individuals exhibit a "paradoxical response" to BZDs. Instead of sedation, they become more agitated and disinhibited.

Abrupt discontinuation of BZDs after chronic use can lead to a withdrawal state that carries a risk of seizures, which can be fatal. Other withdrawal symptoms are similar to alcohol withdrawal: anxiety, agitation, irritability, nausea, insomnia, tremor, headache, hallucinations, and delirium. Withdrawal symptoms may be more severe with short-acting benzodiazepines and the higher-potency drugs (e.g., alprazolam). Longer-acting BZDs (such as clonazepam) are "self-tapering" and should replace short-acting BZDs to stabilize and taper dependent patients.

Abuse Potential

Benzodiazepines are an important class of abused drugs. Some people abuse BZDs in a purely recreational manner, whereas others may develop problems from "quasi-therapeutic" use. Long-term BZD usage generally leads to some form of dependence. Up to half of patients prescribed diazepam for 6 months or more become physically dependent on the drug. Many patients receive BZD prescriptions for years from well-meaning physicians and are unable to discontinue the medication because of physical dependence. Alprazolam is a particularly problematic BZD. The fast onset of action powerfully reinforces the effect, and the short half-life leads to abrupt reemergence of anxiety. These pharmacokinetic properties are a formula for misuse, abuse, and dependence. Alprazolam has incidentally become a popular drug of abuse among adolescents. Clonazepam is perceived as "safer," because of its long half-life, but addiction-medicine specialists have found that it is also frequently abused.

Benzodiazepines are rarely abused alone. Approximately 80% of BZD abuse is polydrug abuse, most commonly with opioids or alcohol. Many alcoholics admit to abusing benzodiazepines to modulate intoxication or withdrawal symptoms. Some individuals experiencing agitation and insomnia after prolonged use of stimulants ("a runner") use BZDs as a tool to "come down" from the stimulant effects.

The problems with BZD dependence, tolerance, withdrawal, rebound, and abuse limit their use for long-term treatment of anxiety disorders. Patients with past or present alcohol or drug addiction have increased levels of risk for developing problems with BZDs or relapsing to a previously abused substance. Many addiction-medicine specialists believe that BZDs are relatively contraindicated in patients with histories of alcohol or drug abuse problems.

Role in Treatment for Addiction

The BZDs (especially lorazepam, diazepam, and chlordiazepoxide) are first-line treatment for the agitation and elevated vital signs that accompany acute alcohol withdrawal. Effective use of BZDs improves comfort and decreases the risk of delirium tremens and seizures in patients during withdrawal. They are also first-line treatment of withdrawal from other BZDs. Benzodiazepines function as comfort measures for stimulant withdrawal, opioid withdrawal, and hallucinogen intoxication. Typically, BZD are not prescribed after the withdrawal is complete in order to avoid the risk of developing a BZD use disorder.

Not all anxiolytic medications have cross, tolerance, or the ability to substitute for alcohol or BZDs in dependent patients during withdrawal. For example, the BZD lorazepam can safely treat alcohol withdrawal if dosed carefully, but the non-BZD anxiolytics such as buspirone and hydroxyzine would have no effect on BZD or alcohol withdrawal symptoms.

Overdose

Benzodiazepine overdose presents with lethargy, somnolence, confusion, decreased reflexes, and coma. Respiratory depression is a common complication of overdose. Benzodiazepines are most dangerous when used with other central nervous system depressants such as alcohol and opioid pain medications. BZD overdose patients are usually hospitalized. Flumazenil is a competitive BZD antagonist that counteracts the effects of the BZDs at the BZD/GABA receptor level. Flumazenil is used empirically in patients presenting with unexplained coma in emergency rooms.

"Z Drugs"

Zolpidem (Ambien)

Zaleplon (Sonata)

Eszopiclone (Lunesta)

"Z Drugs," a new class of hypnotic drugs, were introduced in 1999 for the treatment of insomnia and quickly became among the most widely prescribed medications. Although the medications in this class are structurally similar to the BZDs and have the same clinical target (insomnia), they are thought to act at separate binding sites in the brain and to have less potential for abuse and dependence.

The Z drugs are potent drugs intended for short-term use (2–3 weeks). Eszopiclone is an exception to the rule of short-term use, and patients with chronic insomnia appear to benefit for up to 6 months of use without development of tolerance or dependence. Eszopiclone may also carry less risk of dependence in higher-risk groups such as people with a history of a substance use disorder.

In the years following the release of the Z drugs, published case reports documented problematic use of zolpidem and zaleplon, with dramatic dose escalations and other evidence of dependence. The patients at highest risk for developing problems with Z drugs are those with a history of a substance use disorder

and psychiatric patients. Zolpidem and zaleplon have been reported to cause memory problems, including amnesia. There are also case reports of compulsive behaviors in patients taking zolpidem, such as atypical eating.

Barbiturates

Phenobarbital

Pentobarbital (Nembutal)

Thiopental (Pentothal)

Secobarbital (Seconal)

Barbiturates are anticonvulsant, sedative-hypnotic drugs that act via central nervous system depression at the $GABA_A$ receptor. Dangerous side effects and a high potential for abuse and dependence have resulted in the discontinuation of barbiturates as anxiolytics. Barbiturates often counter the agitation and insomnia from prolonged abuse of stimulants. Occasionally, barbiturates help manage withdrawal from alcohol, other barbiturates, or BZDs. This class of drugs has a very small therapeutic window, with significant risk of death with overdose. In addition, an abrupt withdrawal from barbiturates is associated with a high risk for seizure.

Other Drugs

Buspirone (BuSpar)

Sodium oxybate (gamma-hydroxybutyric acid) (Xyrem)

Ramelteon (Rozerem)

Hydroxyzine (Vistaril)

Meprobamate (Miltown)

Buspirone

Buspirone is a unique anxiolytic that interacts primarily with 5-HT_{1A} serotonin receptors and moderately with brain dopamine receptors. The mechanism of action is unknown. Buspirone has shown to be effective in treating generalized anxiety disorder and has no abuse potential for people with histories of drug or alcohol abuse. It also has few side effects, no withdrawal effects, and a benign overdose potential. The downside to buspirone is the slow onset of action (weeks) and the modest efficacy in treating anxiety disorders, particularly in patients previously treated with BZDs. Buspirone has no impact on alcohol, BZD, or barbiturate withdrawal states.

Sodium Oxybate/Gamma-Hydroxybutyric Acid (Xyrem)

Sodium oxybate, more commonly known as the club drug gamma-hydroxybutyric acid (GHB), is a central nervous system depressant with a recent Food and Drug Administration approval for treatment of narcolepsy. The mechanism of action in unknown, but it helps to reduce daytime sleepiness and may also find application in the treatment of insomnia, opioid withdrawal, and alcohol withdrawal. Because sodium oxybate has an extremely high abuse potential, a central pharmacy controls its distribution.

Ramelteon (Rozerem)

Ramelteon is a selective melatonin receptor agonist that is useful in treating insomnia. It is effective for decreasing the time to falling asleep in patients with chronic anxiety. There is no evidence of potential for abuse or dependence with ramelteon. Unlike many hypnotics, it is not a controlled substance and has demonstrated efficacy with chronic use. Ramelteon is not effective for other symptoms of anxiety and has no efficacy in withdrawal states.

Hydroxyzine (Vistaril)

Hydroxyzine is a sedating antihistamine useful in the treatment of anxiety symptoms and insomnia. Primary benefits of hydroxyzine are that it is non-scheduled and has low abuse potential. The drawbacks are the limited potency, the development of tolerance, and the side effect of dry mouth.

Meprobamate (Miltown, Equanil)

Meprobamate is an older drug that was once very popular for treating anxiety. It binds to $GABA_A$ receptors, but the exact mechanism of action is unknown. The potential for abuse and dependence is high relative to other antianxiety medications, and meprobamate is now very rarely used. Side effects include sedation, psychomotor impairment, and secondary risk of death with overdose.

Conclusion

BZDs are the most commonly used anxiolytics and are safest with short-term use. Long-term use of BZDs risks physiological dependence, which must be managed carefully to prevent medically serious withdrawal states. Other, newer medications such as buspirone and Z drugs have more benign risk profiles but slower onset and different therapeutic actions. Buspirone and antidepressants are the only medications with indications for long-term treatment of anxiety. Many validated behavioral treatments for anxiety disorders, such as cognitive behavioral therapy and progressive muscle relaxation, offer alternative and complementary approaches for treating anxiety disorders.

Nathan Cardon, Samantha Sharp,
and Melissa Piasecki

See also Antidepressant Drugs; Anxiety Disorders; Barbiturates; Benzodiazepines; Co-Occurring Disorders; Pharmacological Approaches to Treatment

Further Readings

Atack, J. R. (2003). Anxioselective compounds acting at the GABA(A) receptor benzodiazepine binding site. *Current Drug Targets. CNS and Neurological Disorders, 2,* 213–232.

Gerada, C., & Ashworth, M. (1997). ABC of mental health. Addiction and dependence—I: Illicit drugs. *British Medical Journal, 315,* 297–300.

Griffiths, R. R., & Johnson, M. W. (2005). Relative abuse liability of hypnotic drugs: A conceptual framework and algorithm for differentiating among compounds. *Journal of Clinical Psychiatry, 66,* 31–41.

Hajak, G., Muller, W. E., Wittchen, H. U., Pittrow, D., & Kirch, W. (2003). Abuse and dependence potential for the non-benzodiazepine hypnotics zolpidem and zopiclone: A review. *Addiction, 98,* 1371–1378.

Krystal, A. D., Walsh, J. K., Laska, E., Caron, J., Amato, D. A., Wessel, T. C., et al. (2003). Sustained efficacy of eszopiclone over 6 months of nightly treatment: Results of a randomized, double-blind, placebo-controlled study in adults with chronic insomnia. *Sleep, 26,* 793–799.

Longo, L. P., & Johnson, B. (2000). Addiction: part I. Benzodiazepines—Side effects, abuse risk and alternatives. *American Family Physician, 61,* 2121–2130.

O'Brien, C. P. (2005) Benzodiazepine use, abuse, and dependence. *Journal of Clinical Psychiatry, 66,* 28–33.

Schatzberg, A. F., Cole, J. O., & Debattista, C. (2007). *Manual of clinical psychopharmacology* (6th ed.). Arlington, VA: American Psychiatric Publishing.

Asian Americans/Pacific Islanders, Issues in Prevention and Treatment

See Racial and Ethnic Minorities, Issues in Prevention; Racial and Ethnic Minorities, Issues in Treatment

Assessment

Assessment of psychopathology, including substance use disorder, plays an important role in the overall care of the client. Accurate and thorough assessment should enable the clinician to (a) reach a diagnosis of the client, (b) develop the client's case conceptualization and treatment plan, and (c) monitor treatment progress and treatment outcome. The overall goal for any assessment should be to better understand the specific disorder from which the client suffers. Assessment also provides a means for clinicians and researchers to share a common language in communicating about the client's diagnosis, case conceptualization, progress, and outcome.

Ideally, the assessment process provides the therapist and patient the opportunity to develop a facilitative working relationship. For that reason, assessment is considered to mark the beginning of the therapeutic relationship. Assessment should also include an evaluation of the client's immediate and longer-term needs. Those needs should be reflected in the development and evaluation of treatment plans.

Pretreatment Assessment

The goals and objectives of the assessment process need to be well defined. In this regard, the Institute of Medicine (IOM) differentiated among three levels of assessment of substance use disorders: (1) screening, (2) problem assessment, and (3) personal assessment. In this listing, screening is the least comprehensive and, accordingly, the least expensive assessment, whereas personal assessment is the most comprehensive and the most costly. The goals of these three levels of assessment differ significantly.

Screening is designed to identify, quickly and inexpensively, individuals who may be at risk for a substance use disorder. This process is sometimes referred to as "case identification." Because substance use and abuse put people at risk for physical, psychological, legal, and social problems, it is important for primary health care professionals to identify individuals who are heavy users of alcohol and other drugs and to initiate early intervention. It is also the case that heavy substance use often interferes with efforts to treat mental, cognitive, and physical disorders, so substance use problems should be identified and evaluated even if the target disorder is not substance abuse.

Unfortunately, substance use disorders are still associated with social stigma, making it difficult for some clients to admit to a problem with alcohol or other drugs until or unless they have lost control over their alcohol or drug use. In addition, the heavy use of psychoactive substances can lead to memory problems, which makes it difficult for those afflicted to provide accurate information. Health care professionals need to be sensitive to these issues and ask about the use of alcohol, tobacco, over-the-counter drugs, and recreational drugs in as nonthreatening a way as possible.

Screening methods are often used in general medical settings, in emergency room settings, and in employee assistance programs. The aim of screening is to determine whether or not the client requires a more in-depth assessment for a substance use disorder, is in immediate need of medical detoxification or psychiatric treatment, or needs advice on how to cut down on the use or abuse of alcohol or other drugs. There are three ways to screen for psychoactive substance use and abuse: (1) laboratory tests, which are often used in medical settings (e.g., blood or urine analysis); (2) self-report screening methods, which are easy to administer, require minimal training, and are easy to incorporate into a comprehensive health assessment; and (3) brief screening interviews.

The second level of assessment according to the 1990 IOM report is often referred to as "problem assessment." It involves the effort both to determine whether the individual merits the diagnosis of a substance use disorder and to identify problems and consequences of substance use or abuse. Problem assessment may also extend to the diagnosis of co-occurring mental health or physical health disorders that may impact the substance use disorder diagnosis. To diagnose a substance use disorder, the clinician may choose to use a semistructured interview or a structured interview, or the clinician may dispense with one of these formats and simply use his or her own interview format. If the client is seen in an emergency room setting and is unable to participate in the interview, the clinician may need to interview a family member, a friend, or a collateral informant to form a preliminary diagnosis.

According to the 1990 IOM report, personal assessment is the most comprehensive assessment in which a clinician engages a client. Hence, the use of the personal assessment encompasses evaluation of the extent of the client's substance use disorder, as well as its full range of medical, emotional, psychiatric, social, vocational, and familial consequences. Biopsychosocial problems often result from substance use disorders and should be addressed in treatment. It is also the case that biopsychosocial problems may serve as antecedents to substance use disorders, in which case they may require an even stronger focus in treatment. Finally, a personal assessment should include an evaluation of the level of care required by a client with a substance use disorder.

Holistic Assessment

According to the IOM, a holistic approach to assessment is recommended for substance use disorders. This recommendation reflects the view that substance use disorders are chronic, relapsing disorders. As such, their treatment should no longer focus on acute care and discharge but, instead, a lifelong plan for dealing with a chronic condition. Thus, the holistic approach to assessment and treatment of substance abuse takes into consideration the client's immediate and short-term needs as well as his or her longer-term needs for treatment, community support, vocational and family support, and involvement with the community.

The holistic assessment of substance use disorders should include an evaluation of the client's motivation to change his or her substance use pattern, as well as determination of the client's stage of change at the time of the assessment. In this assessment paradigm, it is also seen as important to assess the client's imminent and long-term risk for relapse. Holistic assessment should lead to a treatment plan that includes a determination of the function alcohol and other drug use or abuse has played in the client's life. This latter assessment is often referred to as "functional behavioral analysis."

Cultural Factors in Case Conceptualization

Assessment for case conceptualization needs to take into consideration the risk a substance-dependent client runs for physical, psychological, and social problems associated with addiction. In addition, if the client has a physical or mental disorder, consideration must be given to the fact that treatment of this disorder will be negatively affected by the substance use.

Cultural considerations are important in case conceptualizations. Different patterns of substance abuse may characterize different ethnic groups. Some ethnic groups are more reticent than others to access substance abuse services, or they may not have the resources to access services, resulting in substantial health disparities. Many ethnic groups have an understandable historical mistrust of being assessed for health problems by someone from a different ethnic or cultural background and, accordingly, may not be forthcoming with information about their health or substance use. A thorough and comprehensive assessment needs to include an evaluation not only of how the substance use disorder affects the client but also of how it affects his or her role in the community and relationships with, and obligations to, his or her family. Arthur Blume and colleagues recommend that, by asking clients to self-monitor and then report their behavior, they might provide the clinician insight into the context of social, familial, and emotional aspects of the client's life that might help explain the client's addictive disorder.

Treatment planning may also include a specific effort to enhance the client's problem solving, refusal, coping, and communication skills. These skills are all culturally based, so treatment planning should include a thorough evaluation of the extent to which the client is rooted in one or more cultural groups. Connectedness to a client's own culture, as well as to the surrounding world, is a factor in predicting recovery from substance use disorders.

Treatment Monitoring

Assessment of the client's progress in treatment should take place every time the client meets with health care professionals. Often, this is done in collaboration with the client, by informally asking about the problems for which they were referred for treatment. This can be done in a treatment session or by self-monitoring by the client of the target behavior. Clinicians typically rely on self-reports from clients (which may be unreliable) as well as other health care professionals' observations of the client's behavior. Family members can also function as important informants on progress by the client, if this is agreed upon in advance of treatment. If a substance use disorder is the primary focus of treatment, urine tests, breath tests of blood alcohol levels, or other laboratory tests are frequently used.

Anne Helene Skinstad

See also Addiction Severity Index; Assessment Instruments; Diagnosis; Patient Placement Criteria; Screening; Screening Instruments; Substance Use Disorders

Further Readings

Blume, A. W., Schmaling, K. B., & Marlatt, G. A. (2000). Revisiting the self-medication hypothesis from a behavioral perspective. *Cognitive and Behavioral Practices, 7,* 379–384.

Craig, R. J. (2005). *Clinical and diagnostic interviewing* (2nd ed.). Lanham, MD: Jason Aronson.

Donovan, D. M., & Marlatt, G. A. (2005). *Assessment of addictive behaviors* (2nd ed.). New York: Guilford Press.

Hunsley, J., & Mash, E. J. (2008). *A guide to assessments that work.* New York: Oxford University Press.

Institute of Medicine. (1990). *Broadening the base of treatment for alcohol problems.* Washington, DC: National Academies Press.

O'Donohue, W. T., & Cucciare, M. A. (2008). *Termination psychotherapy: A clinician's guide.* New York: Routledge.

Rounsaville, B. J., Tims, F. M., Horton, A. M., & Sowder, B. J. (Eds.). (1996). *Diagnostic sourcebook on drug abuse research and treatment* (NIH Publication No. 96-350). Rockville, MD: National Institute on Alcohol Abuse and Alcoholism.

ASSESSMENT INSTRUMENTS

The use of assessment instruments in an evaluation of a client's substance use pattern, consequences of substance use disorders, and need for services can be very helpful in planning interventions. Whereas the clinical interview often used to form a diagnosis and develop a treatment plan is dependent on the counselor's background and experiences, a standardized assessment instrument is less influenced by these factors and, hence, more objective.

The choice of assessment instruments should be guided by the purpose of and goals for the assessment of the client as well as whether the instrument is normed for the client's gender, age, and ethnicity. The choice of assessment instrument can also be influenced by the client's drug of choice: Some assessment instruments have been developed specifically to evaluate the use of such substances as alcohol, marijuana, tobacco, and opiates.

The assessment instrument's psychometric properties are important to consider before choosing to use it. How should the clinician interpret the findings for various demographic groups? Are there specific cutoff points needed to interpret the data correctly for specific populations? Is the instrument sensitive to changes over time as a result of treatment? Has research shown that the instrument has clinical utility? Is an instrument's clinical utility based on clinical experience or clinical research? To which groups can the instrument's findings be generalized? How reliable is the instrument (i.e., consistency and predictability of scores)? All these questions should be answered by the clinician before he or she chooses to use a specific assessment instrument.

An assessment instrument also needs to show high levels of validity (i.e., measure what it is intended to measure). The instrument should have content validity (the instrument clearly defines what is being measured) and construct validity (the assessment instrument measures the underlying psychological or clinical construct).

Additional issues that might influence the choice of assessment instrument include (a) the client's financial situation or insurance coverage, (b) how much time the clinician has for the assessment, (c) who is requesting information about the client and for what purpose, (d) the potential presence of comorbid mental or medical conditions, (e) the certification or licensure status of the clinician, and (f) the clinician's level of training in the use of the specific instrument. It is important that clinicians use only assessment instruments for which they have had appropriate professional training and are allowed to use these instruments on the basis of their state certification or licensure statutes.

Diagnostic Assessment Instruments

In most clinical settings, clinicians diagnose without using a standardized diagnostic interview. However, if the goal of the diagnostic assessment is to provide an accurate formal diagnosis for certain purposes, including the legal system, use of a standardized diagnostic interview is a recommended practice. Several diagnostic interviews are based on the *Diagnostic and Statistical Manual of Mental Disorders, Fourth Edition or Fourth Edition, Text Revision* (*DSM-IV* or *DSM-IV-TR*) diagnostic systems. For example, the Structural Clinical Interview for the *DSM-IV* Axis I and II (SCID) will produce a comprehensive psychiatric diagnosis, including all five axes in the *DSM*. However, the SCID module covering substance use and substance-related disorders can be used alone. The *International Classification of Diseases* has a Composite International Diagnostic Interview that was developed by the World Health Organization. These instruments are quite comprehensive and time consuming to administer, and advanced training is recommended before clinicians use them. The Diagnostic Interview Schedule (DIS), developed for epidemiological research, also provides reliable *DSM-IV* diagnoses and it is much less time consuming to administer. An electronic version of the Diagnostic Interview Schedule has been developed.

Other assessment instruments are available to evaluate acute withdrawal symptoms and to determine the need for medical treatment to alleviate these symptoms. The Clinical Institute Withdrawal Assessment for Alcohol is an observational checklist of current withdrawal symptoms that has strong psychometric qualities. The Marijuana Withdrawal Checklist was created through research by the developers on the withdrawal symptoms of marijuana.

Two assessment instruments are designed to assess opiate withdrawal: Subjective Opiate Withdrawal Scale, a self-report instrument completed by the client, and Objective Opiate Withdrawal Scale, completed by the clinician.

Personal Assessment and Case Conceptualization

In 1990, the Institute of Medicine introduced the concept, "personal assessment," which was later changed to "case conceptualizations." Both terms refer to a comprehensive assessment intended for detailed treatment planning. Some comprehensive assessment instruments provide information on the issues related to the use of a specific substance, some focus on the consequences of the substance use disorder, and some assess how the client is functioning in different aspects of his or her life, such as family, social, and personal relationships; physical and mental health; education or vocation; and criminal justice involvement. In addition to these areas, some comprehensive assessment instruments examine the client's motivation to change, risk for relapse, and coping skills.

The Addiction Severity Index (ASI) is the most widely used comprehensive assessment instrument. It provides severity scores for alcohol and drug abuse and assesses their impact on five life areas: medical, social, employment, legal, psychological, and social and family functioning. Clinical training is necessary to administer the ASI appropriately. Although the ASI is widely used in treatment settings, some clinicians report that the ASI is too long and cumbersome to use, and many have been unable to use the instrument to develop a treatment plan. In addition, the ASI has been criticized for gender bias. An ASI-female version has been developed to address this criticism.

In addition to the ASI, some other comprehensive assessment instruments include the Comprehensive Drinkers' Profile, which is a comprehensive, semistructured assessment instrument designed to evaluate a client's specific problems controlling alcohol intake. The Global Appraisal of Individual Needs (GAIN) is a semistructured interview that requires 60 to 120 minutes to administer. It is designed as a standardized biopsychosocial assessment and can be used for diagnosis, to determine the need for service utilization, and to measure changes over time. The GAIN can also be administered by paper and pencil or on a computer.

The decision about levels of care for a client with a substance use disorder is important to make accurately in the beginning of treatment. The American Society of Addiction Medicine (ASAM) has developed a set of Patient Placement Criteria (PPC) intended to determine the client's optimal level of care. ASAM-PPC requires patients to be evaluated on six domains: (1) acute intoxication and/or withdrawal potential, (2) health conditions that may require medical supervision, (3) comorbid psychiatric conditions, (4) level of treatment resistance or acceptance, (5) relapse potential, and (6) nature of the patient's social environment. David Mee-Lee has developed a clinical interview called the Recovery Attitude and Treatment Evaluator, which has adequate statistical qualities across all six domains and can increase the validity and reliability of decisions about the ASAM-PPC.

Other Assessment Instruments

There are a number of other assessment instruments designed to provide information in specific areas related to treatment planning, For example, a client's motivation and readiness for change when seeking treatment can be assessed using one of several instruments: the University of Rhode Island Change Assessment, which measures motivation; Stages of Change, which assesses the client's stage of change; the Readiness for Change Questionnaire, which evaluates the client's readiness for change and treatment; or the Stages of Change Readiness and Treatment Eagerness, which is intended to assess problem recognition, ambivalence, and motivation to take action.

A client's treatment history can influence his or her acceptance of and resistance to treatment. The Center for Alcoholism, Substance Abuse and Addiction published an instrument called Lifetime Treatment History Interview to examine treatment history. There is a similar instrument for adolescents: the Teen Treatment Service Review.

Planning treatment for a client with alcohol use disorders needs to include an understanding of the consumption pattern of the client, level of craving for the substance, and high-risk situations for the client. Alcohol consumption patterns can be evaluated by using the Timeline Followback. This instrument provides information about daily, weekly, monthly, and yearly consumption of alcohol by using the past year's calendar for the client to recollect drinking events and levels. Another instrument to assess alcohol consumption patterns is the self-report Quantity-Frequency Index, which is less time consuming to administer than the Timeline Followback.

Several measures to assess craving for alcohol have been developed, including the Alcohol Urge Questionnaire, the Obsessive-Compulsive Drinking Scale, the Adolescents Obsessive-Compulsive Drinking Scale, and the Alcohol Craving Questionnaire.

Assessment of high-risk situations can assist clients in developing skills and strategies to stay sober. Examples of instruments designed to measure high-risk situations include the Inventory of Drinking Situations and the Situational Confidence Scale. Through gathering information about past year's drinking in eight different circumstances, both instruments provide information on the client's ability to cope with difficult situations. Both the Inventory of Drinking Situations and the Situational Confidence Scale have good psychometric qualities and are available in both paper-and-pencil and computerized versions.

Cognitive, emotional, and behavioral coping skills, as well as social networks, have an impact on substance use and abuse. There are a variety of instruments designed to examine these areas. For example, instruments assessing alcohol expectancies, such as the Comprehensive Effects of Alcohol Scale and the Alcohol Expectancy Questionnaire, can provide information about a client's motives for drinking. A client's perceived ability to change, as well as his or her skills to change can be measured with the Drinking Refusal Self-Efficacy Questionnaire or the Situation Confidence Questionnaire. The Coping Behaviors Inventory can help assess a client's cognitive and behavioral coping skills. Finally, a client's network and support can be assessed with the Important People and Activities Interview.

Conclusion

Assessment instruments can play an important role in the evaluation of, and treatment planning for, clients with suspected or already diagnosed substance use disorders. As with the use of any behavioral health assessment tool, it is important to determine that the assessment instrument has adequate psychometric qualities (normative procedures, reliability, validity), the normative population is consistent with the client's demographic characteristics, the purposes of the assessment instrument are congruent with the needs of the client, and the clinician is adequately trained to administer and interpret the assessment instruments. Comprehensive diagnostic assessment instruments can be time consuming but extremely valuable in diagnosis and treatment planning. A variety of instruments exist to measure specific areas related to substance abuse, treatment, and recovery.

Anne Helene Skinstad

See also Addiction Severity Index; Assessment; Diagnosis; Patient Placement Criteria; Psychosocial History; Screening Instruments; Self-Report Inventories; Timeline Followback

Further Readings

American Psychiatric Association. (2000). *Diagnostic and statistical manual of mental disorders* (4th ed., text rev.). Washington, DC: Author.

Committee on Cultural Psychiatry. (2002). *Cultural assessment in clinical psychiatry* (Group for the Advancement of Psychiatry, Report No. 145). Washington, DC: American Psychiatric Publishing.

Craig, R. J. (2005). *Clinical and diagnostic interviewing* (2nd ed.). Lanham, MD: Jason Aronson.

Donovan, D. M., & Marlatt, G. A. (2005). *Assessment of addictive behaviors* (2nd ed.). New York: Guilford Press.

Hunsley, J., & Mash, E. J. (2008). *A guide to assessments that work.* New York: Oxford University Press.

ATHLETES AND DRUG USE

The impact of performance-enhancing drugs in the world of athleticism is garnering more attention than the games that the athletes play. No longer in the locker rooms of muscular professional male athletes, performance-enhancing drugs have infiltrated their way into the lives of both the young and the old, the professional and the aspiring athlete. Drug use among athletes has grown from occasional speculation to full-blown federal investigations. The media have carved a space to inform the public of the result of various athletes suspected drug use whether it be performance enhancing or merely recreational in nature. The term *doping* refers to the use of anabolic steroids and other performance-enhancing drugs that are used to improve cardiovascular endurance, muscle size, or both. Doping, or *juicing*, as it is sometimes called, has garnered attention in the general public, but up until 2003, there were fewer than 30 empirical studies in the area of athletes and drug use. Performance-enhancing drugs, anabolic steroids or their derivatives, usually refer to the following classes of drugs.

Lean muscle mass builders are designed to increase lean muscle while decreasing overall body fat and adipose tissue. This class of drugs includes artificial growth hormones and testosterone-enhanced steroids.

Stimulants are used by athletes in an effort to increase speed, overall endurance, and attention span while training. Drugs classified as stimulants activate the central nervous system to an increased level of functioning and raise the metabolic processes in the body.

Analgesic drugs, drugs that eliminate or mask pain symptoms, are used to assist athletes with acute and chronic pain conditions that result from overtraining or improper training.

Muscle relaxers are often used to calm the tension in an athlete's body that usually results from sprains and strains associated with a high level of sport performance.

Diuretics are frequently used by athletes in an effort to control bloating and weight associated with water retention.

Drug adulteration products are masking agents used to eliminate the presence of other substances; these drugs are perhaps the most critical and sophisticated, as these drugs prevent authorities from detecting if an athlete is involved in the use of banned substances.

Some of the most notable side effects of these substances are heart attacks, strokes, dehydration, erratic behavior, and death. It is also important to note that the use of recreational drugs such as cocaine, marijuana, alcohol, ecstasy, heroin, and tobacco has increased among athletes as well. Reported use of these drugs seems to have diminished in media coverage in the wake of so many steroid scandals.

One of many publicized scandals about drug abuse in recent times was the admission by baseball celebrity Jose Canseco that many of the athletes in major league baseball were doping. The prevalence of such drug use continued to be a media spotlight as Olympic athletes and athletes from all sports and levels, including high school, middle school, and college, are regularly testing positive for such drugs.

There are many sports that have a relaxed drug tolerance policy, whereby career-ending consequences are invoked once a player has committed three or more offenses. Additionally, some major sports franchises have not been rigorous in testing athletes on a regular schedule. The World Anti-Doping Agency maintains a list of banned substances for athletes; however, drug testing and bans are not consistent across sports, making it increasingly difficult to decide which drugs are not considered harmful or worthy of legal sanctions. One of the most popular drugs, human growth hormone, is growing in popularity among users as there is no test that exists to detect its presence.

The detection of performance-enhancing drugs does not seem to be evolving at a rate quick enough to be deemed effective. The doctors, chemists, and laboratories are experiencing increasing difficulties catching the athletes abusing a banned drug that would impose a penalty on them and damage their careers. However, media exposure often convicts the athlete in question through the court of popular opinion. Often, athletes who exceed and break previously held world records are automatically up for media scrutiny and doubt. Barry Bonds has finally beaten out the legendary Hank Aaron and Babe Ruth; however, the sweet victory continues to remain bitter due to a cloud of speculation surrounding him and steroid abuse.

The need to perform at levels never thought possible seems to be the blame for the young athlete to look for the extra edge to beat out other classmates for a spot on a varsity team or squad. The push to ascertain a limited number of priceless scholarships seems to drive both parents and coaches toward sinister means of acquiring a first-string lineup. Even the thought of various side effects and death does not seem to deter those who are determined to run longer, jump higher, and move faster. Researchers are beginning to study the long-term effects of performance-enhancing drugs on both physiological and psychological responses. Recent deaths in the world of wrestling have prompted a renewed interest in the negative impacts that doping has on sports. There are but a handful of athletes that have confessed to using these drugs, because once they confess, it ends their career. One study has found that more than 50% of athletes agreed that they would potentially use a performance-enhancing drug for rehabilitation purposes. More specifically, these athletes were willing to risk using a banned substance if an injury were career threatening. Some researchers have begun to speculate that the use of illicit substances in sports is a tear in the moral fabric of societies, particularly those that are galvanized by their sports (e.g., the World Cup, Olympics), because the younger athletes are no longer driven to success by internal motivation, thereby decreasing the positive impact that is usually attributed to sports involvement. As the topic of athletes and drug use garners more attention, the U.S. government has

reined in top officials and players in sports franchises to testify before the Senate, House of Representatives, and numerous congressional hearings on the scope of banned substances in sports. While the exposure has brought about a few grand jury hearings, the consequences for athletes involved in drug use have been less than devastating. At present, sports franchises are unwilling to enforce any sort of zero-tolerance policy that includes the routine testing of 100% of their athletes.

Ireon Lebeauf

See also Anabolic Steroids; Drug Testing

Further Readings

Meldrum, R., & Feinberg, J. R. (2002). Drug use by college athletes: Is random testing an effective deterrent? *The Sport Journal, 5*(1). Retrieved June 16, 2008, from http://www.thesportjournal.org/article/drug-use-college-athletes-random-testing-effective-deterrent

Naylor, A. H., Gardner, D., & Zaichkowsky, L. (2001). Drug use patterns among high school athletes and non athletes. *Adolescence, 36,* 627–639.

ATTENTION DEFICIT HYPERACTIVITY DISORDER

A growing body of research indicates that there is a connection between attention deficit hyperactivity disorder (ADHD) and substance use disorders (SUD). Of adolescents and adults with with SUD, 30% to 50% and 15% to 25%, respectively, also have ADHD. Compared to individuals with SUD alone, adolescents and adults with ADHD and SUD have greater drug use severity, greater difficulty achieving abstinence, and higher rates of relapse.

The association between ADHD and SUD begs the question of whether treatment of ADHD in childhood lowers the risk of developing SUD. Numerous controlled studies have shown that psychostimulant treatment of ADHD improves school performance, psychosocial functioning, and associated behavior problems. More recent studies show that treatment of ADHD may reduce the risk of adolescent SUD by as much as half compared to children whose ADHD goes untreated.

Whereas the evidence supporting a linkage between ADHD and SUD has strengthened over the past decade, the reasons for the connection are more obscure. The data indicate that the incidence of SUD is highest in youth who have significant behavior problems with ADHD. Twenty-five percent to seventy-five percent of children and adolescents with ADHD also meet *DSM-IV* diagnostic criteria for oppositional defiant disorder or conduct disorder. Conduct disorder, characterized by a chronic pattern of antisocial behaviors that violate the rights of others, is the most common co-occurring disorder in adolescents with SUD (60%–80%), followed by ADHD (30%–50%). Longitudinal studies indicate that the combination of ADHD and conduct disorder imparts the highest risk of adolescent substance abuse as well as higher rates of school failure, risky behaviors (including motor vehicle accidents), and association with a deviant peer group.

In a 19-year longitudinal study conducted by the Mayo Clinic, researchers concluded that psychostimulant medication treatment for childhood ADHD conferred a protective effect (especially for boys) against SUD when the youths were 15 to 21 years of age compared to those whose ADHD went untreated. The findings held even for the subset of children with both ADHD and comorbid conduct disorder, which raises the risk of drug abuse even more than ADHD alone. All untreated children with both ADHD and conduct disorder developed SUD; treatment reduced the number by about half.

Numerous controlled trials support the safety and efficacy of psychostimulant medications—and more recently, nonstimulant (e.g., atomoxetine) medications—for ADHD in children and adolescents without SUD. Because individuals with active substance abuse have traditionally been excluded from medication trials, less is known about the safety, efficacy, or abuse liability of psychostimulants in individuals with both ADHD and SUD. Results from two controlled trials in adults and one trial in adolescents indicate that psychostimulant medication may be relatively safe and effective for ADHD even in individuals who have not yet achieved abstinence. Results also indicate that pharmacotherapy for ADHD alone has little to no impact on active drug use.

More research is needed with larger sample sizes to determine whether pharmacotherapy for ADHD improves treatment outcomes for SUD when treatment for both disorders is concurrent. One such study is currently under way in the National Institute on Drug Abuse Clinical Trials Network. The study is a randomized controlled trial of osmotic-release methylphenidate in adolescents with ADHD receiving concurrent cognitive behavioral therapy for SUD. The aims of the study are to evaluate the safety, efficacy, and abuse liability of the long-acting psychostimulant for ADHD as well as the impact of treating ADHD on drug use and substance treatment retention and outcomes.

Caution must be exercised in drawing clinical implications from limited research. On the other hand, it is important for clinicians and researchers to use the data available to develop empirically based treatment guidelines. Such an approach should include a structured diagnostic interview that generates *DSM* psychiatric and substance diagnoses. Clinical and diagnostic formulations may be enhanced by the use of a lifetime timeline onto which significant events from developmental, family, educational, work, medical, and psychosocial history can be mapped along with the onset and progression of psychiatric symptoms and substance use. This longitudinal lifetime approach is especially useful when evaluating ADHD given the early childhood onset of impairing symptoms and nonepisodic course across development.

If the diagnosis of ADHD is confirmed in addition to SUD, treatment should be initiated with an evidence-based behavioral intervention for SUD that includes regular urine drug screening. Pharmacotherapy for ADHD may be considered once the patient is engaged and compliant with substance treatment, preferably with some evidence of reduction in drug use. Although abstinence is ideal before initiating pharmacotherapy, this may not be a realistic goal for many patients before treatment of their ADHD. Long-acting, sustained-release psychostimulants or nonstimulant medications should be considered over short-acting, immediate-release psychostimulants in dually diagnosed patients. It is important that ongoing drug use be systematically assessed in conjunction with adverse side effects and ADHD target symptom response. Regular clinical monitoring of medication response, ongoing drug use, drug treatment compliance, and careful tracking of prescription refill and dispensing practices are key components of successful treatment and ongoing clinical management of dually diagnosed patients.

Patricia Katherine Riggs and Paula Riggs

See also Antisocial Personality Disorder; Co-Occurring
Disorders; *Diagnostic and Statistical Manual of Mental
Disorders*; Evidence-Based Treatment; National Institute
on Drug Abuse Clinical Trials Network

Further Readings

Kratochvil, C. J., Wilens, T. E., & Upadhyaya, H. (2006).
Pharmacological management of a youth with ADHD,
marijuana use, and mood symptoms. *Journal of the
American Academy of Child Adolescent Psychiatry,
45*, 1138–1141.

Riggs, P. D. (2003). Treating adolescents for substance use
and comorbid psychiatric disorders. *Science & Practice
Perspectives, 2*(1), 18–29.

Riggs, P. D., Mikulich-Gilbertson, S. K., Davies, R. D.,
Lohman, M., Klein, C., & Stover, S. (2007). A
randomized controlled trial of fluoxetine and cognitive
behavioral therapy in adolescents with major
depression, behavior problems and substance use
disorders. *Archives of Pediatrics & Adolescent
Medicine, 161*(11), 1–9.

Wilens, T. E., Faraone, S. V., Biederman, J., & Gunawardene,
S. (2003). Does stimulant therapy of attention-deficit/
hyperactivity disorder beget later substance abuse?
A meta-analytic review of the literature. *Pediatrics,
111*(1), 179–185.

AVERSIVE CONDITIONING

See AVERSIVE THERAPY

AVERSIVE THERAPY

Aversive control is a method for changing or controlling unwanted behavior. In the clinical setting this is
referred to as aversive therapy. With aversive control,
behavior is changed or controlled with the implementation of certain operant conditioning and classical
conditioning techniques that include the use of an
aversive stimulus, one that is unpleasant or painful. In
the case of operant conditioning, this could include
controlling behavior with the removal of a pleasant
stimulus or the presentation of an unpleasant or
painful stimulus. Techniques that exemplify these
operant conditioning approaches are timeout and

delivery of electric shock. Examples of techniques
that involve classical conditioning implemented aversive control involve pairing an unpleasant or noxious
stimulus with a neutral or pleasant stimulus.
Examples include pairing the taste of an alcoholic
beverage with being ill or pairing an imagined aversive event with images of drinking.

Aversive control has been used as a treatment for
drug abuse, as well as a variety of other behaviors
including eating disorders, bed-wetting, self-injurious
behaviors, compulsive gambling, and specific behaviors in psychotic patients. Due to the ethical concerns of
exposing patients to unpleasant or painful stimuli, aversive control is typically used when nonaversive treatments have failed. Also, aversive control measures have
been shown to be most effective when they are incorporated into a broader treatment plan that addresses the
multiple factors that contribute to a problem behavior.

Modern usage of aversive control can be traced to
the conditioning studies of Russian physiologist Ivan
Pavlov that were done in the 1890s and early 1900s.
In what has come to be known as classical conditioning, Pavlov showed that a stimulus that does not elicit
a reflexive response can be trained to do so if it is
paired with a stimulus that does. An example of an
area in drug abuse treatment where these principles
have been applied is treatment for alcoholism. A drug
(e.g., disulfiram) is administered to the patient. If
alcohol is then consumed, unpleasant symptoms such
as nausea, vomiting, and palpitation can occur.
Alcohol consumption is thereby paired with becoming ill and hopefully the patient will be less likely
to drink in the future. This type of learning, however,
tends to be very context specific. For long-term abstinence, measures must be taken to ensure that the
learning is generalized to a variety of settings where
alcohol will be encountered.

The approach of operant conditioning is different
from that of classical conditioning. Whereas classical
conditioning is concerned with pairing of stimuli and
the resulting reflexive behavior, operant conditioning
focuses on controlling the consequences of voluntary
behavior. There are two types of control in operant
conditioning that are considered aversive. Both
decrease the frequency of undesirable behavior. An
undesirable behavior can be decreased by the removal
of a pleasant stimulus when the behavior occurs or
by presenting an unpleasant stimulus.

Some behavior management approaches such as
contingency management have been designed to both

reinforce desired behavior and punish undesired behavior by removal of an appetitive stimulus. Thus, contingency management can include both aversive and appetitive conditioning. For example, clients receive reinforcement at an increasing rate at predetermined intervals for abstinence from a given substance (appetitive). If the client uses alcohol or other drugs, no reward is given, and the amount of reward that would be given in the future is decreased (aversive).

A major theory of how aversive control works is O. H. Mower's two-factor theory, which posits that both classical and operant conditioning are involved in the conditioning process. According to this theory, the aversive stimulus comes to elicit fear by means of classical conditioning. For example, the alcoholic beverage comes to elicit the fear of becoming ill. After this learning has occurred an avoidance or escape response, which is an operant response, will be made to reduce or eliminate contact with the aversive stimulus. Continuing the above example, the patient would avoid contact with the alcoholic beverage and seek to escape it if it were present.

Robert Packer and John M. Roll

See also Antabuse (Disulfiram); Behavioral Therapy; Contingency Management

Further Readings

Brush, F. R. (Ed.). (1971). *Aversive conditioning and learning.* New York: Academic Press.
Sidman, M. (1989). *Coercion and its fallout.* Boston: Authors Cooperative.

B

BARBITURATES

Barbiturates fall under the category of sedative-hypnotics. Barbiturates are used for calming, relaxation, and sedation so they may also be referred to as central nervous system depressants. At higher doses, barbiturates can be used for inducing sleep. Nicknamed after their colorful appearance, slang terms for barbiturates include *phennies, redbirds, tooies, reds, yellow jackets, barbs,* and *yellows.*

History

Adolph von Baeyer is credited with the discovery of barbiturates in 1863. Synthesizing uric acid, he named it *barbituric acid*, or *barbiturates*. It is said the name was derived from the Day of Saint Barbara. Von Baeyer celebrated his discovery at a tavern with army officers commemorating the day in honor of the artillerymen patron saint. Barbital was the first medical application of barbiturates. In 1903, barbital was first used for treating nervousness and anxiety. The brand name of barbital as it was introduced was Veronal. The second barbiturate introduced to the market came in 1912. Called phenobarbital, it also was used to treat anxiety and to induce relaxation. The names of barbiturates all end in *-al*. This indicates a chemical relationship to barbital. These barbiturates soon became the replacement for bromides, and they were used mainly for anxiety. Although barbiturates were first thought of as safe and effective, problems soon surfaced with overdoses and users developing dependence and tolerance. Today, barbiturates are used only in a limited capacity for anxiety.

Sedative-hypnotics have enjoyed widespread popularity, particularly throughout the 1960s and 1970s. Due to overprescription, thousands of people, particularly American women, became dependent upon them. Prescriptions for barbiturates are on the decline recently, however, as other drugs are not as likely to lead to dependency and can be less toxic. Today, barbiturates have been replaced mainly by a separate category of drugs, benzodiazepines, which have a larger margin of safety. With their dwindling popularity, barbiturates account for less than 10% of U.S. depressant prescriptions. Barbiturates are primarily prescribed as sleeping pills, followed by use for specific convulsive disorders. Short-acting barbiturates are indicated for some anesthetic reasons. For example, thiopental can minimize brain swelling and cerebral pressure while improving blood circulation during surgery.

Types

There are four different classifications for barbiturates. Depending on the length of time they act and their potency, they can be ultra short acting, short acting (4 hours or under), intermediate acting (4–6 hours), or long acting (longer than 6 hours). As their name suggests, short-acting barbiturates take less time to begin working than long-acting barbiturates. Additionally, the effects of short-acting barbiturates do not last for very long. Because short-acting barbiturates take effect quickly, their abuse potential is much higher than for slow-acting drugs. Although barbiturates are classified based upon their acting time, other factors can interfere with the effects. Dosage, body composition differences between

113

users, and administration of the drug can all influence the length of time it takes barbiturates to begin working. As a controlled substance, use of barbiturates is illegal without a prescription. Depending on the barbiturate type, they may be classified as Schedule II, III, or IV on the federal classification of controlled substances and can be effective from 1 to 16 hours depending on the dosage.

Effects

Barbiturates resemble alcohol in their short-term behavioral and psychological effects. As a central nervous system (CNS) depressant, barbiturates create a depressed effect on the user. Activities that require hand–eye coordination or concentration are not advised while under the influence of barbiturates. For example, driving a car is not recommended because in addition to other effects, reaction time and energy levels are adversely affected. Emotionally, rage and hostility are often seen after taking barbiturates. However, a variety of factors can affect how barbiturates influence users, including the setting in which the drug is taken and any previous experiences the user has had with the drug. In general, the side effects of barbiturates can include nausea, vomiting, impaired cognitive functioning, reduced attention span, diminished hand–eye coordination, confusion, poor judgment, slurred speech, vertigo, diarrhea, birth defects, respiratory failure, and violent behavior. With some users, barbiturates are taken to counter the effects of stimulant drugs. They can be taken to attempt sleep after amphetamine use or to ease the pain of heroin withdrawal. Chronic barbiturate users can develop a tolerance to their effects. A cross-tolerance to drugs that are chemically similar (such as minor tranquilizers or alcohol) can also develop in users. Dependence can occur in as little as 4 to 6 weeks if barbiturates are taken daily in large quantities (800–1,000 milligrams). Through drug testing, barbiturates can be detected up to 5 days after use.

Dangers

The possible dangers associated with barbiturate use vary greatly from fatigue to death by overdose. On the mild side, effects can include vomiting, diarrhea, nausea, vertigo, and emotional distress. Because barbiturates can depress breathing, oxygen may have difficulty getting to the bloodstream. Additionally,

blood pressure is automatically lowered because the heartbeat is also depressed. Depressed breathing and lowered blood pressure, in combination, can lead to shock, coma, and even death. Barbiturates taken during pregnancy often lead to infant dependency, brain damage, birth defects or fetal death due to lack of oxygen. Newborns going through barbiturate withdrawal experience symptoms similar to adults. Barbiturates taken with any other depressant, especially alcohol, produce a synergistic effect. This means the effects of the barbiturates and the alcohol are intensified when taken together. Accidental or even intentional death can be a side effect of barbiturates taken with alcohol. Withdrawal, which occurs when barbiturates leave the bloodstream of an addicted person, can be life threatening if not medically supervised. Withdrawal is a severe and painful physical and emotional process that includes excessive sweating, paranoia, vomiting, cramps, quick temper, insomnia, muscular twitching, aches and pains, and, in some instances, even seizures, hallucinations, and nightmares. Rebound insomnia is often found in people withdrawing from barbiturates. Although barbiturates are indicated as sleep aids, they actually interfere with rapid eye movement (REM), which is essential for quality and restful sleep. In fact, hallucination and difficulty concentrating can be the result of REM deprivation. Because of this, people who take sleeping pills can actually wake up more tired than before they went to sleep. Over time, barbiturates can be considered damaging to long-term sleep habits.

Maria Theresa Wessel, Jeanne Martino-McAllister,
and Elizabeth C. Gallon

See also Alcohol; Benzodiazepines; Central Nervous System Depressants; Drugs, Classification of

Further Readings

Ballas, P. (2006). *Barbiturate intoxication and overdose.* Retrieved September 18, 2007, from http://www.nlm.nih .gov/medlineplus/ency/article/000951.htm

Goldberg, R. (2006). Sedative-hypnotic drugs. In *Drugs across the spectrum* (5th ed., pp. 169–178). Pacific Grove, CA: Brooks/Cole.

Hanson, G. R., Venturelli, P. J., & Fleckstein, A. E. (2006). CNS depressants: Sedative-hypnotics. In *Drugs and society* (9th ed., pp. 164–174). Boston: Jones and Bartlett.

National Institute on Drug Abuse. (2007, February 28). *Prescription drug abuse chart.* Retrieved October 8, 2007, from http://www.drugabuse.gov/DrugPages/ PrescripDrugsChart.html

Behavioral Couples Therapy

Couples in which a partner abuses alcohol or other drugs often have moderate to severe relationship dissatisfaction, often engage in high levels of marital conflict, and experience frequent instability. Poor interactions and couple stress often contribute to problematic substance use and relapse. As such, behavioral couples therapy (BCT) was adapted for use with substance-abusing couples in an effort to help the family break the cycle of abuse and relapse and teach spouses productive responses to alcohol-related or drug use situations, thereby reducing substance use and decreasing the perpetuating interactions between the user and their partner. BCT involves teaching couples skills that promote partner support for abstinence and emphasize reduction of common relationship problems and improvements in relationship functioning.

Treatment Components, Efficacy, and Cost-Effectiveness

BCT evolved from early behavioral approaches to martial therapy. Early forms of behavior marital therapy incorporated traditional behavioral theory principles, including operant conditioning, positive reinforcement, punishment, negative reinforcement, and behavioral contracting. In operant conditioning, it is assumed that behavior is a function of its antecedents and consequences. Behavior that is rewarded is maintained or increased via positive reinforcement. Negative reinforcement involves the reduction of an undesired behavior in order to eliminate a negative stimulus. Punishment entails an aversive condition to reduce a negative behavior.

In recent years, BCT has assimilated concepts from Bandura's social learning theory (e.g., modeling and cognition) and Thibaut and Kelley's social exchange theory (e.g., negative reciprocity and coercion), as well as other theoretical approaches and techniques. It is important to recognize that several distinct types of therapy have coalesced under the name BCT. As such, behavioral couples therapists employ many different techniques. Each approach focuses on changing concrete behaviors to reduce negative exchanges and increase positive couple interactions by means of building on communication skills and developing positive contingent behavioral exchanges. Although BCT is a common name for this form of therapy, other names, such as behavioral martial therapy, also are used in the literature.

BCT Treatment Elements

In the initial sessions, the therapist delivering BCT works to develop partner support for maintaining abstinence. Together, the couple and the therapist develop a "recovery contract" in which the partners agree to engage in a daily "abstinence trust agreement." In this brief exchange, the substance-abusing partner states his or her intent not to drink or use drugs that day. In turn, the non-substance-abusing partner verbally states his or her support for the partner's intent to remain sober. The non-substance-abusing partner monitors the performance of the abstinence truth discussion (and consumption of the substance-abusing partner's abstinence-related medications or attendance at support group meetings if appropriate) on a recovery calendar, provided by the therapist. The calendar provides a visual daily inspection of recovery progress. An important part of the recovery contract is for partners to agree not to discuss past drinking or drug use or fears of future substance use outside of the therapy sessions. In the beginning of each BCT session, the therapist reviews the BCT recovery contract. To emphasize the importance of the contract, the couples are asked to practice behaviors that are part of the contract.

After the initial sessions that focus on establishing the recovery contract and reducing conflicts about past or future substance use, the counselor adds another key element: relationship-focused interventions. Relationship-focused interventions are designed to increase positive feelings, shared activities, and constructive communication and to reduce negative patterns of interaction. For instance, Catch Your Partner Doing Something Nice asks partners to acknowledge their partner doing something nice each day. In the Caring Day assignment, each partner chooses an activity to demonstrate their care toward his or her partner. In Shared Rewarding activities, the couple plans and engages in mutually enjoyable activities. An equally important aspect of BCT is teaching effective communication skills, especially with respect to areas of conflict.

When abstinence is maintained, the therapist plans for continuing recovery to prevent or minimize relapse and begins to reduce weekly BCT sessions.

Effectiveness of BCT

BCT has been associated with reduced drinking outcomes, improved relationship functioning and stability, and decreased domestic violence among married and cohabitating male alcoholics and their non-substance-abusing female partners. Specific objectives of BCT (i.e., positive communication skills, partner support, shared activities, and negotiation of agreements) have also been positively correlated with marital satisfaction in couples taking part in BCT and post–alcohol treatment abstinence. However, not all couples demonstrate relationship benefits from BCT. In addition, some substance-abusing partners relapse during treatment or follow-up. For this reason, relapse prevention boosters are strongly recommended. Unfortunately, such booster sessions are rarely implemented in practice.

BCT also is effective for many drug-using patients (mostly cocaine and heroin users), methadone maintenance patients, and heroin patients taking naltrexone, as well as the partners of these patients. In 1996, Fals-Stewart, Birchler, and O'Farrell conducted the first study of the effectiveness of BCT for drug use. They showed that, compared to patients who received individual treatment alone, those who received BCT showed decreased drug use, legal involvement, relapse, and hospitalizations. Similar benefits have been shown for female patients. That is, compared to female patients who received an equally intensive individual therapy for drug use, female patients and their non-substance-abusing male partners randomly assigned to receive BCT appeared to have fewer days of substance use; longer periods of continuous abstinence; lower levels of alcohol, drug, and family problems; and greater relationship satisfaction. Studies also have demonstrated that compared to more traditional individual-based interventions, BCT may be more effective in reducing intimate partner violence and HIV-risk behaviors.

Researchers have also demonstrated that BCT, combined with individual counseling for the substance-abusing parent, may have secondary benefits or trickle-down effects for children in their homes. More specifically, studies have shown that children whose fathers participated in BCT for drug or alcohol use, combined with individual counseling, showed greater improvement in emotional and behavioral symptoms at posttreatment and during 12-month follow-up compared to children whose parents participated in individual-based treatment or in a control group. Recently, studies have examined whether parents' participation in BCT for fathers' alcohol abuse or fathers' drug use has equal secondary benefits for children at markedly different developmental stages. Results of both studies demonstrated that reductions in paternal substance use and improvements in couple functioning were related to decreased internalizing and externalizing symptoms for preadolescent children in their homes. However, improvements in parent and couple functioning did not appear to have secondary benefits for adolescent children in their homes. It is critical to understand whether couples-based treatments may have secondary or indirect benefits for children in their homes.

Cost-Effectiveness of BCT

The inflation of mental health care costs has resulted in attention to the cost of various mental health treatments. Unfortunately, the focus of much of this attention has been on cost containment rather than treatment effectiveness. Although standard BCT is more costly to deliver as compared to shortened versions of BCT, individual-based treatment, or psychoeducational attention control treatment, the cost of delivery for standard BCT appears to be offset by some of the improvements in physical and mental health status (e.g., hospital stays) and reductions in legal problems (e.g., jail stays) associated with standard BCT participation. Therefore, BCT appears cost effective (cost of clinical treatment versus clinical outcome).

A growing number of studies have also demonstrated the cost benefits of modified versions of BCT as compared to other types of treatments. For instance, brief relationship therapy (BRT) is a shortened version of the standard BCT treatment with a greater focus on dyadic support and a reduced focus on communication skills training as compared to standard BCT. BRT was found to be of equal clinical effectiveness when compared to standard BCT. Both treatments were more clinically efficacious than individual-based treatment and a psychoeducational control condition, but the cost-effectiveness of BRT was better than that of standard BCT.

Future of BCT

BCT has demonstrated clinical efficacy in reducing drinking and drug use behaviors, decreasing maladaptive relationship functioning, and improving relationship satisfaction for many patients and their families. However, the BCT literature has several limitations. BCT is often part of a comprehensive treatment program that includes individual and group therapy for the substance-abusing individual. In addition, patients and their partners may attend support groups at the time of treatment or after treatment occurs (e.g., AA, NA, Al-Anon). Whether participation in support groups is related to the effectiveness of BCT is not known. Future research should attempt to clarify the impact of each of these interventions for substance use and relationship outcomes.

Also, the focus of BCT efficacy research has been on patient and family outcomes. However, the underlying mechanisms of change are largely unknown (i.e., How does BCT work? What processes are altered within the family?). In addition, little research has examined couples beyond the 18-month to 2-year mark. Moreover, relapse prevention boosters are highly recommended but often not in place. Clearly, long-term follow-up, as well as the effectiveness of "boosters" to prevent or contend with relapse, is critical in this type of research. In addition, BCT is not effective for all couples. A better understanding of couples that may benefit from other treatment approaches is critically needed.

The potential secondary benefits or trickle-down effects of BCT for children in the homes of substance users and abusers is an emerging area of research. Given the risk associated for children in these homes, the importance of BCT for reducing negative child behaviors (e.g., aggression, academic problems, substance use) and improving parent–child interactions (e.g., discipline, child monitoring) is of critical importance. Moreover, how BCT may benefit families by reducing foster care and other types of social services intervention are important avenues for future research. In addition, other family members (e.g., parents or adult children) may be affected by decisions to enter treatment. Little research has examined whether BCT has secondary benefits for extended family members and adult children who may be affected by substance abuse and subsequent recovery.

Although research has demonstrated the effectiveness of BCT for alcoholism and drug use for heterosexual White and African American couples, additional studies of the effectiveness of BCT for gay and lesbian couples are needed. In addition, studies examining the clinical efficacy and cost-effectiveness of BCT have generally compared standard BCT to modified or shorter versions of BCT or to individual-based therapy or psychoeducational control conditions. Clearly, research examining the clinical efficacy and cost-effectiveness of BCT relative to other available treatments (e.g., group treatment) is necessary.

Although BCT is potentially beneficial for couples in which one partner abuses substances, few community programs offer couples-based therapy. In part, this may reflect the reluctance of insurance companies to pay for longer, more structured, couples-based programs. An additional concern is the degree to which training programs teach couples-based therapeutic approaches. Clearly, both of these issues remain problematic.

Michelle L. Kelley, Amanda Jeffrey Platter,
and William Fals-Stewart

See also Counseling Approaches; Evidence-Based Treatment; Treatment Effectiveness; Treatment of Alcohol and Other Drugs; Violence, Intimate Partner and Substance Abuse Treatment

Further Readings

Epstein, E. E., & McCrady, B. S. (1998). Behavioral couples treatment of alcohol and drug use disorders: Current status and innovations. *Clinical Psychology Review, 18,* 689–711.

Fals-Stewart, W., Birchler, G. R., & O'Farrell, T. J. (1996). Behavioral couples therapy for male substance-abusing patients: Effects on relationship adjustment and drug-using behavioral. *Journal of Consulting and Clinical Psychology, 64,* 959–972.

Fals-Stewart, W., Klostermann, K., Yates, B. T., O'Farrell, T. J., & Birchler, G. (2005). Brief relationship therapy for alcoholism: A randomized clinical trial examining clinical efficacy and cost effectiveness. *Psychology of Addictive Behaviors, 19,* 363–371.

Fals-Stewart, W., O'Farrell, T. J., Birchler, G. R, Cordova, J., & Kelley, M. L. (2005). Behavioral couples therapy for alcoholism and drug abuse: Where we've been, where we are and where we're going. *Journal of Cognitive Psychotherapy: An International Quarterly, 19,* 229–246.

Kelley, M. L., & Fals-Stewart, W. (2007). Treating paternal alcoholism using Learning Sobriety Together: Effects on adolescents versus preadolescents. *Journal of Family Psychology, 21*(3), 435-444.

McCrady, B., Stout, N., Noel, N., Abrams, D., & Nelson, H. (1991). Comparative effectiveness of three types of spouse involved alcohol treatment: Outcomes 18 months after treatment. *British Journal of Addiction, 86,* 1415–1424.

O'Farrell, T. J., & Fals-Stewart, W. (2006). *Behavioral couples therapy for alcoholism and drug abuse.* New York: Guilford Press.

Sayers, S. L., & Heyman, R. E. (2003). Behavioral couples therapy. In G. Sholevar & G. Pirooz (Eds.), *Textbook of family and couples therapy: Clinical applications* (pp. 461–500). Washington, DC: American Psychiatric Publishing.

BEHAVIORAL RISK FACTOR SURVEILLANCE SYSTEM

The Behavioral Risk Factor Surveillance System (BRFSS) is a telephone health survey that is conducted by the Centers for Diseases Control and Prevention (CDC) in collaboration with state health departments. The purpose of the BRFSS is to determine the prevalence of health risk behaviors (e.g., alcohol use, tobacco use, obesity) and protective health practices (e.g., using seat belts, routine screenings for cancer) among noninstitutionalized adults age 18 and over, which are related to the onset of chronic illness and injury. The morbidity (prevalence or incidence) and mortality (causing death) of diseases vary widely by geographic area and demographic constituency. Therefore, the survey is stratified by state to gain a more comprehensive understanding of the distribution of health behaviors and statuses across regions. State-level data can later be combined or further stratified to determine national or local rates of health-related behaviors, respectively. The BRFSS aids public health authorities in identifying developing threats to public health, supporting public health legislation, and designing health initiatives and policy with the ultimate goal of promoting well-being and preventing the onset of disease.

The CDC developed the BFRSS in the early 1980s after overwhelming empirical evidence indicated that individuals' health behaviors were associated with injury and the early onset of chronic illness. From 1981 to 1983, the CDC orchestrated the collection of pilot data in 29 states to determine the feasibility of using telephone surveys to gather behavioral health information. In 1984, the CDC officially created the BRFSS and began data collection in 15 states. Since its inception, the surveillance system has rapidly expanded to include all 50 states, as well as the District of Columbia, Puerto Rico, the U.S. Virgin Islands, and Guam. Every month, staff from each state or territory's health department use random-digit dialing methodology to identify potential participants. One adult per household (landline) is contacted and invited to participate in the health survey. No compensation is offered. Worldwide, the BRFSS is currently the largest telephone health survey with information on over 350,000 adults being collected annually.

The BRFSS questionnaire is divided into three parts: the core (fixed, rotating, and emerging), optional modules, and state-added questions. Core questions are asked verbatim in every state and focus on current health status, demographics, health care access, preventative health care practices (e.g., screenings for prostrate and breast cancer, seat belt use), and health risk behaviors (e.g., alcohol use, tobacco use, obesity). They also gather information on the rates of specific illnesses, such as diabetes, asthma, and cardiovascular disease. Fixed core questions are asked yearly, and rotating core questions are asked every other year; rotating questions are available as optional modules in alternate years. Emerging core questions target developing health care concerns. The utility of these questions is evaluated after 1 year, at which point it is decided if the question will be included on future questionnaires and, if so, whether it will remain a part of the core or appear as an optional module. The CDC holds an annual BRFSS meeting during which new questions are proposed and reviewed for their scientific merit and public health value. In general, the purpose of emerging core questions is to evaluate issues of immediate concern. Thus, these questions tend to undergo less rigorous examination prior to inclusion than is typical of less pressing proposed additions.

The BRFSS survey also contains optional modules to be administered at each state's discretion based on its needs. Optional modules are sanctioned by the CDC (i.e., the CDC provides funding, support, and data analysis for these questions) and include topics such as childhood immunizations, domestic and sexual violence, family planning, and smokeless tobacco. In addition, states may elect to supplement the survey with their own state-added questions, which are not officially part of the BRFSS or sanctioned by the CDC. As such, the data and costs resulting from these inquiries are solely the state's responsibility.

Because of its multiple organizational resources and expertise, the CDC is responsible for funding the BRFSS and providing technical support to the state health departments, as well as aggregating each state's data after every collection point. Subsequent to compilation by the CDC, the data are given back to the states to disseminate and use as they see fit. All of the BRFSS questionnaires (including Spanish versions), coding manuals, data, and related information can be accessed by the public at the BRFSS Web site (http://www.cdc.gov/brfss). The Web site also includes the list of the optional modules and state-added questions that were administered in each state by calendar year. Data yielded by the BRFSS can be used by anyone, provided that the source of the data is appropriately acknowledged.

Results from the BRFSS have many applications. For example, research clearly shows an association between hazardous levels of alcohol consumption and the morbidity and mortality of a range of chronic diseases (e.g., cirrhosis of the liver, certain cancers). Furthermore, hazardous drinking is related to bodily injury, such as those injuries sustained in drinking and driving accidents. Accordingly, two sections included in the core of the BRFSS are alcohol consumption and drinking and driving. The first module inquires about the prevalence, frequency, and quantity of drinking, and the latter asks the number of times the participant has driven while under the influence of alcohol in the past 30 days. Taken together, these measures of drinking and related health risk behaviors may help public health officials to gauge the scope of alcohol-related problems and develop health initiatives to promote responsible drinking. Alternatively, the BRFSS can be used to monitor trends in drinking behavior across time to evaluate the impact of public health programs geared at reducing hazardous drinking and consequent problems.

Overall, the BRFSS is a useful research tool that provides a wide range of health-related information in a timely manner. In addition to local, state, and federal health departments, many other organizations, such as the American Heart Association and the American Cancer Society, rely on the BRFSS to provide statistics regarding the morbidity and mortality of various diseases. On the basis of survey results, interventions and health care initiatives targeting specific problem areas can be developed to promote healthy living and prevent health risk behaviors associated with chronic disease, disability, and death.

Katherine W. Follansbee and Gregory L. Stuart

See also High-Risk Behaviors; Monitoring the Future; National Epidemiologic Survey on Alcohol and Related Conditions; National Survey on Drug Use and Health

Further Readings

Centers for Disease Control and Prevention. (2006). *Behavioral Risk Factor Surveillance System Survey questionnaire*. Atlanta, GA: Author.

Centers for Disease Control and Prevention. (2008). *Behavioral Risk Factor Surveillance System*. Retrieved May 9, 2008, from http://www.cdc.gov/brfss

Figgs, L. W., Bloom, Y., & Dugbatey, K. (2000). Uses of Behavioral Risk Factor Surveillance System data, 1993–1997. *American Journal of Public Health, 90,* 774–776.

Stein, A. D., Lederman, R. I., & Shea, S. (1993). The Behavioral Risk Factor Surveillance System questionnaire: Its reliability in a statewide sample. *American Journal of Public Health, 83,* 1768–1772.

BEHAVIORAL THERAPY

See BEHAVIORAL COUPLES THERAPY; COGNITIVE BEHAVIORAL THERAPY; CONTINGENCY MANAGEMENT

BENZODIAZEPINES

Benzodiazepines are a family of psychotropic drugs that produce a hypnotic and sedative effect. They are central nervous system (CNS) depressants that are typically used as minor tranquilizers. Since the 1960s, benzodiazepines have been a popular medication and safer option than barbiturates in treating symptoms associated with anxiety and sleep disorders. Commonly prescribed and well-known benzodiazepines include alprazolam (Xanax), diazepam (Valium), chlordiazepoxide (Librium), temazepam (Restoril), and triazolam (Halcion). As a result of the beneficial anxiolytic and soporific properties, benzodiazepines have a high potential for abuse and dependence. They are among the most commonly abused prescription drugs.

There are many therapeutic uses for benzodiazepines as they safely manage and treat a variety of conditions. Benzodiazepines are most predominantly prescribed for anxiety, elevated stress in fear-evoking situations and other symptoms associated with anxiety disorders (i.e., panic attacks, generalized anxiety disorder, post-traumatic stress disorder). Benzodiazepines are often used to treat insomnia and other sleep disorders. Certain benzodiazepines have been approved as anticonvulsants for seizures caused by forms of epilepsy and delirium tremens related to alcohol dependence. Other therapeutic uses include myorelaxants (muscle relaxation), medication before surgical procedures (as a light anesthetic), and sedation of patients on mechanical ventilation in intensive care. When used correctly, benzodiazepines can be advantageous across a wide range of symptoms and disorders.

Although there are as many as 50 benzodiazepines marketed worldwide, they all have the same mechanism of action, which is associated with affecting the neurotransmitter gamma-aminobutyric acid (GABA). Therefore, all benzodiazepines produce a similar effect within a range of intensity. The variation of intensity among the different benzodiazepines is due to speed of elimination (half-life) and duration of effect. They can be divided into three groups: short-acting, intermediate-acting and long-acting. This classification is based on the half-life of each drug. The half-life is the time it takes for the substance's concentration in the blood to decrease to half its initial level after a single dose. Consequently, the half-life determines the length of time the drug is active (duration of effect).

The three groups are used to determine which benzodiazepine is the best fit for treatment. Short-acting benzodiazepines have a half-life of less than 12 hours and are best utilized for the short-term management of insomnia and related symptoms. These include estazolam (ProSom), temazepam (Restoril), and triazolam (Halcion), which facilitate sleep and assist the individual in staying asleep. Due to the short half-life, they yield little residual effect (hangover) but are quicker to produce tolerance. The intermediate-acting compounds are characterized by a half-life of between 12 and 24 hours, and long-acting benzodiazepines have a half-life greater than 24 hours. The intermediate- and long-acting benzodiazepines, such as lorazepam (Ativan), clonazepam (Klonopin), and diazepam (Valium), are more generally used as anxiolytics. Long-acting compounds accumulate in the bloodstream with use over time. This buildup may ease withdrawal symptoms (which often mimic the initial complaint) or enhance the effect as the drug is compounded. Regardless of the length of the half-life, all benzodiazepines have potential for tolerance and sometimes dependence.

Although the therapeutic advantages are great, benzodiazepines produce side effects. Common side effects, though often mild, include drowsiness, dizziness, weakness, confusion, and other cognitive impairments. Benzodiazepines can also produce slurred speech, ataxia, and impairment of psychomotor skills. Drug interactions can occur, and when used in combination with other substances, the latter mentioned side effects are compounded. A fatality resulting from an overdose of benzodiazepines alone is rare, but the risk of death is greatly increased when benzodiazepines are combined with other CNS depressants (e.g., alcohol, barbiturates).

Tolerance to benzodiazepines may occur, especially with long-term users. Tolerance to the soporific effect develops more rapidly (within days) than do the anxiolytic effects. Long-term use of benzodiazepines leads to a decrease in effectiveness and efficacy as well as an increase in the risk of negative side effects. The optimal therapeutic consumption of benzodiazepines is limited to a few weeks (2–4 weeks), though intermittent and occasional use can still be effective over time. As tolerance develops, some benzodiazepine users will progressively increase their dose to obtain the original result. Increasing the dose or reducing the time interval between doses can lead to dependence.

Physical and psychological dependence to benzodiazepines is a potential risk of use. Dependence can occur after just a few weeks or months as tolerance develops. It is most likely to occur with chronic use. Therapeutic dose dependence develops as patients who are initially prescribed the drug as a hypnotic or anxiolytic continue to use the medication to prevent expected withdrawal effects. The individuals will continue to use the benzodiazepine for months or years, even though they are not experiencing the sedative or anxiolytic corollary any longer. Prescribed high-dose dependence is not as common as therapeutic-dose dependence, but it can develop as patients "need" their prescribed dosage progressively increased. Characteristics of benzodiazepine dependence include feeling as though the drug is needed to get through a regular day, difficulty ending or reducing use, "doctor shopping," and contacting a doctor regularly for prescriptions. As benzodiazepine dependence worsens, the risk of withdrawal upon cessation of the drugs increases.

Symptoms of mild withdrawal are normal when therapeutic benzodiazepine use is reduced or discontinued. The intensity of the withdrawal symptoms is dependent on length of use, dosage, and which benzodiazepine the individual is taking. Short-acting benzodiazepines produce withdrawal symptoms sooner than do long-acting benzodiazepines. Withdrawal from a therapeutic dose typically results in rebound insomnia and mild anxiety symptoms. Uncomfortable symptoms of withdrawal can be diminished or completely eliminated with dosage tapering or switching to long-acting benzodiazepines before tapering.

Dosage tapering is the process of slowly reducing the quantity used until it is completely discontinued. In cases of acute dependence to short-acting benzodiazepines, to combat severe withdrawal symptoms, a long-acting benzodiazepine, like diazepam (Valium), is prescribed as a substitute. Because long-acting benzodiazepines are metabolized slower, withdrawal symptoms are weakened and reduced, making them more tolerable. Once negative symptoms are under control, dosage tapering of the long-acting drug is implemented to terminate use completely. In severe cases of dependence, high-dosage and long-term benzodiazepine users are more likely to experience unpleasant or severe withdrawal symptoms (i.e., muscle pain, mood disturbance, psychosis). With high-dosage use, there is also a higher risk that abrupt cessation of use can result in convulsions and delirium tremens.

Benzodiazepines are seldom used alone as drugs of abuse. According to the U.S. Drug Enforcement Administration, benzodiazepine abuse is particularly high among heroin and cocaine abusers. Benzodiazepines are used to compliment or intensify the intended intoxication of the primary drug of abuse. Recreational abuse of benzodiazepines also includes taking them to "come down" off stimulant drugs (e.g., amphetamine, cocaine) or mixing them with alcohol. Among polydrug users, approximately 50% of individuals commencing substance abuse treatment for opioid or stimulant addiction also confirm benzodiazepine abuse.

Mixing benzodiazepines and alcohol can be fatal as they are both CNS depressants, and when taken concurrently, the affect on the central nervous system is intensified. Under the influence of alcohol combined with benzodiazepines, disinhibition is intensified. With intoxication and unrestraint, engaging in high-risk behaviors is likely. Recreational abusers have diverse means of accessing benzodiazepines. Methods of obtaining the drug include "doctor shopping" (acquiring prescriptions from different doctors for different reasons), forging prescriptions, or buying pharmaceuticals from an illicit market. Benzodiazepines may also be used to facilitate criminal activity, predominantly "date rape."

Flunitrazepam (Rohypnol) is a benzodiazepine with very strong sedative properties that is illegal in the United States. Smuggled into the United States by traffickers, the popularity of flunitrazepam increased in the mid-1990s as it hit the party scene. Known on the street by various slang terms like *roofies*, *Mexican Valium*, and *forget-me-now*, flunitrazepam is a common "date rape" drug. It is used to facilitate rape when it is slipped into the beverage of an unsuspecting victim with the intent of inducing disinhibition, varying degrees of consciousness, or complete incapacitation. After ingesting flunitrazepam, the victim is left defenseless or incapacitated, thus prohibiting him or her from escaping a sexual assault. Often slipped into alcoholic drinks, the effects are compounded and the risk of fatality increases. Due to the amnesiac properties of flunitrazepam, the victim may not remember the attack and consequently does not report the incident to authorities.

A wide variety of psychiatric and medical conditions are treated effectively with benzodiazepines. Benzodiazepines successfully manage anxiety and insomnia, which in some cases may otherwise be debilitating disorders for an individual. With a wide margin between a therapeutic dose and a harmful overdose, benzodiazepines are generally safe and well tolerated. When used for a short interval of time at low doses, side effects are minimal and the benefits are remarkable. As medical research advances, new drugs have been developed, yet benzodiazepines remain one of the most commonly prescribed types of drugs.

Jordana L. Hemberg

See also Anxiolytic Drugs; Central Nervous System Depressants; Pharmacological Approaches to Treatment; Prescription Drugs; Substance Dependence; Tolerance; Withdrawal

Further Readings

Marks, J. (1978). *The benzodiazepines: Use, overuse, misuse, abuse.* Baltimore: University Park Press.

Moeller, H.-J. (1999). Effectiveness and safety of benzodiazepines. *Journal of Clinical Psychopharmacology, 19,* 2S–11S.

O'Brien, C. P. (2005). Benzodiazepine use, abuse, and dependence. *Journal of Clinical Psychiatry, 66,* 28–33.

U.S. Drug Enforcement Administration. (2005). *Drugs of abuse.* Retrieved September 4, 2007, from http://www.usdoj.gov/dea/pubs/abuse/index.htm

BICULTURALISM

See MULTICULTURALISM

BIG BOOK, THE

Alcoholics Anonymous is the name of a book, originally published in 1939, which is central to the worldview of most members of a society commonly going by the same name: Alcoholics Anonymous. The original edition of the book was printed in large type and quickly became referred to as "The Big Book," a moniker that has stuck ever since, even though subsequent editions were printed in normal type. Alcoholics Anonymous refers to itself as a "fellowship," or more commonly a "program," and is most often simply called "AA." The AA Big Book as been in press continuously since 1939, with a fourth edition published in 2001 and distributed by AA World Services incorporated in New York City. Its history and central theses are presented here.

Tradition holds that the work was truly a collaborative effort by the first 100 members of AA, most of whom had been sober less than 2 years. While AA founders Bill Wilson and Bob Silkworth likely had a strong hand in its writing, the book actually lists no authors by name. The structure of Alcoholics Anonymous as an organization is guided by 12 traditions. Among these is the tradition of anonymity, which "is the spiritual foundation of all our traditions, ever reminding us to place principles before personalities" (Twelfth Tradition). Moreover, it is deemed essential that AA members always remain anonymous in the press, radio, and films (Eleventh Tradition). This principle is encapsulated in the very title and authorship of the basic text upon which the program is based.

The original publication of *Alcoholics Anonymous* was slow to catch on, but distribution received a boost when, in September of 1939, *Liberty Magazine* ran an article titled "Alcoholics and God," by Morris Markey. It briefly described Alcoholics Anonymous. The work was endorsed soon afterward by the Rockefeller Foundation and covered in a popular magazine at the time (*Saturday Evening Post*). National interest in both the book and the fellowship has increased ever since then.

The initial 164 pages of the first edition, the preface, forewords, and a chapter called "The Doctor's Opinion" have not been substantially changed since the 1939 edition. Each new edition altered the original works only with simple membership-number updates and common usage language edits. For example, in the eighth chapter, titled "To Wives," there is now a footnote that states that the suggestions given may be adapted to help people who live with women alcoholics. However, in each successive edition, the personal stories, which comprise an additional 400-plus pages, have been changed to reflect a more contemporaneous AA membership, with the result being that stories written by the original members of the 1930s have gradually been replaced with those deemed more likely to attract new members.

The book is divided into 11 chapters, starting with "Bill's Story," a first-person narrative by one of AA's cofounders, and ending with "A Vision for You," an inspirational essay outlining a way of life centered on helping other alcoholics to recover from alcoholism. Other chapters indicate that "There Is a Solution" to alcoholism, provide background information on the condition, and describe "More About Alcoholism" in which mental control strategies to control alcoholism are described as ineffective. There is a chapter titled "We Agnostics," which directly addresses the issue of how people who are agnostic or who are averse to religion may adapt themselves to a deeply spiritual program. The book quickly arrives at what many members of the society see as the heart of the program, chapter 5: "How It Works."

The first three pages of chapter 5 are traditionally read at the start of many meetings where recovering alcoholics gather to help one another and share stories of recovery. In these three pages, the Twelve Steps of Alcoholics Anonymous are found, steps which have spawned additional programs such as Al-Anon/Alateen, Gamblers Anonymous, Narcotics Anonymous, and Overeaters Anonymous. The central thesis of this chapter is that individuals afflicted with alcoholism do not have the personal power to control their drinking behavior and that the experience of the writers is that only God can relieve them of the obsession with alcohol and the compulsion to drink. For the authors of this chapter, regaining the ability to self-regulate or control their drinking has proved impossible. The tenor of this writing, like that of most of the book, is not one of promoting ideas or trying to convince the reader of anything as much as it is one of sharing experience. It seems key to the writers' strategy to avoid arguing or preaching. They remain true to another of the program's traditions, "Our public relations policy is based on attraction rather than promotion . . ." (Eleventh Tradition). After outlining the steps to recovery, chapter 5 goes on to describe how they have been applied in the lives of AA members.

Chapter 6 details the tactics and techniques that members have used and could use to achieve a lasting abstinence from alcohol. Subsequent chapters address repairing relationships with spouses, the family, and employers. All of chapter 7 is devoted to "Working With Others," which indicates that, consistent with the 12th step of recovery, "nothing will so much insure [*sic*] immunity from drinking as intensive work with other alcoholics. It works when other activities fail" (p. 89).

The final two thirds of the book contains 42 first-person stories by recovering alcoholics who have achieved recovery, sanity, and stability by "working the program" of Alcoholics Anonymous. In the end, it is this sharing of personal experience—the practical, real-life application of the principles of the AA program—that Alcoholics Anonymous holds out as most useful for helping others who seek to recover from alcoholism.

Timothy B. Conley

See also Alcoholics Anonymous; Twelve Steps

Further Readings

Alcoholics Anonymous: http://www.aa.org

Alcoholics Anonymous. (2007). *The big book online* (4th ed.). Retrieved May 21, 2007, from http://www.aa.org/ bigbookonline/

K., M. (2006). *Writing of the big book*. Retrieved May 21, 2007, from http://alcoholism.about.com/cs/ history/ a/blmitch8.htm

BILL W.

Bill W., born Bill Wilson, was the cofounder of Alcoholics Anonymous (AA), the largest support group for recovering alcoholics. In keeping with the AA principle of anonymity, Bill Wilson is most often referred to as Bill W. Born in a time when temperance was taught in New England schools, few would believe Bill would struggle with alcoholism for years before becoming sober. His creation of an enterprise that has become an international fellowship of recovering alcoholics may be the single most important contribution to the field of alcohol recovery. His accomplishments earned him a doctorate from Yale University (which he refused) and a cover story in *Time* magazine.

Early History

Born on November 26, 1895, the older of two children (sister Dorothy) in Vermont to parents whose marriage was already crumbling, he spent most of his childhood separated from his parents and living with his maternal grandparents. By the time he was 10 years old, his parents' marriage was over. Shortly thereafter, his mother left to pursue studies in medicine, and his father went to work in the quarry mines. It is believed that Bill's father's womanizing and drinking (he was raised in an inn-keeping family), contributed to the marital strife. Bill's relationship with his parents would remain strained throughout his life. His mother suffered from many "nervous breakdowns" during her life, and it seemed Bill was prone to bouts of depression and solitude, even during childhood.

Young Adulthood

While in Vermont, Bill Wilson met and married Lois Burham, who came from a successful family and was 4 years older than he. Although a good student and naturalist, Bill was fairly aimless. After a series of unsuccessful endeavors, he entered the army at the age of 22, and it was there he is believed to have begun his journey into alcoholism. After his discharge, he was already drinking steadily and struggled to find work. Eventually, he found success as a securities analyst on Wall Street. However, his drinking began to escalate, and when the stock market crashed in 1929, Bill was left penniless and even more despondent.

As a young married couple, Bill and Lois lived in Brooklyn in her family's house for years. Bill struggled to keep a job, and for years they survived on Lois's income as a sales clerk. At times, if it were not for her family's generosity, they would have been homeless. In fact, when the mortgage on that home could not be paid, they were at the mercy of friends for a place to stay.

Getting Sober

Bill was a patient at Towns Hospital in New York on multiple occasions, each time leaving him with a fresh resolve to stop drinking that often would end only hours later. During one stay at Towns Hospital, at age 39, Bill had a spiritual awakening ("a hot flash"), which he credited with his ability to remain sober for the rest of his life. Once released, he took an interest in the Oxford Group, housed in the Calvary Chapel, which emphasized better living by following several basic tenets. Bill was attracted to the Oxford Group members who seemed to achieve sobriety. Although Bill eventually rejected and split from the Oxford Group, it had a profound impact on his development of AA.

In 1935, alone on a trip to Akron, Ohio, for business, Bill found himself tempted to drink. After many desperate phone calls to clergy for support, he was connected with Dr. Bob Smith, a local surgeon struggling with alcoholism. The two talked for hours, and the concept that an alcoholic needs another one for support was forged. It would be years until the two men named their fellowship Alcoholics Anonymous, but the stage was set for a lifetime friendship and commitment to helping other alcoholics recover.

In the early days of AA while it struggled for recognition, the Wilsons lent their Brooklyn home as a meeting site for alcoholics. Bill would host meetings where alcoholics were able to come and get support. From its inception, Bill envisioned an AA that would be open to anyone wishing to recover. Those who were successful at recovery helped "sell" the program to others.

Bill W.: The Author

Bill was prolific throughout his life, eager to put much of the work of AA on paper. His first greatest undertaking was the writing of *Alcoholics Anonymous* in 1939. This was the first publication related to what was then just a movement. Although the book initially was not a best seller, word of its publication spread. Today, *Alcoholics Anonymous* has been translated into many languages and has sold millions of copies. Bill was instrumental in many other texts related to the fellowship, including *Twelve Steps and Twelve Traditions, Alcoholics Anonymous Comes of Age,* and *Twelve Concepts for World Service.*

In keeping with the anonymity tradition of AA, Bill Wilson is still most often referred to as Bill W. Despite his ability to stay sober, he was never able to give up smoking, which ultimately led to his physical demise. Bill W. died of lung disease in 1971 at the age of 76. Survived by his wife Lois, she continued his mission of spreading the word of AA

Conclusion

Despite Bill W.'s incredible influence on the fellowship of AA, he spent most of his life, even sober, as a deeply troubled and depressed man. He was married for more than 50 years to Lois but never had any children and was notoriously unfaithful to his wife. Known as a genius for his innovative approach to helping others get sober, Bill W. was never that comfortable with his celebrity status. However, this much is certain: He forged a legacy of hope and sobriety for millions to follow. Bill W. was a man whose life was destroyed by drinking and who then spent most of his life dedicated to helping others stop drinking.

Maureen C. Kenny and Charles B. Winick

See also Alcoholics Anonymous; Big Book, The; Twelve Steps

Further Readings

B., M. (2000). *My search for Bill W.* Center City, MN: Hazelden Foundation.

Cheever, S. (2004). *My name is Bill, Bill Wilson: His life and the creation of Alcoholics Anonymous.* New York: Simon & Schuster.

Hartigan, F. (2000). *Bill: A biography of Alcoholics Anonymous cofounder Bill Wilson.* New York: Thomas Dunne Books.

Raphael, M. J. (2000). *Bill W. and Mr. Wilson: The legend and life of A.A.'s cofounder.* Amherst: University of Massachusetts Press.

Thomsen, R. (1975). *Bill W.* New York: Harper & Row.

W., B. (2000). *My first 40 Years. An autobiography by the cofounder of Alcoholics Anonymous.* Center City, MN: Hazelden.

BINGE DRINKING

Binge drinking is a pattern of consumption characterized by heavy drinking during a single occasion, leading to intoxication. This pattern of drinking, consisting of at least five drinks per drinking episode for men and four drinks for women, raises concern because of its high correlation with accidents and injuries, such as those incurred when driving while intoxicated. In older adults, binge drinking has significant health implications, such as heart disease. Rates of binge drinking vary by age. It is the most common pattern of alcohol consumption among adolescents, with increasing prevalence through young adulthood, peaking at age 21, and declining through adulthood. For most youth, engaging in binge drinking does not predict the development of alcohol dependence. This pattern changes for older adults, as binge drinking is correlated with patterns of heavy drinking.

Definitions

Historically, "binge drinking" signified the consumption of large amounts of alcohol over extended periods (i.e., several days). The definition of binge drinking currently describes a shorter drinking episode (i.e., several hours) that raises a person's blood alcohol concentration high enough to result in intoxication (0.08). While this definition, proposed by the National Institute on Alcohol Abuse and Alcoholism (NIAAA), indicates both time course and blood alcohol concentration, most research on binge drinking has not included either specifier. To approximate the amount of alcohol necessary to reach this level of intoxication, the NIAAA has defined a binge drinking episode as five drinks per drinking occasion for men and, to account for differences in body size and metabolism, four drinks for women. Similarly, adolescent research has encouraged decreasing the

quantity to three drinks for adolescent girls. In the United Kingdom, binge drinking has been defined as eight or more units of alcohol per drinking episode for men and six or more for women.

Chronology

During adolescence and young adulthood, the majority (90%) of alcohol consumption is in the form of binge drinking. Recently, 11% of 8th graders, 30% of 12th graders, and 40% of college students reported binge drinking within the past 2 weeks to 1 month. These rates have been consistent for the past few decades. However, historically prevalent gender differences are no longer evident across adolescents and young adults. In terms of culture, Native Americans have the highest rates of binge drinking, followed by Caucasian, Hispanic/Latino, biracial/multiracial, Asian American, and African American students.

Around age 22, rates of binge drinking decline. Binge drinking has a low prevalence across adult samples (15%), with the lowest rates found among those age 55 years and above. Nevertheless, of the alcohol consumed by adults, in the United States approximately 75% is in the form of binge drinking. Almost half of all binge drinking episodes occur among adults with alcohol dependence. Of the non-heavy drinkers who engage in binge drinking, most do not have repeated episodes during their adult years.

Clinical Course

The majority of adolescents and young adults who engage in binge drinking do not face alcohol dependence during adulthood. In addition, most people who engage in binge drinking naturally reduce this behavior without formal intervention. However, adolescents and young adults who continue binge drinking into adulthood face a greater likelihood of developing alcohol dependence. Brief interventions, including motivational interviewing and harm reduction approaches, have been found to effectively catalyze reductions in binge drinking and related consequences across people of all age groups. Moreover, reductions in binge drinking achieved during adolescence and young adulthood have been found to have preventive effects during adulthood.

Risk Factors

Adolescents (Ages 13–17)

Several factors place adolescents at increased risk for binge drinking, including early initiation of alcohol use and regular drinking, age, other substance use, peer context, other risk-taking behaviors, parental monitoring, and academic performance. First, early initiation of alcohol use and regular drinking have been found to predict problematic patterns of consumption, including binge drinking, through adolescence, young adulthood, and older adulthood. Second, with increasing age, rates of binge drinking steadily increase. Third, adolescents who use other substances, such as tobacco and marijuana, have evidenced higher rates of binge drinking. Fourth, adolescents who believe that their friends are regular drinkers, frequent drinkers, or binge drinkers are more likely to engage in binge drinking. Fifth, adolescents who exhibit delinquent behaviors, problem behaviors, and high levels of sensation seeking have been found to be more likely to engage in binge drinking. Sixth, adolescents who have parents who do not monitor their behavior have shown increased rates of binge drinking. In contrast, parents who have clearly stated that they expect their child not to drink have adolescents who demonstrate significantly lower levels of binge drinking. Seventh, adolescents who are doing poorly in school, have a negative attitude, or a limited commitment toward school have increased rates of binge drinking.

Young Adults (Ages 18–24)

Several factors have been found to increase the risk of binge drinking during young adulthood, including binge drinking during adolescence, moving away from home, college attendance, peer behaviors, and academic demands. First, studies have found that young adults who engaged in binge drinking during high school averaged 2 to 3 times as many binge drinking episodes per month than those who had no high school binge drinking. Second, moving away from home has been consistently correlated with increases in binge drinking. Third, young adults who attend college evidence higher rates of binge drinking than their non-college-attending peers, particularly when college attendance is coupled with moving away from home. This increase is influenced by several factors within the college environment, including limited parental monitoring, more social environments that encourage heavy drinking, and increased accessibility of alcohol. Fourth, as with adolescents, peer groups influence the binge drinking behaviors of young adults. Specifically, young adults involved with fraternities, sororities, or heavy drinking peer groups have higher rates of binge drinking. Fifth, college semester schedules have been correlated with binge drinking, with increased rates of binge drinking occurring during holidays and school breaks.

Adults

During adulthood, there are several risk factors for increased levels of binge drinking, including age of initiation of binge drinking, gender, cultural patterns of alcohol consumption, and heavy drinking. First, adults who began binge drinking before or during high school have increased rates of binge drinking during adulthood. However, it is important to note that this correlation has been highest among adults who consumed large amounts of alcohol at a high frequency during adolescence. Second, although there are no gender differences in binge drinking rates among adolescents, adult men consistently evidence higher rates of binge drinking than do women. In fact, rates of binge drinking have been found to be 3 times as high for men than for women. In addition, men account for 81% of all binge drinking episodes across adults. Third, increased rates of binge drinking during adulthood have been found in cultures where binge drinking is the predominant pattern of alcohol consumption (e.g., Russia, United Kingdom, Ireland), particularly when contrasted with cultures where alcohol tends to be consumed in smaller quantities and during meals (e.g., Mediterranean cultures, such as Spain, Italy, and France). Fourth, most (76%) heavy drinkers report engaging in binge drinking and doing so more frequently than moderate drinkers.

Correlates

Accidents and Injuries

Most negative consequences of binge drinking stem from accidents and injuries incurred during binge drinking episodes. Specifically, several types of accidents and injuries have been found to correlate with binge drinking, including self-harm (falling, being burned, drowning, overexposure, hypothermia, self-cutting, self-injury, suicide), sexual risk taking (multiple sexual partners, sexual behaviors that were later regretted, inconsistent condom use, forced sexual activities, sexual aggression), and interpersonal harm (physical fighting, assault, domestic violence, child abuse). After binge drinking, adolescents and young adults are 10 times as likely to engage in behaviors that result in accidents and injuries. The high rates of accidents and injuries that occur during episodes of binge drinking appear to be a function of the psychological and physical changes that occur during intoxication, including disinhibition; poor decision making; and impaired judgment, communication, and problem solving. In addition, the setting where binge drinking occurs also factors into the potential risk.

Drinking and Driving

Many of the accidents and injuries related to binge drinking stem from driving during or after the binge drinking episode, while people are still intoxicated. Over 80% of alcohol-impaired driving events occur among people who have been binge drinking. Moreover, adolescents have shown a high acceptability of drinking and driving. Specifically, 17% of high school seniors reported having driven after drinking. By college, that rate increases, with 30% of college students stating that they have driven after binge drinking. In addition, rates of driving after binge drinking are higher for college students who live off-campus.

Health Risks

The consequences of binge drinking upon physical health vary across the life span. For adolescents and young adults, the predominant health risks of binge drinking include alcohol poisoning, unintended pregnancy, sexually transmitted infections (including HIV), physical accidents, and injuries. During adulthood, these risks continue, but additional risks accrue, including heart disease, high blood pressure, and poor diabetes control. While studies have found that moderate alcohol consumption benefits the cardiovascular system, binge drinking counteracts these potential benefits and increases one's chance of mortality. For women, binge drinking during pregnancy may result in fetal alcohol syndrome and fetal alcohol effects.

Prevention and Intervention

When the data on binge drinking are examined, several themes emerge. The greatest risk for binge drinking stems from accidents and injuries, particularly as a consequence of drinking and driving. Brief interventions, such as motivational interviewing and harm reduction approaches, have gained empirical support in reducing the frequency of binge drinking across all age groups. Therefore, the provision of brief interventions may curtail the incidence and correlated consequences of binge drinking. Reducing levels of binge drinking during adolescence and young adulthood has salient protective and preventive effects, both in reducing rates of accidents and injuries and in halting developing patterns of heavy drinking. Therefore, the development of broad-reaching efforts, such as the facilitation of discussions about alcohol use and the provision of brief interventions in medical settings, may help reach the majority of youth who may be engaged in binge drinking but who would otherwise not come to the attention of health professionals. Due to the high concordance between binge drinking and patterns of consistent heavy drinking among adults, assessment and treatment for alcohol abuse and dependence may be the most effective intervention strategy for adults.

Sarah W. Feldstein

See also Adolescents, Substance Abuse and Treatment; Alcoholism; College Students, Alcohol Use and Abuse; Cultural Aspects; Driving Under the Influence; Experimental Substance Use

Further Readings

Centers for Disease Control and Prevention. (2006). Youth risk behavior surveillance—United States, 2005. *MMWR Surveillance Summaries, 55*(SS-5), 1–108.

Hughes, E., McCracken, M., Roberts, H., Mokdad, A. H., Valluru, B., Goodson, R., et al. (2006). Surveillance for certain health behaviors among states and selected local areas—Behavioral Risk Factor Surveillance System, United States, 2004. *MMWR Surveillance Summaries, 55*(SS07), 1–124.

Johnston, L. D., O'Malley, P. M., Bachman, J. G., & Schulenberg, J. E. (2006). *Monitoring the future: National survey results on drug use, 1975–2005: Vol.1. Secondary school students* (NIH Publication No. 06-5883). Bethesda, MD: National Institute on Drug Abuse.

Johnston, L. D., O'Malley, P. M., Bachman, J. G., & Schulenberg, J. E. (2006). *Monitoring the Future: National survey results on drug use, 1975–2005: Vol. 2. College students and adults ages 19–45* (NIH Publication No. 06-5884). Bethesda, MD: National Institute on Drug Abuse.

Miller, J. W., Naimi, T. S., Brewer, R. D., & Jones, S. E. (2007). Binge drinking and associated health risk behaviors among high school students. *Pediatrics, 119*, 76–85.

Naimi, T. S., Brewer, R. D., Mokdad, A., Denny, C., Serdula, M. K., & Marks, J. S. (2003). Binge drinking among US adults. *JAMA, 289*, 70–75.

Substance Abuse and Mental Health Services Administration. (2006). *Results from the 2005 National Survey on Drug Use and Health: National findings* (Office of Applied Studies, NSDUH Series H-30, DHHS Publication No. SMA 06-4194). Rockville, MD: Author.

World Health Organization. (2004). *Global status report on alcohol 2004*. Geneva: World Health Organization Department of Mental Health and Substance Abuse.

BIOPSYCHOSOCIAL MODEL OF ADDICTION

A model of addiction can be viewed as a foundation from which to organize addiction into a set of fundamental intuitive principles. As such, any model allows its adherents to prioritize problems and to search for and discover solutions to these problems within the context or boundary conditions of the model. In recent years, the fields of psychology, social work, and counseling have all begun adopting the biopsychosocial perspective in research. The biopsychosocial model, unlike traditional models of addiction, is atheoretical in that it does not attempt to explain the causality of addiction. However, this model presents a holistic, systems approach and identifies the influence as well as interaction of various dimensions of the biological, social, psychological, spiritual, and cultural environment on the individual. According to the Addictions Foundations of Manitoba (AFM), the etiology of addiction is complex, variable, and multifactorial. The AFM believes that addictive behaviors and experiences arise from complex and ongoing interactions between various biological, psychological, and sociocultural factors. It also believes that the combinations, interactions, and weightings of specific factors will be different for different individuals.

Biological Factors

According to the Center for Substance Abuse Treatment, addiction has biological components including major involvement of the brain. As a result, a number of predisposed characteristics can lay the framework before the use of addictive substances. Additional biological factors related to addiction include genetic components in the etiology of addiction as well as the inevitable physical problems that arise due to addiction. According to Kumpfer and colleagues, the biopsychosocial model includes three clusters of biological variables: (1) genetic inheritance of different alcoholism syndromes (milieu-limited, depression-sensitive), differences in metabolism and reactions to alcohol and other drugs, biochemical and neurological vulnerabilities, and temperament or cognitive structural differences; (2) in utero damage to the fetus that results in central or autonomic nervous system problems and/or physical and biochemical damage that makes a child temperamentally or psychologically more vulnerable to alcohol or drug use; and (3) temperament or other physiological differences that can occur at any time after birth due to sickness, accidents, physical trauma, improper diet, exposure to toxins, or alcohol or drug use.

Psychological Factors

The psychological dimension of addiction explores the thinking that leads a person to engage in substance use in ways that compromise psychological and physical health. Additionally, this dimension examines how addictive behavior affects the psychology of individuals. According to proponents of social learning and cognitive behavioral models, individuals with irrational or unhealthy thought processes often use and abuse substances to cope with existing psychological problems such as depression, self-esteem, life stressors, anxiety, or all of these.

Social Factors

The social component in addiction relates to the setting where substance use takes place as well as where the impact is felt. Related social factors can be categorized into family, peers and social, and community and school. Family variables include family attitudes and values, which interact with family stressors (e.g., conflict, poverty, parent or sibling use of drugs). Peer and social variables includes peer attitudes and values toward prosocial activities and alcohol and drug use, which interact with peer stressors (e.g., peer conformity pressure; developmental adjustment issues, poverty; lack of emotional or material support; depression and poor mental health; lack of opportunities; academic, job, and social adjustment problems). Community and school variables includes community and school attitudes and values toward prosocial activities and alcohol or drug use, which interact with community and school stressors (e.g., poverty, high crime rates, high population density, impersonal climate, discrimination, conflict or noncooperation and support, pressures to use drugs).

Spiritual Factors

This dimension has generally been underemphasized in most discussions of the biospyschosocial model. As this model is viewed as an articulation of "holistic health," it is therefore important to be cognizant of the spiritual elements, which is consistent with holistic health. The spiritual dimension is a critical component in addiction. Spirituality is reported to be a vital aspect of recovery, as it allows addicts to make meaning of their experiences and fosters a sense of interconnectedness. Healing and forgiveness are spiritual concepts that afford addicts to establish or reestablish interpersonal relationships.

Advantages

Researchers propose a number of advantages of the biopsychosocial model. First, the model can viewed as a conceptual framework that allows attention to be focused on all problems related to substance misuse. This allows policymakers, program developers, and service providers to assist people affected by substance abuse to address the broad range of problems, from problems which are just beginning to those that are long standing. Second, the model unifies prior biological, psychological, and social theories of addiction. The beauty of the biopsychosocial model is that is does not refute the validity of existing models. However, it allows for addiction professionals to work toward implementing an Individualized treatment plan that may evolve from one or more traditional models of addiction. Third, the

biopsychosocial model of addiction is congruent with other modern theories of health and education. Many theories, including those in health and education, advocate the matching of individuals with certain characteristics to specific treatments and the measurement of treatment success along more than one dimension.

Disadvantages

According to critics of the model, drawbacks to the use of this model are threefold. First, typically an emphasis is placed on one aspect of the model without a solid integration of the three aspects. Second, it is difficult to make interventions on all aspects at the same time. Third, some factors, such as genetic predisposition, cannot be changed.

Prevention and Treatment

A major implication for prevention as it relates to this model is that prevention interventions targeting any aspect of the person–environment dynamic or the interpersonal system should also affect central determinants in many parts of the system. To this end, addiction professionals do not have to focus solely on the most influential cause that will prevent individuals from using or abusing drugs. Many types of prevention interventions targeted at different points in the person–environment dynamic are more than likely to be effective. However, professionals must understand the total impact of their prevention approach on the person and the total environmental context.

It is of utmost importance that addiction professionals understand the person in relation to his or her total biopsychosocial environment. For example, professionals must understand the potential impact of drug use when a person is at risk for, or suffers from, diseases such as tuberculosis, hepatitis, or HIV. Professionals need to possess a thorough understanding of how the elements of the psychological dimension are involved in addiction as well as how an addict's behavior affects his or her frame of thinking. It is important to understand the roles of the social, political, and economic environments and how these respective roles may contribute to an individual's addictive behavior. Last, and equally important, is for professionals to realize that spirituality is often an integral part of the recovery process for drug abusers, and allowing time for spiritual exploration can produce positive outcomes.

Conclusion

A biopsychosocial model of addiction is a useful conceptual framework for integrating the various etiologies of alcohol and other substance abuse. Training in this framework should enhance communication and mutual respect among professionals in different disciplines working to prevent drug abuse. The biopsychosocial approach strengthens risk assessments for prevention programs and improves diagnosis and treatment of individuals likely to be chemically dependent.

By encouraging addiction professionals to comprehensively assess and develop appropriate interventions across biological, psychological, sociocultural, and spiritual spheres, professionals can remain within one process if the need to change modalities is necessary. Implementing the biopsychosocial model results in a holistically viewed client with individually tailored interventions that hopefully leads to an enhanced quality life for those struggling with addiction.

James Bethea

See also Addiction, Models of; Cognitive-Social Learning Model; Disease Concept; Psychological Models of Addiction; Social Learning Model of Addictive Behaviors; Sociocultural Models of Addiction

Further Readings

Addictions Foundation of Manitoba: http://www.afm.mb.ca/

DiClemente, C. C. (2003). *Addiction and change: How addictions develop and addicted people recover.* New York: Guilford Press.

Kumpfer, K. L., Trunnell, E. P., & Whiteside, H. O. (1990). The biopsychosocial model: Application to the addictions field. In R. C. Engs (Ed.), *Controversy in the addictions field* (pp. 55–66). Dubuque, IA: Kendall/Hunt.

Marlatt, G. (1992). Substance abuse: Implications of a biopsychosocial model for prevention, treatment, and relapse prevention. In J. Gabowski (Ed.), *Psychopharmacology: Basic mechanisms and applied interventions* (pp. 131–162). Washington, DC: American Psychological Association.

Suls, J., & Rothman, A. (2002). Evolution of the biopsychosocial model: Prospects and challenges for health psychology. *Health Psychology, 23,* 119–125.

BLOOD ALCOHOL CONCENTRATION

Blood alcohol concentration (BAC) is the concentrated amount of alcohol within a person's bloodstream. One of three different methods is used to measure BAC: a proportion of a person's size, mass per quantity, or a combination of the two. For example, a BAC of .30% can mean 3 grams of alcohol per 1,000 grams of someone's blood, or it can mean .3 gram of alcohol per 100 milliliters (ml) of blood.

How many drinks someone has had is not the best method for gauging the level of inebriation, primarily because individuals differ in their alcohol tolerance. One drink increases a normal person's BAC by approximately .03%. However, this fluctuates due to the high level of individual differences concerning body mass, gender, and body fat percentage. Moreover, the amount of alcohol a person consumes, a person's BAC, or both, are not always precise guides for level of drunkenness. On average, the more frequently a person drinks, the more his or her body becomes tolerant, though this level depends upon genetics, personal habits, and the synergism of different drugs.

Alcohol is eliminated from the body by metabolism, excretion, and evaporation. While there are individual differences in the percentage of alcohol eliminated from the body through each function, about 90% to 98% is burned through metabolism, 1% to 3% is excreted by the kidneys, and about 1% to 5% evaporates through breathing. A minute amount (less than .5%) leaves the body by excretion in a person's tears and sweat. Approximately 40 to 50 minutes after a person begins drinking, excretion of alcohol by urination begins, while metabolism starts at the moment alcohol is absorbed, even before alcohol's effects have made it to the brain. This means that before a person feels "tipsy," his or her body has already started metabolizing alcohol.

Alcohol is eliminated from the bloodstream at a constant rate. This elimination differs from person to person, but an experienced male alcoholic with an elevated body mass may be able to deal with up to 30 grams (38 ml) per hour, whereas a more average amount is 10 grams (12.7 ml) per hour. Individuals under age 25, females, specific ethnic groups, and anyone with hepatic disease may metabolize alcohol more slowly. Other factors that influence BAC include

- The number of drinks consumed during a drinking episode
- The relative proof (alcohol content) of the alcohol consumed
- Whether or not food was eaten prior to drinking or while drinking
- The person's body fat (people with more body fat can drink more and maintain a lower BAC)

Law enforcement agencies use BAC as a method for defining intoxication levels and as an approximate guide of level of impairment. The level of alcoholic impairment varies from person to person, though they might have identical BAC levels. Even so, BAC can be calculated scientifically and, thus, is usually not easy to dispute in court. In most countries, it is illegal for someone with a high BAC level to operate motor vehicles or heavy machines. Likewise, watercraft and aircraft have restrictions regarding BAC level.

BAC can be calculated in any hospital by a blood test, which is the most accurate method. Most law enforcement agents use a breathalyzer, an instrument in which an individual breathes and receives a breath alcohol concentration. The assumption inherent in the breathalyzer is that the person tested is "average." For instance, with a typical individual, the relative amount of BAC to breath alcohol content is 2,100 to 1. That is, 2,100 parts of alcohol may be found in the average person's blood for every part in his or her inhalation. On the other hand, the precise amount in someone can differ as much as 1,300:1 up to 3,100:1. This percentage changes with each individual, as well as from one moment to the next. Hence, someone possessing a BAC of .08 with a ratio of 1,700:1 at the specific time of the test, would present a BAC of .10 when read by a breathalyzer due to its calibration of 2,100:1. Obviously, this could have serious ramifications for an individual suspected of drunk driving.

A BAC of .08 is the legal standard for driving under the influence (DUI) or driving while intoxicated (DWI) in the United States. Novice drinkers generally pass out with a BAC of .15, and a BAC of .20 results in a severe case of intoxication in most drinkers. Most people would die from alcohol poisoning with a BAC of .40. In fact, the phrase "lethal dose 50" (LD50) refers to the BAC at which 50% of the population would die, and the LD50 is .40. However, someone with a high tolerance for alcohol will vary considerably from these standards. Alcoholics and very heavy drinkers can appear to be only slightly intoxicated with BACs of .20 and can live with BACs much higher than .40.

The following is a guide to interpreting the effects of different BAC levels for average drinkers:

- .02—Initial effects are felt and the face may become flushed.
- .04—Feelings of relaxation and enjoyment begin.
- .06—Behavior and thoughts become mildly impaired.
- .08—Clear-cut impairment regarding movement and reaction time. The ability to operate a motor vehicle safely is disrupted.
- .10—Further deterioration of cognitive and physical abilities.
- .12—Depending on the rate of consumption and tolerance, vomiting may occur.
- .15—Increasingly difficult to maintain balance. At a BAC level this high, an equivalent of one-half pint of alcohol is in the bloodstream.
- .15 to .25—Blackouts occur (i.e., periods of time that cannot be remembered the next day).
- .30—Unconsciousness occurs (i.e., passing out).
- .40 to .45—Respiratory system shuts down and death occurs from alcohol poisoning.

In general, a person can maintain a BAC below .08 by restricting their intake to one drink per hour. Someone who drinks more than this and drives runs the risk of receiving a DUI. More importantly, high BAC levels can endanger the drinker and others as a result of the effects of alcohol on judgment, cognitive abilities, and motor skills.

Cary Stacy Smith and Li-Ching Hung

See also Alcohol; Alcoholism; Alcohol Testing; Driving Under the Influence

Further Readings

Nordegren, T. (2002). *The A-Z encyclopedia of alcohol and drug abuse.* Boca Raton, FL: Brown Walker Press.

Rotgers, F., & Davis, B. (2006). *Treating alcohol problems.* Hoboken, NJ: Wiley.

Stevens, P., & Smith, R. L. (2005). *Substance abuse counseling: Theory and practice* (3rd ed.). Upper Saddle River, NJ: Pearson Education Group.

BORDERLINE PERSONALITY DISORDER

Borderline personality disorder (BPD) is a serious and complex mental disorder marked by a pervasive, chronic pattern of instability and inability to regulate emotions, impulses, self-image, and interpersonal relationships. BPD is an extremely heterogeneous category, ranging from "antagonistic," "volatile" individuals to those who are actively violent and suicidal. BPD has been analyzed from several contrasting perspectives, including psychoanalysis, "traumatology," and biological psychiatry. Current thinking emphasizes that there are multiple causes involved, which vary from individual to individual. BPD is commonly comorbid with substance abuse disorders.

BPD is recognized as a diagnostic entity in the *Diagnostic and Statistical Manual of Mental Disorders, Fourth Edition, Text Revision (DSM-IV-TR)*. The label "borderline" dates from an early concept of an area between "neurotic" and "psychotic." It is sometimes confused with the colloquial "borderline schizophrenic," but BPD has nothing to do with the brain disease schizophrenia. While a minority of BPDs may experience transient psychotic-like conditions, this is not a common or core feature of BPD. There have been proposals for a more descriptive label, such as "emotional regulation disorder" or "interpersonal regulatory disorder."

To diagnose a personality disorder, there must be an enduring, long-lasting pattern of thinking, feeling, interpersonal relations, and impulse control that is maladaptive and causes distress and impairment in functioning. In addition, a personality disorder cannot be accounted for by another major mental disorder, substance abuse, or transient reaction to trauma.

The *DSM-IV-TR* lists borderline personality disorder in its Cluster B (dramatic, emotional, erratic), along with antisocial, narcissistic, and histrionic personality disorders.

It is defined as a "pervasive pattern of instability of interpersonal relationships, self-image, and affects, and marked impulsivity beginning by early adulthood and present in a variety of contexts." Five or more of the following symptoms must be present to diagnose BPD:

1. Frantic attempts to avoid real or imagined abandonment
2. A pattern of unstable and intense interpersonal relationships characterized by alternating between extremes of idealization and devaluation
3. Identity disturbance, that is, markedly and persistently unstable self-image or sense of self
4. Impulsivity in at least two areas that are potentially self-damaging (spending, sex, substance abuse, reckless driving, binge eating)
5. Recurrent suicidal behavior, gestures, or threats, or self-mutilating behavior
6. Affective instability due to a marked reactivity of mood (e.g., intense episodic dysphoria, irritability, or anxiety usually lasting a few hours and only rarely more than a few days)
7. Chronic feelings or emptiness
8. Inappropriate, intense anger or difficulty controlling anger (e.g., frequent displays of temper, constant anger, recurrent physical fights)
9. Transient stress-related paranoid ideation or severe dissociative symptoms

To extrapolate on criteria 1 and 2, persons with BPD typically go to extremes in their attachments, as seen in the book title *I Hate You—Don't Leave Me*. They may alternate between these extremes, inexplicably and unpredictably turning on an intimate, but have an "emotional amnesia" in which they will deny the previous emotional state or attitude (i.e., "I never liked you").

To extrapolate on criteria 6 and 9, persons with BPD show the following:

- An inability to modulate or damp down affects and emotional responses, what has been dubbed an "emotional hemophilia" or an "affective storm"
- An exquisite sensitivity to environmental shifts
- A lower threshold for frustrating stimuli
- Rage, fury, despair, humiliation at small or imagined slights or setbacks

To extrapolate on criteria 5, 6, and 9, in some individuals with BPD, overwhelming negative emotions and affective storms are turned against the self via self-mutilation (cutting) and suicide attempts. Through some as yet unknown mechanism, self-mutilation has the effect of relieving tension, anxiety, and other extreme affects. Other behavioral extremes listed under criterion 4 (i.e., shopping, shoplifting, sexual promiscuity, gambling) also allow them to feel calmer for a short time. BPD with self-destructive behavior is more often found among females than among males.

Other Cluster B Disorders

It is difficult to draw clear distinctions between the Cluster B personality disorders (dramatic/emotional or erratic), which include antisocial personality disorder (ASP), borderline personality disorder, histrionic personality disorder, and narcissistic personality disorder. The criteria overlap:

- Both ASP and BPD show impulsive, reckless thrill seeking. The comorbidity of ASP and BPD is much greater among males than among females.
- Both BPD and narcissistic personality disordered individuals react with rage at criticism, real or imagined.
- Both BPD and histrionic personality disordered individuals are attention seeking and experience rapidly shifting emotions. Fifty percent of individuals with BPD meet criteria for histrionic personality disorder.

Many modern researchers on personality disorders question whether it is valid to grab a bundle of symptoms and posit a concrete "disorder," like strep throat or diabetes, and would like to substitute one of several proposed systems whereby individuals with personality disorders can be rated on a number of personality dimensions.

Mood Disorders

Clinical psychopharmacology studies suggest a link between BPD and mood disorders for at least a subset of patients with BPD. BPD in conjunction with a diagnosed mood disorder is much more common among female patients. However, women are much more likely than men to seek treatment for depression and to self-identify as depressed or in psychological

pain, so a sociocultural component probably figures into these statistics. The mood disorders include dysthymic disorder (mild depression), major depression, cyclothymic disorder, and premenstrual dysmorphic disorder.

Some researchers suggest that BPD reflects an underlying bipolar (manic-depressive) disorder, usually a rapidly cycling variety, or of the bipolar II variety. They cite studies showing improvement in symptoms of patients with BPD who are taking mood-stabilizing anticonvulsants (e.g., topiramate), now commonly prescribed for bipolar disorder. Mania can present as extreme irritability and dysphoria, rather than a euphoric, grandiose "high."

Premenstrual dysmorphic disorder is listed in Appendix B of the *DSM-IV-TR*, as a category that did not warrant official inclusion but was marked off for future research and study. Severe premenstrual dysmorphic disorder is marked by lability of mood, anger, and interpersonal conflicts. It is distinguished from premenstrual worsening of a current mental disorder. However, borderline symptoms worsen premenstrually.

Trauma

Many patients with BPD, especially in hospitalized samples, have a history of childhood abuse and trauma. This alone could result in extreme sensitivity to cues of threat, poor ability to process social information (e.g., they see neutral behaviors as threats, attribute negative intent, and respond aggressively), and a tendency to see their problems as coming from others.

Judith Herman proposes a category of "complex post-traumatic stress disorder (CPTSD)" to identify victims of prolonged trauma and abuse who develop personality changes, which may include problems in affect regulation, suicidality and self-mutilation, disruption in intimate relationships, search for a rescuer, sense of hopelessness and despair, and a sense of complete difference from others. Herman and her colleagues in the "traumatology" movement would abandon the BPD concept entirely and see individuals with BPD symptoms as suffering from a variant of CPTSD. Their view dovetails with earlier psychodynamic perspectives on BPD in that prolonged trauma and abuse could be the source of failure to form stable inner representations of trusted people, consequent inability to self-sooth, fragmentation and unstable sense of the self, and the primitive defense of "splitting" (i.e., disassociation). Splitting can be viewed as a defense against trauma, walling off the image of the abusive figure from the positive one, or the internalization or repetition of the experience of trauma and inconsistent messages. Alternation of idealization and devaluation of others recapitulates or models the paradoxical bonding with an abuser.

Alcohol and Other Drug Abuse

The rhythms of out-of-control addictive behaviors parallel the dysregulation of BPD. BPD intersects and interacts with substance abuse in a variety of ways:

- Alcohol and stimulant abuse can intensify impulsivity and aggressive outbursts.
- Alcohol can intensify behavioral dysregulation by suppressing problem-solving, inhibitory, and decision-making functions.
- Alcohol amnestic disorder ("blackouts") and confabulation resemble the emotional amnesia of BPD.
- Marijuana, alcohol, and sedative use may help individuals with BPD modulate their moods and blunt, sooth, or block out psychic pain, feelings of abandonment, anxiety, and self-loathing.
- Alcoholism in patients with BPD, as in the general population, is associated with more suicide attempts.
- Involvement with alcohol and drugs among patients with BPD is a predictor for poor rates of remission.
- Persons in a multigenerational addictive family may predictably anticipate and fear abandonment.
- Newly recovering addicts may experience intense feelings that had been chemically muted, including strong transference to counselors. They may be overwhelmed, may experience panic and guilt, and may defend themselves by devaluing the counselor.

Biology and Environment

BPD is common among first-degree relatives of BPD patients. There is a neurobiological substrate for affective instability and sensitivity, lower threshold of tolerance to frustrating environmental stimuli, and impulse aggression, which may be inherited. Individuals with BPD also have first-degree relatives with affective disorders. Dysregulation or affective disorder in parents can explain

the chaotic, inconsistent, and neglectful family history of some individuals with BPD. Hypersensitive children have difficulty mastering developmental tasks: They overreact to mothers' leave-taking, are difficult to sooth, and have tantrums if "crossed." The overwhelmed parent may be overprotective, creating unrealistic expectations of relationships that reverberate into adulthood. Conversely, "difficult" children can elicit negative reactions from family members, peers, and teachers, creating the feeling that the social environment is not nurturing but rather rejecting and hostile. As young adults, these individuals will come to anticipate slights, abandonment, and rejection in every interaction and may adopt a combative, almost paranoid, posture.

Some researchers also postulate the development of BPD as stemming from early experience of attention deficit hyperactivity disorder (ADHD); these are children who display an impulsive, disorganized, erratic, and intense temperament. They elicit negative responses from caregivers and peers, which leads to low self-esteem, depression, lack of sense of stable relatedness, mistrust and resentment, and self-medication via psychoactive substance use. BPD is comorbid with ADHD more often with males. Substance-abusing parents, in particular, may scapegoat and abuse their ADHD offspring.

Thus, individuals with BPD can have a constitutional vulnerability and live in an adverse environment. In the etiological mix, some individuals may be pushed by their genetic or neurobiological vulnerability toward a borderline personality organization despite the best parenting, whereas very destructive families may prompt a borderline adaptation with little or no genetic bias. The worst case scenario is the child who has inherited vulnerability, dysregulation, and impulsivity from a parent with BPD and who also experiences an abusive environment among these parents.

Conclusion

Borderline personality disorder is a category that includes persons who, for a wide variety of genetic, biochemical, and environmental reasons, have great difficulty in regulating and modulating their emotions, behavior, and relationships, often leading to self-harm and self-medication with psychoactive substances. Because of their wildly oscillating attitudes toward others, they present a tremendous challenge to clinicians in building and maintaining a therapeutic relationship.

Peter L. Myers

See also Antisocial Personality Disorder; Criminal Justice Populations; *Diagnostic and Statistical Manual of Mental Disorders*

Further Readings

American Psychiatric Association. (2000). *Diagnostic and statistical manual of mental disorders* (4th ed., text rev.). Washington, DC: Author.

Bockian, N. R. (2002). *New hope for people with borderline personality disorder.* New York: Three Rivers Press.

Herman, J. L. (1992). *Trauma and recovery.* New York: Basic Books.

Kernberg, O. (1975). *Borderline conditions and pathological narcissism.* New York: Jason Aronson.

Kreisman, J. J., & Straus, H. (1989). *I hate you—don't leave me.* Los Angeles: Body Press.

Linehan, M. M. (1993). *Cognitive behavioral treatment of borderline personality disorder.* New York: Guilford Press.

Preston, J. D. (2006). *Integrative treatment for borderline personality disorder.* Oakland, CA: New Harbinger.

Skodol, A. E., Gunderson, J. G., Pfohl, B., Widiger, T. A., Livesley, W. J., & Siever, L. J. (2002). The borderline diagnosis I: Psychopathology, comorbidity, and personality structure. *Biological Psychiatry, 51,* 936–950.

Skodol, A. E., Gunderson, J. G., Pfohl, B., Widiger, T. A., Livesley, W. J., & Siever, L. J. (2002). The borderline diagnosis II: Biology, genetics, and clinical course. *Biological Psychiatry, 51,* 951–963.

Stone, M. H. (1986). *Essential papers on borderline disorders.* New York: New York University Press.

Stone, M. H. (1990). *The fate of borderline patients.* New York: Guilford Press.

Yeomans, F. E., Clarkin, J. F., & Kernberg, O. F. (2002). *A primer of transference-focused psychotherapy for the borderline patient.* Northvale, NJ: Jason Aronson.

BRAIN CHEMISTRY AND ADDICTION

Any substance taken into the body results in changes to that body. If the substance is beneficial, such as food or oxygen, the body works better, continues to thrive, lives. If the substance is detrimental, the body's functions are impaired; cell damage and death may ensue. Such is the case with drug use. This entry focuses on the effects of drug use and addiction on the chemistry of the brain.

To understand the effects of drugs on the brain, one must first understand the various structures and neurotransmitters affected. There are a number of areas in the brain affected by drugs and alcohol; one of the main areas involved is the area often referred to as the "reward center": the limbic system, nucleus accumbens, and the ventral tegmental area. This reward center is important because using drugs and drinking alcohol is often pleasurable. If drug use were not so pleasurable, especially at the onset, people would be less likely to engage in these behaviors. In addition to the reward center, the prefrontal cortex, the locus coeruleus, the amygdala, and the hippocampus are activated when someone uses drugs or drinks alcohol and are particularly important in understanding relapse. There are many structures involved in addiction; there also are a few neurotransmitters involved in drug addiction, the main one being dopamine; however, other neurotransmitters, such as serotonin, gamma-aminobutyric acid (GABA), norepinephrine, and glutamine, are also be affected.

Structures and Neurotransmitters

The limbic system consists of a set of structures, located in both hemispheres of the brain, under the thalamus. The limbic system is involved in almost everything one does on a given day—good and bad. It takes the stored memories, sensory input, and information regarding body functions to determine one's mood, which can have an effect on behaviors. Your reaction to someone who cuts you off and takes the last parking space may be different if you are stuck in traffic, late for a class, and have not adequately prepared for the day when compared to a day when you arrive early for class completely prepared. The limbic system is also responsible for the behaviors related to the classic "fight or flight" response. You are walking through the woods and see a bear; your heart rate increases, and you must decide on your course of action. The limbic system will have a lot of input into that decision. And more importantly for the current topic, the limbic system regulates feelings of pleasure, particularly those pleasurable behaviors that are required for the survival of the individual (e.g., eating) and the survival of the species (e.g., sex/reproduction).

The nucleus accumbens is located in the forebrain and consists of a bundle of neurons that are responsible for one's experience of reward and pleasure—making it the perfect target for many drugs to act upon.

The ventral tegmental area (VTA) works closely with the nucleus accumbens especially where the mechanics of drug addiction are involved. The VTA is located in the midbrain at the top of the brain stem. Dopamine is synthesized in the neurons of the VTA. So drugs that affect this part of the brain effect the production of dopamine. The activity in the VTA effects the activity of the neurons in the nucleus accumbens. Thus, the production of dopamine in the VTA results in the stimulation of the neurons in the nucleus accumbens, resulting in the experience of pleasure; that pleasure can be intense if there is an excess of dopamine.

Each neurotransmitter has a specific purpose. For example, dopamine has a role in the way one behaves and thinks, as well as helping to regulate sleep, attention, mood, and learning. Dopamine is also the primary "feel good" neurotransmitter. Serotonin is helpful in regulating desire for sex, aggression, sleep, appetite, and body temperature. Norepinephrine works to control arousal. Gamma-aminobutyric acid (GABA) functions primarily as an inhibitory neurotransmitter, working to reduce or slow the actions of the neurons, and glutamine is an excitatory neurotransmitter, the presence of which results in increased neuronal activity.

The majority of the changes that occur in the brain as a result of drug addiction occur in the synapse—the space between two or more neurons. Specifically, the drug either affects the presynaptic neuron (the neuron that is sending the message) or the drug affects the postsynaptic neuron (the neuron that is receiving the message). All of the drugs presented here affect the neurons and neurotransmitters differently. Dopamine, for example, is either prevented from being reabsorbed (reuptake) into the neuron, or the neuron is excited to the point of secreting excess amounts of dopamine, or some combination of both of these events occurs.

Effects of Drug Addiction

Alcohol

When alcohol is ingested, the effects on dopamine are somewhat indirect. Alcohol has the ability to increase the levels of dopamine in the synapse; however, the exact mechanism for the increase of dopamine is still up for debate. Because dopamine is a "good mood" neurotransmitter, it is the cause of the initial good feeling one experiences when drinking alcohol.

Alcohol increases the effects of GABA, which results in an inhibition of the firing of neurons. Alcohol may also weaken glutamine. The increase in the inhibition of the firing of a neuron coupled with a decrease in an excitatory neurotransmitter results in the slurring of speech, slowed reflexes, clouded cognitive processing, and the sluggish gait of someone who is drunk.

Amphetamines and Methamphetamine

Amphetamines and methamphetamine (MA) use a combination approach when it comes to affecting the amount of dopamine in the synapse. First, MA passes directly into the neuron and is picked up by the vesicles that normally carry dopamine or norepinephrine. The vesicles then release not only the MA but also more of the neurotransmitter into the neural synapse than would normally occur. Second, MA blocks the reuptake (reabsorption) of the drug, resulting in an excess of dopamine residing in the synapse. The result is a rapid increase in the amount of dopamine in the synapse. The increase in dopamine after one takes MA is 5 to 10 times greater than what is released when the body is provided with food or sex.

Both methamphetamine (and cocaine) keep dopamine in the synapse by blocking reuptake. However, because neither drug can impede the enzymes that exist in the synapse to dissolve the neurotransmitters trapped there, the dopamine is destroyed. The nervous system is an efficient machine, and because it requires a substantial amount of energy to create neurotransmitters, instead of creating them, the body, under normal conditions, recycles neurotransmitters. However, if the neurotransmitter remains in the synapse too long and is dissolved by the enzymes found there, the body has to make more of that neurotransmitter. Even worse, if the neurons were forced to expel copious amounts of that neurotransmitter, it is likely that the body will be in short supply for the time it takes to manufacture more. This lack of sufficient neurotransmitters, dopamine in particular, contributes to the "crash" experienced by many who are addicted to these drugs. The crash experienced by methamphetamine addicts can be particularly unpleasant because of the two ways MA increases the presence of dopamine in the synapse.

Cocaine/Crack

Similar to methamphetamine, cocaine also alters the removal of dopamine (as well as serotonin and norepinephrine) from the synapse by blocking the reuptake. The presynaptic neuron releases these neurotransmitters into the synapse, resulting in an action potential at the postsynaptic neuron, but instead of the neurotransmitters then being reabsorbed into the presynaptic neuron, the transporters become blocked by the cocaine. This results in the feelings expressed by those who take cocaine including the high levels of energy, confidence, and euphoria that result from the excess levels of norepinephrine, serotonin, and dopamine, respectively. Chronic use of cocaine can result in changes to the brain whereby the neurons not only habituate to the excess amounts of neurotransmitters, particularly dopamine, but also may create additional receptors to accommodate the additional dopamine. The amount of excess dopamine found in someone who uses cocaine is also greater than that produced when someone is provided with food or sex (perhaps two to three times greater); *however,* it is not as high as when someone uses methamphetamine.

Heroin and Other Opioids

Few drugs have the effect on the body and mind as that of opioids. Because opioids have a structure that closely mimics the body's own chemicals, opioids have the ability to induce levels of pleasure (euphoria) so great that few experiences can compete. This coupled with the delivery system for the drug, most often via injection, provides for an experience of euphoria that is not only intense but occurs within seconds of introduction of the drug to the system.

Opioids act on very specific neurons in the brain, spinal column, and in the gastrointestinal tract, specifically mu and kappa. When the opioids attach to the mu and kappa neurons, pain is diminished, dopamine is released, and euphoria is experienced. The fact that opioids affect not only the brain but also the spinal column and the gastrointestinal tract helps to explain both the utility of the drug to manage pain and the symptoms of withdrawal. Opioids block the transmission of pain messages between the spinal column and the brain. As a result, although the physical state of the person has not changed (e.g., the person with stomach cancer still has cancer), the excruciating pain associated with such an ailment is

alleviated. In addition, the fact that opioids act on the gastrointestinal tract explain why those addicted to opioids experience nausea and vomiting.

A significant danger in the taking of opioids is that these drugs have the ability to reduce respiration; thus, the dosage and administration of the drug should be closely monitored by a medical doctor.

Lysergic Acid Diethylamide (LSD)

Lysergic acid diethylamide (LSD) is unique in that it does not act on dopamine; rather it acts on serotonin. Serotonin, as mentioned earlier, is another important neurotransmitter involved in perception and helps to regulate sleeping, eating, and mood. The effects of LSD on the brain are still being studied. What is known is that LSD may either activate or block serotonin receptors, providing for the distorted perception of reality as well as the improved mood.

Marijuana

The active ingredient in marijuana is delta-9-tetrahydrocannabinol (THC). THC binds to receptors on neurons in the pleasure center in the brain. THC also affects other areas of the brain that control thought, movement, and memory. When THC binds to receptors in the hippocampus, the part of the brain responsible for organizing, accessing, and converting short-term memories into long-term memories, the neurons in the hippocampus cease to function properly. In other words, in addition to affecting dopamine levels, use of marijuana results in the brain's inability to access certain short-term memories and may interfere with the conversion of memories from short-term to long-term.

Methylenedioxymethamphetamine (MDMA)

Methylenedioxymethamphetamine (MDMA, ecstasy) is chemically similar to amphetamine (stimulant) and mescaline (hallucinogen). Much of the research on the effect of MDMA on the brain consists of rat studies and limited nonhuman primate studies. As such, the specific effects of this drug on the brain are not known. What is known or can be inferred from the animal studies is that MDMA produces damage to neurons responsible for the production of serotonin and has been associated with impaired memory functioning. The damage to serotonin-producing neurons is most likely the reason why many users of MDMA suffer from hyperthermia (increase in body temperature) as serotonin is important for body temperature regulation. The impairment to memory processing implies that use of MDMA may affect the hippocampus.

Nicotine

Use of nicotine results in an increase in the amount of dopamine found in the synapse, like the other drugs discussed here (except LSD). However, unlike the other drugs presented, nicotine does not tag along in the vesicles resulting in the increased dispersing of dopamine like MA; nor does it block the reuptake of dopamine like cocaine. Instead, nicotine attaches itself to a receptor on the body of the neuron in the VTA (there are places on the cell body where nicotine attaches and affects the internal operations of the neuron) and stimulates the neuron, which results in more firings of the neuron (action potential). In addition, nicotine also binds to receptors, resulting in the release of a greater amount of dopamine than would normally be secreted. In essence, nicotine increases dopamine by causing the presynaptic neuron to fire more often and to release more dopamine, thereby affecting the synapse in two distinct ways.

Methods of Administration

Each method of administering drugs results in a different concentration of the drug and varying lengths of time the drug is active. For example, injecting and smoking a drug results in a faster and more intense high as compared to inhaling (snorting or snuffing) or ingesting the drug, whereas the highs experienced when someone snorts or ingests a drug are, by contrast, sustained for a longer period of time. This may explain why most drug addicts may start off snorting a drug and move to smoking. A trade is made in that the duration of the "high" is shorter, but the intensity is much greater. This difference may also offer some explanation with regard to why drugs that are injected (e.g., heroin) are so difficult to abstain from—the intensity (and fleeting nature) of the high.

Method of drug administration may offer some explanation as to the difference experienced when someone smokes crack cocaine as compared to an individual who snorts powdered cocaine. Crack, because it is smoked, enters the bloodstream and affects the brain rapidly, essentially traveling from the lungs into the heart, which then pumps the drug to the brain. Drugs that are snorted or snuffed, like cocaine, must be absorbed into the bloodstream by the blood vessels in the nose, which is a slower process. Therefore, it is not necessarily the crack cocaine itself that results in the more intense high; rather, the route of administration determines the intensity of the high.

Why Does Relapse Occur?

One of the most fascinating and frustrating aspects of drug addiction is the difficulty in obtaining and maintaining sobriety. Many who have not experienced addiction to drugs find it difficult to understand why someone would risk their quality of life, relationships, health, even life and limb for an inanimate object. What is important to understand is that the brain changes, often dramatically, when an individual becomes addicted to alcohol or other drugs.

These changes have been noted in various area of the brain, but the prefrontal cortex, locus coeruleus, amygdala, and hippocampus, in particular, appear to play "supporting roles" in drug addiction and relapse. The prefrontal cortex relays information concerning the pleasurable nature of drug use, and it is the prefrontal cortex that motivates the person to obtain more drugs. The locus coeruleus, impacted mainly by norepinephrine, may become stimulated when there are insufficient levels of the drug in the body, rousing the addicted person to find more of the desired drug. The amygdala tells the body that taking the drug will make it feel good, and the hippocampus stores and retrieves all of the positive memories associated with taking the drug. Interestingly enough, the hippocampus stores not only the physical memories associated with drug use but also the place use occurred, the people present, the sights (paraphernalia) and smells, and any number of other memories that become associated with the drug which can trigger relapse. The desire to use drugs becomes something that is no longer under conscious control; rather, the brain will focus a substantial amount of its resources to "will" the person to use drugs again. Professionals should inform treatment participants of the increased likelihood of relapse if participants are in contact with the people, places, or things (e.g., paraphernalia) that were present when they were using drugs.

Conclusion

Drugs have a significant impact on the individual psychologically and physically. The increases in dopamine and other neurotransmitters may result in changes or damage to neurons, forcing the brain to adapt. Once the brain no longer perceives the drug as a foreign, temporary body, it may begin to incorporate it into everyday functioning. What's more, because of the profound effect on dopamine, the brain gives drugs a level of importance that rivals eating, sleeping, and sex. When one considers the motivations behind eating, sleeping, and sex, it becomes clear why, once addicted, an individual may find it exceptionally difficult to refuse the pleasures of that drug's company.

Desirée A. Crèvecoeur

See also Craving; Detoxification; Medical Consequences; Neurobiology of Addiction; Neurotransmitters; Pharmacological Approaches to Treatment; Withdrawal

Further Readings

Hoffman, J., & Froemke, S. (Eds.). (2007). *Addiction: Why can't they just stop?* New York: Holtzbrink.

Leppa, M., Korvenoja, A., Carlson, S., Timonen, P., Martinkauppi, S., Ahonen, J., et al. (2005). Acute opioid effects on human brain as revealed by functional magnetic resonance imaging. *NeuroImage, 31*, 661–669.

NIDA Community Alert Bulletin on Club Drugs. (2004, May). *Some facts about club drugs.* Retrieved September 10, 2007, from http://www.nida.nih.gov/ClubAlert/ Clubdrugalert.html

NIDA Notes. (1996, September/October). *The brain's drug reward system.* Retrieved September 1, 2007, from http://www.nida.nih.gov/NIDA_notes/NNVol11N4/ Brain.html

NIH and NIDA. (n.d.). *The brain: Understanding neurobiology through the study of addiction.* Colorado Springs, CO: BSCS. Retrieved April 29, 2008, from http://science.education.nih.gov/supplements/nih2/ addiction/default.htm

Rawson, R. A. (2006). *Methamphetamine: New knowledge, new treatments.* Center City, MN: Hazelden.

Roiser, J. P., Rogers, R. D., & Sahakian, B. J. (2005). Neuropsychological function in ecstasy users: A study controlling for poly drug use. *Psychopharmacology, 189*, 505–516.

Stimmel, B., & Kreek, M. J. (2000). Neurobiology of addictive behaviors and its relationship to methadone maintenance. *Mount Sinai Journal of Medicine, 67*, 375–380.

World Health Organization. (2004). *Neuroscience of psychoactive substance use and dependence.* Geneva, Switzerland: Author.

BRIEF INTERVENTIONS

Brief interventions refer to the body of practices designed to increase an individual's awareness of the impact of his or her substance use and to motivate the individual toward behavior change. On the spectrum of responses to substance use, brief interventions fall between prevention activities and treatment practices. While specific interventions vary, they have in common a five-step process for engaging substance users in productive dialogue. Brief interventions may be used to intervene with any individual using addictive substances; however, they have been found to be most effective with those who are at mild to moderate risk of substance use disorders, so many brief intervention strategies are targeted to that population. While brief interventions are distinct from motivational interviewing, the skills involved in motivational interviewing are effectively utilized in successful brief interventions. Settings in which brief interventions are used include substance abuse treatment programs, mental health clinics, health offices or clinics in secondary schools and universities, emergency departments, and physicians' offices. Brief interventions are effective and cost-effective means of addressing substance use and fostering behavior change.

Steps in Brief Interventions

Although the specific practices of brief interventions vary with the presenting issues and the setting, the Center for Substance Abuse Treatment and most professionals agree that any brief intervention consists of five basic steps: introducing the issue; screening, evaluating, and assessing; providing feedback; talking about change and setting goals; and summarizing and reaching closure. In initiating the brief intervention, the clinician introduces the substance use issue in the context of the individual's health. The aim is to raise concern about substance use in a nonthreatening manner while acquainting the individual with the focus and intent of the session. This step also gives the clinician the opportunity to begin establishing rapport with the individual and to gain the individual's permission to proceed. Introducing the issue is followed by screening, evaluation, and assessment of the substance use and substance-related consequences experienced by the individual. A wide variety of well-validated screening and assessment tools are available to clinicians, some of which are designed to give a reasonably accurate picture of the severity and sequelae of use without requiring a lengthy history.

Once the clinician has this information, he or she is in a position to provide feedback to the individual. Feedback is neither diagnosis nor confrontation, neither of which is likely to be productive in the brief intervention setting. Feedback consists of a dialogue in which the clinician offers specific information and engages the individual in reflection on and response to the information. The intent of the session is best served if the clinician offers one concrete statement of feedback at a time, each time eliciting the individual's response. The clinician may also ask open-ended questions that allow the individual to broaden his or her understanding of the feedback.

Essential to the step of providing feedback is an assessment of the individual's stage of change with regard to his or her substance use. When an individual is seen in a brief intervention setting, he or she is most typically found to be in the precontemplation, contemplation, or action stage. By utilizing an understanding of the stages of change, the clinician can determine the individual's readiness to act on specific feedback, thus effectively preparing for the next step: talking about change and setting goals. The clinician's feedback and the individual's self-reflection and comments have set the stage to consider possible behavior changes with regard to substance use. If the individual is in precontemplation, the clinician might guide the discussion to helping the individual accept the connection between substance use and unwanted consequences. An individual in contemplation has likely made this connection and may see some benefit in change, but is ambivalent about moving forward into action; in this case, a desirable outcome is resolution of the ambivalence. If the individual is in action, the clinician might assist the individual in identifying and removing obstacles to success. Regardless of the stage of change, this discussion is meant to generate one or more goals that the individual is willing to implement.

Ideally, the chosen goals are short- to intermediate-term goals and are highly specific; the greater the specificity, the better the individual can tell whether or not the goals have been achieved. If, for example, the individual states the goal as, "I will cut down on my drinking," the clinician can help him or her restate the goal with measurable outcomes: "I will reduce my drinking to no more than three drinks per day and drink no more than three days per week." Typically, goal setting involves negotiation, with either the clinician or the individual proposing an action; the clinician's aim is then to work toward a goal that the individual is willing to attempt. While the clinician may have a long-term goal in mind, such as referring the individual to counseling, it is generally unproductive to push this goal on an individual who is just beginning to look at substance use as a possible problem. Attempting to convince the individual is most likely to result in activating resistance and losing the therapeutic opportunity. When the goal is one that the individual helps to devise and agrees to take, the individual may take ownership of it.

The brief intervention session ends with summarizing and reaching closure. The clinician may restate the key points of the session, with particular attention to the goals that the individual has agreed to undertake. The clinician remains supportive and encouraging, affirming the individual's ability to undertake and meet the goals. If (as sometimes happens) the individual has refused to take on any goals, the clinician affirms his or her willingness to engage in the conversation. Also important at this stage is arranging a follow-up session. This allows the clinician to make an additional contact with the individual to ascertain whether the individual has achieved or attempted to achieve the goals, and what the outcomes have been. Follow-up may take place in another face-to-face meeting, over the telephone, or by other means. Ideally, closure is achieved with the individual having gained new perspective on his or her drug use and its consequences, undertaken a specific goal or goals, been supported in his or her sense of self-efficacy with regard to meeting the goals, and been affirmed in what he/she has accomplished during the session.

Counseling Skills and Practices

Many of the counseling skills and practices used in brief interventions are similar to those used in motivational interviewing. At times, brief intervention and motivational interviewing are assumed to be one and the same, but this is inaccurate. Brief interventions are a group of practices that may be undertaken by a variety of clinicians for the express purpose of helping people gain insight into their substance use and its consequences. Motivational interviewing is not an intervention per se; rather, it is a counseling method designed to direct people toward possible change while completely affirming their autonomy. One of the best-known features of motivational interviewing is its nonadversarial approach, in which the counselor views resistance as a natural response to considering change and does not attempt to "break through it."

Although brief intervention and motivational interviewing are not the same thing, it is apparent that the same knowledge base and skill set can foster positive outcomes in either one. Both assume a strong knowledge of the stages of change model and how to assess for readiness to change. Both rely on high levels of empathy for, acceptance of, and positive feedback to the individual being intervened upon or interviewed. Both emphasize active listening and dialogue while eschewing confrontational and prescriptive methods. Both focus on short- to intermediate-term goals and affirm the individual's self-efficacy. Thus, a clinician with a strong grounding in motivational interviewing will have many of the tools needed to make the best use of brief intervention practices.

Applicability

Brief interventions for substance use have wide applicability. In traditional substance abuse treatment programs, clinicians who perform assessments and intakes frequently encounter those who are entering treatment under duress. Using a brief intervention allows such clinicians to begin establishing a positive relationship between the individual and the program, as well as to start fostering ownership of the substance use problem and of the actions needed for recovery. Mental health professionals can utilize brief interventions with their patients when substance use or abuse has emerged as a barrier to mental health and wellness. By helping them to see the impact of substance use on their mental health recovery, psychiatrists and therapists better their patients' chances for improvement in both areas. In addition, especially among the chronically mentally ill, regular contact with the mental health professional offers the opportunity for goal setting and guided self-evaluation with regular follow-up.

In recent years, there has been a strong push for adoption of brief intervention practices in hospital emergency departments and physicians' offices. Personnel in medical settings, particularly nurses, social workers, and physicians, are often the first professionals to encounter the negative consequences of an individual's substance use. An alcohol-related traffic accident, chronic sinusitis due to cocaine use, drug-related domestic violence, and many other conditions can alert medical professionals to the likelihood of a substance use problem. Clinical staff in hospitals, health clinics, and primary care physicians' offices can be trained in brief interventions that facilitate behavior change and provide a context for ongoing monitoring of substance use.

Effectiveness

A substantial body of evidence supports the effectiveness of brief interventions across clinical settings. Substance-involved adolescents benefit from brief interventions by school health nurses and counselors and by emergency department clinicians. Use of brief interventions with alcohol users indicates wide effectiveness; brief interventions consistently produce reductions in drinking in those with mild to moderate alcohol problems and increases in treatment admission and adherence in alcohol-dependent individuals. These results are seen in multiple settings, including hospitals, health clinics, and substance abuse treatment programs. Smoking cessation programs that utilize brief interventions improve quit rates, which are further increased when used together with nicotine replacement therapy. Cannabis users benefit from brief interventions in terms of sustained decreases in use; however, those diagnosed with cannabis dependence generally do not show significant changes in use without longer-term interventions. Even Web-based brief interventions for alcohol use and mental health clinic interventions with chronically mentally ill patients show promise.

An emerging body of research also supports the cost-effectiveness of brief interventions. In some cases, brief interventions show results similar to those of time-limited therapies while requiring fewer sessions (thus fewer staff hours). In overburdened emergency departments, mental health clinics, and substance abuse settings, getting positive outcomes while using staff time efficiently is a powerful argument in favor of using brief interventions. The more rigorously the brief intervention is implemented and the more powerful the study design is, the more strongly the cost-effectiveness is supported. When weighed against the larger costs of substance abuse (according to the National Institute on Drug Abuse and the National Institute on Alcohol Abuse and Alcoholism, $375 billion annually in the United States), it appears that the benefits of brief interventions to individuals and society far outweigh the relatively modest costs.

The benefits of brief interventions are, of course, dependent on their appropriate implementation. Studies suggest that, despite evidence of effectiveness and cost-effectiveness, many medical personnel and facilities either are slow to adopt brief interventions or attempt to do so without proper training. In response, the Center for Substance Abuse Treatment introduced the Screening, Brief Intervention, and Referral to Treatment (SBIRT) initiative. SBIRT funds state, tribal council, and university efforts to expand capacities by including brief interventions for substance use in their services. These and similar efforts not only make brief interventions more widely available but also provide additional data regarding their effectiveness.

Conclusion

Brief interventions are designed to facilitate individuals' awareness of their substance use and to generate behavior change. Brief interventions empower substance-using individuals to understand their substance use and its consequences, choose what changes they will implement, and develop a sense of self-efficacy with regard to such changes. These interventions are successful and cost effective. Ongoing utilization and research will help expand service capacities and understanding of brief interventions.

Therissa A. Libby

See also Client Engagement; Motivational Interviewing; Screening; Stages of Change Model

Further Readings

Babor, T. F., McRee, B. G., Kassebaum, P. A., Grimaldi, P. L., Ahmed, K., & Bray, J. (2007). Screening, brief intervention, and referral to treatment (SBIRT): Toward a public health approach to the management of substance abuse. *Substance Abuse, 28,* 7–30.

Bien, T. H., Miller, W. R., & Tonigan, J. S. (1993). Brief interventions for alcohol problems: A review. *Addiction, 88,* 315–336.

Center for Substance Abuse Treatment. (1999). *TIP 34: Brief interventions and brief therapies for substance abuse.* Rockville, MD: Author.

Kaner, E. F., Beyer, F., Dickinson, H. O., Pienaar, E., Campbell, F., Schlesinger, C., et al. (2007, April). Effectiveness of brief alcohol interventions in primary care populations. *Cochrane Database of Systematic Reviews.* Retrieved April 10, 2008, from http://mrw.interscience.wiley.com/cochrane/clsysrev/ articles/CD004148/frame.html

Miller, W. R., & Rollnick, S. (2002) *Motivational interviewing: Preparing people for change* (2nd ed.). New York: Guilford Press.

Prochaska, J. O., DiClemente, C. C., & Norcross, J. (1992). In search of how people change. *American Psychologist, 47,* 1102–1114.

Saitz, R., Sullivan, L. M., & Samet, J. H. (2000). Training community-based clinicians in screening and brief intervention for substance abuse problems: Translating evidence into practice. *Substance Abuse, 21,* 21–31.

Vasiliki, E. I., Hosier, S. G., & Cox, W. M. (2006). The efficacy of motivational interviewing as a brief intervention for excessive drinking: A meta-analytic review. *Alcohol and Alcoholism, 41,* 328–335.

BRIEF STRATEGIC FAMILY THERAPY

Brief strategic family therapy (BSFT) is a sustainable, problem-focused, family-based intervention designed to help children and adolescents with behavioral problems and substance abuse. The goal of BSFT is to identify and restructure maladaptive family patterns of interaction that perpetuate family-identified problems. The treatment intervention is designed to help the family shift from destructive patterns of interactions that are maintaining the problems to the development of new solutions and processes. Research has found that BSFT reduces adolescent drug use, increases treatment engagement and retention, improves family functioning, and emphasizes the cultural context of the family. This entry provides a discussion of the theoretical underpinnings of BSFT, relevant research findings for BSFT, and an overview of the techniques used for adolescent drug use.

Theoretical Framework

BSFT is an integrated approach combining compatible components from structural and strategic family therapies. As described by Salvador Minuchin, one of the goals of structural family therapy is to restructure the family system when it fails to adapt to various stressors. In structural family theory, family systems are characterized by essential components: boundaries, subsystems, structures, triangles, and coalitions. BSFT incorporates structural theories of family functioning in five structural domains: (1) Structure refers to leadership, communication flow, and subsystems. (2) Conflict resolution identifies the family's style in addressing disagreements. (3) Resonance focuses on boundaries and emotional distance between family members. (4) Development stage refers to the extent to which each family member's roles are consistent with their age and family role. (5) Identified patienthood refers to the extent to which the family views the symptom bearer (e.g., adolescent using drugs) as the cause of all the family problems. Once the structural issues are identified, the focus of treatment shifts to interrupting processes, restructuring, and developing new solutions to solve existing problems.

Research Findings

Research has shown that BSFT may be particularly helpful for more treatment-resistant clients, by employing specialized family engagement techniques for clients with unique challenges. For example, BSFT engagement techniques help temporarily ameliorate problematic family interactions that present obstacles to removing an adolescent's problem behavior. BSFT has also been shown to address stressors faced by Hispanic immigrant families that may influence family functioning, such as differences in attitudes, beliefs, values, and behaviors that develop between parents and children, when children acculturate quickly to a culture that is not the parents' culture. With regard to adolescent behavioral problems and substance abuse, BSFT targets family conflict, lack of support, poor communication, poor limit-setting, inadequate parental monitoring, inconsistent parenting, and parental drug use, which have been shown to be associated with these behavioral problems.

Intervention Techniques

BSFT is a short-term, directive, problem-focused, and structured intervention. The average length of treatment is 12 to 16 sessions, over the course of 3 to 4 months. BSFT may be conducted in the office or in the home, with the latter providing additional insight into the social context of the family. The definition of *family* is broadly defined in BSFT to include anyone who *functions* as family, and thus, the family is not seen in only the traditional biological sense, which makes BSFT culturally sensitive in populations that recognize the importance of the extended family. The clinical intervention is based on the assumption that a family's difficulties often reflect problems in the way the family is interacting. From a structural perspective, assessment includes joining with the client to build an alliance and then setting the family system into action with enactments and in-session conversations. The structural and strategic assessment goes beyond the initial client complaints and focuses on the underlying relational issues in the family.

BSFT includes some of the following research-proven, specialized engagement techniques: (a) treatment engagement techniques, such as allying with the adolescent if the adolescent is the primary source of resistance to treatment; (b) getting permission from the family member seeking treatment to talk to all family members involved in the adolescent's life; and (c) coaching the family member on ways to get other family members into treatment. Other BSFT components central to the effectiveness of the treatment include (a) developing therapeutic alliance through "joining" and respecting each individual family member as well as the way in which the family is organized; (b) asking clarifying, process-oriented questions of the family about the presenting complaint, until family members begin to see that the problems go beyond the symptom bearer; (c) helping family members see how their interactions inadvertently may be perpetuating the problems (e.g., problem-maintaining interactions or family patterns); (d) exploring alternative ways of relating and redefining the problem using reframes (e.g., reframing parents' anger toward the adolescent's behavior as "caring"); and (e) restructuring the family system and actively directing and eliciting new behaviors. The main strength of BSFT is the long-term implications for change with this form of systemic treatment. One of the main criticisms of this approach is that the therapist may not be able to find a function for the current symptoms within the family system. Proponents of the approach say that you only need to find the problem-maintaining patterns to effectively use BSFT.

Current research in the NIDA Clinical Trials Network is under way, testing the effectiveness of BSFT in real-world community settings. Real-world application of family therapy in community treatment settings is important to bridge the gap between research and practice and serves as a point of departure for future research.

Catherine L. Dempsey

See also Adolescents, Substance Abuse and Treatment; Brief Interventions; Counseling Approaches; Evidenced-Based Treatment; Family Therapy; Multidimensional Family Therapy

Further Readings

Minuchin, S., Nichols, M. P., & Lee, W.-Y. (2007). *Assessing families and couples: From symptom to system.* Boston: Pearson Press.

Robbins, M. S., Bachrach, K., & Szapocznik, J. (2003). Bridging the research-practice gap in adolescent substance abuse treatment: The case of brief strategic family therapy. *Journal of Substance Abuse Treatment, 23,* 123–132.

Santisteban, D. A., Coatsworth, J. D., Perez-Vidal, A., Kurtines, W. M., Schwartz, S. J., LaPerriere, A., et al. (2003). The efficacy of brief strategic/structural family therapy in modifying behavior problems and an exploration of the mediating role that family functioning plays in behavior change. *Journal of Family Psychology, 17*(1), 121–133.

Santisteban, D. A., Morales-Suarez, L., Robbins, M. S., & Szapocznik, J. (2006). Brief strategic family therapy: Lessons learned in efficacy research and challenges to blending research to practice. *Family Process, 45*(2), 259–272.

Szapocznik, J., Hervis, O., & Schwartz, S. (2003). *Brief strategic family therapy for adolescent drug abuse.* Bethesda, MD: National Institute on Drug Abuse.

Szapocznik, J., Perez-Vidal, A., Brickman, A. L., Foote, F. H., Santisteban, D., Hervis, O., et al. (1988). Engaging adolescent drug abusers and their families in treatment: A strategic structural systems approach. *Journal of Consulting and Clinical Psychology, 56,* 552–557.

Bulimia Nervosa

As defined by the *Diagnostic and Statistical Manual of Mental Disorders* (*DSM-IV-TR*), bulimia nervosa (usually referred to as "bulimia") is characterized by recurrent episodes of binge eating often followed by compensatory behaviors to prevent weight gain. Some of these behaviors include chemical-, alcohol-, or self-induced vomiting (purging); compulsive exercise; fasting; chewing food and subsequently spitting it out after initially tasting it; using enemas; and using a variety of over-the-counter and prescription drugs, including laxatives (chemical and natural), thyroid hormones, and diuretics. Many individuals will purge with multiple methods. Bulimia is practiced by men and women, girls and boys. At this time, there is much more research on women who practice bulimia than on men who do so. However, purging through laxative and diuretic abuse to regulate weight is not uncommon in male-dominated athletic endeavors such as body building, horseracing, and wrestling. Both males and females with bulimia report body dissatisfaction along with weight and shape preoccupation. This disorder can be life threatening.

Methods of Purging

The most common over-the-counter substance used by individuals engaging in bulimia is Ipecac. This substance is commonly sold in drug stores. When ingested, it causes the individual to vomit. Many will use Ipecac until they become proficient at throwing up without its assistance. Some individuals will eventually become so adept at controlling their muscles that they need only to lean over to vomit.

Laxatives are often used by individuals with bulimia. There are many types of laxatives, but the most commonly used are the stimulant or irritant types with a therapeutic dosage of one per day for constipation. Clients have reported an excess of 30 in a single day, with some taking that many or more on a daily basis. The long-term effects of laxatives can be a dependence on the chemical for elimination. During the withdrawal from long-term usage, medical monitoring is required because the muscles in the intestines atrophy. Recently, there has been a trend to use herbal laxatives with the assumption that cleaning out the colon is good for the body. However, women with laxative abuse problems are likely to also abuse herbal products as well.

Diuretics are also abused by individuals with bulimia, as a way to eliminate "water weight." There are several brands of diuretics available over the counter. Some individuals manage to have their physician prescribe diuretics. However, these individuals may not take the correct dosage as prescribed, often increasing the medication to achieve their desired effect (weight loss).

Nicotine addiction has also been reported in individuals with bulimia. The common reasons given for nicotine usage by these individuals seems to be to help prevent the binge behaviors and to help curb hunger. Because appearance, with emphasis on weight, is the common complaint of individuals with bulimia, many are reluctant to give up smoking and would not normally present for smoking cessation treatment.

Social and Emotional Issues

Many individuals with eating disorders report feeling self-conscious socially, particularly in situations where eating is part of the function. When placed in a situation where they are expected to eat "normally," there is heightened anxiety. They question whether their eating is like everyone else's or if their binging is noticeable. Clients with a primary diagnosis of bulimia have reported that when they go out with their friends and are unable to control their eating behaviors, they will drink alcohol in excess to help them vomit. Unfortunately, it is somewhat socially forgivable to throw up after drinking, but it is humiliating to throw up after eating in excess.

There is a great deal of shame for individuals engaging in binge eating, self-induced vomiting, and in feeling that the individual's body or weight is not acceptable. Often, the binge eating and compensatory behaviors are practiced in private. An exception is exercising. However, the individual, when questioned, often minimizes the amount of time spent exercising. Individuals have reported as much as 8 hours a day at the gym or on their personal equipment.

As with other disordered eating behaviors, the issue for the client with bulimia is not the food. The issue has to do with the client's ability to manage emotions. With bulimia, the most common emotions clients report difficulty with are anger and anxiety. However, careful questioning around the events leading up to the episodes of binging, purging, or both, can assist the client and therapist in discovering the issues and emotions that are experienced by the client as unbearable. Learning other behaviors to substitute for binging and purging can be most useful.

Substance Abuse Issues

When bulimia is suspected, a physical examination and laboratory tests should be conducted by medical professionals. However, it is frequently the case that intake counselors in alcohol and other drug treatment facilities might be the first to suspect that an eating disorder is present.

As part of an intake interview for inpatient or outpatient substance abuse treatment, questions should be asked that would assess for an eating disorder. Bulimia, unlike other eating disorders, may not have visible physical symptoms. If the binge/purge behavior has been recent and chronic, the parotid glands (behind the jaw, below the ear) may be swollen. The client may also appear bloated. If these physical symptoms are present, the client should be asked about binging and purging. As stated earlier, these behaviors evoke shame in many individuals, and it may be difficult for them to volunteer the information. Therefore, it is imperative that a solid rapport be established before some individuals are comfortable in disclosing their self-induced vomiting behaviors. Due to the sensitivity of the admission, asking questions that lead up to disclosure should be considered. For example, questions such as "How comfortable are you with your current weight?" and "Has this always been the case?" can be helpful. It is important to determine the frequency of self-induced vomiting as this can be life threatening should the individual's electrolytes become imbalanced.

Women with both substance use disorders and bulimia are more likely to have other issues with impulse control, such as unsafe sex, self-harm, and suicide ideation or attempts. Therefore, therapists must assess for self-destructive behaviors.

There are online screening tests that can assist counselors and clients to determine if an eating disorder may be present. Two examples are the SCOFF questions for eating disorders (St. George's Hospital Medical School, University of London) and the Are You at Risk for an Eating Disorder? (Dartmouth College Health Services). Other assessment tools can be purchased from commercial vendors.

Treatment

Some individuals may begin binging and purging and add alcohol or drugs later. Others may begin with alcohol or drugs and incorporate disordered eating behaviors. Clients with bulimia and drug abuse issues may present for treatment for only one of the problems. The client may be admitted to an eating disorder treatment facility and have a co-occurring substance abuse problem. The client could present to a drug treatment facility and may or may not report the bulimia. Once it has been determined that a client has both a substance abuse disorder and an eating disorder, it is important to encourage the client to address both issues.

An individual in an inpatient drug and alcohol treatment program could easily be practicing unobserved binge and purge behaviors. Most often, the individual would disappear after meals to engage in self-induced vomiting. The individual might volunteer to work in the kitchen or do food shopping where they would have access to binge foods. If the client presents for inpatient substance abuse treatment and admits to binge behaviors, it is imperative that they not have unmonitored access to the kitchen or food storage.

In the outpatient counseling setting, the counselor may not know that the individual engages in bulimia unless the client discloses this information. The client may present another problem, such as anxiety or depression, without disclosing the bulimia. Consequently, it is imperative that substance-abusing individuals be assessed for problem eating behaviors.

Clearly, the treatment of bulimia requires qualified professionals and a multidisciplinary approach. While some substance abuse treatment facilities have the staff and program to offer both types of services, most do not. Therefore, clients with substance use disorders and bulimia should be treated by professionals and in facilities qualified to treat both conditions. Treatment for bulimia involves medical monitoring; nutritional counseling; individual, couple, and family therapy; group counseling; and support groups.

Conclusion

Bulimia nervosa is an eating disorder that includes binging and purging. It is a medically dangerous condition originating from social and emotional causes. Substance abuse treatment professionals should assess for the possibility of bulimia, particularly in female clients, and should refer suspected clients for a medical evaluation and diagnosis. The treatment for bulimia in conjunction with a substance use disorder should be implemented by qualified, multidisciplinary staff.

Jean E. Griffin

See also Anorexia Nervosa; Co-Occurring Disorders; Cross-Addictions, *Diagnostic and Statistical Manual of Mental Disorders*; Other Addictions

Further Readings

Duncan, A. E., Newman, R. J., Kramer, J. R., Kuperman, S., Hesselbrock, V. M., & Bucholz, K. K. (2006). Lifetime psychiatric comorbidity of alcohol dependence and bulimia nervosa in women. *Drug and Alcohol Dependence, 84*(1), 122–132.

Garner, D. M., & Garfinkel, P. E. (1997). *Handbook of treatment for eating disorders.* New York: Guilford Press.

Steffen, K. J., Mitchell, J. E., Roerig, J. L., & Lancaster, K. L. (2007). The eating disorders medicine cabinet revisited: A clinician's guide to Ipecac and laxatives. *International Journal of Eating Disorders, 40*(4), 360–368.

BUPRENORPHINE

Buprenorphine is a medication to treat opioid dependence. It was approved by the U.S. Food and Drug Administration on October 8, 2002, as a Schedule III narcotic (i.e., it has abuse potential and it is used as a medicine in the United States). This entry describes the pharmacology of buprenorphine, available types, and the drug's safety and efficacy. Buprenorphine is expected to increase access to opioid addiction treatment for an estimated 379,000 current illicit opioid (i.e., heroin) users and approximately 2 million problem users of prescription opioids as reported by the 2005 National Survey on Drug Use and Health.

As a medication that can be prescribed to patients under the Drug Addiction Treatment Act of 2000 (DATA 2000), buprenorphine provides an alternative to patients who are not able to access methadone clinics or who do not meet criteria for treatment in an outpatient treatment program (e.g., patient criteria for methadone treatment clinics often include opioid dependence for 1 or more years). As reviewed by Johnson and colleagues, buprenorphine has unique pharmacological characteristics that provide for a wide margin of safety and long duration of action. Buprenorphine is a partial agonist at the mu-opioid receptor and antagonist at the kappa-opioid receptor. As a partial agonist at the mu-opioid receptor, buprenorphine does not activate the mu-receptor to the same extent as does a full mu-opioid agonist (e.g., methadone), resulting in less than maximal opioid effect (also called a ceiling or plateau effect). Buprenorphine also binds tightly to the mu-receptor, allowing it to displace other opioids (e.g., methadone) from the receptor. Once it occupies the receptor, buprenorphine blocks the effects of other opioids for the mu-opioid receptor. Buprenorphine also disassociates or leaves the mu-opioid receptor slowly and this is thought to account for its long duration of action in the treatment of opioid dependence. It is this partial agonist activity at the mu-receptor, combined with its strong binding to the receptor site, that is believed to be responsible for buprenorphine's ability to block the effects of opioids (e.g., morphine, hydromorphone, heroin). Buprenorphine also has high affinity for, and antagonist action, at the kappa-receptor. As an antagonist at the kappa-receptor, buprenorphine may block increased kappa activity associated with opioid agonist withdrawal and lead to less dysthymia and increased positive mood and feelings. For the purpose of opioid-dependence treatment, the effects produced by buprenorphine at the mu-opioid receptor are the most important. In addition to buprenorphine's unique pharmacology, the safety profile (i.e., less respiratory depression and less overdose risk) for buprenorphine is greater than that of a full mu-opioid agonist (e.g., morphine, heroin, methadone, oxycodone). Additionally, buprenorphine has been reported to have less autonomic associated signs and symptoms of opioid withdrawal upon cessation.

There are two formulations of buprenorphine: a buprenorphine hydrogen chloride (HCl) tablet (Subutex) and a buprenorphine HCl plus naloxone salt combination tablet (Suboxone). As discussed by Mendelson and Jones, Suboxone with a 4:1 buprenorphine-to-naloxone ratio was developed because buprenorphine alone has abuse potential and is abused in many countries. Naloxone is poorly absorbed sublingually; however, when injected into the vein, naloxone can produce a precipitated opioid withdrawal syndrome in persons addicted to full mu-opioid agonists. The addition of naloxone in Suboxone is expected to reduce the abuse liability of buprenorphine alone. These unique characteristics allow for buprenorphine to be used both in new (e.g., office-based practice) and more traditional opioid treatment programs, thus providing opioid-dependent patients greater access to treatment.

The safety and efficacy of buprenorphine has been well studied. Initial research by Jasinski and colleagues showed that buprenorphine produced a profile of signs and symptoms similar to morphine (e.g., constricted pupils, sleepy, itchy skin), yet unlike morphine, it produced little physical dependence or respiratory depression and abruptly stopping buprenorphine produced only mild withdrawal. The potential efficacy of buprenorphine was further demonstrated by Mello and colleagues when chronic buprenorphine–treated subjects failed to self-administer heroin relative to placebo-treated subjects. Subsequently, numerous studies examined the safety and efficacy of buprenorphine maintenance. The only study to directly compare all three agonist medications (buprenorphine, levo-alpha acetyl methadol [LAAM], and methadone versus low-dose methadone) was conducted by Johnson and colleagues and showed that, compared to low-dose methadone, all three medications produced similar reductions in illicit opioid use. Taken together, these studies demonstrate that (a) buprenorphine has efficacy similar to methadone over a broad dose range and (b) the dose response to buprenorphine and methadone maintenance is such that larger doses of either medication are associated with decreases in illicit opioid use.

The treatment objectives for buprenorphine are identical to those of other opioid agonist medications like methadone. Objectives include to first prevent opioid withdrawal signs and symptoms, provide a comfortable induction onto the medication, and then attenuate the motivation (i.e., craving, social interactions) to use illicit opioids. By eliminating illicit opioid use, it is expected that opioid-dependent individuals can begin to focus energy on building balanced lives; this may include repairing family and social relationships, finding positive social support networks, obtaining fulfilling employment, and engaging in novel recreational activities. Buprenorphine, while effective for eliminating illicit opioid use, is not a cure for opioid dependence, but it is a critical component to developing a complete treatment regimen. Whereas buprenorphine effectively addresses the medical aspect of opioid dependence, no drug has been found to change the behaviors associated with illicit drug use. It has been suggested that as adjuncts to medication, behavioral and psychosocial interventions are elements that complete a treatment plan and provide a greater likelihood that patients will achieve and sustain drug abstinence. Thus, it would be expected that buprenorphine will have greatest effects when used in combination with behavioral interventions. On a societal level, buprenorphine treatment has been shown by several research groups, including Kakko and colleagues, to reduce the harmful effects of opioid dependence (i.e., reducing drug use severity, increasing social status, reducing the diffusion of HIV/AIDS or other infectious diseases) and may provide other substantial advantages.

Hendree E. Jones

See also Levo-Alpha Acetyl Methadol; Methadone Maintenance Treatment; Naloxone; Opioids; Pharmacological Approaches to Treatment

Further Readings

Center for Substance Abuse Treatment. (2004). *TIP 40: Clinical guidelines for the use of buprenorphine in the treatment of opioid addiction* (DHHS Publication No. SMA 04-3939). Rockville, MD: Substance Abuse and Mental Health Services Administration.

Jasinski, D. R., Pevnick, J. S., & Griffith, J. D. (1978). Human pharmacology and abuse potential of the analgesic buprenorphine: A potential agent for treating narcotic addiction. *Archives of General Psychiatry, 35,* 501–516.

Johnson, R. E., Chutuape, M. A., Strain, E. C., Walsh, S. L., Stitzer, M. L., & Bigelow, G. E. (2000). A comparison of levomethadyl acetate, buprenorphine, and methadone for opioid dependence. *New England Journal of Medicine, 343,* 1290–1297.

Johnson, R. E., Strain, E. C., & Amass, L. (2003). How to use buprenorphine right. *Drug and Alcohol Dependence, 70,* S59–S77.

Kakko, J., Svanborg, K. D., Kreek, M. J., & Heilig, M. (2003). 1-year retention and social function after buprenorphine-assisted relapse prevention treatment for heroin dependence in Sweden: A randomized placebo-controlled trial. *Lancet, 361,* 662–668.

Mello, N. K., & Mendelson, J. H. (1980). Buprenorphine suppresses heroin use by heroin addicts. *Science, 207,* 657–659.

Mendelson, J., & Jones, R. T. (2003). Clinical and pharmacological evaluation of buprenorphine and naloxone combinations: Why the 4:1 ratio for treatment? *Drug and Alcohol Dependence, 70,* S29–S37.

BUSINESS IMPROVEMENT PRACTICES

The world of addiction treatment organizations is increasingly dominated by business scenarios such as mergers, buyouts, and rising competition. Larger and larger organizations are taking control of what began as independent "mom and pop" treatment agencies.

The result is that addiction treatment organizations (largely nonprofit), which faced few demands in the past for marketing, competition, and performance, are now fighting to keep their identity, financial solvency, and places in communities. In an environment in which agencies are folding, restructuring, and merging with others to stay competitive, it is critical that addiction treatment organizations demonstrate business savvy, not only so that they can remain in compliance with a labyrinth of laws and regulations but even more so to demonstrate good stewardship in doing the most with their limited resources.

Addiction Treatment Organizations

In a special 2006 issue of the *Journal of Substance Abuse Treatment* that was devoted to the "business of addiction treatment," Kimberly and McLellan provided a synopsis of the status and function of the specialty care programs that comprise more than 80% of the nation's treatments for alcohol and drug abuse. They found the following:

- These specialty sector programs are predominantly small (more than two thirds treat fewer than 300 patients per year), community-based, outpatient, and not-for-profit organizations. Most are freestanding and are not affiliated with any general medical institution.
- The great majority of revenues received by these programs (approximately 80%) come from government sources (such as state Medicaid and block-grant allocations and Department of Veterans Affairs and Indian Health Services programs) and funds provided by state and county criminal justice and welfare programs.
- Less than 12% of revenues come from private health care insurance, and this specialty sector treatment system appears to operate outside mainstream health care.

These addiction treatment organizations exist in extremely complex business and clinical environments. They face numerous types of funding, including federal, state, and private sources, each with different eligibility requirements and payment mechanisms. There is increased emphasis on accountability for this funding and demand for improved treatment practices that are based upon scientific evidence. There are numerous regulations that are imposed on virtually all aspects of the treatment delivery process—for example, community restrictions on site licenses for treatment programs, regulations on buildings in which care is delivered, and the requirement for regular inspections at the federal, state, county, and city levels to sustain operation permits. Likewise, there are often particular issues that addiction treatment organizations must address, such as unclear performance expectations, multiple and conflicting stakeholder interests, frequent political influence attempts, and heightened public scrutiny.

Partners for Recovery, a component of the Substance Abuse and Mental Health Services Administration, conducted a survey of current addiction treatment leaders. Survey results emphasized business issues as major themes impacting leaders today and in the near future, including such themes as a tighter funding and regulatory environment, using research as the basis for funding and policy, addiction treatment increasingly blended with mental health and primary care, managed care constraints on treatment practices and quality of care, high-tech efficiencies replacing face-to-face interaction, and greater expectations and accountability for outcomes. Survey respondents stressed the need for current and future addiction treatment leaders to be proficient in both business and clinical arenas.

Sound Business Research

Specific research on the organization, financing, effectiveness, and management of addiction services has not advanced to the same degree as has clinical and pharmaceutical research. Citing a review of the health services research portfolio of the National Institute on Drug Abuse, Kimberly and McLellan identified very little research in the areas of organization, finance, or management practices within the addiction treatment field. Therefore, in seeking a research base, one must look to research conducted in other related industries that have experienced significant problems that are similar, in many respects, to those seen in the addiction treatment realm.

The closest body of research to investigate is that of the nonprofit sector, as the majority of addiction services are delivered through nonprofit organizations. Over the past decade, a growing number of books and nonprofit resource and training centers—such as the Brookings Institution, Harvard Business School, Peter Drucker Institute, National Center on Nonprofit Enterprise, and Johnson Center, to name a few—have become available with the goal of helping nonprofit practitioners to manage their organizations more

effectively and efficiently. Some of these resources attempt to bring business concepts, such as business planning, reengineering, quality management, benchmarking, and measuring return on investment, to bear on the nonprofit sector. It is important to note, however, that there is great diversity among nonprofit organizations both in size and mission, which range from hospitals and human service organizations to charities, foundations, advocacy groups, universities, and chambers of commerce. Therefore, when looking at the research in this arena, one needs to realize that, even in the nonprofit sector, one size does not fit all.

Improved Business Practices

It is not enough to be a competent specialist in today's business world. Successful addiction treatment organizations need leaders and managers that have a broad understanding of strategy, operations, and finance, and how these all interact. Leaders and managers need to be armed with *business acumen,* which includes understanding the organization's business model and financial goals; utilizing economic, financial, and organizational data to build and document the business case for investing in workplace and performance solutions; and using business terminology when communicating with others. More simply put, business acumen is the ability to focus on the business basics, to link these to an insightful assessment of the external business landscape, and then to execute the strategy to acquire the desired results. Business acumen requires skill and practice and demands intense mental activity. Being able to see how the internal and external landscapes are evolving requires a high caliber of qualitative logic and the ability to frame, assess, discard, and adopt many assumptions at once.

The successful operation of addiction treatment organizations requires competency in a remarkable number of business operations. Certain business principles and practices are universal; however, some of these practices must be modified to meet the needs of these types of organizations. For example, decision-making processes generally have to be handled in a more consultative, inclusive style due to the oftentimes disparate concerns of funders, community stakeholders, and boards of directors. Likewise, measuring performance and success in addiction treatment organizations is not simply a financial metric, as these organizations are dealing with the behavioral changes of service recipients and, at times, more intangible issues of social change. Leaders in these organizations need to be more entrepreneurial than the typical chief executive officer in the corporate world, as they have fewer resources, fewer staff, and less certainty.

Striving for Excellence

Addiction treatment organizations, like business and government, must adapt the principles and best practices of excellence and continuous improvement if they are to meet growing public service needs in the face of scarce resources. A commitment to excellence must become ingrained in the basic culture within these organizations if they expect to be successful over time. Paul Light's 2002 book, *Pathways to Nonprofit Excellence,* addresses fundamental business practices that correlate with high performance in nonprofit organizations. These practices include investment in staff training, collaboration with other organizations, diversification of the funding base, maintenance of reserve funds, better integration of electronic technology, and recruitment of talented and motivated staff who are intrinsically rewarded by mission-related accomplishments. Light prioritizes the strengthening of nonprofits' management infrastructure as a key factor in the pursuit of nonprofit excellence and sustainability.

The Nonprofit Handbook: Management, by Tracy Daniel Connors, proposes an excellence equation for nonprofit organizations that seek to renew and revitalize their business practices. It identifies three fundamental elements necessary for nonprofit organizations to achieve and sustain excellence: effectiveness, efficiency, and organizational environment.

1. *Effectiveness* deals with those topics and issues facing an organization that are necessary to ensure it has a valid purpose in accomplishing its customer-focused mission and focused strategies. Business practices in this area encompass strategic planning and development, customer focus and satisfaction, and public service provider (business) results.

2. *Efficiency* addresses the processes and techniques leaders must use to create an organization that performs well and economically, with reduced waste of time, energy, and materials, through efficient resource development, process improvement, and resource conservation. Business practices in this area encompass process management and information and analysis.

3. *Organizational environment* includes a focus on how to create and sustain an organizational environment able to adapt to changing conditions, manage change effectively, transition to new states, and turn in new directions—to constantly evolve. Business practices in this area encompass leadership, change management, and human resource development and management.

Conclusion

It is important that addiction treatment organizations attend to the trends and practices that drive their livelihood and viability. The business practices that have been discussed are not new, nor is their importance particularly surprising or counterintuitive. However, organizations can all too easily forget or ignore the basics. Succeeding in business can be hard work, yet it stands to reason that addiction treatment organizations with the managerial sophistication to adopt state-of-the-art business and clinical practices will have a competitive edge in the marketplace.

Pamela Waters

See also Addiction Technology Transfer Centers; Center for Substance Abuse Treatment; Health Care System and Substance Abuse; Insurance Parity; Qualified Services Organization Agreements

Further Readings

Center for the Organization and Management of Addiction Treatment (COMAT): http://www.Tresearch.org/centers/comat.htm

Connors, T. D. (Ed.). (2001). *The nonprofit handbook: Management* (3rd ed.). New York: Wiley.

Dorothy A. Johnson Center for Philanthropy & Nonprofit Leadership. (2008). *Nonprofit good practice guide.* Retrieved April 12, 2008, from http://www.npgood practice.org

Kimberly, J., & McLellan, A. (2006). The business of addiction treatment: A research agenda. *Journal of Substance Abuse Treatment, 31*(3), 213–219.

Lahey, M. A., Burling, A. S., Shore, K. K., & Schmitt, J. (2003). *The BEST assessment and planning guide: An agency guide for building effective substance abuse treatment organizations.* Palo Alto, CA: American Institutes for Research.

Light, P. C. (2002). *Pathways to nonprofit excellence.* Washington, DC: Brookings Institution Press.

Light, P. C. (2004). *Sustaining nonprofit performance: The case for capacity building and the evidence to support it.* Washington, DC: Brookings Institution Press.

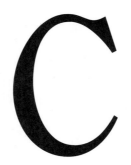

CAFFEINE

Caffeine is the most widely used psychoactive drug in the world. It exists naturally in plants and can also be produced synthetically and added to foods and beverages. Although frequently ingested through food (e.g., chocolate) and sometimes in pain, cold, or diet medication, caffeine is most often consumed through beverages such as coffee, tea, and carbonated soda or sodalike beverages (including many energy drinks). The amount of caffeine in coffee varies based on the size of the serving, the type of coffee, and how the coffee is prepared. According to the U.S. National Institute of Health, a 250-ml cup of coffee can vary in the quantity of contained caffeine from 5 mg in decaffeinated coffee to 30 mg to 120 mg in instant coffee and to 40 mg to 180 mg in brewed coffee. In comparison, brewed tea can contain 20 mg to 90 mg, instant tea roughly 28 mg, common soft drinks 36 mg to 90 mg, and chocolate milk 3 mg to 6 mg of caffeine. In the United States, as well as in many other countries, caffeine does not have to be listed on product labels unless it has been added to the product separately. In other words, if a product contains another substance (e.g., yerba maté) that naturally includes caffeine, caffeine does not have to be listed as a separate ingredient.

Caffeine is not a nutrient that the body requires for optimal healthy functioning. Rather, it belongs to the class of drugs popularly called central nervous system stimulants due to their ability to heighten physical and psychological functioning. Several sources, including the American Psychiatric Association, note that the average daily consumption of caffeine among American adults is at least 200 mg to 300 mg a day (equivalent to about two to three cups of regular coffee) and that roughly 80% of Americans consume caffeine daily. Along with its reported beneficial effects, caffeine carries with it a host of possible adverse consequences. Such consequences, combined with caffeine's prevalent use in North America, have triggered a growing concern over this legally sanctioned drug.

The U.S. Food and Drug Administration (FDA) recognizes caffeine under the category of "Generally Recognized as Safe" for moderate consumption, and the American Medical Association maintains a similar position. However, the concept of moderate consumption is unique to every individual and depends on factors such as an individual's health and body makeup. For example, some individuals can drink several caffeinated beverages in short succession and experience little or no effects while others may experience caffeine's stimulating properties after consuming only one.

Ubiquitous caffeine use raises the question of how much is too much. Whereas the United States does not hold official national guidelines for general caffeine consumption, such principles are available in Canada. For the general adult population, Health Canada recommends a maximum of 400 mg per day, the equivalent of three to four 8 ounce cups of brewed coffee. Health Canada's recommendation for caffeine intake for women of childbearing age who are anticipating pregnancy in the future was lowered in 2003 based on new research. They reported that these women are at increased risk of adverse reproductive effects and should not exceed more than 300 mg per day. This recommendation is inline with those made by the

U.S. National Institute of Health, which stated that caffeine consumption over 300 mg per day by pregnant women results in an increased risk of miscarriage and in slowed growth of a developing fetus. Children are at much greater risk for the negative behavioral consequences that can result from caffeine use. For those age 12 and under, based on average body weight, Health Canada recommends a maximum daily intake of 45 mg for children ages 4 to 6, 62.5 mg for children ages 7 to 9 and 85 mg for children ages 10 to 12.

Once caffeine enters the body, the effects can be felt by some individuals within 15 minutes. Upon consumption, caffeine produces diverse psychological and physiological effects largely through stimulation of the central nervous system. Doses of caffeine under the recommended limits can produce increased energy, alertness, and sociability while also serving to elevate mood. In addition, individuals who have consumed up to such a moderate dose report enhanced cognitive performance, the ability to sustain attention for longer periods, and a partial counteracting of performance detriments associated with sleep deprivation. In light of these desirable effects, many individuals are unaware of the potentially negative consequences of caffeine use. Even within recommended limits, caffeine has been found to result in insomnia and increased blood pressure. In higher doses, caffeine has been shown to produce anxiety, jitteriness, stomach pain, diarrhea, dehydration, dizziness, rapid heart beat, blurred vision, severe confusion (delirium), muscle tremors, nausea, vomiting, increased sensitivity to touch and pain, seizures, and decreased bone density.

Although alcohol and other psychoactive drug use have been closely monitored in national surveys, such is not the case for caffeine. Although caffeine consumption has become an everyday part of many people's lives, caffeine is nonetheless a potential drug of abuse. For example, caffeine use can lead to withdrawal symptoms, the development of tolerance, and other dependence-type symptoms (e.g., preoccupation with thoughts related to its use, unsuccessful attempts to stop usage, using more than intended). Furthermore, caffeine is included in the *Diagnostic and Statistical Manual of Mental Disorders, Fourth Edition, Text Revision* (*DSM-IV-TR*), published by the American Psychiatric Association, by means of the following psychiatric disorders: caffeine-intoxication, caffeine-induced anxiety disorder, caffeine-induced sleep disorder, and caffeine-related disorder not otherwise specified (a catchall category of other caffeine-related conditions). In-line with the *DSM-IV-TR*, the *International Classification of Diseases, Tenth Edition* (*ICD-10*), published by the World Health Organization, lists "mental and behavioral disorders due to use of other stimulants, including caffeine" and "poisoning: psychostimulants with abuse potential," a category that includes caffeine.

When an individual whose body has become accustomed to certain levels of caffeine stops ingesting caffeine, a range of unpleasant physical and psychological consequences may result. The most comprehensive review of the effects of caffeine withdrawal to date, completed by Laura Juliano of American University and Roland Griffiths of Johns Hopkins University, validated the following as the key symptoms of caffeine withdrawal upon abrupt discontinuation of its use (even at doses as low as 100 mg per day): headaches, decreased energy, tiredness, depressed mood, heartburn, sleep difficulty, irritability, general anxiety, decreased alertness, drowsiness, and difficulty concentrating. Withdrawal symptoms tend to peak during the first 12 to 24 hours after the last use of caffeine and typically end within a week. The potential for caffeine withdrawal to cause clinically significant distress or impairment in functioning is reflected by the inclusion of caffeine withdrawal as a diagnosis in the *ICD-10* and as a condition in need of further study for possible future inclusion by the *DSM-IV-TR*.

Robinder P. Bedi and Natalie G. Wuitchik

See also Central Nervous System Stimulants; *Diagnostic and Statistical Manual of Mental Disorders*; Substance-Induced Disorders; Substance Use Disorders

Further Readings

Health Canada. (2006, February). *It's your health: Caffeine.* Retrieved March 11, 2007, from http://www.hc-sc.gc.ca/iyh-vsv/alt_formats/cmcd-dcmc/pdf/caffeine_e.pdf

James, J. E. (1997). *Understanding caffeine: A biobehavioral analysis.* Thousand Oaks, CA: Sage.

Juliano, L. M., & Griffiths, R. R. (2004). A critical review of caffeine withdrawal: Empirical validation of symptoms and signs, incidence, severity, and associated features. *Psychopharmacology, 176,* 1–29.

Nehlig, A. (2004). Dependence upon coffee and caffeine: An update. In A. Nehlig (Ed.), *Coffee, tea, chocolate, and the brain* (pp. 133–146). Boca Raton, FL: CRC Press.

CAGE SCREENING INSTRUMENT

The CAGE Questionnaire is the most commonly used screening instrument for alcohol use disorders. The CAGE was designed to quickly screen adults for drinking problems by asking them four questions about their drinking experiences across their lifetime. The questions were selected because they appeared to be sensitive indicators of covert problem drinking in preliminary studies. Each of the questions has within it a key word that serves to form the CAGE acronym.

The four key CAGE questions are as follows: (1) Have you ever felt you should *cut* down on your drinking? (2) Have people *annoyed* you by criticizing your drinking? (3) Have you ever felt bad or *guilty* about your drinking? (4) Have you ever had a drink first thing in the morning to steady your nerves or to get rid of a hangover (*eye-opener*)?

Individuals complete the CAGE on their own in a written format or the questions may be asked as part of an interview. Individuals answer the questions either *yes* or *no*. Each yes response to a CAGE question is scored as 1. A total score of 0 to 4 results from summing positive answers. A score of 2 or higher is considered clinically significant and raises concern that an individual may have problematic alcohol use patterns or symptoms of alcoholism. The CAGE takes less than 1 minute to complete and score. No special training is required to use the CAGE, and it may be used without permission. The CAGE has been translated into multiple languages other than English, including Flemish, French, Hebrew, Japanese, Polish, Portuguese, and Spanish.

When used in the context of a clinical interview, affirmative answers to CAGE questions may be explored by professionals with additional questions to understand the nature and severity of the patients' potential drinking problems. For patients who report they have tried to cut down their drinking, professionals might ask about the difficulty of this process, how successful they had been in reducing or stopping drinking, and when prior elevated drinking levels resumed. Patients who note annoyance about criticism of their drinking could be asked about the sources and nature of the criticisms and how the criticisms have affected their self-perception. Professionals might ask patients who have indicated feeling guilty about their drinking to describe what caused the guilt, how drinking affects their behavior, and what impact the guilt has had on their current intentions to drink. Finally, with patients who report having had morning eye-openers, professionals could explore the types of alcohol withdrawal symptoms they may have experienced, the recency of the symptoms, and how often they may have been drinking throughout the day.

The extent to which the CAGE items yield consistent responses (i.e., that it is reliable as a measure) has not received much research attention. In a study of underage drinkers treated in emergency departments, however, the CAGE item responses typically varied by differences in respondents' drinking experiences rather than problems in item interpretation or other errors. Moreover, the CAGE has been included in numerous studies with large sample sizes of patients seeking treatment in general medical or psychiatric settings to determine how well it screens for problematic drinking. In general, a cutoff score of 1 or 2 has been found to improve the accuracy of clinicians in identifying patients who have and do not have drinking problems (as determined by independent clinical or structured diagnostic assessments). Studies that compare the CAGE with single items such as "How much do you drink?" or to biological measures such as liver function tests or breath tests for alcohol show the CAGE greatly improves the ability of clinicians to accurately screen patients for alcohol use disorders.

The CAGE has several strengths. It is easy to understand and administer, inexpensive, and can be used by professionals across disciplines and health care settings. In addition, the CAGE works well for detecting harmful lifetime drinking when individuals may have developed more severe alcohol use disorders. It is less effective, however, in capturing individuals at an earlier stage of drinking. The CAGE also has been found to perform less well among females, adolescents, and college students where the severe problems assessed by the CAGE may be less indicative of problematic alcohol use in these populations. If used in these populations, a cutoff of 1 customarily is recommended. The CAGE also does not quantify drinking frequency and quantity. Finally, because the intent of the CAGE questions is obvious, individuals may conceal the extent of the problems they have related to drinking alcohol.

Steve Martino

See also Alcohol Use Disorders Identification Test; Inventory of Drinking Situations; Michigan Alcohol Screening Test; Screening; Screening Instruments

Further Readings

Ewing, J. A. (1984). Detecting alcoholism: The CAGE Questionnaire. *JAMA, 252,* 1905–1907.

Knight, J. R., Sherritt, L., Harris, S. K., Gates, E. C., & Chang, G. (2003). Validity of brief alcohol screening tests among adolescents: A comparison of the AUDIT, POSIT, CAGE, and CRAFFT. *Alcoholism: Clinical and Experimental Research, 27,* 67–73.

Liskow, B., Campbell, J., Nickel, E. J., & Powell, B. J. (1995). Validity of the CAGE Questionnaire in screening for alcohol dependence in a walk-in (triage) clinic. *Journal of Studies on Alcohol, 56,* 277–281.

Mayfield, D., McLeod, G., & Hall, P. (1974). The CAGE Questionnaire: Validation of a new alcoholism screening instrument. *American Journal of Psychiatry, 131,* 1121–1123.

CANNABINOLS

See MARIJUANA

CANNABIS YOUTH TREATMENT STUDY

Cannabis is a substance containing the chemical compound delta-9-tetrahydrocannabinol (i.e., THC), which exists in multiple forms commonly known as hashish, marijuana, and blunts. According to the *Diagnostic and Statistical Manual of Mental Disorders, Fourth Edition, Text Revision (DSM-IV-TR)*, cannabis intoxication is typically associated with symptoms such as euphoria, sedation, lethargy, impaired judgment, distorted sensory perceptions, and impaired motor performance. Cannabis is the most widely used illicit psychoactive substance in the United States, and prevalence rates are high, particularly among adolescents. In 2006, the National Survey on Drug Use and Health estimated that 6.7% of 12- to 17-year-olds used cannabis within the past month.

Due to the growing literature demonstrating significant social, medical, and psychological consequences of cannabis use disorders among adolescents, the Center for Substance Abuse Treatment (CSAT) of the Substance Abuse and Mental Health Services Administration, within the U.S. Department of Health and Human Services, created the Cannabis Youth Treatment Study (CYTS) to identify the cost, effectiveness, and cost-benefit of short-term outpatient treatment programs for adolescents with cannabis use disorders. Grants were awarded to four sites to conduct the study; these sites included the University of Connecticut Health Center; Operation Parental Awareness and Responsibility, Inc.; Chestnut Health Systems; and Children's Hospital of Philadelphia. A 35-member steering committee composed of researchers and clinicians from each grant site, other research collaborators, CSAT staff, and an independent advisory board chose five short-term interventions that showed promise from previous research for implementation in the CYTS. Some of the treatments were subjected to previous randomized controlled trials but were implemented with adults.

The five interventions were evaluated in two trials, which included motivational enhancement treatment and cognitive behavior therapy, 5 sessions (MET/CBT5); motivational enhancement treatment and cognitive behavior therapy, 12 sessions (MET/CBT12); family support network (FSN); the adolescent community reinforcement approach (ACRA); and multidimensional family therapy (MDFT). The first two treatment approaches, MET/CBT5 and MET/CBT12, included a combination of two sessions of MET with either three or seven CBT sessions, respectively. MET was used to decrease ambivalence and increase motivation to change cannabis use, whereas CBT provided the adolescent with skills for refusing cannabis, increasing social support and pleasant activities, and coping with high-risk situations. The FSN intervention was a treatment package combining the MET/CBT12 with six parent education group meetings, four therapeutic home visits, referral to support groups, and case management. The ACRA utilized operant conditioning, skills training, and social systems approaches in a 12-to 14-week intervention, including 10 individual sessions with the adolescent, four sessions involving caregivers, and limited case management. MDFT was a comprehensive intervention based on systems theory and included 12 to 15 sessions with the individual, parents, and entire family, as well as case management over 12 to 14 weeks. Participants of the CYTS included 600 adolescents and their families. To be included in the study, adolescents had to be between the ages of 12 and 18, meet one or more *DSM-IV-TR* criteria for cannabis abuse or dependence based on self-report, used cannabis in the past 90 days, and be appropriate for outpatient treatment. Exclusion criteria included heavy use of alcohol or other drugs within the past 90 days and presence of factors based on participant report that prohibited or limited participation in treatment (e.g., limited cognitive abilities, significant conduct problems). Participants were primarily male (83%), Caucasian (61%) or African American (30%), and from single-parent families (50%). Many of the adolescents were previously involved in the juvenile justice system (62%) and engaged in risk behaviors (e.g., multiple sexual partners). Participants were randomly assigned to one of three treatment conditions within each treatment site due to limited case flow and resources. In Trial 1 (at University of Connecticut Health Center and Operation PAR), treatment conditions were MET/CBT5, MET/CBT12, or FSN; in Trial 2 (at Chestnut Health Systems and Children's Hospital of Philadelphia), treatment conditions were MET/CBT5, ACRA, or MDFT. Therapists were experienced clinicians from diverse educational backgrounds (20% doctoral level, 50% master's level, 30% bachelor's level) and participated in weekly supervision with clinical coordinators.

Participants were evaluated at 3-, 6-, 9-, and 12-month follow-up interviews. The two types of outcomes examined were clinical outcome and cost-benefit. Measures of clinical outcome were (a) the total number of days of abstinence from the randomization date to the 12-month follow-up interview and (b) the adolescent being in recovery, which was defined as the adolescent living in the community (vs. incarceration or inpatient treatment) and self-reporting no problems with substance use at the 12-month follow-up interview. For cost-benefit, treatment costs were combined with the clinical outcomes to estimate (a) the cost per day of abstinence over the 12-month follow-up period and (b) the cost per person in recovery. In both trials, all five treatment conditions showed significant pre/post treatment effects for both days of abstinence and recovery, but there were no significant differences between treatments for these clinical outcomes. The results were stable across the four follow-up assessments, but the effect sizes were generally small. Across all treatments, the average total days of abstinence increased from 52 to 65 days per quarter (of 90 days), and the percentage of adolescents in recovery increased from 3% to 24% across the four follow-up periods. In Trial 1, MET/CBT5 and MET/CBT12 were significantly more cost-effective than FSN, and

in Trial 2, ACRA and MET/CBT5 were significantly more cost-effective than MDFT.

In sum, the CYTS was a multisite randomized trial examining the effectiveness and cost-benefit of five different psychosocial interventions for adolescents with cannabis abuse or dependence. The study addressed a large gap in the substance abuse literature and demonstrated a well-designed effectiveness study that will help improve cannabis treatment for adolescents in clinical practice. Other strengths of the study include the randomized design, large sample size, and examination of cost-benefit. Limitations include reliance on participant self-report, lack of a treatment as usual or no treatment control group, and no differences in clinical outcome among the interventions. Future research could examine treatment for the substantial number of adolescents who were not in recovery following any of the interventions provided in the CYTS. In addition, adolescents with significant alcohol and/or other drug use were screened out of the CYTS, perhaps reducing the generalizability of the results. Given the high comorbidity between cannabis use and alcohol and/or other drug use, it would provide more clinical utility to examine treatment among these at risk youth.

Daniel M. Bagner, Stephen J. Sheinkopf, and Gregory L. Stuart

See also Adolescents, Substance Abuse and Treatment; Evidence-Based Treatment; Marijuana; Research Issues in Treatment; Substance Use Disorders; Treatment of Alcohol and Other Drugs

Further Readings

Compton, W. M., & Pringle, B. (2004). Services research on adolescent drug treatment. Commentary on "The Cannabis Youth Treatment (CYT) Study: Main findings from two randomized trials." *Journal of Substance Abuse Treatment, 27,* 195–196.

Dennis, M., Godley, S. H., Diamond, G., Tims, F. M., Babor, T., Donaldson, J., et al. (2004). The Cannabis Youth Treatment (CYT) Study: Main findings from two randomized trials. *Journal of Substance Abuse Treatment, 27,* 197–213.

Dennis, M., Titus, J. C., Diamond, G., Donaldson, J., Godley, S. H., Tims, F. M., et al. (2002). The Cannabis Youth Treatment (CYT) experiment: Rationale, study design and analysis plans. *Addiction, 97,* 16–34.

Diamond, G., Godley, S. H., Liddle, H. A., Sampl, S., Webb, C., Tims, F. M., et al. (2002). Five outpatient treatment models for adolescent marijuana use: A description of the Cannabis Youth Treatment Interventions. *Addiction, 97,* 70–83.

French, M. T., Roebuck, M. C., Dennis, M. L., Diamond, G., Godley, S. H., Tims, F., et al. (2002). The economic cost of outpatient marijuana treatment for adolescents: Findings from a multi-site field experiment. *Addiction, 1,* 84–97.

CENAPS MODEL

The CENAPS Model of relapse prevention provides a theoretical understanding of factors that contribute to substance dependence, as well as principles that guide treatment interventions of substance dependent individuals. The CENAPS Model has been under construction since the 1970s. This model includes theoretical as well as clinical practice elements from Alcoholics Anonymous and the Minnesota model of treatment. The model also integrates a number of educational materials, clinical procedures, and self-help methods that permit patients and clinicians to utilize theoretical principles to help patients achieve and maintain recovery.

Within the CENAPS Model of relapse prevention, substance dependence is conceptualized to consist of biopsychosocial influences, with significant contributing factors derived from biological, psychological, and social domains. Treatment is thus engineered to target dysfunction in each of these areas. Treatment is separated into three stages; within each of these stages, a focus is maintained on identification and treatment of biological, psychological, and social dysfunction. Stages of treatment include programs for assessment and stabilization, recovery planning, and relapse prevention planning.

Patients are categorized by their history of recovery within the CENAPS Model of relapse prevention. According to the model, patients who are in recovery can be classified as being recovery prone or relapse prone. Those who are relapse prone can be further subdivided into patients who are either motivated or unmotivated. Those who are unmotivated are unwilling to acknowledge chemical dependency; they refuse to follow guidelines of recovery programs that stipulate requirements to maintain abstinence and to make major lifestyle changes. For patients who are unmotivated, treatment will not be effective in instilling motivation to interrupt the progress of the disease.

In contrast, patients who are motivated acknowledge that they are chemically dependent and recognize the need to make lifestyle changes. However, despite efforts of these patients, they relapse into substance use. The distinction between motivated and unmotivated relapse prone patients is notable because many clinicians believe that individuals who relapse are unmotivated with respect to treatment goals. However, the CENAPS Model suggests that patients who are motivated but relapse are in treatment programs that are insufficient in meeting their needs. The CENAPS Model tries to address these deficiencies by providing a systematic method for identifying warning signs of relapse and by providing patients with tools to develop concrete warning-sign management and recovery plans.

Treatment

Within the CENAPS Model, total abstinence and personality and lifestyle changes are viewed as critical in achieving full recovery and maintaining relapse. However, the goal is not simply for abstinence, but rather for improvement in all spheres of biopsychosocial health. This goal is important because health in all areas, even during periods of sobriety, will increase the likelihood of maintaining recovery during times of stress. Specifically, the principles of the CENAPS Model suggest that symptoms that arise during sobriety are a part of the disease because they lead to relapse or to other negative outcomes (e.g., suicide or other self-harm behaviors). For example, within the biological domain, brain dysfunction obstructs clear thinking and decision-making skills. In the psychological domain, self-defeating personality styles that are characteristic of substance dependent individuals lead to decision making that lands individuals in high-risk situations. Given that self-defeating personality styles originate from family of origin, addressing dysfunctional family structures may be a target of treatment. Finally, in the social domain, social influences on substance dependent individuals may also represent a main target for intervention.

The CENAPS Model of relapse prevention aims to teach individuals to identify signs of relapse early on so that they might interrupt the progression and reverse the evolution towards relapse to a state of improvement and recovery. In the first stage of stabilization, the central goals are detoxification and stabilization. This stage also incorporates assessment to determine the most appropriate setting for the patient (i.e., primary treatment or relapse prevention therapy). In the second stage, the primary recovery program, there are four main goals: recognition of the disease, acknowledgement of the need for lifelong abstinence, development and implementation of recovery program, and treatment of any comorbid conditions that might obstruct long-term recovery. Finally, within the third stage of relapse prevention planning, patients are provided with means to identify early warning signs of relapse. Such strategies can be used in primary treatment but also may be applied later on in relapse prevention planning. A set of nine principles, discussed below, guides interventions throughout these stages.

According to the CENAPS Model, criteria for candidates who will do well in relapse prevention planning include the following: patients who are able to integrate information about substance dependence; patients with past successful efforts at recovery; patients with a history of clear warning signs that have arisen during past episodes of recovery; and patients who demonstrate both the ability and the motivation to participate in the treatment.

Basic Principles

There are nine basic principles of the CENAPS Model that guide the tailoring of treatment to patient's individual needs. Each principle is accompanied by clinical interventions that can be used to help patients effectively implement the principle. The nine principles are self-regulation, integration, understanding, self-knowledge, coping skills, change, awareness, significant others, and maintenance. Several examples of the principles and their adjunctive clinical interventions are given below.

According to the first principle, capacity for self-regulation, patients who are able to regulate thoughts, emotions, and behaviors will have decreased risk for relapse. A clinical intervention derived from this principle would be the identification and challenging of patients' irrational thoughts regarding substance use. For example, patients who develop justifications for relapse are encouraged to share such thoughts and to work together with the therapist to challenge thoughts through the use of past experiences of relapse.

Another example of a basic principle and related clinical intervention is the principle of maintenance. This principle suggests that individuals who periodically update their relapse prevention plan are likely to

decrease their risk for relapse. Interventions generated from this principle require that the patient's relapse plan be reviewed and updated periodically. Updates to relapse plans are based on the patient and therapist's observations of ongoing warning signs that have evolved or surfaced following the development of the initial relapse plan. New plans for previously identified warning signs and strategies to manage newly identified warning signs would be added into the relapse plan with each review of the plan.

Conclusion

The CENAPS Model of relapse prevention is based in biopsychosocial theory and involves clinical interventions that address patient needs in areas of biological, psychological, and social domains. Given that the approach in the CENAPS Model provides systematic assessment and planning for relapse prevention, needs of patients who are relapse prone, but who are motivated for treatment, can be addressed. There is little empirical research that supports the efficacy of the treatment CENAPS Model treatment package, although research supports the efficacy of pieces of the model. The evaluation of the efficacy of this model and treatment package remains a task for future research.

Yael Chatav and Gregory L. Stuart

See also Continuum of Care; High-Risk Situations; Minnesota Model; Relapse; Relapse Prevention

Further Readings

Gorski, T. T. (1990). The Cenaps Model of relapse prevention: Basic principles and procedures. *Journal of Psychoactive Drugs, 22,* 125–133.

CENTER FOR SUBSTANCE ABUSE PREVENTION

The Center for Substance Abuse Prevention (CSAP) is the lead federal agency responsible for improving the quality and accessibility of substance abuse prevention services. The CSAP replaced the Office for Substance Abuse Prevention (OSAP), which was established by the Anti-Drug Abuse Act of 1988 as part of the Alcohol, Drug Abuse, and Mental Health

Administration (ADAMHA) under the Department of Health and Human Services. When the Substance Abuse and Mental Health Services Administration (SAMHSA) replaced ADAMHA, through reorganization in 1992, OSAP became the CSAP.

The general mission of the CSAP is to provide national leadership for policies, programs, and services to prevent the onset of illicit drug use and underage alcohol and tobacco use and to reduce the negative consequences of substance use. It is largely by means of the Substance Abuse Prevention and Treatment Block Grant as well as an array of discretionary grants that the CSAP is able to accomplish its mission.

The organizational structure of the CSAP consists of the Office of the Director, the Office of Program Analysis and Coordination, and four major divisions. The respective divisions of the CSAP are the Division of State and Community Assistance, the Division of Knowledge Application and Systems Improvement, the Division of Prevention Education and Dissemination, and the Division of Workplace Programs.

The CSAP requires that only effective, evidence-based programs be funded. Accordingly, CSAP synthesizes peer reviewed prevention research such as through its Prevention Enhancement Protocols System and its National Center for the Advancement of Prevention, both of which are intended to review and synthesize prevention research and to make it more usable and understandable for practitioners and policymakers. The CSAP uses a five-step strategic prevention framework process consisting of assessment, capacity, planning, implementation, and evaluation to achieve its goals of preventing substance abuse.

The CSAP administers the prevention portion of the Substance Abuse Prevention and Treatment Block Grant. By law, 20% of the funds in the block grant (nearly $1.8 billion in FY 2008) must be devoted to prevention. This money is distributed to states, which in turn fund community prevention efforts. The CSAP ensures that these funds are used to support evidence-based prevention and that data on the effectiveness of prevention programs and strategies are gathered.

Beginning in 1990, broad based community prevention initiatives were begun with the awarding of 95 Community Partnership Demonstration Program grants. CSAP awarded 13 demonstration grants in 1994 for female adolescent programs to create gender specific strategies to decrease substance abuse. In 1995, the CSAP awarded 16 replication demonstration program grants that served 24 states. Beginning

in 2004, the CSAP has been awarding State Incentive Grants from SAMHSA as part of a systematic federal effort intended to support prevention capacity and infrastructure at the state and community levels. Also beginning in 2004, the Drug Free Communities (DFC) grants program was moved to CSAP; this program provides grants of up to $100,000 to community coalitions that develop initiatives to prevent youth alcohol, tobacco, illicit drug, and inhalant abuse. These DFC grants allow community coalitions to improve prevention efforts through greater communitywide coordination, as well as by encouraging citizen participation in substance abuse prevention efforts and by disseminating information on effective prevention programs.

Since 1992, the CSAP administers the Synar Amendment, which was intended to decrease access to tobacco products among individuals under age 18. To comply with provisions of the Substance Abuse Prevention and Treatment Block Grant, states must provide detailed information on progress achieved in enforcing youth tobacco access laws.

The CSAP supports the Centers for the Application of Prevention Technologies (CAPTS) program for the application and dissemination of evidence based substance abuse prevention interventions (http://captus.samhsa.gov). The regionally based CAPTS provide states and communities with technical assistance and training on the latest evidence based information on effective substance abuse prevention policies, programming, and practices.

Since 2000, the CSAP has provided various Web-based prevention tools under the Prevention Decision Support System. For instance, the CSAP operates the Workplace Information and Reference Center for SAMHSA's Division of Workplace Programs as a Web portal (http://www.drugfree workplace.gov) for those interested in drug-free workplace resources and strategies. Information can be found pertaining to drug testing, federal and non-federal drug-free workplace programs, young adults in the workplace, and materials on workplace health, wellness, and safety, as well as prevention research and interventions.

The CSAP provides an array of public education initiatives to achieve substance abuse prevention goals. For instance, A Family Guide to Keeping Youth Mentally Healthy and Drug Free is a Web site aimed at educating parents and caregivers of 7 to 18 year olds (http://family.samhsa.gov); Building Blocks for a Healthy Future is another Web site with information on prevention basics that targets parents and caregivers of children ages 3 to 6 years (http://bblocks.samhsa.gov). The Stop Underage Drinking campaign provides directed information for those concerned with underage drinking prevention initiatives (http://www.stopalcoholabuse.gov).

The CSAP produces a variety of prevention publications and other informational materials, such as its Prevention Resource Guides on selected topics, for example, the *CSAP Substance Abuse Resource Guide: American Indians and Native Alaskans,* and other publications, such as its *Technical Assistance Bulletins* and *Tips For Teens* series. These publications and other materials can be ordered from the National Clearinghouse for Alcohol and Drug Information.

Victor B. Stolberg

See also Centers for the Application of Prevention Technologies; National Clearinghouse for Alcohol and Drug Information; Prevention Resources; Substance Abuse and Mental Health Services Administration; Synar Amendment

Further Readings

Building Blocks for a Healthy Future: http://bblocks .samhsa.gov

Center for Substance Abuse Prevention. (1998). *A catalog from CSAP's findings bank of science-based prevention practices.* Rockville, MD: Author.

Center for Substance Abuse Prevention. (1999). *Understanding substance abuse prevention: Toward the 21st century: A primer on effective programs.* Rockville, MD: Author.

Center for Substance Abuse Prevention. (2000). *CSAP's model programs.* Rockville, MD: Author.

Center for Substance Abuse Prevention. (2001). *Principles of substance abuse prevention.* Rockville, MD: Author.

Centers for the Application of Prevention Technologies: http://captus.samhsa.gov

Division of Workplace Programs: http://www.drugfree workplace.gov

A Family Guide to Keeping Youth Mentally Healthy and Drug Free: http://family.samhsa.gov

Stop Underage Drinking: http://www.stopalcoholabuse.gov

Yin, R. K., Kaftarian, S. J., Yu, P., & Jansen, M. A. (1997). Outcomes from CSAP's Community Partnerships Program: Findings from the National Cross-Site Evaluation. *Evaluation and Program Planning, 20*(3), 345–356.

CENTER FOR SUBSTANCE ABUSE TREATMENT

The Center for Substance Abuse Treatment (CSAT) of the Substance Abuse and Mental Health Services Administration (SAMHSA), within the U.S. Department of Health and Human Services, is the federal agency responsible for promoting the quality and availability of substance abuse treatment services for individuals and families who need them. CSAT provides funding for residential and nonresidential substance abuse treatment programs through block grants to states for alcohol and drug treatment services, national demonstration projects, criminal justice system rehabilitation programs, and addiction counselor training programs.

The CSAT replaced the Office for Treatment Improvement (OTI), which was established in January 1990 as part of the Alcohol, Drug Abuse, and Mental Health Administration (ADAMHA) under the Department of Health and Human Services. When the SAMHSA replaced ADAMHA through reorganization in 1992, OTI became the CSAT.

The organizational structure of CSAT consists of the Office of the Director, the Office of Program Analysis and Coordination, and three major divisions. The respective divisions of the CSAT are the Division of Services Improvement, The Division of State and Community Assistance (DSCA), and the Division of Pharmacologic Therapies.

The mission of the CSAT is to increase the availability of effective treatment and recovery services for individuals with alcohol and other drug problems. The primary mechanism to achieve this mission is through the administration of the Substance Abuse Prevention and Treatment Block Grant. This grant is the responsibility of DSCA. In fiscal year (FY) 2008, the Block Grant was $1.8 billion, and 80% is devoted to treatment. This money is distributed to states, which in turn fund community-based treatment programs. The CSAT ensures that these funds are used to support evidence-based treatment and that data on the effectiveness of treatment are gathered.

To help meet its mission, CSAT provides several grant competitions, such as grants for Targeted Capacity Expansion Program for Substance Abuse Treatment and HIV/AIDS Services and State Incentive Grants for Treatment of Persons with

Co-Occurring Substance Related and Mental Disorders, that are designed to help states and other groups meet emerging substance abuse problems and fill in gaps in substance abuse services. Pregnant and Postpartum Women grants are to provide residential treatment services for pregnant and postpartum women. Assertive Adolescent and Family Treatment grants are designed to provide family centered substance abuse treatment for adolescents and their families. Strengthening Treatment Access and Retention–State Implementation Cooperative Agreements promote state-level infrastructure improvement. Treatment for Homeless grants are intended to develop comprehensive alcohol and drug and mental health treatment systems for persons who are homeless. The Recovery Community Services Program is a grants project to design and deliver peer-to-peer recovery support services (http://rcsp.samhsa.gov).

CSAT promotes screening, brief intervention, referral, and treatment as a comprehensive, integrated public health approach to delivering early intervention and treatment services to those with substance abuse disorders, as well as to those who are at risk for developing those conditions (http://sbirt.samhsa.gov). Hospital emergency rooms, primary care centers, clinics, trauma centers, and other community settings are recognized to offer opportunities for early intervention with those at risk for becoming substance abusers before they experience more severe consequences.

CSAT supports the Addiction Technology Transfer Center (ATTC) Network. The ATTC is a regionally based national program dedicated to identifying and advancing opportunities for improving substance abuse treatment (http://www.nattc.org/index.html). The ATTC Network operates as 14 separate regional centers and a national office.

CSAT supports an array of initiatives intended to expand and enhance clinically sound, cost-effective addiction treatment. The Treatment Improvement Exchange is a forum intended to promote information exchange between CSAT staff and state and local substance abuse agencies (http://www.tie.samhsa.gov). The Center for Mental Health Services/CSAT Spending, Organization and Financing Treatment Services project is concerned with how individuals use mental health and substance abuse services across various agencies and provides comprehensive national estimates on spending for mental health and substance

abuse treatment (http://csat.samhsa.gov/IDBSE/index.aspx). The Practice Improvements Collaboratives program is examining factors that impede the adoption of evidence-based treatment practices in community based treatment settings (http://csat.samhsa.gov/pic/index.html). The National Center on Substance Abuse and Child Welfare is improving systems and practices for families with substance use disorders that are involved with the child welfare and family judicial systems (http://www.ncsacw.samhsa.gov). CSAT sponsors the National Alcohol and Drug Addiction Recovery Month held each September to promote the benefits of substance abuse treatment and that recovery from substance abuse is possible (http://www.recoverymonth.gov). The Persistent Effects of Treatment Studies is examining the longer term treatment outcomes of individuals with substance abuse problems (http://alt.samhsa.gov/pets).

CSAT produces an array of treatment publications and other informational materials, such as their Technical Assistance Publications (TAPs) such as "TAP 27: Navigating the Pathways: Lessons and Promising Practices in Linking Alcohol and Drug Services with Child Welfare" and "TAP 26: Identifying Substance Abuse Among TANF-Eligible Families" and their Treatment Improvement Protocols (TIPs) such as "TIP 47: Substance Abuse: Clinical Issues in Intensive Outpatient Treatment" and "TIP 46: Substance Abuse: Administrative Issues in Intensive Outpatient Treatment." Other publication series from the CSAT include Knowledge Application Program Keys, Quick Guides, and Substance Abuse Treatment Advisory. These publications and other substance abuse treatment materials can be obtained from the National Clearinghouse for Alcohol and Drug Information.

CSAT operates SAMHSA's national toll-free referral hotline as a service for locating alcohol and drug abuse treatment programs at (800) 662-HELP (4357) and TDD (telecommunications device for the deaf): (800) 487-4889. CSAT also maintains SAMHSA's Substance Abuse Treatment Facility Locator (http://www.findtreatment.samhsa.gov).

Victor B. Stolberg

See also Addiction Technology Transfer Centers; National Clearinghouse for Alcohol and Drug Information; National Institute of Mental Health; Substance Abuse and Mental Health Services Administration; Treatment Approaches and Strategies

Further Readings

Center for Substance Abuse Treatment. (2006). *TAP 27: Navigating the pathways: Lessons and promising practices in linking alcohol and drug services with child welfare* (Inventory No. BKD436). Rockville, MD: Substance Abuse and Mental Health Services Administration. Available from http://ncadi.samhsa.gov

Center for Substance Abuse Treatment. (2006). *TAP 28: The National Rural Alcohol and Drug Abuse Network Awards for Excellence 2004* (Inventory No. BKD552). Rockville, MD: Substance Abuse and Mental Health Services Administration. Available from http://ncadi.samhsa.gov

Center for Substance Abuse Treatment. (2006). *TIP 46: Substance abuse: Administrative issues in intensive outpatient treatment* (Inventory No. BKD545). Rockville, MD: Substance Abuse and Mental Health Services Administration. Available from http://ncadi.samhsa.gov

Center for Substance Abuse Treatment. (2006). *TIP 47: Substance abuse: Clinical issues in intensive outpatient treatment* (Inventory No. BKD551). Rockville, MD: Substance Abuse and Mental Health Services Administration. Available from http://ncadi.samhsa.gov

Center for Substance Abuse Treatment. (2007). *Alcohol screening and brief intervention for trauma patients* (Inventory No. [SMA] 07-4266). Rockville, MD: Substance Abuse and Mental Health Services Administration. Available from http://ncadi.samhsa.gov

CENTERS FOR THE APPLICATION OF PREVENTION TECHNOLOGIES

The Centers for the Application of Prevention Technologies (CAPTs) are five regional centers funded by the federal government and are dedicated to increasing the utilization of empirically supported substance abuse prevention programs by local and state organizations. CAPTs were established in 1997 by the Center for Substance Abuse Prevention, which operates under the umbrella of the Substance Abuse and Mental Health Services Administration. The development of CAPTs mirrors a wider movement within the helping professions adopt evidence-based programs and strategies in an effort to increase both the quality of care and the cost-effectiveness of services. Consistent with other areas of research, there is often a gap whereby scientifically supported substance abuse prevention programs fail to be widely adopted in applied settings. Common obstacles to the translation of these programs to real world settings include a lack of dissemination of findings that can result, in part, from the shear amount of available information, as well as organizational barriers encountered by prevention providers (e.g., a scarcity of resources, an entrenched program of services, insufficient infrastructure). In response to this problem, CAPTs were developed to facilitate the delivery of evidence-based prevention by individuals within a community, local and state agencies, and policymakers. The centers are divided into five geographic areas: Central (Iowa, Illinois, Indiana, Michigan, Minnesota, North Dakota, Ohio, South Dakota, Wisconsin, West Virginia, Red Lake Nation), Northeast (Connecticut, Delaware, Massachusetts, Maryland, Maine, New Hampshire, New Jersey, New York, Pennsylvania, Rhode Island, Vermont), Southeast (Alabama, District of Columbia, Florida, Georgia, Kentucky, Mississippi, North Carolina, Puerto Rico, South Carolina, Tennessee, Virginia, Virgin Islands), Southwest (Arkansas, Colorado, Kansas, Louisiana, Missouri, Nebraska, New Mexico, Oklahoma, Texas), and Western (Alaska, American Somoa, Arizona, California, Federated States of Micronesia, Guam, Hawaii, Idaho, Marshall Islands, Mariana Islands, Montana, Nevada, Oregon, Palau, Utah, Washington, Wyoming). Through these networks, CAPTs provide technical assistance as agencies develop, apply, and evaluate alcohol and drug abuse prevention programs and policies. The ultimate goal of these centers is to reduce the gap between research and practice while maximizing the impact of effective and comprehensive prevention programs.

CAPTs facilitate the progression of science from clinical research to applied settings by providing resources, guidance, and support in a variety of domains. To increase dissemination of empirically supported prevention research, CAPTs maintain an online library of the current literature in the substance abuse prevention field, as well as manuals for administering specific protocols. Moreover, CAPTs compiled a list of prevention resources categorized by state for efficient referencing, also available online (http://captus.samhsa.gov/national/about/about.cfm). Interested organizations can use the Web site to search and compare evidence-based prevention services, including information about how prevention has previously been implemented, the target population, and data on the effectiveness of various programs. Furthermore, matching the treatment to the intended recipients is critical for maximizing the acceptability and effect of the prevention program. Accordingly, CAPTs help providers choose and tailor evidence-based preventions to best serve their goals by factoring in the demographic constituency of the target population, barriers to services, and available resources.

During the adoption and implementation phases, CAPTs strive to minimize the challenges that may arise by helping the organization anticipate possible obstacles and develop viable solutions. For instance, in order to implement a prevention program, several agencies within a state or community may have to collaborate. Guided by the notion that an overarching commitment to success is imperative to the success of a program, CAPTs strives to increase communication and cooperation among the participating groups. Another example of a potential barrier to a prevention policy is a concern that the initiative will encounter resistance from other interested parties. In this case, CAPTs may help policymakers strategize ways of minimizing opposition or garnering a strong support base among citizens to increase the popularity of the measure. Making efforts to ensure that the prevention is implemented with limited difficulties is important since an early negative experience may discourage both the sponsors and the targets of the prevention from adopting the measure for the longer term. Similarly, some prevention programs may be delivered on a temporary basis as a pilot program and thus must prove to be feasible, sustainable, and successful in reaching the established goals to be adopted permanently; a problematic trial period may effectively end the delivery of that prevention. Following implementation of the prevention program, CAPTs aid the organization in evaluating the performance of the intervention, including helping make any necessary adjustments to the protocol.

In-line with their commitment to promote expertise in applying empirically supported prevention among local, regional, and state providers, CAPTs sponsor professional development opportunities such as workshops, conferences, and fellowships. Examples of specific training opportunities include working in multidisciplinary teams, grant writing, school crisis intervention planning, responding in the case of a natural disaster, budgets and budgeting, conflict resolution, community mobilization, and sustainability. CAPTs encourage prevention practitioners and policymakers to develop specific skills sets that increase their ability to efficiently administer prevention technologies.

In summary, it is imperative that evidence-based substance abuse prevention technologies be made available to the public; however, the translation of these prevention programs is often overwhelmed by difficulties in dissemination and implementation. Thus, CAPTs endeavor to limit these obstacles so that high quality, cost-effective prevention programs can be delivered to prevent and ameliorate substance-related problems at all levels of the population. The Office of National Drug Control Policy reported that CAPTs were successful in meeting their 2004 goals for facilitating the adoption of evidence-based technologies by service providers; however, more outcome research on the effectiveness of the organization is needed.

Katherine W. Follansbee, Jeff R. Temple, and Gregory L. Stuart

See also Addiction Technology Transfer Centers; Center for Substance Abuse Prevention; Evidence-Based Prevention; Evidence-Based Prevention and Treatment, Dissemination and Adoption of; National Registry of Evidence-based Programs and Practices

Further Readings

Centers for the Application of Prevention Technologies: http://captus.samhsa.gov/national/about/about.cfm
Hogan, J. A., Baca, I., Daley, C., Garcia, T., Jaker, J., Lowther, M., et al. (2003). Disseminating science-based prevention: Lessons learned from the CSAP's CAPTs. *Journal of Drug Education, 33*(3), 233–243.
National Registry of Evidence-based Programs and Practices: http://www.nrepp.samhsa.gov

CENTRAL NERVOUS SYSTEM DEPRESSANTS

Depressants (also known as *downers*) affect individuals by reducing the activity of the brain. They do this by inducing sedation, muscle relaxation, and drowsiness. They are often prescribed for those who are overwhelmed with the myriad of stressors associated with everyday life and who therefore need help to reduce anxiety reactions. Depressants are also commonly prescribed to help treat people with insomnia, pain, and seizure disorders. Barbiturates, benzodiazepines, and alcohol make up some of the common central nervous system (CNS) depressants available today. The most common depressant, alcohol, is widely abused throughout the world, and its abuse can lead to disease, addiction, overdose, and death. Unfortunately, depressants are widely prescribed throughout the United States, and many of these drugs are sold illicitly on the streets.

Most depressants generally act in the body by affecting the levels of available gamma-aminobutyric acid (GABA), a neurotransmitter that reduces activation of CNS neurons. GABA produces a calming effect on people and is therefore used to treat those with hypertension and epilepsy. In the brain, GABA helps control impulses, induces muscle relaxation, and is the brain's main neurotransmitter involved with inhibitory responses. This inhibitory effect GABA has on motor neurons slows or stops the brain's neuronal activity, thereby causing a depressing effect on the CNS.

Barbiturates

Barbiturates are one of the oldest classes of depressants and were first synthesized in the mid-1800s. They may be used during the induction of surgical anesthesia as sedative-hypnotic agents to induce a coma, to control seizures, or to relieve intracranial pressure in patients with head trauma. When administering barbiturates, it is often difficult to determine the correct dosage required for a desired effect; unfortunately, even very small doses can lead to death. Barbiturates are extremely addicting and must be prescribed with caution.

Barbiturates are known on the street as downers and work by depressing activity of the entire nervous system. They can produce sedation and reduce motor activity when taken in low doses; however, at high doses, they can distort judgment, decrease cognitive activity, elicit hypnosis, and produce anesthesia (i.e., loss of consciousness) at extremely high doses. Other common effects of barbiturate overdose include respiratory failure, coma, and death. Long-term use of these drugs can cause aggressiveness, severe insomnia, and dependency as the level of intake increases. Ten times the prescribed therapeutic dose of barbiturates can cause death. Given the severe depressive effects of these compounds, many accidental overdoses occur when they are taken with other CNS depressants, most notably alcohol.

The most common barbiturate is phenobarbital, which is used as a sleep aid or for treating disorders such as epilepsy. It is a long-acting barbiturate and can last for up to 24 hours. Phenobarbital helps in depressing abnormal stimulating neurons and improves chemical imbalance within the brain. Although it is widely used to treat epilepsy, it can be habit forming and may result in addiction, cognitive disorders, and mood disorders. Secobarbital (i.e., Seconal) is another common barbiturate and was historically prescribed for epilepsy and insomnia. Because of its intense sedative properties, it is no longer widely prescribed. The drug has been linked to several overdoses and suicides among the famous (e.g., Judy Garland, Jimi Hendrix, and Marilyn Monroe, to name a few).

Benzodiazepines

Benzodiazepines represent the other major class of CNS depressant drugs. These drugs have replaced barbiturates as the prescription of choice among physicians for treating anxiety and insomnia. Benzodiazepines act on the neurotransmitters, GABA, serotonin, and dopamine. Benzodiazepines absorb slowly into the bloodstream, making their effects longer lasting than barbiturates. These drugs are also safer than barbiturates because it takes a much higher therapeutic dose of benzodiazepines to be fatal. For example, 700 times the therapeutic dose would be needed to cause a fatality in someone who has developed a tolerance to these drugs.

Benzodiazepines are one of the most common depressants prescribed and include common medications such as Xanax, Valium, and Ativan. Benzodiazepines have a lower fat-solubility, greater water-solubility, and are absorbed from the small intestine instead of the stomach like barbiturates. Benzodiazepines are administered medicinally to help a patient forget traumatic surgical procedures because they disrupt short-term memory by preventing its transfer into long-term memory.

They have been approved for use in people with obsessive-compulsive disorders and as anxiolytics, muscle relaxants, anesthetic adjuncts, and anticonvulsants. The safety of benzodiazepines is the major advantage of these drugs. However, abuse of these drugs is common because of their sedative characteristics. They have fewer side effects and lower withdrawal symptoms than barbiturates; however, they are often abused concomitantly with methamphetamine, cocaine, or even heroin. Illicit use of benzodiazepines can be found when substance abusers inject the crushed tablets or jelly from the capsules. This injection can be especially dangerous because intravenous use has the potential to cause circulation problems and the potential for loss of limbs. Withdrawal and even seizures are common in people who abruptly stop using these drugs. Long-term use of benzodiazepines can cause many negative side effects, including depression, mental confusion, aggression, and loss of coordination. Benzodiazepines are especially dangerous when concomitantly mixed with other drugs such as alcohol or opioids. They can cause slowed reflexes, euphoria, and hostile behaviors when taken in high doses. Furthermore, they can suppress respiration and circulatory functions. Because benzodiazepines are water soluble and hence may last in body tissues for long periods, they can induce tissue dependence at even low levels. There is therefore a high rate of relapse with these drugs in individuals with a long history of use.

Xanax

Xanax is one of the most widely prescribed drugs to treat anxiety. Anxiety or excessive nervousness is most often a result of deficiency in the neurotransmitter GABA. Xanax works by increasing the effectiveness of the small amounts of GABA that are present in the brain. In addition to treating anxiety, it is commonly prescribed to treat panic attacks, agoraphobia (fear of open spaces), premenstrual syndrome, and tension. This benzodiazepine can be dangerous and may lead to a high level of dependence with strong withdrawal symptoms, such as decreased libido, memory impairment and fatigue.

Valium

Valium has the properties of being a sedative hypnotic, anticonvulsant, and muscle relaxant. It is generally prescribed to treat anxiety and insomnia and is used as a relief for muscle spasms and spasticity caused by disorders such as tetanus or neurological disorders. Intravenously, Valium is used in sedation before surgery. When abused, it is usually used as a secondary drug to maintain the high of another drug. Overdose as a result of intoxication of Valium is usually found when it is mixed with alcohol, which can lead to respiratory arrest and coma.

Rohypnol and Gamma-Hydroxybutyrate (GHB)

Rohypnol causes rapid and intense relaxation, drowsiness, and sedation. It was also historically prescribed to treat insomnia and as a preanesthetic; however, prescription of this drug is prohibited in the United States because of its ability to incapacitate a person, disrupt memory, and lower inhibitions, all of which make it a common drug in date rape. Rohypnol acts by causing anterograde amnesia in which events occurring while under the influence of this medication are often completely forgotten.

Although it is not technically a benzodiazepine, GHB has similar effects. GHB is a fast-acting, CNS depressant and is a metabolite or byproduct of GABA. It has been thought to increase levels of growth hormone in the body and has been used by bodybuilders to help increase muscle mass. It can be synthesized from electrical circuit boards and is available in liquid, tablet, powder, or capsule form. Like Rohypnol, GHB has also been used by sexual predators to decrease inhibitions and defenses of women and has become popular in party clubs. Recently, GHB has resurfaced as an experimental medication (Xyrem) for cataplexy symptoms resulting from narcolepsy.

Alcohol

Alcohol is one of the most commonly abused depressants, and in fact it is estimated that annually over 2 million people die worldwide from alcohol-related incidents. Numerous physiological effects are associated with alcohol consumption, such as gastric irritation, liver disease, cardiovascular effects, sleeping problems, and pregnancy defects such as fetal alcohol syndrome. Many people use depressants such as alcohol to run away from the many ordeals and challenges life brings. Thus, overdose, addiction, and fatalities are potential problems related to this commonly abused depressant.

Motor Vehicle Fatalities

Alcohol is a common psychoactive substance found in the blood of victims involved in motor vehicle crashes. Since it affects the neurotransmitter, GABA, it reduces motor coordination as well as alertness and depth perception. To drive safely, one must be alert and able to make fast decisions. Alcohol, as a depressant, slows the brain and body, which can further limit awareness and coordination. Not only can people become careless when driving under the influence, but also they can become too confident in their driving abilities. Other important driving skills that may be affected by alcohol include speed control, lane control, concentration, and reaction time when braking. There is a direct correlation between blood alcohol concentration and motor vehicle accidents: the risk for accidents increases positively with increases in blood alcohol concentration.

As one of the major causes of mortality, motor vehicle accidents kill around 300,000 people in the world every year. Alcohol, prescription drugs, and illicit drugs can be correlated to many of these unfortunate motor vehicle fatalities.

Crime

Not only does alcohol have detrimental effects on the body, but also there is a relationship between alcohol, drugs, and violence. Studies have shown that violent acts are overwhelmingly associated with alcohol use, more than any other illicit or nonillicit substance.

Increases in aggression have been found with consumption of alcohol because it interferes with the main inhibitory neurotransmitter (GABA). Impulse control may also be inhibited due to decreases in the levels of serotonin.

When an individual is provoked while under the influence of alcohol, he or she is more likely to be aggressive and violent. This is because alcohol causes selective disinhibition and reduced intellectual functioning. Alcohol also causes reduced self-awareness and inaccurate assessment of risks, therefore making it more likely that violence related to alcohol consumption may occur.

Overdose

Alcoholic overdose results from large amounts of alcohol, such as a blood alcohol content (BAC) at a level of 0.40 or higher; however, this BAC can be lower depending on the physiologic characteristics of an individual. When this poisoning occurs, depression of the CNS results, which may lead to death. Although a 0.40 BAC has been noted as the threshold for alcohol poisoning, levels at 0.20 or greater can depress respiration and lead to death in those with low tolerance levels.

Suicide

As alcoholics age, they are more likely to have social, health, and interpersonal problems. Thus, their risk for suicide increases. Furthermore, along with increased age, suicide rates among alcoholics are twice as high as that of the general population. The typical alcohol-suicide victim is a White, middle-aged male. Depression, job loss, living alone, and poor social support are other potential risk factors associated with suicide, all of which are exacerbated by alcohol use and abuse.

Conclusion

Barbiturates, benzodiazepines, and alcohol make up the majority of all depressants that are prescribed and used illicitly throughout the world. When used properly, benzodiazepines and barbiturates can be beneficial in surgery and treating patients with epilepsy or with anxiety disorders. In the eyes of many, then, the therapeutic uses of these drugs far outweigh the risks associated with them. However, dependency, withdrawal, and abuse are common among all these drugs, especially when mixed with other depressants.

Melanie L. Gulmatico-Mullin and Chad L. Cross

See also Alcohol; Barbiturates; Benzodiazepines; Central Nervous System Stimulants; Club Drugs; Drugs, Classification of

Further Readings

Inaba, D., & Cohen, W. E. (2004). *Uppers, downers, all arounders.* Ashland, OR: CNS Publications.

Levinthal, C. F. (2004). *Drugs, behavior, and modern society.* Boston: Allyn & Bacon.

Parker, R. N., & Auerhahn, K. (1998). Alcohol, drugs, and violence. *Annual Review of Sociology, 24,* 291–311.

CENTRAL NERVOUS SYSTEM STIMULANTS

Central nervous system (CNS) stimulants are characterized by their ability to activate systems in the brain including those that regulate mood, motor function, wakefulness, thought processing, and pleasure perception. The most apparent effects of using these drugs include elevated mood, increased movement and fidgeting, suppressed sense of boredom and fatigue and inability to sleep, rapid and sometimes disjointed formation of thoughts and speech, illogical and even dangerous behavior, elevated sense of euphoria and self-confidence, and the ability to persist at a task for longer periods of time. Because some of these effects are perceived as enjoyable and gratifying, it is common to see individuals repeatedly using these substances to enhance performance and to feel better. As a result of these positive effects, for some people- the potent CNS stimulants can be highly addicting and problematic. Although the CNS effects caused by the stimulants are the most common reasons for using these drugs, many of the stimulants can have profound pharmacological influences on other critical body functions as well. Most noteworthy is that many of these drugs are sympathomimetics, meaning that they stimulate the sympathetic autonomic nervous system and related functions. The consequences of such actions are generally increased heart rate, vasoconstriction, elevated blood pressure, and enhanced sensitivity to cardiovascular activation.

Frequent exposure of the brain and other organs such as the cardiovascular system to these drugs can result in what appears to be contradictory responses. Thus, the pleasurable effects often appear to diminish with persistent exposure to these drugs. This tolerance frequently, although not universally, is due to increased metabolism and inactivation of the drugs by the liver. Compensation for this diminished response is typically achieved by increasing stimulant doses and thereby offsetting the elevated liver metabolism. The required increases in drug doses can sometimes be as much as an order of magnitude greater than that used originally. Such increases in stimulant doses will elevate the likelihood of serious side effects. Another, almost paradoxical response to the extended use of some of the psychostimulants is what is called *sensitization*. In some ways, this sensitization is an effect that is opposite to the tolerance described above. Sensitization includes enhanced responses to the stimulant. These exaggerated effects typically are not pleasurable or desirable and may include things such as increased likelihood of seizures or a psychotic episode. Even though tolerance and sensitization appear to be opposite responses, they can express concurrently in the stimulant-dependent user making the response of the user appear bizarre and difficult to understand.

Drug Types

The CNS stimulants are distinguished by their unique pharmacologies (i.e., mechanism of action, especially on the CNS), potencies, and access. Briefly, the stimulants can be classified as major and minor. The major stimulants include drugs such as the amphetamines (e.g., amphetamine, methamphetamine, and ecstasy) and cocaine. These drugs can exert powerful stimulation on both the brain and the cardiovascular systems when used in moderate to high doses. It is common to hear users describe their first exposure to these drugs as "the greatest feeling they ever experienced." This reaction almost certainly reflects the ability of these drugs to dramatically and rapidly activate the brain's pleasure systems and to cause a dramatic release of the neurotransmitter dopamine from brain cell terminals located in a brain region known as the nucleus accumbens. Also interesting is that most of those addicted to these stimulants also claim that they are never able to duplicate the intensity of that first stimulant experience no matter how often they administer the drug or how high a dose they use. In fact, with continual stimulant exposure, the brain's pleasure pathway appears to be compromised even for nondrug-related naturally occurring rewards making it difficult for the user to find enjoyment in activities that used to be pleasurable. The positive properties of the stimulants tend to diminish until the user must repeatedly administer the stimulant just to achieve a normal level of natural reward. Typically, when the stimulant-dependent person reaches this stage, abstinence from the drug can lead to severe depression and in extreme cases, suicide ideation or even attempts. This stimulant-induced downward spiral of pleasure function reinforces continued stimulant use and can lead to severe dependence and even episodes of intense and dangerous bingeing with these drugs. Although there are many similarities between the amphetamines and cocaine, there also are significant clinical and practical differences. For example, cocaine is a naturally occurring substance that is extracted from the coca plant found only in the Andes mountains of South America. Consequently, all cocaine (both legal and illegal) used in the United States must be shipped across the borders of this country. After administration of cocaine (especially intravenous injection or by smoking routes), it enters the brain rapidly and exerts CNS effects within seconds. Cocaine is also metabolized rapidly, and the pharmacological actions disappear after a few minutes. In contrast, the amphetamines such as methamphetamine are synthetics that can be made by relatively unsophisticated chemistry; thus, it is common to see local methamphetamine labs "cooking" this stimulant and selling the products on the streets. These labs use over-the-counter decongestant ingredients such as pseudoephedrine as starter material. The synthesis requires toxic and potentially lethal chemicals. As a result, the methamphetamine labs are a significant hazard to occupants of the building where the lab is located, neighboring buildings, and enforcement or cleanup personnel who enter the premise. In order to close or prevent the methamphetamine labs, law enforcement agencies at the federal, state, and local levels have controlled access by the general public to the precursor decongestant and cold products. This control is achieved by requiring pharmacies and stores that sell such products to keep them behind the counter and to limit the number of boxes sold to individuals. This effort has been extremely effective in shutting down the local "mom and pop" labs, but has had little impact on imported methamphetamine from Mexico, Asia, or other foreign sources. Consequently, methamphetamine is still readily accessible, relatively inexpensive, and its abuse is a major problem for many regions in this country.

Nonmedicinal (e.g., recreational) use of the major stimulants is illegal in the United States, and to discourage this type of abuse, these drugs for the most part are classified as Schedule II substances (i.e., high abuse potential with few accepted medical uses) by the federal government through the Comprehensive Drug Abuse and Prevention Control Act. Consequently, stimulants that are frequently purchased on the street from illicit sources are often associated with both domestic and foreign criminal organizations. Purchasing and using illegal stimulant drugs from street dealers is potentially dangerous because of the likelihood of obtaining and using contaminated and deadly substances as well as because of the individuals and groups one must deal with to obtain these drugs are prone to violence and criminal activities.

The minor stimulants include substances such as caffeine or over-the-counter active ingredients such as minor sympathomimetics (e.g., pseudoephedrine). The ability of these drugs to stimulate the brain and cardiovascular system is considerably less than that of the major stimulants. Consequently, the likelihood of serious side effects, including major dependence, is also considerably reduced. These compounds are found in products such as beverages (e.g., caffeine in coffee, teas, and cola drinks), decongestants and cold medicines (e.g., pseudoephedrine), and stay-awake products (e.g., caffeine). Caffeine is the most frequently used of all of the stimulants but is not considered to be a major addiction problem by the medical community or society in general. For this reason, there have been no significant efforts to prevent access to caffeine-containing products by either law enforcement or public health organizations. Although frequent use of caffeine clearly does cause dependence (both psychological and physical) and abstinence can result in unpleasant withdrawals such as headaches, agitation, and disturbed sleep, there is no indication that routine moderate use of caffeine-containing products poses significant health hazards. For this reason, there is little effort to even discourage the millions of caffeine users in this country, regardless of their age, from consuming this drug. It is viewed by most as an acceptable part of our social customs and is not seen as a reason for concern. However, even these minor stimulants are significant drugs with potential side effects. For some people, their use will disturb sleep patterns, or in extreme cases, they can elevate blood pressure or cause significant stimulation of the heart. Consequently, those people who are especially sensitive to cardiovascular stimulants, even those with minor potency, should avoid the use of these drugs.

Side Effects

Many of the most significant side effects of the stimulants have already been mentioned. The major stimulants can be extremely addicting for some users. Approximately 10% of those people who use these drugs for nonmedicinal purposes (i.e., recreationally or even just for experimentation) will escalate their use and develop addiction. As already discussed, these powerful drugs encourage repeated use and bingeing episodes that can result in extremely high doses entering the body and dangerously stimulating the cardiovascular system. Some severe consequences of these effects are heart attacks, strokes, or cardiac arrhythmias. All of these reactions require immediate medical attention and can be fatal. Intense stimulation of the CNS by high doses of potent stimulants can also cause serious consequences such as extreme anxiety, psychotic episodes that resemble schizophrenia, dangerous antisocial behavior, and even life-threatening seizure episodes.

Frequent high doses of the minor stimulants such as caffeine can also have significant health consequences such as chronic headaches, sleep disruption, anxiety, and persistent agitation.

Clinical Use

Most of the stimulants can be legally prescribed to treat a variety of conditions. These prescription products are mostly administered orally to diminish the likelihood of abuse. Despite this precaution, these medications can be ground up into a powder and snorted, injected, or even smoked by stimulant-dependent people.

Some of the amphetamines are legally prescribed to treat attention deficit disorder (ADD), narcolepsy, and obesity. Treatment of ADD with amphetamines results in a paradoxical reduction of associated symptoms and diminishes the tendency toward distraction, thereby improving the ability of the ADD patient to focus on tasks and interact socially in a productive manner. Amphetamine-related drugs prescribed for this purpose include methylphenidate (Ritalin), dextroamphetamine (Dexedrine) and pemoline (Cylert). Of relevance to this therapeutic effect is the observation that many methamphetamine addicts have an underlying ADD condition. This observation suggests that some stimulant-dependent people may have begun use of amphetamine-related drugs in an attempt to self-medicate the ADD symptoms with the stimulant. It is important to know if a person has self-medicated before establishing a treatment program for a methamphetamine addict with ADD.

The amphetamines are also used to treat narcolepsy (spontaneous sleep disorder) due to the ability of these drugs to suppress sleep centers in the brain and maintain wakefulness. Again, treatment of this condition consists of relatively low doses of the stimulant administered orally and closely monitored by a well-trained clinician.

The final approved use of the amphetamines by the Food and Drug Administration (FDA) is for the treatment of obesity. Amphetamine-like drugs suppress the appetite and reduce the inclination to eat excessively. Obviously, a reduction of eating in combination with increased exercise is a helpful strategy to reduce weight and to diminish associated pathology. However, the use of these stimulants is not considered to be more than a temporary adjunct therapy to help the obese patient establish a pattern of weight loss.

Once a pattern occurs, the clinician will gradually withdraw the stimulant to avoid dependence and long-term addiction. That drugs such as the amphetamine are potent appetite suppressants is well known not only to clinicians but also to the public. Therefore, it is not uncommon to find methamphetamine addicts, particularly women, who are initially attracted to the amphetamines because of their ability to cause weight loss. However, without proper medical management, what can start as an innocent desire to lose a few extra pounds escalates out of control and transforms into a life-threatening addiction.

Cocaine is also a Schedule II drug due to its FDA approval as a local anesthetic. This property to block the activity of pain pathways was originally identified in the 19th century and is still used today in limited clinical settings for minor surgeries such as biopsy procedures. Another clinical use of cocaine takes advantage of cocaine's ability to cause vasoconstriction when applied topically to stop local bleeding. Thus, for conditions such as severe nosebleeds, gauze packs soaked in cocaine solutions can be very effective. However, cocaine's short action and its lack of effect with oral administration limit its practical clinical value.

Vulnerability to Dependence

What makes 10% of those who abuse the major stimulants go on to become severely dependent on these potent drugs? Although there is much that remains to be learned about this issue, researchers do know that genetics and environment contribute equally to addiction vulnerability. Although twin studies have demonstrated that dependence on the stimulants tends to cluster in families suggesting heritability, as of now, there is little evidence to identify the specific genes involved.

It is important to recognize that even if a person does possess genetic factors that cause vulnerability to stimulant addiction, dependence on these substances is not inevitable because the environment is as important as heritability in determining drug dependence outcomes. The factors leading to stimulant abuse likely include (a) mental disorders such as ADD, anxiety, and depression; (b) poor self-image; (c) stressful and abusive past; and (d) easily manipulated. Research continues to identify the predisposing vulnerabilities to stimulant abuse and addiction in order to develop more effective prevention, intervention, and treatment programs.

Treatment and Withdrawal

There are effective therapeutic strategies for dealing with addictions to cocaine and to the amphetamines such as methamphetamine. These consist mainly of behavioral strategies such as contingency management, cognitive behavioral therapy, Motivational Enhancement Therapy, or a combination of these strategies. Currently, there is not an FDA-approved medication for dealing with stimulant dependence, although some candidates are being evaluated, and it is likely that effective medication strategies will be identified. Even when medications are approved for use in stimulant-dependent patients, it is unlikely that the medication alone will be sufficient to manage the addiction. It is almost certain that medications will only be an adjunct to behavioral therapy and that when used together, the two approaches will significantly improve the therapeutic outcomes for stimulant dependence.

Conclusion

In general, CNS stimulants activate many brain and cardiovascular functions. They are perceived as reinforcing by many people and can cause significant and even life-threatening dependence in a significant fraction of the users. The stimulants are divided into major and minor categories based on their likelihood for causing severe dependence and cardiovascular consequences. Addiction to the major stimulants such as methamphetamine and cocaine have, and do, cause major social problems with troubling costs to society. There are distinct pharmacologies among these drugs that should be appreciated to effectively manage their adverse side effects. These drugs can be prescribed for conditions such as ADD, narcolepsy, and obesity but require close monitoring by trained clinicians to avoid adverse consequences.

Glen R. Hanson

See also Amphetamines; Caffeine; Cocaine and Crack; Comprehensive Drug Abuse Prevention and Control Act; Methamphetamine

Further Readings

Barr, A., Panenka, W., MacEwan, G., Thornton, A., Lang, D., Honer, W., et al. (2006). The need for speed: An update on methamphetamine addiction. *Journal of Psychiatry & Neuroscience, 31,* 301–313.

Greenhill, L. L. (2006). The science of stimulant abuse. *Pediatric Annals, 35,* 552–556.

Hanson, G. R., Venturelli, P. J., & Fleckenstein, A. E. (2006). Stimulants. In *Drugs and society* (9th ed., pp. 280–321). Boston: Jones and Bartlett.

Harper, S., & Jones, N. (2006). Cocaine: What role does it have in current ENT practice? A review of the current literature. *The Journal of Laryngology & Otology, 120,* 808–811.

Higdon, J., & Frei, B. (2006). Coffee and health: A review of recent human research. *Critical Reviews in Food Science and Nutrition, 46,* 101–123.

Lopez, F. A. (2006). ADHD: New pharmacological treatment on the horizon. *Journal of Developmental and Behavioral Pediatrics, 27,* 410–416.

National Institute on Drug Abuse: http://www.nida.nih.gov/NIDAhome.html

Runyon, S., & Carroll, F. (2006). Dopamine transporter ligands: Recent developments and therapeutic potential. *Current Topics in Medicinal Chemistry, 6,* 1825–1843.

Westfall, T. C., & Westfall, D. P. (2006). Adrenergic agonists and antagonists. In L. Brown (Ed.), *Goodman & Gilman's pharmacological basis of therapeutics* (11th ed., pp. 237–315). New York: McGraw-Hill.

CERTIFICATION AND LICENSING

The demand for substance abuse counselors continues to grow, as well as the need for counselors in this field to be certified or licensed. Now, more than half of those working in the substance abuse field have a master's degree, and over 80% have a bachelor's degree, according to a report published by the Center for Substance Abuse Treatment (CSAT).

Currently, the U.S. Department of Labor report for 2004 indicates counselors were working in 601,000 jobs, of which 76,000 were in the substance abuse field. The U.S. Department of Labor also reports that a strong demand continues for substance abuse counselors. This demand is further highlighted by NAADAC, the Association for Addiction Professionals, which estimates that in the next 10 years, a 35% growth is anticipated in the addictions-behavioral disorder area for counselors. In addition, certification-licensure requirements will probably continue to increase.

What used to be essentially an apprentice model of learning substance abuse skills has been replaced by a more formal educational model. National certification and licensure credentials are still evolving with various agencies and helping professions proposing standards. In a field that has seen treatment become increasingly sophisticated and complex, it is essential to determine the type of training and experience treatment providers need to provide effective services.

History of the Profession

Until the 19th century, most people considered alcoholism and other forms of substance abuse untreatable. Therefore, resources were not provided for rehabilitation and care of those who suffered from this chronic problem. Rather, as William White points out, addicts were left on their own with no treatment. Alcohol and substance abuse issues in society were often framed as a moral issue; people just needed to exert their will power to quit. As various organizations sprang up in the 19th century to help those with alcohol and other drug problems, no coherent philosophy or central authority arose to create an addictions field. Various fraternal temperance clubs and societies, such as the Sons of Temperance, then began to help alcoholics by focusing on goals of mutual social support to moderate drinking or promote abstinence. Later in the 19th century, some treatment started, and recovering patients stayed on to assist those who came after them. This trend of recovering individuals helping each other in the substance abuse counseling profession continues to this day.

Addictions counseling came into its own as a mental health discipline in the 1960s with the advent of a professional infrastructure based on six major components. The six key features were the development of (1) widespread national and state addictions advocacy agencies, (2) licensing and accreditation of standards for treatment programs, (3) associations dedicated to alcohol and drug counselors at the national and state level, (4) academic and nonacademic counselor programs dedicated to training, (5) certification and licensing credentialing systems, and (6) professional literature and research on addictions. Organizations like NAADAC; the Association for Addicted Professionals; the CSAT; the National Institute on Alcohol Abuse and Alcoholism; and the National Institute on Drug Abuse helped establish advocacy programs and training courses in addictions. Twelve core functions of substance abuse counselors were identified that were required for certification and/or licensing, and these core functions were adopted in

part or whole by various states, agencies, or national organizations. These 12 core functions were a catalyst for the development of the document, *Addiction Counseling Competencies: The Knowledge, Skills, and Attitudes of Professional Practice*, which was produced by the CSAT through the Addiction Technology Transfer Centers.

State Certification and Licensure

In general, certification involves the regulation of a title for a profession while licensure regulates the practice of the profession. Therefore, in a state that has certification for drug and alcohol counselors, a professional must have the certification to use the title drug and alcohol counselor. In a state that has licensure for drug and alcohol counselors, the functions of drug and alcohol counseling are regulated by the licensure law. In other words, it would be unlawful for someone to perform these functions if the person was not licensed as a drug and alcohol counselor or licensed as another mental health professional licensed to perform these functions. It should be noted that other health care and mental health care professionals (e.g., physicians, psychologists, social workers, marriage and family therapists, licensed professional counselors) may be allowed (by state certification and/or licensure laws) to provide screening, assessment, diagnosis, and treatment services for substance use disorders.

Licensure requirements are imposed by each individual state, and these requirements vary. Not all states require a substance abuse counselor to have a license, but most states require certification or a credential of some kind. Licensure tends to be more rigorous, require more course work, and is generally considered to be a higher credential than a certification given by a state or a national organization.

Certification can be awarded by a state government agency, a private national organization, or a college or university. Each has different requirements and implications for scope of practice and responsibilities. Certification, as opposed to licensure, can be achieved at the associate or the bachelor's degree level in drug and alcohol counseling in some states through accredited colleges or universities. To obtain a state license as a substance abuse counselor, formal academic training is required at an accredited college or university. Most states require a substance abuse counselor to obtain a certificate and/or license to practice in their state to do specific tasks without direct supervision such as group or family counseling, individual counseling, and assessments or evaluations.

States also vary in their requirements for formal education. For substance abuse counselors, 32 states (as of June 2007) require some form of formal education or professional training to become certified or licensed to practice in the drug and alcohol area. Almost all states, 94%, require a substance abuse counselor to take a qualification examination before being allowed to practice in the substance abuse profession.

Many states seem to be moving toward a three-tiered educational requirement for drug counselors that include (1) an associate's degree, (2) bachelor's degree, or (3) a master's degree. All three have educational requirements to be completed in the area of mental health with specialized addictions coursework also required. These requirements most often include practicum and internship hours or direct work experience under supervision of licensed mental health practitioners in substance abuse facilities or agencies.

The National Addiction Technology Transfer Web site has information on the certification and licensure requirements for each state (www.nattc.org/get Certified.asp).

National Certification and Licensure

At a broader level, a uniform certification process has been developed by NAADAC, the Association for Addiction Professionals, which is an independent national body certifying educational and training requirements for substance abuse counselors. This organization has developed a three-tiered system: (1) National Certified Addiction Counselor, Level I (NCAC I); (2) National Certified Addiction Counselor, Level II (NCAC II); and (3) Master Addiction Counselor (MAC). Moving upward from Level I, II, and finally MAC (the highest credential) requires more education, more supervised clock hours, and a current state certification or license as outlined below.

To qualify as a National Certified Addiction Counselor, Level I (NCAC I), there are three criteria: (1) certification or license as a substance abuse counselor that is current in the state of practice, (2) at least 270 clock hours of substance abuse counseling training to include ethics and HIV/AIDS training of 6 hours in each area, and (3) 6,000 hours of supervision in substance abuse counseling or full time work experience of 3 years. Qualifications at Level II (NCAC II)

requires that (a) the certification or licensure must be in a health and human services area such as social work or counseling and (b) 450 clock hours of substance abuse education and training must be completed, again with 6 hours each of ethics and HIV/AIDS training as in Level I. Also, there is a requirement to hold a bachelor's degree from an accredited college or university. For Level II, the number of hours of supervised experience climbs up to 10,000 hours or the equivalent of 5 years of full-time experience working as a substance abuse counselor.

NAADAC has also developed an exam for those wanting licensure, the MAC. The MAC requires a master's degree in nursing, social work, psychology, counseling, or another area of the helping professions. It also requires 500 clock hours of training and education with specific training in drug abuse counseling. Individuals must also have current state licenses or certificates in their profession such as a Licensed Professional Counselor, Licensed Psychologist and/or Social Worker. Additionally, applicants for the MAC must have 3 years of supervised clinical experience, of which 2 years are acquired after obtaining their master's degree.

Examination by NAADAC is provided for each of the three levels. Level I and II are tested for certification in four core areas, which are (1) pharmacology of addictive substances, (2) counseling practices, (3) theoretical base of counseling, and (4) professional issues. For the MAC licensure exam, three areas are tested, and they are (1) pharmacology of addictive substances, (2) counseling practices and (3) professional issues.

Physicians, psychologists, substance abuse counselors, social workers, and other helping professions can also receive a NAADAC qualification as a Substance Abuse Professional (SAP), which is not a certification or license. Obtaining a qualification as a SAP allows those in the health and human services counseling field to evaluate Department of Transportation government workers for follow-up care if needed.

Additionally, for licensure, another organization, the National Board for Certified Counselors (NBCC), has developed an Examination for Master Addictions Counselors (EMAC), which consists of 100 questions. The NBCC, a nonprofit agency, is a nationally recognized organization that offers licensure exams that are usually acceptable by states. The NBCC is an agency that helps set the standards for the general practice of counseling professionals to include specialty areas like substance abuse counseling. Five broad areas of content are examined by the EMAC. They are (1) assessment, (2) counseling practices, (3) treatment process, (4) treatment planning and implementation, and (5) prevention.

Another organization of significance is the International Certification & Reciprocity Consortium/ Alcohol Other Drug Abuse, Inc. (IC&RC). It is composed of certifying agencies involved in credentialing or licensing alcohol and other drug abuse counselors, clinical supervisors, prevention specialists, co-occurring professionals, and criminal justice professionals. The importance of the IC&RC's endorsement is that 44 states, other federal government agencies such as the Department of Transportation and the Department of Defense, and 12 global jurisdictions recognize its stamp of approval of substance abuse certification and licensure. Thus, IC&RC endorsement allows portability of certification and license to other jurisdictions. For example, substance abuse counselors from one state in the IC&RC consortium could move to other states or government agencies and have their NBCC MAC exam results accepted without having to retake the exam in the new state. The professional would still have to take the state exam regarding laws and regulations, which varies from state to state.

A somewhat unique aspect of the alcohol and substance abuse counseling field is its inclusion of individuals in recovery serving as counselors. In the past, many recovering counselors could receive state certification without any postsecondary school training. However, the increase in certification requirements has dramatically reduced the number of drug and alcohol counselors who do not have at least a bachelor's degree. Since the recovery experience can be so valuable in treating addicted individuals, many states, colleges, and universities are actively assisting recovering individuals in their pursuit of the training necessary to receive certification or licensure.

Conclusion

Substance abuse is a major health concern of this nation and requires well-qualified individuals to treat it. Career projections indicate a need for more qualified counselors knowledgeable of substance abuse issues as the field continues to grow. The growing professionalism in the field of substance abuse counseling requires higher education programs that train counselors to treat individuals with addictive disorders. Currently, there is no one model of certification or licensure across the country that provides standards for education and supervision. Each state has its own set of standards regarding certification or licensure for drug and alcohol counselors. The national trend indicates that states are instituting more rigorous guidelines, rules, and education and training requirements, both academic and nonacademic, for the practice of substance abuse counseling.

Frank Norton and Rhonda Jeter

See also Addiction Technology Transfer Centers; Clinical Supervision for Addiction Counselors; NAADAC, The Association for Addiction Professionals; State Provider Associations

Further Readings

Center for Substance Abuse Treatment. (2006). *Addiction counseling competencies: The knowledge, skills, and attitudes of professional practice.* Retrieved July 16, 2007, from http://www.treatment.org/Taps/tap21/ TAP21Toc.html

Culbreth, J. R., & Borders, L. D. (1999). Perceptions of the supervisory relationship: Recovering and nonrecovering substance abuse counselors. *Journal of Counseling & Development, 77,* 330–338.

Fisher, G. L., & Harrison, T. C. (2008). *Substance abuse: Information for school counselors, social workers, therapists, and counselors* (4th ed.). Boston: Allyn & Bacon.

Kerwin, M. E., Walker-Smith, K., & Kirby, K. (2006). Comparative analysis of state requirements for the training of substance abuse and mental health counselors. *Journal of Substance Abuse Treatment, 30,* 173–181.

Libretto, S., Weil, J., Nemes, S., Linder, N., & Johansson, A. (2004). Snapshot of the substance abuse treatment workforce in 2002: A synthesis of current literature. *Journal of Psychoactive Drugs, 36,* 489–497.

Mulvey, K. P., Hubbard, S., & Hayashi, S. (2003). A national study of the substance abuse treatment workforce. *Journal of Substance Abuse Treatment, 24,* 51–57.

National Addiction Technology Transfer: http://www.nattc .org/getCertified.asp

White, W. (1998). *Slaying the dragon: The history of addiction treatment and recovery in America.* Bloomington, IL: Chestnut Health Systems/ Lighthouse Institute.

CHEMICAL DEPENDENCY

See SUBSTANCE DEPENDENCE

CHILDREN OF ALCOHOLICS

According to the National Institute on Alcohol Abuse and Alcoholism, approximately 43% of all children in the United States are exposed to someone with alcoholism while growing up, and one in four children is exposed to alcohol abuse and/or dependence in the family at some point before the age of 18. The alcoholic family environment is often characterized by disruption and instability, inadequate supervision and parenting, and dysfunctional parent–child relationships. This type of developmental chaos undermines healthy and normal childhood development and puts children at risk for a wide range of cognitive, emotional, and behavioral problems. According to the National Association for Children of Alcoholics, these problems are often seen in children from alcoholic homes who exhibit more symptoms of depression and anxiety, experience greater physical and mental health problems, and experience more school problems than children growing up in nonalcoholic homes.

The disease of alcoholism tends to run in families; consequently, children with alcoholic parents have approximately 4 times greater risk of becoming alcoholics themselves than the general population. Despite the increased risk, it is important to note that not all children of alcoholics (COAs) become alcoholics or develop other forms of pathology. Although COAs are unquestionably at risk, this does not mean that their risk will inevitably lead to alcoholism and adverse life events. Because there are multiple variables that play a role in the development of alcoholism and functional impairments, it is important to understand the complex interactions among the family, the individual, and the genetic variables that contribute either to increasing risk for or increasing resiliency against the development of alcoholism in COAs.

Family Characteristics

Families play a pivotal and defining role in the development and growth of children. Some of the essential tasks of families include (a) providing food, clothing, safety, and shelter; (b) promoting a sense of right and wrong—fostering a strong moral compass within each child; (c) promoting a sense of individual identity and self-worth; (d) promoting a sense of family connectedness and cohesion; (e) providing appropriate boundaries and limits for each child; (f) supporting educational achievement; and (g) promoting individual competence and positive participation within society. Role confusion, neglect, abuse, or inconsistency in the provision of any of these essential family tasks can lead to damaging and traumatic childhood experiences that result in impaired functioning.

Alcoholic families are often characterized by inconsistent parenting, inadequate supervision of the children's behaviors and activities, a lack of emotional support and good role modeling, impoverished home life, and poor communication within the home. Consequently, children from alcoholic homes typically lack (a) effective problem solving skills that lead to aggressive behavior with peers, (b) understanding of appropriate personal boundaries that lead to dysfunctional friendships and failed relationships, (c) effective communication skills that result in undersocialization, and (d) clear parent–child role assignments that result in confused identity development.

If the alcoholism of the parent progresses, the children and other adults in the family develop defense mechanisms such as denial and minimizing the alcoholism to protect them from the severe social stigma attached to the disease. A distorted family system develops in an effort to protect the parent with the disease. As the children struggle to maintain the illusion of normalcy, they often become isolated from friends, peers, and outside activities. Many clinicians and researchers have identified specific family rules that are developed within the alcoholic home. These include the following rules:

a. *Don't talk.* The alcoholic behavior is never discussed; instead, children learn that it is important to be silent about the drinking and its impact upon the family. This silence often leads to secretive and avoidant behavior throughout the child's life.

b. *Don't feel.* When painful family fights occur or special events are forgotten, children learn to suppress their feelings and to ignore the emotional hurt. Unfortunately, children do not learn how to identify normal feelings, how to describe them, or how to resolve them. Obviously, this lack creates a multitude of interpersonal problems throughout the child's life.

c. *Don't trust.* Many times alcoholics do not follow through on promises they have made to attend sporting games, school plays, or other activities that children may be involved in. Because the parents are often unreliable and inconsistent in their support, children learn not to trust their parents or others. They may also incorporate the idea that they (children) are unworthy, unlovable, or selfish. These negative internalizations can impair the child's ability to maintain successful relationships and careers in adulthood.

Recent research has suggested that observing family rituals provides an important protective element within a child's home and routine. However, if the drinking behavior in an alcoholic home disrupts family rituals such as daily routines, common mealtimes, family vacations, birthday celebrations, and holiday activities, children within this setting are experiencing inconsistency, unpredictability, insecurity, and a decreased sense of parental support. The lack of rituals leads to decreased family cohesion, more disturbed family interactions, and an increased risk that the children will experience maladaptive outcomes.

Research has also suggested that comorbid psychopathology in the alcoholic parents may increase the children's risk for developing alcoholism. Data from the National Comorbidity Study indicate that one third to one half of people diagnosed with alcohol abuse and/or dependence also have a comorbid psychiatric diagnosis such as antisocial personality disorder, depression, anxiety, or bipolar disease. Families with comorbid psychiatric illnesses appear to experience higher levels of family conflict and violence, aggression, inconsistent or harsh discipline, and poor communication skills. In numerous research studies, children from alcoholic homes report experiencing more parental rejection and aggression, feeling less emotional warmth, and having more attention problems than children from nonalcoholic homes. These findings underscore the importance of considering the parent's comorbid psychopathologies, not just the alcoholism, when studying the relationship between parental alcoholism and the behavioral adjustment of the children. Dr. Kenneth Sher's research has consistently demonstrated that parental psychopathology and family dysfunction puts the children at greater risk of developing mental health problems, as does alcoholism. However, Sher is quick to point out that

alcoholics are not a homogenous group of people, and consequently, it is difficult to pinpoint the specific domains and variables that contribute to alcoholism and mental health problems in children of alcoholics.

Individual Characteristics

Children raised in dysfunctional families that do not provide warmth, affection, consistency, and appropriate boundaries are more likely to experience traumatic stressors during childhood as compared to children who are raised in functional families. The Adverse Childhood Experiences Study found that stressful or traumatic childhood experiences such as abuse, neglect, growing up with alcohol abuse, parental psychopathology, and marital discord provide a common pathway to social, emotional, and cognitive impairments. Normal psychological development is seriously compromised under these kinds of family conditions, and the risk of health and mental problems are significantly increased.

Children growing up in alcoholic homes may experience a variety of interpersonal problems including the following:

a. *confusion*—inconsistent interactions with the alcoholic parent who can quickly change from being loving to being hostile creates confusion and fear within the child;

b. *anxiety*—the child may be consumed with fear and anxiety about the anger, violence, and fighting at home;

c. *guilt*—the child may blame him/herself for the parent's drinking;

d. *depression*—the child may internalize anger, guilt, isolation, helplessness, and anxiety and turn it into depression; and

e. *shame*—embarrassment over the alcoholic parent can increase the sense of isolation and loneliness that the child experiences.

These feelings may manifest as academic problems, truancy, lack of friends, bed wetting, aggression toward other children, delinquent behaviors, problems with other drugs, and/or increased physical problems such as headaches or stomachaches.

Children of alcoholics may have increased expectations that alcohol use will be positive and reinforcing—this is in part because they have been exposed to their parents' use of alcohol to reduce stress. Research conducted by Dr. Brook S. G. Molina demonstrates that cognition regarding alcohol develops at a young age before the onset of drinking; consequently, children growing up in an alcoholic home have numerous opportunities to be exposed to parental drinking. This exposure seems to have a negative effect on younger children; however, by middle and high school, the negative effect of parental drinking appears to change into more positive alcohol expectancies. Molina suggests that improved social functioning, social assertiveness, and peer acceptance while using alcohol may contribute to increased alcohol expectancies among adolescent children of alcoholics. Research has also demonstrated that as children of alcoholics move into adolescence and teen years, their beliefs about alcohol became more similar to the beliefs of their parents.

Recent research has demonstrated that children with attention deficit hyperactive disorder (ADHD) and/or conduct disorders are often vulnerable to early use of alcohol that can lead to abuse and later alcoholism. Familial alcoholism has been associated with a childhood history of hyperactivity and conduct disorder; however, the exact nature of this association is unclear. Molina suggests that the impulsivity and behavioral disinhibition associated with these two disorders may be nested with a lack of parental supervision, increased positive alcohol expectancies, improved social functioning, and increased peer acceptance that contributes to the development of alcohol use disorders in the children of alcoholics.

Genetic Vulnerability

The National Institute on Alcohol Abuse and Alcoholism has actively supported research on both the genetic and environmental variables that contribute to the development of alcoholism. Researchers have begun to identify several biological mechanisms that differ between children of alcoholics and children of nonalcoholics. Although these physiologic, genetic, and biochemical markers are distinct, researchers agree that any model of alcoholism is multifactorial with many biological and environmental variables contributing to the development of the disease. Some research has demonstrated that children of alcoholics may metabolize alcohol differently or have decreased feelings of intoxication at the same blood alcohol levels compared to children of nonalcoholics. Additional biological markers that have been identified include brain wave differences (reduced P300 waves) during cognitive processing tasks, increased sensitivity-reactivity to alcohol, and increased levels of relaxation from drinking alcohol.

Physiological markers are genetic variables that may identify individuals who are at risk for developing alcoholism. Physiological markers such as the measurement of brain wave activity during cognitive tasks have been researched for a number of years. The Event-Related Potential (ERP) is a measure of electrical activity on the cerebral cortex surface and provides information about how the brain responds to external sensory stimuli. Two components of the ERP are the P300 positivity and the N200 negativity amplitudes. Numerous studies have demonstrated that alcoholics have significantly attenuated (diminished) P300 amplitude compared to nonalcoholics. This same diminished P300 amplitude has been noted in children of alcoholics even before they begin drinking. This finding may represent a genetic marker that can be used to identify individuals who are at high risk for alcoholism. Current research is also investigating the delta and theta wave event oscillations, which are major contributors to the P300 signal. Another physiological marker that has been researched is static ataxia (body sway), which has been used to measure difference in the response to ethanol in children of alcoholics and children of nonalcoholics. Several studies have noted that individuals with a positive family history of alcoholism have a greater baseline body sway than individuals without a family history of alcoholism.

Biochemical markers include gene products that may predispose an individual to the risk of developing alcoholism. One such biochemical marker that has been researched in relation to alcoholism is the enzyme monoamine oxidase (MAO). At present, two forms of MAO have been identified: MAO A and MAO B. MAO B is typically found in platelets and is under genetic control. Numerous studies have reported that platelet MAO activity is significantly lower in alcoholics than in control subjects. Adenylate cyclase is another enzyme located on platelets that is being researched as a potential biochemical marker. This enzyme, also under genetic control, has demonstrated reduced activity in alcoholics compared to nonalcoholic subjects.

At present, research is being conducted on the neurotransmitters dopamine, serotonin, and GABA to more clearly delineate how they may contribute to the development of alcoholism in children of alcoholics. Although more research is needed on these neurotransmitters and other physiological and biochemical markers, they serve as a foundation for determining who is at risk of developing alcoholism.

Conclusion

Family interaction patterns, individual alcohol expectancies, genetic variables, parental psychopathologies, and adolescent conduct disorders all play a role in the development of alcoholism in the children of alcoholics. Although children of alcoholics are a high risk group, the development of alcoholism is not inevitable. Early identification of high risk children and the provision of effective interventions are critical to stopping the intergenerational transfer of the disease. Whether or not the parents are receiving treatment for their alcoholism, the children and teens can benefit from educational programs, social skills building, multihelp groups such as Al-Anon and Alateen, and positive social activities that reduce their isolation. Because it is common for children of alcoholics to have significant misinformation and misunderstandings about the disease of alcoholism, it is important they understand that they did not cause, they cannot control, and they cannot cure their parents' disease. Efforts to improve self-esteem, autonomy, self-efficacy, communication skills, and decision making skills are important behavioral competencies that children of alcoholics will need to develop. Pediatricians, educators, coaches, and religious leaders are in unique positions to identify children who are growing up in alcoholic homes and provide healthy interventions for these children. Numerous screening tools including the Children of Alcoholics Screening Test, the Family Drinking Survey, the Family CAGE, and the Alcohol Use Disorders Inventory are available to aid in the early detection of children from alcoholic homes.

Barbara Sullivan

See also Adult Children of Alcoholics; Alcohol-Related Birth Defects; Codependency; Family Therapy; Genetic Aspects of Addition; Prevention Strategies; Risk Factors for Addiction

Further Readings

Anda, R. (n.d.). *The health and social impact of growing up with alcohol abuse and related adverse childhood experiences: The human and economic costs of the status quo.* Retrieved November 2007 from http://www.nacoa .org/pdfs/Anda%20NACoA%20Review_web.pdf

Ellis, D. A., Zucker, A. R., & Fitzgerald, H. E. (1997). The role of family influences in development and risk. *Alcohol Health & Research World, 21,* 218–225.

Jacob, T., & Johnson, S. (1997). Parenting influences on the development of alcohol abuse and dependence. *Alcohol Health and Research World, 21,* 204–209.

McCrady, B. S., Zucker, R. A., Molina, B. S. G., Ammon, L., Ames, G. M, & Longabaugh, R. (2006). Social environmental influences on the development and resolution of alcohol problems [Electronic version]. *Alcoholism: Clinical and Experimental Research,30,* 688–699.

Molina, B., & Pelham, W. E. (2003). Childhood predictors of adolescent substance use in a longitudinal study of children with ADHD. *Journal of Abnormal Psychology, 112,* 497–507.

Ohannessian, C., Hesselbrock, V. M., Kramer, J., Kuperman, S., Bucholz, K. K., Schuckit, M. A., et al. (2004). The relationship between parental alcoholism and adolescent psychopathology: A systematic examination of parental comorbid psychopathology. *Journal of Abnormal Child Psychology, 32,* 519–533.

Patel, S. H., & Azzam, P. N. (2005). Characterization of N200 and P300: Selected studies of the Event-Related Potential. *International Journal of Medical Sciences, 2,* 147–154.

Rangaswamy, M., Jones, K. A., Porjesz, B., Chorlian, D. B., Padmanabhapillai, A., Kamarajan, C., et al. (2007). Delta and theta oscillations as risk markers in adolescent offspring of alcoholics. *International Journal of Psychophysiology, 63,* 3–15.

Sher, K. J. (1997). Psychological characteristics of children of alcoholics. *Alcohol Health and Research World, 21,* 247–254.

Tabakoff, B., & Hoffman, P. L. (1988). Genetics and biological markers of risk for alcoholism. *Public Health Reports, 103,* 690–698.

Werner, M. J., Joffe, A., & Graham, A. V. (1999). Screening, early identification, and office-based intervention with children and youth living in substance-abusing families [Electronic version]. *Pediatrics, 103,* 1099–1112.

CHRONICITY

The word *chronicity* can imply many things when related to substance use and addiction. Most typically, it references the chronic nature of addiction and the reoccurrence, or the more stigmatizing term *relapse*, of the illness. Recent studies confirm that the majority of people with severe and persistent substance use disorders (e.g., substance dependence as defined in the revision of the fourth edition of the *Diagnostic and Statistical Manual of Mental Disorders, Edition, Text Revision (DSM-IV-TR)* who achieve a year of stable recovery do so only after three or four treatment episodes over the span of many years. To society, this appears as relapse, is often equated with patient failure in treatment, and is not viewed as a medical reoccurrence of a chronic illness. However, studies of publicly funded addiction treatment document the medical intractability of the illness. For example, William White notes that of all individuals inducted into treatment at a publicly funded agency, 60% have already had one or more prior treatment admissions, and 24% have had three or more prior admissions. Between 25% and 35% of clients who complete addiction treatment will be readmitted within 1 year, and 50% will be readmitted within 2 to 5 years. Viewed from another perspective, in the past 25 years, many researchers have documented the rate of full recovery (abstinence) ranging from 30% to 72% over an individual's lifetime. A 60-year comprehensive study completed by George Valliant reports that 59% of individuals who receive treatment attain full recovery at some point in their life. In this context, Clinton DeSoto and colleagues define recovery as durable after 4 to 5 years of sustained remission (when risk of future lifetime use drops below 15%).

Interestingly, some studies do document a post-treatment return to social drinking in clients; that is, they return to drinking at levels that do not meet *DSM-IV-TR* clinical criteria for dependence or abuse. Deborah A. Dawson reports that in the year following treatment, as many as 49% of individuals return to nondiagnosable use. Treatment of substance use disorders, usually by measures based on a medically acute care understanding of addiction, underscores the need for clarity in defining both chronicity and recovery. Specifically, the chronicity of addiction is often not taken into account when providing treatment and this failure, in turn, can lead to inadequate care. In addition, when the definition of recovery is based solely on abstinence from alcohol and other drugs, there is no flexibility to incorporate instances of reoccurrence into the accepted course of the illness.

Treatment

The term *chronic illness* or chronicity is not a phrase that describes just one illness. It actually describes a group of health conditions that last a long time, often reoccur, and—if left unchecked—lead to other more serious health conditions. The Centers for Disease Control and Prevention report that the leading causes of death or disability in the United States are due to chronic illnesses such as heart disease, hypertension, cancer, HIV/AIDS, and diabetes. Further, chronic illnesses account for 70% of all deaths in the United States, or about 1.7 million individuals each year. Although chronic illnesses are among the most common and costly health problems, they are also among the most preventable. In addition, although not counted in the above data, studies by Brandeis University and the Robert Wood Johnson Foundation indicate that there are more deaths, illnesses, and disabilities from substance use than from any other preventable chronic health condition.

Most addicts and alcoholics will experience chronicity. In fact, a study by M. Douglas Anglin and colleagues indicate that a majority of individuals will experience reoccurrence of symptoms within 6 months after treatment cessation. A reoccurrence typically means that the individual has reinitiated active use and is also experiencing the related physical, psychological, and social conditions of use. This finding has led many, from policymakers to private citizens, to conclude that addiction is not treatable, that treatment is ineffective, or that hope for recovery is possible, but unlikely. This conclusion is based mainly on results from treatments that are more appropriate to an acute illness (e.g. cold, headache, wound) than approaches that are used to address a chronic illness (e.g., continuing medical care, active self-care including peer support, precautions to moderate illness). In fact, chronic care is often impossible or very difficult to implement due to systemic restrictions such as health insurance limits on the number of treatment episodes over a lifetime and restrictive management of the levels and units of care provided. These restrictions are appropriate for acute illnesses but are inappropriate to address illnesses with chronicity because these restrictions do not allow for a continuum of care over time. In essence, the system is effectively fostering treatment failure and the chronicity of addiction by not allowing for adequate care when qualified professionals deem it medically necessary.

Numerous leading researchers in addiction including A. Thomas McLellan, White, Michael Boyle, David Loveland, Charles P. O'Brien, the Institute of Medicine, and many others have demonstrated that addiction is most like a chronic illness in terms of vulnerability, onset, and course. Study after study demonstrate that the failure to properly treat addiction as a chronic disorder leads to increased health costs not only for substance use disorder treatment itself, but also for care to address attendant health problems caused or exacerbated by addiction. Through a lifetime simulation model for treatment of heroin use, Gary Zarkin and colleagues estimated that the benefit-cost ratio of chronic care was $37.72:1 in comparison to a benefit-cost ratio of $4.86:1 for a static or acute-care model. Moreover, according to the results of the 2006 National Survey on Drug Use and Health, only 20% of those needing addiction treatment receive it, and the Schneider Institute for Health Policy at Brandies University estimates that the societal costs for this untreated illness are more than $28 billion dollars each year. These costs are not unexpected when one considers that a majority of patients in the United States do not receive addiction care based on the chronic etiology of the condition.

Recovery

Numerous studies have confirmed that addiction alters the brain and its functioning. However, researchers are still grappling with related questions such as the following:

- Are brain alterations caused by addiction permanent? Are the changes intergenerational?
- Once addicted, do individuals have a lifetime risk of reoccurrence?
- Once individuals become addicted to a certain substances, are they at risk for reoccurrence to only that particular substance or all substances?
- Are individuals at greater risk of reoccurrence if they do not participate in ongoing care that helps support an attitude of recovery and related behavioral changes?

Although science works on these questions and further develops and refines a chronic care model for treatment of addiction, many in recovery have advocated for such chronic care all along, knowing intuitively what science is finally beginning to support—that addiction is a lifetime illness requiring ongoing treatment, peer support (e.g., Alcoholics Anonymous, Narcotics Anonymous, formal or

informal mentors, a recovery coach), an attitude protective of recovery, and active pursuit of behavioral changes (e.g., avoid people, places, and things, i.e., triggers) to reduce the likelihood of reoccurrence or chronicity.

As part of the wide recognition of the scientifically supported view of the chronicity of addiction, all stakeholders must work together to change the language related to prevention, treatment, and recovery in order to destigmatize the illness based on the historical perception of it as an acute condition. For example, *reoccurrence* would replace *relapse, person with addiction* would replace *addict*, and *positive urine screen* would replace *dirty urine*. This revolution further emphasizes the need for an overhaul of addiction terminology where the divide between the current language and the messages clients receive from practitioners remain acute, confusing, and stigmatizing. Practitioners tell clients that addiction is a chronic disorder, but individual treatment episodes continue to get shorter and shorter; recovery is a process over time, but clients are discharged or graduated after one phase of treatment; posttreatment recovery supports are important to sustained recovery, but practitioners do little to facilitate and monitor the recovery process; and if a client experiences reoccurrence, he or she should return to treatment even though those who do return are often shamed for their perceived failure. These statements are especially poignant in light of studies by Robert Hubbard and colleagues, which points out that more than 80% of individuals experience a reoccurrence within 90 days after discharge from treatment. In addition, more than half of these reoccurrences occur within the first 30 days after discharge. Research indicates that recovery can take years; is often attained through multiple attempts, which become cumulative and synergistic; and can be facilitated by posttreatment check-ups and linkage to recovery-support services. Despite these facts, less than 20% of individuals discharged from treatment continue with professionally directed or peer-supported care after discharge.

As with treatment for other chronic illnesses, addiction practitioners need to focus more on the sustained management of the illness instead of its cure. This change in recovery does not mean that recovery is not possible. To the contrary, millions of individuals achieve stable, long-term recovery. The focus on sustained management, however, is a more honest portrayal of the illness and emphasizes that addiction is more complex than a cold or other acute conditions. Further, this treatment perspective affords health professionals the opportunity to identify and intervene earlier with any emerging or related conditions that could lead to reoccurrence, for example, depression, other health conditions, psychological well-being, and so on.

New Understanding

Both medical and recovery experts are beginning to utilize a broader understanding of chronicity. For example, in the foundational diagnostic systems of both the International Classification System and the *DSM-IV-TR*, one aspect of the definition of remission is the time period of improvement. Although not scientifically or experientially equated to recovery, full or partial, early or sustained remission are defined in terms of the amount of clinical criteria evident for dependence (absence of all clinical criteria indicates full remission and presence of some clinical criteria indicates partial remission) and the length of time there are no clinical criteria present to indicate dependence (1–12 months for early remission and more than 12 months for sustained remission). Special criteria are also applied for those on agonist or maintenance therapies, but again, as with other chronic conditions, such pharmacological supports are not the measure of remission or recovery in themselves but a medical adjunct to improve medical outcomes and other measures of remission, for example quality of life, level of functioning, compliance with treatment, and so on. In sum, the time and severity of pathology measured by several criteria define an illness, remission of that illness, and probable chronicity.

Similarly, those in recovery understand chronicity in a broad way when they describe an individual's progress in recovery and measure of personal choice. Specifically, there is a distinction between the stage of the illness (e.g., stage 4 cancer vs. stage 3 cancer) and what Jeffrey Smith describes as the stages in recovery of free will (e.g., the first phase when alcoholics will compulsively seek routes back to active drinking vs. the second phase when alcoholics begin to gain an increasing amount of healthy free will and can clearly weigh positive and negative consequences of returning to drinking). From this perspective, recovery begins with a choice and is measured through one's progressively achieved wellness (vs. pathology) in life as a result of that choice. Recovery then may be said to occur in stages that, like stages of other chronic

illnesses, connote both the level of pathology and wellness present. In this way, when measuring either pathology or wellness, chronicity is unquestionably a major factor in the illness and no longer simply a measure of treatment success or failure or recovery.

Conclusion

Chronicity refers to the chronic nature of a disease. Research indicates that in all aspects, addiction is most appropriately considered a chronic illness similar to diabetes, hypertension, and HIV/AIDS. Unfortunately, the system in place to treat individuals with addiction operates from an acute understanding of the illness and does not support the chronic, continuing care that the vulnerability, onset, and course of addiction take. This leads to high costs to society to treat addicted individuals and the attendant physical health problems that result from inadequate care. Through changing the language associated with addiction to destigmatize the illness and focusing on sustained management instead of a cure, all stakeholders will better understand how to evaluate treatment and the treatment course of an addicted individual.

Michael Flaherty and Debra Langer

See also Addiction, Models of; Continuum of Care; Disease Concept; Evidence-Based Treatment; Peer Recovery Support Services; Recovery; Relapse

Further Readings

Dawson, D. A., Grant, B. F., Stinson, F. S., Chou, P. S., Huang, B., & Ruan, J. (2005). Recovery from *DSM-IV* alcohol dependence: United States, 2001-2002. *Addiction, 100,* 281–292.

De Soto, C. B., O'Donnell, W. E., & De Soto, J. L. (1989). Long-term recovery in alcoholics. *Alcoholism: Clinical and Experimental Research, 13,* 693–697.

Flaherty, M. T. (2006). *A unified vision for the prevention and management of substance use disorders: Building resiliency, wellness and recovery—A shift from an acute care to a sustained care recovery management model.* Pittsburgh, PA: Institute for Research, Education and Training in Addiction.

Hser, Y., Anglin, M. D., Grella, C., Longshore, D., & Prendergast, M. L. (1997). Drug treatment careers: A conceptual framework and existing research findings. *Journal of Substance Abuse Treatment, 14*(6), 543–558.

Hubbard, R. L., Flynn, P. M., Craddock, G., & Fletcher, B. (2001). Relapse after drug abuse treatment. In F. Tims, C. Leukfield, & J. Platt (Eds.), *Relapse and recovery in addictions* (pp. 109–121). New Haven, CT: Yale University Press.

Institute of Medicine. (2006). *Improving the quality of health care for mental and substance-use conditions.* Washington, DC: National Academy Press.

McLellan, A. T., Lewis, D. C., O'Brien, C. P., & Kleber, H. D. (2000). Drug dependence, a chronic medical illness: Implications for treatment, insurance, and outcomes evaluation. *JAMA, 284*(13), 1689–1695.

Moos, R., & Moos, B. (2005). Paths of entry into Alcoholics Anonymous: Consequences for participation and remission. *Alcoholism: Clinical & Experimental Research, 29*(10), 1858–1868.

National Institute on Drug Abuse. (1999). *Principles of drug addiction treatment* (NIH Publication No. 00-4180). Rockville, MD: National Institute of Health and National Institute on Drug Abuse.

O'Brien, C. P., & McLellan, A. T. (1997). Addiction medicine. *The Journal of the American Medical Association, 277*(23), 1840–1842.

Schneider Institute for Health Policy, Brandeis University. (2001). *Substance abuse: The nation's number one health problem.* Princeton, NJ: The Robert Wood Johnson Foundation.

Smith, J. (2005). Commentary: Alcoholism and free will. *Psychiatric Times, 41*(4), 17.

White, W., Boyle, M., & Loveland, D. (2002). Alcoholism/addiction as a chronic disease: From rhetoric to clinical reality. *Alcoholism Treatment Quarterly, 20*(3–4), 107–130.

White, W., & Kurtz, E. (2006). *Linking addiction treatment and communities of recovery: A primer for addiction counselors and recovery coaches.* Pittsburgh, PA: Northeast Addiction Technology Transfer Center.

CLIENT ENGAGEMENT

Individuals who abuse alcohol and/or illicit drugs are notorious for missing scheduled intake and treatment sessions, arriving late to scheduled sessions, and demonstrating poor participation and compliance during treatment sessions. According to a review of the research by Noelle L. Lefforge, Brad Donohue, and Marilyn J. Strada, 50% of all initial scheduled sessions are attended in mental health settings whereas the attendance rates for initial sessions in substance abuse settings are often as low as 30%. There are many contributing factors that have been identified in the literature that contribute to poor clinic attendance rates in those with substance use disorders. Some of these factors have been directly related to substance use (e.g., oversleeping, hangover effects, apathy, poor concentration, memory loss), whereas other influences are either unrelated or indirectly related to substance use (e.g., mistrust of treatment staff, lack of transportation, need for childcare, odd working hours, ambivalence regarding the need for treatment). Of course, missed appointments waste available resources (i.e., therapist time, office space), delay the provision of treatment, and limit treatment opportunities for others. Moreover, low attendance rates have been associated with poor treatment outcomes in substance abuse settings. Therefore, it is critical to implement methods that will enhance treatment compliance, particularly as it relates to session attendance. To address this concern, various enlistment and retention strategies have been developed and favorably evaluated in substance abuse settings. Interestingly, however, these strategies have been grossly underutilized in community settings. Engagement strategies have also been developed to encourage effort and participation of those in substance abuse treatment, such as motivational enhancement strategies. The following sections delineate engagement strategies that have demonstrated effectiveness in enlisting, retaining, and motivating those with substance use disorders to actively participate in treatment.

Enlistment Strategies

Enlistment strategies are primarily focused on encouraging clients to participate in treatment services. The initial enlistment contact with the potential client varies, but it usually includes a telephone call with an employee of the treatment program. Asking clients to review expected therapeutic gains during the enlistment call is a customary practice that will likely increase first session attendance. Similarly, conducting a brief 5-minute telephone call immediately after the initial session is attended provides an opportunity to address concerns that may have spontaneously occurred and can reinforce the need to maintain the appointment. In some situations, postcards or flyers may be utilized to initially enlist participants, although these procedures are less effective than individualized telephone contacts. Although initial enlistment is usually conducted during telephone calls, when client motivation is wanting or ability to attend the clinic is particularly problematic, enlistment sessions may be conducted in the potential client's home or at a nearby public place (i.e., park, busy restaurant). Home visits are less practical than telephone contacts because they are comparatively more involved and costly, but such visits offer a more accessible and relaxed environment in which to engage clients.

It is helpful to identify one or more staff members who can serve as enlistment specialists. Ideally, enlistment specialists will be experienced in the provision of substance abuse services, but at the very least, they must be familiar with the respective treatment program. Given that poor first impressions have been shown to decrease participation of clients in substance abuse treatment programs, it is prudent to extensively train enlistment specialists and ideally, to utilize experienced clinicians in the process to some extent. Although it is impossible to anticipate all of the potential obstacles and excuses that clients will voice during these initial contacts, an effective model of enlistment training involves both didactic components in which common issues are discussed and elaborated and extensive role-playing in real world scenarios. Most evidence-based engagement interventions are initiated with a brief discussion of the presenting problem, delineation of available clinical services, reviewing directions to the treatment center, and facilitating the generation of solutions to potential barriers that may interfere with program participation. Discussion of the presenting problem includes queries that are relevant to the reason for referral and, subsequently, empathizing with solicited concerns. In doing so, the enlistment specialist is provided an opportunity to selectively indicate intervention services that may be offered in the treatment program to assist in resolving identified problems. It is imperative that the client understands when sessions will occur, how long sessions will last, and how many sessions are likely to be prescribed. Indeed, insufficient information about the parameters of treatment may lead to inappropriate expectations and subsequent poor attendance. It is also important to personalize the treatment program to the fullest extent possible (i.e., indicate the treatment provider's name, report positive characteristics of the treatment provider, emphasize treatment

components that are relevant to presenting concerns). Along a different vein, controlled studies have demonstrated significant improvements in session attendance consequent to warning clients that missed appointments will result in treatment delays, and with consent, involving significant others in the enlistment process (e.g., discussing how the significant other can help the client attend treatment sessions or facilitate the client's treatment plan).

Reminder telephone calls are another commonly used enlistment strategy and appear to be most effective when implemented 2 or 3 days prior to the initial session. Although anecdotal, there is some support to suggest that if the call is made 4 or more days prior to the scheduled session, the call does not act as a reminder, and if the call is made the day before the intake, the call increases the likelihood of session cancellation or rescheduling. It is a good idea to confirm the time, date, and location of the respective session. Clients may be unavailable during typical business hours. Therefore, employers should ideally identify enlistment specialists who have a relatively flexible schedule (i.e., can conduct enlistment sessions during weekends and evenings).

Lefforge and colleagues found that promising token incentives for initial session attendance increases attendance rates by about 15% and may be especially effective when used in low-income populations. Although this practice may appear to be costly, token rewards may be donated by community-conscious companies or limited to relatively inexpensive items (e.g., costume jewelry, candy, refreshments, beverages, raffles, combs, pens). Comprehensive approaches (i.e., the Community Reinforcement Approach and the Community Reinforcement and Family Training programs) have been found to engage adults into substance abuse treatment by training their significant others to manage consequences that are relevant to substance use (e.g., permitting the client to experience natural consequences when alcohol is consumed, encouragement, and romantic interactions when abstinent from illicit drugs).

Lefforge and colleagues found that mailing a personalized program orientation letter to arrive 1 to 2 days prior to the initial intake session engages clients by approximately 25%. The content of these letters (e.g., indicating date, time, and location of the initial session; emphasizing program strengths) are similar to reminder telephone calls. Once generic letters are originated, costs are limited to postage and time spent mailing the letters. However, it is difficult to coordinate the mailing to be read by the client 1 or 2 days prior to the scheduled session, and potential clients often mistakenly throw the orientation letter into the garbage, assuming it is unsolicited mail. If an enlistment meeting can be arranged or funding permits mail delivery, Lefforge and colleagues found that orientation videotapes that emphasize optimization of the treatment experience improve session attendance by approximately 15%. Although personalized videos are relatively costly to produce and update, they are relatively easy to maintain.

When reviewing directions to the treatment center, it is important not only to provide directions, but to assess how the client intends on getting to the session. Depending on the clientele served by the treatment center, many clients may not have adequate means of personal transportation and thus may have to rely on a friend or relative to transport them or alternatively, to rely on the local transit system. For those relying on friends or relatives, it will be important for those providing the transportation to be reminded of the appointment, which can be accomplished by having the clients contact them directly or by having the enlistment specialist make this contact. For those using public transportation, ensuring that the clients know the appropriate bus route to the treatment center (including transfers) and the time it will take to get to the treatment facility is of critical importance. Neglecting to address this simple issue contributes to poor session attendance.

Retention Strategies

Attendance rates have been shown to drop precipitously, according to Lefforge and colleagues, after the intake session is attended, usually by as much as 40% in samples involving individuals who have been identified to abuse drugs. Therefore, retention interventions, performed by designated enlistment specialists or treatment providers, have been developed to provide ongoing extra intervention session support to clients throughout therapy to assist them in maintaining active attendance. Enlistment specialists offer certain advantages over treatment providers, including enhanced objectivity and opportunities to mediate disagreements that may exist between the treatment provider and client. Other advantages of enlistment

specialists who are not directly involved in treatment include opportunities to reinforce therapist initiatives and reporting issues to therapists that may be relevant to the treatment plan. Retention telephone calls, or in-person meetings, also provide opportunities to assist clients with difficulties that may occur between therapy assignments, solicit positive aspects of the treatment program, assess quality assurance, and request suggestions for program improvement.

Those with substance user disorders often lack appropriate assertiveness skills that are relevant to negotiating alternative session times when unanticipated difficulties occur. Periodic queries to assure treatment sessions are scheduled conveniently have improved retention. When funding is limited, automatically rescheduling sessions that were previously missed through mail correspondence has been shown to significantly improve retention.

Enhancement of Effort and Participation in Treatment

Coercive and aggressive confrontational therapeutic styles have been shown to be relatively ineffective for individuals with substance use disorders and, in fact, may cause clients to withdraw from therapy prematurely. Alternatively, motivational interviewing techniques have been shown to improve abstinence-oriented activities through enhanced effort and participation in therapy. Consistent with motivational interviewing, the treatment provider follows a directive style that is focused on behavioral change (i.e., abstinence) through resolution of ambivalence. Clients should be guided to appreciate the positive and negative consequences of substance abusive behavior and to determine for themselves the importance of maintaining nonabusive behavior patterns. Other engagement strategies include reflective listening, avoiding diagnostic labels, acceptance and support, carefully monitoring readiness to change, deescalating resistance, and emphasizing the client's freedom of choice. The conservative practice of offering advice only when encouraged to do so is especially warranted during the initial sessions for two primary reasons: (1) substance abusing individuals may think the therapist is providing advice prior to sufficiently understanding their situation and (2) the therapist may suggest a behavior to be changed that the client is not interested, or prepared, to change.

Conclusion

Client participation is relatively poor in substance abuse clinics. However, in controlled outcome studies, various interventions have demonstrated improvements in attendance and promptness to scheduled sessions, as well as engagement of clients during intervention sessions. These interventions have included mail correspondence (e.g., orientation letters, postcard reminders), telephone correspondence (e.g., empathizing with client concerns), and home-based sessions that are focused on program enlistment (e.g., recruitment of significant others). Motivational interviewing strategies have also greatly enhanced compliance of clients to session protocol and have increased retention.

Suzanne Gorney, Mora Kim, Brad Donohue,
and Daniel N. Allen

See also Coercion and Treatment; Community Reinforcement Approach; Motivational Interviewing; Stages of Change Model; Treatment Access and Retention

Further Readings

Lefforge, N. L., Donohue, B., & Strada, M. J. (2007). Improving session attendance in mental health and substance abuse settings: A review of controlled studies. *Behavior Therapy, 38,* 1–22.

Miller, W. R., & Rollnick, S. (1991). *Preparing people to change addictive behavior.* New York: Guilford Press.

CLIENT/TREATMENT MATCHING

Matching, the idea that treatment outcomes can be improved by tailoring treatments to specific client characteristics and needs, is not a new concept. It is a cornerstone of modern medical practice that is becoming even more prominent as recent advances in human genetics have raised the possibility of tailoring treatments for specific diseases to specific patients based on the patient's genetic characteristics. In education, as well, the notion of using instructional methods tailored to specific student learning needs is a longstanding practice. Thus, the idea of matching interventions to client characteristics represents a general approach to human change and treatment efforts.

History of Matching

Two disparate sources of impetus had driven researcher and clinician attempts to develop client-treatment matching formulas. The first was a desire by clinical researchers to develop, test, and disseminate improved treatments for people with alcohol and drug problems. The second impetus came from a more purely financial perspective in the form of the advent of managed care, which imposed increasing restrictions on the provision of substance abuse treatment and produced an increasing need for clinicians to be able to justify the type of treatment they were providing to clients.

Clinical Research on Matching

In 1941, E. M. Jellinek, the originator of the disease concept of alcoholism, suggested tailoring treatments to each of the several types of alcoholics he identified in his research as a way to improve treatment outcomes. Following Jellinek's initial suggestion that matching specific types of alcoholics to specific treatments might improve treatment outcomes, the matching hypothesis (as it has come to be called) fell into a period of relative dormancy. This dormancy resulted in part from the lack of differentially effective treatments for alcohol and drug problems that could be studied with respect to their efficacy with clients of different types. Because the alcohol and drug treatment system in the United States became focused almost exclusively around a single treatment philosophy and approach—one derived from the Twelve-Steps of Alcoholics Anonymous, which was believed by many in the middle years of the 20th century to be the only effective approach to treating substance use disorders—interest in the concept of matching waned.

Nonetheless, a trial was conducted by R.S. Wasserstein at the Winter Veterans Administration Hospital in Topeka, Kansas, in the 1950s in which four treatments were studied (disulfiram [Antabuse]; conditioned reflex therapy, an early form of behavior therapy; group hypnotherapy; and a milieu therapy control group). Wasserstein found that Antabuse was more effective than the other three comparison treatments, but that many of the clients treated were helped by the other treatments offered. Wasserstein reanalyzed the data and found that particular client characteristics (such as compulsiveness or depression) appeared to be associated with differential success across the treatments. This finding was the first strong indication that Jellinek's hypothesis might be a viable one to guide treatment. Despite the fact that Wasserstein published his results, which represented the first large scale attempt at matching research, in the mid-1950s, the dormancy of the matching hypothesis that followed Jellinek's original suggestion continued.

This began to change in last quarter of the 20th century with the establishment of the National Institute of Alcohol Abuse and Alcoholism (NIAAA) and the National Institute on Drug Abuse the two research funding arms of the National Institutes of Health devoted to research in substance abuse. As researchers began to develop additional treatments, the possibility of matching clients to specific treatments became much more of a reality. In the 1970s and 1980s, many studies, particularly in the alcohol treatment field, found that particular types of clients seemed to do better with particular treatments. For example, research in the 1980s found that certain behavioral approaches to the treatment of alcoholics, such as social skills training, appeared to be more effective than traditional Twelve Step–based counseling approaches with clients diagnosed as suffering from antisocial personality disorder.

In the early 1980s, researchers at the University of Pennsylvania and Philadelphia Veterans Administration Hospital published the first prospective study of matching, this time including both alcohol and drug dependent clients. In contrast to Wasserstein's study, which had developed matching variables through a post hoc analysis of the data, the Philadelphia group, led by A. Thomas McLellan, George Woody, Charles O'Brien, and Lester Luborsky, assigned clients to particular treatments based on client characteristics that had been identified in previous research as being associated with positive outcomes in particular treatments. The findings were encouraging in that clients who were appropriately matched were doing significantly better on measures of treatment outcome at a 6-month follow-up assessment than were clients who were inappropriately matched.

In 1987, Helen Annis of the Addiction Research Foundation in Toronto, Canada, suggested at a meeting of an Institute of Medicine group assembled to make recommendations for enhancing the effectiveness of alcohol treatment, that systematic research on client-treatment matching was a major path to enhancing treatment effectiveness. Annis's assertion became a part of the Institute of Medicine's landmark report *Broadening the Base of Treatment for Alcohol Problems*, which devoted an entire chapter to the matching concept. Spurred, in part, by the Institute of Medicine report, NIAAA issued a request for proposals to develop and implement a large scale, multisite study of client treatment matching in alcohol treatment that later became known as Project MATCH (MATCH being an acronym for matching alcohol treatment to client heterogeneity). MATCH will be discussed more fully below.

Managed Care–Focused Research on Matching

At about the same time that the Institute of Medicine assembled its work group on alcoholism treatment, health care funding began to come under the influence of what has come to be known as managed care. The goal of managed care was to reduce health care costs by ensuring that clients received only the treatments that were likely to be effective and that if there was a choice to be made among treatments that were equally likely to be effective with a particular client problem, the least costly should be implemented first.

In response to the increasing incursions of managed care into health care funding, two groups of researchers engaged by the Northern Ohio Chemical Dependency Treatment Directors Association (NOCDTDA) and the National Association of Addiction Treatment Providers (NAATP) developed sets of criteria that were designed to meet the managed care requirements of enhancing treatment effective while containing costs by placing clients in the specific types of treatment that research and clinical experience suggested were most likely to be effective. Under the leadership of Norman Hoffman, the NOCDTDA developed what came to be known as the Cleveland criteria. The NAATP developed the NAATP patient placement criteria. Subsequent research failed to find that appropriate placement of clients using these criteria enhanced treatment outcomes. Nonetheless, workgroups were formed under the aegis of the American Society of Addiction Medicine (ASAM) to develop the ASAM patient placement criteria-1 (PPC), first published in 1991, followed by a revision (the ASAM patient placement criteria-2) published in 1996, with further revision published in 2001. The PPC have become the standard mechanism in clinical settings for assigning clients to specific levels and intensities of care based on a variety of what have been called *complicating factors*. Complicating factors comprise such client characteristics as severity of dependence, presence or absence of social support, housing status, previous treatments, and problem duration.

The PPC have not been without their critics, and a number of alternative sets of criteria for matching clients to appropriate levels of care have also been developed. However, none has achieved the widespread use that the PPC have.

Project MATCH and the PPC

The two most prominent, large scale attempts to develop client-treatment matching criteria to date have been MATCH, which focused exclusively on alcohol treatment, and the ASAM PPC development, which attempts to delineate matching criteria for clients who use both alcohol and illicit drugs.

Project MATCH

Although a full recounting of MATCH is beyond the scope of this article, a brief overview of the guiding principles and intent behind the research as well as the basic outcomes and current status will be presented.

MATCH was conceived as a way of combining research findings that had accumulated over the several decades preceding MATCH's inception and identifying which clients did best with one of three treatments: Twelve-Step Facilitation, Cognitive-Behavioral Coping Skills, and Motivational Enhancement Therapy. These three treatments were selected because they represented both widespread contemporary practice (Twelve-Step based approaches were used in the vast majority of substance abuse treatment programs in the United States at the time, which was in the early 1990s, as almost the exclusive treatment approach for alcohol problems), which had garnered significant research support (cognitive behavioral treatment) and which had both research support and held the promise of being a briefer treatment that would be applicable to people who were not yet fully ready to make significant changes in drinking (Motivational Enhancement Therapy). Two groups of clients were included in MATCH: clients who had just completed an inpatient treatment for

alcohol abuse or dependence (for whom the MATCH intervention was essentially aftercare) and a group of clients for whom the MATCH intervention constituted an outpatient treatment program that was often their initial treatment. Clients were recruited from multiple sites around the United States (to minimize differences in regional effects such as differential quality of local treatment programs in the aftercare group) and randomly assigned within each arm (aftercare and outpatient) to receive one of the three manualized treatments. Two of the treatments were 12 sessions long, the third (Motivational Enhancement Therapy) was 4 sessions, but the amount of time clients met with counselors was the same for all three treatments. Study clinicians were extensively and closely supervised to ensure adherence to the treatment manuals for each treatment.

Clients enrolled in MATCH were extensively assessed on a variety of characteristics that were chosen from among those that had been shown in previous research to be associated with differential effectiveness of one or more of the treatments. Clients were then followed up with and assessed for drinking and other outcomes every 3 months for a total of 39 months. In all, MATCH represented, at the time, what was probably the single largest randomized clinical research trial on alcohol treatment ever conducted, costing approximately $35 million to complete. Data analysis is still continuing at this writing, and the vast data set is available for researchers who wish to perform analyses on the data to test hypotheses not originally part of the MATCH design.

Despite the massive effort and expense devoted to MATCH, the results have ultimately been somewhat disappointing. Although it seemed clear that all three treatments were effective (although critics have maintained that the study was only minimally related to what happens in the real world where clients typically are not followed up with regularly after treatment, where clinicians typically receive minimal supervision and the degree to which treatments are delivered as they should be is rarely monitored, and where treatments are often delivered in the context of oversight and influence by managed care) few of the numerous matching hypotheses that were advanced at the beginning of the study were supported by the data. In fact, only a handful of the matching hypotheses were supported.

ASAM PPC

Beginning with the Cleveland and NAATP patient placement criteria, a number of studies have focused on what should be the key question with regard to any PPC: Is proper placement of clients using the criteria associated with better outcomes and less costly treatment? As with MATCH, the results of studies designed to answer this critical question have been disappointing, at best. Several studies carried out by researchers at the University of Pennsylvania, led by James McKay, have found that while the PPC are reliable (i.e., different clinicians applying the criteria come to the same level of care recommendations for the same client the vast majority of the time), they lack validity. Simply stated, researchers have been unable to find any significant or strong link between appropriate placement of clients using the PPC and treatment outcomes. This inability has led a number of researchers to suggest that the theoretical basis upon which the PPC is based is flawed—that is, that the PPC is focused on assigning clients to fixed levels of care when in fact clients may require different types of treatments in different settings at different points in treatment, and each client's pattern of needs may be different from those of other clients. This "needs to services" model has spurred the development of at least one alternative set of placement criteria, the cumulative block increment (CBI) model in which placements are made to small service units of care (e.g., several hours of social skills training followed by several hours of vocational counseling) by assessing specific client needs at a particular point in time rather than to a global level of care for which it is difficult to determine whether the services provided at that level actually are appropriate for any particular client.

Conclusion

Despite its lengthy history, and significant attempts to realize a set of effective matching prescriptions in actual practice, the current status of client treatment matching is ambiguous, at best. To date, there has been little success in discovering reliable and valid ways of matching specific individual clients to specific tailored treatments. Nonetheless, the concept of matching carries with it significant intuitive appeal, particularly in the current context of increased emphasis not only on cost-effectiveness of treatment, but on development of a variety of new evidence-based treatment approaches.

Frederick Rotgers

See also American Society of Addiction Medicine; Continuum of Care; Evidence-Based Treatment; Fidelity of Prevention Programs; Patient Placement Criteria; Project MATCH; Research Issues in Treatment; Treatment Effectiveness

Further Readings

American Society of Addiction Medicine. (2001). *Patient placement criteria 2* (Rev. ed.). Annapolis, MD: Author.

Institute of Medicine. (1990). *Broadening the base of treatment for alcohol problems.* Washington, DC: National Academy Press.

McKay, J. R., Cacciola, J. S., McLellan, A. T., Alterman, A. I., & Wirtz, P. W. (1997). An initial evaluation of the psychosocial dimensions of the American Society of Addiction Medicine criteria for inpatient versus intensive outpatient substance abuse rehabilitation. *Journal of Studies on Alcohol, 57,* 239–252.

McLellan, A. T., Woody, G. E., Luborsky, L., O'Brien, C. P., & Druley, K. A. (1983). Increased effectiveness of substance abuse treatment: A prospective study of patient-treatment matching. *Journal of Nervous and Mental Disease, 171*(10), 597–605.

Project MATCH Research Group. (1999). Comments on Project MATCH: Matching alcohol treatments to client heterogeneity [Commentaries]. *Addiction, 94*(1), 31–69.

Project MATCH series manuals: http://pubs.niaaa.nih.gov/publications/match.htm

CLINICAL SUPERVISION OF ADDICTION COUNSELORS

Clinical supervision is transtheoretical in nature, encompassing developmental, evaluative, administrative, and interrelational aspects of clinical practice. Most models of clinical supervision evolved from therapeutic theories and focus on the support and training of the counselor according to a specific theoretical practice. Clinical supervision of addiction counselors incorporates therapeutic theory and practice, as well as knowledge of addiction, with management and education skills. Clinical supervision enhances counselor development as well as the treatment team's capacity to function efficiently and effectively so that substance abuse clients receive expert services resulting in positive treatment outcomes. Traditionally, clinical supervision has been viewed as the gatekeeper of the profession by identifying strengths and weaknesses of clinical staff members and through recommending and modeling skill enhancing therapeutic interventions and techniques, as well as providing insight into the counselor's personal reactions to the therapeutic milieu. Clinical supervision's relevance to addiction treatment rests on the impact that effective clinical supervision plays in ensuring the integrity and success of clinical services. This entry describes the parameters and process of clinical supervision of addiction counselors.

The Clinical Supervisor

Most authors agree that clinical supervision is a multidimensional skill set that demands competence in education, administration, relationship building, and counseling

The ideal clinical supervisor has 3 to 5 years of professional experience, at least a master's degree in a clinical discipline, and counseling and case management expertise combined with the ability to navigate internal and external referral systems. In addition, the clinical supervisor is a teacher whose interventions integrate therapeutic process with concrete suggestions for skill development.

Education and Training

Ideally, clinical supervisors learn their craft as part of a graduate school experience. This experience is a learning opportunity that includes both classroom and experiential components and is managed by expert counselor educators who teach clinical supervision to doctoral level and postmasters students. For example, at the Hazelden Graduate School in Minnesota, the clinical supervisor training program incorporates postmasters clinical staff who enroll in a clinical supervision course. During this course, the potential clinical supervisors provide supervision to master's students at a clinical site and participate in a weekly faculty supervision group where they progress from observation to facilitation, with videotaping of their work and appropriate feedback. This process provides the treatment organization with a staff of trained clinical supervisors. After initial training, conference and other training opportunities can enhance knowledge and skill. For those who cannot access a graduate school, continuing education programs covering the basics of clinical supervision are available at conferences and via distance education.

Certifications and Licensure

The International Certification & Reciprocity Consortium/Alcohol and Other Drug Abuse, Inc. (IC&RC) grew out of the certification movement of addiction counselors and provides certification in counseling and clinical supervision. Frequently, state certification and/or licensing boards also offer certification of clinical supervisors.

Because of the inconsistency of clinical supervision certification between the states, individuals seeking certification as a clinical supervisor should check with the state agency overseeing certification and licensure. IC&RC provides a guide regarding state certification and licensing boards for those states belonging to the consortium.

Ethical Guidelines

Along with the Certification of Clinical Supervisors, IC&RC provides standards to guide clinical supervisors of addiction professionals in their practice. The IC&RC has identified the domains of assessment and evaluation, counselor development, professional responsibility, and management and administration in these ethical standards. Supervisors have the responsibility to be guardians of ethical behavior and to be versed in the nuances of the federal, state, and agency ethical standards.

Another source of ethical guidance is the Association for Counseling Education and Supervision (a division of the American Counseling Association) Ethical Guidelines for Clinical Supervisors. Although not specifically designed for alcohol and drug abuse counselor supervisors, these standards provide a behavioral guide for the clinical supervisor's everyday practice. By adhering to these guidelines, professionals have a road map that protects the rights of clients and supervisees; establishes policies, procedures, and standards for implementing programs; and suggests a system for meeting training and professional development needs of supervisees in ways consistent with clients' welfare and programmatic requirements.

Supervision Process

Authors in the field of clinical supervision and codes of ethics are consistent in specifying the areas of competence a clinical supervisor must possess to effectively function. These competencies lay the groundwork for understanding the challenges and processes of clinical supervision of addiction counselors. The areas are management and administration, evaluation, interrelational or clinical, and supportive. The following descriptions of these functions clarify the role of the clinical supervisor and the process of clinical supervision of addiction counselors.

Management and/or Administration

The supervisor sets the tone for the clinical environment by establishing processes and procedures that facilitate a smooth operation that enhances counselor and client satisfaction. Traditionally, clinical supervisors were independent of administrative responsibilities, as their role was to provide clarity and technical direction to clinicians working in a therapeutic relationship according to a specific theory. However, more recently, the clinical supervisor's scope of responsibility includes tasks such as scheduling of employees' time off, office assignment, and patient assignment; determining pay raises and promotions; and providing regularly scheduled clinical supervision to staff members with a variety of levels of formal training.

The key challenge is to create an organizational structure that fosters efficiency and clear communication while allowing for the intimacy of a supervisor–supervisee relationship that delves into deeply personal reactions to clients and situations. Clearly defined documentation of roles sets boundaries for effectively carrying out these conflicting functions by creating an environment that runs efficiently while encouraging professional growth. Effective supervisors follow management practices that support efficient and productive use of time via clearly defined procedures and processes using a clear communication system. Proactively addressing staff issues in terms clearly understood by all involved eliminates confusion and dissention. Because of the timely nature of record keeping and the importance of staff communication to client welfare, systems that facilitate communication must be in place. When management roles, processes, and procedures are clear, the clinical environment is safe for clients and counselors to do their important therapeutic work.

Evaluation

Clinical supervisors of addiction counselors must evaluate the job performance of the staff they supervise. Effective evaluation systems encourage supervisors to identify areas and skills requiring improvement and provide mechanisms for attaining behavioral goals in a timely fashion. Organizational skills such as time management, accurate documentation, and an attitude of professionalism are included in the clinical supervisor's evaluation. Of course, clinical expertise as demonstrated by the ability to engage in a therapeutic alliance, appropriate clinical decision making, and evidence of a willingness to participate in professional growth activities must also be addressed.

The sensitive nature of evaluation process and procedures demand that the clinical supervisor of addiction counselors become comfortable giving administrative and clinical feedback that encourages supervisees to build on their strengths and overcome obstacles in their path. Again, the supervisor must maintain a delicate balance in delivering performance feedback that impacts not only the counselor's job status but also, most importantly, the effectiveness of client care. Organizations that provide a mechanism that incorporates a written professional development plan that is agreed to by both parties and sets out a schedule of attainable goals creates an environment that validates the evaluation process. By integrating evaluation into the organizational structure, performance standards are clearly understood by supervisor and supervisee resulting in an environment where clinical supervision and counselor development is valued.

Clinical supervisor's frequently need mentoring and training around evaluating and communicating such information to supervisees. The skillful supervisor provides clinical critique, demonstrates clinical behavior, partners with supervisees to create workable professional goals and objectives that build on strengths, and supports continued learning and skill development while maintaining a working relationship.

Interrelational-Clinical

Addiction counseling requires expert counselors who are also educated in the unique characteristics of the addicted client and family members. For programs to achieve positive outcomes and to provide clients opportunities for life-changing experiences, this combination of addiction and counseling expertise must permeate the organization. Clinical supervisors of addiction counselors must also be knowledgeable in the transtheoretical nature of addiction and clinical supervision, as well as being well versed in counseling theories and techniques. In order to facilitate clinical growth in supervisees, the clinical supervisor must also be an expert educator whose interventions, demonstrations, and explanations focus on developing supervisee counseling skills necessary to address ongoing clinical dilemmas.

Many supervision models focus specifically on the clinical area and clearly address the supervisor's role in the development of clinical skill. By building on the strengths of the counselor, the supervisor encourages practicing more advanced clinical interventions. By demonstrating appropriate clinical behaviors and techniques, the supervisor sets the standard of clinical expertise. The professional behaviors of the supervisor and the interventions he or she demonstrates serve as models of clinical competency. Ideally, the partnership between supervisee and supervisor strengthens overtime and allows for experimentation and growth of the supervisee. This critical area requires the clinical expertise of the supervisor as well as skill in the art of supervision.

Supportive

Addiction counseling can be a stressful and isolating job that demands sensitivity and compassion combined with time management and crisis intervention skills. Counselors need support and direction throughout their careers. Models of clinical supervision agree that support is an integral part of the supervisor's role. Supervision is the place to explore personal reactions and/or counter-transference to clients and situations. Because most addiction counselors have had personal or family experience with addiction, counter-transference issues frequently arise. Clinical supervisors must develop skill in maintaining a boundary between the supportive supervisor role and the therapist role. When counter-transference consistently emerges, a referral to the employee assistance program or a therapist is in order.

Clinical supervision is the place where counselors learn to deal with their personal reactions to clinical situations. It is also where addiction counselors learn clinical problem-solving skills. Most clinical supervisors were counselors who have followed their own personal and professional journey, are sensitive to these situations, and are uniquely qualified to guide supervisees through the maze. However, addiction

clinical supervisors must also continually develop their skill set to meet the needs of supervisees in demanding clinical settings.

Supervision of Clinical Supervisors

Because clinical supervision of addiction counselors is demanding work with the stressors experienced by middle management and clinicians, every clinical supervisor of addiction counselors should also have a supervisor who can offer them the same support and guidance that they provide the clinical staff. Clinical supervisors must deal with administrative issues as well as their personal reactions to supervisees and situations. Addressing these issues is equally important for clinical supervisors.

When designing a clinical supervision system for an addiction counseling facility or program, it is important to consider failsafe measures to assure clinical integrity of both supervisors and supervisees. The Association for Counselor Education and Supervision ethical guidelines provides a structure for work systems that address situations that foster blurred boundaries and work overload that often leads to errors in clinical judgment, complicating the supervision process for supervisor and supervisee. Addiction counseling clinical supervisors carry complex workloads including a mix of administrative, clinical, and supervisory responsibilities. Often, these roles are conflicting, creating ethical dilemmas for the supervisor. Supervisors, therefore, require their own supervision that encompasses administrative and clinical issues and allows for safe discussion of personal reactions to staff, clients, and the organization as a whole.

Often, a consultant is hired to supervise clinical leaders. This consultant can provide objectivity and ensure the clinical integrity of the services of the organization. Ideally, the supervisor would be an experienced clinician with a minimum of 3 to 5 years in the field, be trained in the art and discipline of clinical supervision, and continue to seek clinical supervision himself or herself. Effective supervision of clinical judgment of both supervisors and supervisees regarding patients and staff issues is critical to program success, preventing staff burnout, and promoting effective patient outcomes. There is evidence that preventing burnout of staff (supervisees and supervisors) enhances treatment outcomes and that patients treated by burned-out staff report feeling as though they had not be adequately treated. Supervision can alert the organization to issues needing interventions and can enhance the flow of work, reduce incidence of burnout, and improve outcomes.

Conclusion

Clinical supervision is the bedrock of professional development and the vehicle that assures patient welfare. Clinical supervision is a multilevel organizational process that demands commitment and support throughout the organization. Providing clinical supervision to every service provider assures the uninterrupted and seamless flow of treatment. It is incumbent upon the organization to include in their strategic plan a philosophical commitment that is substantiated by allocating funds for providing supervision to those responsible for clinical services. Identifying clinical supervision training and continuing education as a professional development issue worthy of funds and time assures clinical supervision's integration into the fiber of the substance abuse treatment and/or prevention organization.

Eileen McCabe O'Mara

See also Certification and Licensing; Confidentiality; Dual Relationships; Ethical Standards for Addiction Professionals; Impaired Professionals; NAADAC, The Association for Addiction Professionals

Further Readings

Bernard, J. M., & Goodyear, R. K. (2004). *Fundamentals of clinical supervision*. New York: Allyn & Bacon.
Forrest, G. (2002). *Countertransference in chemical dependency counseling*. Binghamton, NY: Haworth Press.
Powell, D. (1998). *Clinical supervision in alcohol and drug abuse counseling*. San Francisco: Jossey-Bass.

Club Drugs

Club drugs are a specific classification of drugs characterized as being used primarily among the nightclub, trance, rave, and bar scene. The trance and rave scenes are commonly know for night-long or weekend-long dances that are often held in warehouses or other large and open facilities. Although many who attend these events do not use club drugs, those who do are generally attracted to the minimal cost of the drugs and the stimulating highs that have been said to heighten the trance and rave experiences. Club drugs can include but are not limited to the following drugs: MDMA (methylenedioxymethamphetamine or ecstasy), GHB (gamma hydroxybutyrate), ketamine, amphetamines (particularly methamphetamine), LSD (lyseric acid diethylamide), and Rohypnol.

Club drugs are primarily used by young people. According to the 2006 Monitoring the Future survey of drug use among young people, college students, and young adults, the use of club drugs has decreased since the late 1990s and early part of this decade. For example, from 2000 to 2005, past-month use of ecstasy has fallen more than 50%. Even more dramatic reductions have occurred in past-month use of LSD since the relatively high levels reported in the mid- to late 1990s.

MDMA

MDMA (or ecstasy) was first developed in 1912 by the German pharmaceutical company, Merck. Although Merck did not find a relevant use for the drug, when it later resurfaced in the late 1960s, it found its way into the underground drug culture where it became known as the mellow drug or the love drug because it enhanced feelings of empathy, which tended to last between 6 and 8 hours. As research and experimentation continued on MDMA, brain damage became a recurring side effect found among laboratory rats. On July 1, 1985, MDMA was declared an illegal substance by the federal government.

MDMA has the properties of central nervous system stimulants and hallucinogens. Unlike many other varieties of drugs that often come from plant derivatives, MDMA is synthesized in laboratories. Because of this method of manufacturing, the quality or purity of the drug can vary from laboratory to laboratory, and other contaminants often make their way into the processing such as caffeine, ephedrine, and ketamine (described below). Therefore, some of the danger in the use of MDMA derives from contaminated adulterates used in the manufacturing process. This contamination has led some raves to institute drug checking stations where MDMA can be assessed on site for contaminants. MDMA tends to interfere with the body's ability to regulate temperature. In rare but nevertheless unpredictable instances, this inability to regulate can lead to not only an increase in body temperature but also can result in kidney, liver, and/or cardiovascular system failure and even death. Ecstasy has several street names, including *XTC, Adam, M&M, E, MDEA (Eve), MDA love drug, MBDB, hug,* and *beans.*

GHB

GHB was developed in 1961 when French biochemist Henri Laborit synthesized it for use as an anesthetic. It was quickly discovered that GHB had little use as an anesthetic, as patients given the drug often experienced seizures. Through the 1980s, bodybuilders were exposed to the drug because of its ability to build muscle mass and to produce rapid weight gain. GHB was sold legally in most health food stores until 1990 when the Food and Drug Administration (FDA) discovered the harmful side effects. In response to several deaths linked to the effects of GHB, the drug was labeled as a controlled substance in 2000, making it a crime to possess in the United States.

GHB is a central nervous system (CNS) depressant that tends to be abused for its euphoric, sedative, and anabolic (bodybuilding) effects. When combined with alcohol or other drugs, other effects such as nausea, dizziness, loss of muscle control, loss of consciousness, amnesia, and death can also occur. Withdrawal from GHB can result in tremors, anxiety, insomnia, and sweating. GHB has also been associated with poisonings, overdoses, rapes, and deaths. Common street names for the drug are *liquid ecstasy, soap, easy lay, Vita-G, goob,* and *Georgia home boy.*

Ketamine

In 1956, Parke-Davis, a pharmaceutical company, attempted to find an effective anesthetic that would dull pain and put patients to sleep. The drug they found was termed phencyclidine (PCP). Although originally thought to be a miracle drug, the hallucinogenic effects of PCP became evident quickly. Patients lost touch with their environments and often had violent fits of rage. The Parke-Davis company continued to search for a drug that had the anesthetic effects of PCP without the delirious and delusional side effects. In 1962, ketamine-hydrochloride (labeled as CI-1581) was developed. Ketamine was so unique in its effects that new terminology had to be created to describe what was being witnessed in experimentation. Patients given ketamine were completely disconnected from their surroundings. Although their eyes were open, the patients were in an anesthetic (sedated) and analgesic (pain-free) state said to be like that of zombies.

Although ketamine had hallucinogenic effects, it was approved by the FDA in 1966 and 1970 to be used as an anesthetic in low doses under the names Ketalar and Ketaject. By the 1970s, the underground drug culture was well aware of ketamine's hallucinogenic effects, and it was illegally made available in pill, powder, and liquid forms. Due to a rising increase in ketamine abuse, most physicians stopped prescribing the drug. In 1999, ketamine was labeled as a federally controlled substance. Although some physicians and veterinarians still use forms of ketamine, it is used only in rare circumstances and under strict supervision.

Ketamine abuse is primarily due to the hallucinogenic properties of the drug. It can be taken orally, by injection, or through snorting. In addition to hallucination, the effects of ketamine include vertigo, slurred speech, slow reaction and response time, and euphoria. In higher doses, ketamine can produce amnesia and coma. Some of the street names for ketamine are *Special K, Vitamin K, Lady K,* and *Super K.*

Methamphetamine (Meth)

In 1919, a more potent form of amphetamine was developed in Japan and labeled as methamphetamine (meth). During World War II, meth was used by both Americans and the Japanese to keep soldiers alert and motivated. However, by 1970, the abuse of meth was climbing. As a result of the Controlled Substances Act, there was a temporary decline in the illegal consumption of meth. Although the abuse of meth is widely publicized in the news, the use by young people is actually low compared to other illicit drugs and has been decreasing since 2000.

Because many of the ingredients used to manufacture meth can be found in stores, it can be produced by nearly anyone with the motivation to do so. This ability has resulted in wide availability of the drug. Meth labs are dangerous not only to the "cook" (manufacturer) but also to the surrounding community and to anyone who discovers the lab.

The short-term effects of meth include alertness, euphoria, psychomotor stimulation, and elevation of mood. Long-term effects of the drug can include anxiety, insomnia, irregular heartbeat, and an increase in blood pressure. Strokes and heart attacks can occur. Following long-term abuse, meth users can experience paranoia, other psychotic behavior, and violent episodes. Chronic meth abusers may experience "crank bugs," or the feeling of bugs crawling under their skin. Withdrawal symptoms include fatigue, depression, aggression, and an intense addictive craving for the drug. Some common street names for the drug are *crank*, *speed*, *ice*, *chalk*, and *meth*.

LSD

LSD was first synthesized in Switzerland in 1938 by Albert Hoffman of Sandoz Laboratories. The drug was initially brought onto the American market as a legal psychiatric cure-all, primarily researched to aid in schizophrenia. However, the results of LSD proved to be less medically effective than originally thought, for it tended to bring about schizophrenic tendencies rather than to cure them. In the 1960s and 1970s, LSD became popular in the underground drug culture for its psychotropic hallucinogenic quality. Unlike other drugs, LSD primarily is available in a blotter paper form which is dipped in the LSD chemical formula.

The effects of LSD are often related to the mood of the user. Visual, auditory, and tactile sensations may be enhanced or distorted. These effects may be disconcerting for some users, precipitating a panic attack. In addition, emotional fragile or unstable users may experience a significant escalation of negative emotional states. The negative effects from using LSD are referred to as a bad trip. Some users of LSD have experienced a reoccurrence of the effect of the drug long after using it. These events are called flashbacks. The unpredictability of a flashback has resulted in panic in those who experience them. Some common street names of the drug are *acid*, *trips*, *blotters*, *microdots*, *tabs*, *doses*, *hits*, and *sugar cubes*.

Rohypnol

Although illegal in the United States, Rohypnol (flunitrazepam) is manufactured legally by the Swiss drug maker Hoffman-LaRoche. The drug was introduced in 1975 as a treatment for insomnia. Rohypnol is in a classification of drugs referred to as benzodiazepines, which are considered depressants or tranquilizers, signifying that they slow brain and body functions. It was declared a controlled substance by the Drug Enforcement Administration (DEA) in 1983. By 1992, Rohypnol was a common club drug often found at parties on U.S. college campuses.

Rohypnol is odorless and tasteless, which has been known to be a contributing factor to the drug's active role in date-rapes, as it can be added to a person's drink without his or her awareness of any change in taste or scent. The drug can incapacitate people rendering them victims to their environment. It can also cause anterograde amnesia, which is a type of memory loss where the person who took the drug may not remember events that had occurred while under the influence of the drug. When mixed with alcohol and/or other drugs, Rohypnol can also cause death. Rohypnol is commonly referred to as *forget-me pill*, *roofies*, *rophies*, *ruffies*, *roach*, and *rope*.

Schedule of Controlled Substances

In 1970, Congress passed the U.S. Controlled Substances Act, which designates five schedules under which all illicit drugs are classified. MDMA, LSD, and GHB are categorized as Schedule I drugs that are characterized as having a high potential for abuse and that currently have no medical use in the United States. The DEA has recommended that Rohypnol be classified as a Schedule I drug. Amphetamines and methamphetamine are categorized as Schedule II, which means they also have a high potential for abuse but are accepted for medical use with severe restrictions. Ketamine is a Schedule III drug. Obviously, these placements imply that these drugs have lower abuse potential and more accepted medical uses. Although the schedule of controlled substances is outdated and has been criticized, it does characterize the level to which drugs can be harmful for health reasons and also outlines the levels to which the possession or trafficking of these drugs can be punishable by law.

Conclusion

The label *club drugs* refers to a classification of illicit substances used primarily by young people and associated with clubs or raves. However, some of the drugs considered to be club drugs are also used and abused by other demographic groups and in other settings. Although the use of these drugs has decreased in recent years, there continues to be a subculture attracted to these substances. Some club drugs have dangerous short-term effects and some have significant abuse potential. Clearly, as with all illicit substances, there is a danger of harmful effects from adulterants used in the manufacture of these drugs. Although the decreased use of club drugs can be viewed as a positive development, the history of the use of illicit drugs by young people provides ample lessons in the danger of complacency with regard to club drugs.

Melissa M. Irniger, Sabina Mutisya,
and Thomas Harrison

See also Amphetamines; Central Nervous System Depressants; Ecstasy; Illicit and Illegal Drugs; Methamphetamine

Further Readings

Britt, G. C., & McCance-Katz, E. F. (2005). A brief overview of the clinical pharmacology of "club drugs." *Substance Use & Abuse, 40,* 1189–1201.

Freese, T. E., Miotto, K., & Reback, C. J. (2002). The effects and consequences of selected club drugs. *Journal of Substance Abuse and Treatment, 23,* 151–156.

Marcovitz, H. (2006). *Drug education library: Club drugs.* Stockton, NJ: OTTN.

Maxwell, J. C. (2005). Party drugs: Properties, prevalence, patterns, and problems. *Substance Use & Misuse, 40,* 1203–1240.

National Drug Intelligence Center. (2005). *National drug threat assessment.* Johnstown, PA: National Drug Intelligence Center.

National Institute on Drug Abuse, club drugs: http://www.clubdrugs.gov

National Institute on Drug Abuse, National Institute of Health. (2006). Retrieved February 22, 2007, from http://www.nida.nih.gov/Infofacts/clubdrugs.html

Office of National Drug Control Policy. (2007). Retrieved April 9, 2007, from http://www.whitehousedrugpolicy.gov/drugfact/club/index.html

COALCOHOLIC

See CODEPENDENCY

COCAINE AND CRACK

Cocaine and crack represent major drugs of abuse (about 6.4 million regular users in North America and 4 million in Europe) due to the rapid production of euphoria following administration. Cocaine is probably the oldest known peripheral nerve conduction blocker. It serves as local painkiller by blocking the inward flux of sodium ions during depolarization and is still used in eye, nose, throat, dental, and ear surgery. Cocaine abuse causes many health problems, is very damaging to heart cells, and, depending upon route of administration, has high addiction potential. Cocaine hydrochloride (named by Dr. Albert Neimann in 1860) is a major psychomotor stimulant drug. It is also called benzoylmethylecgoninen, an ester of the tropane alkaloid.

Crack is of a form of cocaine named because of the distinctive sound made as the crystals are heated. Large quantities of cocaine hydrochloride are needed to produce a freebase "rock." Usually an ammonia or sodium bicarbonate base is heated with cocaine to remove the hydrochloride salt leaving base that is about 50% cocaine and is nonwater soluble. Crack is not just purified cocaine as many users believe. Crack rocks are sold in small quantities making crack more affordable than cocaine hydrochloride. Crack is usually smoked with a small glass pipe that can be filled with rum instead of water. Because much of the cocaine is lost through condensation and escapes as smoke, only about 5% of vaporized cocaine is absorbed in the user. When users inhales the vapor, they can experience euphoria in seconds. However, this euphoria fades rapidly over a minute and terminates in about 10 minutes. Crack also produces a greater craving for redosing than cocaine hydrocholoride administered intravenously does.

Cocaine is a natural plant chemical synthesized by many of the genus *Erythroxylum* species, a common looking shrub. The five major cocaine-producing plant species are *laetevirens* (among the newest discovered and the highest cocaine-producing variant); *coca* variety *coca* (grown mainly in Bolivia), *coca* variety *ipadu* (grown mainly in the Amazon Basin), *novogranatense* variety *novogranatense* (grown in Colombia and now accounts for about 85% of all illicit global cocaine grown), and *novogranatense* variety *truillense* (grown in the Western Andes; the common name is Trujillo, and this is the plant the Incas called Royal Coca). Originally, these cocaine-producing plants, which normally grow about a meter tall, were indigenous in South America's moist mountainous regions with the highest amount found in locations corresponding to Bolivia and Peru. Historically, the word *coca* derives from the pre-Incan Tiwanaku tribe word for plant or tree used by peoples that live in the Peruvian Andes and is not related to the cocoa nut.

Today, more cocaine is grown in Colombia than any other country. According to a 2007 World Drug Report, in 2006 an estimated 610 metric tons were produced in Colombia compared to a total South American production of 984 metric tons. In 2005, estimated cocaine sales worldwide exceeded $71 billion while the total global sales of illicit drugs were about $320 billion to $400 billion. Given that profit margin on illicit cocaine is about 300%, drop in cocaine production is unlikely anytime soon.

Administration and Adverse Effects

People first used cocaine by placing waded leaves in between their cheeks and gums; they believed the coca plant to be a gift from the Gods. Leaf use allowed field workers to suppress hunger and increased stamina. The leaves are actually nutritious (in daily vitamins, calcium, iron, and phosphorus) and are also used to treat altitude sickness. In 3,000 BC, the leaves of the coca shrub were found to be psychoactive when storing them in the mouth (for hours with chalk, lime, or wood ash to raise mouth pH and hence liberate more coca alkaloid) as a quid (not by chewing); this action turned saliva green. Natives would move the quid around in the mouth to liberate more fluid to reduce hunger and increase stamina. The leaf also held spiritual importance; in the Inca civilization, dead were buried with a coca leaf pouch.

Today, the most common routes of cocaine administration are by nasal insufflation (or snorting)—the effect peaks in 10 to 20 minutes and diminishes in 40 to 90 minutes—or by intravenous injection (IV). IV administration results in the second quickest (15 seconds) route for cocaine to travel from the blood and penetrate into the brain. Following the act of snorting cocaine (euphoria is delayed for around 3 minutes, a rather slow onset compared to smoking or IV), it is also common for a user to wipe up any remaining crystals with a finger and wipe them onto the gums. This habit does not add measurably to the effects following snorted cocaine, but it does add to the unique experience as the gums feel numb. The numbness is due to cocaine's powerful local anesthetics (by interfering with sodium channels and hence blocking nerve conduction) as well as efficient constriction of blood vessels. Oral cocaine absorption can also result in the user becoming more likely to bite the inner cheeks, lips, and tongue without feeling the damage and in an increase in dental cavities and gum disease.

Other adverse behavioral effects of cocaine include increased irritability, insomnia, psychosis, hallucinations (e.g., an odd feeling of bugs crawling under the skin called parasitosis), anhedonia (the inability to experience natural pleasures), depression and/or suicide, paranoia, sexual dysfunction, memory loss, and violent behaviors.

Cocaine is lipophillic and freely crosses the blood-brain barrier; white matter brain neurons are covered (insulated) with a double lipid (fat) layer called myelin (it is about 80% fat). Another route for cocaine injection is skin popping (injecting between the surface skin and fat layer causing skin to balloon). Skin popping cocaine is rare, as it causes significant tissue death and promotes infection at the injection site due to multiple contaminates.

Smoking cocaine hydrochloride is not common and wasteful, as the temperature needed to vaporize the salt decomposes the cocaine. Smoking is the preferred route for crack since crack does not dissolve in water, but it does vaporize without destruction. Cocaine vapors absorbed directly into the bloodstream following lung inhalation penetrate into the brain in 7 seconds and produces euphoria (described as a whole-body orgasm) intense enough to drop a first-time user to his or her knees (referred to as a cherry high). The quicker the onset of action and penetration into the brain by a given drug of abuse, the more intense the subjective feeling of euphoria (brain reward) as reported by users.

Cocaine Mechanism of Action

Other euphoria-causing drugs include opioids (oxycodone, hydromorphone, fentanly, and heroin) and high purity, smokable methanphetamine (called *ice* or *glass*). But cocaine is used as half of the most preferred two drug combination (in conjunction with heroin) called a speed ball. Speed ball use is alluring because of the synergism of cocaine and opioid euphoria producing brain process and a concurrent functional antagonism of both hyperactivity (produced by cocaine) and depression (leading to opioid-induced stupor or sleep). Thus, the user is kept awake, but not overstimulated. Cocaine's effects can also be enhanced by either pre- or simultaneous-administration of either caffeine or nicotine, as both compounds enhance brain dopamine release. Even in nonsmokers, co-use of crack and nicotine results in chain smoking. When used with alcohol, the liver synthesizes a third psychoactive substance called cocaethylene, which can be detected in urine and blood in about 100 minutes. Cocaethylene lasts considerably longer than cocaine (2.5 hours) is slightly more toxic and produces euphoria similar to cocaine. The cardiac toxicity of cocaine involves a combination of four mechanisms. The psychomotor stimulant effects upon cardiac toxicity are primarily mediated by the blockade of norepinephrine (NE) uptake. Due to enhanced NE levels, cocaine produces increased sympathetic arousal (via beta-adrenergic receptors) and heightened awareness. Prolonged reuptake of NE constricts blood vessels in the heart, and cocaine has a direct effect on calcium release leading to destructive contraction of muscle and produces increased myocardial oxygen demand. Another mechanism contributing to cardio toxicity is cocaine's ability to block sodium channels in motor neurons supplying the heart. And last, cocaine increases platelet stickiness and thrombosis (formation of a blood clot, usually in an artery, which blocks blood flow resulting in ischemia and cell death), resulting in some degree of cardiac cell necrosis.

Once cocaine is in the bloodstream, about 50% is deactivated by hepatic esterases and plasma pseudocholinesterase enzymes and about another 40% is nonenzymatically hydrolyzed. However, the dose of cocaine usually taken to achieve euphoria greatly exceeds the capacity of these enzymes to deactivate a significant amount of cocaine prior to its penetration into brain and heart tissues. About 5% of cocaine is eliminated via the kidney unchanged. Due to a huge number of variables, the average lethal dose of cocaine varies widely among individuals.

Cocaine-Induced Causes of Death

There are many different ways that cocaine may cause death. For example, during binge use, large amounts of cocaine reach the brain, overloading the neurochemistry and triggering neural toxicity, a cascade of reactions involving intracellular calcium and excitatory amino acids (glutamate). Brain hemorrhaging may occur because a major effect of cocaine is to produce a sudden and dramatic increase in blood pressure. If a vessel is weak, a cerebral aneurysm can burst resulting in internal bleeding. Deadly fevers can occur when cocaine users (bicyclists, football players, basketball players, or runners) combine physical exertion with cocaine intake. Cocaine is a sympathomimetic

and increases body temperature to life threatening levels (108–110 degrees Fahrenheit). In addition, spontaneous epileptic seizures can occur as a result of cocaine use. Furthermore, cocaine decreases coronary blood flow, and a person with a marginal blood supply to the heart is in danger of myocardial infarction.

Cocaine deaths also occur as a result of homicide, suicide, and accidents. Cocaine intensifies paranoid thought processes, resulting in impaired judgment. Much of cocaine growing, processing, transporting, and selling is illegal; criminal elements protect their interest with deadly force. When cocaine is not available, users fall below the normal range of mood and can experience depression. The depression can be so severe that suicide is the result. Finally, cocaine produces a sense of power and omnipotence. Irritability and exertion can increase reckless driving and other risk-taking behaviors.

Death from acute cocaine toxicity is a rare event unless massive dose exposure occurs. To transport cocaine, persons (or animals) are often made to swallow cocaine wrapped in protective materials (condoms or finger cots; or inserts rectally or vaginally called body packing). If the packaging ruptures or develops a hole, a massive absorption of cocaine leads to convulsions and death.

Pharmacological Treatment for Cocaine Addiction

Unfortunately, there is no effective antidote to reverse cocaine-induced adverse and overdose effects. In addition, there also are exceedingly few effective drug treatments to reduce cocaine craving. It appears that ongoing cocaine addiction in the United States will continue as 301 million Americans represent only a small fraction of the global population of 6.7 billion; however, even though less than 3% of Americans use, they consume around 50% of the global cocaine supply.

Few drugs suitable for use as anticocaine medications have been identified. They include disulfiram (a dopaminergic), tiagabine and topiramate (GABA NT enhancers), modafinil (a dopamine uptake blocker). In clinical trials are two types of cocaine "vaccines" that slow entry of cocaine into the brain by increasing plasma levels of pseudocholinesterase or selectively attach to cocaine rendering it unable to penetrate the blood–brain barrier.

Daniel J. Calcagnetti

See also Brain Chemistry and Addiction; Central Nervous
System Stimulants; Drugs, Classification of;
Neurobiology of Addiction; Neurotransmitters;
Pharmacological Approaches to Treatment; Physiological
Aspects of Drug Use

Further Readings

Burnett, L. B., & Adler, J. (2006). *Toxicity, cocaine.*
Retrieved September 9, 2007, from http://www.emedicine
.com/med/topic400.htm

Claustre, A., Bresch-Rieu, I., & Fouilhé, N (1993). *Cocaine.*
Retrieved September 9, 2007, from http://www.inchem
.org/documents/pims/pharm/pim139e.htm

Coca Museum: http://cocamuseum.com/main.htm

Karch, S. B. (1999). Cocaine: History, use, abuse. *Journal of
the Royal Society of Medicine, 92,* 393–397. Retrieved
September 9, 2007, from http://www.pubmedcentral.nih
.gov/articlerender.fcgi?artid=1297313

National Highway Traffic Safety Administration. (n.d.).
Drugs and human performance sheets. Retrieved
September 9, 2007, from http://www.nhtsa.dot.gov/
PEOPLE/injury/research/job185drugs/cocain.htm

Stewart, C. (2003). *Cocaine.* Retrieved September 9, 2007,
from http://www.storysmith.net/Articles/Cocaine%201.pdf

UN Office on Drugs and Crime. (2007). *Coca/cocaine
market: Summary trend overview.* Retrieved September 9,
2007, from http://www.unodc.org/pdf/research/wdr07/
WDR_2007_1.3_coca_cocaine.pdf

Wells, S. A. (2000). *American drugs in Egyptian mummies:
A review of the evidence.* Retrieved September 9, 2007,
from http://www.colostate.edu/Dept/Entomology/
courses/en570/papers_2000/wells.html

Cocaine Anonymous

Cocaine Anonymous (CA), created in 1982, is a
Twelve-Step recovery program that was developed in
line with the philosophy of Alcoholics Anonymous
(AA) to treat cocaine addiction. Support groups such
as AA, which follow the Twelve-Step recovery
method, are among the most commonly recommended treatments for alcohol and drug disorders in
the United States. AA, which was created in 1935,
rapidly grew in popularity and consequently, various
other groups were formed including CA, Narcotics
Anonymous, and Methampethamine Anonymous.
Group therapy is one of the primary approaches to

treating alcohol and drug addictions; overall,
Twelve-Step programs such as CA have been associated with positive treatment outcomes. Research has
further shown that active participation in CA facilitates abstinence from cocaine. The National Institute
on Drug Abuse (NIDA) recommends using individual drug counseling in conjunction with group drug
counseling (which stresses involvement in Twelve-
Step programs such as CA) for the treatment of
cocaine dependence. Moreover, the Matrix Model,
an empirically supported treatment for stimulants
such as cocaine, encourages Twelve-Step program
involvement as one of the model's specific strategies
for treatment.

CA groups are now being held regularly throughout
the United States and Europe, and group materials and
literature are available in several different languages.
Membership in CA is free as expenses are paid by voluntary contributions by members. The CA program of
recovery stresses abstinence—not reduction—from all
mind-altering substances. CA is not affiliated with any
organization or institution, does not participate formally in drug addiction research, nor does it provide
medical or psychiatric services as a group, though
members may choose to participate in research or seek
alternative treatments on their own. The dynamic of
each group is comprised of two components: one being
the program itself (i.e., the Twelve-Step philosophy)
and the other being the fellowship-social organization
of the group. The fellowship aspect can vary greatly
depending on the people who comprise the individual
group. For example, the style of the group can vary
(e.g., supportive versus confrontational), and furthermore, groups are available that cater to specific religions as well as sexual orientations.

Several research studies have examined various
patient variables that may predict treatment outcome
for cocaine dependence. Data from the NIDA-funded
Collaborative Cocaine Treatment Study (NCCTS), a
controlled, randomized, multisite project comparing
different forms of psychotherapy and drug counseling
among 487 cocaine-dependant individuals, revealed
that the degree of endorsement of the Twelve-Step
philosophy and willingness to follow the Twelve-Step
recommendations was associated with attendance and
participation in meetings, as well as treatment outcome. Moreover, a belief in the Twelve-Step philosophy was found to be a significant predictor of
sustained abstinence. NCCTS data also shows that
active participation in the CA program (e.g., speaking

at meetings, working on one or more of the Twelve Steps, speaking to a sponsor, and performing meeting duties such as making coffee) as opposed to just meeting attendance, predicted decreased drug use among cocaine-dependent individuals. Those who participated consistently during CA meetings reported fewer days of cocaine use compared to those who participated in meetings inconsistently. Furthermore, those individuals who increased their participation in CA over time had better outcomes compared to those who had high levels of participation in the first half of treatment and gradually decreased over time, as well as those who had low levels of participation overall. NCCTS data also demonstrated that patterns of attendance and participation remained relatively the same over the course of the study, suggesting that a treatment approach that encourages early involvement in CA may be extremely beneficial to treatment outcome. The pilot data from the NCCTS study showed that those who attended Twelve-Step groups were significantly more likely to be abstinent from cocaine during the following month than those who did not attend groups. When varying degrees of participation were measured, it was found that the specific type of participation at meetings (e.g., speaking at meetings, actively working on steps, meeting with members or a sponsor, setting up for meetings) and the degree of participation (e.g., number of days active participation occurred) were not associated with treatment outcome, suggesting that any form of active participation in Twelve-Step meetings is helpful.

Much of the current research suggests that a combination of individual drug counseling and group therapy, including Twelve-Step programs, can yield the best treatment outcomes for cocaine-dependant patients. Research findings, including those from the NCCTS data, suggest that there is an additive effect for individual drug treatment and support group attendance and participation so that patients who utilized individual drug treatment in addition to Twelve-Step groups had higher rates of abstinence than those who participated in only one avenue of treatment. Patients can become involved in CA as part of their individual treatment and can continue their involvement as part of their aftercare. Moreover, Twelve-Step programs offer a no-cost treatment option to maintain abstinence and reduce the possibility of a relapse after individualized treatment has ended.

Many current treatment strategies facilitate and encourage attendance and participation in Twelve-Step groups. The Group Drug Counseling (GDC), approach a manualized psychosocial treatment used in the NCCTS study, maintains that cocaine addiction is a complex biopsychosocial disease that is influenced by many biological, psychological, sociocultural, and spiritual factors. The GDC manual strongly encourages attendance and active participation in Twelve-Step programs such as AA and CA, emphasizing the importance of Twelve-Step groups. The NCCTS data showed that individual drug counseling coupled with GDC yielded the best results for decreased cocaine use and increased abstinence rates among cocaine-dependant participants. In addition to GDC, the Matrix Model incorporates aspects from several different treatment strategies including Twelve-Step program involvement. It is thought that formal, individualized drug counseling can increase a patient's engagement and commitment to the treatment process, thus resulting in longer attendance and greater participation in meetings, which in turn improves treatment outcomes.

Constructed social networks have been shown to decrease relapse rates in substance abusing populations. AA and related programs (e.g., CA) are among the most salient examples of constructed social networks. These programs are easily accessible support networks that satisfy several of the required elements of a behavioral choice model of relapse prevention. Twelve-Step programs provide alternative activities to drinking and/or substance use, constrain access to substances by attending meetings instead of being somewhere else, and reinforce sober behavior by providing an instant social support network of other sober individuals. Research examining changes in treatment outcomes and social networks shows that involvement in Twelve-Step programs helps to decrease substance use, which may be due to the presence of a social network that discourages substance use as well as the replacement of a substance-using network with a sobriety-reinforcing network.

Although many studies examining the effectiveness of AA, and more recently CA, yield promising results for the treatment and prevention of relapse for cocaine addictions, research shows that long-term attendance in Twelve-Step programs and active participation could be improved. Low rates of attendance are consistently found during and after treatment, despite efforts to encourage attendance and participation in Twelve-Step meetings given through group or individual therapy. In spite of these barriers, research indicates that active participation and regular attendance in conjunction with individual drug counseling significantly increases abstinence from cocaine use among cocaine-dependent individuals.

Meggan M. Bucossi, Katherine W. Follansbee,
and Gregory L. Stuart

See also Alcoholics Anonymous; Cocaine and Crack; Narcotics Anonymous; Twelve-Step Facilitation; Twelve-Step Recovery Programs; Twelve Steps

Further Readings

Cocaine Anonymous World Services. (n.d.). *About C.A.* Retrieved September 7, 2007, from http://www.ca.org

Crits-Christoph, P., Gibbons, M. B. C., Barber, J. P., Hu, B., Hearon, B., Worley, M., et al. (2007). Predictors of sustained abstinence during psychosocial treatments for cocaine dependence. *Psychotherapy Research, 17,* 240–252.

National Institute on Drug Abuse. (n.d.) *Drug counseling for cocaine addiction.* Retrieved September 7, 2007, from http://www.nida.nih.gov

Weiss, R. D., Griffin, M. L., Gallop, R. J., Najavits, L. M., Frank, A., Crits-Christoph, P., et al. (2005). The effect of 12-step self-help group attendance and participation on drug use outcomes among cocaine-dependent patients. *Drug and Alcohol Dependence, 77,* 177–184.

Weiss, R. D., Griffin, M. L., Gallop, R., Onken, L. S., Gastfriend, D. R., Daley, D., et al. (2000). Self-help group attendance and participation among cocaine dependent patients. *Drug and Alcohol Dependence, 60,* 169–177.

Weiss, R. D., Griffin, M. L., Najavits, L. M., Hufford, C., Kogan, J., Thompson, H. J., et al. (1996). Self-help activities in cocaine dependent patients entering treatment: Results from the NIDA collaborative cocaine treatment study. *Drug and Alcohol Dependence, 43,* 79–86.

CODEPENDENCY

Codependency can be defined as a pattern of dysfunctional behaviors between an addict-alcoholic and another important adult in his or her life such as a spouse, parent, sibling, or friend. The codependent is the nonaddicted person in the relationship who acts almost as if addicted to and obsessed with the behaviors of the addict-alcoholic.

Sharon Wegscheider-Cruse has described the codependent as one who becomes emotionally and socially dependent on the addicted partner. The codependent becomes more and more involved with trying to control the actions of the other while giving up more and more of his or her needs, desires, or personal behaviors. The codependent submits to the continued goal of trying to observe and influence the actions of the addict-alcoholic. Some, such as Terry Gorski, even use the term to describe any person who displays such controlling, dysfunctional behavior in any close relationship, whether an addiction is involved or not. Nonaddicts may have other mental health issues, out-of-control emotions, or compulsive behaviors like eating or working excessively.

Harold Doweiko points out what he believes are the four common elements to all codependency definitions. There is an over-involvement with the problematic loved one, the codependent is obsessed with controlling the problem person, the codependent sees him- or herself as worthless and tied to the approval of the partner, and the codependent makes extreme personal sacrifices to fix or change the behaviors of the other in the relationship.

Further Characteristics

Timmen Cermak has added other aspects to the descriptions of codependency. He states that it involves an enmeshment with the emotions of others with a poor ability to feel the boundary between oneself and another. The codependent often denies that he or she is displaying behaviors that are clear to everyone else. He or she must be involved in the dysfunctional relationship for at least 2 years without seeking help. Codependents often suffer their own substance abuse disorder of some kind. He believes that the symptoms of codependency substantially match those of post-traumatic stress disorder. Similarities would include symptoms such as emotional numbing, hypervigilance, depressive symptoms, and behaviors where the person freezes up when faced with stress.

Like the alcoholic or addict, the life of the codependent becomes unmanageable. The person feels out-of-control in the constant attempts to affect the behavior of the other. For example, a codependent might be the spouse who constantly searches the house for hidden bottles, marijuana stashes, or other signs of drinking or drugging. It may be the parent who constantly checks up on the adult child by calling at work or by getting others to cut the child breaks if he or she misses work or behaves poorly there.

Melody Beattie has proposed certain unexpressed rules through which the codependent seems to lead life. These rules include thinking things such as "My feelings don't count," "I can't have fun," "I am not loveable or good enough as I am," and "If the addict-alcoholic creates trouble, I am to blame because I should have stopped it somehow." In these rules, one can see the dysfunctional and self-destructive beliefs of the codependent who exists with constant self-denial, low self-worth, and self-blame. The failure of the codependent to change the behavior of the alcoholic-addict only serves to prove that he or she is indeed incompetent, worthless, and a bad spouse, parent, friend, or sibling and deserves low self-esteem. These beliefs then become a self-fulfilling cycle of action and failure leading to lower and lower self-worth resulting in new attempts at action, which lead to more failure, and the downward cycle continues.

The codependent has such low self-esteem that he or she can only feel value in trying the hopeless task of caring for the alcoholic-addict. The codependent may also wrap his or her identity in the noble role of the suffering victim. The addict-alcoholic is happy to reinforce the beliefs of the codependent by regularly blaming the codependent for his drinking or drugging: "If only you weren't such a nag, I wouldn't drink," or "If you made more money, I wouldn't have to relieve my stresses by getting high." The alcoholic-addict may also attack the self-esteem of the codependent by threatening to leave or abandon the individual if his or her behaviors are not perfect or good enough. The codependent may then restrict behavior even more so as not to bother the user and risk abandonment or separation.

Most experts view codependency as a behavior learned in the family of origin. The individual grows up in a dysfunctional family where the relationships are usually poor, criticizing, blaming, and hurtful. The developing child may be dismissed, branded a failure, ignored, criticized, or otherwise taught that he or she is worthless and unlovable. The child gets the message that his or her value can come from only the unpredictable approval of the powerful and harsh parent. The child may also learn that the only way to get approval or love is to please or care for the dysfunctional parent.

The growing child then takes these beliefs about self and others into adult life and manages to connect with relationships that recapitulate this early and harmful family environment. It is all the person knows about relationships, and there is a tendency to repeat what is known. Ironically, the codependent is desperate for healthier, more affirming relationships but does not know how to find them or even know what they look like. They unconsciously connect with people who fit the familiar, if negative, pattern.

The Recovery Process

Most authors on this topic compare the disease of codependence with the disease of alcoholism and other addictions. Some describe it as an addiction to a process as opposed to a substance. As such, much of the literature on recovering from codependency follows the recommendations for recovery from addiction, including a reliance on support groups and the Twelve-Step model. Al-Anon groups often help members work on issues around codependency. A support group called Co-Dependents Anonymous uses the Twelve Steps of Alcoholics Anonymous adapted for the particular problems of its members. Adult Children of Alcoholics is another support group with a national availability that has been founded to help people who have grown up in addicted households and may have codependent issues as well as other needs for support and guidance.

Cermak has proposed a four-stage model of recovery from codependency. The first stage is called survival-denial, when the person's life and relationships feel unmanageable but somehow normal, and there is a sad pride in being able to cope.

The second stage is reidentification, when the individual begins to see him or herself more clearly as a codependent and surrenders to the powerlessness over others. Cermak calls the third stage reintegration, when the codependent begins to be more realistic about life and its problems while discovering a healthier self-efficacy. The final stage is genesis, when the person puts newfound insights and skills into practice as he or she starts a new beginning in life.

The new skills that must be learned by the codependent include learning to detach from the addicted partner while still loving the person. One must learn healthier problem-solving skills and learn to express legitimate feelings in appropriate ways. The codependent learns to recognize and value his or her needs and values while discovering it is acceptable to pursue them. The codependent realizes that selfishness is not the same as self-care, self-efficacy, and self-valuing.

Criticisms of the Concept

The concept of codependency has its critics. They say that the idea relegates a person to a constant state of helplessness, which is then described as a progressive disease just like that of alcoholism or drug addiction. Critics decry the fact that there is no cure expected, but that people can only manage the disease through a one-size-fits-all membership in a support group based on the Alcoholics Anonymous model. This model does not allow for individual differences in a child's development or in the early family structures. It does not allow for the fact that people may change or grow through other means and are not necessarily doomed to repeat dysfunctional family patterns. Many people do show a certain resiliency in coping with past family problems and do develop healthy lives.

Critics also state that the codependency concept lumps all alcoholics and addicts families together and fails to account for different levels of substance abuse and other idiosyncratic family behaviors. A violent alcoholic father would certainly have a different impact on a developing child than one who came home from work, drank, and then fell peacefully asleep watching television every night.

The concept is also described as relieving people of their personal responsibility in the conduct of their relationships. If one has a disease of codependency, then one may be helpless under the influences of the disease. Some have defined codependency so broadly that it could include any relationship where someone remains despite any weaknesses or dysfunctional behaviors by the partner. This description could mean staying with someone despite poor communications, emotional distancing, or inability to hold a job.

The symptoms of codependency also substantially overlap the traits of mental health disorders called dependent personality disorder and avoidant personality disorder. These symptoms are described in the *Diagnostic and Statistical Manual of Mental Disorders, Fourth Edition, Text Revision* of the American Psychiatric Association. Symptoms of the avoidant personality include but are not limited to excessive fear of criticism or disapproval, restraint in intimate relations out of fear of being criticized, inhibitions in relationships because of feelings of personal inadequacy, and seeing the self as inept and as less valuable than others. Symptoms of the dependent personality include but are not limited to an inability to make decisions without the assurance of another,

excessive attempts at getting nurturance from a relationship even if it involves doing unpleasant things, feelings that one cannot care for oneself, and being obsessed with a fear of being alone. Many feel that these diagnostic categories sufficiently account for those traits described in codependency and therefore, the field does not need another classification category.

Others criticize the concept on feminist grounds. It pathologizes typically feminine traits of nurturance, support, and relationship building, especially in someone who is just trying to survive or cope with someone else's problem. The concept of codependency has been described as one that has emerged or evolved from the experience of people who are involved in addicted or dysfunctional families and from their struggles with its negative consequences on the self. This is also a criticism of the concept in that it is not one that has developed from a more professional or objective framework by outside observers. There is always the danger that investigations and writings on the concept are colored by the experiences and biases of those who suffer from the concept of codependency. Some studies have shown no difference in negative traits between self-identified adult children of alcoholics and those who are not.

Conclusion

The concept of codependency does not yet have a single definition in the addictions field. Some have defined it so broadly as to include almost any relationship with unhealthy interactions. Most see it as a relationship issue where one partner is trying to cope with the behaviors of an addicted partner by giving up the self, over controlling the other, and over-identifying oneself with the problems and behaviors of the addict-alcoholic. All seem to agree that the traits of the codependent are learned while growing up in an addicted or dysfunctional family.

Interventions center on the use of support groups, most of which are adapted from the structures of Alcoholics Anonymous. Many professionals outside the field of addictions criticize the concept as being too broad, antifemale, sufficiently described in other diagnostic categories, or limiting on the individual.

David Borsos

See also Al-Anon; Alateen; Children of Alcoholics; Enabling; Family Therapy

Further Readings

Beattie, M. (1989). *Beyond codependency and getting better all the time.* New York: Harper & Row.

Cermak, T. (1986). *Diagnosing and treating codependency.* Minneapolis, MN: Johnson Institute.

Gorski, T. T. (1992). Diagnosing codependence. *Addiction and Recovery, 12,* 14–16.

Wegscheider-Cruse, S., & Cruse, J. R. (1990). *Understanding co-dependency.* Pompano Beach, FL: Health Communications.

Coercion and Treatment

Studies have shown that there is a strong association between drug use and crime. Drug use is directly related to crime in that it is a crime to use, possess, and manufacture illegal drugs. Drugs are also related to crime through the effects they have on the user's behavior (such as committing violent offenses or by committing offenses to get money to support their continued use). Even though treatment is seen as the most effective way of breaking the cycle between drug use and crime, many individuals with drug problems do not receive treatment. The National Survey on Drug Use and Health estimated that in 2006, 21.1 million people ages 12 or older needed but did not receive treatment for an illicit drug or alcohol problem. Some of the reasons why people did not receive treatment were (a) they encountered barriers related to cost, (b) they did not think they had a problem, and (c) they were not ready to stop using. The consequences of an untreated substance use problem can lead to significant costs to society. These include costs associated with drug-related crimes, prison expenses, court and criminal costs, emergency room visits, reduced productivity, and unemployment. In fact, a report released by the Office of National Drug Control Policy estimated that the costs associated with drug abuse in 2002 came to approximately $181 billion, $107 billion of which was associated with a drug-related crime. Based on the evidence supporting that the successful completion of drug abuse treatment helps reduce drug-related crime and the costs associated with it, there has been a push to employ more forceful means of pressuring substance users into treatment through the use of legal coercion.

The use of coercion as a way to get people into treatment has been employed throughout the United States for decades, starting with the morphine maintenance clinics in the early 1920s. The 1960s saw the implementation of civil commitment procedures in the federal system, as well as in New York and California. The civil commitment procedures have since been replaced with the process of providing legal referrals to treatment from various criminal justice sources. The current system, which has been in place since the 1970s, emphasizes community-based treatment as an alternative to incarceration or as a condition of probation or parole. It is estimated that the criminal justice system is responsible for almost half of the referrals to community-based treatment programs. The criminal justice system also provides treatment to offenders while incarcerated, which can also be coercive, depending on whether or not the offender can make the decision to enter treatment. For instance, some states have recently developed prison-based treatment programs where the inmates identified as needing treatment are mandated to participate in the program while other prison-based treatment programs leave it up to the offender to decide if they want to participate in the treatment program.

Coercion through legal pressure can take on many different forms. It can be a recommendation to receive treatment through the criminal justice system; an option of having legal sanctions deferred, reduced, or lifted if a person enters and completes treatment; or even a requirement, sending inmates involuntarily to a prison treatment program. Coercion through the criminal system can also be defined based on the amount of control a criminal agency has over the client. For example, low coercion would be a referral to a treatment program without having to undergo drug testing while enrolled; moderate coercion would be where an offender is formally ordered to enter treatment but not required to submit to drug testing while enrolled; high coercion would take place when an offender is ordered to enter treatment and to undergo drug testing.

Legal pressure to enter treatment through the criminal justice system is not the only source of coercion. Other forms of coercion can come from family members, friends, employers, health care professionals, and other noncriminal justice agencies. Having financial or health problems can pressure people to enter treatment as well. So even though someone may be referred to treatment through a criminal justice source, he or she may actually feel more pressure to enter and complete treatment from these other sources than from the threat of legal sanctions.

Even though the use of legal coercion is popular throughout the nation, some have argued that there is little benefit from forcing an individual into treatment who does not really want to be there. It is believed that motivation is essential to get people to actively participate and engage in treatment and that it is waste of resources to give a treatment slot to someone who is coerced into treatment and is unlikely to change. Another variation of this reasoning is that addicts must hit bottom before they are able to benefit from treatment. But some have argued that coerced treatment is necessary because it gets clients into treatment and keeps them there long enough to allow them to become engaged in treatment and to change their motivation to one of commitment. Others are concerned about protecting the civil rights of the addict, but many believe that it is more important to force the drug-abusing offender into treatment to protect the well-being of the community and to reduce the costs to society associated with drug and alcohol abuse than it is to protect the addict. In addition, some believe that just because people are referred to treatment does not necessarily mean they are under greater coercion than others or that they are not motivated to change. Referrals can be seen as a way to facilitate voluntary entry into treatment.

The outcomes from studies on coerced treatment show quite a bit of variation. Some studies report better outcomes for coerced clients, while others show either a negative outcome for the coerced client or no difference. A lot of the variation can be attributed to the use of different program types, outcome measures, and measures of legal involvement or coercion by the various studies. Further research is needed to determine what factors may moderate the effect of coercion or interact with coercion. In addition, studies are needed to find effective ways to get coerced clients to actively engage in the treatment process.

Stacy B. Calhoun

See also Client Engagement; Court-Mandated Treatment; Crime and Substance Abuse; Criminal Justice Populations; Drug Courts; Resistance in Treatment; Treatment in Jails and Prisons

Further Readings

Farabee, D., Prendergast, M., & Anglin, M. D. (1998). The effectiveness of coerced treatment for drug-abusing offenders. *Federal Probation, 62,* 3–10.

Hiller, M., Knight, K., Leukefeld, C., & Simpson, D. (2002). Motivation as a predictor of therapeutic engagement in mandated residential substance abuse treatment. *Criminal Justice and Behavior, 29,* 56–75.

Klag, S., O'Callaghan, F., & Creed, P. (2005). The use of legal coercion in the treatment of substance abusers: An overview and critical analysis of thirty years of research. *Substance Use & Misuse, 40,* 1777–1795.

Longshore, D., Urada, D., Evans, E., Hser, Y., Prendergast, M., & Hawken, A. (2005). *Evaluation of the Substance Abuse and Crime Prevention Act: 2004 report.* Sacramento: Department of Alcohol and Drug Programs, California Health and Human Services Agency.

Marlowe, D. B., Glass, D. J., Merikle, E. P., Festinger, D. S., DeMatteo, D. S., Marczyk, G. R., et al. (2001). Efficacy of coercion in substance abuse treatment. In F. Tims, C. Leukefeld, & J. Platt (Eds.), *Relapse and recovery in addictions* (chap. 9). New Haven, CT: Yale University Press.

Prendergast, M., Farabee, D., Cartier, J., & Henkin, S. (2002). Involuntary treatment within a prison setting: Impact on psychosocial change during treatment. *Criminal Justice and Behavior, 29,* 5–26.

COGNITIVE BEHAVIORAL THERAPY

Substance use disorders are a complex and debilitating set of conditions. Substance use disorders are highly prevalent, are related to increased morbidity and mortality, and are often comorbid with other psychiatric phenotypes, thereby constituting a major public health concern. Without treatment, substance use disorders confer cost to both the individuals and society in various forms (e.g., lost productivity at work, health care costs, violence, child abuse and neglect, and judicial system costs). Fortunately, addiction is treatable, and therefore, immense effort from researchers and clinicians has been employed to develop and implement successful treatments, both psychological and pharmacological, for individuals afflicted with addictive disorders. Many programs and modalities have been developed such as Twelve-Step Facilitation cognitive therapy (e.g., Beck's cognitive therapy), behavior therapy (e.g., contingency management, Community Reinforcement Approach), and Motiva-tional Enhancement Therapy. Not only are various forms of treatment available today, but often multiple forms of treatment are employed simultaneously. For example, patients often engage in some form of individual therapy as well as attending Twelve-Step programs. Further, many of these modalities of treatment are offered in both individual and group format. Despite differing logistical and theoretical underpinnings, all treatments for substance use disorders share the common goal of helping the patient reach and maintain recovery. The purpose of this entry is to review one of the most frequently employed and effective treatment types for substance use disorders, cognitive behavioral therapy (CBT).

Common Tenets of CBT

Many therapy packages fall under the umbrella of CBT, all of which incorporate elements of both cognitive and behavioral theory to varying degrees. Further, all of the various CBT treatment packages share common tenets. First, psychological distress or difficulties are believed to be caused by maladaptive thoughts and behaviors. These difficulties are remedied through helping the patient identify and change these thoughts and behaviors, leading to a reduction in distress. In this modality, cognitions are believed to play a role such that (a) the individual is exposed to a stimulus, (b) the individual makes a cognitive appraisal of the stimulus, and (c) the cognitive appraisal then affects the resulting emotional response. Thus, it is not the situation, per se, that gives rise to emotional responses, but the individual's appraisal of that situation that leads to the emotional experience. Appraisals are thought to occur near instantaneously and often outside conscious awareness. A key aspect of treatment, therefore, is teaching patients to be cognizant of these automatic thoughts in an attempt to have opportunities to decrease the automaticity of these appraisal processes and alter maladaptive cognitions.

The second shared tenet of CBT treatments is that behaviors are learned through operant or classical conditioning and therefore, are able to be altered. Specifically, CBT therapists assume that (a) any behavior that is followed by a positive outcome will be more likely to be repeated and (b) any behavior that is followed by a negative outcome will be less likely to be repeated. Teaching patients to alter their maladaptive cognitions will lead to more pleasant emotional states, which will be rewarding to the patient, therefore reinforcing this new behavioral pattern. In regard to classical conditioning, CBT therapists share an awareness that stimuli that were previously neutral may be paired with an unconditioned stimulus to give rise to behaviors. Therefore, acute attention to the environments of patients is needed to accurately conceptualize their behavior and to effectively assist patients in altering their behavior.

Finally, the third shared tenet is that CBT is a collaborative treatment process, with patients playing an active role in defining the problem to be targeted for intervention, utilizing new skills learned, and practicing these skills between therapy sessions. During each session, goals or homework are collaboratively decided on and are to be completed during the proceeding intersession days. At treatment onset, therapeutic rationale is clearly explained, and the patient is taught skills to help facilitate changes in thought patterns and behaviors. The onus of change resides with the patients and their willingness to practice and incorporate these new skills outside of sessions.

Outcomes

Treatment outcome in CBT has received an extensive amount of attention in scientific research, with efficacy examined among a wide range of psychological disorders and problems. For example, CBT has shown to be effective in treating various mental health problems including depression, generalized anxiety disorder, panic disorder, social phobia, and post-traumatic stress disorder. There is also evidence to suggest that CBT may be superior to other treatments when used for these disorders and that CBT may produce effects that endure following treatment discontinuation. Although CBT is regarded by many as the most effective and scientifically based form of psychotherapy to date, there are certain conditions in which the research studies have produced mixed results on CBT's efficacy (e.g., marital distress, child conduct problems, patients with lower intelligence). With regards to substance abuse treatment, CBT has shown initial promise for use with certain substances of abuse. However, more scientific research has been conducted with motivational interviewing (MI) treatment of substance use disorders than has been conducted with CBT. It is important to note that many of the non-CBT psychotherapy modalities incorporate CBT techniques into the repertoire of treatment (e.g., MI), making it difficult to gauge the relative efficacy compared to CBT. A brief review of CBT treatment in relation to certain substances of abuse (alcohol, cocaine, nicotine) follows. Finally, an overview of typical substance use CBT treatment sessions is provided.

CBT and Specific Substances of Abuse

Among alcohol use disorders, a landmark, large-scale study (Project MATCH) sought to determine if patient characteristics could be useful predictors as to which form of psychotherapy would be most effective: Twelve-Step Facilitation, CBT, and MI. Overall, the results of this study showed that for alcohol treatment, each modality of therapy was effective in treating alcohol use disorders at a comparable rate. However, there were specific factors that made one form of treatment more effective than others. Patients with high levels of anger tended to fare better with MI. Patients with high levels of dependence tended to do better with Twelve-Step Facilitation. Finally, patients with low levels of dependence tended to do better with CBT. These results suggest that patient characteristics and characteristics of the patient substance use disorder may be relevant to selection of treatment type.

For cocaine use disorders, CBT has also been shown to be an effective treatment. As noted above, homework is an essential component of CBT. With cocaine treatment, rate of homework completion has actually been linked to better outcome. Interestingly, in relation to number of treatment sessions per week, there does not appear to be a dose-dependent relationship, with patients receiving CBT therapy once per week faring just as well as those who receive CBT three times per week. This may be particularly important when considering cost savings in relation to the present day managed health care system. Although there seems to be some specific benefits of concurrent MI with CBT (e.g., greater treatment attendance), when looking at actual cocaine use posttreatment, adding MI does not appear to increase the overall treatment effectiveness. CBT for cocaine use has also been compared to contingency management (CM)— that is, rewarding prosober behaviors. CM tends to show a faster reduction in cocaine use. However, the effects of CM drop quickly after treatment cessation; the effects of CBT can be seen for months postcessation of treatment. Additionally, when CBT and CM

are provided concurrently (in contrast to concurrent CBT and MI), there is some evidence that suggests increased treatment effectiveness.

CBT has also been shown to be effective in the treatment of nicotine addiction. However, in comparison to other drugs of abuse, nicotine addiction has a much higher societal prevalence rate and is frequently comorbid with other psychiatric conditions. Thus, efficacy is often linked to a third variable being studied. In addition, withdrawal from nicotine dependence can often produce symptoms of depression and anxiety. Conversely, individuals who are anxious or depressed are much more likely to be nicotine dependent. Indeed, one of the common pharmacological treatments of nicotine dependence is also marketed as an antidepressant (buproprion). Among the patient with a history of depression, including CBT for depression and CBT for smoking produces greater abstinence rates than CBT for smoking alone. Thus, consideration of these third variables (e.g., comorbid psychiatric conditions) may be particularly important to certain types of substance use disorders.

Overview of CBT Therapy Sessions

As noted earlier, CBT is an effective treatment for numerous substance use disorders. Nonetheless, certain facets of CBT treatment remain consistent across these various substances. Initially, it is particularly important to focus on building rapport, outline the structure of therapy, and stress the importance of homework completion and the patient as an active force in recovery. Education on the nature of addiction is also particularly important.

Subsequent sessions focus on coping skills—that is, teaching the patient methods of dealing with stressors or withdrawal symptoms that would typically precipitate relapse (e.g., progressive muscle relaxation, deep breathing, exercise). Next, the therapist helps the patient identify idiosyncratic triggers of cravings for the substance. These triggers can include specific places where the substance was used, people, situations, and certain emotional states. The patient would use previously learned coping skills when faced with such triggers and/or cravings. Eventually, the patient would learn to predict and avoid such triggers.

Another important component of treatment is to educate patients on how their thoughts can lead to relapse. For example, during the maintenance period of sobriety, it is common for the patient to start having thoughts such as, "I have it under control now. I can use it recreationally." Emotions also play a critical role, with relapse frequently occurring after experiencing negative ones (e.g., anger, sadness).

A common difficulty for patients is distancing themselves from individuals who are actively using the substance that they are addicted to. Indeed, in the case of alcohol use disorders, completely disassociating themselves from individuals who drink can be extremely difficult or impractical. Thus, it is important to teach the patient refusal skills in treatment. It is also important to go above and beyond just education. Role-playing situations in which the patient has to implement these refusal skills can be particularly helpful.

In CBT, termination of treatment is done in a tapered fashion; follow-up sessions are scheduled at longer intervals until ultimately ending treatment. During these follow-up sessions, implementation of learned skills is checked, and booster sessions on particular topics may be warranted. For example, substance refusal skills may again be addressed and practiced if this is a particular difficulty for the patient. In review, the overarching goal of CBT treatment is to teach the patient new skills, increase awareness of thoughts and behaviors, and ultimately engender a sense of mastery in these recovery skills.

Conclusion

CBT has been shown to be effective in the treatment of numerous substances of abuse. In fact, the American Psychological Association has published practice guidelines for treating substance use disorders, stressing the importance of CBT techniques. Although pharmacological advances have produced numerous medications that show promise in the treatment of addictions (e.g., acamprosate, buprenorphine, disulfiram, naltrexone), CBT has been identified in several studies to be just as efficacious and to produce even greater benefit when used in combination with pharmacological treatment. However, it is important to remember that one size does not fit all; the number of treatment sessions and even modality needs to be selected based on the particular patients' presenting needs, characteristics, and life situation. Although CBT has been shown to be effective as an independent treatment, a multidisciplinary approach, incorporating medicine, mental health, and various support groups, is often best. Although it is true that research has identified many third variables that determine if the additional

treatment modality enhances outcome, it is unlikely that additional treatments would be to the detriment of the patient. As it is not practical (or even possible, at times) to link these third variables to one's specific patient, taking a broad spectrum approach to treating this insidious disorder may provide the addicted individual the best chance at maintaining sobriety.

Jared P. Dempsey, Ananda B. Amstadyer, Grace S. Hubel, and Noreen Watson

See also Behavioral Couples Therapy; Brief Interventions; Client/Treatment Matching; Contingency Management; Evidence-Based Treatment; Motivational Interviewing

Further Readings

Gonzalez, V. M., Schmitz, J. M., & DeLaune, K. A. (2006). The role of homework in cognitive-behavioral therapy for cocaine dependence. *Journal of Consulting and Clinical Psychology, 74*(3), 633–637.

Longabaugh, R., Zweben, A., Locastro, J. S., & Miller, W. R. (2005). Origins, issues and options in the development of the combined behavioral intervention. *Journal of Studies on Alcohol*, Supplement No. 15, 179–187.

O'Leary, T. A., Monti, P. M., Hofmann, S. G., & Tompson, M. C. (2002). *Cognitive-behavioral therapy for alcohol addiction.* New York: Guilford Press.

Project MATCH Research Group. (1998). Matching alcoholism treatments to client heterogeneity: Project MATCH three-year drinking outcomes. *Alcoholism: Clinical & Experimental Research, 22*(6), 1300–1311.

Thase, M. E., Dickstein, L. J., Riba, M. B., & Oldham, J. M. (1997). *Cognitive-behavioral therapy for substance abuse disorders.* Washington, DC: American Psychiatric Association.

Waldron, H. B., & Kaminer, Y. (2004). On the learning curve: The emerging evidence supporting cognitive-behavioral therapies for adolescent substance abuse. *Addiction, 99,* 93–105.

COGNITIVE-SOCIAL LEARNING MODEL

The function of biological and genetic factors in the development and maintenance of substance use and substance use disorders has been widely documented. Research has also indicated that cognitive-social learning variables, such as acquired expectations about substance use consumption and self-efficacy, can influence the development and maintenance of substance use and substance use disorders. Substance use researchers have long sought to understand the antecedent events and reinforcing consequences of substance use behaviors in an effort to provide better prevention efforts, intervention and treatment options, and tools for the maintenance of sobriety for substance abusing and substance dependent patients. An antecedent event is an event that precedes a substance use behavior and may tend to cause that behavior to occur. A consequence is the outcome of engaging in the substance use behavior, and if that outcome is reinforcing, it will increase the likelihood that the behavior will occur again. This entry focuses on the development of the cognitive-social learning model of substance use from social learning theory, the role of expectancies about self-efficacy and expectancies about the outcome of substance use, and treatment modalities and relapse prevention techniques that have arisen from the cognitive-social learning model.

Introduction

Albert Bandura's social learning theory proposed that a great deal of human behavior is learned from the environment, particularly the social environment. This theory postulated that human behavior was not controlled solely by the environment or solely by internal drives, but rather by a combination of environmental events, internal processing, and reinforcing feedback. This view of multiple influences on human behavior differed widely from the predominant psychological theories of the time (i.e., psychoanalytic, associative learning).

As it relates to the study of addictive behaviors, social learning theory may be applied to both the development and maintenance of substance use and substance use disorders. Bandura cited social modeling as a major factor in the development and maintenance of substance use. Modeling may be defined as learning that arises by observing the behavior of others and imitating their behavior. Bandura also cited the negative reinforcement of substance use as a major factor in the development and maintenance of substance use via the stress reduction that occurs in the individual's environment due to the physiological effects of alcohol. Coping skills and social resources are also identified as major components of the ability to change problematic substance use patterns and the

ability to maintain these changes. Social learning theory postulates that substance use is largely an effort to reduce stress in the environment. Alcohol researchers have used social learning theory to understand the development of substance use disorders and to devise substance use treatment strategies. Additionally, researchers have built upon existing social learning theory to provide a more comprehensive view of the development and maintenance of substance use.

Expansion of Social Learning Theory

Arising from social learning theory, the cognitive-social learning model incorporates cognitive factors that mediate substance use behaviors in addition to the factors outlined in social learning theory, including self-efficacy expectancies and substance use outcome expectancies. Self-efficacy may be defined as the confidence that an individual can cope effectively with a prospectively stressful situation. Thus, self-efficacy expectancies may be defined as the belief that an individual can execute a specific behavior to attain a desired outcome. Substance use outcome expectancies may be defined as the belief about the probability of achieving a desired outcome if a particular behavior is exhibited. These substance use outcome expectancies are based upon past experiences in which a specific behavior resulted in a specific outcome or consequence. These cognitive factors and their relationship to substance use and substance use disorders are described in greater detail in the next sections.

Role of Expectancies

Self-Efficacy Expectancies

The cognitive-social learning model incorporates self-efficacy expectancies as a cognitive factor that mediates substance use behaviors. An individual's level of self-efficacy dictates that person's confidence that he or she can cope effectively with a stressful situation. Thus, self-efficacy expectancies are beliefs that a specific behavior can be executed to attain a desired outcome. The construct of self-efficacy expectancies has been heavily researched and reliably linked to the development and maintenance of substance use and substance use disorders.

In the case of substance use, individuals typically report that their level of stress arousal (i.e., anxiety symptoms, avoidance) tends to decrease as they begin to feel the effects of the substance. This stress diminishing effect may serve to strengthen an individual's self-efficacy when a particular substance is used (i.e., the belief drinking alcohol will be help the person to cope with stressful social situations). Substance use and its mood-altering effects can also tend to alter the perception of negative social feedback, either via direct misunderstanding or via the production of alternative explanations for the feedback due to lowered anxiety and arousal. These altered perceptions of social feedback from others serve as a protective factor for the individual's level of self-efficacy in situations where they use the substance. Additionally, the cognitive context in which substance use occurs can influence the impact on the level of self-efficacy. If someone is able to attribute perceived social disapproval to the effects of substance use rather than as a direct attack on the person, this may serve to lessen the impact on his or her self-efficacy in these situations. These self-efficacy expectancies may serve to reinforce substance use due to the belief that using the substance will help one to cope in situations that typically produce anxious arousal or avoidance.

Substance Use Outcome Expectancies

The cognitive-social learning model incorporates substance use outcome expectancies as a cognitive factor that mediates substance use behaviors. Substance use outcome expectancies dictate beliefs about the probability of achieving a desired outcome if a particular behavior is exhibited. These expectancies are based upon past experiences in which enacting a specific behavior resulted in a desired outcome or consequence. A large body of scientific research has been devoted to the link between substance use outcome expectancies and substance use and substance use disorders.

As mentioned previously, individuals commonly learn to predict that substance use can serve to lessen their level of stress arousal (i.e., anxiety symptoms, avoidance). This association results in a learned outcome expectation about substance use and resulting stress diminishment, a cognitively mediated expectancy relationship rather than simply a learned association. The person holds the expectancy that substance use can produce a desired outcome (i.e., the belief that when he or she drinks alcohol he or she

will not be anxious in social situations). This substance use outcome expectancy becomes stronger with sustained substance use being paired with the desired outcome. This cognitive process is affected by other factors as well, such as the amount of the substance that is consumed, the duration of substance use, the frequency of substance use, prior experiences with substance use, individual differences based on physiological variables, and the setting in which the substance use typically occurs. The integration of these specific factors may serve to affect the specificity of the substance use outcome expectancies (i.e., the belief that drinking two 12-ounce beers during one's first hour at a bar will reduce social anxiety symptoms and result in positive social interaction). These substance use outcome expectancies may serve to reinforce substance use due to the belief that using the substance will produce a desired outcome.

Treatment of Substance Use Disorders

Several reliable substance use treatment modalities have been derived from the principles of the cognitive-social learning model. Specifically, many cognitive behavioral treatment strategies were developed using this model of the development and maintenance of substance use and substance use disorders. Cognitive behavioral treatments are designed to help patients develop coping skills to deal with anxious and avoidant behaviors, increase self-efficacy, and encourage clients to attribute negative coping outcomes to external factors and attribute positive coping outcomes to internal factors. Treatments to help reduce or cease substance use (i.e., cognitive restructuring, social skills training, and strategies for self-monitoring) are used to develop specific coping skills and to increase self-efficacy during substance use treatment. In the same manner that self-efficacy or substance use expectancies can reinforce substance use and result in problematic patterns of use, treatment providers may utilize these principles of the cognitive-social learning model to help their patients develop alternative coping strategies to decrease anxious arousal and avoidance and to increase their self-efficacy during periods of sobriety.

Relapse Prevention Techniques

G. Alan Marlatt and Denis M. Gordon used the principles of the cognitive-social learning model to develop a model of the cognitive processes that may affect relapse in substance users who have achieved sobriety. Even after successful substance use treatment and cessation of use, many abstinent substance users will encounter high-risk situations that may increase their likelihood of relapse (i.e., going to a setting that serves alcohol, social interactions with people who use the substance). The lack of coping strategies to deal with these high-risk situations may serve to decrease the abstinent user's self-efficacy that may incline him or her to engage in substance use patterns to increase his or her self-efficacy, based largely upon his or her previous belief that substance use would help him or her to cope with the stressful situation. Relapse is also highly probable if the individual has positive substance use expectancies. These positive substance use outcome expectancies may increase the likelihood of use in high-risk situations because the abstinent user still holds the belief that using will decrease the stress associated with being in the high-risk situation. Research examining the role of self-efficacy and substance use outcome expectancies in the prediction of relapse has provided substantial support for the principles of the cognitive-social learning model.

Conclusion

Substance use researchers have built upon the existing principles of social learning theory in order to provide a more comprehensive view of the development and maintenance of substance use. The cognitive-social learning model attempts to explain continued motivation to use a substance despite increasingly negative substance abuse–related consequences that are incurred by incorporating cognitive factors, such as self-efficacy and substance use outcome expectancies, to existing principles of social learning theory. Self-efficacy expectancies may serve to reinforce substance use due to the belief that using the substance will help people to cope in situations that typically produce anxious arousal or avoidance. Substance use outcome expectancies may also serve to reinforce substance use due to the belief that using the substance will produce a desired outcome. Several reliable substance use treatment modalities have been derived from the principles of the cognitive-social learning model, including many cognitive behavioral treatments for substance use and abuse and relapse prevention techniques to reduce the likelihood of returning to problematic patterns of substance use.

Jennifer M. Day

See also Cognitive Behavioral Therapy; Expectancies; High-Risk Situations; Relapse Prevention; Social Learning Model of Addictive Behaviors

Further Readings

Bandura, A. (1969). *Principles of behavior modification.* New York: Holt, Rinehart and Winston.

Bandura, A. (1971). Self-efficacy: Toward a unifying theory of behavior change. *Psychological Review, 84,* 191–215.

Bandura, A. (1977). *Social learning theory.* Englewood Cliffs, NJ: Prentice Hall.

Bandura, A. (1982). Self-efficacy mechanism in human agency. *American Psychologist, 37,* 122–147.

Bandura, A. (1986). *Social foundations of thought and action.* Englewood Cliffs, NJ: Prentice Hall.

Leonard, K. E., & Blane, H. T. (1999). *Psychological theories of drinking and substance useism.* New York: Guilford Press.

Marlatt, G. A., & Gordon, J. R. (Eds.). (2005). *Relapse prevention: Maintenance strategies in the treatment of addictive behaviors* (2nd ed.). New York: Guilford Press.

Wilson, G. T. (1987). Cognitive processes in addiction. *British Journal of Addiction, 82,* 343–353.

Wilson, G .T. (1987). Cognitive studies in alcoholism. *Journal of Consulting and Clinical Psychology, 55,* 325–331.

COLLEGE ON PROBLEMS OF DRUG DEPENDENCE

The College on Problems of Drug Dependence (CPDD), an interdisciplinary research society, is the oldest organization in the United States to address problems of drug abuse and dependence. Formerly called the Committee on Problems of Drug Dependence, it began in 1929 as part of the National Academy of Sciences before becoming an independent organization in 1976. In 1991, the name was changed from Committee to College, and it evolved into a member organization that includes scientists in a wide range of fields from biology, chemistry, and preclinical pharmacology to psychology, anthropology, and epidemiology.

In its mission to serve researchers and policymakers, CPDD provides a link among academic, government, and industrial communities with regulatory and research agencies. CPDD provides updates on research advances that have implications for public health practice. CPDD also is a collaborating center of the World Health Organization. Some of the major foci of CPDD include its Annual Scientific Meeting, support for research and drug dependence testing in animals, drug assessment activities, consultation, sponsorship of the journal *Drug and Alcohol Dependence,* and affiliations with several scientific and professional organizations.

Annual Scientific Meeting

CPDD sponsors a scientific meeting that attracts basic scientists and clinical investigators from industry, academia, and government. Scientists and other professionals interested in biochemical, behavioral, and public health aspects of drug abuse and dependence participate in poster sessions, symposia, workshops, oral communications, invited lectures, and committee meetings. Proceedings of each meeting are published and archived. In recent years, annual meetings have been held in Canada, Puerto Rico, and the mainland United States.

Drug Dependence Testing

CPDD partners with the National Institute on Drug Abuse (NIDA) to provide support for research and for drug dependence testing in animals via its Drug Evaluation Committee (DEC). Testing is conducted at three institutions: The University of Michigan, Virginia Commonwealth University's Medical College of Virginia, and the University of Mississippi. Recently, the CPDD has had a role in developing more broadly based methodologies for testing drug abuse liability and dependence potential in animals and humans.

Drug Assessment Activities

Largely through the DEC, the CPDD provides services to evaluate the dependence potential, abuse liability, or both of new drugs. Some compounds are drugs with current or potential clinical utility. Knowing the dependence potential of a proposed drug for marketing is important to regulatory requirements within the United States and internationally. Street drugs and compounds submitted for research purposes are also tested. Information

obtained by these evaluations provides information to national and international governments, academia, the pharmaceutical industry, and the public.

Publication Sponsorship

Drug and Alcohol Dependence is an international, interdisciplinary, scientific journal sponsored by CPDD publishing original research, scholarly reviews, commentaries, and policy analysis in the areas of drug, alcohol and tobacco use, abuse, and dependence. Articles include laboratory-based and clinical research in humans, substance abuse treatment and prevention research, studies of the chemistry of substances of abuse, their actions at molecular and cellular sites, and studies with methodologies from epidemiology, sociology, and economics. The journal is published 18 times per year, and CPDD invites contributors. CPDD publishes the newsletter, *Newsline,* quarterly. *Newsline* contains a column from the CPDD President, interviews with various scientists, and information about upcoming annual meetings and other relevant topics.

In addition to more formal publications, the CPDD had developed fact sheets, available on its Web site, that include educational information, policy statements, and reports. Fact sheets are available on drug abuse research and the health of the nation, treatment for drug abuse, and medication treatments for drug abuse. Policy statements on tobacco, national drug policy, animal research, and nonmedical use of opioids can also be obtained on the Web site. Reports of the drug evaluation committee and pharmacotherapy consensus statement between NIDA and CPDD are also available.

Awards

CPDD has established and provides six major awards of excellence given either annually or every other year. The Nathan B. Eddy Memorial Award is given for outstanding research efforts that have advanced knowledge of drug abuse and dependence. It was established in memory of one of the field's pioneers after his death in 1973. Awardees receive $10,000 and are invited to provide a major address at the annual meeting. The Marian W. Fischman Lectureship Award recognizes contributions of an exemplary woman scientist in drug abuse or dependence research. Founded in 2001 in memory of an admired scientist and drug abuse researcher, the award provides $1,500 and an invitation to give a lecture at the annual meeting. The CPDD provides a Mentorship Award to a member with excellence in developing new researchers in the field. Awardees receive $1,500. An award named in memory of Joseph Cochin, former Executive Secretary of CPDD, recognizes an outstanding researcher under age 40 who has shown excellence in any facet of the field. The award comes with $1,500. An administrative award is given every other year for exceptional contribution in scientific administration in the field. This award is named for and given as a memorial to J. Michael Morrison, a former administrator at NIDA. The CPDD provides a media award to a member of the media who has substantially contributed to the public understanding of the science of drug abuse and addition. The awardee receives $1,500. All awardees receive travel expenses to attend the annual meeting where awards are presented.

CPDD membership is by application, endorsement by two active members of the CPDD, and an annual fee of $120. Benefits of membership include reduced fees to the annual meeting, a complimentary subscription to *Drug and Alcohol Dependence,* Listserv membership, access to a members only section of the CPDD Web site that contains directory information, mentorship activities, opportunities to serve on CPDD committees, discount on registration fees to attend the Annual Scientific Meeting, and a searchable abstract database of past meetings. Corporate memberships are also available for $1,500. Benefits include attendance of two company participants to the Annual Scientific Meeting at the member rate, a corporate member listing on the program for the corporation, ability to sponsor an unlimited number of abstracts, and subscription to *Drug and Alcohol Dependence.*

Sherry Dyche Ceperich

See also Drug Testing; National Institute on Drug Abuse; Pharmacological Approaches to Treatment; Substance Dependence; Treatment of Alcohol and Other Drugs

Further Readings

College on Problems of Drug Dependence: http://www.cpdd .vcu.edu

May, E. L., & Jacobson, A. E. (1989). The Committee on Problems of Drug Dependence: A legacy of the National Academy of Sciences. A historical account. *Drug and Alcohol Dependence, 23,* 183–218.

Negus, S. S. (2006). Brief history of the Drug Evaluation Committee (DEC) and its role in the college on problems of drug dependence. *Drug and Alcohol Dependence, 82,* 182–183.

College Students, Alcohol Use and Abuse

It is well documented that college students demonstrate high rates of alcohol use and abuse. For example, the annual Monitoring the Future survey conducted by the National Institute on Drug Abuse showed that in 2006, 65.4% of college students had consumed alcohol in the past month. Furthermore, over 40% of college students had five drinks or more in the previous 2 weeks during one drinking episode. This rate was higher than for similar age individuals who were not attending college.

Increased alcohol use during the college years is to a large extent a developmentally based phenomenon that occurs as young adults begin to adjust to heightened levels of personal freedom and easier access to alcohol. Many students are able to successfully avoid developing maladaptive alcohol use. However, for some, maladaptive patterns of alcohol use and consumption do emerge in regard to either quantity or frequency. These drinking patterns can and do result in substantive negative consequences.

With regard to quantity and frequency of use, a number of terms are commonly used to describe college student drinking patterns. Binge drinking refers to consumption of four or more units of alcohol (i.e., 1.5 ounces of hard liquor, one 12-ounce beer, or 5 ounces of wine) for women or five units of alcohol for men within a single drinking occasion. Heavy use is considered to be the occurrence of five or more episodes of binge drinking within a 30-day period. These terms are not utilized in the diagnosis of alcohol-related substance abuse disorders. Nevertheless, a variety of negative outcomes are associated with such drinking patterns.

Consequences

Excessive campus drinking has been associated with negative physical and psychosocial consequences that are sometimes severe. Impaired judgment and motor skills lead to physical injuries while driving and when engaging in other tasks. Indeed, in 2004, there were 1,700 deaths among college students and another 599,000 injuries primarily due to driving while under the influence or due to alcohol poisoning. Many students who engage in heavy drinking experience difficulties completing daily tasks and maintaining motivation for achievement, difficulties which can lead to academic failure. Impaired judgment during intoxication can also lead students to engage in criminal activities that they typically would not engage in and which potentially result in legal sanctions with severe consequences for college completion and future employment. Even behaviors that are not illegal can negatively influence future opportunities, as evidenced by a recent trend to post compromising pictures of intoxicated students on social networking Web sites. Heavy drinking can also exacerbate emotional distress that is sometimes associated with the rigors of academic life and has been found to be associated with increased levels of depression and suicidal ideation. In addition, the lowered impulse control during intoxication can lead to unplanned, unprotected sex, which can lead to increased risk for pregnancy, contraction of sexually transmitted diseases such as HIV, and negative emotional consequences. For a segment of the college population, heavy use leads to more frequent and severe patterns of alcohol use and the eventual development of an alcohol use disorder (i.e., alcohol abuse or dependence). Therefore, although students and the general population may view campus alcohol use as a natural right of passage, many students could benefit from professional guidance and leadership to ameliorate the negative consequences of alcohol misuse and abuse.

Risk Factors

Although alcohol consumption is common in campus settings, several factors are associated with increased risk for heavy use. For instance, compared to individuals in their same age-cohort who are not enrolled in college, students have been found to drink less frequently but to drink significantly greater amounts when they do drink. Individuals enrolled in 2-year schools have lower alcohol consumption rates than students at 4-year institutions. Similarly, students residing off campus with relatives report lower levels of alcohol use than those who live independently, either on or off campus.

Thus, factors such as level of adult supervision and social climate of the campus influence attitudes towards alcohol consumption and should be targeted for specific prevention-based interventions.

Additionally, gender differences place women at greater risk than men for negative consequences resulting from excessive alcohol use. Physically, women have a body composition composed of a greater percentage of fat and lower water content and are generally smaller than males. Alcohol metabolism is thus slowed, as it is not diluted by water. Also, intoxicated women are more likely to be victims of sexual assault or to find themselves in situations in which consent to sexual intercourse may be uncertain. Recent social changes in the acceptability of female alcohol consumption are also increasing female students' risk. Historically, women have delayed onset of alcohol use, which led to lower drinking rates and later onset of alcohol use disorders. However, current popular culture encourages alcohol use among young women in an overt manner through media, specific advertisements, and alcohol discounts, which are powerful factors contributing to increased problem drinking among women. Awareness of these factors can assist in developing campus policies (i.e., enforcing sanctions, regulating advertisements) and identifying segments within the student body for specific or more intensive prevention programs.

Brief Screening Techniques

As with other at-risk populations, an initial step is to identify those requiring professional assistance, and screening techniques have been developed for this purpose. One screening instrument, the CAGE questionnaire, is composed of four items that ask if the individual has ever cut back his or her drinking, been annoyed because others have criticized his or her drinking, felt guilty about his or her drinking, or needed a morning "eye-opener" to alleviate hangover or withdrawal symptoms. Endorsement of two or more items indicates the potential for alcohol abuse or dependence and that further assessment is required. The Alcohol Use Disorders Identification Test is another screening instrument composed of 10 items derived from diagnostic criteria for alcohol use disorders, such as impaired social and occupational functioning, withdrawal, and blackouts. Items are endorsed on a 0-to-4 point scale with higher scores indicating increased frequency of symptoms. Scores of 16 to 19 indicate need for advice and brief interventions with continued monitoring, and scores over 20 indicate need for referral for formal evaluation and treatment.

Brief Interventions to Motivate At-Risk Students

Empirically derived brief interventions have been utilized to motivate at-risk students to participate in prevention and treatment programs. Motivational interviewing is one such intervention successfully utilized to prevent or decrease heavy alcohol consumption. This technique entails conducting interviews with individuals or groups to assist them in identifying the consequences of their heavy drinking and how it is inconsistent with their goals, while at the same time displaying empathy and understanding around resistance to changing attitudes and behaviors. Simply sharing with students the average number of drinks and frequency of drinking that occurs within their social groups (e.g., fraternity members) is an adaptation of motivational interviewing. Heavy drinkers then reframe their view of normative drinking to more appropriate levels, while the attitudes and behaviors of students who drink within normal levels are reinforced.

Characteristics of Effective Prevention Programs

There are both theoretical and practical differences between prevention techniques and intervention techniques, primarily because prevention programs target a broad audience of at-risk individuals prior to the occurrence significant problems. There are several vital characteristics of effective prevention programs. First, such programs should be grounded in empirically derived theories that are directly related to the targeted problem. Second, effective programs must enhance specific skills that assist individuals in addressing the problem behavior. Third, such programs should promote increased positive social interactions and support in relation to the at-risk activities, in this case engaging in activities in which responsible drinking is the norm. Fourth, prevention programs should be briefer than treatment interventions in both session length and number, as the behaviors being addressed are less severe than those seen in treatment settings. Fifth, timing of prevention programming is critical. If conducted

prematurely, effects dissipate prior to when they are most needed. Conversely, if conducted subsequent to onset of heavy drinking, the program may not be effective since, at this point, intervention may be more appropriate. For college students, an optimal time frame for implementing prevention programs addressing problem drinking is during campus orientation or early in the freshman year. Thus, the development of any prevention program must reach the greatest possible number of individuals at the time in which it is most needed utilizing theoretically grounded strategies that have been found to be effective.

Common Prevention Techniques

Several prevention programs follow the aforementioned principles of effective prevention and have demonstrated some efficacy in changing students' attitudes and excessive alcohol use. Although limited when used alone, psychoeducation is a component of most campus alcohol abuse prevention programs and usually includes information regarding consequences for underage and on-campus drinking, university regulations and local laws, how to monitor blood alcohol concentration within legal limits (.08 in the United States), and differences in alcohol metabolization between men and women. Social skills training is also a component of many effective programs and is derived from the theoretical view that maladaptive behavior results from skills deficits. Conducted in groups, this technique teaches strategies for effectively refusing alcohol. These strategies include stating an unqualified no (i.e., rather than hesitating or implying a subsequent offer may be accepted), stating goals and associated reasons clearly (i.e., why one has declined and whether he or she is abstaining from or moderating alcohol use), and planning and engaging in alternative activities. Role-plays in a naturalistic environment are utilized to increase social skills and assess skill level. Ongoing self-monitoring of alcohol use is also utilized as a common behavioral prevention technique. Students use a standardized form to document amount of alcohol consumed over a specific week, including both the precursory event and subsequent consequences that occur. This standardization allows for identification of specific triggers so that the student can implement plans to more effectively avoid or safely engage in high-risk situations. These techniques are taken from empirically derived treatments for alcohol abuse and dependence and modified to fit a prevention model through reducing number and duration of sessions, as well as adapting them to the structure of student life.

Future Directions

Future programs could more effectively address the cognitions around alcohol consumption, including thoughts about external triggers and those that may be emotionally based (i.e., depression, anxiety, general stress). In addition, although the trend to decrease the time involved in prevention programs better fits a prevention model (e.g., several 2-hour sessions to a single 2-hour session), ongoing monitoring could be established, particularly for those individuals initially identified as being at significant risk for alcohol related consequences or disorders. Computer-based dissemination could incorporate the prevention program itself, interactive supplemental materials, and monitoring of at-risk students. More specifically, computer-based techniques might include training and rehearsal materials, interactive self-monitoring alcohol consumption charts and cue lists, message boards, and expedited electronic messaging to supportive professionals. This approach is particularly effective for college populations because such technology is already frequently utilized by students for many college-related tasks and so could be made available in an accessible format with little need for professional assistance or as a component of supervised prevention programs for heavy drinkers. Finally, prevention efforts specific to women and their drinking patterns are also needed due to their increased vulnerability to alcohol related problems and the current trend toward increased alcohol use.

Jennifer D. Karmely, Daniel N. Allen,
Roberto Valdez, and Bradley C. Donohue

Authors' note: This entry was supported by a grant from the National Institute on Drug Abuse (NIDA 1R01DA 020548-01A1).

See also Alcohol Testing; Alcohol Use Disorders Identification Test; Binge Drinking; College Students, Drug Use and Abuse

Further Readings

Donohue, B., Allen, D. N., Maurer, A., Ozols, J., & Destephano, G. (2004). A controlled evaluation of two prevention programs in reducing alcohol use among college students at low and high risk for alcohol related problems. *Journal of Alcohol and Drug Education, 48,* 13–33.

Murphy, J. G., Duchnick, J. J., Vuchinich, R. E., Davidson, J. W., Karg, R. S., Olson, A. M., et al. (2001). Relative efficacy of a brief motivational intervention for college student drinkers. *Psychology of Addictive Behaviors, 15,* 373–379.

Nations, M., Crusto, C., Wandersman, A., Kumpfer, K. L., Seybolt, D., Morrissey-Kane, E., et al. (2003). What works in prevention: Principles of effective prevention programs. *American Psychologist, 58,* 449–456.

COLLEGE STUDENTS, DRUG USE AND ABUSE

The collegiate culture is associated with numerous lifestyle adjustments thereby contributing to a unique set of substance use patterns not seen in other populations. For example, the college environment provides many individuals with their first opportunity to be exposed to a large group of peers with minimal supervision and few adult responsibilities (e.g., full-time employment, childcare, financial pressures). Those who attend college after graduating from high school are more likely to live away from their parents than their same-age peers who do not attend college. Similarly, those in commuter schools who live with parents tend to have lower rates of drug use than those in residential colleges who are isolated from parental supervision. Thus, limited supervision coupled with peer pressure to use substances and to be socially accepted contributes to substance use and abuse on college campuses. In addition, college students perceive that their peers are using substances at higher rates than is actually occurring, which in some instances has been shown to be associated with increases in substance abuse. Similar to all drug populations, the various drug use prevalence rates vary across college campuses. Estimates of substance use also vary across studies, likely due to differences in methodology employed to quantify and verify use (e.g., self-report versus urine analysis).

The best source of information on the prevalence of illicit drug use and abuse among college students is the annual Monitoring the Future (MTF) survey, conducted under a contract issued by the National Institute on Drug Abuse. Although this survey focuses on secondary level students (8th, 10th, and 12th graders), a follow-up survey is conducted each year with a selected sample of college students and other young adults. Since MTF has been conducted annually since 1975, trends in illicit drug use among college students can be ascertained. As of July 2008, the most recent data available for college students are from 2006.

It is no surprise that marijuana is the most popular illicit drug among college students. In 2006, nearly 17% of college students reported past-month use of marijuana. Comparatively, the next most frequent illicit drugs (prescription pain medications) were used by 3.1% of college students in the previous month. Amphetamines were used by 2.5%, tranquilizers by 2.4%, cocaine 1.8%, barbiturates 1.3%, and hallucinogens 0.9%. Contrary to what is reported in the popular press, methamphetamine use among college students is quite low (0.2%). What is clear is that, next to marijuana, prescription drug abuse among college students is the largest problem. Amphetamine use includes drugs used for treating attention deficit hyperactivity disorder, which college students use to stay alert and awake for extended periods of time. When these students use these drugs for this purpose, they gravitate toward tranquilizers and barbiturates in order to counteract the effects of amphetamine drugs (i.e., these drugs must be used in order to sleep).

Just as an examination of current illicit drug use by college students is important, the long-term trends in this population are also instructive. Over an 11-year period, the use of any illicit drugs in the past 30 days among secondary level students has dropped nearly 26%. In this same period, the use of illicit drugs by college students has increased by 9%. (It should be noted that this same increasing trend occurred among young adults not in college.) Although no definitive explanation has been found for this phenomenon, it is logical to assume that young people have been delaying their illicit drug use until they are older. Whether this delay is due to drug prevention efforts, greater parental scrutiny, public policies, or other factors is unclear. However, the data do suggest that young people are not convinced to avoid illicit drug use altogether, but they are influenced to wait to use these substances until they are older.

Although it would be reasonable to suspect that the 10-year trend toward increasing illicit drug use among college students is attributable to marijuana use, the MTF data do not support this. The use of

marijuana in the last 30 days among college students has actually decreased slightly over the 11-year period. The use of any illicit drugs other than marijuana has increased by over 82%. Comparatively, the use of any illicit drugs other than marijuana by secondary level students has decreased by nearly 22%. The increase among college students can almost totally be attributed to increasing prescription drug use (cocaine use has also increased).

The examination of illicit drug use in the past 30 days is the most common method to assess substance use and abuse. However, the trends toward increasing casual illicit drug use among college students are even more pronounced when looking at annual use of illicit drugs. Thirty percent of college students reported using marijuana at least once a year, a decrease of about 9% in the past 11 years. However, 18.5% used an illicit drug other than marijuana, and this usage was an increase of more than 41% in 11 years. Prescription pain medication use was up over 214% in this time period. Amphetamine use in the past year increased nearly 43%. Cocaine use was up more than 76%.

Since experimental illicit drug use precedes drug abuse, this trend is predictive of future increases in illicit drug abuse problems among college students. The only piece of data from MTF related to illicit drug abuse among college students is the daily use of marijuana. In 2006, 4.3% reported daily use of marijuana, an increase of more than 65% in 11 years.

Clearly, an increasing trend of illicit drug use and abuse among college students has been seen in the last 11 years, based on the results of the MTF survey. Little attention has been directed toward this issue in the popular media due to the focus on decreasing illicit use among secondary level students. However, college and university administrators, counselors, and student service professionals are keenly aware of this problem. In particular, the increasing misuse of prescription drugs is of great concern.

Rwida Abdel-Al, Gary L. Fisher,
Ananda B. Amstadyer, and Daniel N. Allen

See also College Students, Alcohol Use and Abuse;
    Monitoring the Future

Further Readings

Gfroerer, J., Greenblatt, J., & Wright, D. (1997). Substance
    use in the US college-age population: Differences

according to educational status and living arrangement. *American Journal of Public Health, 87,* 62–65.

Johnston, L. D., O'Malley, P. M., Bachman, J. G., & Schulenberg, J. E. (2007). *Monitoring the Future national survey results on drug use, 1975–2006:* Vol. 2. *College students and adults ages 19–45.* (NIH Publication No. 07-6206). Bethesda, MD: National Institute on Drug Abuse.

McCabe, S. E., West, B., & Wechsler, H. (2001). Trends and college-level characteristics associated with the nonmedical use of prescription drugs among US college students from 1993 to 2001. *Addiction, 102,* 455–465.

Mohler-Kuo, M., Lee, J. E., & Wechsler, H. (2003). Trends in marijuana and other illicit drug use among college students: Results from 4 Harvard School of Public Health college alcohol study surveys: 1993–2001. *Journal of American College Health, 52,* 17–24.

COMBINE STUDY

The Combined Pharmacotherapies and Behavioral Interventions (COMBINE) study was the first national study to evaluate the effectiveness of behavioral treatments alone and in combination with medications. In the past, the treatment for alcohol dependence consisted of addiction peer counseling and behavioral therapies while pharmacotherapy was basically used for the purposes of detoxification. It was not until 1994 when the Food and Drug Administration approved the use of naltrexone for the treatment of alcohol dependence that pharmacotherapy was prescribed outside the confines of detoxification. Over the years, several behavioral treatments and at least two medications, naltrexone and acamprosate, have shown to be effective in the treatment of alcohol dependence. However, there has never been an evaluation of whether combined pharmacotherapy with or without behavioral therapy could improve treatment outcomes. The COMBINE study was designed to address this lack by uniting pharmacologic and behavioral treatments in a way that had not been undertaken in the field of alcoholism treatment research before.

The National Institute on Alcohol Abuse and Alcoholism awarded federal grant awards to 11 clinical research units and one coordinating center in 1997 to identify the most effective current treatments and treatment combinations for alcohol dependence. The study also sought to evaluate whether taking placebo pills and being seen regularly by a health care professional would enhance addiction specialist counseling. A final goal of the study was to see if improvements observed over 16 weeks of treatment would be maintained for up to 1 year after treatment ended.

The pharmacotherapies were chosen by the COMBINE investigators through a consensus process. They considered things such as evidence of safety, potential drug-drug interactions, management of side effects, optimal dose, treatment duration, the availability of the medication, and integration with psychosocial therapy. They also ranked the various medications giving those with evidence of efficacy in human clinical trials the highest rankings. The full evaluation of this consisted of two pilot studies and the development of an instrument to monitor safety, the COMBINE Systematic Assessment for Treatment Emergent Events. The first pilot study was designed to inform the main trial about the safety and tolerability of the doses of the medications (naltrexone and acamprosate) selected for study, alone and in combination. The second pilot study was conducted as a feasibility study for the main trial, with the goals of assessing the length of and compliance with the research assessments, developing methods for subject recruitment and staff training, and assessing the safety of the medications under less controlled outpatient conditions. Naltrexone, at a dose of 100 mg per day, and acamprosate, at a dose of 3,000 mg per day, were chosen for the main study.

Participants in the main study were recruited by advertisements and from clinical referrals at the 11 participating sites. Around 5,000 potential participants were screened by telephone or in person. Among those screened, 2,928 did not meet the alcohol consumption criteria on the telephone screen. Of the remaining group, 654 individuals who met the initial criteria based on the telephone quick screen were not randomized after they completed their in-person baseline evaluation. The main reasons why these individuals did not make it to randomization were (a) they dropped out of the evaluation after beginning the process, (b) they already established abstinence for a duration that exceeded the maximum threshold for entry into the study, and (c) they were a no-show for any post telephone screening assessment session.

Randomization began in January 2001, and the follow-up ended in January 2004. A total of 1383 patients who met the American Psychiatric Association's *Diagnostic and Statistical Manual,*

Fourth Edition (*DSM-IV-R*) criteria for alcohol dependence were enrolled into the study. Of those, 428 were women and 955 were men. This sample had a mean age of 44.5 and a mean education of 14.5 years. About 77% were non-Hispanic White, 42% were married, and 61% were currently working full-time. The average age of onset of alcohol dependence was 31.9, and about 49% reported having had some previous involvement in treatment for their alcohol problem.

Eligible participants were randomly assigned to one of nine groups for 16 weeks of outpatient treatment after completing the baseline assessment and attaining 4 days of abstinence. Eight of the groups received medical management, which is a nine-session intervention focused on enhancing medication adherence and abstinence. It was delivered by a licensed health care professional (14 physicians, 28 nurses, one physician assistant, and one clinical pharmacist). Four of the groups also received a combined behavioral intervention (CBI), which integrated aspects of cognitive behavioral therapy, Twelve-Step Facilitation, motivational interviewing, and support system involvement external to the study. The CBI was delivered by a licensed behavioral health specialist. Participants in all eight groups received either active-placebo naltrexone or active-placebo acamprosate yielding four medical conditions (placebo, acamprosate, naltrexone, and acamprosate plus naltrexone) within each level of behavioral counseling. The ninth group received the CBI by itself without pills or medical management. All study site personnel along with the participants were blinded to the medication assignment, through the end of the treatment and the 1-year posttreatment assessment period.

Participants completed a baseline assessment prior to randomization to the treatment conditions. Some of the measures included in the baseline assessment were the Structured Clinical Interview for *DSM-IV* disorders, the Alcohol Dependence Scale, the Drinker Inventory of Consequences, the Obsessive-Compulsive Drinking Scale, and the total readiness to change score derived from the University of Rhode Island Change Assessment. After randomization, participants were assessed for alcohol consumption and craving nine times during treatment. Two-hour assessments were performed at weeks 8 and 16 during treatment and again at weeks 26, 52, and 68. Adverse medication effects were assessed at each appointment using the Systematic Assessment for Treatment Emergent Effects. A complete blood cell count and liver and kidney function tests were performed at baseline and every 4 weeks. For the CBI no pill–no medical management group, assessments were made by research assistants at the same postrandomization time points as for the other eight groups.

Findings from this study show that medical management combined with either naltrexone or CBI produced the best outcomes after 16 weeks of active treatment and 1 year later. But the researchers found that there was no extra benefit from combining medical management, naltrexone, and CBI. The researchers also found that most patients showed improvement during treatment and that both the overall level of improvement and the differences between treatment groups diminished during the follow-up period. Acamprosate, shown to be effective in many earlier studies, did not show an effect in this study and naltrexone did not work better when combined with acamprosate. However, naltrexone continued to show a small advantage for preventing relapse at 1 year after the end of treatment. The results show that naltrexone combined medical management could be delivered in health care settings, thus reaching alcohol-dependent patients who might otherwise not receive treatment.

Stacy B. Calhoun

See also Acamprosate; Alcohol; Alcoholism; Naltrexone; National Institute on Alcohol Abuse and Alcoholism; Pharmacological Approaches to Treatment

Further Readings

Anton, R. F., O'Malley, S. S., Ciraulo, D. D., Cisler, R. A., Couper D., Donovan D. M., et al. (2006). Combined Pharmacotherapies and behavioral interventions for alcohol dependence: The COMBINE study: a randomized controlled trial. *Journal of American Medical Association. 295,* 2003–2017.

Miller, W., Locastro, J., Longabaugh, R., O'Malley, S., & Zweben, A. (2005). When worlds collide: Blending the divergent traditions of pharmacotherapy and psychotherapy outcome research. *Journal of Studies on Alcohol and Drugs, 15,* S17–S23.

O'Malley, S., Martin, D., Hosking, J., & Mason B. (2005). How pilot studies improve large-scale clinical trials: lessons learned from the COMBINE Study. *Journal of Studies on Alcohol and Drugs, 15,* S66–S71.

Pettinati, H. M., Weiss, R. D., Dundon, W., Miller, W. R., Donovan, D., Ernst, D. B., et al. (2005). A structured approach to medical management: A psychosocial intervention to support pharmacotherapy in the treatment of alcohol dependence. *Journal of Studies on Alcohol and Drugs, 15,* S170–S178.

COMMUNITY-BASED PROCESSES

Over the past 30 years, the complex field of substance abuse prevention has had some successful prevention strategies. Prevention researchers have made strides in identifying effective programs, policies, and practices. Individuals who are at risk for substance abuse and other negative behaviors are exposed to risk and protective factors in all aspects of the community. Risk factors are the personal and environmental factors that place a person at higher risk for substance abuse and negative behaviors. Protective factors are personal and environmental factors that help reduce the risk of substance abuse and other negative behaviors. Because substance abuse is a phenomenon influenced by multiple risk factors at the individual, peer, family, school, community, and environmental levels, its prevention may be most effectively accomplished with a combination of interventions. Research supports the use and replication of evidence-based approaches that target multiple domains including the community domain. The Center for Substance Abuse Prevention (CSAP) describes community-based processes as school–community team training, systematic community planning and multiagency coordination and collaboration.

Community prevention efforts can affect the entire local environment, including community norms, values, and policies. A communitywide approach promotes the development of strong bonds to family, community, and the school. Because community approaches are likely to involve a wide spectrum of individuals, groups, and organizations, they create a base of support for behavior change. Support and involvement of community leaders and the allocation of resources for evidence-based prevention efforts can reduce risk factors and enhance protective factors and are more likely to lead to long-term behavior change.

The Office of Substance Abuse Prevention, the predecessor to CSAP, conducted a national survey of 26 diverse communities who were selected because they were operating multilevel and multidisciplinary alcohol and other drug community prevention systems. The results of the survey evolved into one of the initial frameworks used for community-based processes. The philosophical assumptions for success stated that the prevention effort must address three factors defined in the public health model of prevention: the host (potential and active users), the agent (sources and availability of drugs), and the environment (social climate). The programs must also reach 100% of the population and be ethnically and culturally relevant. Finally, programs must be inclusive and respectful of all groups; credit for success must be shared, and the community must be seen as the expert.

Vision

The vision is for evidence-based programs and strategies to gradually become integrated into the regular services and activities of local organizations and institutions. The communitywide focus creates a synergy; the whole is more powerful than the sum of its parts. Because many attempts to change families, schools, and other institutions have operated in isolation, they have had limited success. For meaningful change to occur, multiple interconnected forces of the community must share a common vision and agenda.

Readiness

Any community approaching a prevention process must first assess their readiness. According to the National Institute on Drug Abuse, community readiness is the extent to which a community is adequately prepared to implement a drug abuse prevention program. A community must have the support and commitment of its members and the needed resources to implement an effective prevention effort. Because community readiness is a process, factors associated with it can be objectively assessed and systematically enhanced. There are nine stages of community readiness development: (1) community tolerance-no knowledge, (2) denial, (3) vague awareness, (4) preplanning, (5) preparation, (6) initiation, (7) institutionalization-stabilization, (8) confirmation-expansion, and (9) professionalization (see Western Center for the Application of Prevention Technologies for descriptions). As communities realize their level of readiness, they can build their strategies to improve their likelihood of positive results and success.

Collaboration

Collaboration is a mutually beneficial and well-defined relationship entered into by two or more organizations to achieve results they are more likely to achieve together rather than alone. Community, interagency, and intra-agency are three common types of collaborations. Collaborations often begin with just informal networking. Agencies may next develop cooperative agreements and share information but not define a shared mission or structure. They may then move into a phase of coordination that includes some planning and division of roles. Finally, these partners may arrive at a full collaboration, which may include a shared mission statement and set of goals. Interagency agreements can spell out tasks and responsibilities for each member agency, define commitments of resources, and revise policies, procedures, and systems that are compatible and mutually supporting. These formal collaborations may be called consortia or coalitions.

Clear Purpose

Community-based coalitions in more formal situations should begin with a clear understanding of their purpose. Prevention-oriented coalitions can target improvement in their delivery of services to a community (comprehensive service coordination), generate community activism to address substance-related problems (community mobilization), or both (community linkage). Clarity of purpose will facilitate coalition development and, ultimately, success.

Building a Community Process

There are key elements to building and managing a formal, successful community process whether it is called consortia, coalition, partnership, network, alliance, or another named process. Leadership, recruitment, diversity, teambuilding, and sustainability must be considered, as well as the organizational aspects of structure and decision making. Leadership is essential and can be individual or shared. Either way, it must be dynamic, visionary, and inclusive. Membership must be appropriate to the shared purpose (i.e., agency heads or program staff). Members must be recruited from organization-agency leaders to grassroots activists and general citizenry to youth, key leaders, and stakeholders. Coalitions are ideal vehicles for bringing together a diverse representation

of a community. How well people work together is critical to their success. Members who see the importance of team building and who take time to build their trust have a greater likelihood of long-term existence. The organizational structure is important as committees are set and protocols are established for roles and responsibilities, discussion, conflict resolution, and decision making. Committees or task forces with specific purposes within the coalition have proven to be more productive than general committee assignments. Sustainability refers to the continuation of the coalition after the initial resources have ended or community conditions have changed. Evaluation of the coalition efforts should help determine whether the coalition warrants continuation or adjournment.

Conclusion

In today's complex substance abuse prevention environment, community-based processes have emerged as an unparalleled approach to combating substance abuse and its related violence in our neighborhoods. Individuals and individual agencies can no longer afford to work in isolation because resources are too few, programs are too diffused, and personal issues are intertwined. Community coalitions are recognized as a key prevention strategy in the National Drug Control Strategy. Research is beginning to document how many coalitions are impacting substance abuse in their communities, but much remains unknown. The creation of behavioral, environmental and policy changes take time. Evaluation outcomes must be part of any community-based process, and sufficient time must be given to measure the changes.

Jeanne Marie Martino-McAllister,
and Maria Theresa Wessel

See also Center for Substance Abuse Prevention; Centers for the Application of Prevention Technologies; Join Together; National Drug Control Strategy; National Registry of Evidence-based Programs and Practices; National Institute on Drug Abuse; Risk and Protective Factor Theory

Further Readings

Community Anti-Drug Coalitions of America: http://www .cadca.org

National Institute on Drug Abuse. (1997). *Community readiness for drug abuse prevention: Issues, tips and tools.* Rockville, MD: Author.

U.S. Department of Health and Human Services. (1991). *The future by design: A community framework for preventing alcohol and other drug problems through a systems approach.* Rockville, MD: Office for Substance Abuse Prevention, U.S. Department of Health and Human Services.

Western Center for the Application of Prevention Technology Substance Abuse Prevention Specialist Training. (n.d.). *Planning and best practices.* Retrieved April 4, 2008, from http://captus.samhsa.gov/western/resources/bp/index.cfm

COMMUNITY REINFORCEMENT AND FAMILY TRAINING

The 2005 National Survey on Drug Use and Health estimated that only 20% to 25% of individuals with serious substance abuse problems seek treatment within the first year of their diagnosis. One might surmise that access to resources is driving these numbers, but in fact, outright refusal of treatment by substance abusers is the main culprit. Fortunately, recent research has discovered that the family members of treatment-refusing substance abusers can play a critical role in influencing the problem drinker or drug user to enter treatment. An overview of some of the early interventions designed to help these family members is presented first, and a description of a newer program with an impressive scientific base, Community Reinforcement and Family Training (CRAFT), follows.

Traditionally, desperate family members of treatment-refusing substance abusers were offered two options: Al-Anon meetings or the Johnson Institute intervention. Al-Anon teaches family members to detach lovingly from the drinker or drug user. Studies have shown that while Al-Anon is a good source of support for family members, it does not routinely play a role in getting the substance abusers into treatment. The Johnson Institute intervention starts with a series of preparatory meetings with individuals whose lives have been negatively impacted by the substance use and culminates in a "surprise party" at which the substance user is confronted and given a treatment ultimatum. There is a high treatment engagement rate for those families who complete the entire intervention,

and yet, the majority of family members drop out prior to the confrontation session.

Unilateral family therapy is an alternative to these traditional options. This unique family therapy involves treating a family member other than the individual with the identified substance abuse problem. The treatment focuses on teaching the concerned significant other (CSO) how to go home and change her or his interactions with the substance abuser so that abstinence is rewarded and alcohol or drug use becomes associated with the withdrawal of rewards. CRAFT is a unilateral family therapy that has outperformed both Al-Anon and the Johnson Institute Intervention in several studies in terms of its ability to get treatment-refusing individuals to engage in (seek and begin) treatment. For instance, in a large alcohol study that directly compared these three programs, CRAFT-trained CSOs successfully engaged 64% of the resistant problem drinkers, whereas the Johnson Institute intervention and an Al-Anon-based individual therapy engaged 30% and 13%, respectively. Studies using CRAFT to engage illicit drug users have been equally successful, with the largest trial demonstrating CRAFT treatment engagement rates of 67% and Al-Anon/Nar-Anon rates of 29%. Importantly, CRAFT has shown similar positive results across various ethnic groups, regardless of whether the CSO is the substance abuser's spouse, romantic partner, parent, or adult child. Furthermore, treatment engagement occurs, on average, after CSOs have attended only five CRAFT sessions. CRAFT also has been highly successful at achieving its second goal, improving the psychological functioning of the CSOs, and this improvement tends to occur regardless of whether CSOs' substance abusing loved one enters treatment.

CRAFT is an outgrowth of the Community Reinforcement Approach (CRA), a program geared directly for the substance abuser and most often associated with the work of Nate Azrin. Both treatments are built on the premise that an individual's environment plays a significant role in rewarding drinking and drug use. CRAFT was developed by Robert J. Meyers, one of the original CRA therapists, when he recognized that CSOs were in a position to exert a powerful influence over their loved one's home environment and that they simply need to learn the skills to do so.

In terms of the specifics of CRAFT sessions, therapists begin by acknowledging CSOs' difficult home situation and the sacrifices they have made in an attempt to keep their family functioning. CSOs are told that although they will be asked to change some of the ways in which they have been interacting with their loved one, it in no way suggests that the CSOs are responsible for the substance use. The message is one of simply needing guidance and skills training to see that different ways of interacting with their loved one can be more effective. CSOs are assisted in drawing a roadmap of their loved one's drinking or drug use. Given that one objective is for CSOs to make it easier for a loved one to select a healthy behavior over substance use, it is necessary to understand the reasons why their loved one is using in the first place. As part of the roadmap procedure, CSOs are asked about the positive consequences their loved one associates with the drinking or drug use, such as allowing the individual to escape uncomfortable feelings (anxiety, depression) or to experience more enjoyable social interactions with friends. Discovering the function that the substance use serves is a critical step in mapping out a plan for CSOs to influence that behavior. For instance, assume a mother (CSO) reports that her 17-year-old son says he smokes marijuana after school to relax. The mother might be taught how to talk with her son about other methods for relaxing that he has enjoyed in the past, such as collecting and listening to new music. The CSO could then work with the son to gain access to these alternative methods. She might offer the son options for earning money to buy CDs or even a new sound system. The key would be to come up with an alternative method that was enjoyable for the son and served many of the same functions as the marijuana smoking.

Once a picture of the substance abuser's use has been painted, CSOs are asked to generate ideas for regularly introducing rewards for clean, sober behavior and for withdrawing the rewards during using times. For example, a CSO (the wife) might be taught to offer a suitable reward, such as joining her substance abusing husband in a pleasant activity, but only on occasions when the husband is abstinent. The appropriate withdrawal of that reward—namely, not participating in the enjoyable activity when the husband is drinking—would be stressed. Knowing when to deliver and withdraw rewards is critical. These CSO behaviors are clearly contrasted with enabling, which is a CSO behavior that inadvertently makes it easier for the loved one to continue abusing substances.

CRAFT therapists teach CSOs to use positive communication skills to explain their new behaviors. For example, this same CSO might say to her husband, "Honey, I would be happy to watch the 9:00 TV show with you tonight, but only if you haven't been drinking. I love you, but I feel like I need to do these small things to clearly support your sobriety." In addition, CSOs are asked to consider allowing the natural, negative consequences to occur if a loved one abuses substances, as opposed to having the CSO "fix" the situation. For example, instead of helping an inebriated spouse get up from the couch and get ready for bed, the CSO would be encouraged to leave the spouse on the couch for the night. Of course, obvious issues to address as part of this exercise, as well as during the other procedures, are whether there is any concern about domestic violence or the substance abuser's own safety.

In terms of the CRAFT goal of enhancing the CSO's own psychological functioning, the therapist helps CSOs identify areas of their lives in which they would like to aim for greater happiness, such as at work, with friends, or in terms of their own personal habits. Strategies for achieving these goals are developed, and weekly progress is checked through assignments.

Throughout the CRAFT program, time is devoted to recognizing how and when to invite the substance user to enter treatment. The phrasing of the request is addressed as part of the positive communication training, but windows of opportunity also are examined so that the best occasions for making the request are identified. Importantly, having a suitable therapy program lined up for the substance abuser is essential, ideally, one that complements CRAFT (such as CRA). Finally, CSOs are encouraged to remain optimistic if their first (or second) treatment invitation is rejected and to continue to use the CRAFT procedures. The CSOs' new behavior at home should still work to decrease the drinking or drug use, which frequently occurs prior to the substance user making the decision to enter treatment.

Jane Ellen Smith and Robert J. Meyers

See also Behavioral Couples Therapy; Client Engagement; Cognitive Behavioral Therapy; Community Reinforcement Approach; Enabling; Family Behavior Therapy

Further Readings

Meyers, R. J., & Wolfe, B. L. (2004). *Get your loved one sober: Alternatives to nagging, pleading, and threatening.* Center City, MN: Hazelden.

Smith, J. E., & Meyers, R. J. (2004). *Motivating substance abusers to enter treatment: Working with family members*. New York: Guilford Press.

Smith, J. E., Meyers, R. J., & Miller, W. R. (2004). Take the network into treatment. *Drug and Alcohol Findings, 10*, 4–7.

COMMUNITY REINFORCEMENT APPROACH

The Community Reinforcement Approach (CRA) is a comprehensive, cognitive behavior treatment approach that is based in the reinforcement principles of social learning theory. A major premise of the CRA is the idea that environmental conditions play an important role in supporting or discouraging alcohol and other drug abuse. As such, the primary goals of the CRA involve working to rearrange an individual's lifestyle and community in a manner that minimizes positive reinforcement for using behavior and maximizes reinforcement for nonusing behavior. This entry explores the basic principles and treatment components of the CRA as they apply to alcohol, cocaine, and opioids. Further, the entry includes a discussion of current issues and factors related to the effectiveness of the CRA.

Treatment Components

The CRA focuses heavily on the context within which substance abuse occurs and recognizes that this context is different for each individual in the program. As such, the CRA is designed in a way that allows therapists to tailor the program to individual clients by adopting those components likely to be most effective for the specific client. Although not all components are necessary for success, the assessment, treatment planning, and behavior skills components are generally used with most patients. Further, because the CRA recognizes that abuse takes place within the social environment and not within a vacuum, the components are chosen with care to maximize the effectiveness of the consumer's community. In this case, *community* refers to each individual's family, friends, work, social activities, and spiritual affiliations that have the potential to play a part in reinforcing using or non-using behavior. The various treatment components of the CRA are briefly described as follows:

- *CRA Functional Analysis:* Functional analysis is one of the early assessment components that involves taking a closer look at the individualized contexts in which substance abuse occurs. Consumers are encouraged to identify internal and external triggers that lead to abuse and to note both positive and negative consequences of abuse behavior. A focus on the positive consequences of use is especially important because these reinforcements must be effectively minimized if the behavior is to be reduced. This stage lays the groundwork for later treatment planning and behavioral reinforcement.

- *Sobriety Sampling:* The philosophy of sobriety sampling, which refers to negotiated, time-limited periods of abstinence, is not especially popular with many abstinence-based approaches; however, it may be an especially important component of CRA. The sobriety sampling approach is thought to serve two primary functions. The first function of the shorter, negotiated periods of abstinence is that it is a more realistic goal that is not as scary for many clients as is the prospect of never drinking or using again. The second function is that the shorter periods of abstinence can serve as a training ground for longer periods. That is, clients practice behavioral skills for meeting abstinence goals while identifying the newly experienced positive reinforcements for their drug-free behavior, both of which help to build self-efficacy for future drug-free behavior.

- *CRA Treatment Plans:* The treatment planning stage utilizes a Happiness Scale to help the consumer evaluate and identify issues in ten different life domains. The goals of counseling instrument is then used as a framework for developing goals, strategies, and time frames for addressing issues in the priority domains agreed upon by client and counselor.

- *Behavioral Skills Training:* Behavioral skills deficits are often identified naturally through the earlier assessment and treatment planning processes. Deficits are then addressed through behavioral practice and reinforcement. The primary focus of behavioral skills training is generally in one or more of the following three areas: problem solving, communication skills, and drink-drug refusal.

- *Job Skills:* This component focuses on helping individuals find and maintain employment with an additional focus on identifying and seeking job satisfaction. Some approaches structure this component as a job club in which consumers share in educational opportunities and support one another in developing resumes, practicing interview skills, and honing other employment-related skills.

• *Social/Recreational Counseling:* One challenge faced by individuals in treatment and recovery is finding healthy activities to fill the time that was once filled with drug-using behaviors and spent with drug-using friends and acquaintances. The therapist encourages the client to identify and sample new and alternative social activities. Many CRA programs fulfill this component through the use of a social club that offers alcohol and other drug-free environments for socialization and recreation.

• *Relapse Prevention:* This component actually begins with the functional analysis stage during which high-risk situations and triggers are identified. Consequently, behavioral skills are practiced to assist management of current and future high-risk circumstances.

• *Relationship Counseling:* In line with the goal of making the individual's community more reinforcing, significant others are often encouraged to participate in therapy. The Happiness Scale and goals of counseling instruments are also used with this component to help the client and significant other identify relationship issues and set realistic goals. In addition, the significant other may be educated on how to identify and avoid unintentional reinforcement of the client's using behavior.

• *Monitored Disulfiram:* This component is sometimes treated as a fully separate and optional element of CRA and sometimes is incorporated within the other components of treatment. Disulfiram (Antabuse) is often used to facilitate early stages of treatment, especially with clients who may be struggling to achieve even very short-term abstinence goals. It is important that a monitor (usually a family member) is assigned to the client and trained to help facilitate compliance.

These aforementioned components are the primary elements of most CRA interventions though other components may be developed and incorporated depending on the population and individual needs.

Counselor Role

Unique qualities associated with the counselor role could be considered a less obvious, yet necessary, component of success in the CRA. A CRA counselor should strive for a reinforcing style that is defined by empathy, positive response to resistance, and therapeutic alliance. The counselor should be directive and show enthusiasm, constantly finding ways to encourage or reinforce even the smallest client successes (e.g., showing up for counseling). The idea behind the counselor role in the CRA is that the energy and motivation shown by the counselor will facilitate similar qualities in the client. In addition to serving as a cheerleader for the client, the counselor also takes ownership in the progress. The client and therapist work together to help set goals and solve problems. Some of the most important work carried out by client and therapist may be that which takes place in the first few sessions. Although clients usually meet with their counselor or therapist once a week, they may meet two or three times a week in the beginning to complete the functional analysis and to help support early periods of abstinence. As short-term abstinence goals are met, the intervals between sessions may increase. The client will continue to build his or her behavioral skills repertoire, develop efficacy, and increase abstinence periods while he or she is simultaneously weaned from counseling, which may occur weekly for a while before moving to biweekly or monthly sessions.

Effectiveness

The CRA has achieved a variety of positive outcomes in a range of settings and with several populations of individuals. Although specific effectiveness studies will not be reviewed in this entry, a general overview of findings will be provided. In addition, a discussion of factors believed to be associated with treatment effectiveness will follow.

The CRA was first used and tested as an alcohol intervention. The initiation studies took place in the 1970s and involved small sample comparisons of CRA to a Twelve-Step approach. These studies were promising as the CRA was superior to the comparison approach on drinking and employment outcomes. Although the first tests of CRA took place in an inpatient setting, outpatient studies which took place a decade later also found promise in CRA with alcohol. In the 1990s, the CRA performed consistently among the top interventions across at least three systematic reviews of alcohol treatment research. This approach also performed well in cost-effectiveness investigations during the same time frame. Although the CRA has performed consistently across numerous studies of effectiveness, there are still some concerns regarding effectiveness. As is the case in any systematic review of intervention effectiveness, the studies available for comparison vary considerably in terms of population, fidelity, and methodological rigor. Further, it has been suggested that because the majority of research has been performed by a core group of individuals, further research needs to be conducted in different arenas and in different countries.

Outcome operationalization is always an issue when the success of an intervention is being evaluated. In some studies, the CRA has not outperformed other approaches in terms of length of abstinence periods even if it did outperform in terms of number of overall drinking days. In some studies, the CRA performed no better and no worse than other interventions (especially when pharmacological intervention components were included in all of the treatment approaches being compared) in terms of alcohol outcomes, though in these cases CRA often had additional outcomes such as increased employment. Indicators of success, whether directly or indirectly related to use, are likely to be identified with different levels of importance depending upon the audience, making success difficult to establish. Finally, although most of the research has focused on alcohol, the CRA approach has been used with some success with cocaine and opioid-addicted individuals, as well as with homeless and adolescent populations.

In addition to studies that have evaluated the overall CRA, some studies have focused more explicitly on specific components of the CRA. For example, research on the social club aspect has found that structured encouragement of participation in this component has not only increased participation but has also been associated with reduced drinking. Further, many of the CRA programs have found that the addition of a pharmacological component (e.g., disulfiram or methadone) and/or contingency management strategies has boosted performance on use indicators. The couples' therapy component has been successful in increasing marital satisfaction, while the job club component has increased employment prospects, both in terms of decreasing time needed to find a job and increasing initial rates of pay.

Conclusion

Despite some methodological criticisms, the CRA has found consistent support as an effective addiction-focused treatment intervention. However, this consistent success has not been enough to encourage widespread adoption of the CRA. Several reasons have been suggested for the lack of adoption, including (a) it is often thought to be expensive even though outpatient versions of the approach are judged relatively cost-effective and can often adhere to the guidelines of most managed care programs; (b) a therapist may be resistant to the overly enthusiastic reinforcement requirements, especially if he or she typically practices a more confrontational approach; and (c) because many therapists use some cognitive behavioral strategies in treatment, they may think that they are already using the CRA. It may be important for future research to further explore resistance to the CRA and to implement social marketing and technology transfer strategies to facilitate adoption and implementation. Other issues for future research may include a continued focus on defining and measuring CRA effectiveness with different drugs of abuse with a focus on achieving the right recipe of component implementation. Finally, continued research should employ the use of increasingly diverse samples, including dual diagnosis populations.

Samantha S. Clinkinbeard

See also Antabuse (Disulfiram); Community Reinforcement and Family Training; Contingency Management; Pharmacological Approaches to Treatment; Social Learning Model of Addictive Behaviors

Further Readings

Finney, J. W., & Monahan, S. C. (1996). The cost-effectiveness of treatment for alcoholism: A second approximation. *Journal of Studies on Alcohol, 57*(3), 229–243.

Meyers, R. J., & Miller, W. R. (2001). *A community reinforcement approach to addiction treatment.* Cambridge, UK: Cambridge University Press.

Meyers, R. J., Villanueva, M., & Smith, J. E. (2005). The community reinforcement approach: History and new directions. *Journal of Cognitive Psychotherapy: An International Quarterly, 19*(3), 247–260.

National Institute on Drug Abuse. (1998). *A community reinforcement plus vouchers approach: Treating cocaine addiction.* Retrieved September 25, 2007, from http://www.drugabuse.gov/TXManuals/cra/CRA1.html

Roozen, H. G., Boulogne, J. J., van Tulder, M. W., van den Brink, W., De Jong, C. A., & Kerkhof, A. J. (2004). A systematic review of the effectiveness of the community reinforcement approach in alcohol, cocaine and opioid addiction. *Drug and Alcohol Dependence, 74,* 1–13.

Comprehensive Drug Abuse Prevention and Control Act

The Comprehensive Drug Abuse Prevention and Control Act of 1970 (Public Law 91-513) was signed into law by President Richard M. Nixon on October, 27, 1970. This sweeping law, and its many subsequent amendments, combined many different drug laws into a single federal statute that covered substance use and abuse, treatment and prevention, as well as drug traffic interdiction efforts. It was purposely constructed to serve as a broad uniform federal approach to address substance use and abuse. The Comprehensive Drug Abuse Prevention and Control Act still serves as the major legal foundation for drug enforcement efforts in the United States, as well as for guiding the regulation of illicit drug manufacturing in this country.

The Comprehensive Drug Abuse Prevention and Control Act was intended to replace and update a wide array of earlier U.S. drug laws. For example, the law reduced the penalties for marijuana possession for personal use from a felony to a misdemeanor offense. It also broadened the definition of a drug-dependent person and thereby greatly expanded drug abuse treatment programs in the United States by allowing federally funded addiction treatment centers to serve nonnarcotic drug abusers as well as those who are narcotic addicts. The Comprehensive Drug Abuse Prevention and Control Act repealed both the Harrison Narcotic Act of 1916 and the Drug Abuse Control Amendments of 1965, the latter of which were intended to eliminate illicit drug trafficking of stimulants, depressants, and other drugs with the potential for abuse and which also required drugs to be identified by stipulated symbols, primarily for the ease of pharmacists. The pharmaceutical industry is required under this law to maintain strict security over certain substances along with rigorous record keeping responsibilities. The Comprehensive Drug Abuse Prevention and Control Act also amended the Public Services Act, and other related laws, to increase research on drug abuse and individuals who are drug abusers, as well as to conduct research into substance abuse prevention. The act also has mechanisms in it by which new substances can be investigated as to whether they should be placed under regulatory controls. A major accomplishment of the Comprehensive Drug Abuse Prevention and Control Act was that Congress no longer had to pass separate laws to regulate each respective drug.

The Comprehensive Drug Abuse Prevention and Control Act contained, as its Title II, the Controlled Substances Act, which established schedules for manufacturing, regulating, and distributing drugs, such as opioids, depressants, stimulants, hallucinogens, and anabolic steroids, as well as many of the chemicals used in the making of controlled substances, as determined by evaluating their possible medicinal value and their addictive potential. The law also gave much greater powers to the police and other enforcement agencies for conducting searches and seizures for drugs. In fact, the Comprehensive Drug Abuse Prevention and Control Act was amended in 1978 to permit the criminal justice system to seize all assets, including property, money, and other valuables, from anyone either intending to trade such assets for drugs or who acquired such assets as illegal proceeds from the selling of drugs.

The Controlled Substance Act, Title II of the Comprehensive Drug Abuse Prevention and Control Act of 1970, provides the legal basis for the federal war on drugs and related substances. The act divides substances into five schedules, which serves as a drug classification system for enforcement purposes. These five schedules are purportedly based on the varying potentials for abuse, accepted medical uses, and safety issues of respective controlled substances. Schedule I substances are the most dangerous drugs (i.e., they have a high potential for abuse, no currently accepted medical use in the United States, and cannot be used safely even under medical supervision). Heroin, marijuana, methaqualone (Quaalude), GHB, mescaline, peyote, LSD, and other hallucinogens are all listed as Schedule I drugs. Schedule II substances also have a high potential for abuse, but they currently have accepted medical uses for treatment even though they can still lead to severe physical or psychological dependence. Cocaine, amphetamines, methadone, methylphenidate (Ritalin), phencyclidine (PCP), oxycodone, short-acting barbiturates, and methamphetamine are currently listed as Schedule II drugs. Schedule III substances have less potential for abuse than Schedule I or Schedule II substances and thus may cause moderate to low physical dependence or high psychological dependence, but currently have accepted medical uses. Anabolic steroids, buprenorphine, ketamine, Glutethimide (Doriden), and hydrocodone are listed as Schedule III drugs. Schedule IV substances have a low potential for abuse relative to Schedule III substances, but limited physical or psychological dependence can still develop, and they currently have uses for medical treatment. Benziodiazepines (e.g., Librium, Xanax, Valium) and long-acting barbiturates are listed as Schedule IV drugs. Schedule V substances are the least dangerous. They have a lower potential for abuse than Schedule IV substances, although physical or psychological dependence is still possible, and they currently have medical uses. Cough medicines with codeine, medications with small amounts of opium, Robitussin A-C, and Lomotil are listed as Schedule V products. Some Schedule V drugs do not require a prescription, while all drugs on Schedules II, III, and IV require prescriptions.

These five schedules are controlled by the U.S. Department of Justice and the Department of Health and Human Services, including the Federal Drug Administration. The Comprehensive Drug Abuse Prevention and Control Act permits the addition, deletion, or transfer of substances from one schedule to another. The Drug Enforcement Agency can investigate any drug for inclusion into these controlled schedules upon information from criminal justice agencies, laboratories, or other sources. This initiates a review that determines whether the substance should or should not be controlled.

Victor B. Stolberg

See also Drug Laws, History of; National Drug Control Strategy; Public Policy, Drugs; War on Drugs

Further Readings

Parenti, C. (2000). *Lockdown America: Police and prisons in the age of crisis.* New York: Verso.

Rowe, T. C. (2006). *Federal narcotics laws and the war on drugs: Money down a rat hole.* Binghamton, NY: Haworth Press.

U.S. National Archives and Records Administration. (1993). *An act to amend the Comprehensive Drug Abuse Prevention and Control Act of 1970 to control the diversion of certain chemicals used in the illicit production . . . for other purposes* (SuDoc AE 2.110:103–200). Washington, DC: Government Printing Office.

CONFIDENTIALITY

Facts and beliefs disclosed during treatment for alcohol and drug use disorders are confidential in order to prevent the patient from being penalized as a result of seeking help. Information cannot be disclosed to other individuals without the patient's consent except in limited circumstances where (a) law requires mandatory disclosure (e.g., cases of suspected child abuse), (b) the counselor must act to protect the patient or someone else from harm, or (c) there is a valid court order requiring the release of information. Specific federal regulations, moreover, provided added protection for the confidentiality of alcohol and drug treatment records. This section examines four facets of confidentiality: (1) ethics and clinical practice, (2) the federal regulation specific to alcohol and drug treatment records, (3) the Privacy Rule mandated in the Health Insurance Portability and Accountability Act of 1996 (HIPAA; P.L. 104-191), and (4) research on treatment for alcohol and drug disorders.

Practitioner Ethics and Clinical Considerations

Confidentiality is a cornerstone of ethical practice. Basic ethical principles regarding respect for the worth, dignity, and right of self-determination of individuals in treatment inform and guide the process of establishing and maintaining a confidential treatment relationship. Professional trade groups specify confidentiality requirements in the ethics codes that articulate professional standards of care and practice (e.g., American Psychological Association; American Psychiatric Association; NAADC, the Association for Addiction Professionals; National Association of Social Workers). Practitioners use these standards to guide the resolution of confidentiality questions and dilemmas.

Clinically, confidentiality is a foundation for the development of an atmosphere of trust and safety in treatment. During the course of treatment, patients disclose personal, emotionally painful information and may report behavior that is socially stigmatized and illegal. A careful informed consent process at the outset of treatment explains confidentiality to new patients. Counselors define, discuss, and ensure that patients understand confidentiality and the limits of confidentiality. A discussion about confidentiality also initiates the development of a treatment relationship. In situations that require reporting treatment progress as a condition of treatment (e.g., patients referred by the criminal justice system), a clear understanding at the outset of treatment about information that will and will not be released can help promote clear expectations and trust.

During the course of treatment, counselors may receive information that they are required to report, such as information regarding suspected child abuse. Treatment programs usually have established procedures for mandatory reporting. Mandatory reporting is a difficult situation in which the patient's treatment needs, the safety of others, and compliance with law must all be balanced. Clinically, it is important to discuss with patients what, how, to whom, and why it is necessary to disclose this information. It is also appropriate to engage patients in the process to the extent possible. This engagement may include seeking the patient's consent to release the information in addition to explaining that treatment professionals are required to report it regardless. In other cases, it is helpful to all parties involved to encourage patients to voluntarily participate in the reporting process. Skillful clinicians use these situations to strengthen a sense of clinical trust.

Confidentiality, moreover, is more than good clinical practice; it is a legal requirement, and violations of confidentiality can be prosecuted. Federal regulations require clinicians and treatment programs maintain the confidentiality of treatment records (with certain exceptions).

42 CFR Part 2

Section 42, Code of Federal Regulation, Part 2 (42 CFR Part 2), titled *Confidentiality of Alcohol and Drug Abuse Patient Records Regulations,* implemented federal standards to assure and protect the confidentiality of treatment notes and treatment plans included in clinical files for individuals treated for alcohol and drug disorders. Authorization for confidentiality standards for alcohol dependence treatment records was included in the Comprehensive Alcohol Abuse and Alcoholism Prevention, Treatment, and Rehabilitation Act of 1970 (The Hughes Act; P.L. 91-616) and extended to drug abuse treatment records in the Drug Abuse Prevention, Treatment and Rehabilitation Act of 1972 (P.L. 92-255). These acts recognized that alcohol and drug use disorders are

stigmatized and that without a guarantee of privacy, patients might avoid rather than seek treatment services. The regulations protect the privacy of individuals entering care and promote a sense that it is safe to enter alcohol and drug treatment services.

42 CFR Part 2 prohibits disclosure that an individual is in care or has been in care unless the patient provides a valid consent to the release or specific conditions are met for a court-ordered release. The regulations apply to all federally assisted programs. Federal assistance is defined broadly and includes any form of federal funds; a grant of tax exempt status; an authorization to conduct business; or an agency of federal, state, or local government. As a result, the rules apply to all facilities that are licensed or authorized by state regulations. State regulations may be more restrictive than 42 CFR Part 2, but they cannot permit disclosures that are prohibited by the federal regulations.

There were many questions of interpretation when the regulations were first issued, and the Legal Action Center has worked to standardize the implementation of procedures for patient consent and appropriate disclosure of records and continues to train states, providers, and courts in the application of the standards. The Legal Action Center advocates for the rights of individuals in recovery and is widely recognized as the nation's leading authority on effective implementation and enforcement of the confidentiality standards laid out in 42 CFR Part 2. They provide workshops that train counselors and administrators in the basics of confidentiality and publish manuals that provide guidance and standardized forms for the release of confidential information.

Treatment programs have routine procedures to facilitate both the protection of client information and the appropriate release of information. To share information about treatment progress, treatment services ask patients to consent to the release of that information. A proper consent includes nine elements: (1) the name of the treatment program, (2) the name of the organization or individual receiving the information, (3) the patient name, (4) the reason for the disclosure, (5) the amount and kind of information to be released, (6) a notice that the consent may be revoked, (7) the date or reason that consent will expire, (8) the patient signature, and (9) the date of the signature. Standard forms are available to promote compliance. Patient information may be disclosed without consent for research and audit purposes, but the information may not be redisclosed by the researchers or auditors.

Violations of 42 CFR Part 2 may be reported to the local U.S. Attorney. Individuals found in violation of the regulations may be fined up to $500 for a first offense and up to $5,000 for subsequent offenses. 42 CFR Part 2 is generally the most restrictive patient confidentiality regulation. The strict limits on disclosure in the federal regulations are unique to alcohol and drug abuse treatment programs. Treatment programs, however, must also comply with HIPAA.

HIPAA and the Privacy Rule

HIPAA is federal legislation enacted to promote continuation of health insurance coverage when individuals left employment, to facilitate electronic exchange of health information, and to protect the privacy of health information. The U.S. Department of Health and Human Services issued the Privacy Rule (Section 45 Code of Federal Regulations Parts 160, 162, and 164) to guide implementation of HIPAA's confidentiality requirements. The Privacy Rule addresses the use and disclosure of individuals' health information (called *protected health information*), defines how protected health information may be disclosed, and allows individuals to understand and control the use of their health information. The Privacy Rule is designed to be flexible and comprehensive in order to cover the variety of uses and disclosures that need to be addressed in the medical field. Substance abuse treatment programs must comply with the regulations of 42 CFR Part 2 and the HIPAA Privacy Rule. Although there is overlap, the rules contain some different provisions. Programs follow 42 CFR Part 2's general rule of obtaining written consent to release information unless specific exceptions apply. The Privacy Rule requires written consent for disclosures whose purpose is outside treatment, payment, or health care operations. When written consent is required under both regulations, additional elements required by the Privacy Rule (e.g., giving patients a copy of the signed form) are added to the consent procedure.

Confidentiality and Research on Treatment

Confidentiality standards are also applicable to research. In 1979, the *Federal Register* published the Ethical Principles and Guidelines for the Protection of Human Subjects in Research. Commonly known as the Belmont Report, it provides the ethical principles upon which the federal regulations for the protection of research participants are based. The Belmont Report implies that respect for persons includes respect for the confidentiality of information. Confidentiality is defined as ensuring that data or information is accessible only to those authorized to have access. The basic principles of confidentiality are (a) respect for an individual's right to privacy, (b) respect for human relationships in which personal information is shared and gathered, (c) understanding the importance of confidentiality, and (d) expectations that those who commit to safeguard confidential information will maintain this commitment.

Within research, confidentiality refers to agreements with study participants about what may be done with the information that is gathered during the research procedures. Authorization of such agreement is made through an informed consent process. An effective and appropriate informed consent includes language thoroughly explaining the exceptions to confidentiality, potential threats to confidentiality and ways of safeguarding confidentiality. To further protect information collected for research, investigators may also obtain a Certificate of Confidentiality and protect the research data from a court subpoena.

Certificate of Confidentiality

Section 301(d) of the Public Health Service Act (42 U.S.C. 241 [d]) authorizes the issuance of confidentiality certificates. Certificates of Confidentiality are issued to protect investigators and researchers from being forced to release information that could be used to identify individuals that are involved in research. The certificate allows investigators and others to refuse disclosure of identifying information in any civil, criminal, administrative, or other proceeding whether at state, federal, or local levels. Identifying information is broadly defined as any information or combination of information in the research data that can lead to identification of a research participant, either directly or indirectly.

The certificates permit investigators to refuse to disclose identifying information about participants and to provide additional assurances to study participants that their disclosure of illegal acts for purposes of contributing to research cannot be used against them in a court of law. Certificates of Confidentiality help to minimize risks to participants by adding an additional level of protection for maintaining confidentiality of participant information. The certificate protects data maintained during the time that the certificate is in effect. The certificate does not protect against voluntary disclosure, child abuse, threat of harm to self or other, reportable communicable diseases, and/or participants own disclosure. For more information about Certificates of Confidentiality, see http://grants2 .nih.gov/grants/policy/coc/index.htm.

Limits of Research Confidentiality

Although both researchers and clinical professionals make every effort to safeguard confidentiality, there are ethical and legal limits to confidentiality. States commonly require mandatory reporting if there is (a) a clear threat to self or others, (b) there is evidence of recent or ongoing abuse of children, (c) evidence of recent or ongoing abuse of a dependent adult, and (d) a diagnosis of a disease or condition subject to mandatory public health reporting. State laws, however, vary, and it is important to understand the laws that are applicable. The limits of confidentiality should be clearly stated in the appropriate place in the consent to participate in research.

Dennis McCarty, Lynn Kunkel, and
Barbara Campbell

See also Electronic Health Records; Ethics; Health Insurance Portability and Accessibility Act; Informed Consent; Legal Action Center

Further Readings

American Psychological Association. (2002). *Ethical principals of psychologists and code of conduct.* Washington, DC: Author. Retrieved from http://www .apa.org/ethics

Legal Action Center. (2006). *Confidentiality and communication: A guide to the federal alcohol and drug confidentiality and HIPAA, 2006 revised edition.* New York: Author.

Luepker, E. (2003). *Record keeping in psychotherapy & counseling.* New York: Brunner & Routledge.

McGuire Dunn, C., & Chadwick, G. (1999). *Protecting study volunteers in research.* Boston: CenterWatch.

National Association of Alcohol and Drug Abuse Counselors. (2004). *NAADAC code of ethics.* Retrieved from http://naadac.org/documents/index.php?CategoryID=23

Sales, B. D., & Folkman, S. (2000). *Ethics in research with human participants.* Washington, DC: American Psychological Association.

U.S. Department of Health & Human Services. (2003). *OCR privacy brief: Summary of the HIPAA Privacy Rule.* Retrieved from http://www.hhs.gov/ocr/hipaa

U.S. Public Health Service. (2000). Confidentiality of mental health information: Ethical, legal, and policy issues. In *Mental health: A report of the Surgeon General* (Chap. 7). Retrieved from http://www.surgeongeneral.gov/library/ mentalhealth/toc.html

CONTINGENCY MANAGEMENT

When treating substance use disorders (SUDs) there is a tremendous need for interventions that motivate individuals to change their behavior. Indeed, a waxing and waning commitment to and ambivalence about change is a common characteristic of SUDs. Contingency management (CM) is one effective approach to addressing this need. CM interventions are based in operant conditioning, which is an area of psychology that studies how environmental contingencies of reinforcement and punishment alter the probability of future behavior. Interestingly, there is extensive basic scientific research showing that operant conditioning is involved in important ways in the development of SUDs—that is, the mind-altering substances that people abuse stimulate the brain's basic reward centers thereby increasing the likelihood that people will want to take the substance again. In the terms of operant conditioning, that is an example of a positive reinforcement contingency, wherein taking a substance stimulates the brain reward centers thereby increasing the likelihood that the person will again take the substance that produces still further brain reward, and so on. What CM attempts to do is to use similar positive reinforcement contingencies, along with other principles of operant conditioning, to promote therapeutic changes in behavior such as abstaining from substance use, attending therapy sessions, and taking prescribed medications.

Process of Behavior Change

All CM interventions promote behavior change through the use of one of the following generic types of contingencies administered alone or in combination:

positive reinforcement, which involves the delivery of a reinforcing consequence (e.g., monetary-based voucher) contingent on meeting a therapeutic goal (e.g., abstinence from recent alcohol or other drug use); negative reinforcement, which involves the removal or a reduction in the intensity of an aversive event (e.g., job suspension) contingent on meeting a therapeutic goal (successful completion of treatment); positive punishment, which involves the delivery of an aversive event (e.g., social reprimand) contingent on evidence of the occurrence of a therapeutically undesirable response (failure to attend therapy sessions); and negative punishment, which involves the removal of a positive condition (forfeiture of clinic privileges) contingent on the occurrence of an undesirable response (e.g., resumption of substance use).

Reinforcement and punishment contingencies are effective, but by definition, the latter are disliked by patients and staff and can inadvertently increase treatment dropout. CM interventions that comprise high rates of positive reinforcement and judicious use of negative punishment can be effective at retaining patients in treatment, reducing substance use, and improving other therapeutic targets. To be maximally effective, contingencies need to involve objective verification that the therapeutic target response has occurred, relatively minimal delay in delivering the designated consequence once the response has been verified, and a consequence of sufficient magnitude or intensity to function as a reinforcer or punisher. Objective monitoring of the target response in applications with substance abuse and dependence typically involves some form of testing of biological markers of recent substance use (e.g., urine toxicology testing). Delivering the consequence on the same day that testing occurs results in larger therapeutic effects than waiting to the next day or later. The magnitude of reinforcement or punishment necessary to change behavior will depend on the nature of the behavior change involved, patient population, and other factors.

Applications

CM involves an agreement or contract that carefully lays out the desired behavior change, how progress in making the behavior change will be monitored, the consequences that will follow success or failure in making the behavior change, and the duration of the contract. Practical details on the development and use of contracts for CM interventions can be found in

several sources from Stephen T. Higgins and colleagues. Most typically, but not always, CM is used in substance abuse treatment to increase abstinence from recent substance use. However, it can also be used to improve other outcomes as well such as attendance at therapy sessions. Additionally, CM is usually offered as one part of a more comprehensive treatment plan, although not always depending on the nature of the problem being treated.

Although compelling evidence regarding the effectiveness of CM in the treatment of various forms of SUDs has been available since the 1970s and 1980s through the work of Maxine Stitzer, George Bigelow, and colleagues interest in this treatment approach was increased substantially by successes achieved with CM in the treatment of cocaine dependence. In a seminal study on that topic, 38 cocaine-dependent adults were randomly assigned to 24 weeks of behavior therapy including CM or to standard drug abuse counseling. The CM program used in that study was developed by Higgins and colleagues and is the model on which many contemporary CM interventions are based. The CM intervention was 12 weeks in duration and explicitly integrated with routine urine toxicology testing. Urine specimens were analyzed at the clinic to minimize delay between obtaining the specimen and delivering appropriate consequences. Cocaine-negative test results earned points that were recorded on vouchers and provided to patients. Points were worth $0.25 each, with the first negative test result, earning 10 points or $2.50 in purchasing power. To promote sustained abstinence in the outpatient setting where opportunities to resume drug use are ubiquitous, the number of points earned increased by 5 with each consecutive cocaine-negative test result, and each three consecutive negative test results earned a $10 bonus voucher. Moreover, a cocaine-positive test result or failure to provide a scheduled specimen reset the value of the vouchers back to the initial low level from which it could escalate again according to the same schedule. Five consecutive test results following a reset restored voucher value back to where it was prior to the reset. Money was never given to patients because for many cocaine-dependent individuals, cash is a well-established cue for cocaine use. Instead, points were used to purchase retail items in the community, with clinic staff making all purchases. Staff counseled patients to use vouchers to support involvement in healthy activities that could serve as attractive alternatives to cocaine use. Vouchers were often used to purchase retail items such as gym memberships, fishing licenses, or gift certificates to local restaurants. If a patient earned all of the points available across 12 weeks, he or she could earn a total of $997.50 in purchasing power, although average earnings were approximately half of the total possible, which is typical in these interventions.

The majority (58%) of patients in the CM condition remained in treatment for the recommended 24 weeks of treatment compared to only 11% in the comparison treatment using standard drug abuse counseling. Regarding cocaine abstinence, 68% of those treated with CM achieved 2 or more months of continuous cocaine abstinence during the recommended treatment period that was verified by urine toxicology testing. By contrast, among those assigned to standard treatment, the majority either dropped out of treatment or resumed cocaine use, with only 11% achieving 2 or more months of objectively verified abstinence from cocaine use.

Subsequent studies of CM in the treatment of cocaine dependence repeated those findings and also demonstrated continuing benefits after the CM program was discontinued. In one such study, for example, 70 cocaine-dependent patients were randomly assigned to one of two treatment conditions. The counseling was identical in both treatments and all received 12 weeks of vouchers. The only difference was that in one condition patients had to abstain from cocaine use in order to receive the vouchers while in the other condition they received vouchers independent of whether they recently used cocaine. Cocaine use was monitored through urine toxicology testing during the 24-week treatment and for 1 year after treatment termination. Cocaine-abstinence rates were significantly higher during treatment and posttreatment follow-up among patients who earned vouchers contingent on cocaine abstinence compared to those who earned them independent of cocaine use. Those results demonstrated the importance of the reinforcement contingency to promoting cocaine abstinence and showed that therapeutic benefits extended beyond the period when the incentive program operated.

These positive results with CM were particularly encouraging because so few other treatment approaches have been shown to be effective with cocaine dependence. They led to a wide range of subsequent applications of CM to treat cocaine as well as other types of substance abuse and dependence in many different populations. For example, a review was published of all controlled studies using voucher-based or related monetary-based CM to treat substance abuse between January 1991 and March 2004. The review identified 63 reports of studies in peer-reviewed journals where voucher-based and related CM interventions were used to treat substance abusers. The vast majority of those studies involved interventions targeting abstinence from substance use, while a small number targeted clinic attendance or medication compliance. The review provided overwhelming quantitative evidence supporting the efficacy of CM for increasing drug abstinence and somewhat weaker but nevertheless positive support for its efficacy in the other applications as well.

Special Populations

CM is also proving to be capable of improving the success of treatment with important special subpopulations of individuals with SUDs. CM is effective at improving the likelihood of taking medication among those with infectious diseases. Improving compliance with antiretroviral medications for HIV/AIDS patients with SUDs is an example in that area. Another special population with whom there is growing evidence of CM's efficacy is the seriously mentally ill who also have SUDs. CM is effective at reducing substance use in that population and reducing other complicating factors such as rehospitalization rates that often go along with drug abuse among the mentally ill. CM is effective with adolescents with SUDs, with the evidence mostly centering on cigarette smoking and marijuana use. CM is an essential component of a multi-element treatment developed by Jesse Milby and colleagues that is effective in the treatment of homeless crack and other drug abusers. Still another special population for whom CM is effective is drug-dependent pregnant women. For example, Kenneth Silverman and colleagues demonstrated that voucher-based CM treatments increase abstinence from cocaine and heroin use among pregnant women. In another effective CM intervention with pregnant women, voucher delivery contingent on abstinence from cigarette smoking increases quit rates during pregnancy and after delivery.

Conclusion

CM treatments represent an important part of evidence-based treatments for SUDs. CM interventions are effective and sufficiently versatile to be used in many different settings and with many different populations in need of treatment for SUDs. Despite the promise of CM interventions, more research is needed to find ways to increase the effectiveness of the interventions so that they will succeed with even more patients, to develop methods that will ensure longer-term maintenance of beneficial effects over time, and to continue to develop and refine practical applications that will be used widely in society. CM interventions represent a set of procedures that are based on fundamental principles of behavioral science. As such, the further improvement and development of these procedures can be guided by the basic scientific principles on which the interventions are based. The broad success to date should give great confidence in the continuing development and improvement of CM interventions to help address the individual and societal consequences of SUDs.

Stephen T. Higgins and Sarah H. Heil

Authors' note: Preparation of this chapter was supported in part by National Institute on Drug Abuse research grants DA 09378, DA 14028, DA 08076, and DA 018410.

See also Behavioral Couples Therapy; Cognitive Behavioral Therapy; Community Reinforcement Approach; Evidence-Based Treatment; Treatment Approaches and Strategies

Further Readings

Budney, A. J., & Higgins, S. T. (1998). *The community reinforcement plus vouchers approach: Manual 2: National Institute on Drug Abuse therapy manuals for drug addiction* (NIH publication No. 98-4308). Rockville, MD: National Institute on Drug Abuse.

Higgins, S. T., Silverman, K., & Heil, S. H. (2007). *Contingency management in substance abuse treatment.* New York: Guilford Press.

Higgins, S. T., Wong, C. J., Badger G. J., Haug Ogden, D., & Dantona, R. L. (2000). Contingent reinforcement increases cocaine abstinence during outpatient treatment and 1 year of follow-up. *Journal of Consulting and Clinical Psychology, 68,* 64–72.

Lussier, J. P., Heil, S. H., Mongeon, J. A., Badger, G. J., & Higgins, S. T. (2006). A meta-analysis of voucher-based reinforcement therapy for substance use disorders. *Addiction, 101,* 192–203.

Stitzer, M. L., & Bigelow, G. E. (1982). Contingent reinforcement for reduced carbon monoxide levels in cigarette smokers. *Addictive Behaviors, 7,* 403–412.

CONTINUUM OF CARE

The concept of continuum of care responds to the challenge of providing appropriate services at appropriate times to individuals with multiple medical, psychosocial, and material needs. In individual patient care, the continuum of care refers to treatment planning that includes comprehensive, multidisciplinary services at levels that are tailored to individual patient needs. Structuring treatment and services along a continuum of care corresponds to a biopsychosocial perspective on health and is particularly important in the treatment of substance abuse and dependency, which are often accompanied by complex medical, mental health, and socioeconomic challenges. Interventions that address all of patients' salient needs are more likely to lead to optimal individual outcomes, including stable recovery from substance abuse. Continuum of care also refers to a systems-level approach to providing coordinated health and human services for client populations with multiple needs, such as dual diagnosis of substance dependency and mental illness, co-occurring medical conditions for which substance users are at elevated risk (tuberculosis, HIV, and hepatitis C), and homelessness. To promote a continuum of care across service systems, some federal funding organizations and state human services departments have urged or mandated service providers with overlapping client populations to collaborate in strategic planning, funding applications, professional training, client intake and referral processes, and in service provision. The systems-level continuum of care can increase access to and coordination of services, particularly for populations at high risk for falling out of care and services, including the homeless, the mentally ill, and substance abusers. Whether used in reference to individual patient care or in efforts to link various service systems, the concept of continuum of care aims to provide comprehensive, patient-centered treatment and support that improves treatment outcomes and quality of life. The potential benefits are clear; however, the challenges to creating a truly seamless continuum of care are many.

Substance Abuse Patients

Substance abuse disorders develop within a complex constellation of biological, psychosocial, and structural factors, and comprehensive treatment tailored to the patient's unique constellation may increase the likelihood of stable recovery: the continuum of patient care for substance abuse and dependency facilitates such comprehensive treatment. The array of treatment options available may be used sequentially or episodically as appropriate for an individual patient and may be described as ranging from less to more intensive in the nature of the intervention and from brief to long term in their duration. A structured patient assessment allows providers to determine the appropriate level of care and define specific treatment goals. Patient assessment includes signs and symptoms of withdrawal; treatment history; *Diagnostic and Statistical Manual of Mental Disorders* criteria for substance abuse disorders; the Global Assessment of Functioning, which measures social, psychological, and occupational function and level of impairment; general assessment of need, willingness, and cognitive ability to engage in treatment; the presence or absence of family and social support for treatment; and other diagnoses that may impact on the individual's response to substance abuse treatment.

Levels of Intensity

At the low-intensity end of the treatment continuum of care are outpatient interventions for people with moderate levels of substance abuse. These interventions include individual and/or family therapy sessions, group sessions, and support groups for substance abusers and those close to them. Sessions aim to decrease substance use behavior, strengthen coping and problem solving skills, and provide emotional and social support through the process of recovery. For people with dual diagnoses, such treatment may include support for adherence to care for mental illness or other co-occurring conditions. Brief, low-intensity interventions can be delivered in bimonthly sessions, or they may also be offered several times a week, and they may last for several weeks to a few months. Outpatient pharmacological treatments for management of opioid withdrawal, including buprenorphine and methadone, are long term. Day treatment programs, partial hospitalization, and inpatient rehabilitation lasting 2 to 4 weeks represent more intensive interventions for individuals for whom outpatient treatment has failed or who require a more structured intervention and more intensive monitoring. In addition to more intensive individual and group therapy, these interventions may offer comprehensive case management services and planning for appropriate follow-up care. Therapeutic communities provide such structure for sustained periods and are appropriate for people with longer histories of substance use and/or more severe substance use disorders. They offer life skills–building activities, including vocational training, occupational therapy, and general education in a highly structured setting. Medical detoxification, in which continuous medical attention is needed to manage symptoms of withdrawal, represents the most intensive extreme of the treatment continuum of care. Additional assessment criteria, including physical and psychological symptoms, are used to determine the need for medical detoxification. The medical team managing detoxification works in collaboration with medical specialists as necessary.

Continuing Care

Wherever patients find themselves along this continuum of treatment options, ongoing linkage to follow-up services and communication among treatment providers creates a smooth continuum of care. Patients may require different levels of treatment at different times and may undergo treatment several times before achieving stable recovery. Thus, post-treatment assessments and follow-up plans are essential elements of the continuum of care. Follow-up may include additional substance abuse treatment, such as outpatient groups for patients leaving an impatient stay or rehabilitation following medical detoxification.

Follow-up activities also include linking the patient to needed medical, mental health, and human services, and evidence suggests that providing such services along with substance abuse treatment can improve patient outcomes. Integration of care may occur along a centralized model in which multidisciplinary services are colocated at a single site. This model is intended to maximize the accessibility of services to patients and may also facilitate information sharing among service providers. The use in primary medical care settings of pharmacological treatment for dependency, such as naltrexone and buprenorphine, is one example of integrated services. A decentralized model links patients to service providers at separate sites through strengthened referral systems that may include reminder calls for all appointments, transportation and patient navigation among provider sites, and multidisciplinary team meetings to facilitate communication among providers. Both centralized and decentralized models can lead to better informed diagnoses that take full account of medical, mental health, and substance use-related factors. They facilitate coordination of multiple medication regimens, patient retention, and adherence to care, and thus, they strengthen the continuum of care for individual patients.

Challenges

Challenges to sustained integration of services occur at various levels. The enduring stigma of addiction may make some health care providers less willing incorporate treatment for substance abuse disorders. Cross-disciplinary provider education and training is on the rise, but medical providers may still be unfamiliar with the signs of substance use disorders and unaware of the availability of effective treatment options. Substance abuse treatment providers are often similarly unaware of how medical issues and treatment may affect their patients or how to help them access medical and mental health care. Systems for sharing records while safeguarding patient confidentiality are necessary in order for providers to collaborate across health care systems. Finally, differential systems and schedules of payment and reimbursement may create financial barriers to integrated medical, mental health, and substance abuse services.

Many of these barriers to integrated multidisciplinary care transcend the efforts of individual providers and health care organizations. Because of this, several federal and state funding entities, among them the Department of Housing and Urban Development and the Substance Abuse and Mental Health Services Administration, promote coordinated efforts to plan and structure services for populations whose needs significantly overlap. These populations include the homeless, the mentally ill, and people with substance use disorders, as well as the incarcerated, people newly released from correctional institutions, people living with HIV/AIDS, and the uninsured or underinsured.

Systems-Level Continuum of Care

Used in this sense the notion of a continuum of care expands to include the development of infrastructures that support coordinated service provision. The establishment of a systems-level continuum of care begins with the engagement of crucial stakeholders.

Among the stakeholders are representatives of patient populations and their families, funders, regulators, representatives of public and private managed care organizations, institutional administrators, and service providers. Stakeholder collaboration in strategic planning for services, funding applications, and implementation of coordinated care efforts can result in better identification of patient and consumer needs, more efficient use of funds, increased uptake of services, and reduced duplication of efforts. Creating memoranda of understanding among service providers is an effective mechanism to delineate how participating agencies will collaborate and collect and share information. Over time, such collaboration can foster better communication among service providers and the development of shared standards and common goals, in turn creating stronger foundations for integrated care. Examples of shared standards include reimbursement schedules for mental health care and substance abuse treatment that are on par with those for medical care, cross-training of providers to facilitate mental health and substance use treatment in primary care settings, and uniform applications for services and intake or assessment forms so that admission to one service agency facilitates admission to other, related services. Common goals range from shared indicators used for quality assurance and quality improvement to a shared mission statement that all stakeholders can embrace and that articulates the benefits that will accrue to a strengthened continuum of care.

Conclusion

In the 20th century, scientific, medical, and technological advances greatly expanded the range of treatments and services that health care systems can provide, and the pace of medical innovation suggests that advances will continue. Health care systems in turn have become increasingly complex, drawing policymakers, regulators, funders, and payers of health care costs into the delivery of health care. The complexity of these systems provides multiple opportunities for health care to become fragmented, duplicative, partial, and nonresponsive to patient needs. Patients with complex, long-term, and co-occurring conditions are disproportionately likely to receive suboptimal care due to fragmented service delivery. This group includes people with substance abuse disorders, and providers of substance abuse treatment have been among those most active in devising strategies to better coordinate the delivery of health care services. The notion of a continuum of care does not provide a uniform framework for overcoming this fragmentation, but it does suggest specific steps to turn the momentum toward fragmented health care around. These steps include tailor treatment plans to reflect individual patient needs and preferences, educate and cross-train professionals to increase knowledge about common co-occurring conditions and their treatment, promote sustained multidisciplinary collaboration among health care and human service providers, reduce duplication of assessments and services through sharing of information among service providers, promote parity of reimbursement for services along the continuum of care, and collaborate at all levels in policy making and strategic planning for serving communities with complex needs. Taken together, these measures serve to promote more efficient, responsive, and equitable health care systems and improve patient outcomes.

Julie Franks

See also Co-Occurring Disorders; Health Care System and Substance Abuse; Homeless, Substance Abuse and Treatment; Insurance Parity; Medical Consequences; Public Policy, Treatment; Substance Abuse and Mental Health Services Administration

Further Readings

Center for Mental Health Services. (2004). *Building bridges: Co-occurring mental illness and addiction: Consumers and service providers, policymakers, and researchers in dialogue* (DHHS Pub. No. SMA 04-3892). Rockville, MD: Substance Abuse and Mental Health Services Administration.

Grella, C. E., Gil-Rivas, V., & Cooper, L. (2004). Perceptions of mental health and substance abuse program administrators and staff on service delivery to persons with co-occurring substance abuse and mental disorders. *Journal of Behavioral Health Services and Research, 31*(1), 38–49.

Institute of Medicine. (2000). *Crossing the quality chasm: A new health system for the 21st century*. Washington, DC: National Academy Press.

McKay, J. R. (2006). Continuing care in the treatment of addictive disorders. *Current Psychiatry Reports, 8*(5), 355–362.

McLellan A. T., Weinstein, R. L., Shen, Q., Kendif, C., & Levine, M. (2005). Improving continuity of care in a public addiction treatment system with clinical case management. *American Journal on Addictions, 14*(5), 426–440.

Samet, J., Friedmann, P., & Saitz, R. (2001). Benefits of linking primary medical care and substance abuse services: Patient, provider, and societal perspectives. *Archives of Internal Medicine, 161*, 85–91.

Sylla, L., Bruce, R. D., Kamarulzaman, A., & Altice, F. L. (2007). Integration and co-location of HIV/AIDS, tuberculosis, and drug treatment services. *International Journal of Drug Policy, 18*, 306–312.

CO-OCCURRING DISORDERS

Co-occurring disorders are a combination of a substance use disorder (abuse or dependence) and another mental disorder, as established in the fourth text revision edition of the *Diagnostic and Statistical Manual of Mental Disorders* (*DSM-IV-TR*) of the American Psychological Association. It is estimated that 50% to 70% of people diagnosed with either a mental disorder or a substance use disorder will have a co-occurring disorder of the other type; therefore, it is crucial to address the topic of co-occurring disorders. This entry discusses a brief history of co-occurring disorders, incidence and prevalence, screening, assessment, treatment planning, treatment interventions and programs, and evidence-based practices. A list of resources for further information is also included.

Definitions of Terms

A vast number of combinations of disorders have been labeled co-occurring disorders. These include co-occurring substance use disorders in combination with mental disorders, serious mental illnesses, developmental disabilities, health or physical diagnoses, or personality disorders. The term also refers to a combination of substance use disorders (e.g., cocaine dependence and alcohol dependence) or a combination of mental disorders (e.g., depression and schizophrenia or an anxiety disorder co-occurring with a personality disorder). For the purposes of this entry, co-occurring disorders is defined as co-occurring substance use disorders (abuse or dependence) and mental disorders, as established in the *DSM-IV-TR*. A diagnosis of co-occurring disorders can be made when at least one disorder of each type can be established independently of the other, when neither can be documented as a cluster of symptoms resulting from the other.

Substance Use Disorders

Substance abuse, as defined by the *DSM-IV-TR*, is a maladaptive pattern of substance use leading to clinically significant impairment or distress. Substance abuse is manifested by recurrent and significant negative or adverse consequences related to the recurrent use of substances. These negative consequences include repeated failure to fulfill major responsibilities at work, school, or home; repeated use in situations that are physically hazardous; and recurrent legal, social, or interpersonal problems related to the use of the substance.

According to the *DSM-IV-TR*, substance dependence is a maladaptive pattern of substance use, leading to clinically significant impairment or distress. It can be manifested by increased tolerance, a withdrawal syndrome, and/or a number of behavioral symptoms. These symptoms include having a desire to cut down or control the use of the substance; using the substance more than was intended; giving up important social, occupational, or recreational activities; or continuing to use despite knowledge that use affects a recurrent physical or mental health problem. The essential feature of substance dependence is impaired control over the use of the substance.

Mental Disorders

The *DSM-IV-TR* also provides the standard diagnostic criteria for mental disorders that comprise co-occurring disorders. Co-occurring mental disorders fall under a number of different categories. These include affective disorders, anxiety disorders, psychotic disorders, and personality disorders.

Affective disorders (also referred to as mood disorders) are characterized by persistent or episodic exaggerations of emotional states. Some examples of the emotional states include depression, mania, euphoria, dysphoria, anger, and irritability.

Anxiety disorders are characterized by felt anxiety at a frequency or intensity that causes impairment in functioning. Other symptoms may include affective flattening, alogia, apathy, avolition, and social withdrawal. Anxiety disorders include social phobia, panic disorder, and post-traumatic stress disorders.

Psychotic disorders include serious mental disorders, including schizophrenia, in which the person loses touch with reality. Hallucinations and delusions are generally considered symptoms of a psychotic disorder. Delusions are false beliefs that significantly hinder a person's ability to function; hallucinations are false perceptions in which a person sees, hears, feels, or smells things that are not there.

Schizophrenia is one of the most common of the psychotic disorders. Schizophrenia is a persistent, often chronic mental disorder affecting a variety of aspects of cognition, affect, and behavior. In addition to hallucinations and delusions, diagnostic symptoms may include disconnected and illogical thinking, disorganized speech, or catatonic behavior. Peculiar behaviors may be indicative of social withdrawal and disinterest, occupational dysfunction, and poor self-care and hygiene.

Although everyone has a unique personality made up of specific personality traits, people with personality disorders have enduring personality traits that cause impairment in social or occupational functioning or personal distress. The *DSM-IV-TR* defines a personality disorder as an enduring pattern of inner experience and behavior that deviates markedly from the expectations of the individual's culture. This pattern may be manifested in ways of perceiving and interpreting self, other people, and events, as well as the range, intensity, lability, and appropriateness of emotional responses, interpersonal functioning, and/or impulse control. Symptoms are organized into three clusters: Cluster A involves odd or eccentric behavior, including paranoid, schizoid, and schizotypal personality disorders; Cluster B involves dramatic, emotional, or erratic behavior, including antisocial, borderline, histrionic, and narcissistic personality disorders; and Cluster C involves anxious, fearful behavior, including avoidant, dependent, and obsessive-compulsive personality disorders.

Co-Occurring Disorders

Historically, there are a number of terms that have referred to co-occurring disorders. Currently, concern has been expressed among consumer advocacy groups about terminology. People object to being classified and labeled by a diagnosis that does not take into account the entire person. Historically, definitions did not reflect this person-centered terminology.

They also tended to reflect the separation between mental health and substance use disorder professionals and an attempt to argue for the primacy of one disorder over the other.

The following terms have been used to describe co-occurring disorders: dual diagnosis, dual disorders, comorbid disorders, MICA (mentally ill chemical abuser), MISU (mentally ill substance using), MISA (mentally ill substance abuser), CAMI (chemically abusing mentally ill), SAMI (substance abusing mentally ill), MICD (mentally ill chemically dependent), and ICOPSD (individuals with co-occurring psychiatric and substance disorders).

The 2002 Substance Abuse and Mental Health Services Administration (SAMHSA) report to Congress defines co-occurring disorders as individuals who have at least one mental disorder as well as an alcohol or drug use disorder. Although these disorders may interact differently in any one person (e.g., an episode of depression may trigger a relapse into alcohol abuse, or cocaine use may exacerbate schizophrenic symptoms), at least one disorder of each type can be diagnosed independently of the other. SAMHSA's report to Congress also indicated the following:

- Co-occurring disorders may include any combination of two or more substance abuse disorders and mental disorders identified in the *Diagnostic and Statistical Manual of Mental Disorders, Fourth Edition* (*DSM-IV*).
- There are no specific combinations of substance abuse disorders and mental disorders that are defined uniquely as co-occurring disorders.
- Substance abuse and mental health problems (such as binge drinking by people with mental disorders) that do not reach the diagnostic threshold are also part of the co-occurring disorders landscape and may offer opportunities for early intervention.
- Both substance abuse disorders and mental disorders have biological, psychological, and social components.
- Co-occurring disorders may vary among individuals and in the same individual over time.
- Both disorders may be severe or mild, or one may be more severe than the other.

History

Historically, the fields of mental health and substance use disorder treatment have been divided into two separate entities (or silos) resulting in splits in service provisions to consumers with co-occurring disorders. This separation has led to several different approaches to the treatment of those with co-occurring disorders. One approach has been sequential, to treat one disorder first and then treat the second. Another approach has been a separate, but concurrent one in which both disorders were treated at the same time but in different settings. Currently, there is a thrust for an integrated treatment model for co-occurring disorders, in which both disorders are treated simultaneously in the same setting.

Barriers to Integrated Treatment

There have been many far-reaching barriers to integrated treatment. On the local and state governmental levels, there has often been a formal separation of service providers for mental health and substance use disorders. These formal and informal separations have led to separate funding streams, licensing requirements and entities, professional credentials, and education and training. Because of these separations, competition (and often heated debate) has arisen between these areas.

Historically, education and training for alcohol and other drug abuse counselors in the 1960s and 1970s grew out of the experiential philosophy of the Alcoholics Anonymous and Narcotics Anonymous approaches, encouraging people in recovery to become counselors to others. Mental health clinicians focused on educational, academic, and scientific methods. The gap between mental health and substance abuse professionals widened and debates grew with disagreements about prescribing medication.

Recently, the two silos are coming together because of a number of influences. Recent advances in neurophysiology and neuropsychology (i.e., the study of brain-based behavior; the roles of neurochemicals and their effects on learning, cognition, and emotions; and the effects of psychoactive substances on the brain) have led to an increased understanding of the needs of individuals with co-occurring disorders. Research studies are documenting the incidence and prevalence of co-occurring disorders and the disproportionate number of those with a mental disorder having a substance use disorder and vice versa. Finally, from all levels of government and service provision, SAMHSA, state agencies, and local service providers, there are movements toward an integrated model of screening, assessment, treatment planning, and treatment for co-occurring disorders.

Incidence and Prevalence

In a review of studies in the 1980s and 1990s, SAMHMSA found that studies conducted in substance abuse programs typically reported that 50% to 75% of clients had some type of co-occurring mental health disorder (although not usually a severe mental disorder). Studies conducted in mental health settings reported that between 20% and 50% of their clients had a co-occurring substance use disorder. In its 2006 survey of the general population (National Survey on Drug Use and Health), SAMHSA reported the following:

- In 2005, adults who used illicit drugs in the past year were significantly more likely to have a serious psychological distress (SPD) compared to adults who did not use an illicit drug (22% vs. 9.6%).
- Past-year illicit drug use was higher among adults with SPD (26.9 percent) than among adults without SPD (12.1%). Similarly, the rate of past-month cigarette use was higher among adults with SPD (42.8%) than among adults without SPD (24.5%).
- The rate of heavy alcohol use (drinking five or more drinks on the same occasion; i.e., at the same time or within a couple of hours of each other, on each of 5 or more days in the past 30 days) among adults with SPD in the past year was higher (9.4%) than the rate reported among adults without SPD in the past year (6.8%). Similarly, among adults with SPD, the rate of binge alcohol use (drinking five or more drinks on the same occasion on at least 1 day in the past 30 days) was 28.9%, higher than the 23.5% among adults who did not meet the criteria for SPD.
- SPD in the past year was associated with past-year substance dependence or abuse in 2005. Among adults with SPD in 2005, 21.3% (5.2 million) were dependent on or abused illicit drugs or alcohol. The rate among adults without SPD was 7.7% (14.9 million).

Similarly, M. P. McGovern and colleagues reported in their 2006 survey that several co-occurring disorders were extremely common with substance use disorders: mood disorders (40%–42%), anxiety disorders (24%–27%), post-traumatic stress disorder (24%–27%), severe mental illnesses (16%–21%), antisocial personality disorder (18%–20%), and borderline personality disorder (17%–18%). In addition, the prevalence of co-occurring disorders among incarcerated populations is extremely high: 72% of detainees in jails and prisons with severe mental disorders also have a substance use disorder.

Researchers and treatment professionals have also noted the dramatic impact the use of substances (even if it does not reach the diagnostic level of substance abuse) can have on a person with serious mental illness. The difficulties arising during the course of treatment for those with serious mental illness, complicated by a substance use disorder, have also been reported.

Screening, Assessment, and Treatment Planning

According to SAMHSA's Co-Occurring Center for Excellence (COCE), clients with co-occurring disorders are best served through an integrated screening, assessment, and treatment planning process that addresses both substance use and mental disorders, each in the context of the other. In addition, this process informs and guides the provision of appropriate, client-centered services to persons with co-occurring disorders.

Screening

Screening is conducted to determine the likelihood that a client has co-occurring substance use and mental disorders or that his or her presenting signs, symptoms, or behaviors may be influenced by co-occurring issues. The purpose is not to establish the presence or specific type of such a disorder or to make a diagnosis but to establish the need for an in-depth assessment. Screening is a formal process that typically is brief and occurs soon after the client presents for services. There are generally few legal or professional restraints on who may conduct a screening (although proper training is essential), and screening can take place in a wide variety of settings (health and human services, educational, criminal justice, or homeless settings). A vast array of appropriate screening tools are summarized in *Treatment Improvement Protocol (TIP) 42*, published by SAMHSA. Some of the most common include the Mental Health Screening Form-III and the Simple Screening Instrument (SSI) for substance use disorders.

Assessment

Assessment is a process of gathering information and engaging in a process with the client that enables the provider to establish (or rule out) the presence or absence of a co-occurring disorder. It determines the client's readiness for change, identifies client strengths or problem areas that may affect the processes of treatment and recovery, and engages the client in the development of an appropriate treatment relationship. An integrated assessment for co-occurring disorders may be conducted by a qualified mental health or substance use disorder professional who has the necessary specialized training and skills. The co-occurring disorder diagnosis is made by a psychiatrist, psychologist, counselor, or other qualified professional. Assessment is an ongoing process that should be repeated over time to capture the changing nature of the person's status. A comprehensive assessment serves as the basis for an individualized integrated treatment plan.

A number of screening and assessment instruments are summarized and information on ordering them is provided in *Treatment Improvement Protocol (TIP) 42*. Some of these include the Addiction Severity Index (ASI), the Beck Depression Inventory II (BDI-II), the Global Appraisal of Individual Need (GAIN), the Michigan Alcoholism Screening Test (MAST), the Psychiatric Research Interview for Substance and Mental Disorders (PRISM), the Structured Clinical Interview for DSM-IV Disorders (SCID-IV), the Symptom Distress Scale (SDS), and the University of Rhode Island Change Assessment Scale (URICA).

Treatment Planning

An integrated treatment planning process involves a comprehensive set of staged, integrated program placements and treatment interventions for each disorder that is adjusted as needed to take into account issues related to the other disorder. The plan is matched to the individual needs, readiness, preferences, and personal goals of the client.

According to COCE, the components of a client-centered treatment plan include acute safety needs, severity of mental and substance use disorders, appropriate care setting, diagnosis, disability, strengths and skills, availability and continuity of recovery support, cultural context, problem priorities, and the state of recovery or client's readiness to change behaviors relating to each problem. In addition, treatment planning for

people with co-occurring disorders should be designed according to the principle of mental disorder dual (or multiple) primary treatment. Each disorder is considered primary; each has a specific intervention that takes into account the other disorder.

Treatment Programs

Quadrants of Care

The quadrants of care model has been developed by the National Association of State Alcohol and Drug Abuse Directors (NASADAD) and the National Association of State Mental Health Program Directors (NASMHPD). This model provides a conceptual framework that classifies consumers in four basic groups based on relative symptom severity. It provides a classification of service coordination by severity in the context of substance abuse and mental health settings.

The four-quadrant model provides a structure for moving beyond minimal coordination to fostering consultation, collaboration, and integration among systems and providers to deliver appropriate care to every client with co-occurring disorders. The model has two primary uses, as outlined by NASADAD and NASMHPD: to help conceptualize an individual consumer's treatment and to guide improvements in system integration, including efficient allocation of resources.

Overarching Principles

COCE has developed a set of principles to guide services when considering treatment provided to individuals with co-occurring disorders:

Principle 1: Co-occurring disorders are to be expected in all behavioral health settings, and system planning must address the need to serve people with co-occurring disorders in all policies, regulations, funding mechanisms, and programming.

Principle 2: An integrated system of mental health and addiction services that emphasizes continuity and quality is in the best interest of consumers, providers, programs, funders, and systems.

Principle 3: The integrated system of care must be accessible from multiple points of entry (i.e., no wrong door) and be perceived as caring and accepting by the consumer.

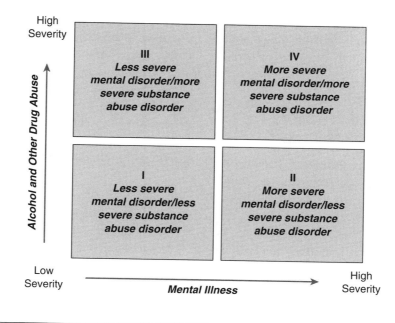

Figure 1   Co-Occurring Disorders by Severity

Sources: Center for Substance Abuse Treatment. (2006). *Definitions and terms relating to co-occurring disorders* (p. 5). COCE Overview Paper 1 (DHHS Publication No. SMA 06-4163). Rockville, MD: Substance Abuse and Mental Health Services Administration, and Center for Mental Health Services. Retrieved April 14, 2007, from http://coce.samhsa.gov/cod_resources/PDF/ DefinitionsandTerms-OP1.pdf; National Association of State Mental Health Program Directors & National Association of State Alcohol and Drug Abuse Directors. (1998). *National dialogue on co-occurring mental health and substance abuse disorders.* Washington, DC: National Association of State Alcohol and Drug Abuse Directors.

Principle 4: The system of care for co-occurring disorders should not be limited to a single "correct" model or approach.

Principle 5: The system of care must reflect the importance of the partnership between science and service and support both the application of evidence and consensus-based practices for persons with co-occurring disorders and evaluation of the efforts of existing programs and services.

Principle 6: Behavioral health systems must collaborate with professionals in primary care, human services, housing, criminal justice, education, and related fields in order to meet the complex needs of persons with co-occurring disorders.

Principle 7: Co-occurring disorders must be expected when evaluating any person, and clinical services should incorporate this assumption into all screening, assessment, and treatment planning.

Principle 8: Within the treatment context, both co-occurring disorders are considered primary.

Principle 9: Empathy, respect, and belief in the individual's capacity for recovery are fundamental provider attitudes.

Principle 10: Treatment should be individualized to accommodate the specific needs, personal goals, and cultural perspectives of unique individuals in different stages of change.

Principle 11: The special needs of children and adolescents must be explicitly recognized and addressed in all phases of assessment, treatment planning, and service delivery.

Principle 12: The contribution of the community to the course of recovery for consumers with co-occurring disorders and the contribution of consumers with co-occurring disorders to the community must be explicitly recognized in program policy, treatment planning, and consumer advocacy.

Finally, it is important to keep in mind that treatment must provide integrated interventions addressing both disorders, that an individual with co-occurring disorders may require recurrent episodes of treatment, and that treatment must be culturally competent.

Evidence-Based Practices for Co-Occurring Disorders

Although most practitioners in the mental health, substance use disorder, and co-occurring disorder fields agree that evidence-based practices (EBPs) improve treatment for consumers, there currently exists a great deal of debate about what constitutes or defines an evidence-based practice. COCE defines an EBP as one which, based on research findings and expert or consensus opinion about available evidence, is expected to produce a specific clinical outcome (measurable change in client status). COCE includes the multiple streams of evidence approach suggested by the Institute of Medicine (IOM). The IOM argues for the integration of three components of EBPs: best research evidence, clinician expertise, and patient values. These three types of evidence can be integrated through evidence-based thinking. Evidence-based thinking may be undertaken to formally designate practices as evidence based or it may be used in day-to-day clinical decision making. Based on the overarching principles outlined above, the following categories and examples of EBP's have been recommended by COCE. At the treatment level, interventions that have their own evidence to support them as EBPs are frequently a part of a comprehensive and integrated response to persons with co-occurring disorders. These interventions include

- psychopharmacological interventions (e.g., desipramine and bupropion for people with cocaine dependence and depression),
- motivational interventions (e.g., Motivational Enhancement Therapy), and
- behavioral interventions (e.g., contingency management).

At the program level, the following models have an evidence base for producing positive clinical outcomes for persons with co-occurring disorders:

- modified therapeutic communities,
- integrated dual disorders treatment, and
- assertive community treatment.

Evidence-based programs and treatment models continue to be developed and research studies replicated. The National Registry of Effective Programs and Practices is a decision-support tool that assesses the strength of evidence and readiness for dissemination of a variety of mental health and substance abuse prevention and treatment interventions. This tool provides an excellent and up-to-date resource for providers to remain current on EBPs.

Laurie J. Rokutani

See also Assessment; *Diagnostic and Statistical Manual of Mental Disorders*; Double Trouble; Evidence-Based Treatment; Screening; Substance Abuse; Substance Dependence; Substance Use Disorders; Treatment of Alcohol and Drug Use Disorders

Further Readings

American Psychiatric Association. (2000). *Diagnostic and statistical manual of mental disorders* (4th ed., text rev.). Washington, DC: Author.

American Society of Addiction Medicine. (2001). *Patient placement criteria for the treatment of substance-related disorders: ASAM PPC-2R* (2nd ed.). Chevy Chase, MD: Author.

Center for Substance Abuse Treatment. (2005). *Tip 42: Substance abuse treatment for persons with co-occurring disorders* (Inventory No. BKD515). Rockville, MD: Substance Abuse and Mental Health Services Administration. Available from http://ncadi.samhsa.gov

Center for Substance Abuse Treatment. (2006). *Overview paper 2: Screening, assessment, and treatment planning for persons with co-occurring disorders.* (Inventory No. PHD1131). Rockville, MD: Substance Abuse and Mental Health Services Administration, and Center for Mental Health Services. Available from http://ncadi.samhsa.gov

Center for Substance Abuse Treatment. (2006). *Overview paper 5: Understanding evidence-based practices for co-occurring disorders* (Inventory No. [SMA] 07-4278). Rockville, MD: Substance Abuse and Mental Health Services Administration, and Center for Mental Health Services. Available from http://ncadi.samhsa.gov

McGovern, M. P., Xie, H. Y., Segal, S. R., Siembab, L., & Drake, R. E. (2006). Addiction treatment services and co-occurring disorders: Prevalence estimates, treatment practices, and barriers. *Journal of Substance Abuse Treatment, 31*(3), 267–275.

National GAINS Center for People with Co-Occurring Disorders in the Justice System. (2001). The prevalence of co-occurring mental illness and substance use disorders in jails. *Fact Sheet Series*. Delmar, NY: Author. Retrieved April 14, 2007, from http://www.gainscenter.samhsa .gov/pdfs/disorders/gainsjailprev.pdf

National Registry of Evidence-based Programs and Practices (NREPP): http://nrepp.samhsa.gov

Substance Abuse and Mental Health Services Administration. (2002). *Report to Congress on the treatment and prevention of co-occurring substance abuse and mental disorders*. Retrieved April 14, 2007, from http://www.samhsa.gov/reports/ congress2002

Substance Abuse and Mental Health Services Administration. (2006). *NSDUH: Results from the 2006 National Survey on Drug Use and Health: National findings* (Inventory No. [SMA] 07-4293). Rockville, MD: Author. Available from http://ncadi.samhsa.gov

COUNSELING APPROACHES

Substance abuse is an important social and public health issue in the United States. As a result of increased public awareness of the negative consequences associated with drug and alcohol abuse, more and more people are entering treatment, both voluntarily and involuntarily (i.e., mandated). Therapists working with substance-abusing clients typically employ strategies, techniques, and skills to guide the treatment process and to help the client deal with his or her concerns. In particular, most therapists conceptualize their clients based on a preferred counseling model, and using this framework, they develop treatment plans based on the presenting client issues and needs. Consequently, a multitude of different approaches have been developed to treat substance abusing patients. In fact, the past 20 years has seen tremendous progress in the development of effective treatments for substance use disorders including individual, couples, family, and group treatments.

Substance Abuse Treatment

Substance abuse is primarily characterized by two symptoms: (1) compulsive drug craving and (2) continued use despite negative consequences. Moreover, many chronic substance users experience relapses, even after lengthy periods of sobriety. Interestingly, substance abusers tend to relapse at rates similar to

those for people diagnosed with diabetes, hypertension, and asthma. Thus, treatment is not believed to be a onetime experience, and clients may reenter treatment several times before finally achieving the desired results. From this vantage, treatment is used as a way to increase the amount of time between relapses, with the goal of decreasing the intensity each time until ultimately abstinence is achieved.

Although the long-term goal of substance abuse treatment is to assist an individual in achieving lasting abstinence, the more immediate goal of this process is to reduce substance consumption, improve the individual's level of functioning, and address any medical and social issues developed as a result of the substance use.

Ingredients of Effective Treatment

Research over the past 30 years has demonstrated that substance abuse treatment can be effective in helping people change unhealthy behaviors, avoid relapse, and successfully refrain from a return to substance abuse and addiction. As stated above, substance abuse treatment may not be successful the first time, and thus, several treatment episodes may be necessary before an individual is able to achieve and maintain abstinence. The National Institute on Drug Abuse recommends the following tenets serve as the foundation for any substance abuse treatment program:

1. treatment must be easily accessed;
2. effective treatment attends to multiple client needs, not just his or her addiction;
3. no single treatment is appropriate for all individuals;
4. individual treatment plans should be frequently reviewed and modified based on client's progress (or lack thereof);
5. client retention is critical for treatment effectiveness;
6. counseling and behavioral therapies are key ingredients of nearly all addiction treatments;
7. in some cases, medications may be an important part of the treatment plan, along with counseling;
8. individuals with comorbid mental disorders should receive integrated mental health and substance abuse treatment;
9. medical management of withdrawal alone does little to change long-term substance use;

10. effective treatment can be voluntary or mandated;

11. substance use during treatment must be continuously monitored;

12. treatment should include information on high-risk behaviors for infection for HIV/AIDS, hepatitis B and C, and tuberculosis; and

13. successful recovery may require multiple episodes of treatment.

Counseling Approaches

There are numerous theories and viewpoints that describe the development and maintenance of substance misuse and abuse. However, most treatment providers would agree that the mainstay of treatment for alcoholism and drug abuse comes in the form of peer support and psychosocial talk therapies. Twelve-Step peer support groups (e.g., Alcoholics Anonymous [AA], and Narcotics Anonymous [NA]) are the largest and most widely known support groups for individuals with drinking and drug problems. Meetings consist mainly of discussions of participants' problems with alcohol and other drugs, with testimonials from those who have recovered. Participants are encouraged to work the Twelve Steps of AA, which include admitting powerlessness over alcohol and drugs, believing that a higher power can restore sanity, making a moral inventory of oneself, and so forth. The program promotes total abstinence from psychoactive substances.

The most commonly used formal treatment approach in the vast majority of community-based treatment programs is derived from the Twelve-Step model; the most formalized version of this approach is referred to as Twelve-Step Facilitation (TSF) treatment. In TSF, substance dependence is viewed not as symptomatic of another illness, but as a primary problem with biological, emotional, and spiritual underpinnings and presenting features. Alcoholism and drug abuse are seen as progressive illnesses, marked largely by denial. The primary goals of treatment are to (a) encourage clients to work through their denial and (b) work the Twelve Steps. These goals are typically accomplished in the context of individual and group therapy, with strong encouragement to attend Twelve-Step support groups on a regular basis. Along with individual and group counseling, medical services and religious services are also considered important parts of treatment because the disease of alcoholism and other drug use is viewed as affecting the biological and spiritual realms, as well as psychosocial functioning.

One of the strongest predictors of success of substance abuse treatment has been the client's motivation to change. According to authors Susan Gray and Marilyn Zide, a treatment intervention that has grown out of this observation is Motivational Enhancement Therapy (MET). Using a technique called motivational interviewing, the goal of MET is to encourage clients to assume responsibility for helping themselves and increasing their desire to change. As such, motivational interviewing incorporates a directive, client-centered approach designed to promote change by assisting clients with exploring and resolving ambivalence about the change process. Several studies (e.g., Bill Saunders and colleagues, J. Douglas Sellman and colleagues) have now demonstrated that MET is an effective treatment for alcoholism and other drug abuse.

Behavioral and cognitive behavioral treatments have been among the most widely used and investigated psychosocial counseling approaches for substance abuse and dependence. From a behavioral perspective, all human behavior, both good and bad (e.g., substance abuse), is learned. Thus, Willliam McCauliffe and Robert Gordon concluded that addiction develops from a conditioned response, which tends to become stronger as a result of the quality, number, and size of the reinforcers. For example, a behavioralist would contend that a client's inability to remain abstinent is a direct result of him or her having a lengthy history of having drinking behavior reinforced, which has contributed to a progressively higher rate of drinking or drug use. In other words, addiction is simply an operantly conditioned behavior which occurs at a high rate.

Cognitive behavioral therapy (CBT) teaches clients coping skills to reduce or eliminate drinking or substance use. For example, common CBT techniques include identifying high-risk situations for relapse, instruction and rehearsal strategies for coping with those situations, self-monitoring and behavioral analysis of substance use, strategies for recognizing and coping with cravings, coping with lapses, and instruction on problem solving.

From a psychoanalytic vantage, substance abuse is considered a symptom of a deficient ego, which according to this model, is responsible for mediating internal demands with the realities of the external world. More specifically, substance abusing individuals are thought to lack the ability to adequately take care of themselves and as a result, expose themselves to a variety of risks (e.g., legal, health, safety). Thus, the goal of psychoanalytic treatment is to help the client improve ego strength to effectively cope with the demands of the outside world so that he or she does not have to resort to unhealthy substance use.

Family-Couples Counseling

More than 25 years ago, the National Institute on Alcohol Abuse and Alcoholism described couples and family therapy as one of the most outstanding advances in the area of treatment of alcoholism. The critical role of the family in the development and maintenance of substance abuse is now widely acknowledged by researchers and practitioners alike. As a result, more and more service providers are intervening with the family as a way to reduce or eliminate abusive drinking or drug use by one or more of its members.

Family treatment for substance abuse disorders considers the alcohol and drug use to have a functional role in the family and that it is an expression of some deeper, unresolved issue. The best known and most widely used is the family disease model. This family disease model views addiction as an illness of the family; it affects not only the substance abuser, but also members of the family. According to the family systems model, addiction is viewed as a major organizing principle of the relationships between family members. The substance abuse represents an unhealthy attempt to cope with difficulties or problems and also serves as a tool to regulate family interactions. Family behavioral models view addiction as a behavior learned through social relations that is reinforced by experience. Thus, substance use can be maintained by triggering cues and postsubstance-using consequences in the family environment.

Behavioral Couples Therapy (BCT) is an evidence-based family treatment for alcoholism and drug abuse. The results of multiple studies conducted during the last 3 decades indicate that participation in BCT by married or cohabiting substance abusing patients, compared to more traditional individual-based interventions, results in greater reductions in substance use, higher levels of relationship satisfaction,

greater reductions in partner violence, and more favorable cost-benefit and cost-effectiveness.

Group Counseling

As Bruce Rounsaville and Kathleen Carroll have noted, the use of one therapist to treat a single client during a given clinical hour has largely given way to group therapy as the most common treatment approach in community-based substance abuse treatment. Several factors have contributed to the widespread use of group therapy in the treatment of substance abusers. Without question, during this time of cost containment and managed care, a fundamental advantage of group therapy is that it is more cost-effective; in particular, group treatment approaches are less costly to deliver. For instance, most groups typically have six members and may have two therapists, thus resulting in a tripling of the number of clients per therapy hour over individual therapy. When one considers the use of a group intervention with eight clients treated by one therapist compared to standard individual treatment with one client treated by one therapist, the group treatment is clearly much less costly to deliver. In addition to economic advantages, Irving Yalom also noted that group treatment capitalizes on the operation of a number of curative factors associated with groups as a form of treatment. However, it is worth mentioning that while surveys have found group therapy is the most common form of treatment in substance abuse programs, most patients are also concurrently involved in one-on-one individual counseling.

Conclusion

From a quality of care perspective, the paramount goal of any therapy is to deliver the most effective treatment available to those seeking help, based on patients' needs and characteristics. The models listed above have been found to be effective approaches to working with clients. Ultimately, the decision to use a particular counseling approach should be guided by the therapist's comfort level and familiarity with the treatment, as well as the client's presenting issues and concerns.

Keith Klostermann

See also Behavioral Couples Therapy; Cognitive Behavioral Therapy; Evidence-Based Treatment: Family Therapy; Group Therapy and Counseling; Motivational Enhancement Therapy; Twelve-Step Facilitation

Further Readings

Gray, S. W., & Zide, M. R. (2006). *Psychopathology: A competency-based treatment model for social workers.* Belmont, CA: Thomson.

National Institute on Drug Abuse. (2000). *Principles of HIV prevention in drug-abusing populations* (National Institute of Health 00-4812). Retrieved from http://www.drugabuse.gov/pohp/index.html

Rounsaville, B. J., & Carroll, K. M. (1997). Individual psychotherapy. In. J. H. Lowinson, P. Ruiz, R. B. Millman, & J. G. Langrod (Eds.), *Substance abuse: A comprehensive textbook* (3rd ed., pp. 430–439). Baltimore: Williams & Wilkins.

Sellman, J. D., Sullivan, P. F., Dore, G. M., Adamson, S. J., & MacEwan, I. (2001). A randomized controlled trial of Motivational Enhancement Therapy (MET) for mild to moderate alcohol dependence. *Journal of Studies on Alcohol, 62,* 389–396.

Saunders, B., Wilkinson, C., & Phillips, M. (1995). The impact of a brief motivational intervention with opiate users attending a methadone program. *Addiction, 90,* 415–424.

Stinchfield, R., Owen, P. L., & Winters, K. C. (1994). Group therapy for substance abuse: A review of the empirical evidence. In A. Fuhriman & G. M. Burlinggame (Eds.), *Handbook of group therapy: An empirical and clinical synthesis* (pp. 458–486). New York: Wiley.

Yalom, I. (1995). *The theory and practice of group psychotherapy* (4th ed.). New York: Basic Books.

COURT-MANDATED TREATMENT

Court-mandated substance abuse treatment uses extrinsic motivators to enforce treatment engagement and compliance, with the underlying premise that personal choice may be important but not essential to treatment success. Proponents of compulsory treatment cite the high relapse rates found in voluntary treatment programs, increases in addiction and drug-related crime rates, and the high economic, health, and emotional cost of illicit drug use to support legal enforcement of substance abuse treatment. Research also supports the use of social control strategies as intrinsic motivation is not universally sufficient to encourage treatment engagement or sustain treatment involvement long enough to result in posttreatment behavior change. Alternatively, opponents of compulsory treatment assert that forced treatment violates U.S. beliefs in individualism and personal choice.

The U.S. legal system, business employers, families, and friends of those with substance use disorders (SUD) utilize various forms of coercion to pressure individuals into substance abuse treatment. Researchers classify these coercive methods as legal, formal, or informal mandates according to the originating source. For example, judges generate legal mandates following adjudication for criminal behavior such as illicit substance use, possession, or sales, and crimes committed while under the influence of illicit substances. Court orders may stipulate that the SUD client must participate in various treatment programs while on parole or probation. These can include inpatient or outpatient treatment, intensive supervision, diversion programs for first-time nonviolent offenders, day-treatment programs, other contingency management programs, and drug courts. Legally mandated programs also include placement in prison-based programs such as therapeutic community programs. These and similar intensive substance abuse treatment programs are available for nonviolent offenders during the last portion of their incarceration and usually involve postrelease monitoring for continued compliance.

Businesses and government social services agencies, for example, the Child Protection Agency, utilize formal mandates to pressure substance abusing employees or clients to participate in treatment. Employers may require drug screening, for example, urinalysis, breathalyzer, saliva testing, or hair cuticle testing, to monitor employee behavior. Employers also may offer drug abuse treatment as a contingency to remaining employed. Social service agencies may compel addicted clients to seek treatment to maintain or gain custody of their children or to qualify for benefits under programs such as the 1996 Welfare Reform Act (Temporary Assistance for Needy Families—TANF).

Informal mandates occur when families and friends apply social pressure in an effort to convince loved ones to seek substance abuse treatment. Family interventions allow family members to voice their concerns regarding substance use in a nonconfrontational, supportive, yet firm manner and to convince the abuser to seek professional help. Families and friends also utilize consequences for refusal to seek treatment, including ostracism and withdrawal of financial and emotional support.

History

Historians trace nonnative psychoactive substance use within the United States to the late 1800s when physicians prescribed cocaine and heroin as medicine. Females constituted the majority of patients receiving these medicines, and society considered their subsequent addiction as the norm for genteel women. By the early 1900s, the population of addicted individuals had expanded to include poor males and societal acceptance of addiction waned. In 1914, the U.S. government passed the Harrison Narcotics Tax Act, the first legal mandate regarding the sale and use of psychoactive substances. This law controlled the amount of narcotics that physicians dispensed and ensured that physicians only dispensed narcotics during their professional practice. Additionally, the law forced heroin addicts to check themselves into hospitals or sanitariums as ill patients in order to receive heroin legally. However, as addiction was not considered a disease during the early 1900s, many addicts resorted to other illegal means to support their addiction. By 1918, a Congressional investigation into the outcome of the Harrison Act revealed that the rate of substance abuse increased rather than decreased and that drug trafficking and use had gone underground due to fear of legal penalties.

Between 1918 and 1957, efforts to stop the abuse of heroin and cocaine changed to punitive legal consequences for use and campaigns designed to demonize drug addicts. Treatment programs that developed between 1914 and 1925 focused on controlling rather than stopping drug use, trying to ensure that clients continued to work and behave as responsible citizens. After 1925, the campaigns to demonize addicts effectively generated mass fear of substance users. In response, federal laws shifted from drug use control to drug abstinence and treatment programs that made controlled use of heroin illegal.

Punitive efforts to curb substance abuse were not effective, and by the 1960s, the rate of drug addiction, relapse, and drug-related crime had risen alarmingly. In response, between 1961 and 1962, California (e.g., California Civil Addict Program) and New York (e.g., Metcalf-Volker Narcotic Addict Commitment Act) passed the first civil laws authorizing compulsory treatment. Following these models, in 1966, the federal government passed a federal civil commitment program, the Narcotic Addict Rehabilitation Act (NARA P.L. 89-793) and in 1972, created the Treatment to Alternatives Street Crime program (TASC). These federal programs initially targeted prison offenders, offered community-based drug treatment as an alternative to incarceration, and acted as precursors to the creation of drug courts in 1989.

Effectiveness

Federally funded national treatment studies, which include the Drug Abuse Reporting Program, from 1969 to 1972; the Treatment Outcome Prospective Study, from 1979 to 1981; and the Drug Abuse Treatment Outcome Studies, from 1990 to 1993, revealed that substance abuse treatment effectively reduces drug use and associated crime. However, self-referral and voluntary engagement in treatment requires client recognition of a substance use problem and the motivation to change. Although, certain therapeutic programs (e.g., Motivational Enhancement Therapy) use strategies to increase problem awareness and encourage motivation for change, many addicts still fail to engage in treatment or leave shortly after treatment has begun. Research reveals that clients who are coerced into treatment exhibit lower levels of intrinsic motivation at intake and lower levels of problem recognition, but treatment outcomes are just as good as or better than the outcomes of self-referred SUD clients. In short, court-mandated treatment forces SUD clients through the treatment door, increasing the probability of successful change.

The national treatment studies also revealed a positive correlation between length of treatment and treatment success. Clients staying in treatment longer than 90 days are less likely to relapse, and the optimum treatment length is 1 year. Self-referred clients who voluntarily engage in treatment are more likely than mandated clients are to leave treatment early. Compulsory treatment legally forces clients to remain in therapy longer, perhaps long enough for extrinsic motivators to build an intrinsic motivation for change.

Conclusion

Court-mandated treatment for substance use disorders coerces SUD clients to engage in substance abuse treatment using extrinsic social control strategies. These strategies can include legal mandates generated through the criminal justice system, formal mandates by employers and government programs, and informal mandates by family members and friends. California and New York civil commitment programs in the early 1960s represented the first legal mandates for treatment. Research shows that mandate treatment is effective at engaging SUD clients in treatment and keeping them in treatment long enough to reduce the likelihood of relapse.

Angela D. Broadus

See also Client Engagement; Crime and Substance Abuse; Criminal Justice Populations; Drug Courts; Treatment in Jails and Prisons

Further Readings

California Civil Commitment Program. (2001–2006). *Encyclopedia of drugs, alcohol & addictive behavior.* Retrieved August 8, 2007, from http://www.bookrags .com/research/california-civil-commitment-program -edaa-01

Jaffe, J. F. (n.d.). *Narcotic Addict Rehabilitation Act (NARA).* Available from http://www.bookrags.com

Leukefeld, C. G., & Tims, F. M. (1988). Compulsory treatment of drug abuse: Research and clinical practice. *National Institute on Drug Abuse, Research Monograph Series No. 86* (Publication No. 94-3713). Retrieved August 19, 2007, from http://www.nida.nih.gov/pdf/ monographs/download86.html

Ragghianti, C. (n.d.). *Coerced treatment for substance offenders.* Retrieved August 19, 2007, from http:// www.bookrags.com/research/coerced-treatment- for-substance-off-edaa-01

Room, R. (1989). The U.S. general population's experiences of responding to alcohol problems. *British Journal of Addiction, 84,* 1291–1304.

Satel, S. L. (2000). Drug treatment: The case for coercion. *National Drug Court Institute Review, 3*(1), 1–22. Retrieved August 19, 2007, from http://www.ndci.org/ ndcirpub.html

Wild, T. C., Roberts, A. B., & Cooper, E. L. (2002). Compulsory substance abuse treatment: an overview of recent findings and issues. *European Addiction Research, 8,* 84–93.

COVERT SENSITIZATION

Sensitization refers to a behavioral treatment designed for myriad problem behaviors including alcohol and drugs as well as obesity, sexual deviance, delinquent behavior, stealing, and compulsions. Sensitization describes building up avoidance to an aversive stimulus, and covert distinguishes this treatment in that neither the stimulus nor the consequence is actually presented. This entry includes the history, rationale and assumptions, implementation, examples, and advantages and disadvantages of covert sensitization.

When covert sensitization is used for alcohol or drug treatment, the client imagines a problem behavior, such as drinking alcohol, and then imagines a negative consequence, such as nausea. The therapist guides the participant through a series of specific situations, increasing the intensity of the consequence based on the proximity to the behavior while at the same time reinforcing escape and avoidance alternatives.

Joseph Cautela developed covert sensitization in the 1960s. It is based on classical and operant conditioning theories, which posit that the problem behaviors evolve from the accidental pairings of stimuli, which are then reinforced by accidental pairings of responses. In covert sensitization, the goal of treatment is to pair an aversive unconditioned stimulus (UCS) with the conditioned stimulus (CS), resulting in negative conditioned responses (CR) as well as unconditioned responses (UCR).

The rationale of covert sensitization posits that the problem behavior is a strongly learned habit, so unlearning can occur through pairing the learned habit with a negative consequence. In this process, cues and urges actually become stimuli to avoid the situations and consequences. The assumptions of covert sensitization include that imaginary actions are homogenous with overt behaviors, that there will be an interaction between the imagined and actual behaviors, and that learning will occur to pair the new consequences to the original stimulus.

To implement covert sensitization, an initial interview takes place between the client and therapist to assess the problem behavior, gather further information about specific settings and cues, create a hierarchy of situations, describe the rationale, and introduce relaxation training. Therapy sessions tend to follow an agenda of relaxation, visualization of the behavior, visualization of the negative consequence, and alternative escape scenarios. Treatment can last between 6 to 40 sessions and is specific to the client's behaviors and negative consequences. In addition, the therapist may assign homework to continue the visualizations between sessions as often as 10 to 20 times per day. Some therapists use audiotapes to record the session so that the client has the therapist's voice as a guide, while others encourage the client to continue the imagination exercises independently. After termination, the client may schedule follow-up or booster sessions to maintain the pairing of the consequence with the stimulus.

When defining the targeted behavior, the therapist identifies a specific behavior that is particular to the client. The client describes the highest risk first, including a specific location, setting, atmosphere, and time of day if applicable. The client describes the visualization in the first-person view, with the goal of depicting the scenario exactly as he or she experiences it. The therapist pays special attention to the experience of temptation and any reinforcing feelings. The therapist then identifies a hierarchy of negative consequences, each specific to the client. The consequences increase in severity as the proximity to the behavior increases and decrease as the client chooses escape or avoidant techniques. The outcome of this intervention is that the problem behavior now elicits a paired negative consequence, and escape from the consequence is negatively reinforced.

For example, in treatment of problem drinking with a goal of abstinence, the client may describe the typical situation of drinking at home after work. The therapist could pair the CS (drinking at home) with the UCS of nausea and vomiting. A detailed scenario would be described to the client where he or she would arrive home feeling good, and as he or she walked toward the liquor cabinet, he or she would start to feel queasy. The closer he or she came to the cabinet, the worse the feeling would get. As he or she reached for the bottle, he or she would experience further discomfort. This description would continue getting more graphic and more undesirable up to a point where he or she took a drink and became sick. Upon pouring out the rest of the drink and retreating from the room, he or she would feel better, thereby negatively reinforcing the escape behavior. The UCR in this description is the client's repulsion to the UCS, which would then be paired with the CS.

Not all consequences need to involve physical responses. In other scenarios, fear of legal problems might be paired with drug use, where the client is arrested and visualizes each of the life problems that might be associated including incarceration, job loss, family problems, and financial trouble. Fear of losing one's children or public embarrassment can also be incorporated into visualizations if those concerns are more relevant for the client. The consequences can also be generalized across situations and targeted toward early behaviors (such as purchasing the alcohol or drugs) in addition to the visualization of actual use.

The principles of covert sensitization are the same as the principles of aversion, or overt sensitization, where the client would be given a nausea-producing drug at the same time as drinking alcohol or given a shock while visualizing drug use. Covert sensitization has some advantages to aversion, including obvious ethical concerns as well as costs of training staff in procedures and the monitoring and administering the drugs or shocks. Sensitization typically has a lower dropout rate, and client buy-in is easier to obtain. In addition, although aversion is contraindicated for medically ill and underage people, sensitization could still be used in a safe environment provided consent has been obtained. On the other hand, covert sensitization is limited to individuals with good communication and visualization skills. Another disadvantage is the potential for undergeneralization in which the client only imagines the consequence in a particular setting or overgeneralization where drinking any liquid from any glass results in nausea.

Although some outcome studies indicate that covert sensitization may be effective, these are based primarily on case studies with a lack of replication. There have been no randomized control trials of covert sensitization to date. Current use of this practice tends to incorporate covert sensitization with other cognitive behavioral techniques such as skills training or mindfulness to effectively treat addictions.

Diane E. Logan

See also Aversive Therapy; Cognitive Behavioral Therapy; Evidence-Based Treatment; High-Risk Situations; Other Addictions; Treatment of Alcohol and Drug Use Disorders

Further Readings

Cautela, J. R. (1977). Covert conditioning: Assumptions and procedures. *Journal of Mental Imagery, 1,* 53–64.

Cautela, J. R., & Baron, M. G. (1977). Covert conditioning: A theoretical analysis. *Behavior Modification, 1,* 351–368.

Emmelkamp, P. M. G., & Kamphuis, J. H. (2002). Aversion relief. In M. Hersen & W. H. Sledge (Eds.), *Encyclopedia of psychotherapy* (Vol. 1, pp. 139–143). New York: Academic Press.

Miller, W. R., & Dougher, M. J. (1989). Covert sensitization: Alternative treatment procedures for alcoholism. *Behavioural Psychotherapy, 17,* 203–220.

Plaud, J. J. (2002). Assisted covert sensitization. In M. Hersen & W. H. Sledge (Eds.), *Encyclopedia of psychotherapy* (Vol. 1, pp. 125–130). New York: Academic Press.

CRACK

See COCAINE AND CRACK

CRAVING

Craving is defined as the desire (of an addict) to experience the effects of a previously experienced psychoactive substance. This definition was established after much controversy in 1992 by an Expert Committee of the UN International Drug Control Programme and the World Health Organization. Shortly after this definition was agreed upon, it was also recommended that drug craving be recognized as a multidimensional phenomenon that consists of subjective, behavioral, physiological, and neurochemical correlates. Current research demonstrate drug craving to be a physiologic response to the absence of drug(s) in a substance dependent individual. The physiologic response consist of increased heart rate and blood pressure, sweating, dilation of the pupils, specific electrical changes in the skin, and even an immediate drop in body temperature. These symptoms are accompanied by the strong emotional and psychological desire to return to drug use, often resulting in relapse.

Science and Treatment

Ongoing recovery work, participation in peer support systems such as the Twelve-Step communities, medical treatments (e.g., naltrexone, acamprosate, varenicline, buproprion), and continued counseling to address life and emotional problems are strategies to prevent craving and relapse. Other important considerations include cognitive impairments, endogenous craving, postacute withdrawal symptoms (PAWS), environmental triggers, relapse prevention, and cue extinction.

Cognitive Impairments

Research has shown that abuse of alcohol, stimulants. and most other drugs of abuse result in significant cognitive impairment due to toxic damage to brain cells. For example, damage to the prefrontal cortex—the area of the brain involved with executive brain functions of decisions making, planning, and response control—results in functional anomalies that correlate to 30% to 80% of substance abusers' having mild to severe cognitive impairments. The abuse of methamphetamine has been shown to result in 11.3% destruction of limbic gray matter. The cingula gyrus, paralimbic cortices, and hippocampus are the brain areas damaged by methamphetamine abuse. These areas are associated with memory, emotions, mood, and craving. The greatest deficit occurred in the hippocampus. Heavy abuse of methamphetamine users results in 7.8% smaller hippocampus volume, which corresponds to the severe cognitive deficits seen in chronic users.

Deficits of cognition impair the ability of addicts to understand what they need to do to prevent cravings that lead to slips and relapse. A public hospital study by A. W. Blume and colleagues found that the majority of substance use disorder patients suffered mild-to-severe cognitive impairments that made it difficult for them to participate in treatment. Reviewing screening exams on neurocognitive functioning at a VA hospital, researchers found that approximately 50% of the patients were mildly to severely impaired.

The most common cognitive impairments associated with substance use disorders consist of problems with attention, memory, understanding, learning, use and meaning of words, problem solving, cognitive inflexibility, abstract thinking and judgment. Abuse of drugs also causes temporal processing problems, which consist of poor understanding of time planning, difficulty processing goals over time, and delayed discounting, the inability to appreciate delayed gratification.

Patients treated for substance use disorders often appear normal during the early phase of recovery treatment, but are actually experiencing an inability to fully understand and process the treatment curriculum. For example, the patient can repeat what he or she hears, but the information and the therapy do not sink in. It may take weeks or months after detoxification for reasoning, memory, and thinking to come back to a point where the individual can begin to fully engage in treatment. Educational strategies during treatment must be tailored to the person's ability to process the information being provided.

Endogenous Craving

A homeostasis paradigm for drug addiction was first proposed by C. K. Himmelsbach in 1941. Homeostasis is the normal balance and functioning of brain chemicals known as neurotransmitters. Abuse of addictive drugs imbalance brain chemistry resulting in allostasis. Allostasis is an abnormal stability of neurotransmitters that reinforces the need or craving to continue abuse of drugs. During the early part of treatment, the addict's brain is in a state of allostasis—usually a depletion of brain neurotransmitters brought about by the drug use. Abuse of psychoactive drugs causes reduction in normal levels of neurotransmitters that users then compensate for by taking increasing doses of the drug(s) they are abusing. When the drug is no longer taken, there is an abnormally low concentration of neurotransmitters in the users' brains and nothing to compensate for their absence. This absence results in a type of drug hunger known as endogenous craving. If recovering addicts again return to drug use to satisfy their cravings, it almost always results in an immediate and severe relapse to addiction.

Also, decreased activity in regions of the brain's neo-cortex also correlates with 90% accuracy in predicting relapse to methamphetamine abuse. Compared to methamphetamine addicts who did not relapse, the relapse group members were noted to have significantly less brain activity in their dorsolateral, prefrontal, parietal, and temporal cortices along with their insula. This is another form of endogenous craving.

Traditional treatments for endogenous cravings consist of counseling, education, discussions with recovery sponsors, stress-reduction therapies, biofeedback, and participation in Twelve-Step meetings. Recent treatments include medications and nutrients such as amino acid (neurotransmitter precursors) that are targeted to restore brain chemistry to a homeostasis that can suppress or reverse the pleasurable effects of drugs and decrease the drug craving.

PAWS

PAWS are a group of emotional and physical symptoms that appear after major withdrawal symptoms have abated. The syndrome can persist for 6 to 18 months or even longer—up to 10 years for some—and may contribute to interrupted abstinence or relapse. It is believed that PAWS result from a combination of brain neuron damage caused by drug use and the psychological stress of living drug and alcohol-free after many years of a drug-using lifestyle. The syndrome usually begins within 7 to 14 days of abstinence and peaks in intensity over 3 to 6 months. Symptoms often occur at regular intervals and without apparent outside stressors. The patterns can be on payday schedules (every 2 weeks or monthly), during holidays, or even annually on recovery birthdays. These are past moments in time that are often associated with drug use or stressful events. PAWS is associated with six major types of problems or symptoms:

1. *sleep disturbances:* difficulty falling or staying asleep, restlessness, and vivid and disturbing nightmares;

2. *memory problems:* short-term memory is most impaired, often making it difficult to learn new skills or process new information;

3. *inability to think clearly:* difficulty with concentration, rigid and repetitive thinking, and impairment of abstract reasoning (non-concrete, theoretical, or philosophical thinking); thoughts become confused and chaotic during stressful situations; decreased problem-solving skills, even with usually simple problems; overall intelligence is not affected, and the thinking impairment is episodic and not continuous;

4. *anxiety and hypersensitivity to stress:* chronic stress with inability to differentiate between low-stress and high-stress situations; inappropriate reaction to situations and difficulty managing stress; all other symptoms of PAWS syndrome become worse during high-stress situations;

5. *inappropriate emotional reactions and mood swings:* overreaction to emotions, resulting in increased stress that then leads to an emotional shutdown or numbness and inability to feel any emotions; and

6. *physical coordination difficulties:* hand-eye coordination issues; and problems with balance, dizziness, and slow reflexes.

Most recovering addicts experience inadequacy, incompetence, embarrassment, lowered self-esteem, and great shame while experiencing PAWS. These are all negative moods states that make them extremely vulnerable to relapse.

Education, individual-group counseling, participation in peer support activities, and isolation from potential sources of alcohol or drug use are the current strategies to prevent drug use and relapse when a recovering substance abuser is experiencing PAWS.

Environmental Triggers

Environmental triggers or cues often precipitate drug cravings. Also known as protracted withdrawal, environmental triggers are a recurrence of the withdrawal symptoms or euphoric feelings associated with abuse of drugs that trigger a heavy craving for drugs long after an addict has been detoxified. The cause of this reaction (similar to a post-traumatic stress phenomenon) often happens when some sensory input (odor, sight, or noise) stimulates the memories experienced during drug use or withdrawal that then evokes a desire for the drug. For instance, the odor of burnt matches or burning metal (smells that occur when cooking heroin) several months after detoxification may cause a heroin addict to suffer some withdrawal symptoms. Any white powder may cause craving in a cocaine addict, a blue pill may do it to a Valium addict, and even attending a barbecue can cause a recovering alcoholic to crave a beer.

Cravings brought about by environmental triggers often causes recovering addicts to slip or renew their drug use, generally leading to a full relapse. These slips are associated with a greater chance of drug overdose because users are prone to taking the same dose they were injecting, smoking, or snorting when they quit. They often forget that their last dose was probably a very high one that they could handle only because tolerance had developed. They do not remember that abstinence allowed their bodies to return to a less tolerant state. Then, once abstinence is interrupted, both tolerance and tissue dependence redevelop at a much faster rate than before. This development results in the accelerated development of a more severe substance dependence problem than previously experienced.

Drug craving triggers also result from mental emotional states. These have been classified into two broad categories: intrapersonal and interpersonal factors. Intrapersonal states (also known as internal influences) that have the greatest impact are negative emotional and physical states or internally motivated attempts to regain control and use. Interpersonal factors (also called external influences) include relationship conflicts, social pressures, lack of support systems, negative life events, and so-called slippery

people, places, and things. Other factors that can lead to relapse are exhaustion, dishonesty, impatience, argumentativeness, depression, frustration, self-pity, cockiness, complacency, expecting too much from others, letting up on disciplines, use of any mood-altering drugs, and overconfidence. Recovering addicts use handy acronyms such as HALT (hungry, angry, lonely, tired) and RID (restless, irritable, discontent) to remind themselves of the triggers that lead to relapse.

Relapse Prevention

Relapse prevention is now a strong treatment focus of substance dependence disorders. There are a number of strategies and themes that are used in this process.

- Addicts must understand the process of relapse and learn to recognize their personal triggers, which can be anything from drug odors, seeing friends who use, having money in one's pocket, and even hearing a song about drugs.
- Addicts must develop behaviors to avoid external cues. These include avoiding old neighborhoods and dealers, changing one's circle of friends, limiting the amount of money that's carried, and voluntary isolation from bars or gatherings where drugs may be readily available.
- Addicts must learn to cope with or be prepared with an automatic reflex strategy to prevent them from using when their craving is activated by internal or external cues. These include networking with the support system they have put together, going to a Twelve-Step meeting, using their developed coping skills for negative emotional states and cognitive distortions, doing something that reminds them of their addiction problems or their reasons for wanting to stay clean, remembering their last binge, creating a balanced lifestyle, and possibly treatment with anti-craving medications.

Cue Extinction

Cue extinction also known as desensitization consists of deconditioning techniques (stress reduction exercises, expressing one's feelings, working out, long walks, and cold showers) that can be used to dissipate the craving response when it arises. A technique such as Dr. Anna Rose Childress's Desensitization

Program retrains brain cells to not react when confronted by environmental cues. The procedure involves exposing an addict to progressively stronger environmental cues over 40 to 50 sessions in a controlled setting. This technique gradually decreases response to the cues until there are no physiological signs of a craving response even when the addict is exposed to heavy triggers. It was noted that every time an addict refrains from using while craving a drug, it lessens the response to the next trigger experience.

Conclusion

Advances in the science of the brain continue to provide a better understanding of Substance Dependence Disorders resulting in more effective prevention and treatment strategies. The discoveries are also starting to erode the stigma, guilt, and shame attached to the concepts of addiction, drug cravings, and relapse.

Darryl S. Inaba and David A. Jones

See also Brain Chemistry and Addiction; High-Risk Situations; Neurobiology of Addiction; Relapse; Relapse Prevention; Withdrawal

Further Readings

Bender, K. J. (1995). Drug craving distinguished from withdrawal symptoms. *Psychiatric Times, 12*(9), 1–5.

Blume, A. W., Davis, J. M., & Schmaling, K. B. (1999). Neurocognitive dysfunction in dually diagnosed patients: A potential roadblock to motivating behavior change. *Journal of Psychoactive Drugs, 31*(2), 111–115.

Brain Activity Patterns Signal Risk of Relapse to Methamphetamine. (2006). *NIDA Notes, 20*(5), 1, 6.

Carter, B. L., & Tiffany, S. T. (1995). Meta-analysis of cue-reactivity in addiction research. *Addiction, 94*(3), 327–340.

Childress, A. R., Mozley, P. D., McElgin, W., Fitzgerald, J., Reivich, M., & O'Brien, C. P. (1999). Limbic activation during cue-induced cocaine craving. *American Journal of Psychiatry, 156*(1), 11–18.

Drummond, D. C. (2001). Theories of drug craving, ancient and modern. *Addiction, 96*(1), 33–46.

Gatch M. B., & Lal, H. (1997). Pharmacological treatment of alcoholism. *Progress in Neuro-Psychopharmacology and Biological Psychiatry, 22*(6), 917–944.

Grossman D., & Onken, L. (2003). *Summaries of NIDA workshop: Developing behavioral treatments for drug abusers with cognitive impairments.* Retrieved May 2, 2007, from http://www.drugabuse.gov/whatsnew/meetings/cognitiveimpairment.html

Inaba, D. S., & Cohen, W. E. (2007). *Uppers, downers, all arounders: Physical and mental effects of psychoactive drugs* (6th ed.). Medford, OR: CNS Productions.

Littleton, J. (1998). Neurochemical mechanisms underlying alcohol withdrawal. *Alcohol Health and Research World, 22*(1), 13–24.

O'Brien, C. P. (1997). A range of research-based pharmacotherapies for addiction. *Science, 278*(5335), 66–70.

Stewart, J. (2003). Stress and relapse to drug seeking: Studies in laboratory animals shed light on mechanisms and sources of long-term vulnerability. *American Journal of Addictions, 12*(1), 1–17.

Taleff, M. J. (2004). Alcohol-caused impairment and early treatment. *Counselor, Magazine for Addiction Professionals, 5*(1), 76–77.

Thompson P. M., Hayashi, K. M., Simon, S. L., Geaga, J. A., Hong, M. S., Sui, Y., et al. (2004). Structural abnormalities in the brain of human subjects who use methamphetamine. *Journal of Neuroscience, 24*(26), 6028–6036.

CRIME AND SUBSTANCE ABUSE

The social problems created by crime date back to the beginnings of organized societies and recorded history. The codes created by rulers such as Hammurabi, the first king of Babylon (1810 BC–1750 BC) and Emperor Justinian in Rome (482 AD–565 AD) outlined acceptable behaviors within their respective societies, and the harms that would be done to persons who violated these codes of conduct.

Similarly, the relationship between crime and substance abuse is both historical and current. The types of crime and the substances of choice have changed from generation to generation, but the problems created for society are constant. For example, the early Greeks banned alcohol-based celebrations of the God Bacchus because they typically resulted in riots. Similarly, the government of the United States upon realizing that opioid use and abuse was threatening to the well-being of the country formed the Brent Commission in 1909, which suggested to President Roosevelt that there should be an international agreement on the control and distribution of opioids. This agreement led to the International Opium Convention of 1912. Following this meeting, U.S. lawmakers drafted legislation, known as the Harrison Narcotics Act of 1914, which regulated the use, distribution, and marketing of opioids. This legislation represented the first attempt by U.S. lawmakers to improve the lives of U.S. citizens through the criminalization of drugs.

In recent years, the relationship between drugs and crime has expanded, and researchers have shown that the effects are more complex than were previously believed, and they may be cyclical rather than linear. For example, the high cost of the war on drugs may be causing funding deficiencies in other areas of social services, such as education. These deficiencies may create problems for those students who require the most support and whose educational success is linked to specialized support services. With these services absent, the student may not succeed in school, and a high school dropout may be much more likely to turn to crime and drug use. Researchers have also found that the relationship between crime and substance abuse is mediated by the type of substance, and the characteristics of the individual taking the substance.

Alcohol and Crime

The relationship between alcohol and crime is long and time honored. It is among the earliest known substance taken for primarily recreational reasons. Like many substances with known cognitive effects, alcohol impacts judgment and physical abilities even at low levels. Alcohol consumption has been linked to all forms of aggression, but has been found to be strongly related to sexual aggression. This link strengthened as alcohol consumption became more frequent, longer in duration, and the amount of alcohol increased. Furthermore, although it has been shown that alcohol affects the decision-making abilities of the sexual assault perpetrators, it also diminished caution and prudence on the part of the victims, leading to increased chances of victimization. The potential for assault was found to be greatest when both the perpetrator and the victim had ingested significant amounts of alcohol over a long period.

Alcohol has also been linked to criminality among juveniles. Because juveniles typically have lower body mass and are less familiar with the effects of alcohol, they are prime candidates for poor decision making as a result of alcohol ingestion. The American Pediatric Association has called underage drinking an "important health risk," and they note that alcohol use dramatically increases the chance of automobile-related injury and death, the probability of suicide, homicide, and other physically injurious outcomes. This problem is compounded by the fact that alcohol drinking is one of the most common activities of juveniles and represents delinquent conduct (or perhaps status offending, depending on the specific laws of the area).

Although the link between various crimes and alcohol is often poorly understood, strong associations have been shown to exist consistently between public disorder crimes and alcohol consumption. This association has been repeatedly studied in both the United States and in the United Kingdom and has been found to be strong. However, it is important to note that cultural traditions and behaviors may be responsible for much of this association. The relationship between alcohol consumption and public disorder is weak in Italy, Spain, and France and is only moderate in Germany and Holland.

Stimulants and Crime

Rarely does a drug gain the attention of the public like methamphetamine (i.e., meth) has in recent years. A few drugs that have garnered great public attention in the past 2 decades were considered interesting because they were "club" drugs, like Ecstasy, GHB, Rohypnol, and Ketamine created in laboratories for a specific purpose and a specific market, or they were performance enhancing drugs like steroids that challenged the public beliefs about the honesty of athletes and the integrity of the records they had broken. Methamphetamine differs from these two examples because it is a drug of wide utility with deep historical roots.

Amphetamine was first synthesized in Germany in 1887. Its effects on alertness and energy were discussed, but the effects were deemed too brief and inconsistent for practical use. In 1919, methamphetamine was synthesized in Japan, but the effects of the compound were not well tested or understood. In 1927, a British researcher Gordon Ailes noted that methamphetamine both increased energy and produced a sense of euphoria, similar to the adrenaline rush created by a stressful situation. As a result of this discovery, methamphetamine became a large part of the war effort in World War II, increasing the production of war-related items for both sides. It has subsequently been estimated that 2% of the entire Japanese population were dependent on methamphetamine at the close of the war. In the United States, methamphetamine use has been a social problem for decades, with the first "epidemic" occurring in the 1950s and the second in the 1960s; the most recent one began in the 1990s and has continued unabated to the present.

Methamphetamine use is related to crime in a multitude of ways. Long-term meth users often develop a form of psychosis (called amphetamine psychosis), which affects their judgment and their ability to self-regulate anger and frustration. When this happens, they can respond to frustration with a level of violence disproportionate to the situation. Methamphetamine users typically purchase the drug from a dealer who either manufacturers the drug or serves as a distribution point for a larger manufacturing or smuggling operation. As in any drug purchase transaction, there is a level of uncertainty, fear, and the potential for robbery or cheating. When this happens, or one of the parties involved perceives that it has happened, a methamphetamine deal can become violent. Deals that have resulted in tragedy have occurred from Texas to New Zealand, and often the perpetrator harms or kills a person that had previously been considered a friend. Law enforcement officers typically find firearms, explosives, and other weapons when they enter a structure where methamphetamine is being sold or manufactured.

Because methamphetamine allows users to work for long periods with less fatigue, it is popular among people who work in service-industry jobs or who are paid by the job rather than hourly or salary. This reality makes methamphetamine users common in the construction industry, where they can augment their wages with the theft of equipment or construction materials. Recently, the price increases in construction materials have created a new wave of construction site thefts, specifically in the area of recyclable metals. When these perpetrators are caught, the majority of them turn out to be methamphetamine users who are looking for a quick way to gather enough cash for the next meth purchase.

Methamphetamine is also related to crime through the addictive nature of the substance. Because it simultaneously produces euphoria and alertness, it has the dual qualities of being functional and desirable. As a result of this admixture, it is exceedingly addictive, and consequently creates significant difficulties for those being released from correctional or incarcerative institutions. Most of these individuals are still under some level of justice system control (probation or parole) at the point of release, and testing positive for drug use may generate new charges or cause them to be re-incarcerated for a violating the terms of their release.

Opioids and Crime

The class of drugs known as opioids is broad, but the primary drug of interest in the relationship between crime and substance abuse within this class is heroin. Heroin accounts for the majority of opioid-related crime. Although data on this claim may be difficult to obtain, most law enforcement professionals would agree that of all of the opioids in society, heroin poses the greatest threat to public safety.

Long-term opioid use creates in the user a physiological tolerance for the drug. This tolerance results in the user requiring increasing amounts of the drug to achieve the same effects as were experienced earlier. This, researchers argue, is one of the reasons that opioids create such a significant impact on society. Chronic, long-term users who support their habits through crime will, over time, commit more and more crime to support their habit, thereby increasing the crime rates in their area of society. Since opioids are physically addictive, chronic users who are forced to choose between the pain of withdrawal and committing additional crimes to maintain their drug habits typically choose to commit more crime and avoid the withdrawal experience.

Because of the nature of the drug and the physiological effects, opioid users are predisposed toward certain criminal activities, and typically less involved in others. Unlike methamphetamines and other stimulants, heroin depresses the central nervous system and induces a sleeplike state coupled with a sense of contentment and euphoria. Because of these effects, heroin users do not tend to engage in violent crimes while under the influence of the drug, but rather when they are in need of another dose of the drug. Heroin users who are experiencing withdrawal may become disoriented, irrational, nauseous, frightened, and potentially violent due to the absence of the drug. Because of these wildly different cognitive states, heroin users are most linked to crimes of gain such as theft and prostitution and less linked to crimes such as robbery and murder. This tendency does not imply that these crimes are never committed by heroin users, but they are less likely since the user is often just interested in the acquisition of sufficient money or property to ensure his or her next fix.

Although heroin and other opioid users are not typically involved in crimes such as robbery or murder, the drug does, in fact, cause these crimes. The cause, however, is related to the manufacturing, processing, and sales of the drug. Opioid production occurs in many areas, from Southeast and Southwest Asia to Central and South America. The gum of the opium poppy is relatively simple to process, and the profit margin for opioid production is quite high. Consequently, smuggling, trafficking, and sales are all very competitive, leading to turf wars, law enforcement bribery and witness coercion and threat, all of which represent crimes at some level. This relationship between opioid production and crime becomes even more apparent in years where crop production is high and competition for market share becomes fierce and potentially violent.

Drugs, Recidivism, and Social Impacts

Substance abuse also has a less direct relationship to crime than those mentioned above. Although less recognized, it is still greatly problematic to those who work within the criminal justice field. This relationship is the result of the addictive nature of many substances, and the difficulty inherent in the process of stopping the use of drugs. When a person is adjudicated by a court for a crime, even one not directly related to drug use (such as theft), and placed on probation, the judge typically makes part of the probation order the requirement that the person refrain from all substance abuse (including alcohol) and obey all the laws of the state and the jurisdiction where the probation order was received. When people who are under this order test positive for drug use, they are in violation of the order of the court and have committed a new crime. Consequently, the addictive nature of certain drugs increases the possibility of relapse and increases the number of cases the justice system is required to adjudicate.

A further relationship between drug use and crime has been posited by theorists who believe that prenatal exposure to certain substances at certain points in prenatal development can lead to the birth of a child with personality characteristics that may predispose him or her to crime later in life. This belief was most prominent when the number of crack-cocaine-addicted mothers increased dramatically in the late 1980s. Social workers noted that the children of these addicts, many of whom were born addicted as well, shared some personality characteristics that if carried into adulthood could make them at risk for criminal activity. Much of that concern was unfounded, but prenatal exposure to certain drugs has been linked to poor school performance, increased chances of dropping out, and has also been linked to both juvenile delinquency and adult criminality. Although this relationship generates controversy among researchers, it is important to note that substance use has direct links to crime for the user; it can also be linked to crime and violence for the producers, the smugglers, the sellers, and the larger society. Evidence suggests that it might be affecting the criminality of the children of the users as well.

Conclusion

The relationship between substance use and crime is a constant in virtually all societies. What seems to change more than the presence of this relationship is the type of substance being abused and the crimes associated with the substance and the users of the substance. The drug-crime relationship is made even more complex by the process of trafficking, cultivating, manufacturing, and selling of the drugs; all of which are crimes to some degree. Use of these substances by people on probation or parole represent additional crimes, and further the relationship between crime and substance abuse. What is clear in all of these relationships is that the best way to control the crime is to first control the use of the substance. Once that has been effectively managed, the crime caused by the substance abuse is virtually eliminated.

Matthew Leone

See also Coercion and Treatment; Court-Mandated Treatment; Criminal Justice Populations; Drug Courts; Treatment in Jails and Prisons

Further Readings

Barton, A. (2003). *Illicit drugs: Use and control.* New York: Routledge.

Bean, P. (2002). *Drugs and crime.* Portland, OR: Willan.

Bowser, L. A. (1969). *Born to raise hell: Case histories on the effects of drinking on crime and violence.* Jericho, NY: Exposition Press.

Dikötter, F. (2001). *The promise of repentance: Crime, punishment and prison reform in modern China.* London: Hurst.

Greenfeld, L. A. (1998). *Alcohol and crime: An analysis of national data on the prevalence of alcohol involvement in crime.* Washington, DC: Office of Justice Programs, Bureau of Justice Statistics, U.S. Department of Justice.

Inciardi, J. A. (Ed.). (1981). *The drugs-crime connection.* Beverly Hills, CA: Sage.

Sommers, I., Baskin, D., & Fagan, J. (2000). *Workin' hard for the money: The social and economic lives of women drug sellers.* Huntington, NY: Nova Science.

CRIMINAL JUSTICE POPULATIONS

Criminal activity and drug abuse are inextricably linked. Criminal drug offenses, as outlined by the National Institute on Drug Abuse, can occur in many ways. These include (a) possession of an illicit drug, (b) sales of an illicit drug, (c) offenses committed owing to drug use or abuse such as theft to obtain money to purchase drugs, and (d) offenses related to illegal activities such as having an association or ties with an illicit drug market. Regardless of how an offense (or offenses) occurs, the criminal justice system is overwhelmed by the ever-growing numbers of inmates, and in particular, those inmates who are imprisoned for crimes related to drug offenses.

Current Size of Population

A wealth of information is reported annually by the U.S. Department of Justice, Office of Justice Programs, Bureau of Justice Statistics (BJS). The statistics available from 2005 indicate that the number of individuals involved in the criminal justice system is immense— over 7 million. At that time, nearly 1.5 million people were in prison, and an additional 750,000 were in local jails. Further, the number of parolees is on the rise at nearly 790,000, and the number of individuals on probation and supervised release is a staggering 4.2 million. Drug arrest rates for the adult population indicate that nearly 1.7 million individuals were arrested for a drug-related crime; for juveniles, the number of arrests for drugs was nearly 200,000.

Drug Use and Crime

Drug-related crime is generally on the rise. In 2004, BJS estimates for state and federal prisoners were nearly identical, with 17% to 18% of convicted criminals stating that they had committed a crime to obtain money to purchase drugs. Of those arrested for such crimes, violent crime accounted for 10% of state and 18% of federal convictions; property crimes accounted for 30% of state and 10% of federal convictions, public order crimes accounted for 7% of both state and federal convictions, and around one quarter of all state and federal prisoners had been convicted of a drug crime. Hence, even if someone convicted of a crime is imprisoned for something other-than-drug offense (e.g., in a plea agreement), there is a relatively high probability that drugs were in some way related to the offending behavior.

Another way to examine the relationship between drugs and crime is to consider those that were under the influence of a drug at the time they committed an offense. The National Crime Victimization Survey estimated that more than 5 million individuals (over 12 years of age) were victims of violent crime in 2004. Perceptions by those victims suggest that nearly one third of the offenders were using alcohol or other drugs at the time the victimization occurred. This estimate increases to around 40% when examining college student victims specifically and to a similar range when examining workplace violence. Interestingly, these estimates of perception did not differ remarkably from surveys of state and federal prisoners, where around one third of this group admitted to having been under the influence at the time that the offense for which they were arrested had occurred. These estimates were slightly higher for prisoners who had been imprisoned for drug-specific offenses.

Offender Drug-Use Behaviors

State and Federal Prisoners

According to data provided by the BJS, drug use among state and federal offenders has remained relatively stable between surveys conducted in 1997 and 2004. Over 80% of these offenders report having used illicit drugs in their pasts, with nearly 50% admitting to use within the month of their offense. Marijuana was by far the most commonly used substance, having been reported by nearly all of those inmates admitting to using drugs. Marijuana use was followed, in order of most prevalent use, by cocaine-crack, hallucinogens, other stimulants (e.g., methamphetamine), opioids, and depressants. Of those who had ever used an illicit drug, a staggering 89% (for both male and female offenders) report having been abused (both sexually and physically) in their pasts.

Jail Inmates

An examination of surveys conducted in 1996 and 2002 suggests that over 80% of jail inmates admit to using illicit drugs in their lifetimes and that 55% admit to use of these substances within the month of their offense. Marijuana was the most prevalent drug used among these offenders (about three quarters of those admitting to using drugs). Marijuana use was followed, in order of most prevalent use, by cocaine/crack, hallucinogens, other stimulants, depressants, opioids, and inhalants.

Probationers

Probationer drug-use statistics are currently available for 1995. According to surveys of probationers, approximately 70% admitted to using illicit drugs in their lifetimes, with nearly one third admitting to use within the month of their offense. Marijuana was the most common drug used by probationers. Marijuana use was followed, in order of most prevalent use, by cocaine-crack and other stimulants; opioids, barbiturates, and hallucinogens had equal prevalence rates.

For those convicted of driving while intoxicated (DWI) offenses, 68% report having ever used an illicit drug, with 17% admitting to using an illicit drug in the month prior to their arrest for DWI. Interestingly, over 55% of DWI offenders admit to using drugs regularly at some point in their lives (defined as drug use at least once a week for at least a 1-month period), suggesting a potential history of risk-taking behaviors. Again, marijuana was the most common drug of choice for these offenders, followed in order by stimulants such as methamphetamine, cocaine-crack, hallucinogens, depressants, and opioids.

Treatment Considerations

The National Institute on Drug Abuse has published a treatment guide for criminal justice populations that outlines 13 research-based principles that treatment providers should consider when working with this population. The following is a description of these 13 principles:

1. *Drug addiction is a brain disease that affects behavior.* Adequate data support the position that chemical use, particularly chronic use, alters the brain's anatomy and neurochemistry; this, in turn, causes changes in behavior. A common argument heard when working with offenders is that the responsibility for inappropriate behaviors is to be blamed on the drugs that were being used prior to or during a crime. It is important to stress throughout treatment that even though drug addiction is considered a brain disease, it is not a disease with an etiology that removes personal responsibility from the decisions and behaviors chosen by those who use drugs. That is, the first poor decision was to use drugs, and this in turn may have led to criminal behaviors.

2. *Recovery from drug addiction requires effective treatment, followed by management of the problem over time.* Substance abuse treatment can only be effective if the condition is treated throughout its entire course, and this may require multiple treatment episodes and monitoring. This principle highlights the importance of including treatment in offender programs, whether that be in jail or prison or while offenders are on parole or probation. Since addiction is accepted as a brain disease, placing someone behind bars or on supervised release does not stop the disease, it may simply delay it. Therefore, it is strongly recommended that the continuum of care include treatment programs for those who are incarcerated and for those who have been released.

3. *Treatment must last long enough to produce behavioral changes.* Breaking old patterns of behavior can take a long time, particularly for a chronic substance abuser; therefore, treatment must be long enough to ensure that patients learn new behaviors. This may mean requiring drug treatment for a long period after release from incarceration or throughout the time that offenders are on supervised release.

4. *Assessment is the first step in treatment.* Comprehensive assessments must be conducted to ensure that the patient receives the appropriate level of care—continuing assessment is necessary for appropriate level-of-care placement. Hence, offenders should be adequately screened for substance use and abuse.

5. *Tailoring services to fit the needs of the individual is an important part of effective drug abuse treatment for criminal justice populations.* A one-size-fits-all approach to treatment will likely not

address the often complex issues of an individual, particularly given their past or concurrent involvement in the criminal justice system. A continuum-of-care approach necessitates that treatment programs be adapted to the environment in which offenders find themselves—whether in prison or while on release.

6. *Drug use during treatment should be carefully monitored.* Triggers leading to potential relapse should be addressed, and appropriate coping mechanisms examined. A relapse, though not to be expected, per se, can be damaging if left undetected owing to the potential of serious continuing use. It is strongly recommended that drug-testing policies be developed both inside prisons and after release since undetected use can rapidly lead to negative consequences.

7. *Treatment should target factors that are associated with criminal behavior.* A cognitive pattern of thinking leading to risky behaviors, failure to acknowledge consequences, and repeated offender behaviors (i.e., criminal thinking) can lead to continued drug use and poor decision making if not addressed.

8. *Criminal justice supervision should incorporate treatment planning for drug-abusing offenders, and treatment providers should be aware of correctional supervision requirements.* It is imperative that treatment providers and parole or probation officers work together in order to enhance the therapeutic outcome of offenders in treatment. The therapist should be recognized as the mental health or substance abuse expert, and the parole or probation officer should be recognized as the criminal justice expert; however, these entities must work in concert throughout the treatment process. It is imperative that appropriate release-of-information documentation be developed that allows communication among entities but that also maintains therapeutic confidentiality.

9. *Continuity of care is essential for drug abusers reentering the community.* It is estimated that from one quarter to one third of inmates participate in substance abuse treatment while in prison—this treatment should be continued outside of prison to assist offenders with their reintegration into the community while maintaining abstinence from drug use. Aftercare programs that allow for continued counseling and follow-up evaluations should be implemented.

10. *A balance of rewards and sanctions encourages prosocial behavior and treatment participation.* There is a tendency to punish offenders, particularly probationers, by revoking their freedom if they relapse. It should be kept in mind, however, that punishments for negative behavior in the absence of rewards for positive behavior rarely produce lasting change. This issue is just as relevant and important when treating the offender population as it is with any other client.

11. *Offenders with co-occurring drug abuse and mental health problems often require an integrated treatment approach.* Offenders with dual diagnoses should be treated by professionals skilled in treating such patients, and referrals should be made when a treatment provider lacks competencies in a given area.

12. *Medications are an important part of treatment for many drug-abusing offenders.* Potential use of medications should be discussed with a prescribing professional to ensure the maximal probability of success. These medications may include anti-craving medications (e.g., naltrexone), medications to address potential anxiety (e.g., benzodiazepines) and/or depression (e.g., SSRI [selective serotonin reuptake inhibitor] or SNRI [selective norepinephrine reuptake inhibitor]), as well as medications that target specific drugs (e.g., antabuse for alcohol and methadone-bupenorphine for heroin).

13. *Treatment planning for drug-abusing offenders who are living in or reentering the community should include strategies to prevent and treat serious, chronic medical conditions.* Communicable diseases caused by past or current drug use (e.g., HIV/AIDS, hepatitis infection) should be addressed and treated appropriately, and referrals to appropriate community agencies should be made.

Conclusion

Given the well-established link between drug use and criminal behavior, it is important that treatment providers gain an in-depth understanding of the offender population. Drug-use rates are often quite high among those involved in the criminal justice system, and many offenders have a long and extensive history of drug use and abuse. Those working with this population must understand the potential for treatment resistance and the special circumstances under which this population must live as they attempt to reintegrate into society.

Chad L. Cross

See also Antisocial Personality Disorder; Coercion and Treatment; Court-Mandated Treatment; Crime and Substance Abuse; Drug Courts

Further Readings

Cross, C. L., & Ashley, L. (2005). The importance of early intervention in diagnosing and treating mentally ill and substance abusing parole and probation clients. *Counselling & Guidance, 20,* 13–21.

Marshall, G. N., & Hser, Y.-I. (2002). Characteristics of criminal justice and noncriminal justice clients receiving treatment for substance abuse. *Addictive Behaviors, 27,* 179–192.

National Institute on Drug Abuse. (2006). *Principles of drug abuse treatment for criminal justice populations: A research-based guide.* Retrieved from http://www .drugabuse.gov/PDF/PODAT_CJ/PODAT_CJ.pdf

CROSS-ADDICTIONS

An individual who abuses or is dependent on a substance will commonly identify a primary substance of abuse. This does not necessarily mean that the individual will not abuse other addictive substances or engage in other addictive behaviors. An individual with addictive tendencies may seek multiple addictive sources of reinforcement throughout their lifetime; this tendency is known as cross-addiction. This behavior typically occurs by successively replacing one addictive behavior with another. These cross-addictions may manifest in the use of another substance within the same drug class, the use of a substance belonging to a different class, or engagement in other addictive behaviors (e.g., compulsive gambling, sexual addiction, Internet addiction, overeating). This entry focuses on the proposed mechanisms behind cross-addictions, subtypes of cross-addictions and their associated risks, and barriers to substance abuse treatment that cross-addictions may present.

Mechanisms Behind Cross-Addiction

A number of mechanisms have been proposed to explain the presence of cross-addictions and the maintenance of addictive behaviors. There is no consensus among substance abuse researchers on the primary underlying mechanism behind cross-addictions. Two processes that have empirical support are impulsivity and genetic predisposition to substance abuse.

Impulsivity

Several researchers have identified a correlation between substance abuse and impulsivity that may serve to explain the presence of cross-addictions. Impulsive behavior involves the pursuit of thrills, adventure, new experiences, lowering of inhibitions, sensation seeking, and avoidance of the mundane. Individuals who display impulsive behaviors are more likely to experiment with drugs at an early age, consume substances at a higher quantity and frequency than nonsensation seeking peers, and experiment with multiple substances of abuse over their lifetime. When the patient decreases use of or ceases to use the primary substance of abuse, his or her impulsive and sensation seeking behaviors will likely be directed toward another source of reinforcement. This commonly results in the presence of a cross-addiction to another substance of abuse or addictive behavior. As such, those patients who demonstrate difficulties with impulsivity and sensation seeking should be monitored closely for the development of a cross-addiction.

Genetic Predisposition to Addiction

Additionally, research has identified a genetic component or predisposition to substance use that may serve to facilitate the tendency to replace one addiction with another. Although perspectives on genetic predisposition to substance abuse have been varied, researchers have presented evidence that a genetic predisposition is commonly a factor in substance abuse and substance dependence, particularly among alcohol use disorders. This genetic predisposition would also increase the likelihood of the patient developing a cross-addiction once they have completed substance cessation treatment for his or her primary substance of abuse.

Substance Abuse Treatment

Once the individual takes steps to obtain sobriety from their primary substance of abuse, many researchers believe that their addictive tendencies may be channeled into other addictive sources of reinforcement. When treating a patient who has successfully ceased use of their primary substance of abuse, the possibility of a cross-addition should be included as a component of relapse prevention education. Substance use treatment providers should be aware of the possible presence of cross-additions in order to monitor for signs of relapse to the patient's primary substance of abuse and to monitor abuse and dependence symptoms that may emerge related to the novel addictive substance or behavior.

Cross-Addiction Within the Same Drug Class

Once a desire for the reinforcing effects of a particular class of drug has emerged, the substance user may seek similar reinforcement after cessation from their primary substance of abuse. Once patients have acquired physiological tolerances to the effects of their primary substance of abuse, they can readily become addicted to other substances, particularly those within the same drug class. This predisposition to addiction occurs due to a decreased sensitivity to the effects of structurally similar drugs within the same drug class, or a cross-tolerance. This cross-tolerance may increase the likelihood that the substitute drug may need to be consumed at an elevated quantity and frequency in order to achieve desired effects. This elevated quantity and frequency of use may place the patient at a higher risk for developing abuse or dependence symptoms to the novel substance.

Cross-Addiction to Other Substances

A cross-addiction may also extend to other classes of drugs, particularly if the patient has expectancies that they cannot control themselves when using a substance similar to their primary substance of abuse. Cross-addictions to legal addictive substances (i.e., alcohol, caffeine, nicotine) are common among former addicts who abused illegal drugs. Although the possibility of a cross-tolerance is markedly lower when using a substance from a different class than the primary substance of abuse, risks of addiction to the secondary substance are still present. Additionally, the decreased inhibitions that typically accompany most substance use may predispose the individual to relapse.

Cross-Addiction to Other Behaviors

For those patients who successfully cease to use addictive substances, the tendency towards addiction may be manifested in another addictive behavior (e.g., compulsive gambling, sexual addiction, Internet addiction, overeating). Although these addictive behaviors do not carry the same physiological consequences as substances of abuse, they can cause similar disruptions in social and occupational functioning. The compulsive engagement in these addictive behaviors is commonly accompanied by the use of alcohol or other drugs, which may also increase the likelihood of relapse to the primary substance of abuse.

Jennifer M. Day

See also Gambling, Pathological; Gambling, Problem; High-Risk Situations; Internet Addiction; Neurobiology of Addiction; Sex Addiction; Substitute Addictions

Further Readings

Gossop, M. (2001). A web of dependence. *Addiction, 96,* 677–678.

Haylett, S. A., Stephenson, G. M., & Lefever, R. M. H. (2004). Covariation in addictive behaviours: A study of addictive orientations using the Shorter PROMIS Questionnaire. *Addictive Behaviors, 29,* 61–71.

Kosten, T. R., Rounsaville, B. J., Babor, T. F., & Spitzer, R. L. (1987). Substance-use disorders in DSM-III-R: Evidence for the dependence syndrome across different psychoactive substances. *British Journal of Psychiatry, 151,* 834–843.

Miller, P. M. (1979). Interactions among addictive behaviors. *British Journal of Addiction, 74,* 211–212.

CULTURAL ASPECTS

Culture is the total way of life of a human group—a learned, shared system of beliefs, behaviors, values, norms, symbols, and customs. Culture profoundly influences how people perceive, define, and regulate intoxicated behavior; the meaning and symbolism of psychoactive substances and their use; and the roles played by persons consuming psychoactive substances.

Integration of Alcohol and Drug Use

Ethnography, the study of culture, reveals that psychoactive substance use is woven throughout the fabric of social life in a large proportion of cultures, especially small-scale, traditional societies. Perhaps most familiar to readers are accounts of southern European societies where alcohol is considered a food, meals and a variety of social and ritual occasions are incomplete without alcohol, people drink daily, alcohol is a social lubricant, but drunkenness is discouraged. Among the Itseo of Western Kenya, there is a highly developed vocabulary pertaining to beer use and beer paraphernalia. Long-lasting relationships between people involve beer-sharing with neighbors defined as people with whom one shares beer. On the other side of the continent, Kofyar of Northern Nigeria make, drink, talk, and think about beer. Beer drinking is pervasive throughout social occasions, relationships, and significant events. Bride-price can be beer and labor, or rent can be paid with beer. The only words for short periods of time in the Kofyar language are based on the brewing cycle. In the South American Andes, coca chewing, an essential ingredient of all ritual activity in the community, makes one a real person and affirms attitudes and values of indigenous Andean culture. At the July 2001 inauguration of President Alejandro Toledo of Peru, the first Native American elevated to that office, coca leaves were among the offerings burned by priests in a celebration of cultural affirmation.

Ritualization of Alcohol and Drug Use

In human groups, eating and/or drinking together represents communal solidarity. Drinking a disinhibitory beverage makes it an even more powerful event. In many cultures, ranging from the Mongols to the Mexicans, the ritual importance of drinking is underscored by the fact that declining a drink is seen as disrespectful and unfriendly. Certain ritual drinking practices, like toasting and buying rounds for the group, are ubiquitous. Chinese cultivate and value the skill of lengthy and loud toasting; in the Republic of Georgia, skilled toastmasters have celebrity status. In Spain, France, Scotland, Israel, Mexico, the United States, and many other cultures, the most common toast is to wish health for those present.

Substance use is also an important aspect of rituals of the sacred and supernatural. An early ethnographic expedition to the Yakut tribe in Siberia in the late 1800s recorded festivals involving fermented mare's milk, a recipe provided by the gods. There is the sacramental wine of the Catholic mass, the traditional Japanese house-building ceremony in which food and sake is offered to the god of the carpenters and a ceremonial cup of sake is poured for all men present, and the familial, sacramental significance of wine in traditional Eastern European Jewish culture. Hallucinogen use is associated with shamanism. In tribal cultures, a shaman is a part-time specialist who has access to supernatural realms which he may manipulate for the purpose of curing, divination, clairvoyance, communication with spirits, among others. Generally a shaman gains access to the supernatural during an altered state of consciousness or trance. The trance state may be induced via fasting, dancing, drumming, sensory deprivation, and by the ceremonial use of hallucinogenic drugs. Often, during the trance, the shaman experiences a journey or encounter with spirits and other supernatural beings. Ethnologists first examined shamanism among native Siberian peoples such as the Koryak, Yakut, Ostyak, Samoyed, and Tungus. The Siberian shamans used the hallucinogenic mushroom *Amanita muscaria* or fly agaric. The psilocybin mushroom and the peyote cactus are used in shamanic and other ceremonial activities by Native American groups. In addition, a religion based on peyote use spread among various North American Indian tribes in the late nineteenth and early twentieth centuries among North Mexican and Plains Indian tribes. Peyote religions had prophetic and millennial aspects for the oppressed reservation-bound native Americans. Rastafarians in Jamaica consider marijuana a sacrament.

Cultural Norms and Settings

In a majority of all cultures, alcohol and drugs are consumed in a specialized, public place. Solitary drinking is uncommon. Social interaction, information exchange, and "play" takes place at these sites. It is inconceivable to imagine European society without the café, or many societies of sub-Saharan Africa without beer gardens and parties. Opium dens in Laos during the 1970s were a social club, café, and a place to eat and sleep. Sociologists and anthropologists have also studied substance-using subcultures from the "skid row" and "bottle gang" alcohol users in classic sociological treatises, to the "crackhouse" and "sex-for-crack" subcultures of the late 20th century.

Cultural Attitudes Toward Alcohol Use

Culture frames alcohol use in several ways. First, cultures vary widely in what is considered an abusive level of drinking, in how badly one may act when intoxicated, and if it is a problem that inebriates become aggressive in a bar, or at home, or drive dangerously, or fail to arrive at work. Next, culture establishes values concerning psychoactive substances. In the "reefer madness" age of the 1930s, many saw marijuana as a "killer" narcotic, while in the 1960s a youth counterculture idealized hallucinogens and marijuana as a psychedelic gate to cosmic consciousness. Today, culture wars are waged over the benefits or dangers of medical marijuana and legalization of drugs. Earlier, the normative use of coca in the Andes was described. This contrasts dramatically with cultural attitudes towards cocaine users in America, seen especially in what sociologists called a moral panic and demonization of "crack moms" in the late 1980s. Finally, culture proclaims the etiology of addictions, whether moral failure, supernatural influence, or soul-loss. A cultural labeling process, applies to deviant categories, who are then scapegoated, segregated, and stigmatized. The new recovery advocacy movement in America is challenging the stigma attached to addiction and recovery. They recognize that some are doubly or triply stigmatized in this culture, such as addicted, minority mothers, and individuals with addiction and co-occurring psychiatric disorders.

Cultural Roots of Substance Abuse Disorders

Many ethnographers have declared that in a majority of small-scale, traditional cultures, alcohol use is not problematic or socially disruptive. Problem drinking is found in cultures with single-sex drinking, the absence of group or community recreation leading to boredom, drinking with strangers, and drinking in secular settings. When alcoholic beverages are defined as a food or medicine, and/or are integrated into the sacred and ceremonial life of a society, problems are rare. Sociologist Robin Room declared that ethnographic studies suffered from "problem deflation," idealizing traditional cultures, while addictions professionals might, conversely, have the bias of problem inflation (i.e., seeing all use as problematic).

The sudden introduction of alcohol into a society that has not had a chance to fully develop a comprehensive set of values and beliefs regarding its use is associated with alcoholism and problem drinking. In the 20th century, many cross-cultural studies were conducted that attempted to show that alcoholism was related to particular features of a culture, such as subsistence anxiety or child-rearing customs that created conflicts about feelings of dependency. Ethnologists have documented alcoholism attendant to rapid cultural change in general, and acculturative stress, in particular which may affect both individuals and entire communities, where traditional culture is fragmented, undermined, diluted, or devalued, or where stress-buffering social networks are weak. Attempting, but failing, to step out and integrate with the dominant or host culture may be stressful in several respects: economic deprivation, loss of status and self-esteem. To lose the role of breadwinner, or having to have children translate language, for example, communicates a loss of face. Social disorganization in general, boredom, solitary and same-sex male drinking, and drinking confined to a secular context are cultural factors associated with excessive and problem drinking. Disruptive drinking almost never occurs in a sacred setting.

Cultural Influences on Intoxicated Behavior

Intoxicated behavior and intoxicated roles are culturally shaped. In 1969, Craig MacAndrew and Robert B. Edgerton proposed that drunken behavior, or as they termed it "drunken comportment," is socially learned and normatively regulated. Beliefs about alcohol and inebriety are also socially learned. Alcohol use is often defined as a time-out, a socially sanctioned time and place for doing many things that would be categorically inexcusable under normal circumstances. The pharmacological disinhibition caused by beverage alcohol, the loosening of constraints on behavior, can mean many different things depending on set, setting, and expectation. Outright feigned intoxication, or pseudointoxicated state, are cited in a wide variety of cultures including the Rarotongans of the Cook Islands; the Truk of Micronesia; the Chippewa of Minnesota; the Yankton, Pine Ridge, and Teton Sioux; the Naskapi; the Aleuts; and the Salish. People become animated and convivial before actually drinking or as a bottle is opened. Some stagger about after a single drink. Conversely, staggers stop staggering when some event or task required their attention and alcoholic aggression carefully misses forbidden targets. Brawlers cease brawling at a ritually defined stage in life. The drunken state is invariably a public drama.

Ethnographers have examined the role of the "drunk" in several traditional societies; showing how socially labeled intoxication provides an opportunity to send information without repercussion. At festive meals and other occasions in the village of Amilpas, in Oaxaca, Mexico, an elaborate, polite front is always maintained. Animosities are denied and hidden behind this façade. But someone is almost always there to play the role of the truth-telling drunk, to everyone's delight. Drunks search out social gatherings, enter uninvited, and are very insistent on getting their information across. Intoxicated Irish Tinkers in mid-20th century engaged in bawdy sexual joking which would otherwise be considered scandalous. This, and antagonistic behavior, is excused with "the drink made him do it," or, "it's the drink talking." Cross-cultural evidence reveals that some groups show little aggression when intoxicated and some are aggressive only in specific kinds of situations.

Information About Culture and Substance Use

Attempts to describe cultural aspects of alcohol and other drug use may suffer from overgeneralizing about broad cultural supercategories such as Hispanic or Asians and may create stereotypes that are perpetuated in cultural competency training. For examples, some studies have shown that Dominicans drink less after migrating but that Guatemalans drink more. Furthermore, alcohol and drug use beliefs and behaviors vary by gender, age, social class, and region, as well as within a particular ethnic group. Among Puerto Ricans in the South Bronx, New York City, in the 1980s, a majority of older women believed that mental illness and addictions were rooted in supernatural causes and would refer an addicted family member to a spiritist, whereas younger and male individuals would more likely refer to conventional treatment. Finally, information about cultural groups goes out of date very rapidly, especially in the globalized, electronic era.

Conclusion

Human beings construct reality using cultural templates. The set, setting, and expectations surrounding drug use provide a framework for people to interpret pharmacological experience. In turn, this shapes their behavior while intoxicated. Cultural categories and social processes concerning normality, deviance, and illness channel the substance user into a moral career as patient, prisoner, fellowship member, or part of a drug-using subculture. Addictions professionals tend to focus on individual or familial aspects of substance use, as well as frame usage as a problem or disease, as opposed to the sociological and anthropological research cited in this article, which tends to emphasize the normative, communal, and ritualized aspects of alcohol and other drug use.

Peter L. Myers

See also Drug Use, History of; Gender Issues; Multiculturalism; Racial and Ethnic Minorities, Issues in Alcohol and Other Drug Use; Sociocultural Models of Addiction

Further Readings

Allen, C. J. (1988). *The hold life has—Coca and cultural identity in an Andean community*. Washington, DC: Smithsonian Institution Press.

Harner, M. J. (1973). The sound of rushing water. In M. J. Harner (Ed.), *Hallucinogens and Shamanism* (pp. 15–27). London: Oxford University Press.

Knipe, E. (1995). *Culture, society, and drugs*. Prospect Heights, IL: Waveland Press.

MacAndrew, C., & Edgerton, R. B. (1969). *Drunken comportment: A social explanation*. Chicago: Aldine.

Marshall, M. (Ed.). (1979). *Beliefs, behaviors, and alcoholic beverages—A cross-cultural survey*. Ann Arbor: University of Michigan Press.

Pittman, D. J., & White, H. R. (1991). *Society, culture, and drinking patterns re-examined*. New Brunswick, NJ: Rutgers Center on Alcohol Studies.

Stewart, O. C. (1987). *Peyote religion.* Norman: University of Oklahoma Press.

D

DECRIMINALIZATION

The decriminalization of drugs refers to a spectrum of laws and law enforcement strategies that are designed to reduce penalties associated with the criminalization of drug-related behaviors. The extent of criminalization varies according to drug type; for many drugs, including alcohol and most opioids, distribution, and use are permitted in some circumstances and sanctioned in others, whereas the manufacture and use of other widely used drugs, such as cannabis and cocaine, are criminalized in almost all contexts. The criteria by which drugs are matched with sanctions have been the subject of controversy, and current criminalization policies have been widely criticized as being arbitrary and counterproductive. Alternatives to criminalization generally fall into the categories of decriminalization or legalization. Advocates of legalization typically envision a system akin to current approaches to alcohol and tobacco wherein drugs are legal, regulated, and taxed. In contrast, those who favor decriminalization aim to reduce negative social consequences related to drug use without explicitly permitting that use. As such, decriminalization might be considered to be an attenuated form of criminalization. Indeed, many decriminalization policies maintain harsh criminal sanctions for a broad array of drug-related behaviors.

Decriminalization policies vary across nations and regions and according to type of drug and type of drug-related behavior. Most jurisdictions that purport to engage in decriminalization require one or more of three approaches to the attenuation of drug-related social consequences. The first approach is *elimination,* in which criminal penalties are eliminated for a subset of drug-related behaviors. The second approach is *replacement,* in which criminal sanctions are replaced with civil sanctions. The third approach is *reduction,* in which sanctions are reduced in severity but retain criminal status. The extent to which a given decriminalization policy conforms to any one of these approaches varies according to the type of drug and the nature of the drug-related behavior. For example, a given decriminalization initiative might eliminate sanctions for possession of cannabis, replace sanctions for distribution of cannabis, and reduce sanctions for possession of cocaine. This diversity of approaches complicates discussion of decriminalization and related consequences.

International Decriminalization Policies

Because much of the discussion surrounding decriminalization centers on the regulation of cannabis, a brief history of cannabis regulation provides a useful backdrop for the discussion of international approaches to decriminalization. The recreational use of drugs has continued in various forms for millennia. In this context, criminalization represents a relatively recent, and anomalous, development in social responses to drug use. Indeed, although cannabis use can be reliably traced back for millennia, the active prohibition of cannabis did not begin in earnest until the early 20th century. The Marihuana Tax Act of the 1930s, which effectively banned cannabis for recreational and medical purposes in the United States, is a seminal document in the history of cannabis criminalization. In the early 1960s, many nations followed the course set out by this document and joined the United Nations Single Convention on Narcotic Drugs, which internationalized the approach set out by the Marihuana Tax Act and expanded it to include most recreational drugs. The wholesale prohibition of these widely used substances quickly drew considerable opposition, and this opposition provided much of the nucleus of the current decriminalization and legalization movements.

Europe

Since the early 1970s, there has been a general trend toward the decriminalization of recreational drug use in Europe. However, as the following examples illustrate, the meaning and scope of decriminalization vary considerably across European nations. In Italy, the possession of small amounts of recreational drugs draws administrative, rather than criminal, sanctions. In Spain, possession of small amounts of recreational drugs is not penalized; however, public use is subject to administrative fines. In Portugal, apprehended drug users have no contact with the criminal justice system and instead appear before an administrative body of medical and legal professionals who administer sanctions ranging from fines to the suspension of driver's licenses and travel rights. In Belgium, cannabis use is technically a crime, but possession of small amounts results in a warning and on-the-spot fine. Russia has decriminalized possession of small amounts of most recreational drugs and has replaced criminal sanctions with fines or community service.

In other European countries, although drug possession is technically illegal, drug laws are routinely not enforced, amounting to de facto decriminalization. The Netherlands provides a well-known example of this approach. Although possession and sale of cannabis is technically illegal, several districts have enacted a formal, written policy of nonenforcement of the possession and sale of up to 30 grams. The sale of small amounts is also tolerated in coffee shops as long as the shops comply with regulations that include not advertising their products, not selling cannabis to persons under 18, and not selling any other drugs. In the United Kingdom, drug possession is a crime, but there is a presumption against arrest for cannabis possession and the common police responses involve warnings, diversions to social services, or no action at all.

In Germany, possession of recreational drugs is criminal, but the Supreme Constitutional Court held that charges for possession of small amounts must be dismissed. These examples illustrate the types of approaches to decriminalization in Europe.

North America

North America has also seen an increase in support for decriminalization over the past several decades. However, the focus has been almost exclusively on cannabis. In the United States, 12 states have decriminalized cannabis. Some decriminalization states, such as Maine and New York, have replaced criminal sanctions with civil fines. Other decriminalization states, including Minnesota and Nevada, have reduced the criminal status of cannabis possession for personal use from a felony to a misdemeanor. Alaska is the only U.S. state that has completely eliminated sanctions for the possession of small amounts of cannabis. This development was a response to a ruling by the Alaskan Supreme Court, which held that the possession of small amounts of cannabis in the home is a civil right that warrants protection under the state's constitutional right to privacy.

In addition to the patchwork of state legislation described in the previous paragraph, some states that do not have recognized decriminalization policies have nonetheless removed sanctions associated with small-scale possession or have enacted legislation that allows for the expungement of cannabis-related offenses. In some of these nondecriminalized states, the legal ramifications associated with cannabis are, in effect, less harsh than those found in states that purport decriminalization. Notably, all state decriminalization laws are, as a class, in conflict with federal drug policy, which emphasizes extensive criminalization. Despite this stance, the federal government has decriminalized the ceremonial use of the potently psychoactive, mescaline-rich peyote plant among members of the Native American Church, which suggests that even the relatively arch position of the federal government allows situations in which sanctioning drug use is appropriate.

Canada and Mexico have also seen increased movement toward decriminalization in recent decades. In Canada, many regions report de facto decriminalization, and there is growing support for formal decriminalization and legalization on the national level. In 2003, the federal government asserted that possession of small amounts of cannabis should not criminalize the behavior of otherwise law-abiding citizens, and it introduced a bill that would have decriminalized small amounts of cannabis across Canada. Under the proposed legislation, possession of relatively small amounts of cannabis would be punishable with a civil fine, and arresting officers could use discretion in determining whether to arrest persons with larger amounts. Although the issue of national decriminalization in Canada has languished subsequent to political change, efforts toward loosening of restrictions of cannabis use proceed at the regional level. The provincial courts of Ontario have held that criminalizing cannabis possession violates the Canadian constitution, thereby effectively eliminating sanctions for cannabis possession. Federal drug prosecutors for the city of Vancouver have stated that they will not pursue charges for cannabis possession that do not involve aggravating factors.

As is the case with Canada, despite growing support for the liberalization of drug laws, national efforts to decriminalize drug use in Mexico have not yet come to fruition. In 2006, the Mexican Senate passed a bill to decriminalize small amounts of drugs, including cannabis, cocaine, heroin, and hallucinogens, for personal use. However, the bill was not signed by Mexican President Vicente Fox. In short, despite legislative failures to establish a coherent decriminalization policy, policies aimed at reducing or eliminating sanctions related to cannabis use continue to enjoy substantial support in Canada and Mexico, and the adoption of decriminalization policies remains a topic of serious intragovernmental debate.

Other Regions

Few nations outside of Europe and North America have enacted decriminalization policies at the national level, and detailed information regarding the status of regional decriminalization efforts is difficult to obtain for many nations outside of Europe and North America. However, reliable information is available for Australia, where several territories have replaced criminal penalties associated with cannabis possession with civil fines. Under these policies, minor possession and cultivation of cannabis are civil offenses punishable by a small fine. This approach to decriminalization has been criticized for having the paradoxical effect of increasing cannabis-related negative consequences due to a policy of criminal prosecution for nonpayment of cannabis-related fines.

Despite considerable variation across nations in the severity of potential sanctions for drug-related crimes, virtually all "non-Western" nations comply with United Nations policies regarding the criminalization of recreational drugs at the level of official policy. Nonetheless, due to variations in enforcement policies and capacities, many regions, particularly in the developing world, have informal or de facto decriminalization for certain drug-related behaviors.

Decriminalization Outcomes

Decriminalization is a divisive issue, and there is substantial disagreement regarding the sequelae of this diverse array of policies. Indeed, as is the case with many drug policy issues, strongly held opinions on both sides are often based on sociocultural values rather than on reliable estimations of potential consequences. Nonetheless, sound empirical investigations of decriminalization-related outcomes have been conducted. The consequences of decriminalization policies can be estimated across several domains. In the following paragraphs, evidence bearing on the impact of decriminalization with regard to rates of drug use and enforcement costs is examined.

Drug Use

A central issue in the decriminalization debate involves the extent to which decriminalization affects rates of drug use, and opposition to decriminalization policies is often based on the assumption that decreased sanctions will lead to increased use. Contrary to this perspective, there is an apparent consensus in the drug policy literature that decriminalization has little effect on drug use. Specifically, studies from several nations that have compared rates of cannabis use before and after the implementation of cannabis decriminalization policies conclude that changes in use could not be reliably attributed to the adoption of decriminalization policies. Although some studies identified increased use subsequent to decriminalization, these studies noted similar rates of change in comparable jurisdictions that did not enact decriminalization policies. Similarly, self-report-based studies have not identified significant differences between U.S. states with and without decriminalization with regard to adolescent attitudes toward cannabis use.

Several explanations have been proposed to account for this somewhat counterintuitive finding. These include the proposal that decriminalization may have little impact on the availability of cannabis, that citizens are unaware of subtle changes in legal status of the drug, and that decriminalization policies merely formalize already low levels of law enforcement. The relative explanatory power of these proposals is an empirical question. However, the apparent lack of effect of decriminalization is generally consistent with literature on the deterrent effects of changes in sanctions for other forms of prohibited behaviors; that is, alterations in sanctions rarely impact rates of target behaviors.

Although the impact of decriminalization on rates of drug use has been the subject of some investigation, consequences for drug users have been less thoroughly examined. Indeed, given that decriminalization might strongly impact individuals who choose to use drugs, the impact of decriminalization on the quality of life for these stakeholders might be an important consideration in the evaluation of such policies. Further research is needed to clarify this important issue.

Enforcement Costs

A frequently cited benefit of decriminalization is an implied reduction in enforcement costs. This intuitively appealing perspective has found support in hypothetical models designed to estimate potential savings. However, given the plethora of factors that impact real-world law enforcement outcomes and given differences across decriminalization programs, a reliable empirical estimate of actual savings is difficult to determine. Nonetheless, studies that have examined real-world outcomes of decriminalization have generally identified results in the expected direction. That is, decriminalization appears to reduce the drug-related burden on the criminal justice system and thereby reduce costs.

Conclusion

Decriminalization includes a variety of policies designed to reduce legal consequences for certain drug-related behaviors by reducing, replacing, or eliminating sanctions. Decriminalization initiatives are increasingly being implemented across Europe and North America. Most of these initiatives are concerned primarily with reducing sanctions related to cannabis use. Decriminalization initiatives differ in substantial ways, and this heterogeneity complicates generalizations regarding the effects. Nonetheless, the best evidence suggests that decriminalization has no impact on use and may reduce social costs.

Tiffany Walsh, Zach Walsh, and Gregory L. Stuart

See also Drug Laws, History of; Economic Costs of Alcohol and Drug Abuse; Illicit and Illegal Drugs; Legalization of Drugs; War on Drugs

Further Readings

Fisher, G. L. (2006). Legalization, decriminalization, harm reduction. In *Rethinking our war on drugs: Candid talk about controversial issues* (pp. 53–69). Westport, CT: Praeger.

MacCoun, R. J., & Reuter, P. (2001). *Drug war heresies: Learning from other vices, times, and places.* Cambridge, UK: Cambridge University Press.

Pacula, R. L., MacCoun, R. J., Reuter, P., Chriqui, J., Kilmer, B., Harris, K., et al. (2004). *What does it mean to decriminalize marijuana? A cross-national empirical examination* (JSP/Center for the Study of Law and Society Faculty Working Paper No. 25). Berkeley: University of California Center for the Study of Law and Society Jurisprudence and Social Policy Program. Retrieved May 23, 2008, from http://repositories .cdlib.org/cgi/viewcontent.cgi?article=1041&context=csls

Single, E., Christie, P., & Ali, R. (2000). The impact of cannabis decriminalisation in Australia and the United States. *Journal of Public Health Policy, 21,* 157–186.

DEMAND REDUCTION

The U.S. National Drug Control Strategy developed by the Office of National Drug Control Policy has two components: supply reduction and demand reduction. Supply reduction involves efforts to lower the amount of illicit drugs available in the United States through interdiction, domestic law enforcement, and international efforts. Demand reduction refers to activities designed to stop young people from using illicit drugs or to intervene in the progression of experimental use of these substances to regular use (called "prevention") and services for people who have already developed problems with illicit drugs (called "treatment").

The demand reduction portion of the federal budget has ranged from nearly $6 billion in 2001 to a proposed $4.6 billion in fiscal year (FY) 2008. As a proportion of the federal drug control budget, demand reduction will be 35.6% in FY 2008 compared to 64.4% for supply reduction activities. The percentage of financial resources devoted to demand reduction has been decreasing since 2002. Nearly 66% of the demand reduction funds are directed toward treatment and the remainder toward prevention.

Prevention

The rationale for substance abuse prevention as a demand reduction strategy is quite simple. If it is possible to prevent young people from experimenting with illicit drugs, then the consequences of drug abuse and addiction can be avoided. Because these consequences are extremely serious (e.g., accidents, health problems, incarceration, family disruption, employment issues, and many others), it makes sense to make prevention a priority.

However, prevention receives a relatively low proportion of federal drug control dollars compared to other initiatives. In addition, there is considerable controversy regarding the best ways to spend these resources. As would be expected, nearly all federal prevention activities are directed toward children and adolescents.

Federal Initiatives

The National Institute on Drug Abuse (NIDA), a part of the U.S. Department of Health and Human Services, provides funding for prevention (and treatment) research. In the past few years, NIDA has supported research on prevention of escalation from early drug use to regular use, prevention of abuse and addiction, and the role of primary health care professionals in drug abuse prevention. NIDA also funds basic research related to prevention, such as understanding the neurobiological consequences of environmental stressors during childhood and adolescence as they pertain to drug use and addiction. This type of research might investigate chemical changes in the brains of young animal subjects that occur in response to a stressful situation (e.g., abuse) and the relationship between these chemical changes and chemical changes that result from drug craving. NIDA has also produced a guide on preventing drug use among children and adolescents.

The Office of Justice Programs in the Department of Justice has administered the Underage Drinking Prevention Program, a grant program for states to support efforts to prohibit the sale of alcoholic beverages to minors and the purchase and consumption of alcoholic beverages by minors. However, the president's budget has recommended the elimination of this program every year since 2004. Up to this time, Congress has ignored this recommendation and maintained this program.

The U.S. Department of Education has had two substance abuse prevention programs: the Safe and Drug-Free Schools and Communities (SDFSC) state grants and the SDFSC national programs. The SDFSC state grant funds are given to governors (20%) and state educational agencies (80%). The state educational agencies are required to distribute 93% of the funds to local education agencies (i.e., school districts) for a wide variety of activities to prevent or reduce violence and delinquency and the use, possession, and distribution of illegal drugs.

The SDFSC national programs provide funding for various grants and national initiatives. Generally, these grants are designed to implement evidence-based drug prevention programs in local educational agencies. One of these grant programs, the Alcohol Abuse Reduction Program, has provided funds to local school districts to implement evidenced-based programs designed to reduce underage drinking. Since 2004, the president's budget has recommended the elimination of these grants, but Congress has not complied. Finally, there have been significant increases in grant money for school-based drug testing programs since 2004. However, it should be noted that there is no empirical evidence that supports drug testing as a method to reduce illicit drug use among school-age youth. Drug testing appears to be part of a political agenda rather than an evidence-based approach to prevention.

The largest amount of federal prevention dollars are administered by the Center for Substance Abuse Prevention (CSAP), a part of the Substance Abuse and Mental Health Services Administration in the U.S. Department of Health and Human Services. CSAP distributes the prevention portion of the Substance Abuse Prevention and Treatment Block Grant (80% of these funds go to treatment and 20% to prevention). The money is given to the single state authority in each state responsible for substance abuse prevention and treatment and distributed to local programs in each state depending on its own structure and system. CSAP requires, under regulation, that the states use their block grant funds to support a range of prevention services and activities in six key areas to ensure that each state offers a comprehensive system for preventing substance abuse. The six areas are information dissemination, community-based process, environmental strategies, alternative activities, education, and problem identification and referral. The block grant funds are the foundation of most states' prevention systems, driving their prevention planning processes and setting standards and priorities for their overall prevention systems.

CSAP's other funding category is called Programs of Regional and National Significance. Since 2004, much of this funding has been directed to the Strategic Prevention Framework State Incentive Grants program. This program incorporates a five-step community development model: (1) Organize the community to profile needs, including community readiness; (2) mobilize the community and build the capacity to address needs and plan for sustainability; (3) develop the prevention action plan (evidence-based activities, programs, strategies, and policies); (4) implement the prevention plan; and (5) conduct ongoing evaluation for quality improvements and outcomes. The strategic prevention framework is based upon the risk and protective factor approach to prevention.

Finally, the Office of National Drug Control Policy, the agency that coordinates federal drug policy, administers two prevention initiatives: the Media Campaign and the Drug-Free Communities Support Program. The Media Campaign is an integrated effort that combines TV, radio, print, and interactive media with public communications outreach to youth and parents. Antidrug messages conveyed in national advertising are supported by Web sites, media events, outreach to the entertainment industry, and the formation of strategic partnerships with public health organizations, nongovernmental organizations, and other government and private sector entities. The Media Campaign focuses the majority of its efforts on educating 14- to 16-year-olds and their parents on the negative consequences of using marijuana. It should be noted that an independent evaluation of the Media Campaign by a federal agency detected no connection between the program advertisements and youth attitudes and behaviors toward drug use.

The Drug-Free Communities Support Program supports the development and expansion of community antidrug coalitions throughout the United States.

Initially created as a 5-year program (FY 1998 through FY 2002) authorized by the Drug-Free Communities Act of 1997, the program has been reauthorized by Congress through at least FY 2008. The program provides up to $100,000 per year in grant funding to local community antidrug coalitions, which must be matched by local communities. Community coalitions typically strive to increase community involvement and effectiveness in carrying out a wide array of drug prevention strategies, initiatives, and activities.

Controversial Issues

The relative emphasis on alcohol in prevention initiatives has been one area of controversy. It was noted in the discussions regarding the Office of Justice Programs and the U.S. Department of Education that programs with a focus on underage drinking have been recommended for elimination. In spite of efforts over the years, alcohol is not included in the congressional mandate for the Office of National Drug Control Policy. Alcohol industry lobbyists have prevented the Media Campaign from focusing on underage drinking. The issue is important because alcohol is the mind-altering substance most often used and abused by young people (and adults) and is normally used by young people before the use of other illicit drugs. Many prevention professionals argue that if alcohol is not the focus of prevention, these efforts have a low probability of success.

Another contentious issue involves "evidence-based" prevention. Although many federal initiatives mention "evidence-based" prevention, a focus on school-based drug testing programs contradicts this. Furthermore, the most widely used prevention program in schools (DARE) has been repeatedly shown to have no impact on the drug use behavior of participants. Although the federal government actively prompts evidence-based programs, it has been difficult for local school districts and communities to secure funding, training, and materials to effectively implement these programs.

Treatment

Most public-sector treatment occurs in freestanding, outpatient settings (i.e., nonresidential treatment programs). In many states, treatment programs serve both public-sector clients and private-pay clients (i.e., clients with medical insurance or their own financial resources). Many programs may have services for special populations, such as adolescents, women with children, and clients with mental disorders in addition to a substance use disorder.

Public-sector treatment also includes methadone maintenance for opioid (i.e., heroin) addicts. Methadone is dispensed through licensed outpatient clinics, and the clients are supposed to receive counseling and support services in addition to methadone.

The services provided by treatment programs may include individual, group, and family counseling; education about addiction and related issues (e.g., HIV); social skills training (e.g., meeting non-drug-using friends); and vocational, educational, financial, and self-care guidance (e.g., nutrition, hygiene). Many programs encourage or require clients to attend support group meetings, such as Alcoholics Anonymous or Narcotics Anonymous. The services provided are supposed to be designed to meet the individual needs of the clients, but there is wide variation in the quality of public-sector programs across the country. So, some programs provide the same services in the same manner to every client. There is also variation among states in the qualifications required for certification as a substance abuse counselor. Whereas some states require at least an undergraduate degree and an extensive internship, others require only a high school diploma or GED (general equivalency diploma).

Federal Initiatives

The National Institute on Drug Abuse is the federal agency that promotes treatment research. The focus in recent years has been on the neurobiology of addiction; dissemination of research-based treatment approaches, materials, and strategies to community-based treatment providers; and the development of medications to be used in treating addictive disorders. NIDA has produced a widely used booklet on the principles of effective treatment, which is based on research.

The federal prison system (part of the U.S. Department of Justice) administers programs that include screening and assessment of all inmates entering the federal prison system, drug abuse education, residential drug abuse treatment (treatment within specialized units), nonresidential drug abuse treatment (treatment integrated within the general prison system), and community-transition drug abuse treatment.

The latter program is a transition from residential drug abuse treatment to a community-based treatment facility following release from prison. The Office of Justice Programs (an agency in the U.S. Department of Justice) oversees drug courts and administers residential substance abuse treatment. Drug courts, a rapidly expanding concept, coordinate treatment services for nonviolent offenders with drug problems as an alternative to incarceration. The residential substance abuse treatment program provides grants to states to operate these programs in state prison facilities.

As was the case in prevention, the Center for Substance Abuse Treatment, an agency in the Substance Abuse and Mental Health Services Administration, is the largest federal agency involved with treatment. The vast majority of its funds are devoted to the Substance Abuse Block Grant. Most of this money is distributed to the state agency in each state responsible for the administration of substance abuse services (called the "Single State Authority"), which then distributes most of this money to community-based treatment providers to serve individuals with substance abuse problems who cannot afford treatment. The Center for Substance Abuse Treatment also has Programs of Regional and National Significance, which generally provide competitive grants for best practices (evidenced-based practices) and targeted capacity expansion (increasing treatment opportunities for special or underserved populations). In 2004, President George W. Bush started a program called Access to Recovery. Competitive grants were awarded to states to establish voucher systems in which individuals with substance abuse problems could get treatment or recovery services from providers of their choice. The idea was to allow faith-based organizations to provide these services and receive reimbursement for them.

Effectiveness of Demand Reduction
Effectiveness of Prevention

It has been extremely difficult to establish the effectiveness (or ineffectiveness) of prevention. The main reason is that most prevention activities are directed toward young people, but substance abuse problems generally do not develop until later in life. Therefore, it is difficult to establish a cause-and-effect relationship between activities that take place in youth and behaviors that occur (or do not occur) later in life.

The federal government has established the National Registry of Evidence-Based Programs and Practices. To be included in this registry, a program must establish significant outcomes on the basis of a rigorous evaluation. Among the many programs on this registry, there are certainly programs that have established effectiveness. This is not to say that the outcomes measured are substance use behaviors. The outcomes are usually self-reports of substance use, attitudes, or behaviors related to substance use (e.g., delinquency).

The federal government has often used national surveys of illicit drug use by youth as documentation of the effectiveness of prevention. However, it is impossible to establish a cause-and-effect relationship between prevention efforts and national surveys of self-reported illicit drug use by youth. As with many types of survey data, it is possible to find support for nearly any position.

In prevention, it is often the case that it is easier to establish what *doesn't* work than what does work. Clearly, the Media Campaign is not effective, nor is the DARE program. Ironically, the prevention activities with the most evidence of concrete effectiveness are those that are called "environmental prevention" and involve tobacco and alcohol. These activities include increases in excise taxes, sting operations, keg registration, reduction in retail outlets, and server training.

Effectiveness of Treatment

In contrast to prevention, there is a great deal of evidence on the effectiveness of treatment. The Center for Substance Abuse Treatment sponsored a congressionally mandated study of treatment outcomes for clients in public-sector treatment programs. The National Treatment Improvement Evaluation Study followed 4,411 clients in 78 treatment sites across the country for 5 years. Clients were from vulnerable and underserved populations, such as minorities, pregnant women, youth, public housing residents, welfare recipients, and those involved in the criminal justice system. Many of the people studied did not complete treatment, which would tend to depress any positive results. In spite of these factors, there were significant reductions in alcohol and other drug use 1 year after treatment regardless of the amount of time spent in treatment or the amount of treatment received. However, in general, stays longer than 90 days were associated with more positive treatment outcomes.

Positive outcomes were found in employment income, mental and physical health, criminal activity, homelessness, and high-risk behaviors for HIV infection. This study also demonstrated that the average cost savings per client in the year after treatment was $9,177, which is significantly more than the average cost of an outpatient treatment episode. The savings occurred in reduced health care and crime-related costs and increased earnings by clients. Outpatient and long-term residential treatment showed the largest cost savings, but short-term residential treatment and outpatient methadone also were cost-effective.

Similar findings resulted from a study sponsored by the National Institute on Drug Abuse of 10,000 clients in nearly 100 treatment programs and in a meta-analysis of 78 separate drug treatment outcome studies. In addition, a summary of 51 published and 17 unpublished reports regarding the costs versus benefits of substance abuse treatment firmly validated the cost-effectiveness of treatment.

Conclusion

Demand reduction activities include prevention and treatment. Although the demand reduction components of the National Drug Control Strategy impact the public most directly, they only receive about one third of the federal drug control funds. While many federal agencies are involved in prevention and treatment, the Substance Abuse and Mental Health Services Administration coordinates the largest source of federal funding: the Substance Abuse Block Grant. Prevention activities have been the most controversial and have the least compelling evidence for effectiveness. In contrast, treatment activities have demonstrated positive outcomes. Certainly, it would seem advisable to reexamine the distribution of federal funding between supply reduction and demand reduction activities.

Tony Clark and Gary L. Fisher

See also National Drug Control Strategy; National Registry of Evidence-based Programs and Practices; Office of National Drug Control Policy; Prevention Strategies; Supply Reduction; Treatment Effectiveness

Further Readings

Fisher, G. L. (2006). *Rethinking our war on drugs: Candid talk about controversial issues.* Westport, CT: Praeger.

Office of National Drug Control Policy. (2007). *The President's national drug control strategy.* Retrieved February 20, 2007, from http://www.whitehousedrug policy.gov/publications/policy/ndcs07

DENIAL

Among the more than six million alcohol and drug addicts who need treatment but do not receive it, the psychological construct of denial may be part of what prevents them from receiving this treatment. Denial is a primitive defense mechanism that originated from the psychodynamic school of psychology. Psychoanalysts generally define denial as an unconscious refusal to accept unpleasant experiences that are occurring. Denial is a way the ego, part of the psyche, protects the individual from experiencing overwhelming emotions and threats to self-identity. An example is when a driver continues to drive under the influence of alcohol or drugs and when he or she gets caught a second time and says, "The cops must have my car tagged." This statement reflects the use of denial as a way the individual's ego protects him- or herself from the unpleasant consequences of drinking and driving.

Most of us, however, use denial in everyday life. It is a universal mechanism in the face of unpleasant and overwhelming sensations. An initial "This is not happening" occurs for individuals in perceived overwhelming situations (e.g., car accidents, fires, deaths, perceived violations of safety or security). When the initial shock is over, denial may diminish as the reality of the situation begins to creep in. Denial can be both an adaptive and a maladaptive defense mechanism. An adaptive use of denial may be when someone's feelings are hurt in a situation and the person may refuse to acknowledge hurt feelings to prevent a scene. Later, the person may think about how his or her feelings were hurt and process these feelings. Eventually, individuals who use denial begin to see the reality of what happened. Facts and evidence help an individual "break through" the magical thinking and acknowledge that reality is different. When this occurs, the individual can see the reality he or she was refusing and begin the process of coping with it.

Denial becomes a maladaptive function when facts and evidence of reality do not "break through" the individual's misperceived reality. A person can become stuck in the distorted reality of denial. Human beings, in general, do not like to see themselves as causing pain to others, and denial is one way to protect this image. Denial severs an individual from reality, and a misconstrued reality takes its place.

Denial comes in many patterns. Absolute denial is the most primitive and global pattern that exists. Statements like "I don't have a problem" or "I can stop anytime I want" suggest an absolute denial pattern, as statements like these reflect a global refusal that substance use is problematic or consequential. Other patterns exist, in which denial is a part of other defense mechanisms. Rationalization is one such mechanism that involves giving reasons for events or reactions. Denial is part of rationalization. There is a refusal to see reality for what it is on a conscious level, but on an unconscious level, reality may be seen for what it is but is "rationalized" away. An example may be the driver under the influence, who, even after a second offense, "rationalizes" he or she can drive, because he or she had seven drinks in 4 hours as opposed to the usual ten. Other common patterns of denial that may be used include minimizing, blaming, intellectualizing, displacing, and repressing.

The disease of addiction was once called the disease of denial. As an addict progresses in the disease, denial takes a stronger hold to continue the misconstrued reality that the person does not have a problem with using substances and that negative consequences are not a result of the using but of something else. Thus, the addict's reality is that it is acceptable to continue using, even though the facts and evidence are to the contrary. As more and more negative consequences accrue as a result of using alcohol and other drugs, denial and its multiple patterns continue to distort reality in order to allow the person to continue to use.

Denial often has been called a core characteristic of addictive disorders. Traditional views of denial were that, when an individual refused to see his or her use as problematic, it was part of the "addictive personality" that required strong confrontation to break through. This concept led to the popular therapeutic communities of the late 1970s, which gave rise to the connotations of what confrontation is. More recent views, however, indicate that denial is not part of an addictive personality. According to research compiled by William Miller and Stephen Rollnick, the authors of *Motivational Interviewing*, there is no scientific evidence for an "addictive personality." Their research also indicates that denial is not a core characteristic of addicts or alcoholics. In the literature of motivational interviewing, denial is suggested to be part of a normal response to statements that threaten an individual's sense of freedom or choice. Denial is viewed as part of the ambivalence and resistance to change when an individual consciously or unconsciously begins thinking that something needs to change. In this regard, "denial" is viewed as a mechanism that reinforces an individual's belief to keep using. Traditional strategies that therapists use to break through this denial often will reinforce the denial, resistance, and ambivalence. When denial is viewed as a mechanism of ambivalence, however, and appropriate strategies are used to help the individual "break through" it on his or her own, resistance decreases.

Thus, the current views of denial indicate that it is not a core defense mechanism inherent in alcoholics or addicts. It may be a general resistance alcoholics and addicts demonstrate in reaction to the loss of the choice and freedom to use. It may also be a general psychological reaction addicts and alcoholics will have when confronted with evidence and facts of the consequences of their use. Both these reactions, however, threaten addicts' and alcoholics' sense of freedom and esteem.

Denial is the initial stage of the grieving process when an individual is protecting the reality of losing something, namely, the choice to use alcohol and other drugs. Literature suggests that when addicts and alcoholics begin the process of recovery, they may still be in denial about the reality of their use. As these individuals continue in the process of recovery and gain sobriety, the consequences of their use tend to surface. If the information is perceived as too overwhelming, there is a chance for the addict or alcoholic to slip back into denial patterns and resume using substances. However, with education and treatment, addicts and alcoholics learn how to cope with this sobering information to continue not only the recovery process but the grieving process as well.

Serena Wadhwa

See also Alcoholic Personality; Counseling Approaches; Motivational Interviewing; Therapeutic Communities

Further Readings

Lowinson, J. H., Ruiz, P., Millman, R. B., & Langrod, J. G. (2005). *Substance abuse: A comprehensive textbook* (4th ed.). Philadelphia: Lippincott Williams & Wilkins.

McWilliams, N. (1994). *Psychoanalytic diagnosis: Understanding personality structure in the clinical process.* New York: Guilford Press.
Miller, W. R., & Rollnick, S. (1991). *Motivational interviewing: Preparing people to change addictive behavior.* New York: Guilford Press.

DEPRESSION

Addiction cannot be studied or discussed without fully understanding the role that psychological disorders and mental illness play in the onset of addiction, the course of the disease, and the outcome of treatment. Specifically, it is important to understand how depression is interrelated with addiction. It must be understood how the interplay of all aspects of both disorders affects the outcome of both. It is not enough to simply understand that there may be a genetic link between the two disorders. Depression can be both a cause of, and an outcome of, addiction. It will impact the path taken by those who suffer from substance use disorders (SUDs). Therefore, it is necessary to understand the complexity of the relationship between the two disorders. Whether depression develops before or after the onset of an SUD, the combination is a deadly one. Among individuals who commit suicide, the coupling of depression and alcohol (along with other drugs of abuse) plays a significant role.

The relationship between affective disorders and substance abuse has been well documented. In a 2004 study of prevalence and co-occurrence of SUD and mood disorders, it was found that in individuals with a current alcohol diagnosis, 40.7% were found to have a co-occurring mood disorder, and in individuals with a drug use disorder, 60% were found to have a mood disorder. The ability to achieve long-term remission of either disorder is compounded by the onset and severity of the other. In particular, those individuals who suffer from a major depressive disorder that precedes an SUD have high rates of relapse. Understanding and differentiating the complex relationships between onset, course, and outcome to both SUDs and depression is important.

Genetic links between alcohol and depression continue to be found in ongoing studies. Yet for drugs other than alcohol, the genetic or biological link to depression, while apparent, is less well understood. However, the association is still evident. In one study with heroin users entering methadone treatment, 28% of patients were found to have major depression. Among cocaine users, it was found that individuals who were depressed had more serious problems across multiple domains than those with cocaine addiction alone.

The literature reflects a strong link between genetics and depression and SUDs. It is also apparent that genetics are not enough to explain depression, addiction, or the interplay between them. Social and environmental factors such as racism, poverty, sexism, ageism, and all other forms of oppression, trauma, and victimization play a significant role in the development of both disorders and can seriously affect the individual's prognosis.

Depression Explained

The term *depression* refers to several distinct disorders that have similar symptoms but vary in intensity and duration.

Major depressive disorder, often referred to as clinical depression, is the most commonly discussed form of depressive mood disorder. It is but one of several forms of affective disorder described in the *Diagnostic and Statistical Manual of Mental Disorders*, *Fourth Edition, Text Revision*. Included in this category of mood disorders is cyclothymic disorder, characterized by short episodes of hypomania and minor depression, and dysthymic disorder, an ongoing minor depression. Also included in the mood disorder category is bipolar disorder I and II.

General symptoms of depression most often appear as a powerful sadness, despair, or a feeling of being "low." Intensity and duration will determine which category of depression is diagnostically assigned. Major depression must last at least 2 weeks, can be a single episode or recurrent, and can be further categorized as mild, moderate, or severe. Some forms of major depression may also have atypical features or be accompanied by psychosis.

Dysthymia is a less severe form of depression but is classed as chronic. Although the individual who suffers from dysthymia may work and participate in the social world, they are generally underfunctioning in most personal and social realms. Individuals who suffer from dysthymia may also develop a major depression.

Bipolar disorder is sometimes referred to as manic-depressive disorder. This disorder is thought to have a strong genetic component and is equally distributed between men and women. Bipolar disorder is characterized by wide swings in mood and a cycling through alternating depressive and manic states. For some individuals, the cycles are rapid and intense, but more often, the mood swings appear gradually. While manic, the individual may simply be considered outgoing, funny, or "the life of the party." They are often talkative, active, and gregarious. In moderate forms of the illness, the individual's judgment is impaired. They are likely to be impulsive and engage in rash decisions that can have serious consequences for themselves and others. In severe cases, mania develops into a complete breakdown of rationality, resulting in a psychotic state.

Treatment

The relationship between SUD and depression can be described in several ways. The SUD can be independent of the depressive disorder. It can occur as a means to cope with the depressive disorder. Conversely, depression can be independent of the SUD, and depression can be a direct result of the use or withdrawal from substances of abuse.

Treatment, therefore, is determined by a number of factors. Etiology is important because the primary illness (addiction or depression) should be established first. This will impact the type of treatment recommended. For example, cessation of heavy drug use in an otherwise nondepressive individual may cause depressive symptoms to occur. Alcohol withdrawal is often accompanied by depressed mood. Withdrawal from cocaine is associated with an anhedonic (i.e., inability to experience pleasure) response that can last for a significant amount of time. Yet, drugs and alcohol are often used as a means to cope with existing depression. The most common epidemiological finding has been that SUDs and depression tend to occur independently yet often coexist. Therefore, knowing whether the depression is a result of substance use withdrawal, or an underlying factor in drug use, or independent of both is important. Understanding the order in which each disorder appeared will improve treatment outcome.

There is no complete agreement about how to proceed with the depressed substance-abusing client. Some professionals use a "sequential approach": One disorder is considered primary and treated first, followed by treatment for the other. Other professionals believe that a "parallel approach" is wiser; that is, treat both problems concurrently. What is critical in treatment is that the mental health system and the substance abuse treatment system should be coordinated. If not, patient diagnosis and care may suffer from competing or conflicting treatments.

Treatment will vary with the types of depression and SUD. Psychotropic medications are often used in the treatment of both addiction and depression. Because of multiple avenues to treatment, careful assessment by an addiction psychiatry specialist should be done with the depressed individual who has an addiction problem. It should be noted that after initial prescription of an antidepressant, improvement can take up to 8 weeks.

In the past, tricyclics and monoamine oxidase inhibitors were the most commonly prescribed antidepressants. However, these drugs—such as imipramine, amitriptyline, nortriptyline, and desipramine—are generally not thought of as first-line treatments primarily because of their side effects. In recent years, a better class of antidepressants called "selective serotonin reuptake inhibitors," or SSRIs, have been developed. Those commonly used for clinical depression include fluoxetine (Prozac), sertraline (Zoloft), fluvoxamine (Luvox), paroxetine (Paxil), and citalopram (Celexa), to name a few. Two drugs that affect the norepinephrine and serotonin neurotransmitters include venlafaxine (Effexor) and nefazodone (Serzone). Bupropion (Wellbutrin), a chemical unlike tricyclics or SSRIs, is often used as a treatment for depression and is sometimes prescribed for smoking cessation as well.

Bipolar disorder often presents special issues for treatment, and lithium is most often used. But due to serious side effects and issues of medical compliance, lithium is not appropriate for all individuals. The anticonvulsant valproic acid (Depakote) is commonly used as an alternative. Other drugs commonly prescribed include carbamazepine (Tegretol), lamotrigine (Lamictal), gabapentin (Neurontin), and topiramate (Topamax).

In prescribing antidepressants to children and youth, special attention needs to be paid. Although the benefits outweigh the risk, there is an increased incidence of suicidal ideation and suicide attempts in youth.

The treatment professional should also be aware that some recovery support advisors, particularly those in Twelve-Step organizations, disparage the use of psychotropic medications. Therefore, individuals prescribed such medications must be fully supported and encouraged to maintain their daily dosages. For many of the medications, abrupt discontinuation can lead to serious withdrawal symptoms.

Special Populations

Certain groups of individuals have unique issues in relation to substance abuse and depression.

Adolescents

There is evidence that adolescents who abuse drugs and alcohol are highly likely to suffer from co-occurring mental health problems. In one study, co-occurring depression in youth was found to be 37.7%, with young women experiencing the most severe distress. It is important to note that a substance use disorder and co-occurring depression raise the risk of suicide. Whereas women are likely to suffer more serious symptoms of addiction and depression, young men suffering from drug abuse, depression, or both are more likely to commit suicide. It has also been reported that youth who are involved in substance use and are depressed have more significant life stressors in their local environment, which increase the likelihood of suicide.

Women

Women are far more likely (2 to 1) to suffer from depression than men. Women who are substance abusers are also more likely to suffer from co-occurring depression. Violence, domestic and otherwise, is interrelated with both addiction and depression. The relationship between women, addiction, depression and violence cannot be overlooked or underestimated. The interrelationship between depression, violence, and addiction is well established, making it a significant area of concern for addiction, mental health, and domestic violence professionals alike. Women who are addicted to alcohol and other drugs are more likely to be victims of domestic violence from an intimate partner than those women who are not addicted. It has also been estimated that up to 75% of women with problems of addiction have been victims of sexual abuse. The evidence is mounting that trauma, and its association with both post-traumatic stress disorder and depression, may be a significant psychological factor in the substance-abusing female client.

Elderly

Depression is a significant problem that affects up to one third of the elderly population. In the elderly, comorbidity of substance abuse problems with depression is common. As individuals age, the likelihood of comorbid alcoholism and depression increases. When depression in the elderly is diagnosed, careful evaluation of substance use is required.

Literature that examines alcohol use and abuse by the elderly can be easily located. Information about the elderly and the abuse of illegal drugs is harder to access. There is some tendency to believe that illegal or street drugs are the province of the young. It is commonly thought that the elderly "age out" of this type of drug use. Unfortunately, this assumption may result in a lack of attention to drug use by the elderly. As the baby boomers of the Woodstock generation reach retirement age, they will enter old age with significant drug histories compared to their parents. This generation's differing attitudes toward drug use may present a challenge to care providers in the next several decades.

As modern medical therapies increasingly rely on prescription drugs for treatment of medical conditions, the risk of drug interactions rises as well. In the elderly, there is a significant danger to concomitant use of alcohol and prescription drugs such as benzodiazepines (i.e., minor tranquilizers). The number of elderly being prescribed antidepressants has increased steadily. Aside from misuse of these drugs, the therapeutic use of these drugs concurrently with alcohol has a potentiating effect that is very dangerous for all age groups, but particularly for the elderly. Suicide is also a serious concern for the elderly, with the rate for this group now shown to be significantly higher than that of the general population.

Conclusion

Depression and addiction are inextricably linked to the onset, progression, and outcome of addiction problems. All co-occurring disorders need to be addressed adequately by treatment professionals. Individuals identified with depressive disorders, addiction issues, or both, should be carefully evaluated and managed.

Nancy Brown

See also Antidepressant Drugs; Anxiety Disorders; Co-Occurring Disorders; *Diagnostic and Statistical Manual of Mental Disorders;* National Institute of Mental Health; Post-Traumatic Stress Disorder

Further Readings

Diamond, G., Panichelli-Mindel, S. M., Shera, D., Dennis, M., Tims, F., & Ungemack, J. (2006). Psychiatric syndromes in adolescents with marijuana abuse and dependency in outpatient treatment. *Journal of Child & Adolescent Substance Abuse, 15,* 37–53.

Grant, B. F., Stinson, F. S., Dawson, D. A., Chou, S. P., Dufour, M. C., Compton, W., et al. (2004). Prevalence and co-occurrence of substance use disorders and independent mood and anxiety disorders. *Archive of General Psychiatry, 62,* 807–816.

Hanna, E. Z., & Grant, B. F. (1997). Gender differences in DSM-IV alcohol use disorders and major depression as distributed in the general population: Clinical implications. *Comprehensive Psychiatry, 38,* 202–212.

Nunes, E. V., Liu, X., Samet, S., Matseoane, K., & Hasin, D. (2006). Independent versus substance-induced major depressive disorder in substance-dependent patients: Observational study of course during follow-up. *Journal of Clinical Psychiatry, 67,* 1561–1567.

Nurnberger, J. I., Foroud, T., Flury, L., Meyer, E. T., & Wiegand, R. (2002). Is there a genetic relationship between alcoholism and depression? *Alcohol Research & Health, 26,* 233–240.

Oslin, D. W. (2005). Treatment of late-life depression complicated by alcohol dependence. *American Journal of Geriatric Psychiatry, 13,* 491–500.

DETOXIFICATION

Detoxification is an initial form of treatment used to eliminate toxins from the body of an individual who is physically dependent on a substance. Substance dependence may occur with regular alcohol or other drug use over a period of time. In cases of physiological substance dependence, patients will experience withdrawal symptoms during the discontinuation of substance use. Programs that are based exclusively on a medical model of detoxification attempt to minimize withdrawal symptoms with medication; in contrast, programs based on social models focus on the psychological and social support of the patient, without the use of medication. Detoxification programs often include a combination of medical and social support from physicians, nurses, counselors, and other clinicians. There are also several types of program settings, including inpatient (e.g., acute care hospital, residential treatment center) and outpatient (e.g., clinic, counseling center). Specific procedures of detoxification vary depending on the severity of the alcohol or drug dependence, the drug(s) used (e.g., central nervous system [CNS] depressants, CNS stimulants, opioids), and preexisting health conditions.

Prior to the development and proliferation of more extended substance abuse treatment programs, detoxification programs were once the sole method of treatment for alcohol and drug dependence. Perhaps because there was no follow-up treatment after the initial detoxification period, people often cycled in and out of such programs, going through periods of substance use, treatment, and recovery. Currently, it is more widely accepted that detoxification is the first step on a continuum of treatment for individuals who are substance dependent. To help prevent alcohol or other drug relapse, detoxification programs often introduce the patient to longer-term treatment subsequent to discharge.

The primary goal of detoxification is to provide a safe and humane environment for the patient to withdraw from a substance of dependence. This includes an attempt to reduce health risks of patients in life-threatening situations. For example, in cases of severe alcohol dependency, there is a risk of fatality during detoxification. Medications (e.g., chlordiazepoxide, clonazepam, diazepam) can be administered to minimize withdrawal symptoms in such cases. Furthermore, there are safety precautions to consider when treating patients with preexisting health or psychological conditions. In circumstances in which patient safety is a significant risk, the individual may be sent to an acute care hospital.

The second goal of detoxification is to provide an opportunity for the patient to cease alcohol and/or drug use in a controlled setting. By removing the patient from his or her environment (e.g., decreasing contact with substance-using friends), he or she will be less likely to continue using substances. This goal is accomplished via provision of an environment that supports the physiological and social needs of the patient.

Because of the diversity among detoxification programs and individual patients, the final goal of detoxification programs is to meet patients' individual needs. Patients enter detoxification for a variety of reasons, including health, job, personal, relational, or criminal problems, and therefore may choose a program based on such circumstances. Furthermore, patients differ in terms of the severity and type of drug dependency, as well as coexisting mental and physical problems, and there are a variety of detoxification programs that cater to such specific conditions. To ensure patients' safety in treatment placement, it is imperative to assess their history of alcohol and other drug use, medical and psychological history, and substance-related medical problems. A thorough evaluation of these issues is critical, as this assessment provides the necessary information for a particular program to meet the patient's individual needs. Validated scales, such as the Addiction Severity Index, have been developed to screen patients and to assist in proper detoxification placement.

Social and Medical Model Programs

One way in which detoxification programs may vary is in terms of the treatment model that they follow. Whereas social model programs are set up to *respond* to severe withdrawal symptoms, medical model programs utilize medications to *prevent* severe withdrawal symptoms during detoxification. Both types of programs provide a caring and supportive environment in which patients can withdraw from their substance of dependence.

The focus of social model programs is to provide the social and psychological means necessary to undergo detoxification without medication. Counselors and other clinicians supply therapeutic support, such as cognitive behavioral therapy. This model is most appropriate for patients with mild substance dependency. Nurses assess patients' health and ensure that their symptoms do not prove too severe for nonmedicated care. They also regularly check vital signs and use validated measures to gauge withdrawal symptoms (e.g., Subjective/Objective Opiate Withdrawal Scale, Cocaine Selective Severity Assessment, Clinical Institute Withdrawal Assessment). To ensure safe withdrawal, patients are typically monitored 24 hours per day during the first few days of detoxification.

Even with proper evaluation, patients may enter social model programs before their withdrawal symptoms reach a level of severity that warrants medication. In serious cases of alcohol or other drug dependency in which physical health risks exist, staff members can assist with administering medication. If patients have more severe health risks than expected, such as those with extreme CNS depressant dependency, clinicians at social detoxification units may refer patients to an acute care hospital or on-call physician. It is necessary for these programs to have backup medical staff for situations of a life-threatening nature.

For individuals who display severe alcohol or other drug dependency, medical model programs may be more appropriate. This type of program employs highly trained medical personnel who administer medication to minimize withdrawal symptoms during detoxification. If a patient is at risk for seizures, tremors, delirium tremens, coma, or death, medication can be administered to prevent such occurrences. Medications are used not only for life-threatening situations, but also they can minimize the risk of withdrawal complications for individuals with preexisting medical conditions (e.g., cardiovascular conditions, psychological disorders) and ease the pain and discomfort of withdrawal symptoms. For instance, medications can prevent insomnia, treat depression, minimize anxiety, or aid in the tapering of drug dosage.

Inpatient and Outpatient Settings

Another way in which detoxification programs differ is in terms of treatment setting (i.e., inpatient or outpatient). Although patients can choose a program that best suits their personal, psychological, and social situation, it is crucial to first assess medical needs when choosing a detoxification treatment program. Severity of withdrawal symptoms and circumstances regarding one's job, family, insurance, support network, and environment are all factors that may influence the patient's choice of detoxification setting. The ideal setting for detoxification depends on each individual's needs.

Inpatient units are typically housed in hospitals (i.e., medical and psychiatric) or residential treatment facilities. Inpatient detoxification would be an appropriate setting for individuals who have preexisting physical or mental conditions, extremely severe chemical dependency, or an unsupportive and unstable home environment. However, such units are often costly and disrupt the patient from his or her daily life.

Outpatient detoxification occurs in a variety of settings, such as at home, in a hospital, clinic, or counseling center. Because the patient is not uprooted from his or her environment, outpatient treatments may be more appropriate for those who have a supportive family or a job with limited flexibility or leave time. Outpatient detoxification is also less expensive than inpatient settings. Unfortunately, outpatient settings do not always have the means to treat serious medical complications and severe chemical dependency. In such cases, patients will be admitted to an emergency room or inpatient unit.

Substances of Specific Drug Classes

Although minimal variation exists for withdrawal symptoms from substances in the same class, greater discrepancies in symptoms can be expected between the substance classes. Clinicians and physicians can employ methods to counterbalance or control withdrawal symptoms. The following is a review of the main substance classes, including common withdrawal symptoms and detoxification strategies of each.

CNS Depressants

CNS depressants are chemicals that slow down activity in the brain and decrease psychomotor activity. Common drugs in this class include alcohol, benzodiazepines, and barbiturates. During the detoxification process from alcohol, for example, a patient may experience anxiety, tremors, seizures, rapid pulse, and delirium tremens. For mild CNS depressant dependency, a patient may abruptly cease drug use with minimal negative consequences. In the treatment of severe dependency, there are two primary strategies. One approach involves a gradual reduction of the drug in the patient's system, and the other involves substitution and gradual tapering of a cross-tolerant drug. Detoxification from CNS depressants holds more health risks than that of other drug classes; therefore, extreme caution is warranted when handling severe cases of dependence.

Because trauma and death are possible, long-acting substitute medication, such as phenobarbital or chlordiazepoxide, will initially minimize withdrawal symptoms and can be systematically tapered throughout the duration of detoxification (e.g., by 10% of dosage per day). The gradual reduction of the substitute medication can take up to 2 weeks, depending on the initial dosage. An appropriate dosage of medication can be determined according to the patient's self-report of substance use, toxin screening, and testing to determine the patient's current tolerance level. When medication is administered, it is important for staff to monitor the patient's intake in order to prevent overdose.

CNS Stimulants

CNS stimulants increase activity in the brain and escalate psychomotor activity. Typical stimulants of dependency include methamphetamine and cocaine. Although there are no life-threatening physiological changes upon elimination of stimulants from an individual's system, there is a more subjective set of withdrawal symptoms that transpire during detoxification. Patients may experience feelings of dysphoria (unpleasant moods), depression, anxiety, insomnia, vivid and unpleasant dreams, and paranoia. There is no standard detoxification method for stimulant withdrawal; however, phenobarbital or chloral hydrate can be used to minimize anxiety and aid in the patient's sleep.

Other reasons for systematic stimulant detoxification are to prevent suicide and manage cravings. Severe depression can lead to suicidal thoughts in extreme cases of stimulant dependency. The lack of stimulants in a patient's system may also cause cravings for up to 12 weeks. For example, cocaine-dependent individuals often report strong cravings for the drug during detoxification, as well as feelings of extreme depression and irritability. Without a supportive environment, the patient may relapse or cause self harm. Therefore, an inpatient setting may be appropriate for severe stimulant detoxification.

Opioids

Opioids are used medically to minimize pain or induce sleep, but they may also induce a feeling of euphoria when they are abused. Well-known drugs in this class include heroin, morphine, codeine, and prescription pain medications such as oxycodone, and methadone. Withdrawal symptoms include gastrointestinal distress, anxiety, nausea, muscle pain, fever, sweating, irritability, and insomnia. Withdrawal symptoms typically last 5 days to 3 weeks, depending on prior usage patterns and the specific drug(s) of dependency.

Pharmacotherapy is a common method to reduce opioid withdrawal symptoms, which includes medications such as clonidine, levo-alpha acetyl methadol (LAAM), buprenorphine, or methadone. Clonidine is used for rapid detoxification from opioids, and it decreases most physiological withdrawal symptoms. However, patients complain that this medication does not decrease subjective symptoms, such as cravings and irritability. Methadone maintenance requires a longer process of detoxification, where the drug of dependence is substituted with methadone (or an alternative, like LAAM) and gradually decreased. The duration of withdrawal from methadone can range from 7 to 180 days. LAAM maintenance is another option, but the health risks of this drug are greater than those of methadone. A relatively newer medication for opioid withdrawal is buprenorphine. This medication is safer than LAAM and methadone if a patient overdoses, and there is a decreased potential for physical dependence on buprenorphine, as compared to most opioids.

Conclusion

Detoxification is an individualized form of treatment that is administered in a variety of settings, with different treatment models and a wide array of strategies. Given that alcohol and drug users are often dependent upon a combination of substances, the development of polysubstance detoxification is expanding. Regardless of the specific detoxification process, appropriate medical attention, a supportive and drug-free environment, and information about long-term treatment should always be provided.

Shawna M. Andersen, Meggan M. Bucossi, and Gregory L. Stuart

See also Continuum of Care; Pharmacological Approaches to Treatment; Rapid Opioid Detoxification; Substance Dependence; Treatment Settings; Withdrawal

Further Readings

Alling, F. A. (1992). Detoxification and treatment of acute sequelae. In J. H. Lowinson, P. Ruiz, R. B. Millman, & J. G. Langrod (Eds.), *Substance abuse: A comprehensive textbook* (2nd ed., pp. 402–415). Baltimore: Williams and Wilkins.

Chang, G., & Kosten, T. R. (1997). Detoxification. In J. H. Lowinson, P. Ruiz, R. B. Millman, & J. G. Langrod (Eds.), *Substance abuse: A comprehensive textbook* (3rd ed., pp. 377–381). Baltimore: Williams and Wilkins.

Mattick, R. P., & Hall, W. (1996). Are detoxification programmes effective? *The Lancet, 347*, 97–100.

McCrady, B. S., & Epstein, E. E. (Eds.). (1999). *Addictions: A comprehensive guidebook* (pp. 75–184). New York: Oxford University Press.

Miller, N. S., & Kipnis, S. S. (Eds.). (2006). *TIP 45: Detoxification and substance abuse treatment*. Rockville, MD: U.S. Department of Health and Human Services.

Wesson, D. R. (Ed.). (1995). *TIP 19: Detoxification from alcohol and other drugs*. Rockville, MD: U.S. Department of Health and Human Services.

DIAGNOSIS

The tradition of diagnosing a patient's illness or disease stems from medical practice. The word *diagnosis* in fact means to classify symptoms with the aim of describing a set of symptoms that the client or patient exhibits. The purposes of diagnosis are to (a) simplify and reduce the complexity of a clinical phenomenon, (b) facilitate communication between clinicians, (c) anticipate outcomes, (d) decide on appropriate treatment for the client, and (e) search for and better understand the etiology of the disorder from which the client suffers.

Diagnostic Systems

There are two diagnostic systems used in different parts of the world to describe mental disorders, including substance use disorders: (1) the *International Classification of Diseases*, now in its 10th edition, developed by the World Health Organization, and (2) the *Diagnostic and Statistical Manual of Mental Disorders (DSM),* developed by the American Psychiatric Association. In the later editions of the *DSM*, psychologists helped develop the diagnostic system, which is currently in its fourth edition, with text revision (*DSM-IV-TR*).

History of Diagnosis of Substance Use Disorders

The history of psychiatric classification started in antiquity. However, the beginning of the modern classification of psychiatric symptoms started with Emil Kraepelin, a German psychiatrist who, beginning in the 1870s, meticulously described schizophrenia, manic-depressive psychosis, and the cognitive disorders, among others. His descriptions were of a clinical nature, and they laid the groundwork for the diagnostic system as it is known today. Diagnostic classifications have been studied since that time. Kraepelin also advocated a thorough diagnostic interview which, today, is an important aspect of diagnosis.

The *International Classification of Diseases (ICD),* now in its 10th edition, is the latest in a series that had its origins in the 1850s. The World Health Organization took responsibility for the development of the *ICD* after World War II; it has now been endorsed by 43 countries. The *ICD* has become the international standard classification for all general epidemiological and health management purposes. It describes diagnostic characteristics for acute intoxication, harmful use of psychoactive substances, withdrawal states with or without delirium, dependence syndrome, and amnesic syndrome associated with substance dependence. There are substantial similarities between the *ICD-10* and the *DSM-IV-TR*. However, the *DSM-IV-TR* is used mostly in the United States, while the *ICD-10* is used around the world, including in developing countries.

After World War II, several state hospital psychiatrists in the United States decided to work together to simplify and unify the then-chaotic diagnostic system. The results, the first two *DSM* editions, *DSM-I*, published in 1952 and *DSM-II*, published in 1968, are considered consensus documents; they were not built on quantitative research. However, in the 1960s and 1970s, support from the National Institute on Mental Health increased funding for diagnostic research on mental disorders, and the more recent versions—*DSM-III*, published in 1980; *DSM-III-R*, published in 1987; and *DSM-IV*, published in 1994—were based far more on research than were earlier versions. The different editions of the *DSM*s have seen many changes for most of the mental health disorders, including the evolution of the diagnosis of substance abuse and dependence.

This evolution in the *DSM* started before the first edition appeared in 1952. In his 1991 overview of the development of the *DSM*, Peter Nathan noted that the diagnoses of alcoholism and drug dependence in the *DSM-I*, considered a subset of sociopathic personality disturbance, were lumped together with antisocial personality disorder and sexual deviations, including homosexuality. The *DSM-II* took a different tack by viewing alcoholism as one of a group of "certain other nonpsychotic mental disorders" together with the sexual deviations and drug dependence. In both instances, alcohol dependence was seen as a voluntary behavior worthy of stigmatization. It was not until publication of the third edition of the *DSM* that the diagnoses of alcoholism and drug dependence moved away from the moralistic burdens that were implicit in the first two editions.

The *DSM-III* was the first of the diagnostic manuals to be based on empirical research. In this diagnostic system, the clinician was given guidelines for reliable diagnostic assessments that had not been provided previously. The *DSM-III* included five Axes, including (1) syndromal diagnoses on Axis I, where the diagnosis of substance abuse or dependence would be completed, (2) diagnosis of personality disorder or mental retardation on Axis II, (3) a summary of medical conditions that might have influenced the psychiatric disorders listed on Axes I and II and on Axis III, (4) assessment of the psychosocial stressors facing the client on Axis IV, and (5) a global assessment of the client's functioning on Axis V. This approach to diagnostic assessment was much more in accordance with clinical experience and rendered a much more reliable and useful diagnosis than its predecessors.

The *DSM-III* also differentiated between physical and psychological dependence and included criteria for psychosocial consequences that are also a part of the most recent diagnostic manual, *DSM-IV-TR*. Alcoholism and drug dependence were seen as similar to each other in the *DSM-III* and so were categorized as substance abuse or dependence disorders, even though some of the specific criteria for abuse and dependence differed from substance to substance. Abuse of a substance was considered less serious than dependence, and tolerance and withdrawal from a substance were included in the diagnostic categories for dependence. Physical dependence on specific substances became a more important characteristic of dependence than it had been in *DSM-I* and *DSM-II*, and physical dependence was one criterion used to differentiate a diagnosis of abuse from a diagnosis of dependence. The *DSM-III* also included several additional diagnostic categories for the substance-induced medical, cognitive, and psychiatric disorders.

In the *DSM-IV*, substance abuse is characterized by pathological use of a substance that is sufficient to lead to adverse social and occupational consequences of that use. Criteria for substance dependence include (a) loss of control over and/or compulsive use of the substance and (b) tolerance and/or dependence. When the client reports tolerance and/or withdrawal, the diagnosis would include "with physical dependence." If the client does not report tolerance and/or withdrawal, the diagnosis would include "without physical dependence."

The new *DSM-IV* has undergone text revision (*DSM-IV-TR*), and the *TR* manual provides more guidelines for use of the diagnostic system than did its predecessors. For example, according to *DSM-IV-TR*, the diagnostician should assess how long the client has abstained from the substance and, in further describing the diagnosis of abuse or dependence, could specify in partial or full remission. If used correctly, the *DSM-IV-TR* provides more clarity and enhances the clinician's ability to communicate with colleagues about a client's symptoms and social as well as personal resources.

Factors Influencing the Diagnostic Process

Even though a diagnostic system is intended to describe a client's symptoms objectively, a range of factors can influence the diagnostic process. For example, cultural factors may contribute to the development of psychiatric symptoms, influence child rearing practices, determine the structure of family-based experiences, and affect coping mechanisms and problem-solving practices. Cultural events such as war, interracial hatred, exposure to violence from an early age, and historic and generational trauma may influence the development of mental health and substance use disorders. In addition, the use of substances may vary from culture to culture: Some substances may be used in religious ceremonies, whereas others may be used strictly for recreational purposes. Culture also may have an impact on how symptoms of a mental health or substance use disorder are expressed, including the content of delusional and hallucinatory states, mirroring current events and current personalities, and the way symptoms are perceived. For example, in North European cultures, it is acceptable to enjoy wandering in the mountains by oneself, and doing so is not a symptom of schizophrenia. Cultural ways of perceiving mental illness and substance use disorders, and the support of family and extended families, may be a protective factor for the client.

Several researchers have advocated assessing a client's cultural/ethnic identity in order to understand his or her mental health and substance use disorders better. One way to assess cultural identity is to elicit the client's perception of his or her demography, social status, and affiliation with different religious communities as well as the behaviors, expectations, and values associated with these same factors. Furthermore, the *DSM-IV-TR* has recommended using "cultural formulation" as a guideline for completing an ethnic identity evaluation and that such an evaluation should take place before the diagnostic evaluation begins. It is also recommended that the clinician not use race as a category for understanding ethnic identity, because the client's ethnic identity may not be related to racial category.

Religious and spiritual beliefs have a profound impact on mental disorders and substance use disorders. For example, Arthur Kleinman suggests that a client's explanatory model of illness that is strongly influenced by religious and spiritual preferences may affect a client's way of explaining their experiences and symptoms. Because these experiences and symptoms are used by clinicians to make diagnostic decisions, it is important to consider these factors.

Age, gender, and sexual identity are also components of cultural identity. Some mental disorders are more prevalent among men than women, and vice versa. Likewise, lesbian, gay, bisexual, and transgender identity development will have an impact on the diagnostic process, as well as the fact that being a member of a sexual minority group is associated with experiences that may make the individual more vulnerable to mental and substance use disorders.

Immigration status and experiences in the country from which the client has emigrated may influence a client's substance use and mental health disorders. Likewise, a client's level of acculturation and assimilation may impact the stress level and social connectedness with the culture in the new country as well as the country from which they come. Level of bicultural competence and ability to integrate two or more cultures successfully, with minimal stress, will impact the clinical picture as well. Closely connected to culture is the use of language, specifically, how comfortable the client is in using language to describe the symptoms they are struggling with. For example, the use of metaphors to describe experiences varies from culture to culture. The challenge becomes even greater when the client does not speak the same language as the diagnostician and an interpreter is required.

Diagnostic Assessment

Diagnostic assessment can be conducted through a nonstandardized diagnostic interview, a standardized interview, the use of specific diagnostic assessment tools, or all of these methods. The classic method used is the nonstandardized diagnostic interview, which can be ill defined, unstructured, unreliable, and invalid.

Research on substance use disorders has resulted in a number of standardized diagnostic interviews which, in addition to substance use disorder, also lead to other Axis I and II diagnoses. These standardized interviews include the Diagnostic Interview Schedule–IV, the Structured Clinical Interview for *DSM-IV,* and the Psychiatric Research Interview for Substance and Mental Disorders. Other semistructured interviews such as Schedule for Clinical Assessment in Neuropsychiatry and a more structured interview like the WHO/NIH Composite International Diagnostic Interview–Substance Abuse Module will give the clinician information about current and lifetime abuse of substances as well as substance quantity and frequency measures for use and abuse over the past year.

Conclusion

The diagnosis of substance use disorders is an essential part of the assessment process. The most commonly used criteria are those included in the *DSM-IV-TR*. The process to reach a diagnosis should include a comprehensive assessment involving a standardized diagnostic interview. Factors that influence the diagnostic process, including culture, ethnic identity, age, gender, and sexual orientation, must be considered in the diagnostic process. Ideally, clinicians who are called upon to diagnose will have had extensive formal training and supervised clinical experience in diagnosis.

Anne Helene Skinstad

See also Assessment; Assessment Instruments; *Diagnostic and Statistical Manual of Mental Disorder*; Substance Abuse; Substance Dependence; Substance Use Disorders

Further Readings

American Psychiatric Association. (2000). *Diagnostic and Statistical Manual of Mental Disorders* (4th ed., text rev.). Washington, DC: Author.

Andreasen, N. C., & Black, D. W. (1995). *Introductory text of psychiatry* (2nd ed.). Washington, DC: American Psychiatric Press.

Committee on Cultural Psychiatry. (2002). *Cultural assessment in clinical psychiatry* (Group for the Advancement of Psychiatry, Report No. 145). Washington, DC: American Psychiatric Publishing.

Craig, R. J. (2005). *Clinical and diagnostic interviewing* (2nd ed.). Lanham, MD: Jason Aronson.

Hersen, M., & Turner, S. M. (Eds.). (2003). *Diagnostic interviewing* (3rd ed.). New York: Springer.

Juhnke, G. (2002). *Substance abuse assessment and diagnosis: A comprehensive guide for counselors and helping professionals.* New York: Brunner-Routledge.

DIAGNOSTIC AND STATISTICAL MANUAL OF MENTAL DISORDERS

The *Diagnostic and Statistical Manual of Mental Disorders, Fourth Edition, Text Revision* (*DSM-IV-TR*) is one of the most widely used diagnostic tools in the field of mental health and is published by the American Psychiatric Association. Its development dates back to the 1950s, and revisions are periodically made to reflect the latest research and changes in the *International Classification of Diseases* (*ICD*). This entry (a) provides a historical background of the *DSM*, (b) explains the implementation of the multiaxial system of assessment, (c) describes the changes made in the *DSM-IV-TR*, (d) gives a brief overview of substance-related disorders within the *DSM-IV-TR*, and (e) outlines several issues in the area of substance-related disorders that deserve further investigation for future publications of the *DSM*.

Historical Background of the *DSM*

The *DSM* is one of the most significant texts used in the field of mental health, impacting clinical practice, research, and education worldwide. The *DSM* is used to classify mental disorders by providing criterion sets for each mental disorder as well as assigning codes to various diagnoses. The *DSM* has been in existence since the publication of the first edition in 1952. Since that time, it has undergone five revisions: the *DSM-II* published in 1968, the *DSM-III* published in 1980, a revision of the *DSM-III* (*DSM-III-R*) published in 1987, the *DSM-IV* published in 1994, and finally, the current text revision, the *DSM-IV-TR*, published in 2000.

Throughout the development of the *DSM*, changes and additions were made to reflect the state of knowledge regarding mental disease. Leading up to the creation of the first *DSM*, there was a need to gather statistical data on mental illnesses as was shown through the 1840 census, which recorded the frequency of "idiocy/insanity." Categories of mental illness continued to increase in number as knowledge in the field expanded. In the beginning of the 20th century, the focus shifted from the collection of statistical information to the development of diagnostic criteria. This occurred when the New York Academy of Medicine and the American Psychiatric Association came together and developed a text used to diagnose patients with neurological and psychiatric disorders known as the *American Medical Association's Standard Classified Nomenclature of Disease.*

According to the *DSM-IV-TR*, the area of mental health was largely influenced by World War II and by the U.S. Army to account for veterans who came back with various acute disorders, broadening the scope of diagnoses. Around the same time, the sixth edition of the *ICD* (*ICD-6*), published by the World Health Organization, also had a considerable impact on the development of the first *DSM*. The publication of the *ICD-6* included a portion for mental disorders providing multiple categories for psychoneuroses and psychoses, as well as behavioral, character, and intelligence disorders. A variation of this section of the *ICD-6* was then adapted by the American Psychiatric Association Committee on Nomenclature and Statistics in 1952 and became the first publication of the *Diagnostic and Statistical Manual of Mental Disorders* (*DSM-I*). The first edition of the *DSM* lent itself to clinical use more than any other mental health text before it. At the time, the term *reaction* was used throughout the text, referring to Adolf Meyer's view that mental disorders were primarily the result of the patients' personality reacting to social, biological, and psychological factors. This term was eliminated with the publication of the *DSM-II*.

After the first edition of the *DSM*, the well-known psychiatrist Erwin Stengel, along with the World Health Organization, conducted an extensive review of concerns surrounding diagnoses. According to the *DSM-IV-TR*, this review considerably influenced the diagnostic advances evident in the *DSM-III* with its inclusion of descriptive details surrounding diagnostic criteria. With the publication of the *DSM-III* came the inclusion of pioneering changes such as the implementation of the multiaxial system of diagnosis along with more explicit diagnostic criteria based on empirical research. Semistructured interviews also were developed during this time to aid clinicians and researchers in making diagnoses. Due to ambiguities discovered in the *DSM-III* edition, the *DSM-III-R* was published in 1987, and after comprehensive reviews and additional research, changes were made in this revision as well, reflected in the *DSM-IV*.

In an attempt to make sense of historical changes in the *DSM*, Lloyd H. Rogler proposed that one of the primary catalysts toward major changes in the *DSM-III* was the neo-Kraepelinian invisible college, consisting of a group of psychiatrists located throughout the United States and Canada. According to Rogler, this group of psychiatrists moved toward making diagnoses more reliable and supported diagnostic criteria through empirical research. Rogler suggested that the shift from a psychodynamic theory of mental illness toward a more medically oriented approach (with the inclusion of the multiaxial system of assessment) was due largely to the influence of the neo-Kraepelinian psychiatrists. Societal changes also affected revisions made in the *DSM*. For example, homosexuality was once a mental disorder in the *DSM-I* and throughout the third publication of the manual. It was then completely eliminated from the *DSM-III-R*, and as suggested by Robert Spitzer, this removal was due to an increase in societal awareness that heterosexual bias may exist.

The Multiaxial System of Assessment

The multiaxial system of assessment was implemented in the *DSM-III* and reflects one of the most important additions made to the *DSM*. The multiaxial system was developed to provide an organized and comprehensive way to assess an individual's mental state. The reasoning behind implementing a multiaxial system of assessment was to aid in examining a patient's mental state as a whole, ensuring a more complete and comprehensive assessment. In addition to assessing mental disorders, the multiaxial system assesses general medical conditions and environmental and psychosocial problems that can impact an individual's overall level of functioning. Although some have argued that this allows for a more holistic approach to assessing an individual, others have asserted that it casts a narrow view of an individual's complexities. Donald Oken refuted the biomedical model on which the multiaxial system is based. He proposed the need for a psychosomatic diagnostic system to help bridge the gap between physical problems and mental disorders. Dr. Oken suggested that this would allow for more holistic diagnostic criteria, accounting for biological, psychological, and social properties, unifying the medical and psychological fields.

The multiaxial system consists of five axes. Axis I involves clinical disorders, which include all psychiatric disorders except for mental retardation and personality disorders. These problems include adjustment, impulse-control, sleeping, eating, sexual and gender identity, dissociative, factitious, somatoform, anxiety, mood, psychotic, substance-related, and cognitive disorders, as well as disorders diagnosed typically in infancy, childhood, or adolescence. Axis II diagnoses include personality disorders, such as paranoid, schizoid, schizotypal, antisocial, borderline, histrionic, narcissistic, avoidant, dependent, and obsessive-compulsive disorders, as well as mental retardation and personality disorders not otherwise specified. This axis is used to account for maladaptive aspects of personality and defense mechanisms. Axis III includes general medical conditions that are relevant to the patient's mental state. This includes medical diseases, immunity disorders, congenital anomalies, neoplasms, injuries, and poisoning. Psychosocial and environmental problems comprise Axis IV. This axis accounts for environmental and social stressors that may have an effect on a patient's level of functioning, such as problems with the primary support system, with one's occupation, interactions with the legal system, access to health care services, or other environmental problems (e.g., exposure to disasters). The fifth and final axis is a global assessment of functioning (GAF). This rating is used for communicating the clinician's assessment of a patient's level of functioning taken as a whole. This can be accomplished by using the GAF scale, which includes functioning within 10 ranges. The clinician takes into account serious symptoms and serious impairments in occupational, school, or social functioning, and with their best judgment, notes the patient's level of functioning ranging from low (0) to high (100).

Changes in the *DSM-IV-TR*

There have been additions and changes made to the *DSM-IV*; the current version of the manual is the *DSM-IV-TR*. In preparation for the release of the text revisions of the *DSM*, review of the fourth edition began in 1996, 2 years after its publication. After extensive literature reviews, careful evaluation of the manual, and consideration of the updates made in the *International Classification of Diseases, Ninth Edition, Clinical Modification* (*ICD-9-CM*), the decision to revise the

DSM-IV was made. However, the American Psychiatric Association was careful to avoid making changes that would merit the publication of an entirely new edition (e.g., changes made to criterion sets). As described by Michael First and Harold Pincus, critics disputed the need to publish a *DSM-V*, as they considered frequent publications of the *DSM* to be disruptive to clinicians, researchers and educators who rely a great deal on the manual. As suggested by First and Pincus, this prompted the plan to publish the *DSM-V* no earlier than 2010, allowing for publication intervals to be approximately every 16 years.

According to the *DSM-IV-TR*, the main objectives for the text revision were to correct inaccuracies in the *DSM-IV*, review the text to ensure that the information was current, update information to be congruent with literature published since 1992, develop the text so that it may be better used as an educational tool, and to make it compatible with *ICD-9-CM* codes that the U.S. government uses to formally report health care. The decision to include changes based on empirically supported information was made in advance; however, according to First and Pincus, to avoid publishing a new edition, no changes were made to criterion sets even if such changes were supported by research.

Additions and changes were made under the following areas within the text, mostly updating information in the "associated features" sections of certain disorders: disorders usually first diagnosed in infancy, childhood, or adolescence; delirium, dementia, amnestic, and other cognitive disorders; mental disorders due to a general medical condition; substance-related disorders; mood disorders; anxiety disorders; sexual and gender identity disorders; eating disorders; sleep disorders; impulse-control disorders not elsewhere classified; adjustment disorders; and personality disorders. According to Michael First and Harold Fincus, the changes in the *DSM-IV-TR* that are notably relevant to clinical practice are the corrections made in the definition of pervasive developmental disorder not otherwise specified, in the clinical significance criterion for tic disorder, in the wording for the paraphilias criteria, psychiatric symptoms occurring in connection with dementia, procedures for using the Axis V GAF rating, and the notion of polysubstance dependence.

The definition of *pervasive developmental disorder not otherwise specified* was clarified by changing the wording to more accurately diagnose the disorder, as the *DSM-IV* wording allowed for the possibility of

more patients to be misdiagnosed. The clinical significance criterion was removed from tic disorders, allowing the possibility for more patients to be diagnosed with these disorders. The patient does not have to be significantly impaired or distressed from their tic, but can have a diagnosis with only the symptoms of the disorder present. Similarly, the wording of the clinical significance criterion for paraphilia and pedophilia was changed back to the wording that was included in the *DSM-III-R*. First and Fincus mentioned that this change was due to confusion caused by the *DSM-IV* wording that some readers thought restricted the possibility of diagnosis by implying that patients must be distressed by their behavior to warrant a diagnosis.

A coding change was made in the *ICD-9-CM* that now places all forms of dementia related to Alzheimer's disease within the same diagnostic code. To incorporate these changes, the *DSM-IV-TR* now instructs the coding of a mental disorder due to Alzheimer's disease to be categorized as Axis I with dementia. In addition, the criterion for *personality change due to a general medical condition* no longer includes delirium.

An additional change made in the *DSM-IV-TR* deemed to have a potential impact on clinical practice involves the clarification of procedures for using the Axis V GAF rating. As reviewed by First and Fincus, confusion surrounding what "current" time frame means prompted clarification, thus operationalizing it to mean the lowest level of functioning for the *past week*. Another issue that needed clarification was that a patient's functioning varies in different aspects of their life; instead of averaging scores taken from these various life areas, the *DSM-IV-TR* instructs the clinician to take the lowest overall score to report for the GAF.

Furthermore, clarifications were made under substance-related disorders, but First and Fincus found the portion on polysubstance dependence to be particularly relevant to clinicians. Clinicians have often misapplied the diagnosis of polysubstance dependence when an individual meets dependence for two or more substances concurrently. In these cases, an individual should be given several substance dependence diagnoses accounting for each class of drug they are dependent on. One interpretation clarified in the *DSM-IV-TR* allows for the diagnosis of polysubstance dependence when an individual does not meet threshold for dependence on various drugs independently but does meet criteria for substance dependence (polysubstance dependence) when combining the symptoms across categories of substances.

Substance-Related Disorders in the *DSM-IV-TR*

In the past, the *DSM* grouped substance use disorders under personality disorders, describing alcoholism primarily in terms of addiction and withdrawal with no structured or detailed criteria. Drug addiction was also listed as a symptom of a personality disorder. It was not until the publication of the *DSM-III* that distinct diagnostic criteria were included for substance use disorders. At that time, there were only three criteria for substance abuse, and substance dependence was defined in terms of tolerance and withdrawal.

In the *DSM-IV-TR*, substance-related disorders refer to disorders associated with the use of toxins, medications, or a drug of abuse. These substances are divided into 11 classes including alcohol, amphetamine (or sympathomimetics), caffeine, cannabis, cocaine, hallucinogens, inhalants, nicotine, opioids, phencyclidine (or arylcyclohexylamines), and sedatives, hypnotics, or anxiolytics. Within the *DSM-IV-TR,* the substance-related disorders are separated into two groups: the *substance use disorders,* which comprised substance dependence and substance abuse of one or more drug categories, and *substance-induced disorders,* which include substance-induced delirium, persisting dementia, persisting amnestic disorder, psychotic disorder, mood disorder, anxiety disorder, sexual dysfunction, and sleep disorder, as well as substance intoxication and substance withdrawal.

Criteria concerning substance dependence, abuse, intoxication, and withdrawal pertain to all classes of substances. The *DSM-IV-TR* criteria for substance dependence include tolerance, withdrawal, increased amount of use or prolonged period of use, continual desire to cut down or unsuccessful efforts to cut down substance use, a lot of time spent in activities associated with the substance, daily activities given up or reduced due to substance use, and continued substance use in spite of knowledge that persistent physical or psychological problems are possibly brought on or intensified by the use of the substance. The individual must endorse three or more of these criteria, all within the same 12-month period, to receive a diagnosis of substance dependence.

In addition, the *DSM-IV-TR* criteria for substance abuse include continued substance use resulting in the incompletion of major obligations at home, school, or work; continued substance use in situations that are physically dangerous; continued substance-related problems with the legal system; and continued use of a substance in spite of recurring social or interpersonal issues resulting from substance use. One of these criteria must be met within a 12-month period for an individual to receive a diagnosis of substance abuse. Substance dependence and abuse cannot exist within the same period. Substance abuse is considered a less severe diagnosis than substance dependence.

The criteria for withdrawal and substance intoxication fall under the umbrella of substance-induced disorders; however, withdrawal and intoxication are components of substance use disorders as well. The criteria for substance intoxication include maladaptive behavioral and psychological changes associated with recent use or exposure to the substance resulting from physiological effects of the substance and not due to a general medical condition or another mental disorder. The criteria for substance withdrawal include behavioral, cognitive, and physiological changes due to the cessation or reduction of substance use, which cause significant impairment or distress in various aspects of life and are not a result of a general medical condition or another mental disorder. The criteria for substance dependence, abuse, intoxication, and withdrawal can be applied across groups of substances.

With the publication of the *DSM-V* projected to be in 2012, research agendas have been implemented to make up-to-date, informed changes within the area of substance-related disorders. When considering future research that may help to integrate the two systems of the *DSM* and the *ICD*, John Saunders suggested that there be more attention paid to the nature of substance use disorders, possibly taking into consideration some of the recent neurobiological research. He also suggested examining the possible undesirable and less foreseeable consequences as a result of substance use and the possible influence of emotional and environmental triggers that may lead to the less severe substance use disorders. In addition, Saunders mentioned the possible incorporation of a condition termed *hazardous use*, which could be a subtype of substance use disorders. Whether this should be combined with substance abuse should be further investigated empirically. Saunders also stated that further examination of the relationship between substance use disorders and other recurring behaviors, such as gambling, is warranted. Furthermore, Saunders argued that there should be an additional investigation of substance dependence, more deeply examining the role of genetics and family history.

Conclusion

The *DSM* outlines what clinicians and researchers currently believe to be mental disorders and the specific symptoms that constitute each disorder. The creation of the *DSM* and the inclusion and exclusion of specific disorders, as well as the criteria that comstitute each disorder, are consistently reevaluated and reexamined in an effort to accurately reflect the most recent body of research. However, it should be noted that the inclusion and exclusion criteria, as well as any disorders that are listed, are constructed by a group of individuals who deem what is important and what is not. Therefore, the material within the *DSM* is influenced to some extent by societal and/or political norms.

Caitlin Diggles, Meggan M. Bucossi,
and Gregory L. Stuart

See also Diagnosis; Substance Abuse; Substance Dependence; Substance-Induced Disorders; Substance Use Disorders

Further Readings

American Psychiatric Association. (2000). *Diagnostic and statistical manual of mental disorders* (4th ed., text rev.). Washington, DC: Author.

First, M. B., & Pincus, H. A. (2002). The *DSM-IV Text Revision*: Rationale and potential impact on clinical practice. *Psychiatric Services, 53,* 288–192.

Oken, D. (2000). Multiaxial diagnosis and the psychosomatic model of disease. *Psychosomatic Medicine, 62,* 171–175.

Rogler, L. (1997). Making sense of historical changes in the *Diagnostic and Statistical Manual of Mental Disorders*: Five propositions. *Journal of Health and Social Behavior, 39*(1), 9–20.

Saunders, J. B. (2006). Substance dependence and nondependence in the *Diagnostic and Statistical Manual of Mental Disorders* (DSM) and the *International Classification of Diseases* (ICD): Can an identical conceptualization be achieved? *Addiction, 101,* 48–58.

Spitzer, R. L. (1981). The diagnostic status of homosexuality in DSM-III: A reformulation of the issues. *American Journal of Psychiatry, 138*(2), 210–215.

Volkmar, F. R., Shaffer, D., & First, M. (2000). PDDNOS in DSM-IV. *Journal of Autism and Developmental Disorders, 30,* 74–75.

DISABILITIES, ISSUES IN PREVENTION AND TREATMENT

Licit drugs (e.g., alcohol and tobacco), illegal drugs (e.g., cocaine, marijuana, ecstasy, heroin), and prescription medications may all be substances of abuse. According to the Office on Disability, alcohol and other drug (AOD) abuse continues to be one of, if not the, most prevalent public health concerns in U.S. society. AOD abuse costs the American economy more than $220 billion per year; these costs directly impact a large portion of the U.S. population. Costs to society include health care expenses, motor vehicle crashes, crime, lost productivity, and death. There is no group more susceptible to AOD abuse than the 54 million Americans who experience a disability. For these individuals, the process of overcoming AOD abuse is increasingly difficult because of barriers that individuals without disabilities do not face. Although AOD abuse varies from disability to disability, it is estimated that people with disabilities (PWD) engage in AOD at a rate that is more than 2 to 4 times that of the general population. It is not widely known that PWD are at a higher risk for misusing alcohol and drugs than the general population.

Risk Factors

PWD are at a greater risk of AOD abuse because of a number of variables. Such variables may include social stigma, easy access to AOD, self-perception, desires to avoid reality, myths, lack of knowledge, medication and health problems, a lack of identification of potential problems, and a lack of accessible and appropriate prevention and treatment services. Additionally, individuals with congenital or acquired disabilities have easy access to prescription drugs for legitimate medical reasons, such as chronic pain or muscle spasms. As a result, the ability of PWD to self-medicate, coupled with other physiological, emotional, or environmental factors, makes the progression from use to abuse quite likely for this group. Other contributing factors appear to be frustration, oppression, or social isolation that some PWD experience, and as a result, they may seek solace through abusing AOD. Lastly, to avoid confrontation, the attitudes of family, friends, health care professionals, and others may implicitly condone

AOD abuse by PWD. Despite their higher risk, PWD access AOD treatment at a much lower rate than people without disabilities. Disability groups that have been associated with an inclination toward AOD abuse include those with (a) mental retardation, (b) learning disabilities, (c) hearing impairments, (d) visual impairments, (e) physical disabilities, and (f) mental illness.

Mental Retardation

There is a noticeable absence in the literature related to individuals with mental retardation and AOD abuse. However, several variables warrant further exploration of this relationship within this group. First, as more people with mild to moderate mental retardation reside in communities with their non–mentally retarded peers, opportunities to engage in high-risk behaviors (AOD abuse) increase. Second, individuals with mental retardation possess cognitive deficits and limitations that may influence their decisions in the social domain. Third, although the research examining individuals with mental retardation and AOD abuse is scarce, the extant data have indicated that people with mental retardation engage in substance use and experience negative consequences. Factors affecting substance use include age, gender, degree of retardation, and residential arrangement (individual, family, or group home).

Individuals who are mentally retarded may experience difficulties processing AOD prevention and treatment materials. To that end, such materials may need to be modified according to the individual's intellectual capacity. Information must be presented in simple, concrete, and clearly defined language.

Learning Disabilities

A paucity of research exists relevant to substance abuse and individuals with learning disabilities. However, this is an issue of much concern. Many individuals with learning disabilities have delayed maturation as well as deficits in attention, psychomotor skills, and memory. Lack of knowledge of the nature and consequences of substance use, social skills deficits, and social ignorance of potential challenges they may face make individuals in this group particularly vulnerable to substance abuse. As individuals with learning disabilities are increasingly encouraged to participate in mainstream activities, their potential to abuse AOD increases.

Individuals with learning disabilities may have difficulty understanding prevention and treatment materials. Therefore, it is important when working with these individuals to (a) stress that ingesting even a small amount of alcohol can be harmful, (b) assist them in developing positive coping skills related to their learning disability, (c) convey the importance of developing stress management skills that do not include AOD, and (d) remind them that the use of AOD can interfere with learning, limit social skill development, and increase isolation. Prevention efforts may focus on teaching them about drugs and the effect of misuse, with developing recreational interests and abilities, enhancing communication skills, and building a strong support system.

Hearing Impairments

Hearing loss, also known as hearing impaired, affects more than 20 million Americans. More than 2 million Americans have no functional hearing and are considered to be deaf. The dearth of literature available indicates AOD abuse among individuals with hearing impairments is about the same, if not more than, for individuals without hearing impairments. Individuals with hearing impairments are usually in communities where their language is the minority language. Communication, or the lack thereof, with friends, family, and the community can be stressful for individuals with hearing impairments. As a result, the potential to abuse AOD is high.

A number of variables exist regarding issues of prevention and treatment of AOD abuse among individuals with hearing impairments. They include (a) a general lack of awareness of the problem and a stigma about having such a problem; (b) inaccessible resources that provide information on AOD; (c) accessible outpatient, inpatient, and aftercare services; (d) relevant training opportunities regarding the hearing impaired for professionals working in the field of AOD; (e) more interpreter training programs in the area of AOD; and (f) more AOD counselors who are fluent in American Sign Language

Blind and Visually Impaired

According to the American Foundation for the Blind, visual impairment (including blindness) affects more than 10 million Americans. A person is considered blind if he or she has the inability to perceive light, whereas a person with a visual impairment has loss of function as a result of visual limitations. It is estimated that at least 25% of the 10 million individuals with visual impairment may require treatment for AOD abuse. Individuals who are visually impaired are usually underemployed, have a lot free time, and isolate themselves from others, all of which increase the risk for AOD abuse problems among this population. Adolescents with visual impairments may face fewer consequences from alcohol and other drug abuse as a result of the enabling of others, social isolation, and constraints imposed by the disability.

There are a number of variables that may impede the treatment of individuals who are visually impaired. They include (a) impact of the visually impaired person's attitude toward service delivery systems, (b) lack of professional preparation in working with visual impairments among AOD professionals, (c) treatment systems, and (d) accessibility of AOD programs. Additionally, as group therapy is an essential component for the treatment of AOD abuse, it may be problematic for an individual with a visual impairment to benefit from this form of treatment because of their inability to follow the flow of dialogue among the group as well as missing the plethora of visual clues that are an integral aspect of the group process.

Physical Disabilities

Many disabilities can constitute a physical disability (i.e., traumatic brain injury, spinal cord injury, quadriplegia, paraplegia, muscular dystrophy, cerebral palsy, etc.) More than 26 million Americans have a physical disability. It is estimated that AOD abuse among people with physical disabilities is much higher than among the general population. However, incidence and prevalence varies depending on the nature and origin of the disability. Individuals with traumatic brain injury, spinal cord injuries, and amputees abuse AOD at much higher rates than other subgroups within this population. These individuals may use AOD to alleviate pain as well as to help them to deal with feelings of anxiety and depression.

A major concern for people with physical disabilities is the AOD and drug interactions. Mixing AOD with prescribed medication, whether analgesics, anti-inflammatory medicines, or both, can cause serious health problems for these individuals. Physical access to community services is probably the most important factor regarding treatment with these individuals.

Mental Illness

It is documented that more than 50% of, or 4 million, individuals with mental illness also abuse AOD. Some common mental disorders associated with AOD abuse include schizophrenia, bipolar disorder, attention deficit hyperactivity disorder (ADHD), generalized anxiety disorder, obsessive-compulsive disorder, post-traumatic stress disorder, panic disorder, and antisocial personality disorder. Individuals with antisocial personality disorder, bipolar disorder, and schizophrenia, in that order, are the most at risk for abusing AOD.

AOD abuse usually disrupts almost every aspect of care for the person with mental illness. These individuals are difficult to assist with seeking treatment. Diagnosis may be difficult because it takes time to decipher the interacting effects of substance abuse and the mental illness. They may have difficulty with home accommodations and may not be tolerated in community residences or rehabilitation programs. They suffer frequent relapses and hospitalizations and, as a result, may lose support systems.

Treatment for these individuals has not been favorable due to a number of variables. First, diagnosis of AOD abuse with this population can be difficult as the symptoms of the mental illness usually mask the symptoms of AOD abuse. Second, professionals are usually not trained to work with AOD abuse and mental illness together. Typically, treatment is available for people with mental illness in one setting and treatment for substance abuse in another. However, in recent years, dual diagnosis programs have evolved to meet the needs of individuals in this group.

Treatment Issues

Treatment of an AOD abuse problem requires accurate identification. Current AOD abuse treatment services are not adequately responsive to the needs of PWD. As a result, access to AOD abuse services can be limited, incomplete, or misdirected. Materials relevant to AOD abuse may be written at too high a reading level for a person with mental retardation or with a learning disability and also might be unavailable in formats accessible to persons with visual impairments (e.g., Braille or interactive technology). Treatment centers are often inaccessible to those with physical disabilities. Transportation issues (distance and location) may hinder access to specialized treatment centers for some PWD. Professionals who exhibit cultural insensitivity may prevent PWD from seeking treatment for substance abuse problems. Potential communication conflicts between professionals and individuals with hearing impairments may disrupt the dynamic as a result of limited availability of assistive supports, such as interpreters for persons who are deaf or hard of hearing.

Prevention

Because health care professionals and health promotion providers alike often focus solely on a person's disability rather than on the full range of health and wellness needs, they may fail to communicate AOD prevention messages that are given routinely to persons without disabilities.

Prevention efforts can be tailored for professionals and human service agencies treating these individuals. Such efforts may include (a) addressing the individual's ability to cope and adjust with his or her disability as well as the potential for increased risk of AOD abuse, (b) assisting PWD to get beyond the denial about the risks that may occur with AOD abuse, and (c) preservice and in-service education regarding early identification of AOD and knowledge of the signs and symptoms of AOD among PWD.

Conclusion

PWD have been linked to higher rates of AOD abuse than in the general population. The risk for abuse among this group can be attributed to a number of factors. PWD need access to substance abuse education and prevention materials that are culturally sensitive, linguistically accessible, and inclusive in order to meet their individual needs. The AOD treatment community should possess a broad range of knowledge of, and sensitivity to, all disability groups. Such awareness may have a profound impact on treatment effectiveness and will help health care professionals better address the needs of PWD.

James Bethea

See also Co-Occurring Disorders; Risk Factors for Addiction; Special Populations

Further Readings

Koch, D. S., Nelipovich, M., & Sneed, Z. (2002). Alcohol and other drug abuse as coexisting disabilities:

Considerations for counselors serving individuals who are blind or visually impaired. *Re:view, 33*(4), 151–159.

Helwig, A. A., & Holicky, R. (1994). Substance abuse in persons with disabilities: Treatment considerations. *Journal of Counseling and Development, 72*(3), 227–233.

Sales, A. (2000). *Substance abuse and disability* Greensboro, NC: ERIC Counseling and Student Services Clearinghouse. (ERIC Document Reproduction Service No. ED440352)

U.S. Department of Health & Human Services, Office on Disability. (n.d.). *Substance abuse and disability*. Retrieved March 15, 2007, from http://www.hhs .gov/od/about/ fact_sheets/substanceabuse.html

Watson, A. L., Franklin, M. E., Ingram, M. A., & Laurie, B. E. (1998). Alcohol and other abuse among persons with disabilities. *Journal of Applied Rehabilitation Counseling, 29*(2), 22–29.

DISCRIMINATION, ADDICTED AND RECOVERING INDIVIDUALS

People seeking help with their addiction or in long-term recovery routinely and consistently encounter public and private policies and laws that make it hard for them to get treatment and recovery support services, jobs, housing, and medical care and to exercise their civic rights. These discriminatory policies and laws are different from attitudes held by people that may or may not stigmatize people with addiction, because laws and polices can be changed and enforced. Discriminatory laws affect the ability of individuals to sustain their recovery, thus affecting clinical treatment outcomes as well as perpetuating addiction, family violence, school dropout rates, crime, injuries, and the spread of HIV and other infectious diseases.

According to the Institute of Medicine, the effects of stigma extend beyond the attitudes and practices of individual members of the public, patients, and clinicians and influence public policy. Discriminatory laws and policies that result from stigma may involve an individual in a position of authority denying employment or housing to an individual who is in recovery. More structurally embedded discrimination can also occur, as when treatment facilities are kept out of certain neighborhoods because of "not in my backyard" pressures and zoning laws.

In 2001, in the first-ever survey of the recovery community for Faces & Voices of Recovery, Peter D. Hart and Associates found that one quarter of people in recovery reported they had been denied a job or promotion or had trouble getting insurance. For people in recovery with criminal records, the legal barriers that they face can be even more daunting. Many leave the criminal justice system still struggling with their addiction, and others in recovery have criminal histories—as a result of their activities while they were still using—that keep them from jobs, housing, and families that would help them get their lives back on track. They often find that they face discrimination for their addiction and criminal justice histories.

Laws

The Americans with Disabilities Act, which protects millions of people with disabilities, offers limited protection to people seeking treatment and recovery from addiction. A 1998 decision by the Fifth Circuit Court found that alcoholics are not protected unless their illness is so extreme that they have permanent, debilitating conditions, such as altered gait, memory loss when sober, or long-term insomnia. Federal laws do not provide any protection from discrimination to people who currently engage in the illegal use of drugs, except when it comes to denying these individuals health services if they are otherwise entitled to those services.

According to the Legal Action Center, many federal and state laws prohibit employers, landlords, schools, government programs, and service providers from refusing to hire, rent to, admit to their schools, or serve anyone simply because he or she is in recovery from alcoholism or drug addiction. Federal laws such as the Americans with Disabilities Act and Fair Housing Act and similar laws in many states outlaw those kinds of across-the-board, stereotyped denial of basic rights to people in recovery.

These laws give people in recovery from addiction the same rights as people who have suffered from other illnesses or "disabilities" (the legal term). They can only be denied jobs, housing, admission to school, or other services or activities for which they are qualified if their addiction history would prevent them from successfully participating.

Insurance Discrimination

One of the most visible forms of discrimination is the more limited health insurance coverage for addiction care. Insurers continue to impose greater limits on health care coverage for people with alcohol and other drug problems by requiring higher co-payments and deductibles, limiting benefits and excluding coverage altogether if an injured individual was under the influence of alcohol or some other drug(s) at the time of injury.

Criminal Justice Issues

Discrimination can be seen in the low levels of treatment for addiction of people who are incarcerated. In 1998, only 20% of convicted jail inmates who were actively involved with drugs prior to their admission to jail had participated in substance use treatment or programs subsequent to their incarceration, although substance use problems and illnesses play a large role in incarceration.

Discrimination is also seen in public policies that impose additional penalties beyond those imposed by the judicial system on individuals with criminal justice convictions related to some types of drug use. These policies are significant barriers to the reintegration of people no longer using alcohol or drugs into families and communities and often make it difficult for individuals to sustain their recovery.

Some state laws prohibit discrimination in certain circumstances based on criminal justice history. The Americans with Disabilities Act and the Fair Housing Act, which protect people from discrimination because they have an addiction history, do not forbid discrimination against someone because of a past criminal record. The Federal Fair Housing Act, passed in 1968 to prevent housing discrimination based on race, color, religion, sex, handicap, familial status, and national origin, does nothing to stop landlords from discriminating against people with criminal records, such as past drug convictions.

According to the Legal Action Center, no federal law specifically prohibits employers or others from discriminating against people based on their past arrests or convictions. While it is illegal for an employer, before making a job offer, to ask questions about whether a job applicant has or has had a disability or about the nature or severity of an applicant's disability, or to discriminate on the basis of a disability, employers can ask about convictions and, in some states, arrest histories. In many states, employers can refuse to hire a person because of that arrest or conviction history.

There are also still some federal laws that specifically target people with drug-related criminal records and bar or limit their eligibility for some public benefits, education aid, and housing. For example, under Section 115 of the Personal Responsibility and Work Opportunity Reconciliation Act of 1996, better known as the Welfare Reform Act, persons convicted of a state or federal felony offense for selling or using drugs are subject to a lifetime ban on receiving government cash assistance and food stamps. Convictions for other crimes, including even murder, do not result in the loss of benefits.

According to the American Bar Association, the drug provision of the Welfare Reform Act applies to all states unless a state legislature elects to either modify or opt out of the provision. Modifications include, for example, ineligibility for welfare benefits limited to persons convicted of a particular drug offense, such as manufacturing or distributing illegal drugs. Other states maintain welfare eligibility provided that a person is participating in a state-approved drug treatment program.

The Anti-Drug Abuse Act of 1988, as amended in 1996, requires that all public housing leases contain a provision that "any drug-related criminal activity on or off such premises, engaged in by a public housing tenant, any member of the tenant's household, or any guest or other person under the tenant's control, shall be cause for termination of tenancy." Eviction does not depend on actual guilt or a criminal conviction; an accusation may be sufficient to evict a family.

The law provides housing authorities with discretion before eviction, including giving authorities the ability to allow people to stay in public housing if they successfully complete a treatment program. Too frequently, though, that discretion is not exercised. Typically, people are summarily evicted or denied housing without individual consideration. It is arguably easier to exclude those who cause problems than to provide them with services. In exercising this discretion, public housing authorities should take into consideration domestic violence concerns.

Some states have laws or licensing restrictions that bar individuals with a drug conviction from certain occupations. According to the National Council on Alcoholism and Drug Dependence–New Jersey, people with a drug conviction, including possession of paraphernalia, regardless of the intervening time frame or rehabilitation, are statutorily barred from obtaining employment as aircraft or airport employees or as school employees, including teacher, substitute teacher, teacher's aide, school bus driver, cafeteria worker, secretary, clerical worker, or maintenance worker. There are also statutory restrictions that deny people employment or prevent them from obtaining certificates or licenses based solely on having an alcohol or drug addiction, even if they have been in recovery. These include but are not limited to administrators and supervisors of the U.S. Department of Conservation, parks and reservations, airfrieghtman, and longshoreman.

Many states do not have laws that regulate how employers should evaluate a criminal record when considering applicants. In states lacking such regulation, employers can deny jobs to applicants solely because of their criminal record, even if the record consists only of arrests that did not lead to conviction or convictions that are old, minor, or unrelated to the job. Other states have laws that prohibit public and private employers and occupational licensing agencies from discrimination. Some states make it illegal for employers and licensing agencies to ask about arrests that did not lead to convictions. Some states also make it illegal for employers to have blanket policies against hiring people with criminal histories. These states require employers to individually consider each person who applies for a job and make a decision about hiring that person based on his or her qualifications and other factors.

Nationally, an estimated 5.3 million Americans are denied the right to vote because of laws that prohibit voting by people with felony convictions, many of whom are in recovery from addiction. There is an extraordinary variety and complexity of state and federal laws that impose a continuing burden on convicted persons long after the court-imposed sentence has been fully discharged. For individuals who have served their time, paid their debt to society, and want to participate in civic life, policies that keep them from voting are counterproductive. In November 2006, Rhode Island voted in a statewide ballot initiative to restore the right to vote to individuals immediately after they leave prison. Before their re-enfranchisement, more than 15,500 Rhode Island residents could not vote.

Conclusion

Despite concerted efforts from the recovery community and certain federal agencies to reduce the stigma of addiction, discrimination against addicted and recovering individuals remains intact in many segments of society. While some discrimination can be attributed to the slow process of changing laws and policies, the relationship between criminal justice involvement and addiction is a significant factor. Furthermore, the discrimination in the health care system remains tied to the stigma of addiction and difficulty in educating policymakers about the disease of addiction.

Pat Taylor

See also Criminal Justice Populations; Drug Courts; Public Policy, Treatment; Recovery

Further Readings

Institute of Medicine. (2006). *Improving the quality of health care for mental health and substance-use conditions.* Washington, DC: National Academies Press. Retrieved June 27, 2007, from http://books.nap.edu/catalog .php?record_id=11470

Join Together. (2004). *Recommendation report: Ending discrimination against people with alcohol and drug problems.* Retrieved May 25, 2008, from http://www.join together.org/aboutus/ourpublications/pdf/discrimination.pdf

Legal Action Center. (2005). *.Advocacy toolkits to combat legal barriers facing individuals with criminal records.* Retrieved June 27, 2007, from http://www.lac .org/toolkits/Introduction.htm

National Council on Alcoholism and Drug Dependence–New Jersey. (2004). *Overcoming addiction discrimination: State experts and policy-makers develop recommendations.* Retrieved May 25, 2007, from http://www.ncaddnj.org/pdf/DescrimFINAL.pdf

DISEASE CONCEPT

This popular and controversial model of addiction is credited to E. M. Jellinek, who presented a comprehensive disease model of alcoholism in 1960. The disease concept has become an implicit component of the Alcoholics Anonymous and Narcotics Anonymous programs, as well as a guiding model for many treatment programs. The World Health Organization acknowledged alcoholism as a medical problem in 1951, and the American Medical Association declared that alcoholism was a treatable illness in 1956. Following Jellinek's work, the American Psychiatric Association began to use the term *disease* to describe alcoholism in 1965, and the American Medical Association followed in 1966. As with many concepts and theoretical models in the addiction field, the disease concept was originally applied to alcoholism and has been generalized to addiction to other drugs.

Characteristics of the Disease Concept

The disease of addiction is viewed as a primary disease. That is, it exists in and of itself and is not secondary to some other condition. This is in contrast to psychological models of addiction in which addictive behavior is seen as secondary to some psychological condition. Jellinek also described the progressive stages of the disease of alcoholism and the symptoms that characterize each stage. The early stage, or prodromal phase, is characterized by an increasing tolerance to alcohol, blackouts, sneaking and gulping drinks, and guilt feelings about drinking and related behaviors. The next stage, the middle or crucial phase, is defined by a loss of control over drinking, personality changes, a loss of friends and jobs, and a preoccupation with protecting the supply of alcohol. The issue of "loss of control" has come to be a central defining characteristic of alcoholism and one of the more controversial aspects of the disease concept. The late stage, or chronic phase, is characterized by morning drinking, violations of ethical standards, tremors, and hallucinations.

It is important to conceptualize these stages as progressive. In other words, the stages proceed in sequence and, in the disease model of addiction, are not reversible. Therefore, an individual does not go from the middle stage back to the early stage of alcoholism. The rate at which this progression occurs depends upon factors such as age, drug of choice, gender, and physiological predisposition. For example, adolescents progress more rapidly than adults, females faster than males, and users of stimulants more quickly than alcohol users. Proponents of the disease concept also do not believe that the progression of addiction disease is affected by a period of sobriety, no matter how long the period of sobriety lasts. Consistent with this concept is the notion that addictive disease is chronic and incurable. That is, if an individual has this disease, it never goes away, and there is no drug or other treatment method that will allow the alcoholic or addict to use again without the danger of a return to problematic use. One implication of this notion is that the only justifiable goal for the alcoholic or addict is abstinence. Furthermore, the idea that addiction is chronic and incurable is the underlying rationale for alcoholics and addicts who are maintaining sobriety for referring to themselves as "recovering" as opposed to "recovered" or "cured."

In addition to the idea that abstinence must be the goal for those with addictive disease, there are other implications to the disease concept. First, if addictive disease is progressive, chronic, and incurable, then it is logical to assume that a person with this condition who does not enter recovery will eventually die. Death occurs as a result of accidents or the physical effects of alcohol and other drugs over time. A further implication of the disease concept of addiction is that, if a person has this disease and, for example, the drug of choice of the person is alcohol, the person will continue to exhibit all the symptoms of the disease if he or she discontinues the use of alcohol and begins to use some other drug. This is true no matter what the drug of choice is. Therefore, alcoholics and other addicts must abstain from all psychoactive drugs.

Evidence to Support the Concept

The primary evidence to support the disease concept is based on the similarity of alcoholism and drug addiction to other chronic diseases. In 2000, Tom McLellan and his colleagues reviewed the literature on chronic illnesses, such as diabetes, asthma, and hypertension, and compared the characteristics of these diseases to addiction. They found that the genetic heritability, established by examining rates of diseases in identical versus fraternal twins, was very similar for alcoholism and drug addiction compared to the other chronic illnesses. In addition, response to treatment is similar. Left untreated, the condition of most alcoholics and drug addicts becomes worse. Remission is unusual. This also occurs with diabetes, asthma, and hypertension. McLellan also showed that the percentages of clients who comply with treatment and the relapse rates of addiction and other chronic illnesses are the same. Addiction, diabetes, asthma, and

hypertension are all conditions in which there is no "cure." However, all these problems can be managed through proper treatment, and this treatment must be followed for life.

McLellan also discussed the issue of the "voluntary" nature of alcohol and other drug use. Again, he compared the choice to use alcohol and other drugs to other chronic illnesses. For example, diet, physical activity, and stress level are all factors affecting hypertension. These factors are all within voluntary control. However, what is not in voluntary control is the person's physiological response to these factors, and the physiological response is strongly influenced by genetic factors. Therefore, addiction is similar to other chronic diseases in that the management of the condition requires voluntary treatment compliance. However, the development of the disease is not due to choice but to factors beyond voluntary control.

Critics of the Concept

Because the disease concept is widely attributed to Jellinek, much criticism has been directed at his research, which was the basis for his conclusions about the disease concept. Jellinek's data were gathered from questionnaires distributed to Alcoholics Anonymous members through its newsletter, *The Grapevine*. Of 158 questionnaires returned, 60 were discarded because members had pooled and averaged their responses. Also, no questionnaires from women were used. Jellinek himself acknowledged that his data were limited. The progressive nature of addiction has also been criticized. George Vailant, a proponent of the disease concept, has suggested that there is no inevitable progression of Jellinek's stages of alcoholism. Vailant reported that as many as one half of the men who abuse alcohol return to social drinking or stable abstinence.

The issue of "loss of control" has also been a contentious issue. Several arguments have been advanced to dispute the notion of loss of control. One critic of the disease concept, Herbert Fingarette, pointed out that if alcoholics lack control only after first consuming alcohol, then they should have no difficulty abstaining. Obviously, however, alcoholics do have difficulty abstaining. If loss of control exists before the first drink (which would explain the difficulty in abstaining), it implies a difficulty in exercising self-control or willpower, which is a much different model of addiction.

Furthermore, experimental studies have demonstrated that alcoholics do exert control over their drinking and that variables such as the amount of effort to get alcohol, the environment in which drinking occurs, the belief about what is being consumed, rewards, and the like influence how much is consumed by an alcoholic. Defenders of the disease concept have responded that loss of control means that the alcoholic or addict cannot predict the situations in which he or she will exercise control and the situations in which he or she will lose control. Therefore, this loss of predictability is thought to define the alcoholic or addict.

Advantages of the Concept

Perhaps the greatest advantage to the articulation that addiction is a disease has been to remove the moral stigma attached to addiction and to replace it with an emphasis on treatment of an illness. People are not punished for having a disease; they are given assistance. In a more functional sense, defining addiction as a disease has also resulted in treatment coverage by insurance companies. Using medical terminology to describe addiction has also led to greater interest in scientific research. Few medical scientists would be interested in investigating the physiological correlates of a lack of willpower or to a moral deficiency. For the individual who has problems with alcohol or other drugs (and for the family as well), the concept of a disease removes much of the stigma and associated embarrassment, blame, and guilt. A person would not feel guilty if he or she was diagnosed with diabetes, and therefore, a person with addictive disease need not feel guilty for having this disease. People who believe that addiction is due to a lack of willpower or to a moral deficiency may avoid treatment, because in their view, the admission of the need for help is an admission that some character flaw exists. Therefore, an acceptance of the disease concept may make it easier for some people to enter treatment. Another advantage of the disease concept is that it is clearly understandable to people and provides an explanatory construct for the differences in their alcohol and other drug-taking behavior compared with others. For example, it is quite clear to the people with diabetes that they cannot use certain foods in the same manner as those who do not have diabetes. If they

do, there will be certain predictable consequences. Knowledge about the disease allows the alcoholic or addict to understand that he or she is physiologically different from others. In the same way that it may be unwise for the diabetic to eat a hot fudge sundae (in spite of the fact that friends may do so without consequences), the alcoholic learns that it would be unwise to drink (in spite of the fact that friends may do so without consequences). Finally, the disease concept has a logical treatment objective that follows from its precepts: abstinence. If a person has a physiological condition that results in severe consequences when alcohol or other drugs are used, these consequences will be avoided by abstaining from alcohol or other drugs. If the alcoholic or addict attempts to use moderately, he or she will eventually lose control, progress through predictable stages, and suffer the consequences. As most individuals who seek treatment for alcohol or other drug problems have experienced some negative consequences already, this argument can be compelling.

Disadvantages of the Concept

As the critics of the disease concept have pointed out, the orthodox precepts of the disease concept may not be accurate. There is neither an inevitable and completely predictable progression of symptoms and stages nor a consistent loss of control. Therefore, individuals with alcohol or other drug problems who may need some form of intervention or treatment may avoid help since they do not fit the "disease model."

The notion that the disease concept removes responsibility from the alcoholic or addict for his or her behavior is frequently cited as a disadvantage of this model. Because the alcoholic or addict is "powerless" over the disease, inappropriate or even criminal behavior may be attributed to the "disease." Relapse may also be blamed on the disease. In other words, if an alcoholic believes the disease concept and the Alcoholics Anonymous slogan "one drink away from a drunk," then a slip (return to use) may result in the alcoholic's giving up responsibility for maintaining sobriety and returning to a previous level of use, as the slip is symptomatic of the loss of control. Proponents of the disease concept counter this argument by saying that the addict is not responsible for the disease but is completely responsible for recovery. In addition, court rulings have rarely allowed a defense of addiction for criminal behavior.

Conclusion

The disease concept of addiction is by far the most popular and widely accepted model of addiction and has been the basis of the most widely used treatment models, including the Minnesota model. The description of the disease concept led to acceptance by the medical community and acknowledgment that alcoholics and addicts require treatment rather than scorn. However, research has established that addiction is a complex condition with biological, social, cultural, and psychological components. No single model of addiction can accurately describe all people who suffer from substance use disorders.

Joyce Hartje

See also Addiction, Models of; Biopsychosocial Model of Addiction; Cognitive-Social Learning Model; Minnesota Model; Psychological Models of Addiction; Social Learning Model of Addictive Behaviors

Further Readings

Fingarette, H. (1988). *Heavy drinking: The myth of alcoholism as a disease.* Berkeley: University of California Press.

Jellinek, E. M. (1960). *The disease concept of addiction.* New Haven, CT: Hillhouse Press.

McLellan, A. T., Lewis, D. C., O'Brien, C. P., & Kleber, H. D. (2000). Drug dependence, a chronic medical illness: Implications for treatment, insurance, and outcome evaluation. *JAMA, 284,* 1689–1695.

DOUBLE TROUBLE

The term *double trouble* refers to a condition that includes dual or multiple diagnoses when one or more diagnoses is for a substance use disorder and one or more diagnoses is for a mental disorder. The term *co-occurring disorder* is used predominantly to describe this condition to further clarify the fact that a disorder of each category (substance use disorder and mental disorder) must not only be present but is also independent of the other. Also known as "coexisting" disorders, double trouble exists when a substance use disorder and mental disorder occur simultaneously, and although they are considered independent of each other, they can have significant influence on each other with regard to illness progression, treatment, and recovery.

Historical Perspective

Traditionally, those with mental health and addiction problems have had, in addition to their illness, the additional burden of shame due to a societal stigma that viewed addiction problems as moral weakness and mental health problems as a result of weak motivation. In spite of this stigma, mental health professionals have historically viewed psychiatric disorders as treatable illnesses. However, while mental health professionals have helped reframe the societal view of mental problems from that of an individual weakness to an illness, many still viewed addiction as a symptom of a mental disorder. Conversely, addiction professionals saw addiction as the primary illness with many firmly believing that once the individual was in recovery, the psychiatric-like symptoms would disappear. It is now known that co-occurring disorders are quite complex, have no common etiology, and, in many cases, are developed independent of each other.

Assessment and Diagnosis

While assessing for a substance use or a mental disorder, the practitioner must be prepared for a majority of cases to be assessed as "double trouble." Therefore, assessments in any mental health or addiction setting must be performed with the assumption that the clients being diagnosed as having co-occurring disorders are the expectation, not the exception. However, accurate diagnoses for co-occurring disorders are complicated by the fact that it is difficult to distinguish between symptoms that are characteristic of a mental disorder and those that are generated by a substance use disorder. Although mental and substance use disorders may occur independent of each other, their bidirectional interaction further complicates the ability to accurately diagnose. Therefore, a precise and thorough differential diagnosis can only be performed over time and under a measured and vigilant approach.

Effective assessments of co-occurring disorders are those that include a welcoming and safe atmosphere with a high degree of empathy and hope. A practitioner who provides an engaging environment can successfully gather information from the client and hence has a better chance of collecting the ingredients necessary to accurately assess the existence of a co-occurring disorder, establish the client's readiness for change, determine strengths as well as challenges to the client's recovery, and engage the client in the development of an appropriate and continuous treatment relationship. Thus, the practitioner is performing an integrated assessment and providing the best means to effectively work with the client to mutually develop a meaningful treatment plan.

Treatment

Effective treatment of "double trouble" can occur with the instillation of empathy, respect, and hope for recovery in a relationship that provides integrated and continual treatment. There is no one prescribed treatment for co-occurring disorders, and the quality of the therapeutic relationship is often the greatest predictor of success in treatment. Due to the uniqueness of each patient's diagnosis, treatment planning must include appropriately intensive diagnosis-specific interventions for each disorder that match the client's individualized needs, readiness for change, and level of care. In addition, the bidirectional nature of co-occurring disorders demands an assessment of each disorder on an ongoing basis with commensurate changes to the treatment plan made when needed.

Treatment planning is most effective when the client is engaged in the process. This collaborative endeavor allows a mutual exploration of the individual's unique needs and goals while focusing on immediate needs, level of motivation, personal goals, culture perspective, and the client's unique combination of disorders. By engaging the client in this process, a sense of ownership and the potential for increased motivation will often result, thus increasing the desire to pursue goals. During this process, the alert practitioner also recognizes cultural differences and respectfully incorporates them into treatment.

Treatment for "double trouble" must be done in such a way that both disorders are treated simultaneously. This integrated dual treatment allows each disorder to receive treatment appropriate for its diagnosis and severity. The first stage of treatment is acute stabilization during which detoxification, if needed, for the substance use disorder is provided along with stabilization of psychiatric symptoms. Once the patient is stabilized, motivational enhancement strategies can be utilized as a means of moving clients toward acceptance and change. This requires an awareness of the client's motivation, level of acceptance of treatment for each diagnosis, and desire to change.

Clinical outcomes for co-occurring disorders are also individualized. By taking a biopsychosocial approach to treatment, the practitioner will view the uniqueness of each individual's co-occurring diagnoses, see causality as multifactorial, help conceptualize the various contributors to the disorders, and determine where and how to intervene with treatment. The biopsychosocial approach to treatment includes the exploration of possible genetic predispositions and biological changes for either disorder (bio); the assessment of the client's cognitive thought process, self-image, and emotional reaction (psycho); and the examination of the client's social and environmental stressors as well and his or her family adaptation (social).

In summary, treatment for each patient, while showing empathic understanding and respect, must be individualized to address readiness for change, medication, treatment of medical complications, supportive counseling, recovery environment, and available support systems.

Recovery

Successful recovery from "double trouble" includes the goal of prolonged stabilization and continued growth and change. It is recommended that the client remain in treatment to ensure ongoing stabilization, consistently attend abstinence support groups, continue any prescribed medication, receive ongoing education about addiction and mental illness, and build skills to prevent relapse. Each client requires a personal relapse prevention plan that includes tools to effectively deal with recurring symptoms and skills, based on the individual's strengths and level of self-esteem, that will help him or her face the unique challenges posed by the continued presence of both disorders.

Successful recovery includes the acceptance by the client of both disorders, ongoing family involvement in its own program of recovery, ongoing assessment by the therapist, and a constant awareness by the client of ongoing risks of relapse for either disease. The client faced with "double trouble" increases his or her success in recovery by taking on the responsibility of continued work on growth and change through therapy, support group involvement, and self-enhanced growth. This, in turn, can lead to an increased capacity to develop positive relationships, self-perpetuating change, peace of mind, and serenity.

Thomas G. Durham

See also Biopsychosocial Model of Addiction; Depression; Pharmacological Approaches to Treatment; Post-Traumatic Stress Disorder; Treatment Plans and Treatment Planning

Further Readings

Minkoff, K. (2005, January). *Comprehensive continuous integrated system of care.* Retrieved September 3, 2007, from http://www.kenminkoff.com/articles.html

Minkoff, K., & Cline, C. A. (2004). Changing the world: The design and implementation of comprehensive continuous integrated systems of care for individuals with co-occurring disorders. *Psychiatric Clinics of North America, 27*(4), 727–743.

Substance Abuse and Mental Health Services Administration. (2005). *Substance abuse treatment for persons with co-occurring disorders: A treatment improvement protocol (TIP 42).* Rockville, MD: Author.

Substance Abuse and Mental Health Services Administration. (2007). *Screening, assessment, and treatment planning for persons with co-occurring disorders.* Retrieved September 10, 2007, from http//:coce.samhsa.gov/products/overview_papers.aspx

DRIVING UNDER THE INFLUENCE

Drinking and driving continues to be a major problem on American highways. The National Highway Traffic Safety Administration estimates that, on average, there are approximately a million and a half driving-under-the-influence (DUI) convictions per year. This is an arrest rate of 1 for every 130 licensed drivers in the United States. In addition, approximately 17,000 deaths per year are attributed to drinking and driving–related crashes. For example, in 2005, there were 16,885 confirmed drinking and driving–related fatalities, which represented 39% of the total traffic-related fatalities during that year. California and Florida had the highest alcohol-related fatality rates in 2005, while North Carolina, Ohio, Texas, and Pennsylvania fall into the second tier of highest fatality rates.

Although there has been greater awareness of the devastating losses brought on by drunk driving by organizations such as Mothers Against Drunk Driving (MADD) and Students Against Drunk Driving (SADD), and the more widespread acceptance of designated drivers, there is still much work that needs to be done to reduce the incidence and prevalence of DUI. It is noteworthy that per capita alcohol consumption does not always correlate with increased incidence of DUI. For example, New Hampshire has one of the highest per capita alcohol consumption rates in the United States, but New Mexico, with lower consumption rates, has higher rates of DUI arrests and fatalities. Although there is a plethora of research that examines blood alcohol levels at the time of arrest, there are few studies that look at individuals who drive under the influence of mood-altering drugs other than alcohol. Usually when drug levels are obtained, it is when an individual has been involved in an accident that requires emergency room treatment. In those instances, a toxicology screen usually is performed, which helps ascertain if the individual was driving under the influence of drugs. It is estimated, therefore, that there are far more individuals driving under the influence of mood-altering substances (both licit and illicit) than is reported in the DUI arrest or fatality statistics.

Characteristics of DUI Offenders

Those convicted of DUI offenses are a rather heterogeneous group composed of individuals from all socioeconomic strata, of all races and ethnicities, of a variety of occupational and educational levels, young and old, male and female, married, divorced and single. This heterogeneity is especially found among first-time offenders, who are often made up of individuals who may have had too much to drink at celebrations such as weddings or parties and exercised poor judgment in their decision to drive after drinking and a second group who drink and drive as a usual pattern of behavior. This second group is more likely to be composed of individuals who may be in the early stages of alcoholism, and their DUI may represent one example of several problems related to their drinking. It is estimated that among first-time offenders, about 50% are probably manifesting symptoms of alcohol dependence, whereas among second-time offenders, it is estimated that approximately 90% are most likely alcoholic. Some research suggests that although not all DUI offenders are alcohol or drug dependent, their drinking and driving may represent one of many problematic behaviors (e.g., occupational and educational problems, financial irresponsibility, relationship difficulties).

Among multiple offenders, a different picture emerges both in terms of demographics and drinking behavior. Multiple offenders tend to be young, single males who work in blue-collar jobs and have, on average, a 12th-grade education. Although men tend to outnumber women among both first and multiple offenders, there has been an increase in the number of women who are convicted of DUI offenses. With regard to race, European males tend to outnumber all other racial groups among first and multiple offenders, although there are some regional differences.

There are a number of personality variables that have been studied that distinguish DUI offenders from nonoffenders. Overall, DUI offenders tend to be more impulsive, more sensation seeking, and more hostile. They also tend to be more depressed and are more likely to manifest an external locus of control. Individuals with an external locus of control are more likely to blame their problems (including the DUI) on chance occurrences rather than to take personal responsibility for their behavior, especially when they experience problems. The need for novel stimulation and sensation seeking may account for increased DUI arrests in this population, as it has been hypothesized that DUI offenders may become bored at one drinking location and will then drive to another location to drink, which places them at high risk for being arrested.

Sanctions

In response to the vast numbers of DUI offender accidents and fatalities, most states have adopted strict laws and penalties for drinking under the influence of alcohol or drugs. For example, every state mandates some period of license suspension (usually a minimum of 6 months for a first offense) and a monetary fine. Many states also impose auto insurance surcharges, which are levied when convicted DUI offenders renew their driver's license following the suspension period. These insurance surcharges are sometimes imposed for several years, based on the fact that convicted DUI offenders fall within a high-risk group for future accidents.

Other sanctions include vehicle impoundment (the DUI offender's car is impounded during the length of his or her license suspension) and ignition interlock devices (the DUI offender must blow into a breathalyzer that is connected to the ignition. If any alcohol is detected by the breathalyzer, the car's ignition will not engage). There are also "zebra sticker" license plates that help to alert police that the owner of the vehicle is a convicted DUI offender. Some states place convicted DUI offenders on probation or on house arrest with television monitoring accompanied by mandatory blood alcohol monitoring. Other states place convicted DUI offenders on house arrest with ankle bracelets.

Screening, Education, and Treatment

Although many states have strict sanctions and penalties for DUI offenders, in the mid-1970s, many states enacted laws that also mandated convicted DUI offenders to attend screening, education, and treatment programs. The screening and education programs were often run by the State, either through the department of motor vehicles or the department of alcohol countermeasures. Individuals convicted of DUI offenses (including those convicted of refusal to submit to a breath chemical test) would be administered a screening questionnaire, a screening test, or both, often along with a screening interview and a review of the DUI offender's driving record. There are a few pencil-and-paper screening measures that have been developed specifically for use with DUI offenders, such as the Driver Risk Inventory and the Research Institute on Addictions Screening Inventory. These screening measures usually include scales that help detect deceptive responses and both direct and indirect questions pertaining to alcohol and drug use and addiction potentiality. The Mortimer–Filkins scale was developed for screening DUI offenders and consists of a structured interview and a questionnaire. The purpose of these measures is to determine who is at high risk for DUI recidivism. High-risk first-time offenders and multiple offenders are usually referred to outpatient treatment programs for periods ranging from 4 to 12 months, on average, while low-risk first offenders are often required to participate in brief educational sessions.

The goal of both education and treatment programs is to reduce the rate of DUI recidivism. Meta-analysis research indicates that treatment is effective in reducing recidivism. It appears that length of treatment is a significant factor, as the longer the DUI offender participates in treatment, the lower is their risk for recidivism. Recidivism rates often range from 22% to 35% on average and vary from state to state. One study found that the average length of time between a first and second offense is approximately 6 years.

One of the difficulties often found in treating DUI offenders (as with other treatment-mandated populations) is that they are resistant to change. Motivational counseling approaches have been found to be effective with this population based on the notion that most DUI offenders enter treatment programs in the precontemplation or contemplation stage (i.e., first stages of the change process). The goal of counseling is then to either raise their awareness that the DUI is a drinking- or drug-related problem or to help tip the balance toward abstinence or toward developing an effective action plan that will successfully prevent another DUI arrest. Another important component of treatment with DUI offenders is the involvement of family members and significant others at various intervals throughout the treatment process. This helps to encourage family members to become allies in the treatment process based on the common goal of preventing DUI recidivism. The majority of treatment programs for DUI offenders offer group counseling as the primary counseling modality. Although individual counseling is advantageous in allowing for more individualized treatment planning, group counseling offers the benefit of reducing the sense of uniqueness that most DUI offenders experience.

Sanctions Versus Treatment

Many law enforcement personnel and politicians are staunch advocates of stronger DUI laws as a means of preventing DUI recidivism and drinking-related crashes. However, from a behavioral perspective, one of the difficulties with punishment is that it only tells a person what they should *not* do. Punishment does not tell a person what to *do*. This appears to be where treatment becomes a valuable tool. Treatment programs often focus on skill development (e.g., learning alcohol and drug refusal skills, learning relapse prevention skills, learning new coping strategies). By learning new skills to reduce abusive drinking or drug use, it is assumed there is less of a likelihood of recidivism. Most researchers agree that strict sanctions need to be combined with education and treatment in order to reduce the rate of drinking and driving accidents and fatalities.

Conclusion

Driving under the influence of drugs and alcohol remains a major problem in the United States as evidenced by the number of highway death and accidents.

As a result, several measures have been adopted to try to ameliorate the rate of DUI, including strict sanctions for drinking and driving along with mandated screening, education, and treatment programs. Each state has adopted various penalties, which often include fines, surcharges, vehicle impoundment, and ignition interlock devices. Treatment for convicted DUI offenders often ranges from brief education for low-risk first offenders to more lengthy counseling for high-risk first offenders and multiple offenders. Meta-analysis research indicates that these treatment efforts are generally efficacious in helping to reduce recidivism rates. However, further research needs to elucidate which specific treatment approaches or treatment factors (other than length of treatment) are most effective.

Alan A. Cavaiola

See also Alcohol Testing; Brief Interventions; Criminal Justice Populations; Coercion and Treatment; Court-Mandated Treatment; Motivational Interviewing; Refusal Skills; Risk Factors for Addiction

Further Readings

Beerman, K. A., Smith, M. M., & Hall, R. L. (1988). Predictors of recidivism in DUI's. *Journal of Studies on Alcohol, 49,* 443–449.

Cavaiola, A. A., Stohmetz, D. B., & Abreo, S. D. (2007). Characteristics of DUI recidivists: A 12 year follow up of first time DUI offenders. *Addictive Behaviors, 32,* 855–861.

Cavaiola, A., & Wuth, C. (2001). *Assessment & treatment of the DWI offender.* New York: Haworth Press.

Donovan, D. M., & Marlatt, G. A. (1983). Personality subtypes among driving-while-intoxicated offenders: Relationships to drinking behavior and driving risk. *Journal of Consulting and Clinical Psychology, 50,* 241–249.

McMillen, D. L., Pang, M. G., Wells-Parker, E., & Anderson, B. J. (1992). Alcohol, personality traits and high risk driving: A comparison of young, drinking drivers. *Addictive Behaviors, 17,* 525–532.

Miller, W. R., & Rollnick, S. (1991). *Motivational interviewing: Preparing People to change addictive behaviors.* New York: Guilford Press.

Mortimer, R. G., Filkins, L. D., Lower, J. S., Kerlan, M. W., Post, D. V., Mudge, B., et al. (1971). *Court procedures for identifying problem drinkers: Report on Phase I* (Report No. DOT HS-800-630). Washington, DC: Department of Transportation.

National Highway Traffic Administration. (2007). *Driver fatalities by state and blood alcohol concentration (BAC) test status 2005: Traffic safety fact sheet.* Retrieved May 25, 2008, from http://www-nrd.nhtsa.dot.gov/pdf/nrd-30/NCSA/TSF2005/2005TSF/810_627/pages/Table6.htm

Nochajski, T. H., & Miller, B. A. (1995). *Training manual for the Research Institute on Addictions Self Inventory (RIASI).* Buffalo, NY: Research Institute on Addictions.

Perrine, M. W. (1990). Who are the drinking drivers? *Alcohol Health and Research World, 14,* 26–35.

Ross, H. L., Howard, J. M., Ganikos, M. L., & Taylor, E. D. (1991). Drunk driving among American Blacks and Hispanics. *Accident Analysis & Prevention, 23,* 1–11.

Wells-Parker, E., Bangert-Drowns, R., McMillen, R., & Williams, M. (1995). Final results from a meta-analysis of remedial interventions with drinking/driver offenders. *Addiction, 9,* 907–926.

Zador, P. L., Krawchuk, S. A., & Voas, R. B. (2000). Alcohol-related relative risk of driver fatalities and driver involvement in fatal crashes in relation to driver age and gender: An update using 1996 data. *Journal of Studies on Alcohol, 61,* 387–395.

Driving While Intoxicated

See Driving Under the Influence

Drug Abuse

See Substance Abuse

Drug Abuse Resistance Education

One of the most debated substance abuse prevention programs in terms of its effectiveness is Drug Abuse Resistance Education (D.A.R.E.), which began in Los Angeles in 1983. This prevention program, which is now being implemented in nearly 75% of U.S. school districts and employs more than 50,000 trained officers, is grounded in the belief that something can be done about delinquency through educational interventions without focusing attention on social forces contributing to delinquency. Traditionally, the program was designed as an educational prevention strategy targeted at fifth-grade students. Currently, however, the D.A.R.E. program has expanded to include many grade levels as well as parenting classes. The central part of the D.A.R.E. program utilizes uniformed police officers to teach children about drugs and the problems they cause. It is the belief of the program that such educational strategies can and will overcome social contributors to drug use in adolescence, such as poverty and poor parental supervision. The literature and debate concerning the D.A.R.E. program largely yield three key conditions that must be met for the program to be effective: (1) police officers who are also excellent teachers, (2) good students willing to participate and learn, and (3) the notion that the program must instill positive memories in the students in order for it to continue to protect the students as they grow older through their adolescent years.

D.A.R.E. was started in 1983 by Los Angeles Chief of Police Daryl F. Gates in response to his relationship with his very troubled son who was addicted to drugs. Chief Gates sought a way in which he could protect the children in Los Angeles from engaging in drug use like his son. By 1984, the program was gaining popularity in the Los Angeles area and was costing the Los Angeles Police Department approximately $5 million per year. In response to the growing popularity, the program spread rapidly across the United States by the late 1990s. As of today, the D.A.R.E. program has been implemented in approximately 75% of U.S. school districts as well as about 50 countries worldwide. The traditional curriculum taught in these schools consisted of 17 weeks of classes that met once per week for 50 minutes and covered the following topics concerning drug education: personal safety practices, drug use and misuse, consequences of using and not using drugs, resisting pressures to use drugs, resistance techniques, building self-esteem, assertiveness, managing stress without using drugs, media influences on drug use, decision making and risk taking, and alternatives to drug use. Currently, officers must accumulate a minimum of 80 hours of training in areas such as child development, communication skills, and teaching techniques prior to stepping forth in front of a classroom as a D.A.R.E. officer; additional training is required for those teaching at the high school level.

D.A.R.E. America

The widespread growth of the program, which led to its establishment in so many schools across the nation, led to the development of D.A.R.E. America, a nonprofit organization led by President and Chief Executive Officer Charlie Parsons, created with the aim of establishing new D.A.R.E. programs as well as improving previously established programs. A community-based project, D.A.R.E. America supplies educational materials for the students, provides training for the officers, and monitors the instructional standards of the D.A.R.E. programs across the nation. Under D.A.R.E. America, the new D.A.R.E. curriculum is based on the traditional program but expands the curriculum to include the elementary school level, the middle school level, the high school level, and parent training; the parent training component assists parents in learning to approach and speak with their children about drugs. It is the hope of the program that this parental education will reinforce the skills learned in the D.A.R.E. classroom. Along with the additions of grade levels and parenting classes, the new D.A.R.E. America curriculum has expanded to include lessons on consequential thinking, self-management skills, social resistance skills, violence prevention, and alternatives. D.A.R.E. America also offers an after-school program known as D.A.R.E.+PLUS (Play and Learn Under Supervision) in which middle school students can engage in a variety of after-school meetings and activities with DARE officers and other community volunteers. Several programs fall under the umbrella of the D.A.R.E.+PLUS program with one of the most popular of these being the D.A.R.E. Dance, an after-school program with over 70 schools participating. This program, which began in 1999, offers dance classes to youth as well as yearly dance assemblies.

D.A.R.E. International

Currently, there are approximately 50 countries participating in the D.A.R.E. program. Some of the major countries that have implemented D.A.R.E. in their school systems (besides the United States) are Canada, Germany, Japan, Italy, Cuba, Mexico, Spain, South Korea, and Turkey.

Effectiveness

Since implementation of the D.A.R.E. program throughout schools in the United States, there has been an increasing amount of debate concerning its effectiveness. Although the D.A.R.E. program may be a good idea in theory, much research suggests that it is not truly effective long term in keeping youth off drugs. In a review of research conducted on the effectiveness of the D.A.R.E. program, D. W. Miller cites a University of Kentucky study of 1,000 individuals age 20, some of whom had participated in the program as sixth graders and some of whom had not. Findings of this study provide an illustration of a majority of D.A.R.E. research studies concluding that there was no significant difference in those who had participated in the program and those who had received other prevention education. In a separate study from the same institution, D.A.R.E. was found to have a very small, insignificant effect on drug use. Although leaders of the program maintain that it is effective in reducing drug use among adolescents, the vast majority of scholarly research has suggested otherwise. Following the research, however, D.A.R.E. announced major changes in the middle school curriculum in 2000. This marked a major effort on the part of program leaders, which is hopeful of future success.

Sherry Lynn Skaggs

See also Evidence-Based Prevention; Prevention Education; Prevention Evaluation, Prevention Strategies; Public Policy, Prevention; Research Issues in Prevention

Further Readings

Drug Abuse Resistance Education: http://www.dare.com

Lundman, R. J. (2001). *Prevention and control of juvenile delinquency* (3rd ed.). New York: Oxford University Press.

Lynam, D. R., Milich, R., Zimmerman, R., Novak, S., Logan, T. K., Martin, C., et al. (1999). Project DARE: No effects at 10-year follow-up. *Journal of Consulting and Clinical Psychology, 67*(4), 590–593.

Miller, D. W. (2001, October 19). D.A.R.E. reinvents itself— With help from its social-scientist critics. *Chronicle of Higher Education, 48,* A12–A14.

DRUG ABUSE SCREENING TEST

The Drug Abuse Screening Test (DAST) is a self-report measure designed to detect lifetime adult drug abuse or dependence across a range of substances other than alcohol. It has been widely used in clinical and nonclinical settings by both professional and non-professional personnel. The items cover drug-related problems (e.g., Item 15: Have you ever neglected your family or missed work because of your use of drugs?), diminished control over drug use (e.g., Item 6: Do you use drugs on a continuous basis?), and symptoms of tolerance and physical withdrawal from drug dependence (e.g., Item 23: Have you ever experienced withdrawal symptoms as a result of heavy drug intake?). The total score serves as a lifetime measure of drug use problem severity.

The original version of the DAST contained 28 yes–no questions that were suitable for a self-report or interview format. Each "yes" answer is scored 1, and each "no" answer is scored 0. The items sum to provide an overall score that is used to determine the likelihood of an individual having a past or present clinically significant drug-related diagnosis. The DAST yields an overall score ranging from 0 to 28 based on the sum of individual items endorsed in the direction of increased drug problems. A cutoff score of 6 or more indicates a probable drug use disorder.

Three alternate versions of the DAST have been developed. DAST-10 has 10 items from the full version (Items 1, 3, 5, 8, 9, 10, 15, 21, 23, and 24). DAST-20 contains 20 items from the original DAST. In addition to the DAST-10 items, the DAST-20 includes items 2, 4, 12, 14, 16, 17, 18, 22, 25, and 27. Some minor wording changes were made to some of the items in both of these briefer versions. Cutoff scores of 2 to 4 have been adopted for the DAST-20 and DAST-10. DAST-A was developed for use with adolescent psychiatric inpatients. Some of the DAST items were modified to make them appropriate for use in an adolescent population. For example, the word *work* was changed to *school*. The word *spouse* was changed to *boyfriend/girlfriend*. The cutoff score for the DAST-A is 7 or above.

The DAST can be completed in a questionnaire or interview format. It takes approximately 5 minutes to complete the DAST and 1 minute to score it. The DAST can be scored by person or by computer. No special training is required for administration. The instrument and scoring procedures are in the public domain and no permission is required for its use.

The DAST items seem to consistently measure lifetime problems related to drug use. Using cutoff scores of between 5 and 10, it also has been shown to be accurate in distinguishing between individuals who have and do not have drug use disorders, regardless of their lifetime problems related to alcohol use or

psychiatric conditions. DAST scores significantly correspond with frequency of drug use in the past 12 months across a host of drugs (e.g., heroin, other opioids, amphetamines, barbiturates, hallucinations, cannabis, and glue). Comparisons between the ability of the 28-item version of the DAST and a 20-item version to accurately identify individuals with lifetime drug use problems have revealed few differences. The 20-item and 10-item DAST versions have been shown to perform equally well as screening measures for drug abuse problems as the 28-item version.

The DAST has several strengths. It covers a wide range of consequences related to drug abuse without being specific about the drug, thus alleviating the need to use different screening instruments specific to different drug categories. The DAST performs well as a screening instrument with a range of different drugs of abuse in a variety of clinical and nonclinical settings and has some support for its use with mentally ill adult and adolescent patients. It is most useful for detecting drug use disorders in settings in which seeking treatment for drug use problems is not the patient's stated goal (e.g., medical clinics or general mental health settings). The DAST can be used to guide further inquiry into drug-related problems and to help determine treatment intensity.

Drawbacks of the DAST include that it relies on lifetime assessment of drug use and, therefore, does not necessarily reflect the status of the respondents' current use or drug-related diagnoses. In addition, it does not ask about drug use amount and frequency or identify which drugs are problematic. As a result, it is not useful as a change measure. Finally, the intent of the DAST questions is transparent. Individuals can falsely answer questions if they are motivated to conceal actual drug-related problems.

Steve Martino

See also Screening; Screening Instruments; Self-Report Inventories; Substance Abuse Subtle Screening Inventory-3

Further Readings

Cocco, K., & Carey, K. (1998). Psychometric properties of the Drug Abuse Screening Test in psychiatric outpatients. *Psychological Assessment, 10,* 408–414.

Martino, S., Grilo, C. M., & Fehon, D. C. (2000). Development of the Drug Abuse Screening Test for Adolescents (DAST-A). *Addictive Behaviors. 25,* 57–70.

Skinner, H. A. (1982). The Drug Abuse Screening Test. *Addictive Behaviors, 7*, 363–371.

Yudko, E., Lozhkina, O., & Fouts, A. (2007). A comprehensive review of the psychometric properties of the Drug Abuse Screening Test. *Journal of Substance Abuse Treatment, 32*, 189–198.

Drug Abuse Treatment Outcome Studies

The Drug Abuse Treatment Outcome Studies (DATOS) were initiated in 1989 under contracts funded by the National Institute on Drug Abuse (NIDA) to evaluate drug abuse treatment outcomes and emerging treatment issues in the United States. This was NIDA's third national outcome evaluation study of publicly funded treatment. The research plan for the adult component of DATOS was based on studies and findings about drug abuse treatment outcomes over the past 30 years. Much of this knowledge came from previous national, multisite longitudinal evaluation studies funded by NIDA. The two previous studies—the Drug Abuse Reporting Program (DARP) and the Treatment Outcomes Prospective Study (TOPS)—helped shape the direction and research questions for the DATOS of treatment outcomes and drug abuse patterns. The companion adolescent study began in 1991. Four collaborating research centers were funded by NIDA as part of a cooperative agreement in 1995 to pursue independent but coordinated programs of research based on DATOS.

1. The National Development and Research Institutes at North Carolina focused on trends in service delivery, client populations, access and utilization, and costs and benefits of treatment (Robert L. Hubbard, Principal Investigator).

2. Texas Christian University in Fort Worth examined factors related to treatment engagement and retention, with focus on treatment for cocaine dependence (D. Dwayne Simpson, Principal Investigator).

3. The University of California at Los Angeles addressed addiction and treatment careers (M. Douglas Anglin, Principal Investigator).

4. The NIDA Services Research Branch considered policy implications related to the changing nature of drug abuse treatment and effectiveness (Bennett W. Fletcher, Principal Investigator).

The collaborating research centers emphasized four variable domains within the contexts of their programs of study. The domains, selected in accord with their significance for the drug abuse field, included cocaine use, HIV risk behaviors, psychiatric comorbidity, and criminal justice status.

Objectives of DATOS

The overall goal of DATOS was to advance scientific knowledge about the effectiveness of drug abuse treatment as it is typically delivered in community-based settings. Issues of importance included shifting public concern and expectations for treatment, changes in the funding and organization of treatment programs, increases in co-occurring mental health and substance use disorders, and significant changes in patterns of illicit substance use. With these issues in mind, DATOS researchers studied a wide range of questions of scientific and policy relevance. These included the following:

- Studies of contemporary treatment delivery, especially long-term client outcomes and how they relate to phases of addiction and treatment
- Examination of the evolving drug abuse treatment system, including delivery and utilization of primary and ancillary services
- Research on the components of effective treatment, including factors that engage and retain clients in programs

To date, more than 85 studies have been published under the DATOS research project. Others continue to appear in the literature because data sets have been archived at the Inter-University Consortium for Political and Social Research and are easily available for both online analyses and download without charge. Key publications describing some of the highlights and major findings from this project have appeared as special journal issues and single articles in journals such as the *Psychology of Addictive Behaviors, Archives of General Psychiatry, Drug and Alcohol Dependence, Journal of Adolescent Research,* and *Journal of Substance Abuse Treatment.*

Summary of Sampling Design

Treatment programs in 11 large U.S. cities were selected to represent typical community-based treatment services broadly available to the public. Geographic location and type of program as well as the type of clients they served were considered in designing the sampling plan. Participating programs were located in Chicago, Houston, Miami, Minneapolis, Newark, New Orleans, New York, Phoenix, Pittsburgh, Portland, and San Jose. The overall methodology used to compile the database, including client samples and program characteristics, is described in a 1997 special issue of the *Psychology of Addictive Behaviors*. Clients were assessed at treatment admission, and data reflecting during-treatment progress were collected at 3 and 6 months. Follow-up data were collected from a sample of approximately 3,000 clients at 12 months posttreatment. An extended follow-up gathered data on clients over a 5-year period after discharge from their index DATOS treatment episode.

Intake Sample

A total of 10,010 clients entered the 96 treatment programs that participated in DATOS from 1991 to 1993. Overall, this treatment sample was 66% male, 47% African American, and 13% Hispanic, with a mean age of 33 years. However, these and other client characteristics varied across modalities, reflecting their different therapeutic and operational characteristics.

One-Year Follow-Up Sample

Of the eligible clients who completed the two-stage intake interviews, 4,229 were selected for follow-up (using a stratified random design). Altogether, 74% ($n = 3,147$) were located, including 70% ($n = 2,966$) who were successfully interviewed, 1.5% ($n = 64$) who were deceased, and 2.7% ($n = 117$) who refused to participate. Gender, ethnicity, and average age were not significantly different between the intake and follow-up samples.

Five-Year Follow-Up Sample

Of the clients interviewed at 1-year posttreatment, 2,041 were targeted for the 5-year follow-up. Altogether, 79% were located, including 68%

($n = 1,393$) who were interviewed, 7% (128) who were deceased, and 3% ($n = 65$) who refused to be interviewed.

Treatment Modalities Represented

Outpatient Methadone Treatment

Outpatient methadone treatment (OMT) programs administered pharmacotherapy (methadone) to reduce cravings for heroin, in addition to providing counseling and case management services. Some provided long-term methadone maintenance for clients, and others used methadone to taper to abstinence. The overall planned length of stay was around 2 years. Private for-profit methadone clinics, nonprofit community-based programs, hospital-based outpatient clinics, and county-managed programs were represented. There were 29 OMT programs with 1,540 clients in the sample.

Long-Term Residential

Long-term residential (LTR) programs offered drug-free treatment in a residential setting, with planned stays ranging from 4 months to 2 years. LTR programs in DATOS included traditional therapeutic communities, modified therapeutic communities, and other programs requiring in-residence treatment. There were 21 LTR programs with 2,774 clients in the sample.

Outpatient Drug-Free

Outpatient drug-free (ODF) programs are characterized by a wide range of therapeutic approaches such as cognitive behavioral, insight-oriented, supportive, and Twelve Step. Planned lengths of stay in treatment were for 3 months or longer. Therapeutic community-managed outpatient programs, nonprofit community programs, mental health and short-term managed programs, and private for-profit programs were included. There were 32 ODF programs with 2,574 clients in the sample.

Short-Term Inpatient

Short-term inpatient (STI) programs generally kept clients in-residence about 21 days, with a focus on medical stabilization, abstinence, and lifestyle changes. They included freestanding nonprofit and for-profit short-term programs, public and nonprofit hospital programs, and county-managed programs. Due to changes in insurance coverage and a national trend toward "managed care" during the time this project was being conducted, planned duration of treatment became shorter over time. Most of the STI programs studied have now closed or have been converted to other types of facilities. There were STI 14 programs with 3,122 clients in the DATOS sample.

Overview of 1-Year Follow-Up Findings

Clients treated in all four modalities studied—that is, OMT, LTR, ODF, and STI—showed large and statistically significant improvements during the 1-year follow-up. Overall, major outcome indicators for drug use, illegal activities, and psychological distress were each reduced on average by about 50%. However, there were notable distinctions between clients admitted to different types of treatment (and there were further variations even between programs of the same general type) as well as in the length of time they remained in treatment. The length of time clients stayed in treatment was directly related to improvements in follow-up outcomes, replicating findings from previous national treatment evaluations (DARP and TOPS). These findings applied to OMT, LTR, and ODF treatment programs in DATOS but not to the brief STI services. A "treatment process model" was developed in previous work by scientists from Texas Christian University to represent essential elements of treatment readiness and engagement indicators as predictors of retention and outcomes. This model was tested using different therapeutic settings represented in DATOS, including LTR (n = 1,362), ODF (n = 866), and OMT (n = 981) treatments. Findings supported the model and included the following:

- Motivated clients developed better relationships with their counselors and stayed in treatment longer.
- Clients who attended more counseling sessions and discussed a broader range of topics in sessions stayed longer in ODF and LTR.
- Clients with more severe background problems (like hostility or cocaine use) had difficulty developing a working relationship with their counselors, attended fewer sessions, and discussed fewer topics.

Treatment of Cocaine Dependence

Cocaine use was the most common drug problem of clients entering treatment for illicit drug use in DATOS. In a national sample from 55 treatment programs, problem severity of clients at admission was found to be directly related to cocaine relapse in the year following discharge, and treatment retention also was a significant predictor among moderate-to-high problem groups. Among the highest severity clients, 90 days or longer in residential programs was needed to improve outcomes. Findings suggest client assessments should play a central role in the selection of appropriate settings and duration of treatment to maximize outcomes. One-year follow-up interviews with 1,605 clients treated for cocaine dependence in 55 programs showed (again) that longer treatment stays are related to better outcomes. Overall, approximately one of four (24%) reported relapses to weekly cocaine use, and another 18% obtained further treatment in the year after discharge in DATOS due to continuing problems. The sample included 542 from 19 LTR, 548 from 24 ODF, and 605 from 12 STI treatment programs.

Five-Year Outcomes Following Cocaine Treatment

Only one of every four clients interviewed 5 years after discharge from a national sample of treatment programs still used cocaine on a weekly basis—similar to rates reported in the first year after treatment. Greater severity of drug use and related problems at intake, as well as more limited treatment contact, were related to poorer outcomes on drug use and criminal activity.

Interviews were conducted at 1 and 5 years after treatment for 708 subjects (from 45 programs in eight cities) who met *DSM-III-R* criteria for cocaine dependence when admitted in 1991 through 1993. Primary outcome measures included drug use and criminality. Self-reported cocaine use showed high overall agreement with urine (79% agreement) and hair (80% agreement) toxicology analyses.

Weekly cocaine use was reported by 25% of the sample in the fifth year of follow-up, slightly higher than the 21% for the first year after treatment. (Similarly, 26% had cocaine detected in urine specimens at follow-up.) Improvements were also reported for other measures.

- Daily alcohol use decreased from 22% before intake to 8% in Year 5.
- Illegal activity declined from 40% before intake to 25% in Year 5 (up slightly from 16% in Year 1).
- Arrests in the past year dropped from 34% before intake to 18% in Year 5 (down slightly from 22% in Year 1).

Costs and Benefits of Cocaine Treatment

Before, during, and after treatment interviews with a national sample of 502 clients treated for cocaine dependence in LTR and ODF treatments from 10 U.S. cities showed (again) that significant returns are realized from public investments in treatment. Overall, reductions in costs of crime to society during and after treatment substantially surpass the cost of treatment in both LTR and ODF. These findings demonstrate the value of public investments to treat cocaine addiction. Clients in each modality showed different levels and associated costs of crime before and after treatment. Justification for the public support for both modalities exists in their effectiveness in treating distinctly different clientele.

Costs and Benefits of Methadone Treatment

In a sample of 395 subjects treated in 16 programs from 8 medium to large cities, methadone treatment benefits from tangible crime cost savings during treatment and at follow-up were greater for continuing patients than those discharged before completing 1 year of their index treatment. Overall, significant returns were provided for treatment investments for both continuing and discharged patients. Upon examining gender differences, it was concluded that greater economic benefits to society were accrued by women than men.

Evaluation of Drug Treatments for Adolescents in Four U.S. Cities

A total of 1,732 consecutive adolescent admissions to 23 treatment programs in four major U.S. cities (Pittsburgh, Pennsylvania; Minneapolis, Minnesota; Chicago, Illinois; and Portland, Oregon) from 1993 to 1995 were interviewed and followed a year after discharge. Treatment modalities included residential (RES),

ODF, and STI. The average client age was 15 to 16 years, primary sources of treatment referral were by family or friends (42%) or the legal system (39%), and the majority were in trouble with the law (i.e., 58% were on parole, on probation, or awaiting trial).

- Significant reductions (before-to-after treatment) were found in weekly or more frequent use of marijuana and other illicit drugs, heavy drinking, criminal activities, and arrests.
- Adolescents reported better psychological adjustment (i.e., reduced suicidal thoughts and hostility, and increased self-esteem), better school attendance, and average or better than average grades after treatment (as compared with the year before).
- Longer time in treatment (greater than 90 days in RES and ODF programs, and 21 days in STI programs) was significantly related to lower drug use and lower arrest rates following treatment.

Conclusion

The DATOS findings illustrate consistent behavioral and psychological improvements for adults and adolescents during residential and outpatient treatments and following discharge across the domains of alcohol and drug use, criminality, social performance, and psychological functioning. Improvements during treatment and first year after discharge also were largely sustained in the 5-year follow-up results. Poorer outcomes were associated with lack of engagement in treatment and inadequate retention, especially for clients reporting more serious drug histories and related problems at admission. More intensive and sustained services are therefore indicated for drug users with greater needs, and this type of systematic adaptation of therapeutic care to client needs can optimize the cost-effectiveness of treatment. However, there were program variations in client engagement and retention that reflect variations in quality of services in practice. Thus, organizational-level factors that influence treatment quality and efforts to adopt and sustain innovations deserve special attention in future studies of treatment effectiveness.

D. Dwayne Simpson and Patrick M. Flynn

See also Client Engagement; Client/Treatment Matching; COMBINE Study; Methadone Maintenance Treatment; National Institute on Drug Abuse; National Treatment

Improvement Evaluation Study; Outpatient Treatment; Project MATCH; Public Policy, Treatment; Residential Treatment; Therapeutic Communities; Treatment Effectiveness; Treatment Settings

Further Readings

Drug Abuse Treatment Outcome Studies (DATOS): http://www.datos.org

Flynn, P. M., Porto, J. V., Rounds-Bryant, J. L., & Kristiansen, P. L. (2003). Costs and benefits of methadone treatment in DATOS–Part 1: Discharged versus continuing patients. *Journal of Maintenance in the Addictions, 2*(1/2), 129–149.

Flynn, P. M., Porto, J. V., Rounds-Bryant, J. L., & Kristiansen, P. L. (2003). Costs and benefits of methadone treatment in DATOS–Part 2: Gender differences for discharged and continuing patients. *Journal of Maintenance in the Addictions, 2*(1/2), 151–169.

Franey, C., & Ashton, M. (2002). The grand design lessons from DATOS. *Drug and Alcohol Findings, 7,* 4–7, 16–19.

Grella, C. E., & Hser, Y. (Eds.). (2001). Drug Abuse Treatment Outcome Studies for Adolescents (DATOS-A) [Special issue]. *Journal of Adolescent Research, 16.*

Hser, Y., Grella, C. E., Hubbard, R. L., Hsieh, S. C., Fletcher, B. W., Brown, B. S., et al. (2001). An evaluation of drug treatment for adolescents in four U.S. cities. *Archives of General Psychiatry, 58*(7), 689–695.

Inter-University Consortium for Political and Social Research: http://www.icpsr.umich.edu

Simpson, D. D. (2003). Introduction to 5-year follow-up treatment outcome studies. *Journal of Substance Abuse Treatment, 25*(3), 123–124.

Simpson, D. D., & Brown, B. S. (Eds.). (1999). Treatment process and outcome studies from DATOS [Special issue]. *Drug and Alcohol Dependence, 57*(2).

Simpson, D. D., & Curry, S. J. (Eds.). (1997). Drug Abuse Treatment Outcome Study (DATOS) [Special issue]. *Psychology of Addictive Behaviors, 11*(4).

Simpson, D. D., Joe, G. W., & Broome, K. M. (2002). A national 5-year follow-up of treatment outcomes for cocaine dependence. *Archives of General Psychiatry, 59,* 538–544.

Simpson, D. D., Joe, G. W., Fletcher, B. W., Hubbard, R. L., & Anglin, M. D. (1999). A national evaluation of treatment outcomes for cocaine dependence. *Archives of General Psychiatry, 56,* 507–514.

Simpson, D. D., Joe, G. W., Rowan-Szal, G. A., & Greener, J. M. (1997). Drug abuse treatment process components that improve retention. *Journal of Substance Abuse Treatment, 14*(6), 565–572.

DRUG ABUSE WARNING NETWORK

The Drug Abuse Warning Network (DAWN) is a public health surveillance system that monitors drug-related emergency department (ED) visits for the nation and for selected metropolitan areas. DAWN estimates pertain to the entire United States, including Alaska, Hawaii, and the District of Columbia. It was implemented nearly 30 years ago to support a specific set of federal policy-making purposes. Its first findings were published in 1973. It was administered by the Drug Enforcement Administration and the National Institute on Drug Abuse (NIDA). Since 1992, the Office of Applied Studies of the Substance Abuse and Mental Health Services Administration (SAMHSA), U.S. Department of Health and Human Services, has been responsible for DAWN operations. SAMHSA is required to collect data on drug-related ED visits under section 505 of the Public Health Service Act.

DAWN is designed to track the impact of drug use, misuse, and abuse on metropolitan areas across the United States. It collects substance use and abuse-related information from data on visits to hospital EDs and drug-related deaths reviewed by medical examiners and coroners (ME/Cs). Information on the demographic characteristics of substance users and the specific drugs involved in each drug-related ED visit or death is also collected.

Drug use–related ED visits, or "episodes," are obtained from a representative sample of 24-hour EDs operating in nonfederal, short-stay general medical/surgical hospitals throughout the coterminous United States. ED-related data provide estimates of the total number of drug use–related ED episodes and the total number of drug mentions for each of 21 selected metropolitan areas and for the nation. DAWN monitors episodes, not individuals. The DAWN report prepared by SAMHSA in 2002 indicated that, in 2000, about 470 EDs participated in DAWN.

Data on drug-related deaths are reviewed by, and obtained from, participating ME/Cs. In 2000, about 140 jurisdictions in 43 metropolitan areas provided these data to DAWN. The number of jurisdictions participating in DAWN varies by location of metropolitan areas. Because the participating jurisdictions are not based on a representative sample, data on drug-related deaths *cannot* provide estimates of the total number of drug-related deaths for the metropolitan areas or for the nation.

According to the DAWN methodology report prepared by SAMHSA in 2002, DAWN data have been used for purposes of drug scheduling and drug labeling, quantifying the extent of the nation's drug problem, assessing effectiveness of local antidrug efforts, guiding resource allocation decisions, tracking local area drug trends, documenting drug problems and trends, and as a data source for academic research on drug abuse. More detailed information about the use and designs of DAWN can be found in the DAWN's methodology report.

The *New* DAWN

The value of DAWN for federal and local policy making is considerable, but it also has limitations. In particular, the U.S. health care system has undergone substantial changes since DAWN's inception in 1972. There are questions regarding the impact that the ongoing changes in the health care system have had on DAWN's ability to gather complete, accurate, and valid data from EDs.

In 1997, the Office of Applied Studies convened two review panels to consider the uses and limitations of DAWN as well as the implications of health system change for DAWN. The two groups agreed that DAWN was a valuable system and identified several issues that needed to be addressed in a redesign of DAWN, including the following:

- How could DAWN be made more timely?
- How could DAWN more rapidly gather, identify, and disseminate information about emerging drug trends?
- Were there local audiences for DAWN data, and how could DAWN be designed to better meet their needs?
- How might DAWN provide useful, timely feedback to facilities and communities?
- To what extent were ED data appropriate for identifying meaningful changes in drug abuse patterns?
- How could DAWN's case definition be improved?

In 2003, a new, redesigned DAWN expanded beyond drug abuse. The *New* DAWN helps communities and member facilities identify emerging problems, improve patient care, and manage resources. There were many changes made to DAWN, such as the following:

- Restructuring the ED sample to reflect changes in the health care system, to update metropolitan area boundaries, and to improve its geographic and population coverage
- Adopting new recruitment strategies to recruit communities, build on community leadership, and provide benefits for participation
- Linking morbidity and mortality components, recruiting all jurisdictions in ED target areas, and adding selected statewide systems
- Using a new, broad and simple case definition to yield a diverse set of drug-related cases
- Improving DAWN data content for both ED and mortality data (e.g., adding data items to describe types of cases and to elucidate health consequences)

The *New* DAWN provides new baseline data for trends and is managed by Westat, a private research corporation, under a contract with SAMHSA.

Who Uses the *New* DAWN?

The primary users of the *New* DAWN data are the following:

- *Federal agencies:* The White House Office of National Drug Control Policy (ONDCP) uses DAWN to assess progress and pinpoint problems in controlling drug abuse in the United States. The Food and Drug Administration uses data from *New* DAWN for postmarketing surveillance and to identify adverse reactions and other health consequences of prescription drugs. SAMHSA uses DAWN to identify emerging drug abuse problems, new populations affected, and needs for prevention and treatment services.

- *Communities and the private sectors:* Communities use DAWN to detect emerging drug problems, to support grant applications for treatment and prevention services, and to assess the need for public health resources. Pharmaceutical firms use DAWN data to track the use, misuse, and abuse of their products.

- *Members of the network:* DAWN provides member hospitals and ME/Cs immediate access to its own data through a secure Internet-based query system ("DAWN *LIVE*"). The DAWN data help members work with public health authorities to address problems related to the use, misuse, and abuse of drugs. They also are utilized to monitor drug-related cases seen in their facilities, recognize sentinel events, and train staff to respond to such cases and to manage resources and staffing to respond to changing caseloads.

Findings From the *New* DAWN Publications

DAWN ED Data

DAWN relies on a national sample of general, non-federal hospitals operating 24-hour EDs, with over-sampling of hospitals in selected metropolitan areas. According to the DAWN report prepared by SAMHSA in 2007, estimates from 2005 are based on data submitted by 355 hospitals, and they provide the first opportunity since the redesign of DAWN to examine changes over time in drug-related ED visits. However, with only 2 years' estimates to compare, caution is needed when interpreting data related to trends. Because of the redesign, comparisons with years prior to the redesign are not possible.

For ED data, ED medical records of participating hospitals are reviewed retrospectively to find drug use–related ED visits. All types of drugs are considered, including illegal drugs, prescription and over-the-counter pharmaceuticals, dietary supplements, and nonpharmaceutical inhalants. Alcohol is included for patients younger than age 21 when it is the *only* drug implicated in a visit. Alcohol is included for patients of all ages when it is present in combination with another drug.

The ED data from the 2005 DAWN are summarized below. In 2005, hospitals in the United States delivered a total of 108 million ED visits, and DAWN estimates that 1,449,154 ED visits were associated with drug misuse or abuse. Of those ED visits,

- 31% involved illicit drugs only (heroin, cocaine, marijuana, methamphetamine, and other illegal drugs),
- 27% involved pharmaceuticals only,
- 7% involved alcohol only in patients under the age of 21,
- 14% involved illicit drugs with alcohol,
- 10% involved alcohol with pharmaceuticals,
- 8% involved illicit drugs with pharmaceuticals, and
- 4% involved illicit drugs with pharmaceuticals and alcohol.

Between 2004 and 2005, there were no significant changes in the total number of ED visits attributable to drug misuse and abuse. However, ED visits related to nonmedical use of pharmaceuticals increased 21% from 2004 to 2005. For example,

- benzodiazepines increased 19%,
- opioids increased 24% overall, with unspecified opioids increasing 33%, and
- methadone increased 29%.

DAWN Mortality Data

The 2003 DAWN mortality report is the first publication of mortality data from the *New* DAWN. This report describes drug-related deaths reported to DAWN by participating ME/Cs for 2003. The mortality component of DAWN is not national in scope. Therefore, it cannot be used to derive national estimates. DAWN mortality data for 2003 are not comparable to those for any prior years. Comparisons of data from the "old" and "new" DAWN cannot be made.

The mortality data from the 2003 DAWN are summarized as follows.

For 2003, 122 jurisdictions in 35 metropolitan areas and 6 states submitted mortality data to DAWN. The response rate varied by areas ranging from 8% of jurisdictions in Louisville and Dallas–Fort Worth–Arlington to 100% in 9 metropolitan areas and the 6 states.

Participating jurisdictions within the 32 metropolitan areas reported between 0 and 389 deaths related to drug misuse or abuse. Seven jurisdictions had rates of drug-related deaths that exceeded 200 per 1,000,000 population: Baltimore City, Maryland; Denver County, Colorado; Bernalillo County, New Mexico; Jefferson Parish, Louisiana; St. Louis City, Missouri; the District of Columbia; and Manassas City, Virginia. Particularly, St. Louis City, Manassas City, and the District of Columbia had rates 3.1, times, 3.8 times, and 4.1 times the metropolitan-area rate, respectively.

Characteristics of decedents vary by gender and age group. In the average metropolitan area, males were reported to constitute 68% of drug-related deaths, ranging from 52% in Louisville to 77% in Phoenix. After adjusting for population size, the rate of drug-related deaths per 1,000,000 population for males was 2.4 times that for females.

There were few drug-related deaths among children and youth ages 6 to 20. This young age group accounted for only less than 4% of DAWN cases in 20 of the 32 metropolitan areas and greater than 10% in only two areas (Chicago and Miami). In general, rates of drug-related deaths tended to be highest in the 35 to 54 age group. Decedents ages 35 to 54 accounted for more than half of the drug-related deaths in 30 metropolitan areas and fell below half in only two metropolitan areas (Ogden–Clearfield and Provo–Orem, both in Utah).

In the metropolitan areas, nearly half of drug-related deaths, on average, involved a major substance of abuse (i.e., cocaine, heroin, marijuana, stimulants, club drugs, hallucinogens, or nonpharmaceutical inhalants). Cocaine was the most frequently reported illicit drug. In drug-related deaths, cocaine was among the top 5 drugs in 28 of the 32 metropolitan areas and all of the 6 states.

In 2003, DAWN started collecting information about place of death. In 21 of the 32 metropolitan areas, and 5 of the 6 states, more than half of the drug-related deaths occurred at home.

Conclusion

DAWN utilizes survey designs that allow for analyzing longitudinal trends in drug-related ED visits. To keep the sampling frame representative of the current population of hospitals, annual updates must be performed. Future *New* DAWN reports will help elucidate changes over time in drug-related ED visits and identify drugs of misuse and abuse for intervention.

Li-Tzy Wu and Daniel J. Pilowsky

See also Medical Consequences; National Epidemiological Survey on Alcohol and Related Conditions; Office of National Drug Control Policy; *Pulse Check*; Substance Abuse and Mental Health Services Administration

Further Readings

Ball, J. K. (2004). *Redesign of the Drug Abuse Warning Network*. Retrieved March 14, 2007, from https://dawninfo.samhsa.gov/files/dawn_redesign.ppt

Bartels, J. R. (1973). *Drug Abuse Warning Network (DAWN I Analysis)* (Interim Report under BNDD Contract No. 72–47). Washington, DC: Drug Enforcement Administration.

Drug Abuse Warning Network (DAWN): https://dawninfo.samhsa.gov/default.asp

Substance Abuse and Mental Health Services Administration, Office of Applied Studies. (2002). *Drug Abuse Warning Network: Development of a new design (methodology report)* (DAWN Series M-4, DHHS Publication No. SMA 02–3754). Rockville, MD: Author.

Substance Abuse and Mental Health Services Administration, Office of Applied Studies. (2005). *Drug Abuse Warning Network, 2003: Area Profiles of Drug-Related Mortality* (DAWN Series D-27, DHHS Publication No. SMA 05-4023). Rockville, MD: Author.

Substance Abuse and Mental Health Services Administration, Office of Applied Studies. (2007). *Drug Abuse Warning Network, 2005: National estimates of drug-related emergency department visits* (DAWN Series D-29, DHHS Publication No. SMA 07-4256). Rockville, MD: Author.

Substance Abuse and Mental Health Services Administration, Office of Applied Studies. (n.d.). *Who uses data from the New DAWN? Federal agencies.* Retrieved March 14, 2007, from https://dawninfo.samhsa.gov/ files/dawn_fact_sheet_4.pdf

Substance Abuse and Mental Health Services Administration, Office of Applied Studies. (n.d.). *Who uses data from the new DAWN? Communities and the private sectors.* Retrieved March 14, 2007, from https://dawninfo.samhsa.gov/about/whousesdawn/communities.asp

Substance Abuse and Mental Health Services Administration, Office of Applied Studies. (n.d.). *Who uses data from the new DAWN? Members of the Network.* Retrieved March 14, 2007, from https://dawninfo.samhsa.gov/about/whousesdawn/members.asp

DRUG ADDICTION

See SUBSTANCE DEPENDENCE

DRUG COURTS

Drug court programs began in the late 1980s in response to the nation's escalating problem of drug possession, use, sales, and drug-related criminal offenses. Traditional judicial efforts to stem the escalation of drug use included harsher legal penalties for drug use and drug-related crimes, court-mandated treatment for criminals upon release from incarceration, and increasingly severe court-ordered sanctions for relapse, recidivism, or failure to follow mandatory treatment. Unfortunately, these traditional efforts at reducing drug use and drug-related crimes proved to be ineffective.

Harsher penalties equated to increased levels of incarceration in jail and prison while awaiting trial and upon adjudication. In 1999, almost 33% of all offenders released from state prisons had drug use histories, and by 2004, 37% of defendants in criminal cases were adjudicated for drug-related offenses. The result was that the nation's jails and prisons quickly overflowed with criminals convicted of "minor," nonviolent crimes; 7.4% of all arrests in 1987 and 13.1% of all arrests in 2005 were attributed to drug-related crimes. State such as Texas and California were unable to safely house the massive numbers in custody and faced federal fines for overcrowding and the use of temporary housing options such as tents. The nation's courts also experienced severe backlogs, as crimes that previously received little or no sanctions now required court hearings and jury trials. This backlog threatened individual rights to a speedy trial, swamping city and county jails with offenders awaiting adjudication and threatening cities' and counties' ability to house those arrested for more violent offenses or career criminals.

These increasingly severe legal sanctions in America's "War on Drugs" also failed to reduce drug use in general. Court-ordered treatment stipulations often were ineffective because of delayed offender assessment and implementation of treatment, lack of available treatment resources, sanctions of insufficient length to address the chronic nature of substance dependence, and failure to address the drug abuse issue from a comprehensive standpoint (e.g., including issues such as co-occurring disorders, domestic violence, mental illness, physical illness, unemployment, and lack of education). From 1998 to 2005, the percentage of all persons over the age of 12 admitting to current use of illicit drugs rose from approximately 6% to just over 8% of the U.S. population, while the percentage of the U.S. population admitting to alcohol use remained just over 50%. Finally, a corollary to the failure in America's "War on Drugs," traditional judicial methods failed to reduce recidivism and stop the offenders' revolving door in and out of custody. Between 1990 and 2000, the rate of offender recidivism from state parole remained at approximately 59%, and the estimated numbers of arrests for drug abuse violations increased from 322,300 in 1970 to 1,654,600 in 2005.

In 1989, the Miami-Dade County's 11th judicial circuit, including Florida's State Attorney General Janet Reno, Public Defender Bennett Drummer, and Judges Gerald Wetherington and Kerbet Klein responded to the county's rising levels of cocaine-related arrests by designing and implementing the first "Expedited Drug Case Management" system, now known as the "drug court" (http://www.nadcp.org/whatis). This program reflected a change in correctional philosophy from incapacitation, punishment, and deterrence toward rehabilitation and restoration. Additionally, the program followed the general move toward team-oriented and community-based programs promoted by custodial agencies such as the states' parole and probation departments, and other partnerships, including TASC (Treatment Alternative to Street Crime). The mission of this program was to provide drug treatment to nonviolent offenders, while reducing the influx of these types of criminals into jail and prison beds, and to provide for a reduction in time from arrest to conviction for nonviolent offenders.

Drug court designers believed that a combination of criminal justice and therapeutic models of addiction treatment utilized in collaboration between community justice and service providers would be more effective than traditional judicial methods. Criminal justice models rely on external forms of motivation such as punishment and reward to curb illegal behavior. Offenders who comply with court orders may be rewarded with reduced time in custody, while those who refuse to comply may receive jail sanctions ranging from 30 days to a year, parole violations and return to prison, or increased fines. Alternatively, therapeutic addiction treatment models rely on the development of a therapeutic relationship with the treatment provider and efforts to increase internal motivation for personal change. Thus, the collaboration was to provide the external motivating factor inherent in punishment and reward, plus the internal motivator that would arise out of a therapeutic relationship with a treatment team, including the judge, the addiction counselor, the criminal justice case manager, the offender's attorney, and other service personnel. Thus, this innovative program would keep offenders under a structured treatment program longer than would traditional methods and prove to be more effective in reducing both substance abuse and drug-related criminal activity.

In 1994, Congress passed the Violent Crime Control and Law Enforcement Act to authorize federal support for state drug courts and evaluation and research into the effectiveness of these programs. That same year saw the birth of the National Association of Drug Court Professionals. By 2007, of the 3,154 total U.S. counties, 1,227 counties supported a total of 1,699 drug court programs with 349 in the planning stages. In addition to adult drug courts, the nation's community justice system now includes juvenile drug courts, family drug courts, tribal drug courts, domestic violence courts, DUI (driving under the influence) courts, and neighborhood courts.

Key Components

By 1997, drug court structure was found to vary from county to county based upon the target population characteristics, available community resources (e.g., addiction treatment and ancillary resources), drug use, and arrest patterns for a particular community, and community and justice authority beliefs about addiction. Additionally, some programs had evolved to access a wider target population. Drug courts originally targeted only nonviolent offenders arrested for minor drug-related offenses such as possession or being under the influence. Over time, some counties expanded their target focus to include probationers and offenders with substance abuse histories who had been charged with non-drug-related charges.

This county-to-county variability reduced the reliability of drug court evaluation research, making it difficult for the government to continue support of unproven programs. In an attempt to generate program consistency, the National Association of Drug Court Professionals and the Office of Justice Programs of the U.S. Department of Justice compiled a list of 10 key components of drug courts, along with performance benchmarks (see Table 1). Although not evidence-based or theory driven, these 10 components have remained a major asset in the development of all drug court programs.

1. Drug courts integrate alcohol and other drug treatment services with justice system case processing.

2. Using a nonadversarial approach, prosecution and defense counsel promote public safety while protecting participants' due process rights.

3. Eligible participants are identified early and promptly placed in the drug court program.

4. Drug courts provide access to a continuum of alcohol, drug, and other related treatment and rehabilitation services.

5. Abstinence is monitored by frequent alcohol and other drug testing.

6. A coordinated strategy governs drug court responses to participants' compliance.

7. Ongoing judicial interaction with each drug court participant is essential.

8. Monitoring and evaluation measure the achievement of program goals and gauge effectiveness.

9. Continuing interdisciplinary education promotes effective drug court planning, implementation, and operations.

10. Forging partnerships among drug courts, public agencies, and community-based organizations generates local support and enhances drug court program effectiveness.

Drug Court Process

In spite of continued variability between drug court programs, certain intercourt processes have remained consistent. These include the roles played by the various drug court team members and the systematic, comprehensive nature of the program.

The drug court team includes one or two judges, defense or prosecuting attorneys, a probation or parole officer, law enforcement, mental health and substance abuse treatment providers, and social services providers. An assumption of the model is that participant association with a maximum of one or two judges is considered to be the key to client success. The model also assumes success is enhanced if the judge exhibits the following essential characteristics: consistency, flexibility, willingness to use a nontraditional approach, and willingness to use direct communication with the offender. The judge must maintain a nonadversarial approach, meet frequently with the offender, and serve as the source of external motivation.

In addition to the judge, law enforcement personnel, attorneys, probation or parole officers, and treatment and social services providers play important roles in the drug court process. This group determines the initial offender eligibility criteria, develops the intake screening and assessment process, determines the in-program evaluation procedures, and determines how the phased treatment will interact with the judicial process to effectively keep the participant in treatment for as long as is necessary. This group determines appropriate incentives for

(Text continued on page 323)

Table 1 Drug Courts: Key Components and Performance Benchmarks

Key	Component	Performance Benchmarks
1	Drug courts integrate alcohol and other drug treatment services with justice system case processing.	1. Initial and ongoing planning is carried out by a broad-based group, including persons representing all aspects of the criminal justice system, the local treatment delivery system, funding agencies, the local community, and other key policymakers. 2. Documents defining the drug court's mission, goals, eligibility criteria, operating procedures, and performance measures are collaboratively developed, reviewed, and agreed upon. 3. Abstinence and law-abiding behavior are the goals, with specific and measurable criteria marking progress. Criteria may include compliance with program requirements, reductions in criminal behavior and alcohol and other drug (AOD) use, participation in treatment, restitution to the victim or to the community, and declining incidence of AOD use. 4. The court and treatment providers maintain ongoing communication, including frequent exchanges of timely and accurate information about the individual participant's overall program performance. 5. The judge plays an active role in the treatment process, including frequently reviewing treatment progress. The judge responds to each participant's positive efforts as well as to noncompliant behavior. 6. Interdisciplinary education is provided for every person involved in drug court operations to develop a shared understanding of the values, goals, and operating procedures of both the treatment and justice system components. 7. Mechanisms for sharing decision making and resolving conflicts among drug court team members, such as multidisciplinary committees, are established to ensure professional integrity.
2	Using a nonadversarial approach, prosecution and defense counsel promote public safety while protecting participants' due process rights.	1. Prosecutors and defense counsel participate in the design of screening, eligibility, and case-processing policies and procedures to guarantee that due process rights and public safety needs are served. 2. For consistency and stability in the early stages of drug court operations, the judge, prosecutor, and court-appointed defense counsel should be assigned to the drug court for a sufficient period of time to build a sense of teamwork and to reinforce a nonadversarial atmosphere.

(Continued)

Table 1 (Continued)

Key	Component	Performance Benchmarks
		3. The prosecuting attorney does the following: • Reviews the case and determines if the defendant is eligible for the drug court program • Files all necessary legal documents • Participates in a coordinated strategy for responding to positive drug tests and other instances of noncompliance • Agrees that a positive drug test or open court admission of drug possession or use will not result in the filing of additional drug charges based on that admission • Makes decisions regarding the participant's continued enrollment in the program based on performance in treatment rather than on legal aspects of the case, barring additional criminal behavior 4. The defense counsel does the following: • Reviews the arrest warrant, affidavits, charging document, and other relevant information, and reviews all program documents (e.g., waivers, written agreements) • Advises the defendant as to the nature and purpose of the drug court, the rules governing participation, the consequences of abiding or failing to abide by the rules, and how participating or not participating in the drug court will affect his or her interests • Explains all of the rights that the defendant will temporarily or permanently relinquish • Gives advice on alternative courses of action, including legal and treatment alternatives available outside the drug court program, and discusses with the defendant the long-term benefits of sobriety and a drug-free life • Explains that because criminal prosecution for admitting to AOD use in open court will not be invoked, the defendant is encouraged to be truthful with the judge and with treatment staff; also informs the participant that he or she will be expected to speak directly to the judge, not through an attorney
3	Eligible participants are identified early and promptly placed in the drug court program.	1. Eligibility screening is based on established written criteria. Criminal justice officials or others (e.g., pretrial services, probation, treatment alternative to street crime [TASC]) are designated to screen cases and identify potential drug court participants. 2. Eligible participants for drug court are promptly advised about program requirements and the relative merits of participating. 3. Trained professionals screen drug court-eligible individuals for AOD problems and suitability for treatment.

Key	Component	Performance Benchmarks
		4. Initial appearance before the drug court judge occurs immediately after arrest or apprehension to ensure program participation.
		5. The court requires that eligible participants enroll in AOD treatment services immediately.
4	Drug courts provide access to a continuum of alcohol, drug, and other related treatment and rehabilitation services.	1. Individuals are initially screened and thereafter periodically assessed by both court and treatment personnel to ensure that treatment services and individuals are suitably matched.

- An assessment at treatment entry, while useful as a baseline, provides a time-specific "snapshot" of a person's needs and may be based on limited or unreliable information. Ongoing assessment is necessary to monitor progress, to change the treatment plan as necessary, and to identify relapse cues.
- If various levels of treatment are available, participants are matched to programs according to their specific needs. Guidelines for placement at various levels should be developed.
- Screening for infectious diseases and health referrals occurs at an early stage.

2. Treatment services are comprehensive.

- Services should be available to meet the needs of each participant.
- Treatment services may include, but are not limited to, group counseling; individual and family counseling; relapse prevention; 12-step self-help groups; preventive and primary medical care; general health education; medical detoxification; acupuncture for detoxification, for control of craving, and to make people more amenable to treatment; domestic violence programs; batterers' treatment; and treatment for the long-term effects of childhood physical and sexual abuse.
- Other services may include housing; educational and vocational training; legal, money management, and other social service needs; cognitive behavioral therapy to address criminal thinking patterns; anger management; transitional housing; social and athletic activities; and meditation or other techniques to promote relaxation and self-control.
- Specialized services should be considered for participants with co-occurring AOD problems and mental health disorders. Drug courts should establish linkages with mental health providers to furnish services (e.g., medication monitoring, acute care) for participants with co-occurring disorders. Flexibility (e.g., in duration of treatment phases) is essential in designing drug court services for participants with mental health problems.

(Continued)

Table 1 (Continued)

Key	Component	Performance Benchmarks

- Treatment programs or program components are designed to address the particular treatment issues of women and other special populations.
- Treatment is available in a number of settings, including detoxification, acute residential, day treatment, outpatient, and sober living residences.
- Clinical case management services are available to provide ongoing assessment of participant progress and needs, to coordinate referrals to services in addition to primary treatment, to provide structure and support for individuals who typically have difficulty using services even when they are available, and to ensure communication between the court and the various service providers.

3. Treatment services are accessible.

- Accommodations are made for persons with physical disabilities, for those not fluent in English, for those needing child care, and for persons with limited literacy.
- Treatment facilities are accessible by public transportation, when possible.

4. Funding for treatment is adequate, stable, and dedicated to the drug court:

- To ensure that services are immediately available throughout the participant's treatment, agreements are made between courts and treatment providers. These agreements are based on firm budgetary and service delivery commitments.
- Diverse treatment funding strategies are developed based on government and private sources at national, state, and local levels.
- Health care delivered through managed care organizations is encouraged to provide resources for the AOD treatment of member participants.
- Payment of fees, fines, and restitution is part of treatment.
- Fee schedules are commensurate with an individual's ability to pay. However, no one should be turned away solely because of an inability to pay.

5. Treatment services have quality controls.

- Direct service providers are certified or licensed, where required, or otherwise demonstrate proficiency according to accepted professional standards.
- Education, training, and ongoing clinical supervision are provided to treatment staff.

Key	Component	Performance Benchmarks
		6. Treatment agencies are accountable. • Treatment agencies give the court accurate and timely information about a participant's progress. Information exchange complies with the provisions of 42 CFR, Part 2 (the federal regulations governing confidentiality of AOD abuse patient records) and with applicable state statutes. • Responses to progress and noncompliance are incorporated into the treatment protocols. 7. Treatment designs and delivery systems are sensitive and relevant to issues of race, culture, religion, gender, age, ethnicity, and sexual orientation.
5	Abstinence is monitored by frequent alcohol and other drug testing.	1. AOD testing policies and procedures are based on established and tested guidelines, such as those established by the American Probation and Parole Association. Contracted laboratories analyzing urine or other samples should also be held to established standards. 2. Testing may be administered randomly or at scheduled intervals but occurs no less than twice a week during the first several months of an individual's enrollment. Frequency thereafter will vary depending on participant progress. 3. The scope of testing is sufficiently broad to detect the participant's primary drug of choice as well as other potential drugs of abuse, including alcohol. 4. The drug-testing procedure must be certain. Elements contributing to the reliability and validity of a urinalysis testing process include, but are not limited to the following: • Direct observation of urine sample collection • Verification temperature and measurement of creatinine levels to determine the extent of water loading • Specific, detailed, written procedures regarding all aspects of urine sample collection, sample analysis, and result reporting • A documented chain of custody for each sample collected; quality control and quality assurance procedures for ensuring the integrity of the process • Procedures for verifying accuracy when drug test results are contested 5. Ideally, test results are available and communicated to the court and the participant within 1 day. The drug court functions best when it can respond immediately to noncompliance; the time between sample collection and availability of results should be short.

(Continued)

Table 1 (Continued)

Key	Component	Performance Benchmarks
		6. The court is immediately notified when a participant has tested positive, has failed to submit to AOD testing, has submitted the sample of another, or has adulterated a sample. 7. The coordinated strategy for responding to noncompliance includes prompt responses to positive tests, missed tests, and fraudulent tests. 8. Participants should be abstinent for a substantial period of time prior to program graduation.
6	A coordinated strategy governs drug court responses to participants' compliance.	1. Treatment providers, the judge, and other program staff maintain frequent, regular communication to provide timely reporting of progress and noncompliance and to enable the court to respond immediately. Procedures for reporting noncompliance are clearly defined in the drug court's operating documents. 2. Responses to compliance and noncompliance are explained verbally and provided in writing to drug court participants before their orientation. Periodic reminders are given throughout the treatment process. 3. The responses for compliance vary in intensity and include the following: • Encouragement and praise from the bench • Ceremonies and tokens of progress, including advancement to the next treatment phase • Reduced supervision • Decreased frequency of court appearances • Reduced fines or fees • Dismissal of criminal charges or reduction in the term of probation. • Reduced or suspended incarceration • Graduation 4. Responses to or sanctions for noncompliance might include the following: • Warnings and admonishment from the bench in open court • Demotion to earlier program phases • Increased frequency of testing and court appearances • Confinement in the courtroom or jury box • Increased monitoring and/or treatment intensity • Fines • Required community service or work programs • Escalating periods of jail confinement (however, drug court participants remanded to jail should receive AOD treatment services while confined) • Termination from the program and reinstatement of regular court processing

Key	Component	Performance Benchmarks
7	Ongoing judicial interaction with each drug court participant is essential.	1. Regular status hearings are used to monitor participant performance: • Frequent status hearings during the initial phases of each participant's program establish and reinforce the drug court's policies and ensure effective supervision of each drug court participant. Frequent hearings also give the participant a sense of how he or she is doing in relation to others. • Time between status hearings may be increased or decreased, based on compliance with treatment protocols and progress observed. • Having a significant number of drug court participants appear at a single session gives the judge the opportunity to educate both the offender at the bench and those waiting as to the benefits of program compliance and consequences for noncompliance. 2. The court applies appropriate incentives and sanctions to match the participant's treatment progress. 3. Payment of fees, fines, and/or restitution is part of the participant's treatment. The court supervises such payments and takes into account the participant's financial ability to fulfill these obligations. The court ensures that no one is denied participation in drug courts solely because of an inability to pay fees, fines, or restitution.
8	Monitoring and evaluation measure the achievement of program goals and gauge effectiveness.	1. Management, monitoring, and evaluation processes begin with initial planning. As part of the comprehensive planning process, drug court leaders and senior managers should establish specific and measurable goals that define the parameters of data collection and information management. An evaluator can be an important member of the planning team. 2. Data needed for program monitoring and management can be obtained from records maintained for day-to-day program operations, such as the numbers and general demographics of individuals screened for eligibility; the extent and nature of AOD problems among those assessed for possible participation in the program; and attendance records, progress reports, drug test results, and incidence of criminality among those accepted into the program. 3. Monitoring and management data are assembled in useful formats for regular review by program leaders and managers. 4. Ideally, much of the information needed for monitoring and evaluation is gathered through an automated system that can provide timely and useful reports. If an automated system is not available, manual data collection and report

(Continued)

Table 1 (Continued)

Key	*Component*	*Performance Benchmarks*

preparation can be streamlined. Additional monitoring information may be acquired by observation and through program staff and participant interviews.

5. Automated manual information systems must adhere to written guidelines that protect against unauthorized disclosure of sensitive personal information about individuals.

6. Monitoring reports need to be reviewed at frequent intervals by program leaders and senior managers. They can be used to analyze program operations, gauge effectiveness, modify procedures when necessary, and refine goals.

7. Process evaluation activities should be undertaken throughout the course of the drug court program. This activity is particularly important in the early stages of program implementation.

8. If feasible, a qualified independent evaluator should be selected and given responsibility for developing and conducting an evaluation design and for preparing interim and final reports. If an independent evaluation is unavailable, the drug court program designs and implements its own evaluation, based on guidance available through the field:

   • Judges, prosecutors, the defense bar, treatment staff, and others design the evaluation collaboratively with the evaluator.

   • Ideally, an independent evaluator will help the information systems expert design and implement the management information system.

   • The drug court program ensures that the evaluator has access to relevant justice system and treatment information.

   • The evaluator maintains continuing contact with the drug court and provides information on a regular basis. Preliminary reports may be reviewed by drug court program personnel and used as the basis for revising goals, policies, and procedures as appropriate.

9. Useful data elements to assist in management and monitoring may include, but are not limited to the following:

   • The number of defendants screened for program eligibility and the outcome of those initial screenings

   • The number of persons admitted to the drug court program

   • Characteristics of program participants, such as age, sex, race/ethnicity, family status, employment status, and educational level; current charges; criminal justice

Key Component	Performance Benchmarks

history; AOD treatment or mental health treatment history; medical needs (including detoxification); and nature and severity of AOD problems

- Number and characteristics of participants (e.g., duration of treatment involvement, reason for discharge from the program)
- Number of active cases
- Patterns of drug use as measured by drug test results
- Aggregate attendance data and general treatment progress measurements
- Number and characteristics of persons who graduate or complete treatment successfully
- Number and characteristics of persons who do not graduate or complete the program
- Number of participants who fail to appear at drug court hearings and number of bench warrants issued for participants
- Rearrests during involvement in the drug court program and type of arrest(s)
- Number, length, and reasons for incarcerations during and subsequent to involvement in the drug court program

10. When making comparisons for evaluation purposes, drug courts should consider the following groups:

- Program graduates
- Program terminations
- Individuals who were referred to, but did not appear for, treatment
- Individuals who were not referred for drug court services

11. At least 6 months after exiting a drug court program, comparison groups (listed above) should be examined to determine long-term effects of the program. Data elements for follow-up evaluation may include the following:

- Criminal behavior or activity
- Days spent in custody on all offenses from date of acceptance into the program
- AOD use since leaving the program
- Changes in job skills and employment status
- Changes in literacy and other educational attainments
- Changes in physical and mental health
- Changes in status of family relationships
- Attitudes and perceptions of participation in the program
- Use of health care and other social services

(Continued)

Table 1 (Continued)

Key	Component	Performance Benchmarks
		12. Drug court evaluations should consider the use of cost–benefit analysis to examine the economic impact of program services. Important elements of cost-benefit analysis include the following: • Reductions in court costs, including judicial, counsel, and investigative resources • Reductions in costs related to law enforcement and corrections • Reductions in health care utilization • Increased economic productivity
9	Continuing interdisciplinary education promotes effective drug court planning, implementation, and operations.	1. Key personnel have attained a specific level of basic education, as defined in staff training requirements and in the written operating procedures. The operating procedures should also define requirements for the continuing education of each drug court staff member. 2. Attendance at education and training sessions by all drug court personnel is essential. Regional and national drug court training provide critical information on innovative developments across the nation. Sessions are most productive when drug court personnel attend as a group. Credits for continuing professional education should be offered, when feasible. 3. Continuing education institutionalizes the drug court and moves it beyond its initial identification with the key staff who may have founded the program and nurtured its development. 4. An education syllabus and curriculum are developed, describing the drug court's goals, policies, and procedures. Topics might include the following: • Goals and philosophy of drug courts • The nature of AOD abuse, its treatment and terminology • The dynamics of abstinence and techniques for preventing relapse • Responses to relapse and to noncompliance with other program requirements • Basic legal requirements of the drug court program and an overview of the local criminal justice system's policies, procedures, and terminology • Drug testing standards and procedures • Sensitivity to race, culture, ethnicity, gender, and sexual orientation as they affect the operation of the drug court • Interrelationships of co-occurring conditions such as AOD abuse and mental illness (also known as "dual diagnosis") • Federal, state, and local confidentiality requirements

Key	Component	Performance Benchmarks
10	Forging partnerships among drug courts, public agencies, and community-based organizations generates local support and enhances drug court program effectiveness.	1. Representatives from the court, community organizations, law enforcement, corrections, prosecution, defense counsel, supervisory agencies, treatment and rehabilitation providers, educators, health and social service agencies, and the faith community meet regularly to provide guidance and direction to the drug court program. 2. The drug court plays a pivotal role in forming linkages between community groups and the criminal justice system. The linkages are a conduit of information to the public about the drug court, and conversely, from the community to the court about available community services and local problems. 3. Partnerships between drug courts and law enforcement and/or community policing programs can build effective links between the court and offenders in the community. 4. Participation of public and private agencies, as well as community-based organizations, is formalized through a steering committee. The steering committee aids in the acquisition and distribution of resources. An especially effective way for the steering committee to operate is through the formation of a nonprofit corporation structure that includes all the principal drug court partners, provides policy guidance, and acts as a conduit for fundraising and resource acquisition. 5. Drug court programs and services are sensitive to, and demonstrate awareness of, the populations they serve and the communities in which they operate. Drug courts provide opportunities for community involvement through forums, informational meetings, and other community outreach efforts. 6. The drug court hires a professional staff that reflects the population served, and the drug court provides ongoing cultural competence training.

Source: National Association of Drug Court Professionals. (1997, January). *Defining drug courts: The key components.* Washington, DC: U.S. Department of Justice, Office of Justice Programs. Retrieved July 20, 2007, from http://www.ojp.usdoj.gov/BJA/grant/DrugCourts/DefiningDC.pdf

(Text continued from page 312)

participant compliance (e.g., dismissal of charges, reduced penalties, or reduced sentences), and non-compliance (e.g., increased jail time, remanding to prison, or increased time under supervision), as well as setting the frequency of court hearings and drug court expectations for each participant. Finally, this group develops a personalized comprehensive plan to meet each participant's substance abuse needs as well as other needs such as employment, housing, medical treatment, and educational or vocational training. After creation of this comprehensive plan, the drug court team meets regularly with each participant to assess client needs and progress.

Offender entry into the drug court system differs according to the prosecutorial policy of the county and the perceived benefits to the offender. For example, in 1994 Las Vegas' Clark County judicial system decided that offenders must plead guilty in order to gain admittance to the drug court system. While this decision resulted in greater drug court recommendations by the prosecuting attorneys, it also resulted in fewer offenders requesting the program. Policies allowing offenders to avoid prison time for drug-related felonies, and receive probation in conjunction with drug court participation, also resulted in increased drug court recommendations by the prosecuting attorneys because it reduced prison overcrowding.

Drug Court Research Evaluation

The most salient question for drug court funders (e.g., the federal government) is whether drug courts work. Are they effective in reducing substance abuse and recidivism? Do they reduce the jail and prison populations, freeing bed space for criminals who might be considered more dangerous to society?

Belenko's 2001 review of drug courts found positive outcomes, including a program completion rate of 47%, a reduction in drug use and criminal activity during program participation, lower in-program than nonprogram re-arrest rates, lower in-program recidivism rates, and a cost savings compared to traditional judicial methods. Although promising, Belenko suggested that further analysis is needed with improved and consistent evaluation measures and a multiyear analysis to better capture postprogram recidivism data. A 2003 review of drug court programs also revealed significant barriers related to lack of funding for software, automation, and essential equipment; lack of training in the use of automated case management; and difficulties in connecting the various program information services.

In 2006, the U.S. Department of Justice, Office of Justice Programs/National Institute of Justice (NIJ) released an NIJ special report, *Drug Courts: The Second Decade*. Researchers compiled multiple independent studies into the effectiveness of the drug court model and factors salient to their success. A summary of the findings follows.

Effectiveness

1. Research supports that drug courts can reduce recidivism. In several studies, successful drug court graduates exhibited significantly lower re-arrest rates than did nongraduates for more than 2 years after completing the program. To date, however, causal information regarding the processes key to success has not been found.

2. Drug court programs are less costly than "business as usual." Cost analysis per participant revealed a cost savings of $1,400 in investments costs, $2,300 saved in avoided law enforcement and court costs, and $1,300 saved in victimization costs.

Factors Salient to Success

1. Successful treatment programs must use evidence-based practices, theories, and tools, with a goal of helping participants to build cognitive skills.

2. Ancillary services to address mental health, housing, educational and vocational, and medical issues are essential.

3. All drug court team members should be educated in addiction theory, evidence-based treatment, and relapse prevention. Additionally, all team members should be concerned with the integrity and consistency of the treatment planning, delivery, and assessment even if they are not the actual treatment providers.

4. A good interpersonal relationship between the drug court judge and the participant increases compliance with treatment demands.

Conclusion

The adult drug court model is an innovative, team-oriented, rehabilitative approach to offenders with substance use disorders, which has spawned other team approaches, including those for juvenile drug courts, family drug courts, and DUI (driving under the influence) courts. The adult model, in existence since 1989, has proved to lower recidivism rates and costs associated with the adjudication of convicted felons. Additionally, the model has produced a sixfold increase in drug treatment retention with approximately 70% of drug court participants completing the program. In spite of these promising results, further empirical research is needed to fully evaluate what specific processes within drug courts are causally related to success.

Angela D. Broadus

See also Coercion and Treatment; Court-Mandated
Treatment; Crime and Substance Abuse; Criminal Justice
Populations

Further Readings

American University. (n.d.). *Summary of drug court activity
by state and county: March 19, 2008.* Washington, DC:
Bureau of Justice Assistance. Retrieved May 25, 2008,
from http://spa.american.edu/justice/documents/
2150.pdf#page=105

Ashcroft, J., Daniels, D. J., & Nedelkoff, R. R. (2003,
February). *Drug court monitoring, evaluation, and
management information systems: National scope needs
assessment.* Washington, DC: U.S. Bureau of Justice
Assistance. Retrieved July 21, 2007, from
http://www.ncjrs.gov/pdffiles1/bja/195077.pdf

Bureau of Justice Assistance & National Association of Drug
Court Professionals. (1997, January). *Defining drug
courts: The key components.* Washington, DC: Author.
Retrieved July 20, 2007, from http://www.ojp.usdoj.gov/
BJA/grant/DrugCourts/DefiningDC.pdf

Bureau of Justice Statistics. (2007). *Drug use and crime.*
Washington, DC: Author. Retrieved July 20, 2007, from
http://www.ojp.gov/bjs/dcf/duc.htm#attime

Bureau of Justice Statistics. (2004). *Federal justice statistics.*
Washington, DC: Author. Retrieved July 20, 2007, from
http://www.ojp.usdoj.gov/bjs/fed.htm#Adjudication

Gebelein, R. S. (2000, May). The rebirth of rehabilitation:
Promise and perils of drug courts. *Sentencing &
Corrections: Issues for the 21st Century,* No. 6. Retrieved
July 21, 2007, from http://www.ncjrs.gov/pdffiles1/
nij/181412.pdf

Goldkamp, J. (1995, July). *The drug court movement* (NCJ
Report No. 149260). Washington, DC: National Institute
of Justice. Retrieved July 20, 2007, from
http://www.ncjrs.gov/pdffiles/drgctmov.pdf

Gonzales, A. R., Schofield, R. B., & Schmitt, G. R. (2006,
June). *Drug courts: The second decade.* Washington, DC:
National Institute of Justice. Retrieved July 20, 2007,
from http://www.ojp.usdoj.gov/nij/pubs-sum/211081.htm

National Association of Drug Court Professionals:
http://www.nadcp.org

*What's new: Latest data on alcohol, tobacco, and illegal
drugs.* (2007). Washington, DC: Office of Applied
Studies. Retrieved July 20, 2007, from http://www
.drugabusestatistics.samhsa.gov/newpubs.htm#New

Wright, D., Sathe, N., & Spagnola, K. (2007). *State estimates
of substance use from the 2004–2005 National Surveys on
Drug Use and Health* (DHHS Publication No. SMA 07-
4235, NSDUH Series H-31). Rockville, MD: Substance

Abuse and Mental Health Services Administration, Office
of Applied Studies. Retrieved July 20, 2007, from
http://www.drugabusestatistics.samhsa.gov/2k5state/pdf/
2k5state.pdf

DRUG-CRIME CYCLE

See CRIME AND SUBSTANCE ABUSE

DRUG-FREE SCHOOLS AND COMMUNITIES ACT

The safe and drug-free schools and communities program is the federal government's major initiative to prevent drug abuse and violence in and around schools. The Drug-Free Schools and Communities Act of 1986 (20 U.S.C. 3181) was amended in 1989 by Public Law 101-226 to become the Safe and Drug-Free Schools and Communities Act. In 2001, the Safe and Drug-Free Schools and Communities Act was amended and reauthorized by the No Child Left Behind Act (Public Law 107-110) as Part A, Title IV, 21st Century Schools. The Safe and Drug-Free Schools and Communities Act is intended primarily to support prevention programs and activities. It provides formula grants to states to support local educational agencies, consortia of agencies, and community-based organizations in developing and implementing programs to prevent drug use and violence among American children and youth. The Safe and Drug-Free Schools and Communities Act supports the development of comprehensive drug and violence prevention programs for students from preschool through to the postsecondary educational level. These prevention programs include health education, early intervention, student services, mentoring, referrals for treatment and rehabilitation, and other related activities.

The purpose of the Safe and Drug-Free Schools and Communities Act is to support programs and activities that prevent violence in and around schools; that prevent the illegal use of alcohol, tobacco, and other drugs; that involve parents and communities in drug and violence prevention; and that are coordinated with relevant federal, state, school, and community efforts and resources to promote a safe and drug-free learning environment that fosters enhanced student learning and outcomes. The Safe and Drug-Free Schools and Communities Act is a central part of the federal effort to encourage the creation of safe, disciplined, and drug-free learning environments that will help all children and youth meet challenging academic standards.

Under the provisions of the Safe and Drug-Free Schools and Communities Act, authorized by the Elementary and Secondary Education Act, the U.S. Department of Education administers the Safe and Drug-Free Schools and Communities State Grants Program. These consist of formula grants awarded through states to local educational agencies and consortia of agencies to establish, expand, and conduct local prevention programs. Funded programs provide support for both school and community-based programs designed to help communities prevent alcohol, tobacco, and other drug use, as well as prevent youth violence. These programs and their activities must be based on an assessment of objective data on the incidence of drug use and violence in elementary and secondary schools, as well as the communities they serve. They must be designed in accordance with evidence-based practices. Analysis of the data must consider conditions and consequences related to problem areas, such as delinquency and serious discipline problems. The evaluation of these programs must demonstrate how they achieve measurable performance results. The Safe and Drug-Free Schools and Communities Act also stipulates that there be meaningful and ongoing consultation with, and input from, parents concerning drug and violence prevention activities and programs. The Safe and Drug-Free Schools and Communities Act also provides for the training of teachers, counselors, and other school personnel, and it also provides funding for national leadership activities that directly support classroom teaching.

The Uniform Management Information and Reporting System is required under the Safe and Drug-Free Schools and Communities Act. The Uniform Management Information and Reporting System provides the public with information on youth drug use and school violence at national, state, and local levels. States must provide data on a school-by-school basis. These data include the frequency, incidence, and seriousness of drug- and violence-related offenses that resulted in suspensions or expulsions from elementary and secondary schools in the respective states; truancy rates; and the incidence and prevalence, age of initiation,

perception of health risks, and perception of social disapproval of drug use and violence by children and youth in schools and communities.

The Drug Free Schools and Communities Act Amendments of 1989 require that, as a condition of receiving funds or any other form of financial assistance from any federal program, an institution of higher education (e.g., vocational, technical, business, or trade school, college or university) must certify that it has adopted and implemented a program to prevent the unlawful possession, use, and/or distribution of alcohol or illicit drugs by students and employees. It is also required under the Drug Free Schools and Campuses Regulations (Education Department General Administrative Regulations [EDGAR], Part 86) that there be, in writing, an annual distribution describing to each student and employee of the institution of higher education the expected standards of conduct related to substance use and abuse; a listing of the legal alcohol and drug criminal offenses, penalties, and fines; specific institutional disciplinary sanctions related to substance use, misuse, and abuse; a description of the health risks of substance use and abuse; and available alcohol and drug counseling, treatment, rehabilitation, and reentry program resources for students and employees. There is a mandated biennial review of the institution of higher education's substance use policy and prevention program effectiveness required under the Drug Free Schools and Communities Act (EDGAR, Part 86); this review must also examine whether institutional substance use sanctions are enforced consistently.

Victor B. Stolberg

See also Prevention Education; Prevention Resources; School-Based Prevention Programs; Violence Prevention

Further Readings

Brandon, P. R. (1992). State-level evaluation of school programs funded under the Drug-Free Schools and Communities Act. *Journal of Drug Education 22,* 25–36.

Gorman, D. M. (2002). Defining and operationalizing "research-based" prevention: A critique (with case studies) of the U. S. Department of Education's Safe, Disciplined and Drug-Free Schools Exemplary Programs. *Evaluation and Program Planning, 25,* 295–302.

Hantman, I., & Crosse, S. (2000). *Progress in prevention report on the national study of local education agency activities under the Safe and Drug Free Schools and*

Communities Act. Washington, DC: U.S. Department of Education, Planning and Evaluation Service.

U.S. Department of Education, Office of Safe and Drug-Free Schools: http://www.ed.gov/about/offices/list/osdfs/index.html

DRUG LAWS, HISTORY OF

The history of drug laws is characterized by great variability across time and cultures. This variability is particularly evident in the selection of substances for prohibition; drugs that were unregulated for centuries are now widely prohibited, and substances that are now virtually unregulated were subject to strict prohibitions in the past. The aims of drug regulation are also diverse and are often controversial. Whereas proponents of drug regulation typically refer to the protection of the vulnerable and the maintenance of cultural values, critics of drug policy cite institutionalized racism and the indirect pursuit of sociopolitical interests. Indeed, societal efforts to regulate the use and distribution of psychoactive substances can be traced back to antiquity, and no single attribution captures the confluences of social, political, and individual forces that influence policy. However, across eras, the creation of drug laws has surely been subject to social influences and biases that are unrelated to the psychoactive properties of the prohibited substances. Indeed, a historical examination of drug laws provides a fascinating reflection of the aspirations, conflicts, and bigotries of the eras in which those laws were created.

The Ancient World Through the 19th Century

Attempts to regulate psychoactive substances date back to antiquity. In the 5th century BC, the Greek philosopher Plato recommended prohibiting alcohol use for men younger than 18 years and regulating use for men younger than 30. Likewise, Roman custom restricted alcohol consumption to men older than 30. With the Christianization of the Roman Empire and Europe in the 4th through 9th centuries, a variety of nonalcoholic psychoactive substances fell into official disfavor. This attitudinal shift is thought to have reflected religious rivalry, as these drugs were associated with pre-Christian "pagan" religious traditions. Indeed, following the adoption of Christianity in Rome, a succession of Roman councils persecuted individuals accused of distributing drugs. Antagonism toward users of nonalcoholic intoxicants continued as the Church consolidated its power in the Middle Ages, and by the 10th century, drug use was considered heretical. Drug prohibitions continued throughout the Inquisition, which outlawed cannabis use in the 12th and 13th centuries. Travel to the Americas in the 15th and 16th centuries brought Europeans into contact with new peoples and new psychoactive substances. However, these early immigrants to the New World superimposed European beliefs regarding drugs and witchcraft upon indigenous behaviors. This imperialistic attitude is reflected in the activities of the Inquisition of the Americas, which prohibited indigenous peoples from the ceremonial use of psychoactive drugs. Indeed, in many parts of Europe and the colonies, the association between psychoactive substances and witchcraft persisted beyond the Renaissance, and drug users continued to endure persecution as witches until the late 17th century.

Of the drugs encountered by European explorers in the Americas, coca and tobacco had the greatest impact. Early attempts to regulate coca were religiously based; the Church condemned ceremonial coca use among Native Americans as impeding conversion to Christianity. However, this condemnation was not without exception; the chewing of coca leaves by indigenous slaves was encouraged by Spanish Conquistadors to aid stamina for toil in the mines. Like coca, tobacco was first met with suspicion and repression. In the early 17th century, many European status prohibited tobacco use, as did Turkey, Japan, and China, and by mid-century, several papal edits had been issued against tobacco. These early anti-tobacco prohibitions were often accompanied by harsh punishments; Russia, Germany, Turkey, and China all executed tobacco users. However, despite these widespread and severe prohibitions, the use of tobacco remained popular and was permitted across many nations in Europe, the Near East, and Asia by the late 17th century.

The African stimulant coffee was first introduced to the Middle East in the 15th century and to Europe in the 16th century. As had been the case with other novel psychoactive substances, coffee was initially greeted with widespread prohibitions. In 16th-century Arabia, coffee was considered to be an intoxicant and was therefore prohibited under religious law. However, there is evidence that Arabic coffee prohibitions may have also reflected political concerns; coffee houses were purported to be meeting places for political dissidents. Coffee was likewise banned in Egypt around the same time, and coffee establishments and warehouses were ransacked. However, coffee was soon accepted in Middle Eastern culture and even found sacred use as a stimulant during prolonged religious vigils. There is also documentation of attempts to repress coffee when it arrived in Europe from the Middle East. This repression may have reflected the association between coffee and Middle Eastern culture, as priestly entreaties for the Church to ban coffee cited its status as a beverage of "infidels." However, by 1600, the Vatican declared coffee to be sacrosanct and coffee drinking was established throughout Europe by the 17th century.

The 18th century, the "Age of Reason," was a period of relative tolerance with regard to drug use. Perhaps the most significant development of that era involved the Chinese ban on opium in the early 1700s. This prohibition displeased the British, who reaped considerable profit from the importation of Indian opium to China, and British resistance to Chinese opium regulations led to two Opium Wars between China and Britain in the mid-1800s. Soon after the second Opium War, China legalized opium imports, and by the end of the century, China was producing sufficient quantities of opium to satisfy domestic demand.

The relative tolerance that characterized 18th-century drug regulation continued throughout much of the 19th century. During this period, opium was used widely for medicinal and recreational purposes. Despite this tolerance, the relatively unregulated use of opiates was somewhat controversial, and to better examine this issue the British government convened two commissions on opium and hemp in India in the late 1800s. These commissions concluded that moderate use of these drugs resembled moderate alcohol use and, in most situations, did not give rise to extreme negative outcomes. Nonetheless, public concern surrounding opium addiction and overdose in Britain led to the establishment of the Pharmacy Act of 1868, which restricted the sale of opium to professional pharmacists. This regulatory response was relatively strict compared to practices in the United States, where opiates, cocaine, and cannabis were largely unregulated until the 20th century.

The 20th Century

The history of drug laws in the 20th century reflects the growing global dominance of the United States, and international drug policy was largely directed by the United States for most of the century. Attitudes toward drug regulation in the United States at the beginning of the 20th century stand in stark contrast to regulatory practices at the end of the century. In the early 1900s, most psychoactive drugs were available in pharmacies and, in many cases, could be bought directly from manufacturers. Indeed, it was during this period that the Bayer Corporation introduced heroin as a cough suppressant. Likewise, cocaine was an ingredient in the popular drink Coca-Cola until 1903 and was used in medicines to treat respiratory ailments and fatigue until the 1920s. Despite this apparent tolerance, U.S. attitudes toward drug use were undergoing a transformation in the early part of the 20th century, and by the 1930s, the stage was set for national and international prohibitions of many psychoactive drugs. This change was, in part, a response to negative consequences related to drug use and addiction and an increased awareness of the dangers of unscrupulous manufacturers and unregulated markets. However, there is also substantial evidence that policy was strongly influenced by religious, social, and economic interests.

The Shanghai Opium Commission in 1909 represented an important turning point in the development of U.S.-led international drug policy. The commission was largely the creation of American missionaries who had successfully campaigned to outlaw opium sales in the Philippines in the 1890s and who aimed to extend this prohibition internationally. Although the commission was unsuccessful at establishing international prohibitions, it nonetheless had a substantial impact on domestic policy in the United States. To demonstrate a commitment to global narcotics control, the United States began strictly regulating domestic opium production while the commission was in progress. The Shanghai Opium Commission was followed by several related attempts at international drug prohibitions including the 1912 Hague Opium Convention, in which 12 nations, including the United States, Britain, France, China, and Japan, resolved that the use of opiates and cocaine should be confined to medical purposes. Following the Hague Convention, American antidrug activists worked to broaden domestic drug prohibitions, and in 1914, these interests were central to the passage of the Harrison Narcotic Act (HNA). The HNA required distributors of opium and cocaine to register and pay a tax on each transaction; this requirement dramatically limited the availability of these drugs for nonmedical purposes. The strict penalties for drug offenses that characterized the HNA set the stage for the incarceration crisis that continues to plague the United States. By the late 1920s, there were more people in federal prisons for HNA offenses than for any other crime.

The social control of distinct subgroups, from traditional healers to dissidents in coffee shops, has long inspired drug policy. Consistent with this tradition, concern about the influence of immigrant and minority populations has been a prime mover of U.S. drug policy from the end of the 19th century to present time. One of the earliest substances to receive substantial sanctions in the United States was opium. Opium was first criminalized locally in San Francisco in 1875 due to concerns that European American youth were smoking the drug in shops frequented by Chinese laborers. Yet, opium-related prohibitions were confined to the distinctly Chinese practice of opium smoking, whereas other forms of opium ingestion were permitted. As had been the case with these early prohibitions against opium, the broader sanctions specified a few decades later in the HNA were also supported by popular prejudices relating opium and cocaine to miscegenation and criminality. Specifically, there is substantial evidence of efforts to relate opium use to concerns that European American women would frequent opium dens and mingle with Asian American men. Similarly, with the assistance of the U.S. media, hysteria spread regarding the role of cocaine in fueling sexual rampages by African American men.

The prohibitionist sentiment in the United States soon extended beyond substances included in the HNA to include tobacco, alcohol, and cannabis. In the early 1920s, a short-lived tobacco prohibition was enacted in several U.S. states, and alcohol was prohibited nationally in 1920. Although it was more successful than attempts at tobacco prohibition, alcohol prohibition was nonetheless a failure by all accounts. It was unpopular, ineffective, and criminogenic, and by 1933, federal prohibition was repealed. Yet cannabis, which was introduced to the United States by migrant Mexican farm workers, did not concern drug reformers in the 1920s and early 1930s. Indeed, during this period, the U.S. Department of Agriculture encouraged Americans to cultivate cannabis crops, and the Federal

Bureau of Narcotics downplayed the intoxicating properties of cannabis. Anticannabis sentiment rose during the mid- to late 1930s, as the economic insecurity of the Great Depression focused anger on Mexican workers who favored the drug. As was the case with cocaine and opium, sentiment was fueled by bigoted fears of miscegenation and crime; cannabis use was purported to provoke violence and sexual disinhibition among these already-suspect migrant workers. Moreover, there is evidence that powerful interests in the petrochemical and paper industries lobbied for cannabis prohibition because of its potential as an alternative source of paper and plastics. The distribution of cannabis was severely restricted by the Marihuana Tax Act of 1937, which prohibited the recreational use of cannabis and included jail sentences of up to 20 years for violators. Severe penalties for drug crimes were further entrenched in 1951 with the passage of the Boggs Act, which mandated 2 years of imprisonment for first-time drug offenders. The trend toward increasing penalties continued with the 1956 Narcotics Control Act, which included possible life sentences and capital punishment for drug crimes.

With its harsh domestic drug laws entrenched, the United States continued to pressure other nations to implement punitive drug laws. In 1961, the United States led the United Nations (UN) Single Convention on Narcotic Drugs, which internationalized this punitive approach. Under the Single Convention, a diverse host of nations agreed to criminalize the production, sale, and, in many cases, possession, of opiates, cocaine, and cannabis for nonmedical purposes. Today, virtually all nations comply with UN policies regarding the criminalization of recreational drugs. Although there is widespread compliance at the level of official policy, nations differ dramatically with regard to enforcement. Indeed, many nations that endorse strict prohibitions do little to enforce these laws, and so the impact of official policy on local patterns of substance use varies widely.

The War on Drugs and Beyond

Popular attitudes toward drug use in the North America and Europe softened somewhat in the late 1960s and early 1970s, and the shift toward cultural liberalism that characterized that era led to increased pressure for less-punitive policies, particularly with regard to cannabis. Many critics noted that, like the 1930s U.S. experiment in alcohol prohibition, drug

4 plays4444444

prohibition was counterproductive and criminogenic, and in the 1970s, several U.S. states reduced penalties, or decriminalized, possession of small amounts of cannabis for personal use. This recognition was mirrored by several European regimes, which decriminalized or legalized possession of small amounts of psychoactive substances. Despite these international and local movements, the U.S. federal government remained committed to a policy of strict prohibitions. In 1970, U.S. Congress passed the Comprehensive Drug Abuse Prevention and Control Act, which classified drugs into five schedules with escalating penalties based on potential for abuse. This legislation forms the basis of current U.S. drug laws. In that same year, President Richard Nixon declared a "war on drugs" and included drug use among the most pressing threats to the well-being of the American public.

Despite consistent criticism across the political spectrum, and robust evidence that punitive policies have little impact on levels of drug use and related negative consequences, the United States maintains its position as a world leader in prohibiting the use of select drugs and punishing violators of these prohibitions. Indeed, the United States is the world's leader in incarceration; over 2 million Americans are currently imprisoned, which represents a more than 500% increase since the beginning of the war on drugs. Drug-related incarceration accounts for more than half of all federal inmates, and the number of drug offenders in state prisons has increased more than tenfold since 1980. As has been the case throughout the history of drug laws, current efforts at drug regulation are inextricably tied to class and ethnicity. African Americans, in particular, are dramatically overrepresented among drug-related offenders, despite levels of drug use that are comparable to other ethnic groups. Indeed, persons of color account for as much as three quarters of all drug-related prisoners, and social critics have identified the war on drugs as a significant factor in the perpetuation of racial inequality in U.S. society.

Conclusion

The use of psychoactive substances can be traced back to antiquity, and efforts to regulate drug use are also ancient. As is the case in present times, past regimes selected some substances for prohibition and allowed relatively free access to others. Throughout history, the determination of which substances warrant prohibition has been influenced by factors unrelated to the properties of the specific substances. Rather, drug laws have largely represented support for some cultural traditions and derogation of others. Indeed, drug laws have frequently been enacted as a means of social control, and contemporary critics have proposed that these laws disproportionately impact vulnerable ethnic and social groups.

Tiffany Walsh, Zach Walsh,
and Gregory L. Stuart

See also Cultural Aspects; Drug Use, History of; Illicit Drugs and Illegal Drugs; National Drug Control Strategy; Office of National Drug Control Policy; War on Drugs

Further Readings

Bewley-Taylor, D. R. (1999). *The United States and international drug control, 1909–1997*. London: Pinter.

Brecher, E. M. (1972). *Licit & illicit drugs: The consumers union report on narcotics, stimulants, depressants, inhalants, hallucinogens & marijuana—Including caffeine, nicotine and alcohol*. Mount Vernon, NY: Consumers Union.

Davenport-Hines, R. (2002). *The pursuit of oblivion: A global history of narcotics*. New York: Norton.

Fisher, G. L. (2006). *Rethinking our war on drugs: Candid talk about controversial issues*. Westport, CT: Praeger.

Herer, J. (2000). *The emperor wears no clothes* (11th ed.). Van Nuys, CA: Ah Ha Publishing.

Legal Frameworks Group of the King County Bar Association Drug Policy Project. (2005). Drugs and the drug laws: Historical and cultural contexts. In *Effective drug control: Toward a new legal framework: State-level regulation as a workable alternative to the "war on drugs"* (pp. 7–30). Retrieved October 22, 2007, from http://www.kcba.org/ScriptContent/KCBA/druglaw/pdf/EffectiveDrugControl.pdf

Musto, D. F. (1999). *The American disease: Origins of narcotic control* (3rd ed.). New York: Oxford University Press.

Provine, D. M. (2007). *Unequal under law: Race in the war on drugs*. Chicago: University of Chicago Press.

Szasz, T. (1974). *Ceremonial chemistry: The ritual persecution of drugs, addicts, and pushers*. New York: Anchor/Doubleday.

DRUGS, CLASSIFICATION OF

Although there are different methods that are used to classify drugs, the most common scheme groups drugs by their pharmacological similarity. However, this scheme does not work well for "club drugs," which are discussed as a separate classification. This entry describes, for each drug classification, the common drugs contained in the classification, some common street names, major effects, signs of intoxication, signs of overdose, tolerance, withdrawal, and acute and chronic effects. It should be noted that the term *drugs* includes both legal and illegal mood-altering substances.

Central Nervous System Depressants

Central nervous system (CNS) depressants (also referred to as sedative-hypnotics) depress the overall functioning of the CNS to induce sedation, drowsiness, and coma. The drugs in this classification include the most commonly used and abused psychoactive drug, alcohol; prescription drugs used for anxiety, sleep disturbance, and seizure control; and over-the-counter medications for sleep disturbance, colds and allergies, and coughs. In general, CNS depressants are extremely dangerous. According to the Centers for Disease Control, excessive alcohol consumption is the third-leading cause of preventable death in the United States. Alcohol in combination with other drugs accounted for about one third of drug abuse–related emergency room episodes in 2005.

Drugs in This Classification

Alcohol is the best-known CNS depressant because of its widespread use and legality. The alcohol content of beer is generally 3% to 6%; wine, 11% to 20%; liqueurs, 25% to 35%; and liquor (whiskey, gin, vodka, etc.), 40% to 50%. Barbiturates are prescription drugs used to aid sleep for insomniacs and for the control of seizures. These drugs include Seconal (*reds, red devils*), Nembutal (*yellows, yellow jackets*), Tuinal (*rainbows*), Amytal (*blues, blue heaven*), and phenobarbital. There are also nonbarbiturate sedative-hypnotics with similar effects but with different pharmacological properties. These include Doriden (*goofballs*), Quaalude (*ludes*), Miltown, and Equinil.

The development of benzodiazepines, or minor tranquilizers, reduced the number of prescriptions for barbiturates written by physicians. These drugs were initially seen as safe and having little abuse potential. Although the minor tranquilizers cannot be used easily in suicide as can barbiturates, the potential for

abuse is significant. The benzodiazepines are among the most widely prescribed drugs and include Valium, Librium, Dalmane, Halcion, Xanax, and Ativan.

Finally, certain over-the-counter medications contain depressant drugs. Sleep aids such as Nytol and Sominex, cold and allergy products, and cough medicines may contain scopolamine, antihistamines, or alcohol to produce the desired effects.

Major Effects

The effects of CNS depressants are related to the dose, method of administration, and tolerance of the individual. At low doses, these drugs produce a feeling of relaxation and calmness. They induce muscle relaxation, disinhibition, and a reduction in anxiety. Judgment and motor coordination are impaired, and there is a decrease in reflexes, pulse rate, and blood pressure. At high doses, the person demonstrates slurred speech, staggering, and, eventually, sleep. Phenobarbital and Valium have anticonvulsant properties and are used to control seizures. Benzodiazepines are also used to clinically control the effects from alcohol withdrawal.

Overdose

Alcohol overdose (being "drunk") is common. The symptoms include staggering, slurred speech, extreme disinhibition, and blackouts (an inability to recall events that occurred when the individual was intoxicated). Generally, the stomach goes into spasm, and the person will vomit, helping to eliminate alcohol from the body. However, the rapid ingestion of alcohol, particularly in a nontolerant individual, may result in coma and death. This happens most frequently with young people who participate in drinking contests.

As these drugs depress the central nervous system, overdose is extremely dangerous and can be fatal. Since the fatal dosage is only 10 to 15 times the therapeutic dosage, barbiturates are often used in suicides, which is one reason they are not frequently prescribed. It is far more difficult to overdose on the minor tranquilizers. However, CNS depressants have a synergistic or potentiation effect, meaning that the effect of a drug is enhanced as a result of the presence of another drug. For example, if a person has been drinking and then takes a minor tranquilizer such as Xanax, the effect of the Xanax may be dramatically enhanced. This combination has been the cause of many accidental deaths and emergency room visits.

Tolerance

There is a rapid development of tolerance to all CNS depressant drugs. Cross-tolerance also develops. This is one reason why overdose is such a problem. The tolerance that develops to the CNS depressants is also one reason that the use of the minor tranquilizers has become problematic. People are given prescriptions to alleviate symptoms such as anxiety and sleep disturbance that are the result of other problems such as marital discord. The minor tranquilizers temporarily relieve the symptoms, but the real problem is never addressed. The person continues to use the drug to alleviate the symptoms but tolerance develops and increasing dosages must be used to achieve the desired effect. This is a classic paradigm for the development of addiction, overdose, or both.

Withdrawal

The withdrawal syndrome from CNS depressants can be medically dangerous. These symptoms may include anxiety, irritability, loss of appetite, tremors, insomnia, and seizures. In the severe form of alcohol withdrawal, called delirium tremens (DTs), additional symptoms are fever, rapid heartbeat, and hallucinations. People can and do die from the withdrawal from these drugs. Therefore, the detoxification process for CNS depressants should include close supervision and the availability of medical personnel. Chronic, high-dosage users of these drugs should be discouraged from detoxifying without support and supervision. For detoxification in a medical setting, minor tranquilizers can be used, in decreasing dosages, to reduce the severity of the withdrawal symptoms.

Acute and Chronic Effects

In terms of damage to the human body and to society, alcohol is the most dangerous psychoactive drug (tobacco causes far more health damage). Alcohol has a damaging effect on every organ system. Chronic effects include permanent loss of memory, gastritis, esophagitis, ulcers, pancreatitis, cirrhosis of the liver, high blood pressure, weakened heart muscles, and damage to a fetus, including fetal alcohol syndrome. Other chronic effects include family, social, occupational, and financial problems. Acutely, alcohol is the cause of many traffic and other accidents and is involved in many acts of violence and crime. The yearly monetary cost to the United States attributable to alcohol is estimated to be more than $200 billion based on a report prepared for the National Institute on Alcohol Abuse and Alcoholism.

Certainly, the other CNS depressants can cause the same acute problems that are the result of injury and accident and chronic effects on the individual and family due to addiction.

Central Nervous System Stimulants

CNS stimulants affect the body in the opposite manner as do the CNS depressants. These drugs increase respiration, heart rate, motor activity, and alertness. This classification includes highly dangerous, illegal substances such as crack cocaine, medically useful stimulants such as Ritalin, drugs with relatively minor psychoactive effects such as caffeine, and the most deadly drug used, nicotine. Cocaine was mentioned in 55% of the drug abuse–related emergency room episodes.

Drugs in This Classification

Cocaine (*coke, blow, toot, snow*) and the freebase or smokeable forms of cocaine (*crack, rock, base*) are the most infamous of the CNS stimulants. Cocaine is found in the leaves of the coca shrub that grows in Central America and South America. The leaves are processed and produce coca paste. The paste, in turn, is processed to form the white hydrochloride salt powder most people know as cocaine. Of course, before it is sold on the street, it is adulterated or "cut" with substances such as powdered sugar, talc, arsenic, lidocaine, strychnine, or methamphetamine. Crack is produced by mixing the cocaine powder with baking soda and water and heating the solution. The paste that forms is hardened and cut into hard pieces or rocks. The mixing and heating process removes most of the impurities from the cocaine. The vaporization point is lowered so the cocaine can be smoked, reaching the brain in one heartbeat less than if it is injected. Therefore, crack is a more pure form of cocaine than is cocaine hydrochloride salt powder.

Amphetamines are also CNS stimulants, and one form in particular, methamphetamine, is a major drug of addiction. The amphetamines include Benzedrine (*crosstops, black beauties*), Methedrine or methamphetamine (*crank, meth, crystal*), and Dexedrine (*dexies*). There are also nonamphetamine stimulants with similar properties such as Ritalin and Cylert (used in the treatment of attention deficit hyperactivity disorder) and Preludin (used in the treatment of obesity). These drugs are synthetics (not naturally occurring), and the amphetamines were widely prescribed in the 1950s and 1960s for weight control.

Some forms of CNS stimulants are available without a prescription and are contained in many substances used on a regular basis. Caffeine is found in coffee, teas, colas, and chocolate, as well as in some over-the-counter products designed to help people stay awake (e.g., NoDoz, Alert, Vivarin). Phenylpropanolamine is a stimulant found in diet-control products sold over the counter (e.g., Dexatrim). These products are abused by individuals who chronically diet (e.g., individuals with anorexia).

Although it has mild euphoric properties, nicotine is the highly addictive stimulant drug found in tobacco products. According to the Centers for Disease Control and Prevention, an estimated 440,000 Americans die each year from smoking-related illnesses.

Major Effects

The uses of CNS stimulants have an interesting history. As many people know, Sigmund Freud wrote "Uber Coca," which described the use of cocaine to treat a number of medical problems. Originally, Coca-Cola contained cocaine. In the 1980s, cocaine was depicted in the popular press as a relatively harmless drug. Amphetamines were used in World War II to combat fatigue and were issued by the U.S. Armed Forces during the Korean War. These drugs have a long history of use by long-distance truck drivers, students cramming for exams, and women trying to lose weight.

As with most of the psychoactive drugs, some of the CNS stimulants (cocaine and amphetamines) have a recreational use. The purpose is to "get high," or to experience a sense of euphoria. Amphetamine and cocaine users report a feeling of self-confidence and self-assurance. There is a "rush" that is experienced, particularly when cocaine is smoked and when cocaine and methamphetamine are injected. The high from amphetamines is generally less intense but longer acting than the high from cocaine.

CNS stimulants result in psychomotor stimulation, alertness, and elevation of mood. There is an increase in heart rate and blood pressure. Performance may be enhanced with increased activity level, one reason why athletes use CNS stimulants. These drugs also suppress appetite and combat fatigue.

Overdose

CNS stimulants activate the reward center of the brain. The most powerful of these drugs result in the body's not experiencing hunger, thirst, or fatigue. There is no built-in satiation point, so humans can continue using cocaine and amphetamines until there are no more or they die. Therefore, the compulsion to use, the desire to maintain the high, and the unpleasantness of withdrawal make overdose fairly common. There may be tremors, sweating and flushing, rapid heartbeat (tachycardia), anxiety, insomnia, paranoia, convulsions, heart attack, or stroke. Death from overdose has been widely publicized because it has occurred with some famous movie stars, musicians, and athletes. However, far more people experience chronic problems from CNS stimulant addictions than from overdose reactions.

Tolerance

There is a rapid tolerance to the pleasurable effects of cocaine and amphetamines and the stimulating effects of tobacco and caffeine. If you drink five or six cups a day of combinations of coffee, tea, and colas, you probably know this with regard to caffeine. You will find that if you stop using caffeine for a couple of weeks and then start again, the initial doses of caffeine produce a minor "buzz," alertness, or restlessness.

The rapid tolerance to the euphoric effects of cocaine and amphetamines leads to major problems with these drugs. The pleasurable effects are so rewarding, particularly when the drugs are smoked or injected, that the user is prone to compulsively use in an effort to recapture the euphoric effects. When injected or smoked, the effects are enhanced but of relatively short duration. Continual use to achieve the high leads to rapid tolerance. The user is then unable to feel the pleasure but must continue to use the drug to reduce the pain of withdrawal.

A sensitization or reverse tolerance can occur, particularly with cocaine. In this instance, a chronic user with a high tolerance has an adverse reaction (i.e., seizure) to a low dose.

Withdrawal

Unlike the withdrawal from CNS depressants, the withdrawal from CNS stimulants is not medically dangerous. However, it is extremely unpleasant. The withdrawal from cocaine and amphetamines is called "crashing." The severe symptoms usually last 2 to 3 days and include intense drug craving, irritability, depression, anxiety, and lethargy. However, the depression, drug craving, and an inability to experience pleasure may last for several months as the body chemistry returns to normal. Suicidal ideation and attempts are frequent during this time, as are relapses. Recovering cocaine and amphetamine addicts can become very discouraged with the slow rate of the lifting of depression; therefore, support is very important during this time.

Acute and Chronic Effects

As previously stated, the acute effects of CNS stimulants can be dramatic and fatal. These effects include heart attacks, strokes, seizures, and respiratory depression. However, the results of chronic use cause the most problems. The addictive properties of these drugs are extremely high. Individuals with addictions to cocaine and amphetamines spend a tremendous amount of money to obtain drugs, and they encounter serious life problems related to their addiction. Also, there is an increased risk of strokes and cardiovascular problems, depression, and suicide in chronic users. Symptoms of paranoid schizophrenia can occur. If cocaine or amphetamines are snorted, perforation of the nasal septum can occur. Injection of CNS stimulants has the same risks (e.g., hepatitis, AIDS) as injecting other drugs. Because these drugs suppress appetite, chronic users are frequently malnourished.

Opioids

The opioids are naturally occurring (opium poppy extracts) and synthetic drugs that are commonly used for their analgesic (pain relief) and cough-suppressing properties. Opium was used by early Egyptian, Greek, and Arabic cultures for the treatment of diarrhea because of its constipating effect. Greek and Roman writers such as Homer and Virgil wrote of the sleep-inducing properties of opium, and recreational use of the drug in these cultures did occur. Morphine was isolated from opium in the early 1800s and was widely available without prescription until the early 1900s when the nonmedical use of opioids was banned. Opioids accounted for 20% of drug abuse–related emergency room episodes in 2005.

Drugs in This Classification

The opioids include opium, codeine, morphine, heroin (*smack, horse*), Vicodin, Dilaudid, OxyContin, Percodan, methadone, Darvon, Demerol, Talwin, buprenorphine, and levo-alpha acetyl methadol ([LAAM] long-acting methadone).

Major Effects

Opioids have medically useful effects including pain relief, cough suppression, and constipation. Obviously, there is also a euphoric effect that accounts for the recreational use of these drugs. They can produce nausea and vomiting and itching. A sedating effect occurs, and the pupils of the eyes become constricted.

Methadone, or Dolophine, is a synthetic opioid that does not have the dramatic euphoric effects of heroin, has a longer duration of action (12 to 24 hours compared with 3 to 6 hours for heroin), and blocks the symptoms of withdrawal when heroin is discontinued. This is the reason for the use of methadone in the treatment of opioid addiction. The action of LAAM has an even longer duration. Buprenorphine is now being prescribed in an office setting to treat opioid dependence.

Overdose

Death from overdose of injectable opioids (usually heroin) can occur from the direct action of the drug on the brain, resulting in respiratory depression. Death can also occur from an allergic reaction to the drug or to substances used to cut it, possibly resulting in cardiac arrest. Overdose of other drugs in this classification may include symptoms such as slow breathing rate and decreased blood pressure, pulse rate, temperature, and reflexes. The person may become extremely drowsy and lose consciousness. There may be flushing and itching skin, abdominal pain, and nausea and vomiting.

Tolerance

Frequency of administration and dosage of opioids is related to the development of tolerance. Tolerance develops rapidly when the drugs are repeatedly administered but does not develop when there are prolonged periods of abstinence. The tolerance that does develop is to the euphoric, sedative, analgesic, and respiratory effects of the drugs. This tolerance results in the individual's using doses that would kill a nontolerant person. The tolerant individual becomes accustomed to using high doses, which accounts for death due to overdose in longtime opioid users who have been detoxified and then go back to using.

Cross-tolerance to natural and synthetic opioids does occur. However, there is no cross-tolerance to CNS depressants. This fact is important, because the combination of moderate to high doses of opioids and alcohol or other CNS depressants can (and often does) result in respiratory depression and death.

Withdrawal

When these drugs are used on a continuous basis, there is a rapid development of physical dependence. Withdrawal symptoms are unpleasant and uncomfortable but rarely dangerous. The symptoms are analogous to a severe case of the flu, with running eyes and nose, restlessness, goose bumps, sweating, muscle cramps or aching, nausea, vomiting, and diarrhea. There is significant drug craving. These symptoms rapidly dissipate when opioids are taken, which accounts for relapse when a person abruptly quits on his or her own ("cold turkey"). When the drugs are not available to the dependent individual, the unpleasant withdrawal symptoms also result in participation in criminal activities in order to purchase the drugs.

Acute and Chronic Effects

There is an acute danger of death from overdose from injecting opioids, particularly heroin. Also, the euphoric effects of opioids rapidly decrease as tolerance increases, and as this tolerance occurs, the opioid use is primarily to ward off the withdrawal symptoms.

Compared with the chronic use of CNS depressants, chronic use of opioids is less dangerous to the body. However, the route of administration and the lifestyle associated with chronic opioid use clearly has serious consequences. Obviously, there is the risk of communicable disease from the intravenous use of opioids and sharing needles. The lifestyle of heroin addicts often includes criminal activity to secure enough money to purchase heroin. Women may participate in prostitution, which adds the associated risks of diseases and violence. Nutrition is frequently neglected. However, those individuals who have been

involved in methadone maintenance programs for long periods do not experience negative health consequences from the use of methadone (which is taken orally).

Hallucinogens

Many of the hallucinogens are naturally occurring and have been used for thousands of years. Some have been (and are currently) used as sacraments in religious rites and have been ascribed with mystical and magical properties. Today, many types of hallucinogens are synthetically produced in laboratories. Some of the hallucinogens became very popular in the 1960s and 1970s, with a drop in use in the 1980s. While there was a resurgence of use from 1992 to 2001 among youth, recent surveys have shown the lowest use of hallucinogens since the surveys were started in 1975.

Drugs in This Classification

This classification comprises a group of heterogeneous compounds. Although there may be some commonality in terms of effect, the chemical structures are quite different. The hallucinogens include LSD (acid, fry), psilocybin (magic mushrooms, shrooms), morning glory seeds (heavenly blue), mescaline (mesc, big chief, peyote), STP (serenity, tranquility, peace), and PCP (angel dust, hog). PCP is used as a veterinary anesthetic, primarily for primates.

Major Effects

These drugs produce an altered state of consciousness, including altered perceptions of visual, auditory, olfactory, and/or tactile senses and an increased awareness of inner thoughts and impulses. Sensory experiences may cross into one another (e.g., hearing color). Common sights and sounds may be perceived as exceptionally intricate and astounding. In the case of PCP, there may be increased suggestibility, delusions, and depersonalization and dissociation. Physiologically, hallucinogens produce a rise in pulse and blood pressure.

Overdose

With the exception of PCP, the concept of "overdose" is not applicable to the hallucinogens. "Bad trips" or panic reactions occur and may include paranoid ideation, depression, undesirable hallucinations, and/or confusion; these effects usually are managed by providing a calm and supportive environment. An overdose of PCP may result in acute intoxication, acute psychosis, or coma. In acute intoxication or psychosis, the person may be agitated, confused, and excited and may exhibit a blank stare and violent behavior. Analgesia (insensibility to pain) occurs, which may result in self-inflicted injuries and injuries to others when attempts are made to restrain the individual.

Tolerance

Tolerance to the hallucinogenic properties of these drugs occurs, as well as cross-tolerance between LSD and other hallucinogens. No cross-tolerance to cannabis has been demonstrated. Tolerance to PCP has not been demonstrated in humans.

Withdrawal

There is no physical dependence that occurs from the use of hallucinogens, although psychological dependence, including drug craving, does occur.

Acute and Chronic Effects

A fairly common and well-publicized adverse effect of hallucinogens is the experience of flashbacks. Flashbacks are the recurrence of the effects of hallucinogens long after the drug has been taken. Reports of flashbacks more than 5 years after taking a hallucinogen have been reported, although abatement after several months is more common.

With regard to LSD, there are acute physical effects, including a rise in heart rate and blood pressure, higher body temperature, dizziness, and dilated pupils. Mental effects include sensory distortions, dreaminess, depersonalization, altered mood, and impaired concentration. "Bad trips" involve acute anxiety, paranoia, fear of loss of control, and delusions. Individuals with preexisting mental disorders may experience more severe symptoms. With regard to chronic effects, the rare but frightening experience of flashbacks may occur. PCP use results in significant adverse effects. Chronic use may result in psychiatric problems, including depression, anxiety, and paranoid psychosis. Accidents, injuries, and violence occur frequently.

Cannabinols

Marijuana is the most widely used illegal drug. Nearly 17% of adults in the 18- to 25-year range reported using marijuana in the previous month. The earliest references to the drug date back to 2700 BC. In the 1700s, the hemp plant (*Cannabis sativa*) was grown in the colonies for its fiber, which was used in rope. Beginning in 1926, states began to outlaw the use of marijuana because it was claimed to cause criminal behavior and violence. Marijuana use became popular with mainstream young people in the 1960s. Some states have basically decriminalized possession of small amounts of marijuana although, according to the federal government, it remains a Schedule I drug. However, emergency room episodes in which marijuana was mentioned constituted 30% of the total drug abuse–related emergency room visits in 2005.

Drugs in This Classification

The various cannabinols include marijuana (*grass, pot, weed, joint, reefer, dube*), hashish, charas, bhang, ganja, and sinsemilla. The active ingredient is delta-9-tetrahydrocannabinol (THC). Hashish and charas have a THC content of 7% to 14%; ganja and sinsemilla, 4% to 7%; and bhang and marijuana, 2% to 5%. However, recent improvements in growing processes have increased the THC content of marijuana sold on the street. For simplicity, the various forms of cannabinols will be referred to as "marijuana."

Major Effects

Marijuana users experience euphoria; enhancement of taste, touch, and smell; relaxation; increased appetite; altered time sense; and impaired immediate recall. An enhanced perception of the humor of situations or events may occur. The physiological effects of marijuana include increase in pulse rate and blood pressure, dilation of blood vessels in the cornea (which produces bloodshot eyes), and dry mouth. Motor skills and reaction time are slowed. Marijuana may be medically useful in reducing nausea and vomiting from chemotherapy, stimulating appetite in AIDS and other wasting-syndrome patients, treating spasticity and nocturnal spasms complicating multiple sclerosis and spinal cord injury, controlling seizures, and managing neuropathic pain. However, further clinical studies are necessary to reach conclusions on the value of marijuana in medical treatment.

Overdose

Overdose is unusual because the normal effects of marijuana are not enhanced by large doses. Intensification of emotional responses and mild hallucinations can occur, and the user may feel "out of control." As with hallucinogens, many reports of overdose are panic reactions to the normal effects of the drug. In individuals with preexisting mental disorders (e.g., schizophrenia), high doses of marijuana may exacerbate symptoms such as delusions, hallucinations, disorientation, and depersonalization.

Tolerance

Tolerance is a controversial area with regard to marijuana. The difference of opinion as to whether tolerance develops slowly or quickly may be due to type of subject studied and various definitions of "dosage." For example, tolerance rapidly occurs in animals but only with frequent use of high doses in humans. At the least, chronic users probably become accustomed to the effects of the drug and are experienced in administering the proper dosage to produce the desired effects. Cross-tolerance to CNS depressants, including alcohol, has been demonstrated.

Withdrawal

A withdrawal syndrome can be observed in chronic, high-dosage users who abruptly discontinue their use. The symptoms include irritability, restlessness, decreased appetite, insomnia, tremor, chills, and increased body temperature. The symptoms usually last 3 to 5 days.

Acute and Chronic Effects

Marijuana has been and continues to be controversial. Ballot measures in several states have involved marijuana laws. This controversy is related to the facts and myths regarding marijuana's acute and chronic effects. The professional community has as many views of the "facts" regarding marijuana as does the general public. However, marijuana should clearly not be a Schedule I drug, although no psychoactive drug is safe. Marijuana can and does result in significant life problems for many people.

If death is the measure of dangerousness, marijuana is not acutely or chronically dangerous. However, the effect on motor skills and reaction time certainly impairs the user's ability to drive a car, boat, plane, or other vehicle, and marijuana use has also been detected in a significant number of victims of vehicular and nonvehicular accidents.

Chronic use of marijuana does seem to have an adverse effect on lung function, although there is no direct evidence that it causes lung cancer. Although an increase in heart rate occurs, there does not seem to be an adverse effect on the heart. As is the case with CNS depressants, marijuana suppresses the immune system. Chronic marijuana use decreases the male hormone testosterone (as does alcohol) and adversely affects sperm formation. However, no effect on male fertility or sexual potency has been noted. Female hormones are also reduced, and impairment in ovulation has been reported.

Inhalants and Volatile Hydrocarbons

Inhalants and volatile hydrocarbons consist largely of chemicals that can be legally purchased and that are normally used for nonrecreational purposes. In addition, this classification includes some drugs that are used legally for medical purposes. As psychoactive drugs, most of these substances are used mainly by young people, particularly in low socioeconomic areas. Because most of these chemicals are accessible in homes and are readily available for purchase, they are easily used as psychoactive drugs by young people who are beginning drug experimentation and by individuals who are unable to purchase other mind-altering substances due to finances or availability.

Drugs in This Classification

The industrial solvents and aerosol sprays that are used for psychoactive purposes include gasoline, kerosene, chloroform, airplane glue, lacquer thinner, acetone, nail polish remover, model cement, lighter fluid, carbon tetrachloride, fluoride-based sprays, and metallic paints. Volatile nitrites are amyl nitrite (*poppers*), butyl, and isobutyl (*locker room, rush, bolt, quick silver, zoom*). Amyl nitrite has typically been used in the gay community. In addition, nitrous oxide ("laughing gas"), a substance used by dentists, is also included in this classification.

Major Effects

The solvents and sprays reduce inhibition and produce euphoria, dizziness, slurred speech, an unsteady gait, and drowsiness. Nystagmus (constant involuntary movements of the eyes) may be noted. The nitrites alter consciousness and enhance sexual pleasure. The user may experience giddiness, headaches, and dizziness. Nitrous oxide produces giddiness, a buzzing or ringing in the ears, and a sense that the user is about to pass out.

Overdose

Overdose of these substances may produce hallucinations, muscle spasms, headaches, dizziness, loss of balance, irregular heartbeat, and coma from lack of oxygen.

Tolerance

Tolerance does develop to nitrous oxide but does not seem to develop to the other inhalants.

Withdrawal

There does not appear to be a withdrawal syndrome associated with these substances.

Acute and Chronic Effects

The most critical acute effect of inhalants is a factor of the method of administration, which can result in loss of consciousness, coma, or death from lack of oxygen. Respiratory arrest, cardiac arrhythmia, or asphyxiation may occur. Many of these substances are highly toxic, and chronic use may cause damage to the liver, kidneys, brain, and lungs.

Club Drugs

Rather than sharing pharmacological similarities, the drugs discussed in this section are grouped together because of the environment in which they are commonly used. The use of these drugs is primarily by youth and young adults associated with dance clubs, bars, and all-night dance parties ("raves").

It would not make sense to discuss the common characteristics of overdose, tolerance, withdrawal, and acute and chronic effects because these drugs are not related pharmacologically. However, it is important to reference these drugs as a separate class because of the wide media coverage of club drugs. The most appropriate pharmacological classification for each drug is referenced.

Rohypnol (*roofies*) is a benzodiazepine (CNS depressant) that is illegal in the United States but widely prescribed in Europe as a sleeping pill. When used in combination with alcohol, Rohypnol produces disinhibition and amnesia. Rohypnol has become known as the "date rape" drug because of reported instances in which women have been unknowingly given the drug while drinking. When women are sexually assaulted, they cannot easily remember the events surrounding the incident.

MDMA (ecstasy) has the properties of the CNS stimulants and hallucinogens. It is taken in tablet form primarily but can also be found in powder and liquid forms. It is relatively inexpensive and long lasting. The euphoric effects include rushes of exhilaration and the sensation of understanding and accepting others. Some people experience nausea, and depression may be experienced following use. Deaths have been reported from ecstasy use primarily as a result of severe dehydration from dancing for long periods without drinking water. Ecstasy can be used compulsively and become psychologically addictive.

Ketamine (*K* or *special K*) is generally considered to be a hallucinogen. It is used as a veterinary anesthetic and is usually cooked from its liquid form into a white powder and snorted. The euphoric effect of ketamine involves dissociative anesthetics or separating perception from sensation. Users report feeling "floaty" or outside their body. Higher doses expand this experience. They may have some numbness in extremities. Ketamine is very dangerous in combination with depressants, as higher doses depress respiration and breathing. Frequent use may lead to mental disorders due to the hallucinogenic properties of the drug. Psychological dependence also occurs in frequent users.

GHB (gamma hydroxybutyrate) is actually a synthetic steroid originally sold over the counter in health food stores as a bodybuilding aid. GHB is usually sold as an odorless liquid that has a slight salty taste. The effects are similar to those of CNS depressants, with low doses resulting in euphoria, relaxation, and happiness. However, higher doses can cause dizziness, drowsiness, vomiting, muscle spasms, and loss of consciousness. Overdoses can result in coma or death, as can mixing GHB with other CNS depressants such as alcohol. Physical dependence can occur.

Other drugs, such as LSD, PCP, mescaline, and marijuana are sometimes classified as club drugs. However, because these drugs have a wider use, they were discussed in other drug classifications.

Gary L. Fisher

See also Central Nervous System Depressants; Central Nervous System Stimulants; Club Drugs; Hallucinogens; Inhalants; Marijuana; Opioids

Further Readings

Abadinsky, H. (2007). *Drug abuse: An introduction* (6th ed.). Chicago: Nelson-Hall.

Centers for Disease Control. (2004). Alcohol-attributable deaths and years of potential life lost—United States, 2001. *Morbidity and Mortality Weekly Report, 53,* 866–870. Retrieved June 2, 2008 from http://www.cdc .gov/MMWR/ preview/mmwrhtml/mm5337a2.htm

Hanson, G., Venturelli, P. J., & Fleckenstein, A. E. (2006). *Drugs and society* (9th ed.). Boston: Jones & Bartlett.

Harwood, H. (2000). *Updating estimates of the economic costs of alcohol abuse in the United States: Estimates, update, methods, and data. National Institute on Alcohol Abuse and Alcoholism.* Retrieved June 2, 2008, from http://pubs.niaaa.nih.gov/publications/economic-2000/ alcoholcost.PDF

Inaba, D. S., & Cohen, W. E. (2000). *Uppers, downers, all arounders* (4th ed.). Ashland, OR: Cinemed.

Inciardi, J. A., & McElrath, K. (2007). *The American drug scene: An anthology* (5th ed.). Los Angeles: Roxbury.

Julien, R. M. (2005). *A primer of drug action: A concise, nontechnical guide to the actions, uses, and side effects of psychoactive drugs* (10th ed.). New York: W. H. Freeman.

Schuckit, M. A. (1998). *Educating yourself about alcohol and drugs: A people's primer.* New York: Plenum Press.

DRUG TESTING

Drug testing occurs in a wide variety of settings across the United States, including workplaces, the military, schools, treatment programs, and the criminal justice system. This includes both public and private settings in the United States. Large numbers of individuals are tested every year, such as drug addicts in treatment, individuals on parole, employees in a variety of industries, and students involved in an extracurricular activity in school. Drug testing that occurs in schools and workplaces across the United States is widely debated. Federal drug testing rules authorize testing for the following five types of drugs: marijuana, opioids, cocaine, amphetamine and methamphetamine, and PCP. This list does not include club drugs such as ecstasy. Furthermore, there is no current standard testing procedure that can detect inhalant usage, which is popular among adolescents. There are five types of drug testing currently in practice in the United States: urine testing, hair testing, blood testing, sweat testing, and oral fluid testing.

Urine testing is the most common form of drug testing in practice in schools and in the workplace. It is the least expensive, most widely used, and most accepted form of testing in the United States. The biggest concern about urine testing is the potential for adulterated or substituted samples. Urine testing has a 1- to 5-day window of detection. Urine testing is a fairly cost-effective form of testing, with an individual test costing under $50.

Hair testing is frequent in some industries, such as the gambling industry. It has a longer period of detection but is generally less accurate due to hair treatments and environmental effects. Hair testing can also measure chronic drug use and can detect combination use of alcohol and cocaine. The biggest concerns about hair testing are that it is more expensive than other forms of testing, and it does not have the capability of testing recent drug use. The window of detection for hair testing varies depending on the length of hair, but hair testing does have the longest window of detection of all types of testing, as 1½ inches of hair shows approximately a 3-month usage history.

Blood testing is commonly used in drug overdose cases and in hospitals during postaccident investigations. Almost all drugs can be detected through blood testing, although it is extremely difficult to detect marijuana usage through this method.

Sweat is tested through the use of a waterproof adhesive pad and can be used to test a number of substances, including cocaine, morphine, methamphetamine, heroin, PCP, and marijuana. Sweat patch testing also has a longer period of detection than does urine testing. There are several concerns with this type of testing, however, including the fact that individuals with skin conditions and those with excessive hair cannot wear the patch. Furthermore, passive exposure to drugs can affect the results by contaminating the patch. The patch can detect drug use for up to 7 days.

Oral fluid tests are done by swabbing saliva from the inside of the cheek, which can show usage of amphetamine, barbiturates, cocaine, marijuana, opioids, and PCP. It is more efficient than urine testing for recent use but is not very effective past a window of 3 days. There is a minimal risk of tampering with oral fluid testing samples; however, oral fluid testing is less efficient in detecting marijuana usage than some other forms of testing. Oral fluid testing has only a 10- to 24-hour window of detection.

Drug Testing in the Workplace

Workplace drug testing is commonplace in the United States, as many employers have some form of testing policy in place. Starting in the late 1980s, employers began to recognize a need for drug testing in the workplace due to a concern of employee intoxication, reliability, and drug-seeking behavior. From an employer point of view, drug use results in the following problems: safety hazards, chronic health problems, increased absenteeism, job turnover, reduced productivity, decreased learning ability, and security issues. As a result of these safety and productivity concerns, President Ronald Reagan signed an executive order on September 15, 1986, requiring federal agencies to establish an employee drug-testing program. As per this order, a comprehensive drug testing program was developed by the Department of Transportation and the U.S. Coast Guard. The Drug-Free Workplace Act of 1988 mandated that all federal contractors with a contract of $25,000 or more to have programs for a drug-free workplace. In the 1990s, drug testing in the workplace became more and more common. Publicizing the need for drug testing in the workplace, the National Survey on Drug Use and Health found that there were 6.3 million illicit drug users among the 81.8 million people in the U.S. workforce.

With regard to additional legislation concerning drug abuse, past drug addiction is considered a disability under the Americans with Disabilities Act. As a result of this, employers cannot ask about former drug use prior to employment. Employers are, however, allowed to ask about, and test for, current use. This serves as a protective factor for employees, as it protects their privacy and any previous usage or addiction history. This can also be viewed as a protective factor ensuring that employees are not discriminated against based on previous history with experimentation, recreational drug use, or even drug addiction.

With regard to the practice of testing in the workplace, there are generally six types of drug testing. These include preemployment tests, reasonable suspicion tests, postaccident tests, random tests, return-to-duty tests, and follow-up tests. Preemployment tests are given while an applicant is being considered for employment; reasonable suspicion tests follow a supervisor observing actions or behaviors causing a reasonable suspicion of drug use; postaccident tests are conducted after an accident in the workplace; random drug tests occur without warning; return-to-duty tests are given after a previous positive test and before the employee is allowed to return to work; and follow-up tests are conducted subsequent to a return-to-duty test. Follow-up tests are frequently unannounced. Perhaps one of the most common forms of testing that occurs in the workplace is random testing, which supporters argue deters employees from usage as they may be tested at any point in time during employment.

Drug Testing in Schools

Drug testing in schools is a controversial subject in this area. This debate was fueled in June 2002 when, in a 5-to-4 decision concerning the case of the *Board of Education of Independent School District No. 92 of Pottawatomie County et al. v. Earls et al.,* the Supreme Court ruled that random drug testing for all middle and high school students participating in extracurricular activities is allowable. Prior to this decision, only student athletes could be tested. There remains a serious debate as to the appropriateness of drug testing students in the United States. Supporters argue that students who use drugs do not perform as well academically as other students. Drug testing deters drug use among students and provides them with a reason to say no to drugs. This could result in improved academic performance and a reduction in school dropouts. Critics, however, argue that drug testing is not effective in deterring use among adolescents. Furthermore, drug testing may actually drive students away from participating in extracurricular activities, which have shown to serve as a protective factor in keeping adolescents away from drugs and criminal activity. Critics are also concerned that drug testing may lead to unintended consequences, such as encouraging adolescents to use substances that are harder to detect such as alcohol, inhalants, and ecstasy.

While it is clear that there are reasonable arguments to both sides of this debate, it remains up to local communities to determine if there is a need for testing in the schools. Furthermore, it remains the responsibility of these communities to determine what specific substances present a problem for that area, as well as what type of testing program, if any, will be implemented in the school district. Also, who is tested may vary among school districts. For example, some school districts only test student athletes during the athletic season for that sport. Others test students who participate in extracurricular activities including sports, band, choir, theater, and other clubs and activities at that school. There are also a number of schools that have implemented drug testing programs in the past but have discontinued these programs as a result of change in perceived need, cost-effectiveness, or other reasons. For the most part, schools that have testing programs in place typically have a system in which students who test positive receive a subsequent test to ensure reliability. These students usually receive sanctions such as suspension from the sport or activity for a time. Parents are also notified, and schools generally refer these students and families to treatment resources.

Tampering of Testing Results

Specimen tampering is a major concern for drug testing in any setting. Tampering with urine specimens is the most common and easiest form of tampering, as there are many ways of attempting to conceal drug usage on the test. These methods include diluting urine by drinking excess amounts of water, drinking products designed to dilute urine, placing products in the urine sample in attempt to disguise usage, and substituting urine samples by buying "clean urine" or having a drug-free friend provide a sample. The problem is so widespread today that a simple Google search on the topic produces over 3 million results on products designed to cover up drug usage to pass a urine test. Tampering with the urine sample is generally suspected when the urine sample is outside of the permissible temperature range (within one degree of body temperature), the individual is observed substituting the urine specimen or using a product to disguise drug usage in the specimen, the specimen is diluted (either through excess water or other products designed to dilute urine), or when the laboratory cannot analyze the sample due to contamination through one of these available products or some other

source. While these products rarely work to disguise drug usage, they are still frequently used by individuals trying to disguise their usage to pass a test. Furthermore, even if the product is successful in disguising the drug in the urine sample, the product itself is easily detected in the laboratory. As a result of the concern over these products, however, four states (Texas, Nebraska, Pennsylvania, and South Carolina) have prohibited the sale or possession of these products.

False Positives

Among critics of drug testing, there is a strong concern about false positives. Individuals may test positive on a drug test not because of illicit drug use but because of legal use of different types of medicines. Among the many medicines that may result in a false positive, some of the most commonly used are Tylenol with codeine, Vicks inhaler, Adderall, and Robitussin. Subsequent follow-up tests to the initial positive test are generally able to detect whether the positive test was the result of illicit drug use or the result of the legal use of one of these types of medications.

Conclusion

While drug testing in the United States continues to remain a controversial issue, it has become increasingly popular in both school systems and workplaces throughout the country. As the number of individuals in prisons and jails across the nation as a result of drugs continues to rise, it is easy to anticipate that the popularity of testing will continue to grow. Further, as the number of lawsuits in the country increases, employer liability has resulted in increased interest in the testing of employees. Some argue that drug testing serves as a deterrent, but the number of young people who continue to use drugs regardless of the testing practices in their schools and the number of individuals (both children in schools and adults in the workplace) who use strategies to attempt to "fool" the test is particularly disturbing. Because drug testing can be costly for school districts and employers and because drug testing raises important civil liberty issues, it is important to gather accurate data on the effectiveness of drug testing in reducing drug use and in increasing productivity in school and workplace settings.

Sherry Lynn Skaggs

See also Employee Assistance Program; School Drug Policies; Student Assistance Program; Urine Toxicology Testing; Workplace Drug Policies; Workplace Drug Use; Workplace Prevention

Further Readings

Gahlinger, P. M. (2001). *Illegal drugs: A complete guide to their history, chemistry, use and abuse.* Salt Lake City, UT: Sagebrush Press.

Goldberg, R. (2006). *Taking sides: Clashing views in drugs and society* (7th ed.). Dubuque, IA: McGraw-Hill.

Lundman, R. J. (2001). *Prevention and control of juvenile delinquency* (3rd ed.). New York: Oxford University Press.

Office of National Drug Control Policy. (2006). *What you need to know about drug testing in schools.* Retrieved September 10, 2007, from http://www.whitehouse drugpolicy.gov/publications/drug_testing/index.html

Office of National Drug Control Policy. (2006). *What you need to know about starting a student drug-testing program.* Retrieved September 10, 2007, from http://www.whitehousedrugpolicy.gov/publications/student_drug_testing

Drug Use, History of

Certainly one, among many things, at which humans consistently excel is the willingness and desire to alter our consciousness and augment our sensory experiences. The vehicle for humans from prehistoric time to current day is the use of drugs to quickly accomplish this goal (although there are a host of nondrug practices to equally alter consciousness, such as meditation). The large majority of humanity does not suffer from drug addiction; yet, members of every human culture (from Aboriginal to Indian, Chinese, Egyptian, South American, Aleuts, Chukchi, and Eskimo) use psychoactive drugs on a daily basis for a variety of reasons (i.e., pain relief, religious, vision seeking, consciousness expansion, entertainment, as a food source, healing disease, and even seeking immortality).

Historically, the vast majority of drugs used by humans were hallucinogens, and few were central nervous system stimulants or depressants. A mere 300 years ago, plants and fungi were the major sources of psychoactive chemicals, as humans had not yet become clever enough to reproduce complex synthesis routes that plants accomplish with only water, earth, and sunlight. There are over 800,000 species of plants living today; a small fraction of these species (about 4,000) are the best producers of psychoactive substances on the planet, and they were most convenient for human discovery and use.

Why Plants and Fungi Produce Psychoactive Substances

One theory about the purpose underlying the variety of psychoactive chemicals synthesized by plants is believed to be as a chemical defense against organisms that would consume them. Eating a plant or fungus containing psychoactives would disrupt the central nervous system of the animal via stimulant (organism becomes hyperactive, or anorectic and ceases eating the plant) or depressant (organism becomes sleepy and eating ceases). If additional plant substance continued to be consumed, the dose could rise to lethal levels in the case of stimulant and depressant plant substances. Plants and fungi producing hallucinogens (the main effect is to disrupt sensory systems) and eaten by mammals would most likely result in an aversive event for the mammal. Again, the organism would discontinue eating.

According to Ronald K. Siegal, practically all animals consume plants and fungi that contain psychoactive substances. Humans could have watched animals eat plants with psychoactive properties and imitated them to develop drug use patterns in neolithic ages. Elephants, koalas, goats, cows, cats, reindeer, rabbits, mice, and birds, respectively, eat fermented fruit (alcohol), eucalyptus leaves, caffeine, locoweed, catnip, mushrooms, belladonna in wild lettuce, and hempseed. An interesting observation is that animals do not seem to prefer the effects of hallucinogens (as demonstrated by drug self-administration research studies). Only humans are known to regularly consume hallucinogens voluntarily and for entertainment purposes.

Drugs of Abuse: Ancient Use History

The study of drug use in humans before the common era (BC) overlaps several areas of study and can include ethnobotony, archeopharmacology, ethnopharmacology, and the history of drug use with regard to tracing prehistoric, neolithic medicinal and religious plant use in humans. Note that the "factual" dating of evidence in excess of 300 years prior to the common era is considered imprecise and, in many instances, are simply good guesses based on some empirical evidence (i.e., radiocarbon dating, uncovering burial remains, chemical analyses of residue for pottery). For instance, among the oldest reports of evidence in the family *Hominidae* is archeological evidence of *H. neanderthalensis* burial sites in Iraq from 50,000 years ago. Examination of plant remains reveals the presence of the natural stimulant herbal ephedra. This evidence seems to support the conclusion that Neanderthals used psychoactive drugs. However, the oldest drugs used by humans, that today are considered drugs of abuse, include depressants, stimulants, and hallucinogens.

Depressants

Prehistoric drugs, now classified as drugs of abuse, include the oldest drug used by humans, alcohol. Alcohol was probably consumed as long ago as 10,000 BC (cave drawings suggest its consumption), and its original name was *aqua vitae* (translated water of life). The word is derived from the Arabic word *alkohl* meaning, "subtly divided spirit." The first instance of human intoxication was probably when a cave person knelt down and drank the remains of yeast-fermented fruit resting in a pool of liquid on the rock floor. Archaeological evidence suggests humans consumed berry wine in about 6400 BC. Wine was considered a medicine; it was also the fluid in which most herbal remedies were dissolved. Ancient Egyptian medical preparations commonly included foods (onions, figs, garlic, anise, juniper berries), and the mixtures prescribed were to be consumed in wine or beer.

Among the oldest (dated about 6500 BC in Turkey) evidence for beer consumption in humans includes homely beer made in sieve-pots. Babylonian clay tablets (6000 BC) were used to record and save detailed recipes for brewing beer. The Sumerians (5500 BC) were accomplished brewers. The remains of an ancient brewery were found in Egypt (3700 BC). Beer is among the oldest forms of alcohol beverages (others include fermented yeast and honey, Cyser, Braggot, and grape wine). In Egypt, barley was crushed and fermented by yeast to make beer. Evidence suggests that, at about this time, many Asian cultures made and consumed beer as food and for its psychoactive effects. There are numerous examples from varied cultures of what was used to make beer: Germans (wheat); Russian (rye); Africans (millet and sorghum); Tibetans (barley); Peruvians (corn); South Americans (manic root); Mexicans (pulque [fermented sap] from agave); Chinese and Japanese (rice).

Distillation is accomplished by gentle boiling in a sealed container. The process of distillation to achieve an alcohol content greater than 45% is attributed to two Arabic alchemists, Gerber (800 AD) and Rhazes (900 AD). Today, alcohol is consumed in the billions of gallons yearly and is second in consumption only to caffeine-containing beverages, caffeine being the most consumed drug by humans worldwide.

Another major depressant class of abusive drugs include the alkaloids (morphine and codeine) found in the juice of the opium poppy. The word *opium* is derived from the Greek word for juice. This is rather fitting, since the poppy seed capsule of the poppy weeps a milky-white juice when cut. The early cultivation of poppies (probably first as food using the oil and seeds rather than consumed for pain relief and euphoria) and preparation of opium dates back to about 5000 BC, as evidenced from Sumerian clay tablets. Opium is mentioned in the Assyrian medical tablets under the name *arat pa pa,* and in Egypt (Luxor, 1550 BC), it is mentioned in the Ebers Papyrus, a document among the oldest written records of medicine. Use of opium has a long recorded history employed in the service of performing magic and religious rituals and as a sedative and sleep potion. Perhaps, it was Arabian traders that introduced opium to the Middle East from the Orient, where opium was used primarily to treat dysentery as opioids produce constipation.

The opium poppy, whose petals may be white, red, mauve, or purple, is one of a hundred species of poppy, along with corn poppy, Oriental poppy, and California poppy. The harvest of opium begins with slicing the unripened seed capsule to release the milky-white alkaloid-rich latex after the petals fall off. The gum darkens, and then it is scraped off with an iron paddle and dripped into wood form about the size of bricks. With each successive lancing of the capsule, up to 10 times each, more gum is obtained. The raw gum smells like just cut grass, and it is about 70% solid and 30% water. The gum is allowed to sit 28 days in the sun to facilitate evaporation and, with occasional stirring, produces a 90% solid. In this form, the gum retains its potency for hundreds of years if wrapped and buried. Opium gum recovered from 2,000-year-old burial sites has been shown to remain psychoactive using animal tests for analgesia.

Stimulants

Among the oldest used stimulant drugs now considered drugs of abuse are nicotine (in tobacco, used by Peruvian Aguaruna aboriginals 6,000 years ago), areca nut (the psychoactive substance is arecoline and used mainly in India and Thailand), and cathinone in the khat shrub (used in Yemen, Ethiopia, and East Africa). Chewing the young khat leaves produce effects indistinguishable from low doses of amphetamine and cocaine.

Cocaine is a strong, naturally occurring stimulant, an alkaloid ester with a rigid structure that is extracted from the leaves of the coca plant. Each leaf of the *Erythroxylum coca* plant contains about 1% of cocaine. Chewing the coca leaves probably predate the Incas. It is believed that as long ago as 1500 BC, the Incas of Peru were wrapping coca leaves for slow mouth consumption (not just chewing leaves). Peruvian and Ecuadorian grave statues, created in 200 BC, display puffed cheeks, indicating wads of coca in the mouth. It is believed that Incas absorbed cocaine into the bloodstream via mouth tissue absorption for its stimulant effects, as a social ritual, as a dietary supplement, and was brewed as a tea by the upper class.

The Incas had two myths to account for the origin of the coca plant. One myth states that coca was an herb created by the God Inti. Inti instructed the moon mother to plant the coca in the humid valleys of the Andes Mountains and stated that only the descendants of Gods should eat them. This herb provided them the enduring strength and, in times of famine or drought, would help to reduce hunger. Another myth is that a woman convicted of adultery was put to death by being drawn and quartered. It is told that the first coca plant blossomed from where her body was buried, and the coca leaf was to be consumed by males in memory of her. Cocaine also played a critical role in the Incas' religious ceremonies. Its use was reserved for members of the highest classes. The Inca priests placed the coca leaf on the royal emblem and named the first Inca queen, Mama Cuca.

Hallucinogens

Hallucinogens represent, by far, the most diverse and most frequently occurring psychoactive substances used by humans over wide geographical locations to alter consciousness and behavior. Hallucinogens include seven major chemical classes:

1. Phenylethylamines (peyote). Mescaline grows naturally in northern Mexico. Traditional users include Native American tribes in Mexico and Central America. The Aztecs used peyote and ololiuqui, a small lentil-like seed containing lysergic acid.

2. The indole derivatives include bufotenine, psilocybine, 3-ring harmines, and ergots (the backbone of LSD-25).

3. Tropanes (piperidine derivatives: belladonna, atropine, scopolamine)

4. Phenylpropene, myristicin (found in nutmeg, a relative of mescaline). Evidence suggests Arab physicians used nutmeg as a drug in the first century AD.

5. Isoxazoles (muscimol and ibotenic acid).

6. Quinolizidines (cryogenine).

7. Dibenzopyrans (tetrahydrocannibinols found in marijuana)

The mythical Chinese Emperor Shen Nung in 2737 BC wrote of marijuana as a euphoriant and a medicine. The major psychoactive substance in marijuana is Δ9-tetrahydrocannabinol, a relatively insoluble compound that was first isolated and synthesized in 1964. There are three species of hemp plant. These plants are believed to have originally grown in China, India, and Eastern Russia, respectively.

Traditional consumption of *Cannabis sativa* and *Cannibis indica* is now global, with references made to the plants dating as far back as the second millennium BC; *Cannibis ruderalis* was used in Siberia, with earliest recorded use 450 BC. Cannabis contains more than 426 chemicals, 61 of which are unique to cannabis. Among the oldest verifiable uses of hallucinogenic plants come from evidence of cultivation in Australia. It is believed that 2,000 years ago, Aboriginal toolmakers mass-produced granite blades and cutting tools and traded them for a mildly hallucinogenic drug, Pituri. This drug was used by Aborigines to reduce hunger pains during a hunt that could cover traveling long distances. Red mescal beans (containing a hallucinogenic alkaloid called cytisine related to nicotine and unrelated to mescaline) suggest hallucinogen use in approximately 1500 BC, as they were found in rock-shelter sites in Texas and Mexico.

Humans (identified as Aleuts, Chukchi, and Eskimo ancestors) migrated to the plateaus of the Chukotka area, North America, and Beringiya, now flooded by the waters of the Bering Sea. Recently, late Neolithic period rock drawings have been found depicting dancing figures and huge mushrooms believed to be fly-agarics. Fly-agarics are capable of growing in Arctic conditions. Other fungi have been used in sacred and shamanistic rites for thousands of years (as far back as 7000 BC); they share in common the psychoactive substance psilocybin, and this drug shares a mechanism of action and effects similar to lysergic acid diethamide (LSD-25).

Daniel J. Calcagnetti

See also Cultural Aspects; Drug Laws, History of

Further Readings

Austin, G. A. (1999). Perspectives on the history of psychoactive substance use. Retrieved October 2, 2007, from http://ibogaine.org/drugmain.html

McGee, H. (2004). *On food and cooking: The science and lore of the kitchen.* New York: Scribner.

Rudgley, R. (1999). *The lost civilizations of the Stone Age.* New York: Free Press.

Schaffer Library of Drug Policy. (n.d.). *Some events in the history of drugs: A summary of historical events.* Retrieved October 2, 2007, from http://www.druglibrary .org/SCHAFFER/History/histsum.htm

Schultes, R. E., Hoffman, A., & Ratsch, C. (1998). *Plants of the gods: Their sacred, healing and hallucinogen powers.* Rochester, VT: Healing Arts Press.

Trager, J. (1995). *The food chronology.* New York: Henry Holt.

DRY DRUNK SYNDROME

Dry drunk syndrome is a term coined by Alcoholics Anonymous (AA) that describes characteristics of someone who is no longer consuming alcohol but is experiencing several behavioral and emotional symptoms of alcoholism, such as irresponsible behavior, impatience, impulsivity, "black and white" thinking, and a rigid, judgmental outlook. These individuals may portray an exaggerated sense of self-importance and grandiose behavior, such as seeking the center of attention for both positive and negative reasons. Additionally, characteristics such as dishonesty, indecisiveness, mood swings, and overreaction may be displayed. They may experience nostalgia or fantasize about drinking, and they may limit alcohol treatment attendance or drop out altogether. These features are seen as being more chronic in nature rather than temporary fluctuations in mood or behavior.

To understand the significance of the dry drunk syndrome, it is important to understand why this term was conceived by AA. An integral component of AA is to work through the Twelve Steps, principles for recovery that aim to guide individuals seeking sobriety to create a worthy life, not only through abstinence from alcohol but also by making a spiritual transformation. These steps include admitting powerlessness over alcohol and reliance on a Higher Power (defined by the individual) for removal of character defects, guidance, and spiritual care. By following the 12 guidelines set forth by AA, individuals can begin to make a spiritual change that inspires a life worth living. AA posits that individuals who abstain from alcohol without fully integrating the lessons taught in the Twelve Steps, will continue to experience spiritual, emotional, and relational difficulties brought about by using "alcoholic" strategies for managing their lives. While these individuals may be "dry," or abstinent from alcohol, they will remain symbolically "drunk," continuing to experience pathology caused by alcoholism and living an alcoholic life. According to AA, they cannot achieve true sobriety without acceptance and implementation of the 12 principles of AA, which leads to spiritual change. The slang term *dry drunk* is typically a derogatory way to refer to someone who is abstinent from alcohol without working the steps.

The symptoms related to the dry drunk syndrome have also been viewed as warning signs of relapse for alcohol use. Much research has been conducted on factors that predict relapse from alcohol or other substance use. Common high-risk situations that precede relapse that also define dry drunk syndrome include experiencing negative emotions such as frustration, anger, hostility, aggression, hopelessness, and loneliness; relationship concerns and interpersonal conflicts; and believing or wishing alcohol use would enhance positive emotional states such as pleasure, joy, and freedom. Combined, these symptoms leave individuals vulnerable for relapse, and AA would argue that without spiritual change, the risk for relapse and dry drunk syndrome will remain.

Additionally, persons with dry drunk syndrome may experience several signs related to depression, such as sadness, tiredness, agitation, poor concentration, hopelessness, and suicidal ideation. Research has also found alcohol relapse to be subsequent to signs of depression. It has been suggested that some individuals who are currently experiencing symptoms of depression but are also abstinent from alcohol may respond better to alcohol treatment (versus depression treatment) if the underlying cause of depression is related to dry drunk syndrome.

There is a dearth of empirical research that has been conducted on the validity or impact of the dry drunk syndrome. However, one study by Edvard Johansson and colleagues in Finland evaluated the relation between alcohol use and labor status. They were interested in seeing if there was a difference in employment between those who did not meet criteria for alcohol dependence and those who were currently abstinent because of past alcohol dependence. The researchers found that individuals who were moderate drinkers or abstained from alcohol by choice (i.e., their abstinence was not related to prior alcohol problems) were more likely to have a full-time job compared to individuals who were abstainers but met criteria for alcohol dependence in the past. Although this research did not directly test the validity of the dry drunk syndrome, these results lend credence to the difficulties experienced by ex-drinkers. According to the definition of dry drunk syndrome, one possible explanation for the study results is that ex-drinkers were still experiencing difficulties related to alcoholism because they had not followed the Twelve Steps toward making the necessary spiritual changes for true sobriety. However, this study did not assess participation in AA or acceptance of the Twelve Steps of AA; thus, it is difficult to support this explanation within the confines of this study.

In conclusion, the dry drunk syndrome is a series of emotional, behavioral, and spiritual problems seen in individuals who no longer consume alcohol but have not made necessary spiritual changes to avoid living an alcoholic life. The Twelve Steps of AA have been provided as a guide for individuals with alcohol problems to make

these changes. Although little empirical work has been conducted on the syndrome, several characteristics, such as negative affect, interpersonal problems, and feeling that life would be better with alcohol, have been found to predict additional difficulties, such as depression and relapse to alcohol use. The symptoms of dry drunk syndrome may be indicative of larger or impending problems. These symptoms may signal individuals, friends, and family members that someone who has a history of alcohol-related problems may still be experiencing problems related to alcohol use despite abstinence.

Tiara M. Dillworth

See also Alcoholics Anonymous; Alcoholism; Relapse; Sobriety; Spiritual Issues; Twelve Steps

Further Readings

Alcoholics Anonymous. (1939). *Alcoholics Anonymous.* New York: Works Publishing.

Davis, D. R., & Jansen, G. G. (1998). Making meaning of Alcoholics Anonymous for social workers: Myths, metaphors, and realities. *Social Work, 43*(2), 169–183.

Johansson, E., Alho, H., Kiiskinen, U., & Poikolainen, K. (2006). Abstaining from alcohol and labour market underperformance—Have we forgotten the "dry" alcoholics? *Alcohol & Alcoholism, 41*(5), 574–579.

Solberg, R. J. (1983). *The dry drunk syndrome.* Center City, MN: Hazelden.

DUAL RELATIONSHIPS

Dual relationships (also known as *multiple relationships*) has more than one definition depending on the setting and the nature of the relationships. James Meyer suggests a working definition of dual relationships such that one exists when there is a combining of incompatible professional roles and behavior to the detriment of someone to whom the helping professional owes a fiduciary duty. Dual or multiple relationships with a client, whether they be social, financial or sexual, can interfere with a mental health practitioner's ability to provide therapy.

Various mental health professionals, such as addiction counselors, pastoral counselors, psychiatrists, clinical social workers, marriage and family therapists, and licensed professional counselors, have codes of ethics developed by professional organizations that they are required to follow. Each of these professional ethics codes addresses the issue of dual or multiple relationships. For the sake of simplicity, only two of these organizations are discussed here: the American Psychological Association and NAADAC, the Association for Addiction Professionals.

American Psychological Association Code of Ethics, 2002

An example of a code of ethics that addresses the issue of dual relationships is the 2002 American Psychological Association (APA) Ethics Code—Section 3.05 that describes "multiple relationships" as occurring when a psychologist is in a professional role with a person and (1) at the same time is in another role with the same person, (2) at the same time is in a relationship with a person closely associated with or related to the person with whom the psychologist has the professional relationship, or (3) promises to enter into another relationship in the future with the person or a person closely associated with or related to the person. It is strongly advised that a psychologist refrains from entering into any multiple relationship if that multiple relationship could reasonably be expected to impair the psychologist's objectivity, competence, or effectiveness in performing his or her functions as a psychologist, or otherwise risks exploitation or harm to the person with whom the professional relationship exists. The APA Ethics Code goes on to state that "multiple relationships" that would not reasonably be expected to cause impairment or risk exploitation or harm are not unethical.

If a psychologist discovers a situation where a dual relationship could be potentially harmful, the psychologist should take reasonable steps to resolve that issue with due regard for the best interests of the affected person and maximal compliance with the APA Code of Ethics. For example, a potential client seeks treatment at a psychotherapeutic agency, and the potential client turns out to be a family member of one of the psychologists. It would be unwise for the psychologist to treat that family member. Another example might be, without prior knowledge, a client in treatment shows up at the helping professional's house one day to fix the roof. At the next opportunity, the issue should be discussed with the client and documented. The client should be given the option to seek treatment with someone else.

However, there are times when psychologists are required by law, institutional policy, or other extraordinary circumstances to serve in more than one role in judicial or administrative proceedings. Under those circumstances, the psychologist must clarify role expectations and the extent of confidentiality to both the client and to those involved in the judicial or administrative proceedings.

It is important to keep in mind that psychologists are not the only mental health service providers that are required to abide by a code of ethics regarding dual or multiple relationships. Professionals who work in the field of substance abuse treatment are also mandated to follow similar codes of ethics. One such organization, NAADAC, is discussed next.

Comparing Other Helping Professions' Ethics Codes

NAADAC, the Association for Addiction Professionals, has the following principle, regarding dual relationships, stated in their Code of Ethics:

> Principle 7: Dual Relationships I understand that I must seek to nurture and support the development of a relationship of equals rather than to take unfair advantage of individuals who are vulnerable and exploitable. * I shall not engage in professional relationships or commitments that conflict with family members, friends, close associates, or others whose welfare might be jeopardized by such a dual relationship. * Because a relationship begins with a power differential, I shall not exploit relationships with current or former clients for personal gain, including social or business relationships. * I shall not under any circumstances engage in sexual behavior with current or former clients. * I shall not accept substantial gifts from clients, other treatment organizations, or the providers of materials or services used in my practice.

Unavoidable Situations

Situations can, and do, arise where multiple relationships may be unavoidable, such as in a small, rural community, where everyone knows each other. To deal with such dilemmas, a decision-making model is suggested. This decision-making model is based on three dimensions: (1) amount or degree of power that the helping professional possesses over the other individual; (2) duration of relationship, which also is an aspect of power; and (3) clarity of termination, the length of obligation the helping professional has to a client. With regard to clarity of termination, it may be safest for any helping professional to assume the adage of "once a client, always a client," just as a doctor may follow a similar ethic of not getting into a dual or multiple relationship with a patient, which could prove harmful to the patient or preclude the patient from returning to that doctor for further treatment. This decision-making process needs to be clearly documented, including the consultations with other professionals regarding this issue, in the event the decision is called into question.

Patricia A. McCoy

See also Confidentiality; Ethical Standards for Addiction Professionals; Ethics; Informed Consent; NAADAC, the Association for Addiction Professionals

Further Readings

American Psychological Association. (2002). *American Psychological Association code of ethics.* Washington, DC: Author.

Koocher, G., & Keith-Spiegel, P. (1998). *Ethics in psychology: Professional standards and cases* (2nd ed.). New York: Oxford University Press.

NAADAC, the Association for Addiction Professionals. (2004). *NAADAC code of ethics.* Retrieved July 15, 2007, from http://naadac.org/documents/index.php? CategoryID=23

Younggren, J. N. (2002). *Dual relationships: Ethical decision-making and dual relationships.* Retrieved June 7, 2004, from http://www.kspope.com/dual/younggren.php

E

EATING DISORDERS

See ANOREXIA NERVOSA; BULIMIA NERVOSA

ECONOMIC COSTS OF ALCOHOL AND DRUG ABUSE

"Costs" of alcohol and drug abuse may be defined as the monetary expenditures necessitated as the result of consequences of alcohol and other drug use. Financial costs include decreases in potential gains; for example, substance abuse impedes productivity of workers and can result in high rates of absenteeism, drug-related illnesses and injuries, increased health care expenditures, low employee morale, theft, and premature death. Costs of drug abuse are also associated with lost production due to drug-related crime careers, incarceration, and correctional services. In addition, often the pursuit of obtaining or purchasing drugs, as well as the time spent using drugs, causes financial problems. Strangely enough, in making drugs harder to obtain or use, it is likely that costs (e.g., financial, time, or addiction) of drug abuse increase, giving drug users reasons to engage in income-generating crimes as a means of supporting drug habits. Consequently, drug abuse also results in costs incurred on the mental and physical health of significant others and coworkers who share the burden of coping with or accommodating the consequences incurred by drug abuse.

Costs of alcohol and other drug abuse are embedded in socioenvironmental contexts. For example, loss of productivity or increases in the cost of medical care may have relatively little meaning in societies in which many individuals do not work, work in areas where drug use is likely to have relatively little impact at least for awhile (e.g., picking rice versus driving a car), or have little access or availability of quality health care. Internationally, though, it appears that drug abuse is considered a problem when an individual's role (e.g., as coworker, spouse, parent) is not fulfilled.

For recreational drugs, abuse can be associated with the production of psychotic symptoms (e.g., paranoid ideation) or injury (e.g., accidents, violence, overdoses). Several drugs of abuse may result in cardiovascular, respiratory, digestive, or excretory dysfunction, problems in cognitive function, or all of these things. One study found that within 32 years of treatment, 49% of a large sample of heroin addicts had died (on average, prior to 60 years of age) and 28% had died within 20 years of treatment. In a small sample of alcoholics, it was found that within 10 years of treatment, approximately 10% of alcoholics were dead prior to 60 years of age. Thus, some drugs of abuse lead to notable mortality-related cost (e.g., productive years lost as employee or parent).

Some costs of alcohol and other drug abuse are difficult to explain in financial terms. Obviously, in conjunction with financial costs, there are the emotional costs of alcohol and other drug abuse to family members, significant others, and the users themselves, and the enduring burden of these costs is difficult to assess.

Neglect of responsibilities as a parent, medical consequences hidden within other diagnoses (e.g., cardiovascular disease), therapy requested by family members to cope with the drug abusers' behavior, and general decrease in social morale are further examples of outcomes that may be difficult to quantify in terms of a direct consequences of drug abuse. Given the burden of these types of costs, it is likely that costs estimated as a result of substance misuse are underestimates. Still, attempts to obtain at least a "ballpark" figure on costs of drug abuse have been made.

Cost of Illegal Drug Use in the United States

In the United States, the Office of National Drug Control Policy estimated the overall cost of drug abuse (i.e., of illegal drugs; tobacco, alcohol, and prescription drugs are not included in calculations) to society was $181 billion in 2002. The cost was estimated to have increased an average of 5.3% per year from 1992 to 2002. In 2002, nearly 60% of the costs involved crime-related issues, including productivity losses due to incarceration and crime careers; local, state, and federal corrections; police protection; legal adjudication; and the National Drug Control Strategy supply reduction expenditures. The remaining 40% involved health care costs (approximately 8%) and productivity losses due to premature death and drug abuse–related illnesses (approximately 32%). According to this study, there were an estimated 23,500 drug-related deaths in 2000. These deaths were caused by overdose, poisoning, homicide, AIDS, and hepatitis.

In the 2008 budget, U.S. federal funding for treatment was 23.6% of the "drug war" budget while prevention was allocated 12.9%. On the supply side, the remaining 63.5% of the budget was devoted to domestic law enforcement, international efforts, and interdiction. Yet, treatment has a large impact on subsequent crime, whereas interdiction does not.

Cost of Legal Drug Use in the United States

In addition to the costs associated with illegal drugs of abuse, it is important to consider costs of legal drugs that are misused or abused. Nearly one quarter of adults throughout the world (approximately 2 billion people) smoke cigarettes. If current trends continue, 8.4 million smokers are estimated to die annually of smoking-related deaths by the year 2020. Despite the adverse health outcomes and enormous costs associated with smoking (e.g., lung cancer, heart disease, and chronic obstructive pulmonary disease), approximately 3 million children and adolescents begin smoking daily. Even smoking as few as one to four cigarettes per day leads to a 50% increase in overall prevalence of disease, including a 400% and 275% increase in prevalence of lung cancer and ischemic heart disease, respectively. (A pack a day or more leads to a 300% increase in overall prevalence of disease, 3000% increase in lung cancer, and 400% increase in ischemic heart disease.)

A surgeon general's report indicated that total costs of tobacco use (cigarette smoking) are approximately $157.7 billion per year. Direct treatment of tobacco use in the United States costs approximately $75.5 billion annually, the loss of productivity from smoking yearly is approximately $81.9 billion, and neonatal costs are approximately $366 million. Thus, the total costs from cigarette smoking are as much as the total costs of all illegal drugs combined.

Likewise, a National Institute on Alcohol Abuse and Alcoholism report indicated that the total costs of alcohol use were $184.6 billion in 1998, including $29 billion in medical or treatment costs, $36.5 billion in lost productivity due to premature death, $86 billion of lost earnings due to alcohol-related illness, and $34 billion due to alcohol-related crimes. Also, although males have more alcohol-related problems and dependence symptoms than females, *among heavy drinkers,* females are equal to or surpass males in problems resulting from alcohol use. Consequences of alcohol consumption are accelerated in females, with chronic alcohol abuse exacting greater physiological impairment (e.g., alcohol-related organ damage) earlier in females, despite consuming less alcohol than males. Female alcoholics (and abusers of other drugs) have death rates 50% to 100% higher than those of male alcoholics, and a greater percentage of female alcoholics die from suicides, alcohol-related accidents, circulatory disorders, and cirrhosis of the liver. In addition, fetal health risks related to female alcohol use during pregnancy are a serious consequence that is extremely difficult to quantify in terms of financial costs.

Cost of Illegal and Legal Drug Use in Australia

On the international front, an econometrics study conducted in Australia provided comprehensive analyses of separate categories of drugs (e.g., tobacco, alcohol, and illegal drug costs) and the associated social costs, which were divided into tangible (e.g., crime, health, productivity, accidents, and fires) and intangible costs (loss of life, pain and suffering). The total social cost of drug use in Australia from 1998 to 1999 was more than $34 billion. Of these costs, 53% were tangible and 47% were intangible. A total of 61% were tobacco related, 22% were alcohol related, and 17% were illegal-drug related. Among the tangible costs, tobacco use accounted for none of the crime costs, 79% of the health costs, 46% of productivity costs (at the workplace or at home), no road accidents, but all of the drug-related fires. Alcohol use accounted for 29% of the crime costs, 16% of the health costs, 18% of productivity costs, 82% of drug-related road accidents, but no fires. Illegal drug use accounted for most of the crime costs (71%), 5% of the health costs, 36% of the productivity costs, 18% of road accidents, but no fires.

In calculating costs this study attempted to estimate lives lost and lives saved as a result of different drug use. Some positive health effects of alcohol but not other drugs were discussed. Ninety-four percent of benefits of alcohol use were from light drinking among individuals 60 years old or older. A total of 23% of social costs in Australia were estimated as crime related. Of the tangible crime costs, all were related to enforcement efforts.

Summary of Cost Data

In summary of these data, in the United States, the total costs of illegal drug abuse averaged to $715 per person living in the United States in 1998. Excluding crime enforcement costs, these costs were $286 per person. Including tobacco and alcohol abuse, the total costs increase to approximately $2,429 per person in 1998, and excluding crime enforcement, costs would be $1,818 per person. In Australia, total costs of drug abuse (which also included tobacco and alcohol use) averaged $1,811 per person in 1998, and $1,378 excluding crime enforcement efforts. Costs due to crime enforcement are high in both countries ($500 to $600 per year per person). Some individuals have argued that legalization might reduce costs or perhaps reduce use of some legal drugs.

Conclusion

Controlling for enforcement efforts, there are many specific costs of drug abuse that add up to a total of $1,400 to $1,800 per person annually. There are several possible means to reduce these costs. For example, one way is to decrease drug misuse. Another might be to impose a tax on citizens. A third means would be to impose a tax on the tobacco and alcohol industries that would offset the costs incurred by the abuse of these substances. It is not clear to what extent taxation would or could be enforced. But annual costs, which are likely higher now than when the costs were calculated, appear to amount to approximately 5% of the average family income in the United States. This is a substantial burden considering other potential monetary needs and purchases, and the likelihood that the costs noted here are underestimates of the true financial impact drug abuse has on the economy.

Costs of drug abuse do need to be differentiated from potential confounders. For example, while it is true that drug misuse may result in environmental costs (stressors), such as violence, vandalism, and deteriorating housing, environmental stressors may perpetuate the use of drugs as a means of coping with these stressors. Order of precedence between costs and drug misuse needs to be carefully examined. Also, to the extent that costs are defined by public institutions that are created and that express disapproval of drug use (some law enforcement or education efforts), as opposed to protecting individuals and society from clear and present danger, calculations may need to made for the costs of relatively value-laden factors separately. Finally, in costs of drug abuse, what also needs to be considered are other potential scenarios of costs that might occur if the drugs were not being used (e.g., increases in obesity or other substitute addictions, other avenues of dependence on public welfare). In other words, the benefits and costs of both using and not using drugs need to be fully considered. Although there are several unknowns, it is clear that drug abuse is a notable economic cost to the world economy.

Steve Sussman and Susan L. Ames

See also Crime and Substance Abuse; Harm Reduction, Public Health; Medical Consequences; Public Policy, Alcohol; Public Policy, Drugs; Workplace Drug Use

Further Readings

Bjartveit, K., & Tverdol, A. (2005). Health consequences of smoking 1–4 cigarettes per day. *Tobacco Control, 14,* 315–320.

Collins, D. J., & Lapsley, H. M. (2002). *Counting the cost: Estimates of the social costs of drug abuse in Australia in 1998–9* (National Drug Strategy Monograph Series No. 49). Canberra, Australia: Commonwealth Department of Health and Ageing.

Galea, S., Ahern, J., & Vlahov, D. (2003). Contextual determinants of drug use risk behavior: A theoretical framework. *Journal of Urban Health, 80,* 50–58.

Harwood, H. (2000). *Updating estimates of the economic costs of alcohol abuse in the United States: Estimates, update methods, and data* (NIH Publication No. 98-4327). Rockville, MD: National Institutes of Health.

Miller, W. R. (1992). Building bridges over troubled waters: A response to "Alcoholism, politics, and bureaucracy: The consensus against controlled-drinking therapy in America." *Addictive Behaviors, 17,* 79–81.

Office of National Drug Control Policy. (2004). *The economic costs of drug abuse in the United States, 1992–2002* (Publication No. 207303).Washington, DC: Executive Office of the President. Retrieved May 20, 2008, from http://www.whitehousedrugpolicy.gov/publications/economic_costs/economic_costs.pdf

Rydell, C. P., & Everingham, S. S. (1994). *Controlling cocaine: Supply vs. demand programs* (Research Rep. No. MR-331-ONDCP/A/DPRC). Santa Monica, CA: RAND.

Sussman, S., & Ames, S. L. (2001). *The social psychology of drug abuse.* Buckingham, UK: Open University Press.

U.S. Department of Health and Human Services. (2004). *The health consequences of smoking: A report of the Surgeon General.* Atlanta, GA: Centers for Disease Control.

Ecstasy

Understanding the social and scientific relevance of the drug ecstasy (MDMA) is made simpler by considering it as one substance with two discrete identities. As a compound worthy of serious scientific inquiry in the lab and in research clinics, MDMA is an intriguing phenethylamine with yet unknown potential as a therapeutic agent. Its "alter ego" reputation as a possible brain toxin on the street and in the club scene, where it is commonly known as ecstasy or simply "E," has led to a premature stifling of methodologically sound research and clinical investigations. Controversies in the political, legal, media, and public health sectors around its perceived threats and benefits remain unresolved. Widespread confusion, gross errors in reporting on MDMA's effects and side effects, and ignorance about serious risk factors have all contributed to a murky collective understanding of which policies and approaches are optimal regarding regulation and research. Despite sensationalized reports of severe damage resulting from just one dose, ecstasy is still commonly regarded by recreational users as a safe drug for inducing a few hours of euphoria. Even though it has been illegal since the mid-1980s, recent surveys show an increase in use among young people ages 18 to 25. Informed insight into the facts about this drug that has inspired both hope and fear is as relevant to clinicians, researchers, the public, and policymakers now as in any earlier point in its remarkable history.

MDMA (3,4-methylenedioxymethamphetamine) in its pure form was developed as a by-product of a styptic compound at Merck in pre–World War I Germany. University- and industry-based medicinal chemists started conducting initial scientific investigations with human subjects during the 1970s after chemistry professor Alexander Shulgin began exploring MDMA's potential to create controllable altered states of consciousness. Although they often lacked formal psychological credentials, early investigators noted MDMA's capacity to help people open up and talk honestly about themselves and their relationships, without defensive conditioning intervening. For several hours, anxiety and fear appeared to melt away, even in subjects who were chronically constricted and apprehensive. Hailed as "penicillin for the soul," MDMA was said to be useful in treating a wide range of conditions, including post-traumatic stress, phobias, psychosomatic disorders, depression, suicidality, drug addiction, relationship difficulties, and the psychological distress of terminal illness. Of particular interest to psychiatric researchers were patients with disorders generally considered to be nonresponsive to conventional treatment models. Beginning in the mid-1970s, hundreds of therapists and psychiatrists quietly provided the still legal MDMA to thousands of clients as an adjunct to therapy.

The transition from an experimental empathogenic agent to the illicit substance that fueled the burgeoning all-night dance party "rave" scene transpired primarily in Texas, thanks largely to the efforts of a former Catholic seminary student, Michael Clegg. Part MDMA evangelist and part entrepreneur, Clegg was inundating the city of Dallas with an estimated 500,000 doses per month by the mid-1980s. Incidentally, he is also credited with naming the new drug "ecstasy" after considering the more accurate but less marketable moniker, "Empathy." As more people sought the novel new high in the United States and abroad, reports of a sinister side to the bliss-inducing pill began to surface.

Although it is not considered physically addicting, MDMA can cause mild to severe side effects and, in rare instances, death. It is a powerful serotonin-releasing catalyst, so temporary depression due to altered neurotransmitter levels affects some users. Elevated blood pressure and increased cardiac load, malignant hyperthermia, and dehydration are dangers that can be exacerbated by vigorous dancing in hot, confined spaces for hours without adequate access to water and proper ventilation. First-time users with congenital heart defects are especially vulnerable. In rare but sometimes lethal cases, naive users have consumed too much water without ingesting required amounts of salt, leading to water intoxication (hyponatremia). Taking MDMA with monoamine oxidase inhibitors (MAOIs) or with certain antiretroviral medications can induce a life-threatening hypertensive crisis. Two additional significant hazards include polydrug use in dangerous combinations and "macho" ingestion of high doses.

Predictably, instances of severe adverse events and preventable deaths related to ecstasy use in suboptimal conditions began to draw public attention, prompting intervention on the part of law enforcement and legislators. Formal hearings commenced in 1985 to determine MDMA's fate. Weighing the interests of the therapeutic community against MDMA's growing abuse liability and the threat it posed to public health and safety, the U.S. Drug Enforcement Administration (DEA) eventually ordered that it be placed in the most restrictive category of drugs, Schedule I. In the wake of the highly publicized scheduling hearings, however, use among young people escalated in the absence of effective harm-reduction measures.

Capitalizing on the growing demand, black-market distributors began introducing increasing degrees of substituted compounds. These impurities range from benign substances like aspirin or caffeine to more dangerous adulterants, such as methamphetamine, phencyclidine (PCP), and dextromethorphan (DXM). The potent stimulant paramethoxyamphetamine (PMA) has been associated with a number of ecstasy fatalities. Batches in pill and powder form can vary widely in both purity and dose. To a regrettable degree, mainstream policymakers resisted harm reduction and pill-testing efforts, thereby maximizing the potential damage likely to be incurred through recreational ecstasy use.

In the decades following the DEA scheduling, discord and divisiveness escalated in the research world, as well. At the center of the debate was the question of whether MDMA use caused brain damage, neurotoxicity in particular. Histopathological findings in animal studies with repeated injections demonstrated that distal serotonergic axonal degeneration could result with doses much higher than those that recreational users consume. Implications of such preclinical findings are further confounded by observations of proximal axonal regeneration, cell body sparing, and absence of standard laboratory markers of neurotoxicity. Other studies suggested that even modest use could lead to irreparable brain damage, including emotional and memory deficits, although these reports were often marred by flawed research methodologies, questionable data analyses, and biased conclusions. The debate reached its zenith with the high-profile retraction in 2003 of highly publicized findings from a government-funded study published in 2002 that concluded MDMA could cause damage to the dopamine system, thereby potentially causing Parkinson's disease. No definitive record of MDMA's tested and confirmed effects on the central nervous system has been established to date.

Progress toward rectifying earlier lapses in methodological integrity and questionable data analysis is advancing quietly through several privately funded research projects. In spring 2004, researchers at the University of South Carolina commenced a clinical trial (approved by the U.S. Food and Drug Administration) with human volunteers to investigate MDMA's potential as a treatment for post-traumatic stress disorder. Protocols for additional studies are currently in development. It is hoped that further efforts to objectively and honestly investigate the full range of effects of MDMA will be successful. By adhering to strict standards of scientific ethics and by being insulated from political pressures and agendas, it should be possible to finally establish the full range of potential risks and benefits. Only in this way will it be possible to address the serious public health concerns that have been raised, as well as to investigate the potential of developing an entirely new and novel psychiatric treatment.

Alicia L. Danforth and Charles S. Grob

See also Club Drugs; College Students, Drug Use and Abuse; Drugs, Classification of; Harm Reduction, Public Health; Neurotransmitters; Substance Abuse

Further Readings

Grob, C. S. (2000). Deconstructing ecstasy: The politics of MDMA research. *Addiction Research, 8,* 549–588.

Grob, C. S. (2005). The enigma of ecstasy: Implications for youth and society. *Adolescent Psychiatry, 29,* 97–117.

Holland, J. (Ed.). (2001). *Ecstasy: The complete guide.* Rochester, VT: Park Street Press.

Kish, S. J. (2002). How strong is the evidence that brain serotonin neurons are damaged in human users of ecstasy? *Pharmacology, Biochemistry and Behavior, 71,* 845–855.

U.S. Department of Health and Human Services, Substance Abuse and Mental Health Services Administration. (2007). 2006 National Survey on Drug Use & Health: Detailed tables. Retrieved September 8, 2007, from http://oas.samhsa.gov/NSDUH/2k6NSDUH/tabs/Sect1peTabs1to46.htm

ELDERLY POPULATIONS, TREATMENT ISSUES

The evaluation and treatment of substance-related problems vary by life phase. As such, understanding the special needs of elders with regard to substance use issues has increased significantly in recent times. In 1900, people 65 years of age and older constituted 4% of the U.S. population, whereas today they are approximately 13%. By the year 2010, *baby boomers* (e.g., the exceptionally large birth cohort born from 1946 and 1964) will start to turn 65, magnifying this aging trend. By 2045, the number of elderly persons will likely exceed the number of children (15 or younger) for the first time in history. Despite this marked shift in demographics, research on elder substance use treatment has not increased at the same rate. This causes concern because of the increasing number of elderly individuals likely to require substance-related treatment services and a number of factors putting these individuals at higher risk for developing substance-related disorders.

Risk Factors Unique to the Elderly

Individuals over the age of 65 disproportionately consume approximately 30% of all prescribed drugs and are the largest consumers of nonprescribed over-the-counter medications. They are three times as likely to use prescription drugs as younger individuals and spend more than $15 billion on these medications each year. This expenditure is fourfold greater per capita than that of younger generations. Furthermore, 22% of elders who receive Medicare use at least one prescription medication with addiction potential. For example, prescriptions are commonly written for opioid analgesics and for central nervous system depressants (e.g., benzodiazepines such as Valium or Ativan). In fact, approximately 40% of benzodiazepine prescriptions go to the elderly. And because these medications may rapidly produce psychological and physical dependence, they have great potential for problems. Such problems may then be complicated because the drugs may interact with the large number of other medications taken by elderly individuals. Over the course of one month, 60% to 70% of individuals 65 years of age or older take one or more medication combinations that put them at risk for experiencing an adverse drug reaction.

Another factor contributing to increasing risk is medication noncompliance or misuse. Substance misuse broadly refers to erratic use, underuse, or overuse, with the most common form being missed doses. Forgetting to take medication or intentionally skipping doses are sometimes to blame, complicated further when individuals try to compensate by doubling the amount at the next dosing. In fact, approximately 10% of elderly individuals report taking extra doses, and only about half of elderly individuals take their medications as prescribed. Even worse, medication compliance decreases as the number of prescribed medications increases.

Increased risk also develops from age-related changes in physiology (e.g., body composition and vital organ function changes). These can alter the metabolism, excretion, and distribution of drugs. For instance, drugs may become more potent and their effects less predictable with such physiological changes. For example, relative to youth, elders have higher blood alcohol levels after consuming similar amounts of alcohol.

Elder baby boomers may further be at increased risk for substance-related disorders because of social characteristics of their birth cohort. Increased exposure to recreational substance use and more tolerant attitudes toward use, compared to prior generations, are anticipated risks. The prevalence of illicit drug use among these individuals has consistently remained higher than age-matched samples from previous generations.

Issues in Establishing Prevalence

The *Diagnostic and Statistical Manual of Mental Disorders, Fourth Edition, Text Revision (DSM-IV-TR)*, published by the American Psychiatric Association, divides substance-related disorders into substance use disorders, including the diagnostic classes of abuse and dependence, and substance-induced disorders, including conditions that mimic other psychiatric disorders, such as anxiety, depression, dementia, delirium, but are caused by substance use. Substance abuse and dependence diagnoses have been developed and well validated for younger individuals. However, currently available diagnostic criteria may not properly characterize the prevalence of substance-related disorders among elderly persons across most of these classes of diagnoses. This is because criteria were developed with individuals of other ages in mind, rather than elders, and obvious age-related differences between individuals across the life span may affect their applicability to the elderly. For example, the criteria of tolerance for diagnoses of dependence is understood to mean that there is increased consumption to achieve the same effect or decreased effect when consuming the same amount of the substance. However, changes in physiology and pharmacokinetics may cause elders to achieve the same effects with less of the substance than used in years past, and so interpretation of reports of tolerance symptoms may need further consideration among elders. Similarly, examples of adverse consequences listed as possible indicators of substance-related problems include absences or poor work performance, suspensions or expulsions from

school, and neglect of children or household, consequences that pertain to young and middle-age individuals, much more so than elders. Also, other factors may limit how these problems are expressed or how they develop. For instance, medical problems that limit desirability and accessibility of alcohol and other drugs may affect the frequency and quantity consumed. Similarly, less financial flexibility and fewer social events with a theme of substance use may be available to elders than younger people.

Unlike the substance use disorders, much less information is generally available for the substance-induced disorders, including such basic information as prevalence rates, reliability of diagnosis, and validity. As such, these disorders may be underidentified in the elderly when standard diagnostic criteria are used, or identified in a way that may not accurately reflect the true prevalence of problems. This may be especially true for prescription medication–related problems. Prescription medication problems are often underdetected in the elderly and often go unrecognized by health care providers. One factor contributing to this underdetection is the masking of substance-related symptoms by coexisting psychiatric disorders, health disorders, or both. Similarly, substance-related conditions may simply be overlooked or misdiagnosed.

Age of Onset and Gender Issues

To date, some distinctions have proven useful with regard to gender and age among elders with substance-related problems. For instance, there are at least two types of individuals with problems related to alcohol: individuals with early onset of alcohol problems and individuals with later onset. Those with early onset account for two thirds of elderly alcohol problems. Some attrition from alcohol-related deaths may occur among this group, but most persons with early-onset alcohol problems eventually develop alcohol-related illnesses that amplify with changes associated with aging. Members of this group usually have a family history of alcoholism, as well as a higher prevalence of antisocial behavior. Early-onset problems are frequently associated with estrangement from family members and declines in socioeconomic status that continue with aging.

In contrast, individuals with late-onset problems generally have a higher level of education and income. The cause of late-life substance use problems, specifically late-life alcohol problems, may have to do with psychosocial factors. There has been considerable research done on the relationship between late life coping and alcohol problems. Loss of one's spouse, retirement from job, loss of physical strength, isolation, and other stressors may be responsible for late-onset cases of alcohol problems. Family who offer support, rather than discouragement, rejection, and resistance, often surround individuals with late-onset alcohol problems. This, paired with heightened levels of resources, makes them more likely to complete treatment and have better outcomes than early-onset individuals.

One complication of late-life onset is that health care providers may not be as likely to detect substance use in elderly individuals simply because these elders have no apparent prior history of substance-related disorders. A number of studies have examined incidence of late-life onset problem drinking in individuals reporting for treatment of alcohol use disorders. These studies have found that between 15% and 68% of elderly individuals treated for alcohol problems were late-onset drinkers.

In terms of gender issues, problems with drugs other than alcohol tend to be more common in women, those who live alone, those who had a greater number of physical illnesses, and those who took multiple prescription drugs simultaneously. In contrast to men, older women who have problems with alcohol are more often widowed. Women are more likely to consult physicians and receive prescriptions for psychoactive drugs and more likely to experience problems with prescribed psychoactive agents than men. Further, women are more likely to request drugs for treatment of intrapsychic problems, whereas men are more likely to request them for what are described as social problems.

Some speculate that without intervention, the incidence of late-life onset substance-related problems will increase as the population ages and advancing medical technology prolongs the average life span. While younger individuals normally experience some "maturing out" from substance use problems, the biological, psychological, and social aspects of aging are suggested to offer a plausible "maturing in" process to problems. Essentially, where the unique and novel challenges of late life combine with increased access to prescription medications and increased potency of substances secondary to physiological changes that accompany the aging process, a new set of contingencies may cause an increased incidence of substance-related disorders among elderly individuals.

Treatment Issues

Underestimation of substance-related disorders and inappropriate screening techniques may be causes for low numbers of elderly entering treatment. Factors such as inability to pay for treatment and meager social support may also "hide" elderly individuals affected by substance use problems.

A potential complication for treatment is cognitive impairment, such as problems with learning and remembering new information. It may render patients unable to fully utilize treatment that requires higher-order cognitive functioning, resulting in poor prognosis for recovery. As such, assessment of cognitive functioning is important for treatment planning, and treatments to enhance cognitive functioning are highly valuable. In the case of dementia, when cognitive functioning is unlikely to improve, intervention strategies tailored to the abilities of the person with dementia are required. In many cases, it may also be appropriate for treatment to include the use of pharmacological agents. Issues related to comorbidity (e.g., the coexistence of an alcohol problem and an anxiety problem) may require the use of such medications.

Treatment programs for elderly populations must take into account specific issues associated with aging. Programs should consider more time for recovery as well as treatment for comorbid psychiatric and physical health disorders. In terms of group-based treatments, homogeneity of group members is valuable and should be utilized whenever possible. Age-specific groups designated to treat older individuals also can cater to issues associated with elder populations, such as isolation and depression, while emphasizing socialization and support.

There are also practical issues that may remedy problems related to elder prescription misuse. Helping elders develop a routine of how and when to take medication may be useful, along with written instructions. Use of monitoring systems to count pills to stay on track may also be helpful, as is working to overcome labeling deficiencies to decrease compliance problems among elderly individuals with impaired vision. Often, labels on prescriptions are crowded with information that is printed in exceedingly small font and is quite condensed (this is particularly true for over-the-counter medications). So enlisting the help of pharmacists to provide more appropriately presented information may be a useful strategy to aid the elderly.

Kristina Wood and Nancy A. Piotrowski

See also Diagnostic and Statistical Manual for Mental Disorders; Prescription Drugs; Special Populations; Substance-Induced Disorders; Substance Use Disorders

Further Readings

Barry, K. L., Oslin, D. W., & Blow, F. C. (2001). *Alcohol problems in older adults: Prevention and management.* New York: Springer.

Colleran, C., & Jay, D. (2002). *Aging and addiction: Helping older adults overcome alcohol or medication dependence.* Center City, MN: Hazelden.

Colliver, J. D., Compton, W. M., Gfroerer, J. C., & Condon, T. (2006). Projecting drug use among aging baby boomers in 2020. *Annals of Epidemiology, 16,* 257–265.

Gurnack, A. M. (1997). *Older adults misuse of alcohol, medicines, and other drugs: Research and practice issues.* New York: Springer.

Simoni-Wastila, L., Zuckerman, I. H., Singhal, P. K., Briesacher, B., & Hsu, V. D. (2006). National estimates of exposure to prescription drugs with addiction potential in community dwelling elders. *Substance Abuse, 26,* 33–42.

ELECTRONIC HEALTH RECORDS

Health informatics is the investigation and application of computing and other information technology (IT) to health care, health education, and biomedical research. Primary uses of IT in providing health care are customized software designed for practice management; services integration through the use of regional computer networks for client referrals and provider communications; direct provision of services on computers in the form of interactive interventions for clients; providing information via Web sites or e-mails; and business management of, and quality assurance for, treatment modalities.

A key link in many of these IT applications in health care is the electronic health record (EHR), an extension of the electronic medical record out of the hospital or medical practice into the wider community health care environment where most substance abuse treatment occurs. The client health record is central to electronic practice management, referral networks, and quality assurance. The role of EHR in quality assurance is highlighted in the 1999 report issued by the Institute of Medicine estimating that up to 100,000 Americans die each year as a result of medical errors, more than of

breast cancer or of motor vehicle accidents. One in every five of those fatal errors results from a lack of immediate access to patient health information.

The U.S. health care industry has been late in adopting IT compared to other economic sectors in the United States and compared to health care providers in other industrialized countries. For example, U.S. financial and banking services typically spend 5% to 6% of revenues on IT, whereas health care organizations spend 3% to 4%. Denmark provides universal health care to its citizens with most of their health information kept in a single system that can be accessed and updated by an individual's primary care doctor and other medical professionals. Despite a late start, U.S. spending on health care IT now exceeds $30 billion annually, and IT has achieved clear priority status in health care policy throughout all levels of government and in health care organizations.

Implementation of EHRs for clients receiving treatment for addiction entails several barriers beyond those that have slowed implementation in other areas of health:

1. The legal and regulatory environment for substance abuse services is more restrictive and complex.

2. Due to the social disapproval of substance abuse, confidentiality and security of health records are particularly critical.

3. Most substance abuse treatment is provided outside the main system of medical care.

4. Substance abuse is comorbid with mental and physical health problems as well as social problems, including homelessness, unemployment, interpersonal violence, and incarceration.

5. Many substance abuse clients as well as providers are on the wrong side of the "digital divide."

In terms of the regulatory environment, EHR for substance abuse clients requires significant additional efforts in terms of the Health Insurance Portability and Accountability Act (HIPAA) requirements, information security, client management regulations and procedures, mandatory reporting, and interface with the criminal justice system. The information that an individual is in treatment for addiction can affect employment, insurance, housing, social relationships, and other aspects of that individual's personal well-being beyond the addiction itself. Therefore, confidentiality is a paramount concern for clients who risk significant life losses if their addiction becomes known to people important in their lives.

Most substance abuse treatment occurs in dedicated community-based clinics or residential treatment facilities rather than in mainstream physician private practice or hospital-based care. Resources available to the mainstream health care system, such as health insurance, private philanthropy, and recruitment and training of personnel in major universities and medical centers, are much less available to substance abuse treatment providers. Lack of funds is the primary reason given for low levels of IT development.

People who live with addictions are frequently dually diagnosed with a serious mental illness. Others suffer from physical complications of the substance abuse, such as HIV or liver disease. These particular comorbidities are just as challenging as the substance abuse treatment itself in terms of confidentiality, out-of-mainstream care systems, and lack of financial resources. Social problems or "wreckage" from the substance abuse, such as unemployment, poverty, violence, and incarceration, also complicate the process of keeping track of clients and maintaining complete and accurate records.

The "digital divide" refers to differential access to computer technologies due to socioeconomic disadvantage. Because substance abuse treatment facilities frequently serve homeless men and women and racial or ethnic minorities, many clients and many providers are on the side of the digital divide that has less access to computers and related IT.

Despite multiple barriers to use of EHRs and other health computer applications, substance abuse treatment providers have succeeded in adopting IT at various levels of government and local organization. A few examples suggest the variety in both the nature and scope of the applications. Applications that circulate EHRs on a regional computer network to integrate services that include substance abuse treatment include (a) a network of homeless services in Boston and (b) a 17-agency network of HIV/AIDS care providers who integrated methadone maintenance, residential drug treatment, substance abuse case management, and a prison transition facility providing both mental health and substance abuse treatment into an electronic referral network of comprehensive HIV care in northern Los Angeles County. The Texas Department of State Health Services introduced a statewide Web-based application for addiction treatment that includes EHR and received the 2006 award from the Healthcare

Information and Management Systems Society for excellence in the public health category. The state of Tennessee tracks substance abuse treatment patients in a state-level database. The Vancouver Island Health Authority was the first health care organization in Canada to use EHRs to improve care for people with addictions and mental health problems.

Judith Resell

See also Business Improvement Practices; Confidentiality; Healthcare System and Substance Abuse; Health Insurance Portability and Accountability Act

Further Readings

Chang, B., Bakker, S., Brown, S. S., Houston, T. K., Kreps, G., Kukafka, R., et al. (2004). Bridging the digital divide: Reaching vulnerable populations. *Journal of the American Medical Informatics Association, 11,* 448–487.

Gaylin, D., Goldman, S., Ketchel, A., & Moiduddin, A. (2005). *Community health center information systems assessment: Issues and opportunities.* Chicago: National Opinion Research Center.

Henrickson, M., & Mayo, J. (2000). The HIV cybermall: A regional cybernetwork of HIV services. *Journal of Information Technology in Human Services, 17,* 7–26.

EMPIRICALLY BASED PREVENTION

See EVIDENCE-BASED PREVENTION

EMPIRICALLY BASED TREATMENT

See EVIDENCE-BASED TREATMENT

EMPLOYEE ASSISTANCE PROGRAM

Employee assistance programs (EAPs) are among several policy-based activities that address alcohol and drug abuse in the workplace. At present, EAPs are singular in that they are designed to provide constructive assistance to personnel with such problems and also to encourage job retention rather than detection and punishment as is the case with other policies.

The basic form of EAPs emerged from industrial alcoholism programs, the latter dating back to the early

1940s. Industrial alcoholism programs endeavored to introduce employees with alcohol dependence to Alcoholics Anonymous (AA). Company employees who had become affiliated with AA outside their employment were often instrumental in initiating or staffing these programs. Nearly all of these early programs were based in company medical departments and supervised by company physicians.

Upon the founding of the National Institute on Alcohol Abuse and Alcoholism in 1970, the workplace became a key target for its sponsored intervention projects and for some of its funded research. During the 1970s, the industrial alcoholism model was transformed to a broader-based EAP model, a change that eventually led to EAPs' diffusing widely in the United States and being adopted internationally. While the focus of EAPs on many workplace problems has increased their attractiveness, it has at the same time deflected many of them from devoting adequate resources to address workplace substance abuse problems. Nonetheless, their identity with substance abuse intervention remains significant.

Within a workplace, an EAP should have two main components: (1) access to qualified personnel who can implement the specific techniques of EAP intervention (i.e., identification, intervention, motivation, referral, and follow-up) and (2) written policies and procedures whereby the core techniques of EAP work are integrated with the workplace such that employees and supervisors will utilize program services when appropriate.

Such service provision varies considerably. In most worksites, access to assistance is provided by an external contracted organization. Such contracts vary greatly in their scope of services and in the managerial control that the contracting worksite exercises over the provider. In other, but increasingly rare instances, fully staffed EAP units are incorporated into the worksite's human resource management or medical function.

EAPs are found in nearly 60% of American workplaces, with their presence directly correlated with workplace size. Thus, on a nationwide basis, EAPs offer a clear potential for addressing employee substance abuse problems. This is, however, a potential that may not be achieved without a concerted effort to overcome the natural barriers to managing substance abuse when there are abundant opportunities to focus attention elsewhere.

Identification and referral to an EAP can occur through supervisory documentation of deteriorated job performance or through self-referral. Evidence from many sources indicates that self-referrals dominate caseloads, accounting for up to 90% of those who use EAP services. After entry into the program, it is the task of the designated EAP coordinator to identify the nature of the presenting problem or to send the individual to a qualified diagnostic facility. The coordinator needs to perform basic screening, for it is critical to determine whether (a) the employee's per-formance difficulties reflect an underlying behavior problem (such as substance abuse) that fits or approximates a diagnostic category, (b) the performance difficulties are an outcome of a poor fit between abilities and job demands, or (c) the referral is a consequence of underlying interpersonal conflicts or work-group politics. Thus, along with clinical expertise, workplace familiarity and knowledge of organizational behavior are critical for the effective performance of EAP coordinator roles.

After the problem is identified, the EAP coordinator links the individual with the intervention that is most appropriate for managing the problem. At this juncture, critical ingredients are the coordinator's knowledge of community resources, insurance coverage, and whether the employee can be absent from work to undergo treatment. The EAP coordinator then functions as a case manager from this point on.

It is evident that this approach maximizes the extent to which the problem is dealt with by appropriate professional resources. This once was how most EAP cases were handled. However, under norms that have emerged over the past decade in response to managed care, EAP coordinators try to minimize external referrals. Instead, they offer a limited number of counseling sessions with the expectation that these will result in a resolution of the problem. This approach may be a reasonable adaptation in the face of limits on the use of behavioral health services imposed by managed care.

Despite some suggestive case studies, there are no studies with acceptable scientific designs that have assessed the efficacy of short-term counseling provided directly by EAP counselors. Several questions are of interest. First, what is the extent to which such counseling addresses substance abuse problems, and under what conditions does it lead to problem resolution? The notable impact of such brief interventions in other settings suggests potential efficacy for work-based brief interventions, but more recent data are less promising. A second issue concerns external referrals.

At what point in the brief counseling process (particularly involving substance abusers) is a decision made to seek external assistance, and what is the role of the EAP counselor once such a referral is made? Again, no available research data address these questions.

Efficacy questions about EAPs cannot be answered as directly as one might expect. As has been described, EAPs can be used to address a wide variety of workplace issues that trouble employees, their supervisors, or both. EAPs are not publicly funded but rather funded by their sponsoring workplace. Thus, their goals are established internally, and effectiveness is relative to their workplace settings, their integration within these settings, and the extent to which the EAPs attract the investment of organizational resources. Whereas those outside the workplace can design models that produce different patterns of outcome and market these models to workplaces, the internal design cannot be imposed from outside. The same holds true for the utility of EAPs in addressing workplace substance abuse. If this is the employer's choice, then such an emphasis can be structured into EAP design by a qualified contractor, but it cannot be mandated.

EAPs continue to hold great potential for addressing substance abuse problems among both employed people and their dependents. The extent to which they are used in this manner has moved out of the public policy arena and into the realm of private decision making. Reversing the pattern will depend on a change in the ideological leadership that defines workplaces' social responsibilities to include helping their employees conserve their employment should they develop dependence on psychoactive substances.

Paul M. Roman

See also Brief Interventions; Confidentiality; Student Assistance Program; Workplace Drug Policies; Workplace Drug Use; Workplace Prevention

Further Readings

Blum, T. C., & Roman, P. M. (1995). *Cost effectiveness and preventive impact of employee assistance programs* (Center for Substance Abuse Prevention Monograph 5). Washington, DC: Department of Health and Human Services.

Hartwell, T. D., Steele, P. D., French, M. T., Potter, F. J., Rodman, N. F., & Zarkin, G. A. (1996). Aiding troubled employees: The prevalence, cost and characteristics of employee assistance programs in the United States. *American Journal of Public Health, 86,* 804–808.

Roman, P. M. (2002). Missing work: The decline in infrastructure and support for workplace alcohol intervention in the United States, with implications for developments in other nations In W. Miller & C. Weisner (Eds.), *Changing substance abuse through health and social systems* (pp. 197–210). New York: Kluwer/Plenum.

Sonnenstuhl, W. J., & Trice, H. M. (1986). *Strategies for employee assistance programs: The crucial balance.* Ithaca, NY: ILR Press.

Trice, H. M., & Roman, P. M. (1978). *Spirits and demons at work: Alcohol and other drugs on the job.* Ithaca, NY: ILR Press.

Zhang, Z., Huang, L., & Brittingham, A. M. (1999). *Worker drug use and workplace policies and programs: Results from the 1994 and 1997 NHSDA.* Washington, DC: Substance Abuse and Mental Health Services Administration, Office of Applied Studies.

ENABLING

Although substance abuse often has substantial physical, social, and psychological effects on individuals who engage in this behavior, alcoholism and drug addiction also have significant effects on the families of those individuals. Family members of substance abusers frequently experience emotional distress, financial strain, and relationship problems as the result of their association with an alcohol or drug abuser.

A focus of research in this area has been the extent to which family members engage in enabling behavior. Enabling behaviors have been defined as learned behaviors that positively and negatively reinforce a loved one's drinking or substance use behavior. Enabling has also been described as naturally occurring attempts to cope with the stress of a loved one's addiction. Regardless of why these behaviors occur, enabling behaviors are actions that inadvertently perpetuate a loved one's continued alcohol or drug abuse. It is important to note that recent definitions of enabling differ from the traditional characterizations of family members of substance abusers as codependent. Individuals who engage in enabling behavior are no longer considered to be active contributors (i.e., a cause) of the user's substance abuse.

Family Members of Alcohol and Drug Abusers

Although partners, parents, children, friends, and coworkers often are impacted by a family member or colleague's addiction, the extant research is based heavily on spouses and partners of substance-abusing men. Therefore, this entry focuses on enabling behaviors among female partners of substance-abusing men. Common enabling behaviors include denying or minimizing the extent of the substance abuse; nagging, pleading, or threatening the substance abuser; making excuses for their partner's behavior, compensating for their partner's inability to perform household and family responsibilities; distancing or disengaging from the substance abuser; and isolating from other family members and support networks.

Spouses of substance-abusing men often engage in enabling behavior in an attempt to cope with or reduce their immediate stress; however, over time, enabling behaviors often reinforce the substance abuser's continued alcohol and drug use. For example, compensating for a partner's inability to perform a household chore may resolve an immediate problem but reinforce the substance abuser's lack of accountability. In turn, reduced family responsibility may serve to escalate the loved one's use of alcohol or drugs. Compensating for the substance abuser may also result in task overload, anger, and resentment in the non-substance-abusing partner.

It is important to recognize that enabling behavior is not always unidirectional (from the non-substance-abusing spouse to the substance abuser). Rather, enabling is often a cycle from which both partners have difficulty escaping. For instance, if the non-abusing partner discontinues an enabling behavior (e.g., buying alcohol for their partner), relationship problems may escalate. In some cases, the non-abusing partner may choose to continue or resume enabling behavior to avoid conflict with the substance-abusing partner and reduce any additional stress in the family system. In other cases, the non-substance-abusing partner may be reluctant to discontinue enabling behaviors because family routines may have to change. For instance, the couple may no longer be able to attend family functions or parties where alcohol is served. Enabling behavior may occur despite the non-substance-abusing partner's awareness of their behaviors and recommendations by mental health professionals and others that they discontinue these types of behaviors.

Assessment of Enabling Behaviors

A number of questionnaires are available for assessing enabling behavior. These include the Enabling Behavior Inventory (EBI), developed by Dittrich and Trapold; the Spouse Enabling Inventory (SEI), developed by Thomas and colleagues; the Significant Other Behavior Questionnaire (SBQ), developed by Love and colleagues; and the Behavioral Enabling Scale (BES), developed by Rotunda.

The EBI asks partners to rate 90 enabling behaviors (e.g., "Helped conceal your spouse's drinking or drug use from business associates"). Similarly, the SEI asks individuals to rate the degree to which they engage in ineffective strategies with the alcohol abuser (e.g., "How many times have you avoided social contact with the extended family to cover up his drinking?"). The SBQ requests that partners rate the extent to which they exhibit the following categories of behaviors: withdrawing from the alcohol-abusing loved one when they are drinking, punishing the alcohol abuser for drinking, supporting the drinking, or supporting sobriety. The BES has partners rate their behaviors toward and beliefs about their substance-abusing loved one (e.g., "I assured my partner that his/her drug use wasn't that bad").

It is important to recognize that most enabling measures were designed for spouses and partners of alcohol or drug abusers. Although understanding the nature and frequency of enabling responses among spouses is essential, it is critically important to examine enabling behavior among parents, children, friends, and coworkers affected by substance abuse. Whether the existing measures of enabling can be adapted for use with extended family members, friends, and coworkers is not known. Moreover, additional validity information is needed on these instruments, as well as studies that reveal the unique and overlapping information provided by these instruments.

Treatment for Family Members

Although the importance of family support for abstinence is well established, drug and alcohol abusers remain a large but relatively untreated population. Interventions that exist for those affected by a loved one's substance abuse frequently focus on helping the spouse engage the substance abuser in treatment and teaching the partner to decrease his or her enabling behaviors, rather than dealing with the psychological needs of these individuals.

The forms of treatment available for family members and significant others of substance abusers include, but are not limited to, the community reinforcement technique, ARISE intervention (i.e., A Relational Intervention Sequence for Engagement), community reinforcement and family training, unilateral family therapy, network therapy, pressures to change procedure, and the Johnson intervention.

Although the specific treatments differ by program, each of these programs focuses on teaching the family member strategies to engage the substance abuser in treatment. For instance, under the community reinforcement technique, family members are taught communication techniques and participate in role-playing situations in which they confront the substance abuser about the addiction. Family members also are taught how to employ nonconfrontational responses (e.g., no threatening) when faced with substance-related relationship stresses. These programs also educate family members about substance abuse. Family members often benefit from forming a social alliance with professionals and others who are concerned about their loved one's addiction. Specific benefits of these programs for family members include reductions in enabling behaviors, less stress and anxiety, and fewer depressive symptoms. Although these programs were generally devised for spouses, they have benefits for others. For instance, the community reinforcement technique has demonstrated effectiveness for nonspouses, particularly when combined with aftercare support for the family member.

Although these programs show promising outcomes for the family members of alcohol and drug abusers (e.g., reductions in enabling, depressive symptoms, and anxiety), they tend to be expensive and not widely available. Moreover, many programs tend to focus on the substance abuser, rather than the significant others affected by the substance abuse.

In contrast to the previously mentioned programs, Al-Anon, Nar-Anon, Alateen, and Adult Children of Alcoholics are widely available open groups that focus on friends and family of substance abusers. Those affected by addiction typically attend weekly group sessions that emphasize the traditional Twelve-Step model philosophy and reliance on a higher power. Family members and friends of substance abusers are encouraged to network with other members experiencing similar stress and recognize their

powerlessness in changing the loved one's alcohol or substance abuse behavior. Goals for recovery include recognition of enabling behaviors, detachment from the problems of the drug or alcohol user, and improvement in the family member's personal feelings of self-esteem and adjustment. Participation in Al-Anon has demonstrated benefit in terms of greater happiness, improved coping, higher family cohesion, and relationship satisfaction.

Recently, standardized programs have been developed to aid primary health care professionals in counseling family members of addicted loved ones. One such program, developed by Copello and colleagues is the 5-Step approach. This program was designed to help affected family members cope with the stress of a substance-dependent loved one. Individuals are given a 58-page self-help manual and meet 4 times with a primary health care professional, health visitor, or practicing nurse. The manual comprises five steps: listening nonjudgmentally, educating about drugs or dependence, counseling on adaptive ways to cope, increasing social support, and considering further options for health and support. Exercises and case examples are also provided throughout the text. Both the full and brief versions of this program have demonstrated effectiveness in terms of reductions in tolerant coping (i.e., one form of enabling) and improvements in anxiety and depression.

Another intervention available to family members and friends in health care settings is the "empowering family members and friends via primary health approach." This approach is characterized by four main goals: listening in an objective manner, providing educational information on the nature of substance abuse and coping, counseling about coping strategies, and encouraging support within the family.

Conclusion

Although enabling behavior has been well established, particularly among female partners of alcohol-abusing men, much less research has examined enabling behavior among male partners of alcohol or drug-abusing women or gay and lesbian partners of substance abusers. In addition, far fewer investigations have examined enabling behavior among extended family members (e.g., parents, children, other relatives) or friends and coworkers of alcohol and drug abusers. It is plausible that enabling behavior and the consequences of such behavior may differ as a function of the specific type of relationship one has or the form of the substance abuse. To understand these differences and derive acceptable measures of enabling behavior, qualitative research with different groups affected by substance abuse may be necessary.

Although a number of programs have been developed to address the needs of partners of substance-abusing men, the effectiveness of structured treatment programs have received modest empirical information. For instance, promising treatments have been designed to facilitate primary health care providers' ability to treat their patients affected by a loved one's substance abuser. Clearly, research is needed that examines the effectiveness of programs offered by primary health care providers. Programs such as Al-Anon and Nar-Anon are widely available, are open to nonfamily members, are continuous, and have nonstop admission. Although these programs may benefit many individuals, the effectiveness of these programs for nonfamily members is less well understood. Moreover, to date, few studies have examined how Al-Anon and Nar-Anon work or what the long-term outcomes are for program participants and their substance-abusing loved ones.

In addition, it is important to identify individuals that may benefit from different treatment modalities. For instance, some programs ask friends and family affected by substance abuse to study psychoeducational manuals or initiate program attendance in nonstructured groups. Although many individuals benefit from these types of treatment modalities, identification of those who may profit from more structured programs or individual treatment is important. Related to this, research is needed to assess how the mental health of the family member (e.g., depression, anxiety), family environment (e.g., family cohesiveness), and personal characteristics (e.g., readiness for change, level of education) may be associated with success in various treatment modalities. At present, little work has attempted to identify whether different treatment modalities may benefit some individuals or some groups more than others. Clearly, a better understanding of the nature of enabling behavior among various groups and the unique characteristics associated with enabling behavior is an important goal for future research.

Amanda Jeffrey Platter and Michelle L. Kelley

See also Adult Children of Alcoholics; Al-Anon; Codependency; Community Reinforcement and Family Training; Family Therapy

Further Readings

Ablon, J. (1982). Support system dynamics of Al-Anon and Alateen. In E. M. Pattison & E. Kaufman (Eds.), *Encyclopedic handbook of alcoholism* (pp. 987–995). New York: Gardner Press.

Barber, J. G., & Crisp, B. R. (1995). The pressures to change approach to working with the partners of heavy drinkers. *Addiction, 90,* 269–276.

Dittrich, J. E., & Trapold, M. A. (1984). A treatment program for wives of alcoholics: An evaluation. *Bulletin of the Society of Psychologists in Addictive Behaviors, 3,* 91–102.

Fernandez, A. C., Begley, E. A., & Marlatt, G. A. (2006). Family and peer interventions for adults: Past approaches and future directions. *Psychology of Addictive Behaviors, 20,* 207–213.

Love, C. T., Longabaugh, R., Clifford, P. R., Beattie, M., & Peaslee, C. F. (1993). The Significant-Other Behavior Questionnaire (SBQ): An instrument for measuring the behavior of significant others toward a person's drinking and abstinence. *Addiction, 88,* 1267–1279.

Meyers, R. J., Miller, W. R., Smith, J. E., & Tonigan, J. S. (2002). A randomized trial of two methods for engaging treatment-refusing drug users through concerned significant others. *Journal of Consulting and Clinical Psychology, 70,* 1182–1185.

Orford, J. (1994). Empowering family and friends: A new approach to the secondary prevention of addiction. *Drug and Alcohol Review, 13,* 417–429.

Orford, J., Templeton, L., Patel, A., Copello, A., & Velleman, R. (2007). The 5-step family intervention in primary care: Strengths and limitations according to family members. *Drugs: Education, Prevention and Policy, 14,* 29–47.

Rotunda, R. J., West, L., & O'Farrell, T. J. (2004). Enabling behavior in a clinical sample of alcohol dependent clients and their partners. *Journal of Substance Abuse Treatment, 26,* 269–276.

Yoshioka, M., Thomas, E., & Ager, R. (1992). Nagging and other drinking control efforts of spouses of uncooperative alcohol abusers: Assessment and modification. *Journal of Substance Abuse, 4,* 309–318.

ENVIRONMENTAL APPROACHES

People make decisions about using mind-altering or mood-altering substances in the context of environments which may incite, ignore, or enable their behavior and in the context of environments which may prevent, discourage, or sanction their behavior. These environmental influences may occur in the surroundings closest to the individual, such as family, school, or faith community. Or, they may occur in the broader societal context, including the physical, economic, social, and political aspects of culture. Environmental approaches to prevention view substance abuse as a systemic issue and follow the public health model, which seeks to reduce the risk and harm for all people rather than for specific individuals or subgroups. Therefore, environmental strategies for the prevention of alcohol problems, tobacco use, and illicit drug involvement do not act directly on individuals, groups, or families. Rather, they target (a) the norms of the communities in which they live, (b) the rules and regulations of the social institutions to which they belong, and (c) the availability of alcohol, tobacco, and illicit drugs.

Norms, regulations, and availability do not act independently of each other. For example, the norms may impact which laws get created or enforced, the laws may determine how available a substance is to the community, and availability may influence the community norms regarding what is acceptable. Although this complex interrelationship is acknowledged, each concept is addressed separately in this entry for ease of discussion.

Norms

Norms are the unwritten, but generally agreed upon, notions a group or community has about what is an acceptable attitude or behavior, regardless of what the written laws or regulations stipulate. In the practice of substance abuse prevention, these norms often express themselves in the answers to such questions as the following: Is it all right for minors to drink if they are under the supervision of an adult? Is it an acceptable "right of passage" for youth to have unsupervised parties at which alcohol is available? Should athletes, politicians, or other high profile community members be provided the same treatment or sanctions as others for alcohol and other drug violations? Are there circumstances under which it is tolerable for law enforcement to confiscate open alcohol containers found in moving vehicles and not cite the drivers?

Community norms can be created or changed through such strategies as community organizing and coalition development, public education, media campaigns, social norms marketing, and policy change. The purpose of community mobilization is to bring the power of community leaders and stakeholders to bear on the problem at hand through such interventions as advocating for change in local public policies and in the

practices of major community institutions, such as law enforcement, licensing departments, community events, civic groups, churches and synagogues, schools, and local mass media. Public education about the prevalence, incidence, and consequences of a problem behavior can increase the community's readiness and motivation to change. Media campaigns (television, radio, or print) may be used to disseminate information and attempt to change attitudes. For example, social norms marketing is one form of public education using the media. It attempts to correct people's (often students') tendencies to overestimate the alcohol consumption of peers by providing current use data, thereby reducing perceived peer pressure to drink. Media advocacy is also a tool used in advancing environmental strategies. Community groups can use media advocacy to communicate statistics or anecdotal information for the purpose of influencing or evaluating changes in the tax laws, school rules, industry promotional practices, or community norms associated with the problem behavior of concern. The goal of media advocacy is not media coverage but a change in norms, laws, or policies.

Regulations

The term *regulations* refers to all written guidelines, including federal, state, and local laws; school rules; and organizational policies. Some important aspects of effective regulations, in addition to their actual existence and content, are whether (a) they are enforced, (b) they contain sufficient sanctions to deter behavior, and (c) people are aware of the laws and the consequences. Lack of enforcement may occur for many reasons. It may be that the law does not match the norms in the community or that some other barrier exists to enforcing the law. For example, a police officer may be reluctant to cite an underage drinking driver if the officer must travel out of the area to deliver the youth to a crisis residential center, which would entail the officer being out of his or her jurisdiction for the balance of the shift, leaving some rural districts without law enforcement during those hours. Another challenge to the effectiveness of regulations is that, although they may be in concert with the norms of the community, they may not have sufficient sanctions attached to have an effect on community behavior. For example, if a driving under the influence (DUI) law is instituted involving a relatively minor fine and no other significant consequence, treatment option, or rehabilitation effort, DUI rates would not be expected to go down when the law is put in place. One of the most effective prevention strategies for law enforcement is to combine sufficient sanctions and a media campaign informing the public regarding the enforcement effort and potential consequences of getting caught.

Table 1 provides examples of regulations, also referred to as environmental policies, for alcohol, tobacco, and illicit drugs.

Availability

Availability refers to the retail, social, and economic accessibility of a substance. Retail availability can be measured in the density of vendors of the substance in the community, or it can refer to the likelihood of retail establishments selling to minors or overselling to adults (serving alcohol to inebriated patrons, e.g.).

Table 1   Examples of Environmental Policies for Alcohol, Tobacco, and Illicit Drugs

Environmental Strategy	Alcohol	Tobacco	Illicit Drugs
Environmental policies to limit access			
Purchase laws	Minimum legal drinking age for purchasing and consuming alcohol	Youth access laws prohibiting retail sales of tobacco to minors	Laws prohibiting possession and use of illicit drugs
Price controls	Sales taxes; bans on drinking discounts and other price specials	Excise taxes; bans on rebates after purchase	Using supply reduction efforts to drive up drug prices
Restrictions on retail sales or sellers (number, location, density, days and hours of sale)	Ordinances establishing minimum distance between outlets and schools and churches	Limits on the number of tobacco vendor licenses	Civil actions to eliminate places where drugs are sold (e.g., drug house abatement); physical barriers to sales (gates, increased lighting)
Environmental policies to influence the culture and contexts of use			
Legal deterrence	Lower blood alcohol concentration for young drivers; administrative license revocation for driving under the influence	Fines for selling tobacco to minors; media advocacy efforts to increase vendors' perceptions of risk of apprehension	Use (drugs)–Lose (driver's license) laws for youth; workplace drug testing; asset forfeiture
Controls on advertising and promotion	Bans on alcohol sponsorship of sporting and cultural events; advertising restrictions	Surgeon general's warning on cigarette packs; restrictions on distribution of free samples and coupons	Public service announcements regarding hazards associated with drug use
Environmental policies to reduce negative consequences of use			
Measures that reduce consequences of excessive use	Safe rides for intoxicated patrons; nonbreakable drinking glassware	Designated nonsmoking areas to reduce nonsmokers' exposure to secondary smoke	Distribution of bleach for disinfecting drug paraphernalia
Substitution of less-damaging products	Low-alcohol beer	Low-tar and self-extinguishing cigarettes	Methadone maintenance

Source: Stewart, K. G., & Carmona, M. G. (2006). *Environmental prevention strategies: Evidence of effectiveness.* Retrieved March 18, 2007, from http://wch.uhs.wisc.edu/docs/SIG/fisher-EnvironmentalPreventionStrategies.pdf

Retail availability can be reduced by such environmental strategies as zoning changes, licensing control, and server training. Social access refers to the ease by which minors are able to attain a substance through family, friends, or other individuals. Examples of strategies that are used to reduce social access are public education regarding personal liability and sanctions for adults who provide alcohol to minors ("social host liability" laws) or media campaigns that educate parents as to the actual consumption levels of teens, which are consistently higher than parents estimate. Economic availability is based on the tenet that as price rises, purchases (and, therefore, consumption) go down, and, as price is reduced, purchases increase. Therefore, an effective strategy to reduce alcohol consumption, for instance, is to successfully lobby to create a law increasing the tax on beer.

In addition to actual availability, perceived availability is also a risk factor for use, as when students think "everyone is drinking," but data show that to be far from the truth. If students in one school perceive that alcohol is easily attainable, they will be more likely to drink than will students in another school in which the students perceive alcohol is less easily attainable, even when actual availability in the two schools is exactly the same. This is a similar logic as that behind social norms marketing. It attempts to change the perception of the availability of, or numbers of people using, drugs or alcohol to a lower, more accurate level in order to reduce the actual level of consumption.

Advantages and Disadvantages

Environmental approaches have several potential advantages. First, they typically reach entire populations compared to the handful of persons targeted by individually focused prevention strategies. For example, training convenience store clerks to check identifications reduces the availability of tobacco for all neighborhood youth. Second, strategies aimed at the shared environment often produce more rapid results than do strategies aimed at individual environments. For example, increases in alcohol prices can produce more or less immediate reductions in youth alcohol use. Third, shared environment strategies may produce larger reductions in substance use. For example, according to the National Highway Traffic Safety Administration, over a 20-year period, an estimated 17,000 lives were saved in impaired driving highway crashes alone by raising the minimum age for alcohol purchase to 21. Fourth, environmental approaches may have more enduring effects, because they are built into the systems of the culture, which are less prone to rapid change. Fifth, environmental strategies are often easier to maintain and more cost-effective, in part because they change the system or culture and do not need to be so intensively repeated with each cohort of youth.

Potential disadvantages of using environment approaches also exist. One difficulty is that it may take longer to accumulate data showing community-level results (e.g., savings in highway deaths over several years) than to show program-level outcomes (e.g., behavior change for a cohort of people attending a parenting class). In addition, strong popular resistance may be generated among community members, especially youth and alcohol- or tobacco-related businesses, when challenging existing norms, laws, and availability issues.

Conclusion

A comprehensive approach to prevention should include strategies that target both the surroundings closest to the individual (such as school and family) and the larger shared physical, economic, social, and political environment (further defined as community norms, regulations, and availability of the substance). Because environmental strategies target the powerfully influential context in which individuals make decisions about their involvement in substance abuse, environmental strategies are a promising complement to programs and other approaches that target individuals and their most immediate surroundings. However, attempting to change the larger community system may also result in potential barriers to change: resistance from within the system and longer and sometimes more challenging data collection efforts.

Table 2 notes the prevention effects known to date of some categories of environmental strategies.

However, conclusive evidence is lacking as to the efficacy of many environmental strategies. For example, current research is insufficient to determine the effectiveness of such strategies as the prohibition of consumption in public places, social norms campaigns, restrictions on locations of outlets, counteradvertising, media advocacy, laws against adult provision, and teen party ordinances. Further, more research would be helpful in determining the efficacy of environmental approaches in a variety of racial and ethnic communities.

Andrea L. S. Dugan

Table 2 The Prevention Effects of Environmental Strategies

Environmental Strategy	Sales/Use	Traffic Crashes	DWI	Violent Crime[1]	Suicide	Long-Term Health Consequences[2]
Price controls	X	X	X	X[3]	X	X
Density restrictions	X	X		X	X	X
Minimum purchase age laws	X	X		X[4]	X	
Impaired driving laws		X	X			
Restrictions on use	X					
Selling or serving controls		X	X			
Counteradvertising	X[5]					

Source: Stewart, K. G., & Carmona, M. G. (2006). *Environmental prevention strategies: Evidence of effectiveness.* Retrieved March 18, 2007, from http://wch.uhs.wisc.edu/docs/SIG/fisher-EnvironmentalPreventionStrategies.pdf

1. Violent or assaultive offenses (i.e., rape, robbery, assault, and homicide)
2. Cancer or cirrhosis mortality
3. Rapes and robberies
4. Youth homicide
5. Effects for tobacco only

See also National Media Campaign; Public Policy, Alcohol; Public Policy, Drugs; Public Policy, Prevention; Social Norms Marketing

Further Readings

Bonnie, R., & O'Connell, M. E. (Eds.). (2004). *Reducing underage drinking: A collective responsibility.* Washington, DC: National Academies Press.

Center of Substance Abuse Prevention, Northeast Center for the Application of Prevention Technologies. (n.d.). *Changing the larger environment: Critical components.* Retrieved May 18, 2007, from http://www.northeastcapt.org/products/critical/envicr/envicr.html

Fisher, D. A. (2006). *Environmental prevention strategies: An introduction and overview.* (pp. 1–3). Retrieved March 18, 2007, from http://wch.uhs.wisc.edu/docs/SIG/fisher-EnvironmentalPreventionStrategies.pdf

Holder, H. D. (1997). Prevention aimed at the environment. In B. S. McCrady & E. E. Epstein (Eds.), *Addictions: A comprehensive guidebook* (pp. 573–594). New York: Oxford University Press.

Imm, P., Chinman, M., Wandersman, A., Rosenbloom, D., Guckenburg, S., & Leis, R. (2007). *Preventing underage drinking: Using Getting to Outcomes™ with the SAMHSA strategic prevention framework to achieve results* (pp. 29–37). Santa Monica, CA: RAND. Retrieved July 30, 2007, from http://www.rand.org/pubs/technical_reports/2007/RAND_TR403.pdf

Klitzner, M. (1998). *Integrating environmental change theory into prevention practice.* Northeast CAPT Regional Summit: Environmental Strategies to Reduce Youth Substance Abuse, Providence, RI, December 2–3. Retrieved May 18, 2007, from http://wch.uhs.wisc.edu/docs/PDF-Pubs/envchangetheory.pdf

Stewart, K. G., & Carmona, M. G. (2006). *Environmental prevention strategies: Evidence of effectiveness* (pp. 4–9). Retrieved March 18, 2007, from http://wch.uhs.wisc.edu/docs/SIG/fisher-EnvironmentalPrevention Strategies.pdf

Treno, A. J., & Lee, J. P. (2002). Approaching alcohol problems through local environmental interventions. *Alcohol Research & Health, 26,* 35.

ETHICAL STANDARDS FOR ADDICTION PROFESSIONALS

Ethical standards are rules and guidelines for the behavior of professionals in the performance of their duties. Most behavioral health care professionals (addiction professionals, marriage and family therapists, professional counselors, social workers, and psychologists) have ethical standards as a part of their professional organizations. Knowledge of and adherence to these standards are usually requirements for certification or licensure by a state or by a national organization. For addiction professionals, NAADAC, the Association for Addiction Professionals, is the primary national professional organization for the field, and the organization has a code of ethics for members. However, addiction professionals who have certification or licensure in another discipline (e.g., social work, marriage and family therapy, professional counseling) may also be required to adhere to the ethical guidelines for this discipline as well.

Generally, there are no conflicts between the ethical standards for various mental health professional disciplines, but it is the responsibility of the clinician to be familiar with all ethical standards for their certification or licensure. In addition, state standards guide the professional practice for most addiction professionals, and any ethical guidelines for addiction counseling developed by states must be followed by state-certified or licensed addiction professionals.

Although the following information covers most of the ethical standards for addiction professionals, it is not meant to substitute for a thorough knowledge of the ethical standards governing the practice of addiction counseling in the state an addiction professional is certified or licensed.

Need for Ethical Standards

Certification and licensure ensure that professionals have a minimum set of knowledge and skills to competently practice. Ethical standards are established to help ensure that the behavior of professionals does not deviate from proscribed parameters. Therefore, the public should have a reasonable expectation that certified or licensed addiction professionals practice within these proscribed parameters. In addition, addiction professionals may be accused of unethical behavior. Ethical standards provide the guidelines to discipline (or not discipline) certified and licensed professionals accused of improper or inappropriate behavior by supervisors, peers, or the public.

Client Welfare

Mental and behavioral health care counselors should always act in the best interests of the client. Addiction professionals may not take any action that is in the self-interest of the counselor or someone other than the client (e.g., agency, parent, or intimate partner). For example, the addiction professional cannot recommend longer or more intensive treatment to make more money when such treatment is not justified. As another example, addiction professionals who like to hug should not hug clients who would interpret physical affection as an indication of romantic interest.

Just like all other helping professionals, addiction professionals are prohibited from discrimination based on age, gender, ethnic/racial background, sexual orientation, religious and political beliefs, socioeconomic status, or disability.

Addiction professionals must fully explain all recommendations for services in terms of approaches, strategies, expected length, involvement of others (e.g., parents, intimate partners, other family members), and fees.

Clients must provide informed consent for all of the services recommended, including fees. If a report to outside agencies or individuals is required, the client must give informed consent prior to the initiation of treatment. The nature of the report that will be submitted (i.e., simple participation in treatment or a report of diagnosis, progress, or both) must be disclosed. If a client is a minor or cannot give consent due to a disability, the addiction professional acts in the best interest of the client. This can mean refusing to treat a minor client who refuses to consent to treatment and the addiction professional believes that treatment is not in the client's best interest. Court-ordered clients who refuse to consent to treatment or refuse to consent to reports to the court should not be treated. The lack of consent can be reported to the court.

Prohibition of sexual relationships is the most common ethical violation. Yet it is least ambiguous of any ethical standard. Addiction professionals are prohibited from engaging in any type of romantic or sexual relationship with clients. It is irrelevant as to whether a sexual invitation was initiated by an adult client. The complete responsibility lies with the addiction professional to avoid a romantic or sexual relationship. Furthermore, addiction professionals should refrain from any type of physical contact that may be interpreted as sexual (e.g., excessive hugging, massage). Addiction professionals are prohibited from treating clients with whom they once had a sexual relationship. Most professional ethical standards have some guidance regarding romantic or sexual relationships with former clients. Generally, at least 2 years should pass between the termination of a professional relationship and the initiation of a personal relationship.

Addiction professionals should not treat anyone with whom they have a close personal or business relationship. This includes students or supervisees. In some cases, a dual relationship cannot be avoided. For example, without prior knowledge, a client in treatment shows up at the addiction professional's house one day to fix the roof. At the next opportunity, the issue should be discussed with the client and documented. The client should be given the option to seek treatment with someone else.

If a client is seeing another addiction professional, consent should be secured from the client to inform the other addiction professional of the treatment arrangement and to avoid duplication of services or conflicting treatment. Addiction professionals avoid enhancing their own status with a client at the expense of another professional. If an addiction professional believes that another professional is behaving unethically with a shared client, the addiction professional must take the appropriate action. (This is discussed further under "Professional Responsibilities.")

Addiction professionals must fully disclose all financial arrangements related to professional services, including any procedures and services that may be used to collect unpaid fees and the ramifications on continued treatment if fees are not paid. The financial status of the client must be considered before establishing fees and beginning services. Clients must be assisted with finding comparable services if they cannot afford the fees of the addiction professional. All professional ethics standards strongly discourage bartering (trading professional services for other goods or services), and most prohibit the practice.

If a conflict of interest occurs between the client and the addiction professional's employer, the addiction professional acts in the best interest of the client. For instance, an addiction professional works for a publicly supported agency. The agency wants to have as many clients as possible in group counseling to save money. The addiction professional has a client who is not ready or in need of group counseling but continues to need individual counseling. The addiction professional's ethical responsibility is to the client and the client's needs rather than to the needs of the agency. If the agency's policies (communicated to the client prior to the initiation of services) limit services (e.g., only five individual sessions), the addiction professional is

ethically responsible to refer the client to an agency or individual who can provide the needed services at a comparable cost to the client.

Addiction professionals terminate services when it is reasonably clear that the client is no longer benefiting from services, when services are no longer needed, when clients have not fulfilled agreed upon arrangements (e.g., payment of fees, arriving at sessions without using alcohol or other drugs), when services no longer meet the needs and interests of the client, or when there are agency or institutional restrictions on continuing services. In cases in which the client needs continued services, the addiction professional is responsible for making a referral to an agency or individual who can perform the needed services at a price the client can afford. Whenever possible, addiction professionals should attempt to secure the client's agreement with a decision to terminate and the reasons for doing so.

Addiction professionals do not initiate services or continue to provide services when the services are not beneficial to the client. Addiction professionals are responsible for being knowledgeable regarding referral sources and for attempting to ensure that clients are referred to an agency or individual who may be better able to provide beneficial services. Even if a client refuses a referral, addiction professionals should not provide services they believe are not benefiting the client.

Professional Competence and Scope of Practice

Except for inappropriate sexual relationships, the most common ethical violations involve addiction professionals who operate outside their professional competence or the scope of practice as defined by the state certification or licensure board. Professional competence refers to the knowledge, skills, and abilities acquired through formal education or other training (i.e., continuing education). Since scope of practice is defined by state certification and licensure rules and regulations, an addiction professional must not provide any service outside the scope of practice of their discipline *regardless* of training or experience. For example, a licensed addiction professional may be restricted by state statutes from diagnosing any condition other than a substance use disorder. So, regardless of how many courses in diagnosis the addiction professional has taken, he or she cannot diagnosis any other condition except substance use disorders.

Addiction professionals must fully disclose to prospective clients their formal educational training, degrees, licenses and certifications, and other training that qualifies them to provide services according to state laws, rules, and regulations. Any attempt to mislead the public about these qualifications is unethical. For example, most states do not recognize national certification in a discipline to be sufficient for state certification in that discipline. Therefore, an addiction professional would be acting unethically if he or she implied that he or she was authorized to provide addiction counseling services solely on the basis of certification by NAADAC, the Association for Addiction Professionals in a state requiring state certification.

Addiction professionals can only conduct assessment procedures for which they have been trained to conduct *and* are included in their scope of practice. This generally impacts individually administered screening and assessment instruments in the areas of intelligence, personality, interests, attitudes, and behavior (e.g., alcohol and other drug use). States differ in the assessment procedures allowed in the scope of practice for various disciplines, and the definitions can be ambiguous. Addiction professionals are strongly urged to ensure that they are qualified and allowed to administer assessment instruments before doing so. In one state, an agency was sanctioned for allowing certified drug and alcohol counselors to administer a self-report depression inventory because, in that state, only psychologists were allowed to administer personality tests.

Diagnosis is a similar situation to assessment. Again, states differ in diagnoses that are within the scope of practice of various disciplines. Drug and alcohol counselors may be allowed to diagnose substance use disorders but no other mental disorders. Addiction professionals are advised to limit diagnostic statements to those allowed in their scope of practice, for ethical reasons and to avoid liability.

Treatment is another area of concern. This may involve specific therapeutic approaches or strategies, including the provision of individual, group, couple, or family counseling or therapy. Whether or not the scope of practice of a discipline allows certain approaches (e.g., family therapy), an addiction professional uses only those strategies and approaches for which they have been trained. For clinical services, the training should involve supervision. Addiction professionals should not provide services to clients with diagnosed conditions they are not trained to treat. For many addiction professionals, this includes clients with co-occurring conditions. The field of co-occurring mental disorders has led to ethical issues in diagnosis and treatment. Many agencies that provide addiction treatment services are offering "dual diagnosis" programs for the many clients suffering from coexisting substance use disorders and other mental disorders such as post-traumatic stress disorder, depressive disorders, and anxiety disorders. Certified and licensed addiction professionals are almost always precluded from diagnosing and treating conditions other than substance use disorders. Therefore, for ethical practice, agencies must employ (as staff or consultants) licensed mental health professionals who are able, by scope of practice in their discipline, to diagnose and treat mental conditions other than substance use disorders. The level of involvement of the addiction professional in the treatment plan of clients with co-occurring substance use and other mental disorders may vary. However, a mental health professional who is qualified by training and state standards to diagnose and treat substance use disorders and other mental disorders should coordinate the treatment plan.

Addiction professionals are ethically obligated to (and usually required to) participate in continuing education activities, including courses, trainings, online training, and reading professional literature. In addition, addiction professionals must not imply in any advertising (e.g., yellow pages) that they are qualified to provide services beyond the ones they have been trained to provide *and* are within their scope of practice.

Confidentiality

This material is about the *ethics* of confidentiality. It should be noted that addiction professionals who provide diagnosis, treatment, or referrals to treatment for alcohol and other drug abuse and who receive any form of federal assistance (e.g., Medicaid or CHAMPUS) are bound by federal confidentiality law 42 CFR, Part 2. These regulations are complex, and an addiction professional should complete training on federal confidentiality law for alcohol and drug abuse clients if these services are provided.

A client's written consent is required to disclose any information regarding the client to third parties. Exceptions are discussed later in this entry. Only information that is relevant, necessary, and verifiable should ever be disclosed.

Before providing any services, addiction professionals must inform clients of their rights in regard to confidentiality, including circumstances in which an addiction professional must disclose confidential information without the client's written consent. Addiction professionals must tell clients about the limits of confidentiality in their state.

Addiction professionals must comply with all state and federal laws with regard to mandated reporting of suicidality, homicidality, child abuse and neglect, elder abuse and neglect, and abuse of people who are unable to protect themselves (i.e., severely disabled).

When a client is a danger to him- or herself or to others, or in cases of the abuse or neglect of minors, the elderly, or people unable to protect themselves (i.e., severely disabled), the addiction professional is obligated to report the client to the appropriate legal authority regardless of written consent by the client. The disclosure should be limited to the purpose of reporting. A court order (not a subpoena) normally requires disclosure without the written consent of the client. Of course, the legal representative for an addiction professional may appeal a court order. When a minor or a person who is not capable of providing informed consent is the client, the addiction professional considers the welfare of the client in all issues involving confidentiality.

It is the responsibility of the addiction professional to ensure that client records that contain personally identifiable information and confidential information are secure and only accessible to the addiction professional or other staff members who must have access to the records for the performance of their duties. This includes written records and computer files. Clients shall be informed of, and give written permission for, access to confidential information by staff members other than the addiction professional. Records should be destroyed when the information can no longer reasonably be expected to be useful to the client.

It is the responsibility of the addiction professional to fully discuss confidentiality with members of a counseling, therapy, or treatment group and to take all reasonable measures to ensure that the confidentiality of group members is protected. The addiction professional must also fully disclose limits to confidentiality.

Professional Responsibilities

Addiction professionals are responsible for maintaining records relating to services provided to clients and progress notes for continuing services provided. Documentation is expected to be objective and to be free of pejorative terms or slang. The professional opinion of the addiction professional is appropriate. From a review of the documentation, it should be possible for another addiction professional to determine what services have been provided, when they were provided, and what the outcomes of these services were.

An addiction professional should seek professional assistance for any personal issue that has the potential to interfere with their job duties. It is recommended that addiction professionals consult with professional colleagues to determine the need for professional assistance.

It is unethical for an addiction professional to provide or receive money or anything of value for referrals. It is also unethical for an addiction professional to encourage clients to see him or her for treatment when the addiction professional is engaged in an unrelated activity. For example, an addiction professional who is giving a lecture to a group should not solicit clients for a treatment program.

Addiction professionals are responsible for acting upon any unethical behavior they become aware of on the part of other addiction professionals. The action to be taken is dependent upon the ethical infraction and the policies of the agency or institution. Addiction professionals must use their professional judgment. Unethical behavior that is impacting the welfare of a client in an ongoing manner should be immediately reported to the offending addiction professional's supervisor, licensure board, or both. In matters not immediately affecting client welfare, it may be appropriate to initially discuss the matter with the addiction professional informally. However, an addiction professional should become familiar with agency or institutional policies regarding the unethical behavior of colleagues.

Conclusion

Ethical standards for addiction professionals are designed primarily to protect the public. Like the ethical standards for other mental health professionals, the requirements are generally common sense. However, situations do arise in which the proper ethical behavior is not clear. Addiction professionals have an obligation to consult with colleagues and supervisors to determine the ethical response in such cases.

Gary L. Fisher

See also Certification and Licensing; Clinical Supervision of Addiction Counselors; Confidentiality; Ethics; NAADAC, the Association for Addiction Professionals

Further Readings

NAADAC, the Association for Addiction Professionals. (2004). *NAADAC code of ethics*. Retrieved October 11, 2007, from http://naadac.org/documents/index.php? CategoryID=23

ETHICS

Ethics is defined as the rules or standards governing the conduct of a person or the conduct of the members of a profession. Developing and practicing ethics is an active process that continues from preservice education throughout the career of the addiction professional. Ethical issues have always been a central feature in addiction counseling, and more recently, with the trend among the states in moving from certification to licensure of addiction professionals, the issue of ethical practice takes on a more important role as the field is transformed. Addiction professionals encounter a variety of ethical dilemmas which create serious conflict among the professional duties and obligations of daily operations involving clinical practice. Moral issues greet professionals each morning from the perspective of society as reflected in the newspaper, on radio, and in conversations around the office. Addiction professionals are faced with ethical dilemmas on a daily basis during the practice of assessment, case planning, and management. Ethical issues fall into two categories: Macro ethics are those from a global or societal perspective, such as program design, policy, and administration, and micro ethics are those based on individual characteristics and conditions. This entry concentrates on models and approaches that will help practicing addiction professionals deal with ethical dilemmas.

Dealing with ethical issues is never without many perplexing questions that must be answered in the quest for a course of action that rests upon moral reason. Thinking through ethical issues appropriately will lead to the process of self-analysis within the context of the issue and the elements that are considered. It is truly the process of going through an ethical reasoning plan that is so valuable to the outcome and to the professional growth of the addictions practitioner.

Initiating the Ethical Inquiry

Beginning with the most obvious question that needs to be asked, "What are the facts to be considered?" gives the ethical inquiry wings. This first step in analyzing moral issues is not always easy. One of the reasons that moral issues create controversy is simply because all of the facts of the situation are not fully verified. This first step of gathering all of the facts, although obvious, is also among the most important and the most frequently overlooked step in the ethical decision-making process. Looking further, the practicing addiction professional must conclude that having the facts is insufficient in sorting through ethical dilemmas, because resolving an ethical issue typically requires one to review personal, cultural, and societal values, which may not be consistent. A typical example involves conflict between a client's right to confidentiality and the professional's duty to protect an individual that has been threatened by the client. Other examples may involve a decision about whether to accept a client's gift or a client's invitation to attend a wedding or some other social or religious event where boundaries or dual relationships threaten the professional association. Often clients in substance use counseling have violated not only their personal values but they also may have legal offenses that come to the forefront as recovery begins, and ethical issues abound in how the addiction professional guides the client in resolving the issues of concern. Addressing ethical issues of all kinds requires some type of consistency to navigate the uncertain ground of ethical dilemmas.

Consistency constitutes the lack of contradiction and serves as a guide for principled living. In what has become the major feature of ethics, consistency provides a moral living guide. The plan is that professionals learn to apply a consistent process that is unbound by contradiction and that has a rational foundation. When ethical principles and practices lack consistency, they also lack a sense of rationality, and it is rationality that must exist in the ethical decision-making process or there will remain a division in what action is taken and about how individuals live their lives. All societies and organizations have a consistent set of principles that are used to protect human rights and to measure actions that are valued as harmonious with the values of society. However, ethical guidelines cannot address all situations that a professional is forced to confront. Therefore, the professional must have a clear set of moral principles and values to guide actions.

Moral Principles

Karen Strohm Kitchener posits that there are five moral principles that contribute to moral development and that are viewed as the foundation of ethical guidelines. The five principles—autonomy, justice, beneficence, nonmaleficence, and fidelity—are absolute truths, and exploring any moral dilemma in relation to the principles leads to a more succinct understanding of the issues in conflict. These principles are essential for addiction professionals to apply to ethical dilemmas.

Autonomy is the principle that addresses the concept of independence of the client, and the fundamental nature of this principle is allowing an individual the freedom of choice and action. The principle of autonomy addresses the responsibility of the addiction professional to encourage clients, as fitting, to be consistent and to make their own decisions and to act on their own values. First, to be consistent with this principle, the professional assists clients to understand how their personal decision making and value system may have a disconnect with the values of society in general and may in fact infringe upon the rights of others. Secondly, the professional must assist clients to make both balanced and rational decisions, and when clients are incapable of making competent choices, they must be guided not to make decisions that might be harmful to themselves. This group includes those with mental handicaps and developmental disabilities, as well as individuals who may make rash decisions as they move through the recovery process.

Nonmaleficence is the concept of not causing harm to others (i.e., "Above all, do no harm.") This principle is critical and reflects the idea of not inflicting intentional harm and not engaging in actions that risk harming others. This includes such behaviors as working within the scope of practice, protecting confidentiality, and maintaining accurate recordkeeping.

Beneficence is the counterpart of nonmaleficence and is the notion that, in order to act ethically, the addiction professional must also "do some good" and is a based on the professional's responsibility to contribute to the welfare of the client in a general sense. This is one good reason for measurable data that come from the outcome of counseling. The professional counselor must be an advocate on behalf of the client to prevent harm to the extent that it is possible.

Justice is the notion that professionals must exercise reasonable judgment to ensure that any potential biases, competency limitations, and lack of experience do not engender any practices that may be unjust in relation to the client. Being just demands that when the addiction professional takes a different course of action with a particular client, there must be justification that clarifies the necessity of doing so.

Fidelity encompasses counselor loyalty, faithfulness, and honoring of commitments to the client. The concept of fidelity has to do with the intent of the professional to lay a foundation of trust for clients. It is imperative that clients have implicit trust in the counselor and have confidence in the therapeutic relationship if growth is to occur. The counselor is responsible for maintaining the therapeutic relationship by making sure that all obligations to the client are addressed.

Ethical Problem–Solving Approaches

When exploring an ethical dilemma, there is a need to examine the situation and see how each of these moral principles relates to the dilemma being examined, which may be enough to at least clarify the issues initially so that a resolution becomes more obvious. When situations are more complex, there is additional guidance based on philosophy that is instructive to addictions practitioners. These notions, rather than providing answers, give a basic set of approaches to ethical problem solving: utilitarianism, rights, fairness and justice, common good, and virtue.

The utilitarianism approach was conceived in the 19th century by Jeremy Bentham and John Stuart Mill in an attempt to assist legislators in the determination of choosing the morally appropriate laws. These authors state that truly ethical actions provide the greatest balance of good over evil, and the steps are as follows: (a) Identify the various courses of action available, (b) ask who will be affected by each action and what benefits or harms will be derived from each, and (c) choose the action that will produce the greatest benefits and the least harm. In this approach, the ethical action is the one that provides the greatest good for the greatest number.

The rights approach has its foundation in the work of those who focus on the rights of the individual to have freedom of choice. This approach takes the view that what makes humans different from animals is that people have dignity based on their ability to choose freely what they will do with their lives. The critical issue here is that humans have a fundamental moral right to have their choices respected, rather than to be treated as objects that are manipulated. It is a violation of human dignity to use people in ways they do not freely choose. Rights include the right to truth and to be informed about matters that significantly affect people's choices; the right of privacy, to have personal beliefs, and to express them so long as they do not violate the rights of others; the right not to be injured or harmed unless freely and knowingly choosing the risk or doing something to deserve punishment; the right to what is agreed and what has been promised by others in contracts or agreements. In this approach, the focus is to examine individual rights to see if the actions violate these rights. If so, then it is said the actions are morally wrong, and the more serious the violation of the rights is, the more wrongful is the action.

The fairness or justice approach to ethics comes from the teachings of the Greek philosopher Aristotle. It was Aristotle who initiated the concept that equals should be treated equally and unequals treated unequally. The moral questions examined in this approach are asking about the level of fairness or discrimination in each situation and pointing out that both are unjust and immoral as each of these positions imposes burdens on people. Favoritism gives benefits to some people without a justifiable reason for singling them out, and discrimination imposes burdens on those who are no different from those on whom burdens are not imposed.

The common good approach to ethics assumes that society is made up of individuals whose own good is inextricably linked to the good of the community. In this approach, community members are tied together by the search for values and goals that are universal. The common good approach is based on the writings of Plato, Aristotle, and Cicero. More recently, ethicists have defined this approach as being the general conditions that are equally to everyone's advantage. In this worldview, individuals are seen as members of the same community who reflect on broad questions concerning the type of society that is desired. While respecting and valuing the freedom of individuals to pursue their own goals, the common good approach challenges professionals to recognize and further those shared goals. The focus of this approach is

ensuring that social policies, social systems, institutions, and environments are beneficial to all individuals. This includes such things as affordable health care, effective public safety, peace among nations, a just legal system, and an unpolluted environment.

Finally, the virtue approach to ethics assumes that there are certain ideals toward which professionals should strive and that these ideals are concerned with the actualization of humanity and are discovered through personal reflection on what kind of people humans have the potential to become. Virtues are attitudes or character traits that enable individuals to be and to act in ways that develop their highest potential. Virtues enable professionals to pursue personal ideals such as honesty, courage, compassion, generosity, fidelity, integrity, fairness, self-control, and prudence. This approach views the virtuous person as an ethical person. Further, the virtues approach promotes the development of character within persons and their communities.

Use of Ethical Problem-Solving Approaches

These approaches lead to a five-question model that assists in the resolution of moral issues suggesting that once the facts are ascertained, the following questions should be asked when trying to resolve a moral issue:

1. What benefits and what harms will each course of action produce, and which alternative will lead to the best overall consequences?

2. What moral rights do the affected parties have, and which course of action best respects those rights?

3. Which course of action treats everyone the same, except where there is a morally justifiable reason not to, and does not show favoritism or discrimination?

4. Which course of action advances the common good?

5. Which course of action develops moral virtues?

This method is not meant to provide an automatic solution to moral problems; rather, it is meant to help identify most of the important ethical considerations. Professionals must deliberate on moral issues for themselves, keeping a watchful eye on all considerations of the ethical problem. For a practical set of guidelines, there are three relatively simple assessments to the selected course of action to ensure that the action is appropriate:

1. *The test of justice*: Assess your own sense of fairness by determining whether you would treat others the same in this situation.

2. *The test of publicity:* Ask yourself whether you would want your behavior reported in the press.

3. *The test of universality:* Ask yourself to assess whether you could recommend the same course of action to another counselor in the same situation.

If the course of action selected presents new ethical issues, then the professional needs to return to the beginning and reevaluate each step of the process. Further, it is suggested that after passing the tests of justice, publicity, and universality, and the professional is satisfied that the course of action selected is appropriate, then the plan of action can be implemented. Taking the appropriate action in an ethical dilemma can be complex, and it takes courage to proceed. Finally, after implementation of the course of action, the ethical practitioner evaluates the course of action to assess the consequences. It is this process that leads to the professional and personal growth that is intended to take place in the ethical decision-making process.

The Association for Addiction Professionals

NAADAC, the Association for Addiction Professionals, focuses on professionals who are active in prevention, intervention, treatment, and education and who serve the field addressing issues in tobacco, gambling, and substance use. The NAADAC Code of Ethics is updated regularly and is an essential guide to addictions practitioners.

Conclusion

Becoming an ethical practitioner takes experience and courage. In addition, it takes the action of the professional to question himself or herself and to make sure to communicate with other professionals to examine ethical issues that present themselves in the practice of addictions counseling. Colleagues will be a benefit as the ethical dilemmas rise to the forefront of nearly every case that comes before the practice of addictions counseling.

Kathryn J. Speck

See also Clinical Supervision of Addiction Counselors; Confidentiality; Dual Relationships; Ethical Standards for Addiction Professionals; NAADAC, the Association for Addiction Professionals

Further Readings

American Psychological Association. (2003). *Ethical principles for psychologists and code of conduct.* Retrieved September 11, 2007, from http://www.apa.org/ethics/code2002.html

Forester-Miller, H., & Davis, T. (1996). *A practitioner's guide to ethical decision making.* Alexandria, VA: American Counseling Association.

Forester-Miller, H., & Rubenstein, R. L. (1992). Group counseling: Ethics and professional issues. In D. Capuzzi & D. R. Gross (Eds.), *Introduction to group counseling.* Denver, CO: Love Publishing.

Kitchener, K. S. (1984). Intuition, critical evaluation and ethical principles: The foundation for ethical decisions in counseling psychology. *Counseling Psychologist, 12,* 43–55.

NAADAC, the Association for Addiction Professionals. (2004). *NAADAC code of ethics.* Retrieved May 20, 2008, from http://naadac.org/documents/index.php?CategoryID=23

Reamer, F. (1998). The evolution of social work ethics. *Social Work, 43,* 488–500.

Stadler, H. A. (1986). Making hard choices: Clarifying controversial ethical issues. *Counseling & Human Development, 19,* 1–10.

Velasquez, M., Andre, C., Shanks, T., & Meyer, M. J. (1996). Thinking ethically: A framework for moral decision making. *Issues in Ethics, 7.* Retrieved September 11, 2007, from http://www.scu.edu/ethics/practicing/decision/thinking.html

Walden, S. L., Herlihy, B., & Ashton, L. (2003). The evolution of ethics: Personal perspectives of ACA ethics committee chairs. *Journal of Counseling & Development, 81,*106–111.

EVIDENCE-BASED PREVENTION

Prevention efforts against substance use have focused primarily on children and adolescents because initial substance use is most likely to occur during adolescence and young adulthood. Primary prevention efforts include planned actions that help adolescents prevent predictable problems, protect existing states of health as well as healthy functioning, and promoting desired goals. This entry focuses on evidence-based prevention programs, which by definition have been developed and evaluated using well-controlled scientific methods.

Prevention Efforts

Although there are many substance use prevention programs, few have been evaluated in controlled experiments. The Substance Abuse and Mental Health Services Administration (SAMHSA) maintains a list of prevention programs that have been evaluated in the National Registry of Evidence-based Programs and Practices (NREPP). The NREPP defines evidence-based programs as those that (a) are conceptually sound and internally consistent, (b) have activities related to the conceptualization of the program, and (c) are reasonably well implemented and evaluated. The NREPP divides programs into three categories: promising, effective, and model programs. Promising programs have some positive outcomes but have not been fully evaluated or proven effective across replications. Effective programs have consistently positive outcomes and have been strongly implemented and evaluated. Model programs are those that are widely effective and have provided SAMHSA with materials, training, and technical assistance for nationwide implementation.

The Office of National Drug Control Policy (ONDCP) also provides guidance on evidence-based prevention programs. These guidelines include (a) addressing appropriate risk and protective factors for substance abuse in a defined population, (b) using approaches with demonstrated efficacy, (c) intervening early at important stages and transitions, (d) intervening in appropriate settings and domains, and (e) managing programs effectively. Taken together, federal guidelines indicate that prevention programs should be theoretically based, have demonstrated efficacy, and be tailored to specific factors, including risk, age, and sociocultural status. In the following section, a number of evidence-based substance abuse prevention programs are reviewed, the key attributes are identified, and recommendations for best practice in terms of substance abuse prevention efforts are provided.

Prevention Efforts With Demonstrated Efficacy

Recent research and reviews of the literature have identified characteristics that are associated with effective prevention programs that target low- and high-risk youth. Excellent reviews in this area are listed in "Further Readings" at the end of this entry. A number of risk and protective factors for substance use and abuse have been identified that vary along a continuum of individual, family, school, and community characteristics. Individual factors associated with risk for substance abuse include comorbid psychiatric disorders and impulsivity. Living in a single-parent home, parental drug use, and lax parenting style represent family factors that are associated with substance abuse risk. School factors that are associated with greater risk for substance abuse include poor performance or lack of engagement in school activities. Positive peer attitudes toward substance abuse and cultural norms that do not prohibit drug use represent community factors that contribute to substance abuse risk. Of course, while these factors represent risk for substance use, they vary along a continuum and their converse may be seen as protective factors against substance use. Many effective prevention programs are aimed at reducing risk factors or promoting protective factors.

While earlier prevention programming focused on single behaviors, more recent substance use prevention interventions focus on comprehensive efforts involving schools, communities, mass media, policy changes, and enforcement. These prevention interventions have been more successful by incorporating broader health-promotion and competence-enhancement strategies, which target reductions in risk factors and enhancement of protective factors.

Given that school-based factors contribute to risk for, and resilience against, substance abuse and dependence, many prevention programs are school based. One example of a comprehensive, school-based program is the Midwestern Prevention Project. Initially implemented in Kansas City, Missouri, and later in Indianapolis, Indiana, this program included mass media, school-based skills training, parent programming, school policy changes, and community organization to address changing local ordinances on the availability of alcohol and tobacco products. Adolescent alcohol, cigarette, and marijuana use decreased significantly from baseline to 1-year follow up, and reduced rates of cigarette and marijuana use among high- and low-risk youth were maintained over 3 years.

Another school-based project with multiple prevention activities was Project Northland, which targeted middle school–age children with four program components—parental involvement, educational activities, peer leadership, and community task force activities—that were implemented in randomly selected school districts. By the end of eighth grade, intervention participants showed decreased alcohol use, even among the regular drinkers, as well as reduced cigarette and marijuana use. Because of its demonstrated efficacy, Project Northland has since been adapted for use in urban youth in the United States, as well as in youth outside the United States. Thus, prevention programs such as the Midwestern Prevention Project and Project Northland have demonstrated that comprehensive strategies, which use consistent messages from multiple social contexts, can delay or prevent adolescent substance use and abuse.

Prevention researchers advocate using varied and interactive teaching methods in school-based programs to enhance important life skills, which include assertiveness, communication, and coping. However, educational approaches alone, particularly those that use didactic teaching methods, have demonstrated limited decreases in drug use among youth.

Family participation in programs is another cornerstone of an effective prevention program, given that family factors contribute to risk for, or protection against, substance use. Specifically, research consistently suggests that strategies for improved family relations, communication, and parental supervision are critical links to improved outcomes. Consequently, the National Institute on Drug Abuse endorses family-based interventions and therapy because family relationships are associated with risk factors, mediators, or protective factors in the literature. Programs like Preparing for the Drug Free Years and the Strengthening Families Program, which target substance-abusing parents of 6- to 10-year-old children and families with young children as well as preteens, are examples of family programs. Both of these family preventive programs (a) target reducing familial risk factors, such as poor familial communication; (b) provide parenting skills training; and (c) enhance protective factors associated with teen substance use. An evaluation of the Preparing for the Drug Free Years reported significant reductions in the rate of increases in teen alcohol use at 1-, 2-, and 3½-year follow-ups. Several evaluations have reported the efficacy of enhanced parenting skills, family conflict, and family communication across different ethnic groups, in both rural and urban settings. These programs have also recently demonstrated efficacy in groups with varying risk factors—particularly in preventing methamphetamine use for those at risk.

Prevention efforts are not entirely school or family based, however. Environment-based prevention efforts have also been developed and evaluated. For example, Challenging College Alcohol Abuse is a SAMHSA model program that has been shown to reduce problem drinking and related risks in college students through education about social norms and modification of university policies and practices. This program engages college students ages 18 to 24 and is multimodal in that it uses mass media, policy development, faculty education, and survey techniques to promote healthy behaviors but does not have a traditional, school-based component. Importantly, this environment-based program demonstrates that prevention efforts need not only be delivered at a young age to be effective. Moreover, the multifaceted nature of this program fits well with ONDCP guidelines described earlier.

Other studies have shown that sufficient intervention dosage, such as the quantity and quality of intervention contact hours, is a critical part of successful prevention interventions. Specifically, in a longitudinal, randomized trial of a school-based prevention program (Life Skills Training), a multicomponent approach in the seventh grade with booster sessions in the eighth and ninth grades reduced alcohol and drug use for the intervention group, and these gains were maintained at a 6-year follow-up. Another school-based program, Project ALERT, used booster sessions in the eighth grade to reinforce what youth had learned in the previous year and demonstrated, in a large randomized study in 30 schools in California and Oregon, that Project ALERT reduced drug use among high- and low-risk students.

Studies also indicate that prevention programs must be age-appropriate and socioculturally relevant to be successful. In addition, studies have shown that an antidrug program's message to adolescents is more effective when discussion is focused on the short-term effects of substance use, such as diminished attractiveness, rather than the long-term adverse effects, such as poor health.

Prevention Efforts Without Demonstrated Efficacy

As mentioned earlier, there are a number of prevention programs that have not been tested for efficacy or have not demonstrated efficacy when tested in controlled conditions. An example of a popular but not effective prevention program that uses didactic teaching is the D.A.R.E. (Drug Abuse Resistance Education) curriculum. D.A.R.E. is a school-based curriculum taught by police officers and aimed at familiarizing students with problems associated with drug use, as well as to introduce students to police officers in a relatively nonthreatening environment. At least 15 evaluation studies have reported that D.A.R.E. does not have long-term effects on adolescent drug use. In addition, a revised iteration of the D.A.R.E. curriculum (D.A.R.E.+PLUS) has shown limited efficacy. The proliferation of the D.A.R.E. program exemplifies the need for theory and research support before program implementation. Although prevention researchers have developed and identified effective prevention programs, recent studies have shown that effective programs are rarely implemented, and at least one study suggests that rural communities in particular are in low stages of prevention program readiness. The reasons for this lack of transfer from research to practice are not fully understood but may be related to the availability of training and resources. Fidelity in replication of evidence-based prevention programs may also represent a reason for low rates of implementation. Emshoff and colleagues suggest that fidelity in replication is possible but that fidelity is dependent upon technical assistance in implementation and mandate by funding agreements.

Recommendations for Best Practice

Interactive prevention interventions, which target families, schools, and communities with consistent "no use" messages, are more effective, particularly when planned booster sessions are used after implementation. Rather than using didactic teaching methods and focusing on single behaviors, the hallmarks of effective prevention programs are interactive educational and environmental approaches, which include targeting multiple behaviors, specific ages, and culturally appropriate values. Moreover, the implementation of evidence-based programs needs to be increased, including enhancing message delivery methods. Finally, given the number of adolescents who continue to experiment with drugs, additional research is

needed to better understand adolescence issues and vulnerability to substance abuse and dependence and to examine innovative approaches to prevent and treat drug misuse and abuse.

Carl G. Leukefeld and William W. Stoops

Authors' note: This entry was adapted from Leukefeld, Smiley McDonald, Stoops, Reed, & Martin, 2005.

See also Center for Substance Abuse Prevention; Fidelity of Prevention Programs; National Registry of Evidence-based Programs and Practices; Prevention Evaluation; Prevention Strategies; Public Policy, Prevention; Research Issues in Prevention

Further Readings

Emshoff, J., Blakely, C., Gray, D., Jakes, S., Brounstein, P., Coulter, J., et al. (2003). An ESID case study at the federal level. *American Journal of Community Psychology, 32*(3–4), 345–357.

Ennett, S. T., Ringwalt, C. L., Thorne, J., Rohrbach, L. A., Vincus, A., Simons-Rudolph, A., et al. (2003). A comparison of current practice in school-based substance use prevention programs with meta-analysis findings. *Prevention Science, 4*(1), 1–14.

Kumpfer, K. L., & Alvarado, R. (2003). Family-strengthening approaches for the prevention of youth problem behaviors. *American Psychologist, 58,* 457–465.

Leukefeld, C. G., Smiley McDonald, H., Stoops, W. W., Reed, L., & Martin, C. (2005). Substance misuse and abuse. In T. P. Gulotta & G. R. Adams (Eds.), *Handbook of adolescent behavioral problems* (pp. 439–465). New York: Springer.

Nation, M., Crusto, C., Wandersman, A., Kumpfer, K. L., Seybolt, D., Morrissey-Kane, E., et al. (2003). What works in prevention. *American Psychologist, 58,* 449–456.

Office of National Drug Control Policy. (2007). *Evidence-based principles for substance abuse prevention.* Retrieved March 7, 2007, from http://www.ncjrs.gov/ondcppubs/publications/prevent/evidence_based_eng.html

Paglia, A., & Room, R. (1999). Preventing substance use problems among youth: A literature review and recommendations. *Journal of Primary Prevention, 20,* 3–50.

Substance Abuse and Mental Health Services Administration. (2005). *SAMHSA model programs: Effective substance abuse and mental health programs for every community.* Retrieved March 2, 2007, from http://www.modelprograms.samhsa.gov

Tobler, N. S., Roona, M. R., Ochshorn, P., Marshall, D. G., Streke, A. V., & Stackpole, K. M. (2000). School-based adolescent drug prevention programs: 1998 meta-analysis. *Journal of Primary Prevention, 20,* 275–336.

Evidence-Based Prevention and Treatment, Dissemination and Adoption of

For the past 15 years, health disciplines have focused on improving the quality of care and services by promoting the use of practices guided by research. Many practitioners perceive that this quality care movement, which has steadily gained popularity, has helped create the terms *evidence-based practices, empirically supported treatments,* and *research-based interventions.* These terms typically are used interchangeably, although some professions prefer one term over another. For purposes of this entry, the term *evidence-based practices* (EBPs) will be utilized. However, researchers, practitioners, and policymakers have identified a gap between these EBPs and practice. To close this gap, activities that promote the dissemination and adoption of EBPs have been implemented. Both terms—*dissemination* and *adoption* (of EBPs)—are used frequently in the substance abuse prevention and treatment literature. Dissemination most often refers to the distribution or circulation of materials, manuals, articles, and newsletters in hard copy or electronic formats, while adoption refers to changes in practitioners' behaviors and skills. Whereas dissemination and adoption are seen and discussed as separate activities, they actually are parts of a larger process called *technology transfer.* As such, the initial section of this entry includes a brief review of EBPs (provided as background information), and the remaining sections provide a comprehensive discussion of technology transfer.

Evidence-Based Practices

Former Surgeon General David Sackett is considered the innovator of the term *EBP.* He described evidence-based medicine as the manner in which physicians make thoughtful decisions about patient care, guided by the current science. This definition highlights the importance of the connection between quality care and use of EBPs in guiding treatment and prevention decisions and practices. Currently, an extensive portfolio of substance abuse treatment and prevention research exists that demonstrates the efficacy of particular approaches and activities, which was not always the case. Therefore, it becomes even more important that EBPs are utilized; in fact, some researchers advocate that professionals have an ethical duty and professional obligation to do so.

Many professionals caution against creating a definitive list of EBPs because the science is always changing. However, there exists a core group of EBPs that appear consistently in literature reviews, efficacy studies, dissemination libraries, and national registries for substance abuse prevention and treatment services. Specifically, the Substance Abuse and Mental Health Services Administration (SAMHSA) hosts a national registry for EBPs in substance abuse prevention and treatment and mental health services. This site, the National Registry of Evidence-based Programs and Practices ([NREPP] http://www.nrepp.samhsa.gov/), offers a searchable database of prevention and treatment interventions for mental health and substance use disorders. The NREPP site serves two purposes: (1) It affords researchers and practitioners the opportunity to submit their intervention for review and consideration as an EBP, and (2) it provides practitioners and the general public access to a single online source for EBPs in the substance abuse and mental health fields. Specifically, the NREPP database (a) rates each intervention, (b) describes its intended outcomes, (c) assesses the intervention's readiness for dissemination, (d) evaluates the quality of the research for the intervention, (e) provides access to the list of studies submitted for the intervention as part of the review, and (f) offers contact information for the innovator(s) of the intervention. Given that NREPP's searchable database is voluntary, some EBPs may not be included, as the innovator(s) of the intervention must submit the appropriate documentation and meet the designated criteria for inclusion. Finally, in addition to the database, the NREPP Web site offers a brief description and discussion of EBPs.

Two other excellent resources for EBPs related to prevention and treatment of substance use disorders are available online. The National Drug Abuse Treatment Clinical Trials Network Dissemination Library is sponsored by the National Institute on Drug Abuse (NIDA). This Web site (http://ctndissemination library.org) offers an electronic repository of research articles, journal abstracts, products, and PowerPoint presentations pertaining to EBPs generated by NIDA's 16 clinical trial nodes. These nodes include university-based research centers partnering with community-based treatment providers across the United States. Contact information for both researchers and community treatment providers is included as part of this Web site. Another excellent online resource is hosted by the State of Oregon, Department of Human Services, and includes an exhaustive compendium of EBPs for substance use and mental health disorders prevention and treatment. Oregon was one of the first states in the nation whose legislature mandated that five state agencies, including the Department of Human Services, spend the majority of its public prevention and treatment dollars to fund providers that utilize EBPs. According to Oregon's Department of Human Services, 75% of its funds must be distributed to providers that utilize EBPs by the 2009–2011 budget period. To facilitate this process, a comprehensive Web site was developed and implemented that includes EBP definitions; Oregon's 2007 EBP inventory; fidelity tools for approved EBPs; methods for fidelity measurement; and EBP-related reports, publications, and research articles and links. Oregon's EBP Web site can be accessed at http://www.oregon .gov/DHS/mentalhealth/ ebp/main.shtml.

Dissemination and Adoption

As with most other professions, the difficulty for the substance abuse prevention and treatment fields does not lie in the development of new practices based on rigorous scientific research but on the dissemination and adoption of these new practices by practitioners. Experts estimate that it takes more than 20 years for an innovation to move from the research laboratory to widespread use by practitioners. For example, Everett Rogers discussed the original diffusion of an innovation study that examined the farming practices of corn farmers in Iowa. In this study, farmers were educated about a new hybrid corn seed that researchers found produced superior crops. Results showed that it took 13 years for farmers to change their practice (i.e., using the new hybrid corn seed) and another 7 years for them to use the new hybrid seed exclusively. In 1998, the Institute of Medicine's seminal report, *Bridging the Gap Between Practice and Research: Forging Partnerships With Community-Based Drug and Alcohol Treatment,* identified the chasm that

exists between science and service and brought this issue to the forefront for funders, policymakers, and substance abuse prevention and treatment providers. According to this report, the substance abuse treatment field cannot afford to wait 20 years for practitioners to adopt evidence-based practices. Therefore, activities need to be designed and technology transfer activities employed because the natural diffusion of knowledge can be a slow and tedious process.

Technology Transfer and Diffusion of Innovations

Two terms are used to describe the process of closing the gap between science and practice: *technology transfer* and *diffusion of innovations.* Although these terms represent different processes, individuals tend to use the terms interchangeably. Technology transfer refers to the process whereby the innovator creates strategies to encourage the use of the innovation, while diffusion of innovation refers to the process by which users become aware of an innovation and its use spreads. Simply stated, technology transfer is planned, whereas diffusion occurs naturally. For example, the use of cell phones has diffused rapidly with little attention paid to activities that will help promote its use (diffusion of innovation); in contrast, high rates of underage drinking by college students remain almost intractable despite the millions of dollars being spent annually on activities to reduce the prevalence (technology transfer). The theory of diffusion of innovation, which was created by Rogers, serves as the foundation of all activities that seek to bridge the gap between science and practice. A majority of Roger's work focused on five characteristics of an innovation that helped or hindered its diffusion. These characteristics are (1) how easy was it to use (complexity), (2) could you try to use it on your own before adopting it (triability), (3) was it better than what you were currently using (relative advantage), (4) how consistent was it with your values (compatibility), and (5) does it have tangible results (observability). Today, these five characteristics are used by SAMHSA to help providers review the characteristics of prevention EBPs that may inhibit their utility.

Among numerous definitions for technology transfer, NIDA researcher Barry Brown developed a practical definition that seems to provide the best fit for the substance abuse prevention and treatment fields.

He suggested that technology transfer is more than the transmission of information and is actually a behavioral change process. This definition stresses the impact technology transfer has on both behavior and cognition (i.e., modifying the practices, policies, behaviors, and attitudes of individuals and organizations). From the perspective that technology transfer is a behavior change process, activities that aid the dissemination and adoption of EBPs must be specifically implemented in order to affect the practitioners' actions and thoughts. Historically, institutions have trained practitioners in a new innovation and crossed their fingers that the new information would "stick" (e.g., be adopted). To avoid this old process of hoping that training will change professionals' or students' behavior, technology transfer theories and research must be utilized.

The seminal technology transfer study in the substance abuse treatment field was conducted by James Sorenson and his colleagues in 1988. The adoption of a job-seeking skills curriculum by substance abuse treatment providers was the focus of the study. Results showed that adoption rates increased when providers attended workshops or received technical assistance as compared to other conditions (e.g., general and targeted dissemination of the job-seeking skills manual). In addition, personal contact with a trainer or consultant made a significant difference in adoption rates. Recent studies confirm Sorenson and colleagues' original findings regarding the importance of personal contact in speeding the adoption of a substance abuse treatment practice. These studies demonstrate that dissemination of educational materials alone does not promote the adoption of new knowledge or skills. The adoption of new practices occurs more readily when a series of educational opportunities, rather than a single event, are offered. Specifically, these studies found that counselors who participated in face-to-face training workshops, received booster sessions, and engaged in coaching sessions had higher rates of adoption than those counselors who participated in a single training workshop or just received written materials. Currently, there is ample evidence to demonstrate that a series of connected learning events that include clinical supervision or performance feedback are the most efficacious because they reinforce previous learning while building new knowledge.

Technology Transfer Model

Many technology transfer experts have recommended specific steps that result in adoption of an innovation or EBP. However, until recently there have been few comprehensive technology transfer models. Nancy Roget and her colleagues developed one such model, called the cycle of technology transfer, which was based on a thorough review of the literature. This model proposes that technology transfer occurs in a cyclical rather than a linear manner, with the cycle containing the following processes: (a) knowledge dissemination, (b) knowledge transfer, (c) knowledge adoption, (d) knowledge adaptation, and (e) knowledge reinvention.

Based on this cycle, all technology transfer activities have a specific goal (e.g., knowledge adoption or knowledge transfer) and should be used accordingly. For example, if the goal is to change a practitioner's skill level, then knowledge adoption activities would be more appropriate than knowledge dissemination activities. Knowledge dissemination activities provide an initial exposure to an evidence-based practice (e.g., 1-day training workshops or research briefs like NIDA Notes), while knowledge transfer activities translate EBPs into more user-friendly formats (e.g., training manuals, CD-ROMs). Knowledge adoption activities include the most intensive activities, like technical assistance and consultation (which includes performance feedback on a new skill). Knowledge adaptation occurs more naturally, although it can be facilitated through peer-led expert group activities. Finally, in the last stage of the cycle, knowledge gained from both the technology transfer process and application to clinical practice is imparted back to researchers (e.g., counselors disliked online courses that did not include some sort of personal contact, or counselors found that motivational interviewing worked better in outpatient settings than inpatient programs). New research questions are generated and studies launched based on this process. This cycle helps differentiate between different knowledge processes and is used to plan technology transfer activities to ensure that multiple exposures, over time, with increasing depth and level of intensity are in place.

Lessons Learned

Because it is just as important to know what doesn't work in technology transfer as what does works, Thomas Backer wrote an influential article about lessons learned in the substance abuse prevention field from failed technology transfer activities. His article identified six common mistakes that organizations or governmental entities make when attempting to promote the adoption of an EBP: (1) choosing an innovation that is not user-friendly; (2) choosing numerous innovations for adoption; (3) using a top-down, authoritative approach (mandating the adoption of an EBP without input or choice); (4) failing to anticipate and plan for resistance; (5) ignoring the importance of context and organizational culture; and (6) failing to build the organization's capacity for the innovation. These "failures" provide an excellent guideline for providers and policymakers who want to avoid costly implementation errors.

Two federally funded projects that have expertise in closing the gap between research and practice are the Centers for the Application of Prevention Technologies and the Addiction Technology Transfer Centers. These regional centers offer training and technical assistance activities to practitioners in the substance abuse treatment and prevention fields. Rogers coined the term *boundary spanners*, referring to entities that bridge the gap between the researchers and practitioners by translating research results and creating exposure opportunities and adoption activities. The Centers for the Application of Prevention Technologies and the Addiction Technology Transfer Centers naturally fit into the role of boundary spanners.

Conclusion

Today, most health professionals readily accept the importance of using EBPs. However, a gap still exists between science and service. To lessen this divide, effective dissemination and adoption strategies are required, which include an understanding of the technology transfer process and cycle, access and multiple exposures to EBPs, and research-based implementation strategies. The technology transfer science is sufficient to reduce the time it takes for an innovation to be adequately diffused into practice and which ultimately benefits individuals affected by substance use disorders and their family members.

Nancy A. Roget

See also Addiction Technology Transfer Centers; Centers for the Application of Prevention Technologies; Evidence-Based Prevention; Evidence-Based Treatment; National Registry of Evidence-based Programs and Practices

Further Readings

Backer, T. E. (2000). The failure of success: Challenges of disseminating effective substance abuse prevention programs. *Journal of Community Psychology, 28*(3), 363–373.

Brown, B. S. (2000). From research to practice: The bridge is out and the water's rising. *Advances in Medical Sociology, 7,* 345–365.

Lamb, S., Greenlick, M. R., & McCarty, D. (Eds.). (1998). *Bridging the gap between practice and research: Forging partnerships with community-based drug and alcohol treatment.* Washington, DC: National Academy Press.

Miller, W. R., Zweben, J., & Johnson, W. (2005). Evidence-based treatment: Why, what, where, when and how? *Journal of Substance Abuse Treatment, 29,* 267–276.

Rogers, E. M. (2004). A prospective and retrospective look at the diffusion model. *Journal of Health Communication, 9,* 13–19.

Roget, N. A., Horvatich, P. K., Skinstad, A. H., & Storti, S. A. (2004). *The active ingredients of technology transfer: Activities and strategies that promote the adoption of evidence-based practices.* Poster session presented at the annual meeting of the College on Problems of Drug Dependence, June 12–17, San Juan, Puerto Rico.

Sackett, D. L. (1997). Evidence-based medicine. *Seminars in Perinatology, 21,* 3–5.

Sorensen, J. L., Hall, S. M., Loeb, P., Allen, T., Glaser, E. M., & Greenberg, P. D. (1988). Dissemination of a job seeker's workshop to drug treatment programs. *Behavior Therapy, 19,* 143–155.

EVIDENCE-BASED TREATMENT

As scientific understanding of substance abuse prevention, treatment, and recovery grows, researchers continue to identify more effective interventions and treatments. Interventions that are shown to be effective through research are called evidence-based treatments.

Importance

As recently as two decades ago, what happened during the course of addiction treatment was somewhat of a mystery. There were few empirical studies showing which treatments worked, and what *was* known took decades to trickle from research studies to clinical practice. A gap, not unlike the gap in medical practice, existed between scientific evidence and addiction treatment.

For addictions, which have historically been stigmatized disorders, the gap was especially wide because treatment tended to be isolated from other medical or mental health practice and because practitioners were often peers who were in recovery themselves and practiced from a base of what had worked for them. Sometimes, these approaches worked, and other times, they did not. In general, there was no compelling scientific rationale to support most approaches.

In contrast, the field has recently been moving into another paradigm, propelled by scientific inquiry. The process of scientific inquiry continues to advance understanding of substance abuse and effective ways to prevent, treat, and recover from it. As scientific knowledge is translated from the research arena to practice, adoption and implementation of evidence-based treatment by frontline practitioners is critical if the gains in scientific understanding are to be realized by the millions of Americans at risk for, suffering from, or recovering from substance abuse.

Organizations that fund substance abuse treatment, from federal grant agencies to state organizations to private foundations, have begun to demand that treatments be evidence-based because they hold promise of efficiency and effectiveness—two traditionally important factors in deciding where resources should be allocated. Furthermore, third-party insurance often requires documented use of evidence-based treatment for reimbursement.

Process

Evidence can be determined in a number of ways including expert opinion panels based on clinical observation, on blending of expert opinion with empirical evidence in consensus reviews, and increasingly, on multiple studies (i.e., meta-analyses) of published scientific evidence. For this latter standard, before a treatment can be called evidence-based, a series of steps takes place in the research domain using the scientific method.

To plan and prepare for a research study, researchers first scour published scientific literature, typically in peer-reviewed journals, to find out what already is known from previous research. They may set out to replicate, disprove, or elaborate on past findings. Or, they may aim to investigate a more novel approach. From there, researchers create hypotheses about how certain treatments (i.e., independent variables) may impact or relate to target outcomes (i.e.,

dependent variables). Researchers carefully specify the independent and dependent variables, data collection procedures, and plans for statistical analyses.

One of the most rigorous ways to determine scientific evidence is through the use of a randomized controlled trial (RCT) study design. In an RCT, a given treatment is tested against another treatment, no treatment, or treatment as usual in an attempt to determine how the given treatment compares with the others.

With data gathered from RCTs and other research designs, researchers use statistical analyses to examine the relations between independent and dependent variables and decide if hypotheses were confirmed or not. Researchers determine if participants who receive a certain treatment changed in significant and systematic ways. Treatments that are consistently associated with significant and systematic desirable changes in dependent variables are deemed evidence-based.

While the RCT has arisen as the gold standard for determining whether a treatment is evidence-based, the evidence base on addiction treatment is informed by other methodologies, which may be more difficult to analyze in as clear-cut a fashion as the RCT. These include longitudinal observational studies where changes and associations can be assessed over time; cross-sectional observational studies, such as surveys, to identify associations between variables across participants; and hypothesis-generating studies that utilize qualitative methods, such as case studies and focus groups, which can provide foundational questions for inquiry using other methodological means. Over time, as the evidence-based treatment movement continues to grow, it is likely that advances in science and practice will come from a blending of these methods that include behavioral, physical, environmental, and contextual variables.

Practice

While there is still much to be learned regarding effective substance use treatments, the National Institute on Drug Abuse (NIDA) reviewed decades of research and created a list of guiding principles that characterize the most effective treatments and the process of delivering them. The principles include the following:

1. No single treatment approach is appropriate for all individuals.

2. Treatment needs to be readily available.

3.   Effective treatment attends to the multiple needs of the individual, not just his or her substance use.

4.   An individual's treatment plan needs to be assessed continually and modified as necessary.

5.   Remaining in treatment for an adequate time is critical for effectiveness.

6.   Counseling and other behavioral therapies are critical components of effective substance abuse treatment.

7.   Medications are an important element of treatment for many people, especially when combined with behavioral therapies.

8.   Substance-abusing individuals with coexisting medical disorders should have the disorders treated in an integrated way.

9.   Medical detoxification is only the first stage of substance abuse treatment and by itself does little to change long-term drug and alcohol use.

10.   Treatment does not need to be voluntary to be effective.

11.   Possible substance use during treatment must be monitored continuously.

12.   Treatment programs should provide assessment for HIV, hepatitis B, hepatitis C, tuberculosis, and other infections and provide counseling to help people change their risk for infection.

It is easier to create a list of principles that characterize evidence-based practice broadly than to develop an exhaustive list of evidence-based treatments. For example, evidence may be determined for specific populations and under certain conditions but not for others. Also, individual patients and practitioners have various preferences and personal characteristics. Additionally, new treatments become evidence-based as research accumulates; thus, a continual updating of any such list is required. However, several well-researched treatments have been deemed evidence-based by NIDA and the National Institute on Alcohol Abuse and Alcoholism; seven (not an exhaustive list) will be briefly described here: (a) Motivational Enhancement Therapy, (b) cognitive behavioral therapy, (c) Twelve-Step Facilitation, (d) structured family and couples therapy, (e) community reinforcement therapy, (f) contingency management, and (g) pharmacological therapies. *Motivational Enhancement Therapy* is a program based on the principles and practices of motivational interviewing, an approach to helping people make behavior change that is based on a client-centered, goal-oriented way of increasing a person's intrinsic motivation to change, capitalizing on his or her readiness. *Cognitive behavioral* approaches help people recognize, avoid, and cope with situations in which they are likely to use substances by using awareness-raising and skill-building activities. *Twelve-Step Facilitation* is a structured, individualized approach to introducing a person to a Twelve-Step program that typically helps the person have a better understanding of his or her role in therapy and what is expected. *Structured family and couples therapy* such as Multidimensional Family Therapy, addresses a variety of influences on the substance-abusing patterns of the person and includes family members in the therapy sessions so as to treat people within their natural social environment. *Community reinforcement therapy* is an approach of connecting a person who has substance abuse problems with a range of services within his or her community. *Contingency management*, also known as motivational incentives, is an approach that uses positive reinforcement (e.g., special rewards such as gift certificates) to increase positive behaviors (e.g., not using substances for a specified period of time). *Pharmacological therapies* include the use of medications like naltrexone, disulfiram (Antabuse), methadone, and buprenorphine to help stabilize a person's life during treatment.

Challenges to Implementation

Although more practitioners are using evidence-based treatments and funding sources often require doing so, various barriers to their implementation slows the process of adoption for the field as a whole. One barrier is the perceived lack of definitive knowledge about what constitutes evidence-based treatment. The reality is that many clinicians in the field are consumed with providing therapy and have little time to read scientific research, which typically is written in a technical manner geared for other researchers rather than for practitioners. Clinicians may not have access to manualized treatment protocols or to trainings in treatments covered in the manuals. Practitioners also may not have the authority to make decisions about types of treatments methods and practices to use and may be bound by regulations and approved adopted practices in their agency. Additionally, with rapid changes in technology (such as computerized assessments), new treatment paradigms, and new medications emerging with increased frequency, it can be difficult for practitioners who are busy providing care to stay abreast of these ongoing innovations in the field. Needed resources to provide evidence-based treatment may also be lacking for some practitioners. Specialized training and ongoing clinical supervision are necessary to move from awareness and understanding of new practice to implementation and adoption. Follow-up training and supervision requires investment of time and money for agencies and practitioners, which may not be available. Similarly, access to physicians for medications or other resources may not always be available or timely. Additionally, although third-party payers prefer evidence-based treatments, there is often a time lag between when new treatments are discovered to be evidence-based in the scientific literature and when third-party payers learn about them and begin to routinely reimburse for their provision.

Resources for Practitioners

Clearly, widespread integration of evidence-based treatment across providers and treatment modalities is highly challenging and may constitute systems change for organizations, which can involve a monumental effort of administration and practitioners. One of the most essential steps in this process is that practitioners receive the training and support they need. Multiple resources on evidence-based practice have become available in recent years at little or no cost to practitioners from various sources.

In particular, the U.S. federal and state governments are committed to disseminating what is known about evidence-based practice in digestible print and online formats. The U.S. Department of Health and Human Services oversees the Substance Abuse and Mental Health Services Administration (SAMHSA). In turn, SAMHSA oversees several centers and programs with the aim of coordinating dissemination efforts. SAMHSA's National Registry of Evidence-based Programs and Practices (NREPP) offers a searchable directory of up-to-date information on evidence-based practice in mental health and substance abuse prevention and treatment. The NREPP is accessible in an online format. Other, specific information regarding evidence-based practices for substance use prevention and treatment is available

through SAMHSA's Center for Substance Abuse Prevention and Center for Substance Abuse Treatment. Two recent examples of print and online resources from SAMHSA's Center for Substance Abuse Treatment are resource kits and treatment improvement protocols.

Additionally, 14 SAMHSA-funded Addiction Technology Transfer Centers (ATTCs) are making inroads into helping practitioners and administrators learn about and, ultimately, adopt evidence-based practices. The ATTCs train practitioners in evidence-based treatment in general as well as in specific treatments via live and online courses and conferences. The ATTCs also work with state and other funding organizations to dedicate time and money to implement evidence-based treatments.

Conclusion

While there is still much to be discovered regarding the effectiveness of substance abuse interventions, the research process continues to yield new evidence-based treatments. Although an investment in training is required to learn evidence-based treatments, and there are many challenges involved in implementing these treatments in practice, many practitioners are dedicated to providing effective substance abuse treatments. At this exciting time in the field of substance abuse treatment practitioners are equipped with more tools than ever.

Leah Farrell and Sherry Dyche Ceperich

See also Addiction Technology Transfer Centers; Center for Substance Abuse Treatment; Evidence-Based Prevention; Evidence-Based Prevention and Treatment, Dissemination and Adoption of; National Institute on Alcohol Abuse and Alcoholism; National Institute on Drug Abuse; Research Issues in Treatment

Further Readings

Addiction Technology Transfer Center. (2003). *Best practices in addition treatment: A workshop facilitator's guide.* Retrieved June 19, 2007, from http://www.nattc.org/resPubs/bpat/index.html

Addiction Technology Transfer Center. (n.d.). *About us.* Retrieved June 19, 2007, from http://www.nattc.org/aboutUs.html

American Psychological Association, Division 12, Society of Clinical Psychology. (n.d.). *A guide to beneficial psychotherapy.* Retrieved June 19, 2007, from http://www.apa.org/divisions/div12/rev_est

Miller, W. R., Sorensen, J. L., Selzer, J., A., & Brigham, G. S. (2006). Disseminating evidence-based practices in substance abuse treatment: A review with suggestions. *Journal of Substance Abuse Treatment, 31,* 25–39.

National Institute on Drug Abuse. (1999). *Principles of drug addiction treatment. A research-based guide* (NIH Publication No. 99-4180). Rockville, MD: Author.

Power, E. J., Zadrozny, S., Nishimi, R. Y., & Kizer, K. W. (Eds.). (2005). *Integrating behavioral healthcare performance measures throughout healthcare: National Quality Forum workshop proceedings.* Retrieved June 19, 2007, from http://www.qualityforum.org/pdf/reports/behavioral_health.pdf

SAMHSA/CSAT Treatment Improvement Protocols. Retrieved June 19, 2007, from http://www.ncbi.nlm.nih.gov/books/bv.fcgi?rid=hstat5.part.22441

Tucker, K. T., & Roth, D. L. (2006). Extending the evidence hierarchy to enhance evidence-based practice for substance use disorders. *Addiction, 101,* 918–932.

EXPECTANCIES

From first experimentation to addiction, substance use is a decision. That is, individuals who use alcohol, tobacco, or other drugs choose to do so (although this choice is not always the result of careful thought). *Expectancies* are powerful motivators of this choice. With regard to drug use, expectancies are the effects that an individual anticipates from the use of any given substance. Examples include "Drinking alcohol makes me drunk" and "Smoking cigarettes make me feel relaxed." Substance-related expectancies are among the most potent predictors of the range of drug use behavior. For instance, they predict the initiation of substance use, onset of problematic patterns of use, current levels of consumption, and treatment outcome. This entry provides overviews of the expectancy concept; expectancy measurement; and alcohol-, smoking-, and illicit drug–related expectancies.

The Expectancy Concept

In the broadest sense, expectancies are the cognitions that individuals hold regarding the consequences of their actions. Statements such as "If I do not eat, then I will be hungry" and "Drinking water quenches my thirst" represent expectancies with which almost everyone is quite familiar. Notice that these statements refer to behaviors (eating and the consumption of water) that are essential to survival. This is not coincidental, as expectancies are crucial for the continuation of life. Consider, for instance, an individual who is incapable of learning that eating food satiates hunger and that drinking water slakes thirst. He or she would not be expected to live long without significant assistance. Indeed, at the core of the expectancy concept is the evolutionary mandate that behavior be guided by the anticipation of the future. In other words, across the millennia of human history, it was vital that humans develop expectancies concerning what was safe to eat, which predators to avoid, how to live through harsh climate changes, and so on. In the modern world, it is similarly critical that humans understand the importance of avoiding dark alleyways, obeying traffic laws, obtaining a steady flow of income, and so forth.

Expectancies are not static. Rather, they are dynamic information processing templates that adapt in response to the demands of the environment. In this sense, expectancies embody the accumulated lifetime of learning history. This includes the guidance of parents, the lessons of teachers, exposure to various media, and direct and vicarious life experience. Humans develop and modify expectancies from birth to death, with the ultimate goal of enhancing their ability to interact more effectively with the world.

The expectancy system is especially oriented toward immediate and biologically meaningful rewards, and it is less influenced by the long-term effects of behavior. Unfortunately, because of this orientation, humans are subject to making decisions that feel good now but may be costly later. This is why, for example, it may be especially difficult to adhere to dietary guidelines when in the presence of pizza, french fries, ice cream, and the like. The immediate incentives associated with eating these foods are more salient than the harmful long-term consequences of unhealthy eating habits. This same unfortunate by-product of the otherwise adaptive expectancy system may be why, for many people, drug use is an especially intractable problem.

Expectancy Measurement

Instrument development is an area in which the field of psychology has truly distinguished itself, as psychological measures have proved to be invaluable tools in a variety of research and clinical settings. Expectancy measurement is no exception. A number of self-report questionnaires have been used to measure substance-related expectancies, including the Alcohol Expectancy Questionnaire, the Smoking Consequences Questionnaire, the Marijuana Effect Expectancy Questionnaire, the Cocaine Effect Expectancy Questionnaire, and the Stimulant Effect Expectancy Questionnaire.

One important function of expectancy questionnaires is to identify and develop interventions for those who are at risk for subsequent substance use. For instance, adolescents who expect fewer negative effects from marijuana have been found to be more likely to use the drug. If stronger expectancies for negative effects protect against initiating use, educators may wish to investigate ways to increase negative expectancies as part of drug prevention programs. Another valuable purpose of these measures is to help clinicians tailor treatment to their patients' expectancies. For example, a counselor might help an abuser who expects cocaine to make him or her more sociable learn to achieve this outcome through nondrug means.

Although these questionnaires have demonstrated their ability to predict substance use behavior, they may not characterize the full complexity of the expectancy construct. Self-report instruments rely on information that is available to conscious awareness, or *explicit* cognition. However, current theory suggests that expectancies are primarily guided by processes that occur outside of conscious awareness, or *implicit* cognition. Thus, explicit cognition may not capture the primary motivational forces that underlie substance use. A helpful analogy is that of an iceberg: The top portion, above water for all to see, corresponds to explicit expectancies, whereas the remainder of the iceberg, underwater and exponentially larger than the top portion, exemplifies implicit expectancies. Expectancies are not simply what people verbally predict will happen if they use tobacco, alcohol, or other drugs, but a sophisticated psychobiological process that unfolds in the presence of substance-consistent stimuli.

Implicit measures of expectancies typically assess changes in task performance following experiences that are below an individual's level of awareness. Such measures have become increasingly popular with researchers over the past 3 decades. Several types of implicit tasks have been used, including the Stroop, false memory, free association, and the Implicit Association Test. For the most part, these tasks have shown that people who use more of a particular substance (e.g., alcohol) have more positive expectancies (e.g., happiness) about that substance than do people who use less. Implicit tasks also show that these expectancies can be activated in people without their awareness and lead to consumption of the substance. In sum, mounting evidence supports the influence of implicit processes in the operation of alcohol-, smoking-, and drug-related expectancies.

Alcohol-Related Expectancies

Alcohol expectancies are extremely wide-ranging. Some expectancies for alcohol include sociability, happiness, sexual effects, relaxation, sleepiness, nausea, and violence, among many others. Interestingly, most people hold many of these expectations simultaneously—even contradictory ones. An individual may expect alcohol to make them happy in some situations and depressed in others, or sexy now and sick later. Although people have many different alcohol expectancies, most expectancies fall on two emotional dimensions: (1) valence (positive/negative) and (2) arousal (aroused/sedated). People who exhibit different patterns of drinking show different levels of these alcohol expectancy dimensions. For instance, whereas heavy drinkers tend to expect a greater degree of positive and/or arousing effects of alcohol, light drinkers tend to anticipate more negative and/or sedating consequences of drinking.

Current alcohol expectancy research focuses on the mechanisms by which people acquire their expectancies. Variables of interest have included advertising, parental and peer influences, personality traits, and genetics. All of these factors have been associated with alcohol expectancies in children, even before drinking begins.

Expectancy Challenge

Perhaps one of the most exciting methods in alcohol expectancy research is a procedure known as the expectancy challenge. This procedure involves giving participants either an alcoholic beverage or a placebo alcohol beverage (e.g., tonic water with vodka rubbed on the rim of the glass) and having them interact socially. Based on the behaviors of others, participants are asked to guess who consumed alcohol and who consumed the placebo beverage. Studies using this procedure have shown that participants are no better at guessing than chance. When presented with this feedback, participants' expectancies for the effects of alcohol are confronted via direct experience. Those whose expectancies are challenged show decreased drinking over time. Moreover, these individuals show a greater decrease in alcohol consumption than those who receive a treatment consisting of a didactic presentation about the potential consequences of drinking alcohol. The expectancy challenge procedure supports a causal role of expectancies on alcohol use behavior, in that experimentally manipulated expectancies lead to changes in drinking. Furthermore, this procedure demonstrates the promise of the role of expectancies in treatment.

Smoking-Related Expectancies

Smoking-related outcome expectancies among adults appear to comprise four broad categories: (1) negative consequences, (2) negative reinforcement, (3) positive reinforcement, and (4) appetite/weight control. Expectancies for negative consequences include the health complications associated with smoking (e.g., heightened risk for lung cancer, shortened life span), unpleasant physical feelings (e.g., the need to cough), and negative social implications (e.g., stigmatization). Negative reinforcement expectancies involve the reduction of aversive emotional states (e.g., feeling less sad, anxious, or angry). Expectancies for positive reinforcement consist of the induction of pleasurable affective states (e.g., feeling "buzzed"), coping with tedium (e.g., smoking gives you something to do when bored), enjoyable sensorimotor experiences (e.g., the taste and smell of tobacco smoke), and the facilitation of social interaction (e.g., feeling more at ease with others when smoking). Finally, expectancies for appetite/weight control include weight loss and the restraint of hunger. Generally speaking, the more positive expectancies and the fewer negative expectancies an individual holds about cigarettes, the more likely he or she is to smoke.

Current smoking expectancy research is exploring expectancies among adolescents, as well as expectancies for appetite/weight control among women, who may be especially likely to smoke for these reasons. Additional topics of contemporary investigation include the way in which smoking-related expectancies vary as a function of internal contexts (e.g., during smoking abstinence), and alcohol and other drug use.

Expectancies for Illicit Drugs

In addition to expectancies for smoking and alcohol, expectancies for the effects of marijuana and cocaine have been examined for their role in initiating and maintaining the use of these drugs. Expectancies for marijuana include (a) cognitive and behavioral impairment (e.g., difficulty thinking and the slowing of activity), (b) relaxation and tension reduction (e.g., feeling calm and peaceful), (c) social and sexual facilitation (e.g., feeling sociable and flirtatious), (d) perceptual and cognitive enhancement (e.g., music sounds better; feeling creative), (e) global negative effects (e.g., feeling sad or angry), and (f) craving and physical effects (e.g., feeling thirsty and hungry). Expectancies for cocaine also include global negative effects and relaxation and tension reduction factors, as well as three other factors not found for marijuana: (1) global positive effects (e.g., feeling confident and powerful), (2) generalized arousal (e.g., feeling animated and hyperactive), and (3) anxiety (e.g., feeling tense and edgy). Expectancies for illicit drugs have not been studied as extensively as have alcohol- and smoking-related expectancies. Nevertheless, consistent with the findings from the alcohol and tobacco literature, the more positive expectancies and the fewer negative expectancies an individual holds for marijuana or cocaine, the more likely he or she is to use the drug.

It remains to be seen whether challenging drug users' expectancies results in reduced marijuana or cocaine use, as has been shown for alcohol. Another topic that remains to be addressed in expectancy research on illicit drugs is the question of whether global positive or negative expectancies are superior to more specific expectancies in predicting the behavioral effects of the drug, or the initiation, change, and maintenance of use. Expectancy researchers are currently addressing these topics.

Conclusion

Expectancy is a fundamental construct relating to alcohol, tobacco, and other drug use. It is therefore essential that substance abuse prevention and treatment programs carefully consider the substance-related expectancies of those they serve. As the field broadens its understanding of substance-related expectancies, such programs will be afforded the opportunity to improve the efficacy of their interventions.

*Peter S. Hendricks, Richard R. Reich,
and J. Lee Westmaas*

See also Alcohol Marketing; Assessment Instruments; Biopsychosocial Model of Addiction; Experimental Substance Use; Risk Factors for Addiction; Tobacco Marketing and Countermarketing

Further Readings

Brandon, T. H., Herzog, T. A., Irvin, J. E, & Gwaltney, C. J. (2004). Cognitive and social learning models of drug dependence: Implications for the assessment of tobacco dependence in adolescents. *Addiction, 99*(Suppl. 1), 51–77.

Brandon, T. H., Juliano, L. M., & Copeland, A. C. (1999). Expectancies for tobacco smoking. In I. Kirsch (Ed.), *How expectancies shape experience* (pp. 263–299). Washington, DC: American Psychological Association.

Darkes, J., & Goldman, M. S. (1993). Expectancy challenge and drinking reduction: Experimental evidence for a mediational process. *Journal of Consulting and Clinical Psychology, 61*, 344–353.

Goldman, M. S. (2002). Expectancy and risk for alcoholism: The unfortunate exploitation of a fundamental characteristic of neurobehavioral adaptation. *Alcoholism: Clinical and Experimental Research, 26*, 737–746.

Goldman, M. S., Reich, R. R., & Darkes, J. (2006). Expectancy as a unifying construct in alcohol-related cognition. In R. W. Wiers & A. W. Stacy (Eds.), *Handbook on implicit cognition and addiction* (pp. 105–119). Thousand Oaks, CA: Sage.

Rohsenow, D. J., Sirota, A. D., Martin, R. A., & Monti, P. M. (2004). The cocaine effects questionnaire for patient populations: Development and psychometric properties. *Addictive Behaviors, 29*, 537–553.

Schafer, J., & Brown, S. A. (1991). Marijuana and cocaine effect expectancies and drug use patterns. *Journal of Consulting and Clinical Psychology, 59*, 558–565.

EXPERIMENTAL SUBSTANCE USE

There is no single set of criteria for classifying substance use as experimental. Rather, the meanings and implications of experimental substance use vary according to the context in which the classification is made. There are at least two contexts in which substance use may be classified as experimental. In the first context, experimental use describes a temporally constrained period of light substance use, most commonly occurring in adolescence and early adulthood, which does not develop into more frequent or problematic use. In this context, the category of experimental use is often contrasted with the more extreme categories of abstinence and habitual use. A second context in which substance use is typically described as experimental involves the use of substances to probe aspects of experience that may be relatively inaccessible to normal consciousness. In contemporary Western cultures, this form of experimental substance use is most often associated with nontraditional forms of psychotherapy and religion that emerged in the latter half of the 20th century.

Developmental Phase

Substance use early in life has been related to a plethora of negative outcomes, and the desire to prevent substance use among adolescents and young adults has led to the development of large-scale antidrug interventions. Interventions aimed at reducing substance use among adolescents generally propose a linear relationship between substance use and maladjustment, such that greater levels of substance use are related to greater levels of undesirable outcomes. Such proposals advocate abstinence as the primary means to avoid negative outcomes. This understanding is reflected in the "Just say no" movement created during the Reagan administration and has been widely propagated by abstinence-oriented organizations. However, despite considerable efforts on the part of abstinence advocates, the majority of adolescents and young adults in the United States use substances for the purpose of intoxication at some point. Moreover, the majority of these young substance users do not experience substantial negative outcomes. This finding is incongruent with a proposed linear relationship between level of substance use and negative outcomes, which predicts that even low levels of substance use will result in proportionate levels of negative outcomes. This apparent incongruence has led researchers to expand taxonomies of substance users to include a category labeled experimental users. Experimental substance users are characterized by relatively infrequent substance use and by a relative absence of use-related negative outcomes.

The boundaries of experimental substance use have not been consistently defined, and the construct has been criticized for insufficient specificity. Nonetheless, the category is generally composed of individuals for whom substance use is limited to fewer than three substances, most often including marijuana and alcohol, and whose frequency of use is limited to once per month or less. Several studies have compared substance experimenters to abstainers and habitual users. An early study of this sort produced the controversial finding that experimenters were characterized by generally better psychological functioning than were abstainers or habitual users. According to that study, whereas habitual substance users were under-controlled, socially alienated, and emotionally distressed, substance abstainers were overcontrolled, anxious, and socially unskilled. In contrast, experimenters appeared to find a happy medium; they were neither excessively controlled nor excessively impulsive. Subsequent studies have challenged these findings, and evidence for superior psychological adaptation among experimenters, relative to abstainers, is scarce. However, most studies report that experimenters are generally more similar to abstainers than to habitual users. That is, they generally exhibit relatively low levels of psychopathology and other negative outcomes. There is evidence that the impact of experimentation may vary according to contextual factors such as age and community norms, such that experimentation among older adolescents and young adults in communities where such experimentation is relatively normative may be particularly innocuous.

Self-Exploration

In the latter half of the 20th century, the use of substances for the explicit purpose of gaining personal and spiritual experience rose to cultural prominence in Western society. This category of substance use has been described as experimental, in order to emphasize an epistemological or didactic focus, relative to the more hedonistic aims associated with recreational substance use. The determination of the extent to which a given instance of use can be classified as experimental is largely reliant on the a priori intent of the user, as many substances that are proposed to have edifying properties are also widely used for their euphoric effects. There are no established criteria for determining whether a given instance of substance use is experimental. Nonetheless, experimental use in this context most often involves hallucinogens derived from substances that have historically been used in shamanic and mystical traditions. In addition, to maximize the edifying elements of the intoxication, experimental use often emphasizes establishing control of the "set and setting" in which the experience proceeds. Substances most commonly used in an experimental manner include psilocybin (magic mushrooms), mescaline, LSD (lysergic acid diethylamide), and DMT (dimethyltryptamine).

Among the most prominent proponents of the potential benefits of drug experimentation include the author Aldous Huxley and the former Harvard psychology professor Timothy Leary. Dr. Leary coined the well-known phrase "Tune in, turn on, drop out," which purported to describe a process by which experimentation with hallucinogens might engender profound changes in values and lifestyle. The experimental use of hallucinogens remains highly controversial, due largely to the criminalization of possession of most of these substances and to the association of drug experimentation with the 1960s counterculture. However, prior to the prohibition of many hallucinogens in the late 1960s, these substances were the objects of considerable empirical attention based on their potential as therapeutic agents for a broad array of psychopathological conditions. Research on the efficacy of psychedelic drugs in this context is scarce, and results are generally inconsistent. Because of this, the clinical utility of these substances remains largely undetermined. Nonetheless, several organizations remain dedicated to exploring the potential psychological benefits of experimental drug use, and the experimental use of hallucinogens retains a prominent role in contemporary counterculture.

Zach Walsh and Gregory L. Stuart

See also College Students, Alcohol Use and Abuse; College Students, Drug Use and Abuse; Cultural Aspects; Moderation in Use; Social Drinking

Further Readings

Huxley, A. (1954). *The doors of perception.* London: Granada.

Leary, T. (1983). *Flashbacks.* Los Angeles: Tarcher.

Milich, R., Lynam, D., Zimmerman, R., Logan, T. K., Martin, C., Leukefeld, C., et al. (2000). Differences in young adult psychopathology among drug abstainers, experimenters and frequent users. *Journal of Substance Abuse, 11,* 69–88.

Shedler, J., & Block, J. (1990). Adolescent drug use and psychological health: A longitudinal inquiry. *American Psychologist, 45,* 612–630.

F

FAMILY BEHAVIOR THERAPY

Family Behavior Therapy for drug abuse (FBT) is one of the most scientifically supported treatments available for substance abuse and its associated problems (e.g., depression, unemployment, conduct disorders, family discord, child maltreatment). More than a decade ago, this intervention was the only comprehensive scientifically based intervention listed in National Institute on Drug Abuse's (NIDA) *Principles of Drug Addiction Treatment: A Research-Based Guide* to demonstrate improved outcomes in both adolescent and adult substance abusers and has received exemplary ratings in Substance Abuse and Mental Health Services Administration's National Registry of Evidence-based Programs and Practices. In a review by National Institute on Alcohol Abuse and Alcoholism, FBT was mentioned as one of the few evidence-based, developmentally sensitive approaches emerging for addressing alcohol, nicotine, and other drug use problems among adolescents.

Historical Context

FBT is conceptually similar to the Community Reinforcement Approach (CRA), which was pioneered by Nathan Azrin and his colleagues in the 1970s. In this approach, substance abuse is conceptualized to occur because of its strong inherent reinforcing properties. Therefore, CRA therapists reinforce addicted individuals for their performance of behaviors that are incompatible with substance use and teach skills to assist them in building strong relationships with individuals who do not use substances. Now one of the most widely utilized treatments for the addictions, CRA was unique to existing treatments when it was developed. It was the first approach to involve multiple significant others of the substance abuser into the treatment plan, one of the first interventions to assist significant others in responding to abusive behavior exacerbated by drug use, is aimed at eliminating stressors that make substance abuse more likely, and teaches communication skills training to enhance the general tone of the relationship.

In the late 1980s, Azrin received funding from NIDA to develop the first behavior therapy for adolescent drug abuse. This study was also the first controlled trial to employ both significant others and self-reports of adolescent substance use in addition to objective urinalysis testing as measures of treatment outcome. Due to initial difficulties in the recruitment of adolescents, adults were also enrolled in the initial clinical trials. This fortuitous event resulted in a robust and developmentally sensitive family-based intervention capable of treating the addictions across the life span. More than 3 decades after the development of CRA, federal funding from NIDA and the National Institute of Mental Health has permitted FBT for substance abuse to evolve into one of the premier evidence-based treatment programs in the world, incorporating standardized treatment plans that are consumer-driven treatment manuals with accompanying step-by-step protocol checklists that may be utilized during sessions to guide treatment implementation and measure program fidelity. Measures of treatment outcome are also now more sophisticated and include standardized methods of conceptualizing assessment results to family members. As the name implies, this cost-effective intervention approach utilizes innovative, easily learned behavioral therapies to treat substance abuse and associated problems within a family context.

Overview

Therapy typically consists of 16 60-minute outpatient sessions scheduled to occur across 6 months. Up to 20 home-based sessions are conducted when target populations are particularly problematic, such as child welfare recipients. After a battery of psychometrically validated assessment measures are completed by the client and adult significant other, standardized methods are utilized to assist therapists in conceptualizing the assessment information for family members and for guiding the family in the selection of their own treatment plan from a menu of alternatives. Selected therapies are implemented successively and cumulatively. That is, after each intervention is implemented for the first time, it is reviewed in all subsequent sessions to a lesser extent as relevant skills are developed. Immediately after treatment, assessment measures are again administered, and comparisons are made to evaluate treatment effects. Almost exclusively in research settings, follow-up assessments occur up to 6 months posttreatment to evaluate treatment outcomes. Recent developments include the incorporation of assessment and prevention programming targeting HIV risk behaviors, child management skills training, and protocols specific to home-based implementation for clients in child protective services. For instance, there are tours of the home to ameliorate safety hazards, teach substance abusing parents to stimulate the cognitive and social development of their children, and monitor adverse events. Controlled trials of FBT are presently testing models that teach children how to reinforce parents for their participation in nondrug associated activities.

Assessment Approach

To examine the effects of treatment, several standardized assessment measures are administered pretreatment, posttreatment, and sometimes up to 6 months after the termination of treatment. These assessments include both objective (e.g., urinalysis, behavioral observation checklists) and subjective (e.g., self and collateral reports, structured interviews, behavioral satisfaction scales, behavioral rating scales) measures of substance use, stress, strength of the family relationship, mood, and conduct. First, a brief standardized screening assessment is administered over the phone to determine the client's appropriateness for FBT and to assist in providing an initial orientation to the program. The time to administer the comprehensive battery is highly relevant to the presenting concerns of the client, but it generally lasts between 1 hour and 2.5 hours, which includes up to 15 minutes with an adult significant other. Questionnaires are usually read to clients due to unusually high rates of poor reading abilities. After pretreatment assessment measures are administered, information is carefully recorded in a database, and the results are summarized for the therapist's review. The therapist utilizes results from client satisfaction scales (measures aimed at assessing client satisfaction in various life and relationship domains) and the Timeline Followback (a standardized measure of drug use frequency) to assist the client in obtaining consumer generated goals for treatment.

Intervention Approach

There are currently about a dozen FBT intervention options that may be implemented. Several interventions are implemented initially in treatment and are capable of handling a variety of contextual factors relevant to substance abuse (e.g., age of substance abuser, number of significant others in the home, presenting problem). These interventions include the development of behavioral goals, treatment planning, stimulus control, urge and self-control, positive exchange of reinforcers within the family, and communication skills training. Other interventions are tailored to address behavior problems that may coexist with some substance abusers, but not with others. For instance, substance abusing parents who reside in low-income communities may derive benefits from the Assurance of Basic Necessities and Safety intervention, which attempts to regularly screen and prevent significant stressors, such as violence, bills, and eviction. Child management (e.g., catching my child being good, positive practice, compliance training) is particularly effective with parents of children who have behavior problems. Financial management and planning and job club assist in gaining desired employment, and contingency management assists in building motivation.

Methods of Enhancing Motivation

Several strategies have been developed to assist FBT therapists when their clients have insufficient motivation for treatment (i.e., refusal to do role-plays, cancelation of sessions, incomplete therapeutic assignments). First, FBT supervision includes agendas. These agendas include prompts for the supervisor to solicit feedback regarding issues that are relevant to nonadherence of clients to prescribed treatment protocols. The selected cases are then given top priority in supervision meetings. Agendas are also utilized by therapists during treatment sessions with their clients. These agendas include prompts for clients to indicate how helpful the interventions were to them (1, *extremely unhelpful,* to 7, *extremely helpful*). When clients indicate therapies were not helpful, the therapist assesses what can be done to enhance their treatment. Proactively, therapists are taught to solicit negative consequences of substance use from their clients, provide empathy for expressed concerns, and review alternative positive consequences that are likely to occur with abstinence. Another method involves informing substance abusers that their compliance with therapeutic procedures will be measured at the end of each session, utilizing a Likert-type scale (i.e., 1, *refused to attempt intervention component,* to 7, *completed intervention exactly as required*). Clients are told these ratings can be provided to caseworkers, with their consent, to support their efforts in therapy. Similar compliance ratings have been shown to closely correspond with clinical outcomes. Thus, clients know what is expected of them, and the ratings may be utilized to provide feedback relevant to effort in the therapeutic process.

Noncompliance with homework assignments between treatment sessions often occurs because clients feel unprepared to implement skills that were reviewed in therapy sessions or because clients attempt the interventions without success due to insufficient practice opportunities with professional instruction. Therefore, role-playing and behavioral rehearsal is utilized extensively to improve the confidence of clients and to prepare them for difficult in vivo problem situations. Assuring success early on increases the likelihood of subsequent assertiveness in future sessions. Similarly, competence is enhanced due to implementing treatments successively and cumulatively—that is, after one intervention skill is implemented, it is usually implemented in all remaining sessions to a lesser extent. Therapists are taught to

manage clients when they are being noncompliant during sessions utilizing motivational interviewing procedures, and solutions to commonly experienced difficult clinical scenarios are included in FBT treatment manuals. Therefore, therapists are primed to expect client noncompliance and to effectively manage noncompliance when it occurs. When noncompliance repeatedly occurs during sessions, even after therapists have attempted procedures that were recommended during supervision, the supervisor will co-lead the next available session with the therapist. These co-led sessions offer the therapist in vivo (onsite) supervision in difficult cases and facilitate their future ability to manage difficult cases.

Administrative Protocols

To facilitate the full adoption of FBT, various standardized administrative protocols have been developed that expeditiously, and efficiently, facilitate service delivery. These protocols are constructed as basic templates that may be quickly and easily adapted to fit the unique needs of agency administrations. For instance, protocols are available to guide the process of recruitment, obtain referrals, and process the necessary paperwork that may be utilized to prepare clients to be admitted to the clinic. There are also protocols available to assist in determining if clients meet the established clinic criteria, to guide pretreatment assessment, record program data, and prepare and implement posttreatment assessments. Finally, the standardized method of FBT permits progress notes, treatment plans, releases of and for information, and termination reports to be reduced to quick and easy fill in the blank forms.

Treatment Integrity

Several strategies are employed to ensure the integrity of FBT, including (a) intervention manuals and therapist step-by-step protocol checklists to be utilized during sessions; (b) written documentation by the therapist of techniques used during the session, ratings of the extent of client participation, and client progress toward treatment goals; (c) audio taping of all sessions; (d) ongoing clinical supervision of treatment sessions, review of selected audiotapes, and corrective feedback to therapists; and (e) detailed protocol checklists by therapists that indicate the materials needed for each session, specific tasks to be completed, and the order in which treatment tasks will be completed. These checklists assist in determining therapist adherence and competence. Therapists indicate on each protocol checklist whether each therapy task was performed. Independent raters then listen to the audiotapes and indicate on a separate protocol checklist the extent the therapy tasks have been completed. The therapists' and raters' lists are compared and a reliability estimate is computed. Reliability is calculated by dividing the total number of agreements by the total number of agreements plus disagreements and multiplying the resulting dividend by 100. The validity estimate is based only upon the lists completed by therapists and is calculated by dividing the number of tasks completed by the total number of possible tasks and multiplying the dividend by 100. This method of protocol adherence has been utilized in controlled treatment studies funded by National Institutes of Health. To be judged satisfactorily competent in the administration of FBT protocol, therapists are customarily required to have a 90% therapist adherence.

Quality assurance is extremely important and is thus monitored in a number of ways. First, a client satisfaction questionnaire is completed immediately posttreatment to assess the extent to which clients are satisfied with the services they received during treatment sessions. This assessment permits consumers the ability to influence the quality of service to future clients. Second, an extensive protocol adherence method has been developed to assure therapists are implementing FBT as intended. Third, clinic procedures, program charts, and data management are routinely evaluated utilizing standardized checklists that depict customary responsibilities. Quality assurance is maintained by monitoring approximately 5% to 10% of client charts of therapists, as well as various clinic procedures, on a random basis. To assist in this process, a chart has been developed to record all necessary quality assurance data that closely corresponds with the detailed step-by-step protocol checklists. All forms are standardized, so the process takes less than a couple of minutes per chart. Therapists who evidence errors are required to fix all problems, and the issues are brought to the attention of supervisors. The charts of these therapists are also examined more frequently in future reviews. When a database is established, it is necessary to ensure that the data are accurately managed as protocol dictates. Therefore, data for approximately 15% to 20% of clients are monitored on a random basis. When errors

are detected, the database is checked more frequently, and feedback is provided to data management specialists so future errors are less likely to occur. Standardized clinic operations assist therapists in managing their cases more efficiently and reduce liability issues that are a great concern in mental health settings, particularly when inexperienced staff members are involved.

Conclusion

Similar to several evidence-based interventions for substance abuse that are currently available, FBT has evolved over the years across randomized controlled trials. For instance, its assessment and intervention strategies are now sophisticated and capable of handling a broader array of clientele, and its standardized clinic protocols provide a context in which to more efficiently manage clientele. Indeed, consistent with the dissemination movement of evidence-based treatments from research settings to community settings, FBT investigators have developed easy-to-implement standardized methods of quality assurance, treatment integrity, and training.

Bradley C. Donohue, Nathan Azrin, Daniel N. Allen, and Vincent Van Hasselt

See also Behavioral Couples Therapy; Community Reinforcement Approach; Evidence-Based Treatment; Family Therapy; Multidimensional Family Therapy

Further Readings

Achievement Center: http://www.unlv.edu/centers/achievement

Azrin, N., Acierno, R., Kogan, E. S., Donohue, B., Besalel, V., & McMahon, P. T. (1996). Follow-up results of supportive versus behavioral therapy for illicit drug use. *Behaviour Research and Therapy, 34,* 41–46.

Azrin, N. H., Donohue, B., Besalel, V., Kogan, E., & Acierno, R. (1994). Youth drug abuse treatment: A controlled outcome study. *Journal of Child and Adolescent Substance Abuse, 3,* 1–16.

Azrin, N. H., Donohue, B., Teichner, G., Crum, T., Howell, J., & DeCato, L. (2001). A controlled evaluation and description of individual-cognitive problem solving and family-behavioral therapies in conduct-disordered and substance dependent youth. *Journal of Child and Adolescent Substance Abuse, 11,* 1–43.

Azrin, N. H., McMahon, P., Donohue, B., Besalel, V., Lapinski, K., Kogan, E., et al. (1994). Behavior therapy of drug abuse: A controlled outcome study. *Behaviour Research and Therapy, 32,* 857–866.

Donohue, B., & Azrin, N. H. (2001). Family behavior therapy. In E. Wagner & H. Waldron (Eds.), *Innovations in adolescent substance abuse intervention* (chap. 10). Tarrytown, NY: Pergamon Press.

Donohue, B., Azrin, N. H., Lawson, H., Friedlander, J., Teichner, G., & Rindsberg, J. (1998). Improving initial session attendance in conduct disordered and substance abusing adolescents: A controlled study. *Journal of Child and Adolescent Drug Abuse, 8,* 1–13.

Donohue, B., & Van Hasselt, V. B. (1999). Development of an ecobehavioral treatment program for child maltreatment. *Behavioral Interventions, 14,* 55–82.

National Institute on Drug Abuse. (1999). *Principles of drug addiction treatment: A research-based guide.* Retrieved October 1, 2008, from http://www.nida.nih.gov/ PDF/PODAT/PODAT.pdf

FAMILY COUNSELING

See FAMILY THERAPY

FAMILY THERAPY

Family therapy for addiction consists of interventions that are aimed at eliciting the support of an individual's family network to foster improved addiction treatment outcomes, as well as to provide assistance to family members who may be experiencing difficulties as a result of living in an environment that is impacted by addiction. As a field, family therapy for addictions emerged during the 1960s and 1970s to augment treatment approaches that had previously been focused at the individual level. The involvement of family members in addiction treatment was initiated to a greater extent by practitioners in the field of addiction treatment rather than by traditional marriage and family therapists. Family therapy has now become a typical component in many addiction treatment programs and is commonly provided by both social service agencies and practitioners in independent practice.

For the purpose of brevity in this entry, the terms addiction, substance abuse, drug abuse, alcohol abuse, and alcoholism will be considered synonymous. Similarly, references to alcoholism treatment and substance abuse treatment are used synonymously to connote interventions that can be applied to addiction in general rather than to the treatment of specific substances of abuse.

Theoretical Underpinnings

The theoretical underpinnings of family therapy for addiction contrast with many individually oriented treatment approaches, particularly with regard to the issue of etiology. Whereas individually oriented theories may identify singular causal factors in the development of addiction (e.g., disease process, faulty thinking), family therapy practitioners employ systems-oriented concepts to conceptualize addiction. For instance, in family systems approaches, the concept of *reciprocal determinism* may be used to describe how addiction both affects and is affected by all other family members, while the concept of *circular causality* may similarly be used to explain how interpersonal dynamics and communication patterns could initiate or support addictive behavior (e.g., through complaints about current or previous substance use). It is further posited that family members continually attempt to establish and maintain a sense of equilibrium or balance in the family system so that if one member is abusing substances, that individual's behavior serves as a *central organizing principle* that ends up providing stability to the family system. Addiction, then, can be understood as a *homeostatic maintaining force* that provides the family with stability and counteracts efforts to change.

In the literature pertaining to family treatment for addiction, a distinction can be made between two general approaches: family systems-oriented therapies and behaviorally based family therapies. Family systems-oriented therapies focus on changing the organization and functioning of the family system by improving interpersonal relationships, communication, and interactions within the family. It is assumed that improved family functioning will circumvent supporting addiction as a homeostatic maintaining force, which in turn will result in a change in substance abusing behavior. Many family therapies for addiction are also grounded in behavioral principles and techniques. Although there is much overlap in the underlying principles and applications of these two broad categories (e.g., in the attention paid to cognitive processes, reciprocal determinism, and homeostasis), behavioral family therapies emphasize the role of operant and classical conditioning in the development of addiction. From this perspective, substance use is considered to be reinforced by physiological effects, increased opportunity for social interaction, and by family members when they attend to addictive behavior or when they protect the user from the negative consequences of his or her actions. The overall therapeutic goal is to reinforce positive interactions among family members and decrease negative behaviors or interactions associated with addiction.

Treatment Planning

There are a number of potential areas for clinical focus in treatment planning, and family therapy practitioners may utilize various methods to intervene at different levels. For example, the therapist may primarily attend to the needs of the addicted individual and focus on helping the client abstain from substance use or reduce the harms associated with substance use. Alternatively, the therapist may work with family members (with or without the involvement of the addicted individual) to promote the addicted individual's entry into a formal treatment program. The therapist may also attempt to improve family functioning to help reduce the addicted individual's involvement in maladaptive behavior. Finally, the therapist may focus on the needs of other family members in and of themselves and provide support and assistance that is separate from interventions focused on treating the addicted person.

Family Systems-Oriented Therapies

Although some traditional family therapy approaches did not develop methods to specifically address addiction, many practitioners utilize various family therapy orientations to treat addictive behavior in the same way that these respective orientations would treat any other presenting problem. Some notable exceptions are multigenerational family therapy, structural therapy, and strategic therapy, which have linked specific theory to the practice of addiction treatment. Murray Bowen (the founder of Multigenerational Family Therapy) conceptualized alcoholism using the concepts of stuck-togetherness, emotional cutoff, emotional fusion, and differentiation of self to describe how alcoholism can pull a family together in times of crisis and serve a homeostatic function. From the view of structural

family therapy, addiction is understood in terms of problematic family organization (e.g., family roles), and concepts such as boundaries, enmeshment, and disengagement are used to explicate how addiction is promoted or maintained. From the strategic family therapy perspective, addictive behavior is reframed as something that may once have served an adaptive function but is no longer desirable. Therefore, whereas Bowenian therapists treat addiction by promoting differentiation among all family members, structural therapists challenge inappropriate roles and coalitions, and strategic family therapists alter the family organization using paradoxical interventions in order to provide members with the opportunity to create positive change.

In 1995, Martha Edwards and Peter Steinglass published a meta-analysis of the efficacy of family treatment for alcoholism and described four types of family systems-oriented therapy. One method, known as couples treatment, consists of brief multiple-couple therapy sessions, discussions of transactional analysis game playing, participation in Alcoholics Anonymous or Al-Anon meetings, and involvement in recreational activities. In another longer term method (weekly sessions for 3–6 months), couples focus on the expression of feelings, improving communication, and enhancing problem solving. In a third method, termed couples involved treatment, patients in a psychiatric hospital and their spouses participate in multiple-couple group therapy sessions where several topics are discussed, such as the impact of alcohol on the marriage, how each of the partners may have contributed to alcohol abuse, and how the couple could improve their life circumstances. The couples also work on problem solving issues regarding sex, finances, children, occupation, and leisure time. Similarly, in the fourth family systems model outlined, couples explore how alcohol may have served an adaptive role in family functioning over the course of about eight conjoint sessions. In this type of systems-oriented family therapy, the therapist assists couples to assess problematic communication and interaction patterns—especially as these patterns are linked to drinking—and helps clients become more effective in the areas of problem solving and communication.

Behaviorally Based Family Therapies

There are many variations in behaviorally based family therapies, including behavioral family counseling, alcohol behavioral marital therapy, relationship-enhanced cognitive behavior therapy, behavioral marital family therapy plus relapse prevention, community reinforcement and family training, a relational intervention sequence for engagement, and social behavior and network therapy, to name some examples.

An example of behaviorally based family therapy that is specifically designed to assist the cooperative, nonaddicted spouse in influencing the uncooperative partner to enter into treatment is unilateral family therapy. Initially, the therapist attempts to reduce anxiety and self-blame in the cooperative spouse that may result from being in a relationship with an addicted individual. The therapist then educates the nonaddicted spouse on topics such as behavioral contracting, neutralizing controlling behaviors, relapse prevention, and how to support the maintenance of treatment gains in order to facilitate change in family functioning and alter interactions that are thought to contribute to the addictive behavior. The therapist also assists the nonaddicted spouse to disengage with his or her addicted spouse if appropriate and provides emotional support when necessary.

An example of behaviorally based family therapy that is specifically designed to focus on the addicted individual's behavior and involves the spouse and other family members is alcohol behavioral marital therapy. In this approach, the therapist begins by conducting a functional analysis of the antecedents, accompanying events and consequences of drinking, before working with clients to set goals such as self-monitoring urges and actual drinking behaviors. Other behavior modification interventions are employed, including drink refusal training, assertiveness training, relaxation training, cognitive restructuring, and education about the effects of alcohol. Spouses are taught how to decrease behaviors that cue drinking, as well as how to reinforce abstinence and avoid protecting the alcohol abuser from the consequences of drinking behavior. Additional techniques that are designed to improve relationships are also utilized, such as communication training, planning and implementing shared activities, and problem-solving training.

Family Therapy for Adolescents

It should be pointed out that there are interventions specifically designed to assist families in the treatment of addiction among adolescents. For instance, in the publication titled *Principles of Drug Addiction Treatment: A Research-Based Guide*, the

U.S. National Institute on Drug Abuse (NIDA) lists Multidimensional Family Therapy for adolescents (MDFT) as a scientifically based approach to adolescent addiction treatment. MDFT utilizes both individual and family therapy sessions that can be held in the home, at school, or at some other location. The method involves working with the adolescent on important skills such as problem solving, decision making, negotiation, communication, and stress-management. MDFT also assists parents with parenting style, issues of control, and promotes positive role-modeling, and prosocial influence on an adolescent's life. NIDA also provides a therapy manual for Brief Strategic Family Therapy for adolescent drug abuse, which focuses on an adolescent's drug abuse within the context of broader family dynamics and other problematic behaviors of the drug-abusing adolescent.

Outcome Studies

There have been several outcome studies conducted that compare individual treatment modalities to family interventions for addiction, and on the whole, family interventions have yielded encouraging results. For example, the preponderance of evidence indicates that involving a nonaddicted spouse in a treatment program can improve participation in therapy and increase the likelihood that the addicted individual will alter drinking and/or other substance use behavior.

In the meta-analysis conducted by Edwards and Steinglass mentioned earlier, family systems approaches produced higher rates of abstinence for problem drinkers as compared to individual treatment approaches in three separate studies and in one study that compared family systems intervention to a no-treatment control group. Behaviorally based family therapy interventions, on the other hand, have received more research attention owing to better research methodologies, greater measurement precision, and a strong relationship between research and practice. For instance, studies of behavioral couples therapy (BCT) report that BCT is superior to individual treatment in terms of producing more abstinence, fewer substance-related problems, happier relationships, reduced violence, fewer couple separations, and lowering the risk of divorce.

Despite considerable empirical support for family therapy for addiction, it is important to acknowledge that there are methodological limitations to research in this area, such as a lack of consensus regarding theoretical constructs and treatment goals, as well as the fact that few researchers utilize control groups or conduct long-term follow ups. Moreover, in their meta-analysis of treatment outcomes for alcoholism, Edwards and Steinglass noted a treatment limitation whereby therapeutic gains diminish over time, and family treatment no longer appears to be superior to individual treatment when follow-up periods exceed 1 year. Notwithstanding, these researchers highlight the following three factors that may mediate the effectiveness of family treatment. First, the gender of the identified patient is important since males may benefit more from family treatment than females. Second, the level of family members' investment in their relationships is an important factor because family therapy may not be effective or appropriate for couples and families who are not committed to strengthening these relationships. Third, an increased level of family support toward the goal of abstinence is considered to be an influential factor in the success of family treatment. In a more general sense, they concluded that family treatment can only be considered to be marginally more effective than interventions that focus on the individual.

James G. Chan and Robinder P. Bedi

See also Adolescents, Substance Abuse and Treatment; Community Reinforcement Approach; Counseling Approaches; Johnson Model Intervention; Multidimensional Family Therapy; Treatment of Alcohol and Drug Use Disorders; Treatment Approaches and Strategies

Further Readings

Bowen, M. (1974). Alcoholism as viewed through family systems theory and family psychotherapy. *Annals of the New York Academy of Science, 233,* 115–122.

Chan, J. G. (2003). An examination of family-involved approaches to alcoholism treatment. *The Family Journal: Counseling and Therapy for Couples and Families, 2,* 1–10.

Collins, R. L. (1990). Family treatment of alcohol abuse: Behavioral and systems perspectives. In R. L. Collins, K. E. Leonard, & J. S. Searles (Eds.), *Alcohol and the family: Research and clinical perspectives* (pp. 338–355). New York: Guilford Press.

Copello, A. G., Velleman, R. D. B., & Templeton, L. J. (2005). Family interventions in the treatment of alcohol and drug problems. *Drug and Alcohol Review, 24,* 369–385.

Edwards, M. E., & Steinglass, P. (1995). Family therapy treatment outcomes for addiction. *Journal of Marital and Family Therapy, 21,* 475–509.

National Institute on Drug Abuse. (1999). *Principles of drug addiction treatment: A research based guide.* Retrieved June 2, 2007, from http://www.nida.nih.gov/PDF/PODAT/PODAT.pdf

O'Farrell, T. J., & Fals-Stewart, W. (2000). Behavioral couples therapy for alcoholism and drug abuse. *Journal of Substance Abuse Treatment, 18,* 51–54.

Steinglass, P. (1992). Family systems approaches to the alcoholic family: Research findings and their clinical applications. In S. Saitoh, P. Steinglass, & M. A. Schuckit (Eds.), *Addiction and the family* (pp. 155–171). New York: Brunner/Mazel.

FENTANYL

Fentanyl is a synthetic opioid analgesic that is approximately 80 times more potent than morphine. As such, it is a Schedule II controlled substance, which means there are specific regulations regarding its use. The intravenous formulation of fentanyl was approved by the Food and Drug Administration (FDA) in the 1960s under the trade name of Sublimaze. Since that time, several other dosage forms have been FDA approved under different trade names (see Table 1). Fentanyl is not absorbed well when taken by mouth and swallowed, thus the other dosage forms are designed to allow fentanyl to be absorbed either though the skin

Table 1   Fentanyl and Its FDA-Approved Dosage Forms

Generic Name	Trade Name	Route of Administration	Clinical Use
Fentanyl	Sublimaze	Intravenous or Intramuscular	Surgical Pain; Acute Severe Pain
Fentanyl	Duragesic	Transdermal Patch	Chronic Pain Management
Fentanyl	Fentora	Buccal (Cheek)	Break Through Cancer Pain
Fentanyl	Actiq	Lozenge	Break Through Pain

(transdermal) or through the mucous membranes in the mouth (buccal).

Clinical Uses

Fentanyl is extensively used for anesthesia and analgesia, and it is generally given intravenously in the operating room or intensive care unit. The fentanyl transdermal patch is attached to the skin and is used for chronic pain management. Both the buccal formulation and the lozenge are used for break through pain in individuals who have tolerance to opioids.

Dosage Forms

Intravenous and Intramuscular Injection

Intravenous and intramuscular are the typical routes of administration for the perioperative use of fentanyl.

Transdermal Patch

The patch works by releasing fentanyl into body fats, which then slowly release the drug into the bloodstream over the course of approximately 72 hours, allowing for long-lasting relief from pain. Body temperature, skin type, and placement of the patch can have a major impact on the rate of fentanyl absorption. Patches should be placed on a flat, dry, hairless area of the chest, back, or side of the upper arm. Soaps, oils, lotions, alcohol, or other chemicals should not be used on the skin where the fentanyl patch will be placed. After removing the patch, it is important to fold the patch in half, sticky side in, and flush it down the toilet. Pets or children who accidentally chew or suck on a used patch may still receive a fatal dose of fentanyl. Used and unused fentanyl patches should be kept out of the reach of children and pets.

Buccal Formulation

The buccal formulation should be placed between the upper cheek and gum above the back tooth. The tablet is left in place until it dissolves. It should not be chewed, sucked, or swallowed whole. The tablet should also not be cut in half. Because the buccal formulation is made to dissolve quickly, it is very fragile. Thus,

it should be removed from its blister pack by peeling back the foil to expose the tablet. The tablet should be used right away after opening the blister unit. The opened tablet should not be stored for future use.

Lozenge

The lozenge is a solid formulation of fentanyl citrate in the form of a lollipop that dissolves and is absorbed directly in the mouth. The lozenge should be swabbed on the mucosal surfaces in the mouth—inside cheeks, under and on the tongue, and on gums to release fentanyl quickly into the system. It is most effective if the lozenge is consumed in 15 minutes. It is important to note that individuals who have a dry mouth cannot use this route of administration.

Side Effects

Side effects to fentanyl depend in part on the dosage form used. All forms of fentanyl can cause allergic reactions, including hives difficulty breathing, or swelling of the face, lips, or tongue, as well as fentanyl toxicity (see overdose below). Other fentanyl side effects include gastrointestinal problems such as nausea, vomiting, stomach pain, gas; central nervous system effects such as dizziness, drowsiness, anxiety, and sleep problems; muscular effects such as muscle stiffness and back pain; as well as other problems such as increased sweating and urinating less than usual. There have been several cases of sudden respiratory depression leading to respiratory death with fentanyl. Individuals who are using the transdermal fentanyl patch may have itching, blistering, redness, or swelling where the patch is worn.

Tolerance and Physical Dependence

When used for long periods or at high doses, tolerance to fentanyl may develop. If tolerance develops, fentanyl may not work as well or may require higher doses for pain relief. Also, with chronic use of fentanyl, physical dependence may develop. Individuals who have physical dependence to fentanyl are likely to experience withdrawal symptoms if fentanyl is abruptly discontinued. These withdrawal symptoms associated with fentanyl are the same as those from any opioid and include anxiety; diarrhea; fever; runny nose; sneezing; abnormal skin sensations;

nausea; vomiting; pain; muscle rigidity; rapid heart beat; seeing, hearing, or feeling things that are not there; shivering; sweating; and trouble sleeping. It is important to note that physical dependence is a physiologic response to chronic use. It is not the same thing as addiction in which there is generally physical dependence, but there is loss of control and compulsive use of fentanyl. Individuals may be physically dependent without being addicted.

Illicit Use

Several synthetic analogues of fentanyl have been manufactured illicitly for recreational use, particularly in the United States. Fentanyl itself is also abused. Fentanyl is structurally unrelated to morphine and does not react to urine drug screens testing for morphine-like compounds. Fentanyl and its analogues are highly potent, and respiratory depression and death can occur very rapidly. They have been snorted, smoked, as well as injected intravenously. Used fentanyl patches may contain significant amounts of fentanyl and have been subject to abuse.

Overdose

Fentanyl overdoses can be fatal. Symptoms of a fentanyl overdose may include slowed breathing, extreme weakness or dizziness, pinpoint pupils, cold and clammy skin, or fainting. Alcohol or other central nervous system depressants may intensify this effect. If an overdose or inadvertent exposure to fentanyl is suspected, emergency medical attention is required.

Drug–Drug Interactions

Fentanyl is metabolized by the liver, and its metabolism may be affected by other medications that are also metabolized by the liver. Some medications such as benzodiazepines may enhance the respiratory depressant effect of fentanyl. It is important that individuals receiving fentanyl tell their prescribers all the medications they are taking to decrease the risk of a drug–drug interaction.

Susan Sonne

See also Central Nervous System Depressants;
    Drugs, Classification of; Morphine; Opioids; Pain
    Management

Further Readings

American Society of Health-System Pharmacists, Inc. (2008). *Fentanyl transdermal.* Retrieved November 1, 2007, from http://www.nlm.nih.gov/medlineplus/druginfo/medmaster/a601202.html

Drugs.com. (2007). *Fentanyl.* Retrieved November 1, 2007, from http://www.drugs.com/pro/fentanyl.html

FETAL ALCOHOL SYNDROME

Fetal alcohol syndrome (FAS) and fetal alcohol spectrum disorders are caused by the ingestion of alcohol during pregnancy, which exposes the developing fetus to alcohol. Although the true prevalence rate of FAS in the United States is believed to be underestimated, it is reported to occur in .2 to 1.5 per 1000 births. The percentage of births affected by maternal alcohol consumption increases to around 1 in 100 when the larger category of fetal alcohol spectrum disorders is included. These prevalence rates vary based on such factors as socioeconomic status and race, with for example, very high prevalence reported for some Native American populations. Although it is fortunate that FAS and related disorders are 100% preventable, the prevalence rates indicate that they continue to represent a substantial health risk. Indications of this health risk are clear from reports by such agencies as the Centers for Disease Control, which indicate that FAS is one of the leading causes of birth defects and is the single most common cause of mental retardation, accounting for as much as 40% of the new cases each year.

From a historical perspective, it is apparent that many early civilizations such as the Greeks and Romans believed that alcohol consumption was dangerous during conception and pregnancy. However, it is not fully known whether these early civilizations understood the true relationship between alcohol consumption and the resulting problems exhibited by infants born to mothers who consumed alcohol during pregnancy. In fact, it was not until the late 1960s that patterns of maternal alcohol consumption and abnormalities in fetal development were identified and reported in France, and it was not until the 1970s that the initial diagnostic criteria for FAS were established by a group of physicians in the United States. However, because alcohol is known to be a pervasive neurotoxin and a teratogen, it has the potential to impact all areas of development of the fetus, a potential which explains the various physical abnormalities that are characteristic of FAS.

In fact, physical abnormalities called *dysmorphologies* are hallmark features of FAS. Some of the more prominent facial abnormalities include a flattened mid face, narrow eye openings, lack of a defined philtrum (the vertical groove in the upper lip between the upper lip and bottom of the nose), and a thin upper lip. FAS is also associated with a lower than average birthweight in full-term infants, developmental delay, a variety of medical disorders, and abnormal brain development. Developmental delays in walking, talking, and toilet training are common. Medical disorders that commonly occur include abnormal immune system function and heart defects, among others. Alcohol can also have devastating effects on the developing brain. Indeed, recent research has suggested that alcohol can differentially impact specific areas of the brain, and the apparent susceptibility of these brain areas is believed to be responsible for the cognitive, behavioral, and emotional problems seen in children with FAS. Cognitive problems with learning and memory, problem-solving ability, and response inhibition are common, as are behavioral and emotional disturbances such as hyperactivity, agitation, impulsivity, and emotional instability. Individuals with FAS often lack normal motor abilities including fine motor coordination and tend to have an awkward, unsteady gait.

The diagnosis of FAS is a medical diagnosis, although it is listed as a potential cause of mental retardation (which is a psychiatric diagnosis) in the *Diagnostic and Statistical Manual of Mental Disorders, Fourth Edition, Text Revision*. The medical diagnosis of FAS is based on the previously described physical and behavioral abnormalities and requires that the following criteria be present: (a) the typical pattern of facial dysmorphologies described above, (b) retardation in growth (e.g., low birthweight), and (c) abnormal development of the central nervous system, specifically the brain. The diagnosis of FAS can be further classified as to whether the maternal use of alcohol is known. Because alcohol can affect the developing fetus even if the resulting abnormalities may not meet full criteria for FAS, a number of other disorders have been identified that fall under the more general classification of fetal alcohol spectrum disorders. Such spectrum disorders include partial fetal alcohol effects, alcohol related neurodevelopmental disorder, and alcohol related birth defects. partial fetal alcohol effects is a fairly recent

classification for a disorder with symptoms that do not meet diagnostic criteria for FAS but is the result of alcohol consumption during pregnancy. It can include symptoms such as motor problems, irritability, hyperactivity, low birthweight, and behavioral or cognitive impairment, to name a few. Alcohol related neurodevelopmental disorder is another alcohol related disorder that occurs when the mother consumes alcohol during the gestational period of her child. Alcohol related birth defects are those birth defects that are known to be associated with the toxic effects of alcohol consumption during the gestational period.

Although research has shown that many of the behavioral and cognitive deficits of FAS can be partially alleviated, none of them can be cured, so FAS is the cause of lifelong disability. After the child is born, structuring the environment, behavioral interventions, and dietary changes may alleviate some of the cognitive and learning deficits as well as some of the behavioral problems associated with FAS. Much of the research in this area has focused on enhanced learning environments, with stable and structured school and home environments being critical components. Some have also suggested that dietary supplements that are precursors to neuron development in the brain may also be helpful. Applied behavioral analysis has also been effective in treating a number of common problems such as delays in toilet training.

Finally, although FAS and fetal alcohol spectrum disorders are totally preventable, their high incidence indicates that active education and prevention efforts are warranted. Because consumption of alcohol is legal for those who are of age, women often recognize that they may have consumed alcohol during the early stages of gestation before they were aware that they were pregnant. Although animal research has demonstrated experimentally that there are extremely critical periods of pregnancy for which alcohol seems to have a greater impact than others, researchers have failed to identify any so-called safe period during which alcohol can be consumed when pregnant. Therefore, it is important for women to reduce the risk to their infant by ceasing any alcohol use when pregnant or when there is a likelihood of becoming pregnant, as is the case for sexually active women who are capable of conceiving and are not using some method of birth control.

Brian D. Leany, Daniel N. Allen,
Amanda Villamar, and Bradley C. Donohue

Authors' note: This entry was supported by a grant from the National Institute on Drug Abuse (NIDA 1R01DA020548-01A1).

See also Alcohol-Related Birth Defects; Fetal Effects of Alcohol and Other Drugs; Indian Health Services; Maternal Drug Use; Medical Consequences;

Further Readings

Calhoun, F., & Warren, K. (2007). Fetal alcohol syndrome: Historical perspectives. *Neuroscience and Biobehavioral Reviews, 31,* 168–171.

Hannigan, J. H., O'leary-Moore, S. K., & Berman, R. F. (2007). Postnatal environmental experiential amelioration of neurobehavioral effects of perinatal alcohol exposure in rats. *Neuroscience and Biobehavioral Reviews, 31,* 202–211.

Wass, T. S., Mattson, S. N., & Riley, E. P. (2004). Neuroanatomical and neurobehavioral effects of heavy prenatal alcohol exposure. In J. Brick (Ed.), *Handbook of the medical consequences of alcohol and drug abuse* (pp. 139–169). New York: Haworth Press.

FETAL EFFECTS OF ALCOHOL AND OTHER DRUGS

The effects of alcohol and other drugs on the developing fetus can be devastating both in terms of fetal development and the potential for postpartum complications. The National Institute on Drug Abuse has estimated that during gestation nearly 20% of infants were exposed to alcohol, 17% were exposed to marijuana, nearly 5% were exposed to cocaine, and nearly 40% were exposed to tobacco. The rates of exposure to opioids and amphetamines are less well known, but according to A. Nobel and colleagues perinatal exposure studies conducted in California suggest exposure in the 1% to 2% range. It should be noted, however, that when neonatologists and other specialists selectively screen infants who are considered high risk, rates of exposure are dramatically higher (e.g., perinatal rates of exposure to cocaine have been estimated to be as high as 25%). Regardless of variable estimates of exposure, it is important to keep in mind that any exposure to alcohol or other drugs during pregnancy potentially can have grave consequences.

Embryogenesis, generally between weeks 3 and 8, is considered the most vulnerable period for exposure to alcohol and other drugs for the fetus. Unfortunately, many women do not learn that they are pregnant until several weeks into the pregnancy, and hence, they may inadvertently expose the fetus to harmful substances. Regardless of when exposure occurs, however, it must be remembered that since drug and alcohol toxins act directly on the brain and that the brain develops throughout pregnancy, exposure at any time can result in damage.

Alcohol

The most widely researched drug relative to pregnancy is alcohol. The term *fetal alcohol syndrome* (FAS) was first used in 1973—scientists at this time believed that the biggest danger of alcohol consumption by mothers was that the fetus would be malnourished. However, further research has confirmed that direct toxicity of alcohol on the developing fetus was the cause of FAS (though it should be mentioned that malnutrition is also of concern in mothers who consume alcohol during pregnancy). Hence, the greatest danger to the fetus from alcohol exposure is brain damage, the full effects of which may not be realized until the child begins school when developmental learning deficits are recognized. It is important to note that exposure to alcohol is the primary cause of mental retardation in the United States.

Diagnosing FAS as a clinical disorder is not always an easy task, though diagnostic standards were established in the 1980s. Even though FAS is the third leading cause of birth defects in the United States, only very severe cases of FAS are diagnosable at birth, and there is no particularly definitive newborn test for FAS. Growth anomalies, such as failure to reach normative developmental milestones may indicate that the fetus was exposed to a toxin, but many exposures, and even simple genetic propensities for below-average fetal development, can appear in the same way. Most diagnoses, therefore, occur later in development. Robert Sokol and Sterling Clarren outline the diagnostic criteria for an FAS diagnosis, namely (a) *developmental retardation*—most notably in height, weight, head circumference, and brain size; (b) *central nervous system problems*—this may include visual/hearing problems, balance and/or gait problems, and neurological problems; and (c) *physical development problems*—these problems can be seen as facial deformities and sometimes problems with organs (e.g., the heart) and in limb development. If not all of these effects are seen, the terms *fetal alcohol effect* and/or *alcohol-related birth defects* may be used.

The incidence rate of FAS births has been estimated to approach, on average, 3 to 5 per 1,000 births in the United States. However, this estimate varies widely relative to race and ethnicity. Rates among Whites, Asians, and Hispanics are generally the lowest (1–2 per 1,000 births), African Americans have rates approaching 6 per 1,000 births, and American Indians average around 30 per 1,000 births (though rates over 100 per 1,000 births have been documented in some tribes).

Marijuana

The prevalence of marijuana use during pregnancy is relatively high (estimated to be between 5% and 20%). Perinatal exposure studies indicate that marijuana use is highest among African American mothers during pregnancy. The neurotransmitter, anandamide, has been suggested to be of importance during the early stages of pregnancy. This neurotransmitter, not discovered until 1995, acts on the limbic system and has been implicated as affecting emotions, motor coordination, and learning. It is generally found in high concentrations in mammalian uteri and may help regulate the early stages of pregnancy. Interestingly, delta-9 tetrahydrocannabinol, the active component in marijuana, attaches to the same receptor sites as anandamide, potentially disrupting the developmental process.

Marijuana exposure in newborns generally leads to diminished growth rates. This rate is owed to somewhat shorter gestation times and reduced fetal weight gain in utero. However, little evidence exists to suggest that developmental effects related to motor skills are related to fetal exposure to marijuana. Some studies have suggested, however, that short-term memory, verbal learning, and executive-function tasks may be somewhat impaired in children who had intrauteral marijuana exposure.

Cocaine and Amphetamines

An estimated 250,000 to 300,000 regular cocaine and crack abusers in the United States are women in their early 20s. Unfortunately, this statistic means that a large number of women are using these drugs when they are in the most fertile years for childbearing—leading to the unfortunate potential consequence of accidental pregnancies among this group of drug users.

The effects of central nervous system stimulants (including caffeine) are well known and include constriction of blood vessels, increased heart rates, and elevated blood pressure, among other effects. Blood vessel constriction can reduce oxygen and nutrient flow to the fetus, therefore causing developmental delays. In addition, dramatic increases in blood pressure are particularly dangerous to the mother and can also cause blood vessel damage and stroke in the fetal brain. For habitual users who exhibit elevated blood pressures, spontaneous abortions owing to abruptio placenta can result.

Physical signs of amphetamine and cocaine exposure are rare in newborns. However, some infants chronically exposed to these stimulants will develop withdrawal symptoms after birth. These symptoms can be as mild as general agitation in the newborn or as severe as seizure activity. Continued exposure via breast milk is also of concern and should be monitored by physicians.

Exposure to amphetamines, such as methamphetamine, by pregnant women can lead to high mortality rates in newborns, low birthweight, various health complications, and neurological abnormalities. Exposure to cocaine by pregnant women can also lead to several issues, as highlighted by the National Institute on Drug Abuse. There is ample evidence of developmental abnormalities in fine and gross motor skills and a myriad of central nervous system effects. In addition, effects on attention, alertness, and intelligence, particularly performance on tests, has been demonstrated in children exposed to cocaine.

Opioids

Use of opioids (e.g., heroin) generally develops into long-term use patterns (whereas in alcohol, for example, binge use may be common). The implication on the fetus, then, is that there is more likely to be prolonged exposure to opioids throughout development than one may see with other drugs, and hence, the impacts may be quite severe. A higher number of stillborn births and miscarriages may be seen, as well as higher incidence of abruptio placenta. In addition, because opioids are often injected, there is an increased risk for the development of fetal infections (e.g., septicemia or endocarditis).

Owing to the often severe withdrawal symptoms associated with opioid use, newborns of opioid-addicted mothers are at risk for severe withdrawal symptoms upon birth. These symptoms can be mild (e.g., agitation, sneezing, or runny nose) or severe (e.g., hypertonicity, vomiting, diarrhea, respiratory alkalosis, or seizures). Long-term effects of fetal opioid exposure are neurobehavioral development problems, abnormal sleep patterns (resulting in up to a sixfold increase in the risk of sudden infant death syndrome), and learning difficulties.

Prescription Drugs and Over-the-Counter Medications

The majority of pregnant women (between 60% and 75%) take medications during pregnancy. These may be simple vitamins or supplements or nonsteroidal anti-inflammatory drugs (e.g., acetaminophen). A striking number of women take a vast array of over-the-counter medications or are prescribed medications by their physicians.

The FDA has developed a standardized system of labeling medications based on their presumed safety when taken during pregnancy. Category A drugs have well-established clinical investigations that have demonstrated harmlessness to the fetus. Category B drugs do not have adequate controlled studies, but reproductive studies have demonstrated no fetal harm. Category C drugs have been shown to cause fetal effects in animal studies, but there are no adequate controlled human studies. Category D drugs have been demonstrated to pose fetal risk, but benefits of the drug may outweigh the risks for some pregnant women. Category X drugs also have been demonstrated to cause fetal harm. The costs of using the drug outweighs the potential benefits, and therefore these drugs should not be used by nor prescribed for pregnant women. Pregnant women should always insist that their prescribing physicians explain the relative risks and benefits of any prescription medication.

Anxiolytic medications are increasingly being prescribed for pregnant women. The most common of these, benzodiazepines (e.g., diazepam or alprazolam), have been demonstrated to accumulate in fetal blood at levels much higher than in the mother; in addition, excretion of benzodiazepines by the fetus is also slower. This effect increases the risk for abnormal heart patterns and congenital abnormalities. Barbiturates are also taken by some pregnant women and have been demonstrated to increase the risk of fetal abnormalities. Withdrawal symptoms can also be quite severe, and newborns must be closely monitored.

Nicotine

Smoking has increased dramatically in women over the last few decades. Smoking during pregnancy has been shown to range somewhere between 5% and 30%, with tobacco use among African American women being highest. Research has demonstrated that smoking can greatly increase the risk of miscarriage or spontaneous abortion and results in a higher number of stillbirths.

One of the greatest risks to the fetus from tobacco is exposure to more than 2,000 different chemical compounds that can be found in tobacco smoke. Many of these compounds (e.g., carbon monoxide and nicotine) have been shown to cross the placental barrier. Birth defects are relatively rare in children exposed to nicotine, but cleft palate and congenital heart defects are more commonly found among children exposed to tobacco in utero. Additionally, smoking is a known risk factor for sudden infant death syndrome. Some researchers have argued that cognitive impairment is also evident in some children of smoking mothers (e.g., lower scores on reading and math achievement tests).

Conclusion

Use of alcohol and other drugs during pregnancy can have a remarkably deleterious effect on fetal growth and development. Use of certain substances during pregnancy—cocaine, amphetamines, and opioids in particular—are most highly associated with miscarriage, stillbirths, and fetal death. If a birth occurs in an alcohol- and/or drug-using mother, several negative conditions may immediately be seen (e.g., low birthweight and abnormal development), whereas others conditions may not be recognized until much later (e.g., central nervous system deficits, learning abnormalities, and behavioral disorders). Inasmuch as many mothers do not learn of a pregnancy until late into the first trimester or even into the second trimester, mothers may not cease alcohol and drug-using behaviors until after damage has been done. Therefore, educational opportunities and prevention efforts should be made a high priority for women of childbearing age.

Chad L. Cross

See also Alcohol-Related Birth Defects; Children of Alcoholics; Fetal Alcohol Syndrome; Maternal Drug Use

Further Readings

Inaba, D. S., & Cohen, W. E. (2004). *Uppers, downers, all arounders: Physical and mental effects of psychoactive drugs* (5th ed.). Ashland, OR: CNS Publications.

Nobel, A., Vega, W. A., Kolody, B., Porter, P., Hwang, J., Merk, G. A., et al. (1997). Prenatal substance abuse in California: Findings from the perinatal substance exposure study. *Journal of Psychoactive Drugs, 29,* 43–53.

Sokol, R. J., & Clarren, S. K. (1989). Guidelines for use of terminology describing the impact of prenatal alcohol on the offspring. *Alcoholism: Clinical and Experimental Research, 13*(4), 597–599.

Woods, J. R., Jr. (1998). Translating basic research on drugs and pregnancy into the clinical setting. In C. L. Wetherington & A. B. Roman (Eds.), *Drug addiction research and the health of women* (pp. 187–196). Retrieved from http://www.drugabuse.gov/PDF/DARHW/187-196_Woods.pdf

Zickler, P. (1999). NIDA studies clarify developmental effects of prenatal cocaine exposure. *NIDA Notes, 14*(3). Retrieved from http://www.drugabuse.gov/NIDA_Notes/NNVol14N3/Prenatal.html

Zuckerman, B. (1997). *Developmental consequences of maternal drug use during pregnancy* (NIDA Monograph No.164, pp. 96–106). Retrieved from http://www.drugabuse.gov/pdf/monographs/monograph164/277-287_Zuckerman.pdf

FIDELITY OF PREVENTION PROGRAMS

In outcome research, fidelity has typically been described as the ability to show that manipulation of the independent variable has occurred as designed. Assessment of prevention program fidelity—that is, the delivery of a manualized program as prescribed by the developer—is useful to providers in determining the level of quality of a given implementation and to offer assurances to providers that services are, in fact, impacting the intended populations. This entry will discuss salient issues regarding fidelity of prevention programming, including the evaluation and measurement of fidelity, elements that may serve to enhance fidelity, and the tension between fidelity and adaptation of programs to specific needs and populations.

Importance of Program Fidelity

As a result of the development of prevention curricula and practices becoming increasingly evidence driven in recent years, more prevention programs are being deemed efficacious in either preventing the development of negative behaviors or enhancing the growth of protective factors in terms of one or more substance use outcomes. With the increase in the dissemination of a variety of community- and school-based prevention programs, researchers have concluded that the success of any program depends a great deal on the fidelity of the implementation of the program's components. When there is a failure to implement a program as planned, there is the possibility to mistakenly conclude that the observed lack of desired outcomes can be credited to the program itself. Fidelity measures have been utilized to explain if, why, and how new programs are successful and to provide salient information about how fidelity may moderate the effects of program components. Information about fidelity enhances the ability of the developers to improve upon future work and aids in replicating successful programs without wasting valuable time and resources on portions of the program that are not working. Research has highlighted the fact that half-hearted implementation of programs designed for high-risk youth fare no better than no program at all.

Evaluation and Measurement

Historically, the empirical literature describing studies evaluating the effectiveness of prevention programs provided little in terms of the assessment of implementation fidelity or much consideration of fidelity as a predictor of outcome. Evaluations of substance use prevention programs are beginning to measure fidelity, and it is not uncommon that they depend on the self-reports of providers or on observations of a single session. In substance use prevention research, there have been studies that have assessed fidelity under real world conditions, and many such programs were found to be lacking in achieved delivery.

Elements of fidelity have typically included organizational elements, process elements, and content elements. Organizational elements include evaluating the precision of the implementation such as on the time starting and ending of each session. Process elements include evaluating the providers' communication, listening, and facilitation skills and whether the provider has set the context and reflected upon the session. Content elements include assessment of whether the provider has followed the lesson plan and has distributed the necessary materials at each session.

Researchers have described constructs and associated measures in which fidelity has been considered. The most common means is by examining program adherence. Here, the degree to which the program provider is following the curriculum manual is measured. In addition, the comfort of the provider with the manual and materials is also examined. Often observers who have training in the content and model of program delivery will be used to document the degree to which particular activities and methods are delivered consistent with the program manual.

Measuring program dose can contribute important information about fidelity. Documenting the number of sessions or modules completed during the course of the program as well as the duration of each of the sessions are measures of dosage. Ideally, measures important in a calculation of dose include self-reported checklists by providers about each of the lesson plans as well as attendance data for each participant.

The interactive methods that are part of many of the more recent evidence-based prevention programs also deserve attention. As such, the quality of delivery is important to assess. Many prevention programs include interactive and role-play techniques that help recipients learn skills or promote specific attitudes. These methods rely on the provider to act as a facilitator of curriculum delivery, often times conveyed in group settings. As such, the level of engagement among participants during the program delivery is important to examine. Frequently, the interactions between the leaders and recipients within a program are observed, and these interactions are rated in order to document the ability of the prevention message to be both relayed and received. The teaching and facilitation skills on the part of the provider can also be observed.

Participant response to the prevention program can be documented by observing the way in which the participants appear engaged and are involved in the activities and subject matter of the session being delivered. Self-report measures, as well as observations, have been used to provide evidence that those who report that sessions were meaningful and interesting

subsequently fared better on desired program related outcomes.

Elements Related to Program Fidelity

The prevention program evaluation literature has pointed to a number of salient elements that appear to enhance the probability of obtaining high levels of program fidelity. Several important ones are described in this entry.

Support of a Stakeholder Team

A number of organizational characteristics have been shown to be related to program fidelity—most importantly, the support of leaders within the organization. This level of support can impact on the provider's morale and sense of self-efficacy to deliver the prevention program elements. In addition, a team of committed leaders can provide a proactive approach in problem solving as well as the organization's readiness to adopt innovative programs.

Training of Program Providers

Published studies, reviews, and guides have all strongly emphasized the importance of extensive and comprehensive training to ensure effective implementation. Although there is only modest empirical research examining which specific features of training promote effectiveness, it has been documented that recipients of prevention program training prefer concrete instruction in addition to user-friendly manuals. Studies have identified that providers value the following: sufficient initial training to convey a curriculum's purpose and content, practice in key teaching techniques, ongoing Web support, proactive and ongoing technical assistance, on-site training, high standards for performance, opportunities for practice, and an understanding of possible latitude that may be allowed for program modification. Findings from studies have been equivocal in determining if live training versus video training is more efficacious. Research on the dissemination of prevention programs suggests that highly detailed protocols have low success rates in terms of institutionalization. Organizations are not necessarily proactive when it comes to planning for continuity of program supporters or implementers, and as a result, curriculum viewed as burdensome is unlikely to be fully implemented or followed entirely.

Provider Characteristics

Provider characteristics that have been shown to increase fidelity include involvement in programmatic decision making, general receptivity to change, discretion in evaluating program components, adequate time to attend training, adequate time to prepare for sessions, prior experience in conducting prevention programming, and perceived overall effectiveness of the particular curriculum.

Program Fidelity Versus Program Adaptation

A controversy has been unfolding in prevention science regarding the importance of fidelity versus program adaptation; that is, the modification of program content or delivery in order to accommodate the needs of specific groups. Currently, the Substance Abuse and Mental Health Services Administration's National Registry of Evidence-based Programs and Practices lists model programs that have been scientifically evaluated, and it has been estimated that more than half of these programs have been adapted in different venues in one form or another. Program developers and prevention researchers have been understandably concerned that any modification in a proven program will temper its desired effect. Program adaptation may include substantive deletions and additions as well as changes in the method or concentration with which various components are delivered. There is increasing documentation that providers have been liberally adapting curricula, either by truncating the number of lessons or by modifying content or instructional methodologies. Some of the reasons for these instances of incomplete or inappropriate adoption of programs reported by providers include the following: inadequate time to deliver all of the components; disagreement with some of the components based upon culture, gender, or developmental stage of recipients; judgments that group dynamics were not conducive to the particular session; and being uncomfortable with the material at hand.

It is generally agreed that program developers often possess a unique understanding that has guided the program's development. They have presumably researched the critical elements of substance use behaviors, the activities that have been shown to be both essential and nonessential, and what might be adaptable. Although reinvention has the potential to change the critical nature of the intervention, time constraints, community norms, availability of resources, and regulatory restrictions may all play a role in program adaptations. Emerging guidelines have been posted on Web sites to encourage thoughtful approaches to resolving these controversies.

Conclusion

Effective substance use prevention programs have been identified, and there are resources to help educators and community providers select the most appropriate programs. Unfortunately, recent research has found that only fractions of organizations are implementing research-proven programs with a high degree of fidelity. Although the importance of examining fidelity during prevention program implementation is increasingly seen as a vital aspect of program evaluation, it is nevertheless an activity that is in need of additional attention. The prevention field, while struggling with its own issue of defining terms, needs to develop a consistent methodology for measuring what is described as fidelity, including instrumentation proved to be valid and reliable.

The empirical literature has generally, but not unanimously, supported the importance of maintaining a high degree of fidelity in prevention programs. Rigid fidelity may result in programs that are inappropriate for meeting the needs of the intended targets. The prevention field is struggling with identifying what components are essential for fidelity and what program adaptations may be fitting. Important issues in considering adaptation strategies include the level of information processing capability of the recipient, as measured by language or developmental stage. Other considerations are intrapersonal motivations and emotions as they are related to gender or background, as well as the ecological aspects of the environment in which the recipients reside. Adaptation strategies that are guided by a clear and informed theory, model, or framework will make the strongest contributions to the design of hybrid interventions that take the essential parts of a proven curriculum and fit them to the needs of the local school or community implementing the prevention or intervention agenda. Here, it is hoped that both fidelity and outcome can be maximized.

Valerie L. Johnson

See also Evidence-Based Prevention; National Registry of Evidence-based Programs and Practices; Prevention Evaluation; Research Issues in Prevention; School-Based Prevention Programs

Further Readings

Castro, F. G., Barrera, M., & Martinez, C. R. (2004). The cultural adaptation of prevention interventions: Resolving tensions between fidelity and fit. *Prevention Science, 5*, 41–45.

Dusenbury, L., Brannigan, R., Falco, M., & Hansen, W. B. (2003). A review of research on fidelity of implementation: Implications for drug abuse prevention in school settings. *Health Education Research, 18*, 237–256.

Dusenbury, L., Brannigan, R., Falco, M., & Lake, A. (2004). An exploration of fidelity of implementation in drug abuse prevention among five professional groups. *Journal of Alcohol and Drug Education, 47*, 4–19.

Dusenbury, L., Brannigan, R., Hansen, W. B, Walsh, J., & Falco, M. (2005). Quality of implementation: Developing measures crucial to understanding the diffusion of preventive interventions, *Health Education Research, 20*, 308–313.

Hill, L. G., Maucione, K., & Hood, B. K. (2007). A focused approach to assessing program fidelity. *Prevention Science, 8*, 25–34.

Mowbray, C. T., & Holter, G. B. (2003). Fidelity criteria: Development, measurement and validation. *American Journal of Evaluation, 24*, 315–340.

Sobeck, J. L., Abbey, A., & Agius, E. (2006). Lessons learned from implementing school based substance abuse prevention curriculums. *Children and Schools, 28*, 77–85.

Substance Abuse and Mental Health Services Administration. (2002). *Finding the balance: Program fidelity and adaptation in substance abuse prevention. A state-of-the-art review.* Retrieved May 7, 2007, from http://www.nrepp.samhsa.gov/resources-legacy-documents.htm

Substance Abuse and Mental Health Services Administration. (2008). *SAMHSA model programs.* Retrieved June 18, 2007, from http://modelprograms.samhsa.gov

G

GAMBLERS ANONYMOUS

Gamblers Anonymous (GA) is a Twelve-Step program designed to help problem gamblers recover from their addiction to gambling. GA has no affiliation to religious organizations, political parties, or special interest groups. The guiding principles are very similar to those of other Twelve-Step programs, such as Alcoholics Anonymous. GA welcomes people with any type of gambling problem to its meetings. As outlined in their Unity Program, the only requirement for membership is an honest desire to stop gambling. Gamblers Anonymous describes a compulsive gambler as someone whose gambling has caused growing and continuing problems in any area of his or her life, including, but not limited to financial, relational, legal, and vocational. GA has adapted the Twelve Steps and Twelve Traditions of Alcoholics Anonymous to gambling.

The first GA meeting was held in 1957 in Los Angeles, California. Since then, Gamblers Anonymous has grown into a fellowship that hosts more than 1,000 weekly meetings across the United States and currently has chapters in more than 30 countries throughout the world.

Most GA meetings take place in community centers, churches, and schools and are scheduled throughout the week during the day and evening hours to accommodate different schedules. Most new members of Gamblers Anonymous arrive after suffering a major setback in their personal lives, including divorce, job loss, bankruptcy, or other legal problems. The majority of GA members tend to be males in their 30s and 40s, with many years of gambling problems, large debt, and serious family conflicts.

Upon arriving at a meeting for the first time, new members are given a self-assessment questionnaire titled "The 20 Questions." This "yes or no" questionnaire is designed to help the person determine whether he or she is a compulsive gambler. Per GA guidelines, most compulsive gamblers will answer "yes" to at least 7 of the 20 questions.

Gamblers Anonymous, as the name implies, provides their members with as much anonymity as they desire. GA contends that this anonymity has great value in attracting new members who feel there is a stigma attached to their gambling problem. They also credit anonymity with the lack of power struggles within the fellowship and with reminding members that they must always place principles above personalities.

GA programs are supported through monetary contributions from their members; to prevent external influences on the Fellowship, they do not accept outside financial assistance or contributions. Although there are no membership fees required to join or be part Gamblers Anonymous, members are encouraged to accept financial responsibility for the expenses related to the meetings and service facilities.

GA does not have a formal hierarchy. Although there are service boards that determine different assignments with the programs, these boards have no formal authority, voting, or veto power and are directly responsible to the entire membership.

Gamblers Anonymous is a nonprofessional entity, and all meetings are led by recovering gamblers. GA does not discourage their members from seeking outside help for their addiction, but they believe that having professional therapists or counselors within their fellowship would interfere with their core principles.

Similar to Al-Anon and Alateen, the significant others and children of compulsive gamblers can receive support from Gam-Anon and Gam-A-Teen. As with any addictive disorder, this support can be helpful in the recovering process for the compulsive gambler, but, just as important, is the support Gam-Anon and Gam-A-Teen provide for those loved ones impacted by compulsive gambling.

The GA program has come under scrutiny for high attrition rates, the abstinence-only principle, the failure to deal with other co-occurring substance addictions, and a perceived gender bias. There is a perception that pressure tactics are utilized to help new members get honest with themselves and their loved ones. These tactics have been blamed for GA's high dropout rate, as many gamblers are not ready to disclose the extent of their problem even to their spouses or closest friends. Of course, the high attrition rate may also be a function of the nature of addiction, similar to what is observed in alcohol and other drug addiction.

The GA insistence on total abstinence from gambling may also contribute to the high attrition rate. Several studies have found that less than 10% of attendees become active GA members, less than 8% reach gambling abstinence after 1 year on the program, and less than 7% achieve it after 2 years of meetings. However, abstinence is the hallmark of all Twelve-Step recovery programs, so GA's stance on this issue is consistent with other groups.

Because GA focuses strictly on gambling and the effects this addiction has on the life of members, it has been difficult to pinpoint exactly what percentage of GA members have other, co-occurring substance addictions that might need attention. However, studies have shown that problem gamblers tend to have much higher levels of co-occurring substance abuse issues than the general population. For this reason, some speculate that GA is most effective for problem gamblers who are free of any other addiction or mental health issue.

Although female membership has been increasing steadily through the years, most GA meetings are still male-dominated. This could be due to several factors, including the fact that problem gambling has been mostly a male issue and that the GA program is not designed to meet certain "special needs" that are often reported by women as factors in their problem gambling.

Studies have found that male gamblers are more likely to report external issues such as finances, job security, and legal problems as important in their recovery, whereas women cite more emotional and social issues, which leads many females to seek more specific counseling and psychotherapy.

Geography also seems to play a major role in determining the participation of females at GA meetings. For example, some Las Vegas GA meetings report that over half of their members are women. States like Arizona and Connecticut have started women-only GA groups because of the rising demand for these types of meetings. However, in areas where casinos are not prevalent, the percentage of females at GA meetings tends to be much lower, some in single digits.

One thing that many critics agree on is that GA works best in conjunction with other treatment programs. The program's "20 Questions" have also been praised as one of the best self-assessment instruments available. Many professionals also agree that GA's social support system is difficult to imitate in a private practice setting.

Regardless of the criticisms, the popularity of GA continues to grow, as does the number of problem gamblers in America. For many people, GA is the only recovery option, considering the lack of treatment services available across the country, the fact that most insurance policies do not pay for compulsive gambling treatment, and the inability of many problem gamblers to pay for private services. Therefore, it is likely that GA will continue to be the most utilized form of support for compulsive gamblers who want help.

José Pacheco and Gary L. Fisher

See also Alcoholics Anonymous; Gambling, Pathological; Gambling, Problem; Narcotics Anonymous; Twelve-Step Recovery Programs

Further Readings

Ciarrocchi, J. W. (2001). *Counseling problem gamblers and their families: A self-regulation manual for individual and family therapy.* Burlington, MA: Academic Press.

Gamblers Anonymous. (1984). *Sharing recovery through Gamblers Anonymous.* Los Angeles: Author.

Gamblers Anonymous. (1994). *A day at a time.* Center City, MN: Hazelden.

Petry, N. M., & Armentano, C. (1999). *Prevalence, assessment, and treatment of pathological gambling: A review.* Retrieved February 10, 2008, from http://ps.psychiatryonline.org/cgi/content/full/50/8/1021

Stewart R. M., & Brown, R. I. F. (1988). An outcome study of Gamblers Anonymous. *British Journal of Psychology, 152,* 284–288. Retrieved February 10, 2008, from

http://bjp.rcpsych.org/cgi/reprint/152/2/284?ijkey=53fa97
612ec57e2c4b7f63c9167ba595c048e56b

Volberg, R. A. (1994). The prevalence and demographics of
pathological gamblers: Implications for public health.
American Journal of Public Health, 84, 237–241.
Retrieved February 10, 2008, from http://www.ajph.org/
cgi/reprint/84/2/237?ijkey=17f60a7420bf7d7f9bdded1113
9f3bcf0745d0b1

GAMBLING, PATHOLOGICAL

Gambling is a common feature of American life as a form of recreation. In addition, it has become an expedient source of revenue for governments and is an attractive entertainment investment for tourism companies. New technologies make gambling even easier to access. Research has demonstrated that the number of gamblers rose throughout the end of the 20th century in the United States.

Due to the prevalence of gambling, many individuals develop a pattern of severe problem gambling called pathological gambling (PG). In 1980, PG was first introduced as a disorder of impulse by the American Psychiatric Association in the third edition of the *Diagnostic and Statistical Manual of Psychiatric Disorder (DSM)*. The newest edition of this manual, *DSM-IV-TR*, provides a widely accepted definition of PG as persistent and recurrent maladaptive gambling behavior that disrupts personal, family, or vocational pursuits. According to the National Council on Problem Gambling, approximately, 3 million people or 1% of adults in the United States meet the criteria for PG in a given year.

Demographics of Pathological Gambling

The issue of PG has developed into a public health phenomenon in the United States because it negatively impacts individuals, their families, and society. The most vulnerable groups for the development of PG are men, adolescents, the elderly, minorities, and people in low socioeconomic status groups or with low education levels. However, no demographic group is immune to the development of PG.

Pathological gamblers can be found throughout the general U.S. population. With regard to gender, more males than females are reported to have issues relating to PG. Males tend to be stimulated by the excitement of winning money, whereas females are more likely to engage in gambling to escape problems. Due to new technologies in gaming, adolescents can easily access gambling through the Internet and video games. As a result, this group is increasingly at risk for developing gambling problems because they have not yet developed the capacity to moderate their behaviors. Therefore, as the National Research Council has pointed out, adolescent gamblers are more apt to develop PG than are adult gamblers. Furthermore, the elderly are also at risk to begin gambling and to consequently develop PG. The Gambling Impact and Behavior Study (a large federal study of gambling behavior and attitudes) found that adults from age 50 to 64 were more likely to engage in problem gambling than other age groups. However, it is difficult to identify special gambling behaviors in the elderly because there is so little research on the subject. Other studies have found that ethnic minorities are involved in high rates of gambling and PG. In the Gambling Impact and Behavior Study, African Americans were reported to be more likely to develop PG when compared with Hispanics and Native Americans. Additionally, this study provided evidence that individuals who have a high school education or less and whose income was less than $24,000 presented higher rates of PG.

Risk Factors for Pathological Gambling

Several risk factors that impact the development and maintenance of PG have been identified. For example, genetics is a factor in the development of PG. Studies of families have revealed an incidence of PG of about 20% in first-degree relatives. Access is another risk factor. Along with widespread legislated gambling, individuals are able to access illicit gambling with ease. Using telephone and patron surveys, the National Opinion Research Center (NORC) at the University of Chicago found that the presence of a gambling facility within 50 miles roughly doubled the prevalence of problem and pathological gambling in a community. With regard to adolescents, technological advances have an impact on gambling. Young people, compared to adults, may be more attracted to technologically advanced gambling venues. Furthermore, family and peers have a significant impact on adolescent PG. For example, the severity of fathers' gambling problems is related to adolescent gambling.

Individual risk factors are also related to PG. About 90% of pathological gamblers have a least one personality disorder. In addition, personality traits such as sensation seeking, impulsivity, neuroticism, irrational thinking, cognitive distortions, erroneous perceptions, and moods may act as risk factors for developing PG. For example, many gamblers have an irrational belief that they can directly or indirectly control the outcome of a game. Superstitious beliefs are also important factors in the maintenance of gambling behavior. Furthermore, manic and depressive disorders occur with high frequency among those with PG, with about 25% of the PG population exhibiting some form of manic disorder and over half demonstrating a depressive disorder. Of course, it is difficult to determine if these mental disorders preceded the development of PG or are the result of PG.

Assessment and Diagnosis

Gambling assessment measurements are utilized to screen or diagnose individuals for PG. Several brief screening instruments for PG have been developed, such as the Early Intervention Gambling Health Test, the South Oaks Gambling Screen, and the Gambler Anonymous' Twenty Questions. The Massachusetts Gambling Screen was designed to screen and assess gambling problems among adolescents and adults. The NORC DSM-IV Screen for Gambling Problems was developed according to *DSM-IV* criteria. It includes 17 lifetime items and 17 corresponding past-year items.

The diagnostic criteria for PG in the *DSM-IV-TR* includes the following: (1) *preoccupation with gambling*—constant thinking and planning regarding past and future gambling and ways to get money to gamble; (2) *tolerance*—needing to gamble with increasing amounts of money in order to achieve the desired excitement; (3) *withdrawal*—feeling restless or irritable when attempting to cut down or stop gambling; (4) *escape*—gambling as a way of escaping from problems or of relieving a distressed mood; (5) *chasing*—after losing money gambling, often returning another day to get the losses back; (6) *lying*—lying to family members, therapists, or others to conceal the extent of involvement with gambling; (7) *loss of control*—unsuccessfully attempting to reduce gambling; (8) *illegal acts*—committing illegal acts such as forgery, fraud, theft, or embezzlement to finance gambling; (9) *risked significant relationship*—jeopardizing or losing a significant

relationship, job, or educational or career opportunity because of gambling; and (10) *bailout*—relying on others to provide money to relieve a desperate financial situation caused by gambling. If gamblers display five or more of the ten-item criteria, they may be diagnosed as PG; fewer than five items is regarded as problem gambling.

Additionally, Howard Shaffer and his colleagues at Harvard have designed a system of levels to indicate the degree of gambling involvement and related problems. Level 0 describes individuals who have never gambled. Level 1 depicts social or recreational gambling. Level 2 is associated with at-risk gambling, in-transition gambling, problem gambling, and disordered gambling. This level does not meet the diagnostic criteria in the *DSM-IV-TR* for PG. Level 3 is identified as compulsive gambling. Individuals involved in Level 3 gambling meet the criteria in the *DSM-IV-TR* for PG.

Prevention and Treatment

With the increased availability of gambling and new gambling technologies, PG is potentially more widespread than ever before and has become a public health problem. The social, emotional, and behavioral consequences of PG are severe and include suicide attempts, bankruptcy, divorce, alcohol or drug abuse, and domestic violence. In addition, desperate pathological gamblers may participate in illegal activities including forgery, embezzlement, and shoplifting to support their gambling. Therefore, prevention and treatment for PG are urgently needed.

For the prevention of PG, educational initiatives are typically prescribed. Education increases individuals' awareness and knowledge about PG, which may affect their attitudes toward gambling behaviors. Programs include television commercials, billboards, bus tails, posters, postcards, and other means of increasing public awareness. The impact of gambling access and availability should be considered in formulating prevention plans. This is vital because legalized gambling has rapidly expanded in the United States over the past several decades.

Government efforts have been involved in prevention and treatment of PG. The first state-funded treatment program was established in Maryland. Several states—such as Minnesota, Iowa, Washington, Connecticut, and Oregon—have been funding gambling prevention and treatment programs by gaming tax receipt or lotteries revenue. For example, the Iowa Gambling Treatment Program educated the public to be aware of PG and provided assistance through its helpline.

Compared to other impulsive disorders, PG is difficult to treat. According to the National Gambling Impact Study Commission Report, treatments are costly and time consuming, results are often difficult to see, and relapse is frequent. The goal of treatment may be abstinence or controlled gambling (i.e., reduce the harm to gamblers and to others around them).

The various types of treatment include the following:

1. *Helplines*—Many states have a gambling helpline number. Individuals with gambling problems can access professional information and help by calling a 24-hour, toll-free number. Also, the National Council on Problem Gambling (NCPG) provides a national 24-hour helpline.

2. *Support groups and organizations*—Gamblers Anonymous (GA) is a Twelve-Step support group program based on the format of Alcoholics Anonymous designed to assist individuals to recover from PG. Similar to other Twelve-Step support programs, GA is a peer-led program that encourages abstinence from all gambling as the method for recovery. The NCPG is a nonprofit organization designed to educate people, research gambling as a public health issue, and provide programs to aid individuals with gambling problems.

3. *Formal treatment*—Just as in treatment for substance use disorders, treatment for PG can occur in outpatient or inpatient settings and may be in publicly supported treatment programs or private treatment programs. Because private health care insurance policies do not normally pay for PG treatment, publicly financed treatment is vital since, by the nature of the disorder, most people with PG have limited financial resources.

Conclusion

With the greater accessibility to gambling, the prevalence of PG has become a public health issue due to the negative impacts of excessive gambling on individuals, families, and society. The vulnerable groups related to PG are men, adolescents, the elder, minorities, and people of low socioeconomic status or with lower levels of education. Although risk factors for PG have been identified, a cause-and-effect relationship between these risk factors and PG has not been established. Screening and assessment instruments have been developed to aid in the identification of PG, with the diagnosis of PG generally made on the basis of criteria in the *DSM-IV-TR*. Given the serious nature of PG, prevention and treatment are essential, and states have increasingly devoted resources to these areas.

Yan Shu, Sabina Mutisya, and Thomas Harrison

See also Gamblers Anonymous; Gambling, Problem; National Council on Problem Gambling; National Gambling Impact and Policy Commission

Further Readings

Committee on the Social and Economic Impact of Pathological Gambling, Committee on Law and Justice, Commission on Behavioral and Social Sciences and Education, & National Research Council. (1999). *Pathological gambling: A critical review*. Washington, DC: National Academy Press.
Gamblers Anonymous:
http://www.gamblersanonymous.org/index.html
Grant, J. E., & Potenza, M. N. (2004). *Pathological gambling: A clinical guide to treatment*. Washington, DC: American Psychiatric Publication.
Marotta, J. J., Cornelius, J. A., & Eadington, W. R. (2001). *The downside: Problem and pathological gambling*. Reno: University of Nevada, Institute for the Study of Gambling and Commercial Gambling.
National Council on Problem Gambling:
http://www.ncpgambling.org
National Gambling Impact and Policy Commission (U.S.). (1999). *National Gambling Impact Study Commission: Final report*. Washington, DC: Author.
Petry, N. M. (2005). *Pathological gambling: Etiology, comorbidity, and treatment*. Washington, DC: American Psychological Association.
Raylu, N., & Oei, T. P. S. (2002). Pathological gambling: A comprehensive review. *Clinical Psychological Review, 22*, 1009–1061.
Shaffer, H. J., Hall, M. N., & Bilt, J. V. (1999). Estimating the prevalence of disordered gambling behavior in the United States and Canada: A meta-analysis. *American Journal of Public Health, 89*, 1371.
Vachon, J., Vitaro, F., Wanner, B., & Tremblay, R. (2004). Adolescent gambling: Relationships with parent gambling and parenting practices. *Psychology of Addictive Behaviors, 18*, 398–401.

GAMBLING, PROBLEM

Problem gambling and *pathological gambling* are terms used to describe gambling behaviors that are negatively impacting normal activities. The technical diagnosis for these behaviors is known as pathological gambling, which is an impulse-control disorder characterized by certain criteria involving maladaptive gambling behaviors. The term *problem gambling* is different in that it generally refers to someone who has maladaptive gambling behaviors but does not fully meet the criteria for the pathological gambling disorder.

The first time problem gambling appeared in the *Diagnostic and Statistical Manual of Mental Disorders* (*DSM*) was in the third edition, published in 1980. However, concern involving maladaptive gambling behaviors started long before then with the establishment of Gamblers Anonymous in 1957. This organization was founded on similar principles as the Alcoholic Anonymous Twelve-Step program. Research on maladaptive gambling behaviors has helped distinguish problem gambling from pathological gambling. Generally, gamblers who do not experience negative interruption in their lives from gambling are labeled "recreational" or "social" gamblers. Some of these gamblers may become "at risk" if they meet one or two of the ten *DSM-IV-TR* criteria for pathological gambling. Although problem gambling is not a technical diagnosis, a person that is classified as a problem gambler would generally meet three or four of the criteria in the *DSM-IV-TR* for pathological gambling. A person diagnosed with pathological gambling must meet five or more of the criteria. Although pathological gambling generally entails more serious gambling issues than problem gambling, both types can benefit from treatment because problem and pathological gamblers alike experience a significant negative impact on their lives because of gambling behaviors. Surveys of gambling behavior have established the prevalence of problem and pathological gambling at anywhere between 1.2% and 4.0% of the population.

To determine if gambling behavior can be described as problem or pathological, most clinicians utilize either the South Oaks Gambling Screen (SOGS) or the NORC DSM-IV Screen for Gambling Problems (NODS). Although there are other assessment instruments available, the SOGS and the NODS are generally the most used and most cited in published articles about problem and pathological gambling.

The SOGS is used mainly in conjunction with an intake interview to detect possible problem or pathological gamblers. Also, it provides the clinician with a better view of a client's gambling habits and gives additional useful information such as what type of betting games a client prefers, how often a client gambles, where money is obtained for gambling, and other instances of problem gambling in a client's family.

Twenty points is the maximum score on this assessment, with a score of 3 or 4 suggesting at-risk gambling behaviors, a score of 5 or above suggesting a probable gambling problem, and 9 or above is labeled a severe gambling problem. Although the SOGS is easy to use and allows for quick administration to get a better idea of gambling habits, there have been criticisms of the SOGS. Some items on the SOGS are easily misunderstood, and a high rate of false positives (i.e., diagnosis of a problem when one does not exist) occurs. Therefore, the SOGS may overestimate how many problem and pathological gamblers there actually are in the population.

The NODS was developed to carefully match the criteria for pathological gambling contained in the fourth edition of the *DSM*. Although it is similar to the SOGS in providing a clinician with valuable information about gambling habits, the NODS differs from the SOGS in that the questions ask about both lifetime gambling behavior and gambling behavior in the past year. This allows clinicians to differentiate between people who have ever met the criteria for pathological gambling and those who currently meet the criteria. This assessment also asks more questions, specifically about the *DSM* criteria.

The treatment of problem gambling is similar to the treatment for pathological gambling. Due to the more serious nature of pathological gambling, treatment may be more intensive or of longer duration. Most treatment occurs in outpatient settings. While many substance abuse treatment programs offer treatment for problem and pathological gambling, some treatment programs for gambling problems are independent of alcohol and drug treatment programs. However, much of the current treatment for problem and pathological gambling incorporates the same components as substance abuse treatment. That is, there is education about problem and pathological gambling; individual, group, and family counseling; and attendance at support groups, usually Gamblers Anonymous. Because most problem and pathological gamblers have experienced vocational, legal, or financial problems, there should be assistance in these areas as needed. Whereas many insurance policies do not currently cover problem gambling treatment, states with legalized gambling are increasingly providing public support for treatment.

Given the continuing proliferation of gambling, it is inevitable that there will be more and more attention given to problem and pathological gambling. In the near future, it is hoped that researchers will establish sufficient data to justify a diagnosis of problem gambling as an addition to the diagnosis of pathological gambling. This would be consistent with the current status of substance use disorders and would help justify more public and private support for treatment.

Megan V. Webster and Larry Ashley

See also Gamblers Anonymous; Gambling, Pathological; National Council on Problem Gambling; National Gambling Impact and Policy Commission

Further Readings

Ciarrocchi, J. W. (2002). *Counseling problem gamblers: A self-regulations manual for individual and family therapy.* San Diego, CA: Academic Press.

Gerstein, D. R., Hoffmann, J., Larison, C., Engelman, L., Murphy, S., Palmer, A., et al. (1999). *Gambling impact and behavior study: Report to the National Gambling Impact Study Commission.* Chicago: NORC at the University of Chicago.

Ladouceur, R., Sylvain, C., Boutin, C., & Doucet, C. (1998). *Understanding and treating the pathological gambler.* West Sussex, UK: Wiley.

Petry, N. (2007). Gambling and substance use disorders: Current status and future directions. *American Journal on Addictions, 16,* 1–9.

GATEWAY DRUGS THEORY

Initiation of substance use usually occurs in nonrandom but trivial temporal order. Unsurprisingly, the use of any substances is preceded by nonuse, and the first use of illicit drugs is *usually* preceded by consumption of licit substances. The use of "hard" drugs, such as cocaine and heroin, is *usually* preceded by "soft" drugs, such as marijuana. The sequential order becomes even less consistent beyond the initiation of involvement with illicit compounds, to the degree that the illicit drugs other than marijuana, that is, hard drugs, are usually collapsed in one class in research modeling use sequences. Moreover, a substantial proportion of drug users initiate their drug involvement with illicit rather than licit drugs, or use hard drugs before marijuana.

Gateway Theory

The temporal order observations gave rise to the "gateway theory" (also known as "gateway hypothesis" and "stage hypothesis"), which was predated by the similar "stepping-stone" theory that first appeared in the 1930s. The latter assumed that consumption of a "soft" drug, such as marijuana, inexorably sets an individual on a trajectory to addiction to hard drugs. The gateway hypothesis (GH) relaxes the inevitability assumption, but postulates a progressive and hierarchical sequence of "stages," whereby the use of a drug at a "lower" stage (a softer drug) is necessary for progression to a harder drug. This sequence applies only to the use of different drugs rather than different levels or extent of drug involvement (from use to dependence). Originally, as proposed by Denise Kandel in 1975, the "gateway" substances were considered to be beer or wine, which later was changed to marijuana.

Gateway Hypothesis Controversy

The few testable components of the GH include its premise that initiation of use of various drugs is not opportunistic but follows certain stages and pathways, and that the use of a drug at a lower stage is necessary for progression to a higher stage. The GH perspective has been presented as a theoretical antithesis to the concept of nonspecific problem behavior outcomes such as substance use disorders.

The "stages," however, are defined in a circular manner: A stage is said to be reached when a certain drug(s) is used, but that drug is supposed to be used only upon reaching that stage. In effect, the drug is identified with the stage. In other words, there is no process, separate from drug use per se, which is hypothesized to underlie the supposed developmental staging indicated by drug milestones. Moreover, the notion of "stage" itself is redefined from its common denotation, such that the later stages are assumed to be reachable before the earlier ones, apparently to accommodate the need in relating the GH to the conventional biological developmental framework. Any explicit causal proposition for the observed sequence is avoided. The numerous implicit statements of causation from the proponents of GH merely restate the observation of a sequential order. Indeed, it is hard to discern a falsifiable element in the GH beyond that observation, as is characteristic of inductive theories. The vagueness of a gateway drug itself is admitted by the originator of the GH. Virtually every proposition of the GH is qualified by a disclaimer, effectively engulfing and neutralizing possible arguments to the contrary. All possible deviations from the hypothesized "basic" sequence are automatically relegated to the category of error, or random, or nonsystematic patterns. Because the "stage," the main component of the gateway hypothesis, is defined by the drugs used at this stage, it is not surprising that the "stage" sequence parallels ranking of the prevalences of use of respective drugs.

It is important, nevertheless, to submit the GH to analysis, because its statement of the sequential order has had a significant influence on policy formation, intervention, and research. The latter, whose purpose is to inform both intervention and policy, may be hindered or misdirected if a concept lacking substance, validity, and utility is accorded prominence. In turn, the targets for policy and intervention may be shifted or insufficiently focused to produce an optimal impact.

The arguments against the substance of the GH, however difficult it is to define, can start from its logic. In addition to the faulty circularity of the definition of "stages," the GH appears to fall into the "false cause" category of logical fallacies, including the ordinary *post hoc ergo propter hoc* ("after that, hence because of that") fallacy. Although the GH proponents avoid statements of causation, the claim of necessity to reach a "lower stage" before progressing to a higher one pertains to causality, developmental sequence, or both. To illustrate the problem with this claim, consider growth in stature. To grow to the height of 6.1 feet, one needs to first reach the 6.0-foot mark and cannot skip it. It is not necessary, however, to hypothesize any causation or, as observed in developmental staging, any difference between the mechanisms involved in reaching these two heights (one of the postulates of the GH for drug use sequence). Nor is it likely that these two points will be called "stages." Nevertheless, these consecutive height values better qualify to be called stages than the "stages" of drug use because (a) they reflect a true developmental process and (b) there are no exclusions, stage reversals, and stage skipping, so common for time-related patterns of drug use. "Stage," however, usually

implies a distinct step in a developmental process (e.g., embryonic stages), which indeed involves activation and deactivation of various mechanisms. It is well known that a considerable proportion of drug users and addicts initiate their substance use with illicit and hard drugs, instead of proceeding from licit to illicit or from soft to hard drugs. Stage skipping and stage reversals in the consecutive use of various drugs illustrate the lack of necessity for the "stages" that are designated to be "lower" and make the "stage" designation dubious.

The conclusion of association between the "stages" in the sequence—necessary to unite them into a meaningful process—is made from the fact that cocaine and heroin users, more frequently than not, have used marijuana before. Even a larger number, however, have drunk water before using any drugs, from which hardly anybody would attempt to derive a meaningful sequence. It is thus not surprising that, as calculations show, when the frequency of marijuana use in the population is taken into account, the actual association between marijuana and cocaine use becomes negligible—and this is assuming that *all* cocaine users have used marijuana. It is even lower for heroin. The high correlations encountered in the literature and establishing the association between marijuana use and other drug use are artifactual because they are estimated among hard drug users, without taking into account the large population of those who try or even habitually use marijuana but never transition to harder drugs. Marijuana is likely to be the first illicit drug offered to the noninitiated person not only because it is likelier to be available from the peers but also because it is likelier to be accepted than, for instance, intravenous heroin. The route of administration is uncomplicated and is as familiar, and thus perceivably innocuous, as tobacco smoking, whose legality is limited only by age.

The alternative explanation of the frequent order of drug use initiation is the common liability model, subsuming, to a large degree, the concept of "problem behavior." The high comorbidity of substance use disorder (SUD) as well as familial aggregation of these disorders, which are heterogeneous in substances used and in symptoms, are parsimoniously explained within the framework of common liability to SUD, a complex (multifactorial) latent trait underlying the risk for SUD. The liability concept was introduced to human genetics for disorders that do not follow Mendelian (single-gene) patterns of inheritance but nevertheless have nonrandom familial distribution. In contrast to Mendelian traits, where risk varies in relation to the genotypes for a single gene, variation in the risk for multifactorial traits depends on multiple genetic and nongenetic factors. The liability phenotype (manifest as risk for and severity of the disorder) is determined by all factors, genetic and nongenetic, that influence the likelihood of the development of the disorder. Significant genetic correlations (correlation between genetic components of phenotypic variance), cotransmission, or both, have been shown between the liabilities to alcohol and drug use disorders, substance use and smoking, as well as nicotine and alcohol dependence. Liabilities to use or abuse of different categories of illicit drugs (marijuana, stimulants, sedatives, heroin, and psychedelics) have been shown to share most of their variance and comprise a group genetically somewhat distinct from the risk to abuse licit substances. The genetic factors are mostly nonspecific to drugs.

At the neurochemical, neuroanatomical, and physiological levels, these commonalities involve the mechanisms of drug reward and dependence, known to be shared in common for various drug classes. These mechanisms are also involved in natural reward and, at the psychological level, are reflected in behavioral or affect dysregulation, frequently preceding drug involvement. No relationship is detected between preferred substance (heroin, cocaine, alcohol) and personality, whereas the extent of polysubstance involvement correlates with an increase in dysregulation, consistent with commonality in psychological mechanisms of liability as well as with the development of liability phenotype. Liability to substance use disorders is a dynamic trait; its development unfolds from the moment of conception and is influenced by numerous factors directing the trajectory to or from substance use and, ultimately, the diagnostic threshold. From the liability concept perspective, there appears to be no more meaning and causation in the temporal sequence of drug use initiation than in the opportunistic order in which dinner is served at a restaurant: first hors d'oeuvres, then soup, and so on, any of which can be skipped or, conceivably, changed in order. In fact, appetizers, intended exactly to arouse appetite, may have more to do with causation than any of the "gateway" drugs for the continuation of the respective sequences. Generally, however, regardless of appetite changes during a meal—or, by analogy, of whether sensitization (a possible increase of sensitivity

to the effect of a drug due to the action of another drug) plays any role in drug use progression—it is the basic need for food that causes food consumption rather than any element of the dinner sequence. This basic need is analogous to the reasons why people use psychoactive substances in general and differ from each other in the risk for using and abusing them. These reasons and differences have been shown to involve all substances, particularly illicit ones, regardless of their class and pharmacological effect. These reasons are likely to be related to behavioral deviancy predating drug abuse, generally described as behavioral dysregulation or disinhibition, manifesting in problem behavior. Thus, the problem behavior concept substantially overlaps with the notion of common liability to SUD, particularly in liability mechanisms preceding drug involvement, as well as its changes—the domain pertaining to the focus of the GH.

Proportions of those who used drugs among those who had the opportunity are strikingly similar for marijuana and the hard drugs, consistent with opportunistic use that is opposed by the GH. The GH would predict that augmenting availability of a "gateway drug" such as cannabis will lead to an increase in cocaine and heroin use. This, however, has not happened in countries where marijuana use is de facto legalized, which is fully consistent with the common liability model, interpreting the predominant sequential order as opportunistic. Like other inductive theories, however, the GH renders arguments against it as ever-incomplete as arguments in its support. For instance, the finding of no differences between the individuals following typical and nontypical sequences on a large number of characteristics can be countered by the "white swans" argument: All swans could be assumed to be white until the black ones were discovered. The stage-specificity of risk factors as a possible argument for the validity of the GH is not testable, because of the circularity of the stage definition. Because different drugs denote different stages, specificity, along with commonality, is expected, because of the existence of drug-specific mechanisms. Nevertheless, an increasingly large body of data in violation of the major postulate of the GH, namely, that of a nonopportunistic order of drug use initiation, seriously compromises the GH's validity. Clearly, what defines the "stages" (licit, marijuana, other illicit drugs) is not their pharmacological properties or differences in the individual's response to them but the obvious socioeconomic boundaries determined by the combined public perception of the "hardness" of drugs (with consequent legal barriers needed to be overcome in order to use a drug) and their price—both subject to change. If the drug use initiation is opportunistic, the likeliest among the possible sequences of drug use initiation are those that correspond to the gradation in the prevalences of drug use. Indeed, taking into account that marijuana is commonly the first illicit drug on offer, common liability has been shown to be more than sufficient to explain the associations and the ordering between marijuana and other illicit drug use. Even stronger associations would still be fully consistent with the common liability model. The high comorbidity of drug addictions is grounded in the evolutionarily very old and conserved system underlying reward and incentive motivation. It is largely common to various drugs exactly because this common system determines their addictive property.

Conclusion

The GH has exerted considerable influence on the field of substance abuse, affecting research, intervention, and policy. In research, it has been presented as antithetical to the "problem behavior" perspective. Research concerned with corollaries from the GH during the 30 years since it was advanced has commanded substantial resources and has been a subject of numerous publications. To a large degree, this attention is explained by the high practical value that has been ascribed to the attractively simple proposition of a sequential order in drug use initiation, which is the essence of the GH. Nevertheless, the GH remains controversial. The hypothesis provides few testable assumptions, which are not supported by empirical evidence. The causal implications of the GH are unsubstantiated and may be based on a logically faulty premise. The temporal order and transitions in drug use initiation, as well as their inconsistency that is ignored by the GH, can parsimoniously be accounted for by an alternative explanation: the common liability model. Importantly, that model also explains the relationships between the liabilities to SUDs, to which the GH, limited to drug use initiation, does not extend.

Preventing drug use by delaying first use of any drug as long as possible, as would follow from the GH, misdirects attention from causes to the effects, manifestations of factors determining the liability

phenotype. As a predictor, alcohol, tobacco, or marijuana use may have good sensitivity, but its specificity and positive predictive value are low.

The GH appears redundant juxtaposed with the parsimonious and empirically proven concept of common liability of the disorder. Considering the abundant exclusions from, and the triviality of, the typical substance use initiation sequence, its utility is uncertain. Taking into account the danger that the typical sequence's presentation as a theory may be (and has been) erroneously interpreted in causal terms, it may be harmful for both research and intervention.

Michael Vanyukov and Ralph Tarter

See also Experimental Substance Use; Genetic Aspects of Addiction; Neurobiology of Addiction

Further Readings

Falconer, D. S. (1965). The inheritance of liability to certain diseases, estimated from the incidence among relatives. *Annals of Human Genetics, 29,* 51–76.

Jessor, R., & Jessor, S. (1977). *Problem behavior and psychosocial development: A longitudinal study of youth.* New York: Academic Press.

Kandel, D. (1975). Stages in adolescent involvement in drug use. *Science, 190,* 912–914.

Kandel, D. (2002). Examining the gateway hypothesis: Stages and pathways of drug involvement. In D. B. Kandel (Ed.), *Stages and pathways of drug involvement: Examining the gateway hypothesis* (pp. 3–15). Cambridge, UK: Cambridge University Press.

Kandel, D., & Yamaguchi, K. (1999) Developmental stages of involvement in substance use. In P. Ott, R. Tarter, & R. Ammerman (Eds.), *Sourcebook on substance abuse: Etiology, epidemiology, assessment, and treatment* (pp. 50–74). Boston: Allyn & Bacon.

Morral, A. R., McCaffrey, D. F., & Paddock, S. M. (2002). Reassessing the marijuana gateway effect. *Addiction, 97,* 1493–1504.

Tarter, R. E., & Vanyukov, M. (1994). Alcoholism: A developmental disorder. *Journal of Consulting and Clinical Psychology, 62,* 1096–1107.

Tarter, R. E., & Vanyukov, M. (1999). Re-visiting the validity of the construct of resilience. In M. D. Glantz & J. L. Johnson (Eds.), *Resilience and development: Positive life adaptations* (pp. 85–100). New York: Plenum Press.

Tarter, R. E., Vanyukov, M., Kirisci, L., Reynolds, M., & Clark, D. B. (2006). Predictors of marijuana use in adolescents before and after licit drug use: Examination of the gateway hypothesis. *American Journal of Psychiatry, 163,* 2134–2140.

Vanyukov, M. M., & Tarter, R. E. (2000). Genetic studies of substance abuse. *Drug and Alcohol Dependence, 59,* 101–123.

Vanyukov, M. M., Tarter, R. E., Kirisci, L., Kirillova, G. P., Maher, B. S., & Clark, D. B. (2003). Liability to substance use disorders: 1. Common mechanisms and manifestations. *Neuroscience and Biobehavioral Reviews, 27,* 507–515.

GAY, LESBIAN, BISEXUAL, AND TRANSGENDER ISSUES

Lesbian, gay, bisexual, and transgender (LGBT) people have patterns of substance use and abuse that differ from the general population and also require treatment services tailored to their specific experiences, that is, "culturally competent" services for sexual minority populations. It is also important to keep in mind that there are significant subgroup variations within the LGBT category.

There are three main differences between LGBT people and others that contribute to differences in substance use and abuse: (1) LGBT people face lifelong harassment, discrimination, social rejections, and increased likelihood of interpersonal violence due to their natural sexual and gender preferences; (2) LGBT people deal with sexual orientation and gender identity issues that significantly complicate personal development; (3) LGBT people tend to congregate in social enclaves or form social networks to find sexual partners, social support from compatible and accepting friends, and refuge from harassment and discrimination.

Many people turn to alcohol, tobacco, and other drugs to cope with emotional pain in its various forms. In any population, elevated rates of alcohol and other drug use and abuse are associated with lower levels of psychological well-being, such as depression, anxiety, and post-traumatic distress. LGBT people are no exception to this association. However, LGBT people live with stressors and threats to their well-being that are unique to being LGBT. These include harassment, multiple social rejections (including the particularly emotional painful and psychologically consequential rejections some experience from family members, professional colleagues or workmates, close friends, and community leaders such as clergy and government), interpersonal violence, increased likelihood of child abuse,

employment discrimination, housing discrimination, discrimination in receipt of public services, discrimination in parental custody or adoption procedures, and heterosexist belief systems that deny the acceptability of LGBT individuals as persons. Clearly LGBT people are at greater risk of substance use than the general population because they experience these stresses. These stresses are frequently experienced by the most visible subgroups: transgenders (who historically have experienced particularly debilitating rates of interpersonal violence and economic discrimination), gay men, and lesbians. Bisexuals are least likely to experience these types of stressors.

The developmental path of a LGBT individual is more complicated and arduous than for a heterosexual individual. Richard A. Isay refers to becoming gay as a journey to self-acceptance. The phrase "coming out," used to refer to disclosing LGBT identity to others, expresses the fact that it must also be a journey to acceptance by others, a significant complication to individual development as well.

A concept frequently used to assess the level of internal difficulty the individual faces in this journey to self-acceptance is the notion of "internalized homophobia," a complex psychosocial phenomenon that can be characterized as decreased self-esteem caused by negative social messages about homosexuality and subconscious fears of homoerotic attractions produced by widely held but erroneous belief systems regarding such attractions. Everyone, LGBT or not, has some degree of internalized homophobia to deal with in their personality development. Among lesbian, gay, and bisexual individuals, numerous studies have linked elevated rates of alcohol and drug use to internalized homophobia. As with the external stresses of interpersonal violence, economic discrimination, and social rejections, transgenders are most likely to experience internal conflict and confusion in their journey to self-acceptance, given the extreme lack of knowledge of gender identity issues in the general population and the related extremity of social rejection of individuals with fluid, ambiguous, or transitioning gender. This puts them at high risk for substance abuse.

Identity formation, self-acceptance, and social acceptance can be further complicated for LGBT individuals with ethnic minority status. International studies have found that gay individuals are born into all cultures at what seems to be a similar rate; the cultures differ a great deal in how they respond to this group in their midst. Within American cities, ethnic minority

LGB individuals face a double discrimination and also may face social and sexual rejection or even exploitation by White LGB individuals.

As for most individuals, adolescence and young adulthood are watershed years in terms of sexuality and identity exploration and consolidation among LGBT people. For many LGBT people, these can be the most difficult years, as evidenced by elevated rates of suicide and suicidality among LGBT youth as compared to other youth, the prevalence of gay-baiting and gay-bashing among young people, and the public disapproval of many adults in positions of authority in the lives of young people. Research studies have found substantially higher rates of cigarette, alcohol, and marijuana use among LGB youth than among non-LGB youth.

Throughout modern and postmodern history, gay men, in particular, but also lesbians, bisexuals, and transgenders, have sought each other out for social support, sexual partnering, and personal security. Most often this connecting takes the form of social networks within predominantly heterosexual communities. However, as LGBT individuals waged a public fight for their civil rights and for recognition of the validity and decency of their romantic and sexual relationships, they began to settle together in openly gay and lesbian enclaves or communities. The best known of these gay enclaves are in major cities, such as the Castro in San Francisco, Le Marais in Paris, West Hollywood in Los Angeles, or the Village in New York.

These openly gay or lesbian communities offer much to their residents: social support; business opportunities; support for personal pride and self-confidence; churches that accept rather than condemn LGBT people and therefore offer a spiritual home and place of worship; health care providers culturally competent to serve LGBT people; opportunities for creative self-expression through art, drama, writing, music, and design; professional associations; LGBT publications; cultural events like Gay Pride and Halloween; and gay-owned and gay-friendly restaurants and hotels. They also offer a highly developed party scene and lively entertainment strip with gay and lesbian bars, lounges, and performance spaces. This entertainment scene makes alcohol and club drugs like ketamine, ecstasy, GBH (gamma-hydroxybutyric acid), and crystal methamphetamine available to gay and bisexual men. When drugs are available, use increases. The availability of alcohol and club drugs in gay communities has contributed to problem drinking and drugging. The communities have responded with a network of treatment services and support groups such as Alcoholics Anonymous, but bars and club drugs remain a significant problem.

Most LGBT people do not reside in visible enclaves but live scattered throughout cities and in small towns. Here, patterns of use differ. Among some African American gay and bisexual men living in low-income African American communities, for example, crack cocaine is more likely to be used than crystal meth, and private house parties are more common than public venues like dance clubs or gay bars.

The epidemiology of substance use and substance abuse disorder among LGBT people is difficult to determine. When studying lesbians, gays, bisexuals and transgenders, defining and locating the total population has always been almost impossible. Venue sampling (at clinics, organizations, bars), street intercept surveys, and other convenience samples are frequently used but cannot adequately calculate population rates. For example, early work estimating substance use and dependence among gay men at 30% were distorted by oversampling of heavy users. Improved design produced better estimates indicating higher rates of alcohol and drug use among homosexual versus heterosexual men and a similar rate among lesbian women. Research also indicates a decline in substance abuse among LGBT individuals over the past 2 decades. However, there remains no clear consensus on the actual prevalence of substance use and abuse among the various subgroups of the LGBT population, due largely to the underlying problem of identifying the population base for a representative sample. The same problem exists in studies of other aspects of psychological well-being that relate to substance use and other risk behaviors. As with substance abuse, most studies find depression levels elevated among LGBT people, with the usual caveat that the overall population prevalence is elusive.

Dealing with substance abuse has urgency in the LGBT community beyond the general population: Substance abuse is strongly linked to the spread of the human immunodeficiency virus (HIV), the virus that causes acquired immune deficiency syndrome (AIDS). Although most AIDS cases worldwide have always been among heterosexuals, the LGBT population is the best example of a subpopulation disproportionately impacted by HIV. That is, gay men have a much higher rate of HIV than the general population, and so any unprotected penetrative sex carries a much higher probability of transmitting the virus than is true among heterosexuals. When ethnic minority status and gay or bisexual behavior are combined with substance abuse, the rates of HIV are particularly high. Numerous studies have linked the use of drugs or alcohol to both sexual risk behavior and the spread of HIV/AIDS. For example, almost all of the transmission of HIV in the gay community in West Hollywood, California, has been tied to the use of methamphetamine over the past decade. In South Central Los Angeles, HIV has spread among African American men who have sex with men and also among African American women who have sex with men who have had sex with other men. Drug and alcohol treatment and HIV prevention thus go hand in hand.

Evaluations of treatment programs for methamphetamine abuse, alcoholism, and other drugs have indicated that treatment programs that are tailored to the experiences of LGBT individuals and take into account both external and internal stressors unique to the LGBT population can be effective in modifying behavior. As with the non-LGBT population, most LGBT individuals who need alcohol or drug treatment are not currently receiving that treatment. However, the AIDS epidemic has pushed those who provide health care to gay and bisexual men, in particular, to increase the availability of substance abuse treatment that works for these individuals to reduce their risk behaviors and increase their ability to manage their illness. Successful substance abuse treatment can become a matter of life and death for an individual infected with HIV.

Judith Resell

See also Club Drugs; HIV/AIDS; Special Populations

Further Readings

Bockting, W., & Kirk, S. (2001). *Transgender and HIV: Risks, prevention and care.* New York: Haworth Press.

Isay, R. A. (1996). *Becoming gay: The journey to self-acceptance.* New York: Henry Holt.

Mills, T., Paul, J., Stall, R., Pollack, L., Cacchola, J., Chang, Y. J., et al. (2004). Distress and depression in men who have sex with men: The urban men's health study. *American Journal of Psychiatry, 161*(2), 278–285.

Weber, G. N. (2008). Using to numb the pain: Substance use and abuse among lesbian, gay and bisexual individuals. *Journal of Mental Health Counseling, 30*(1), 31–48.

GENDER ISSUES

Contemporary substance abuse prevention and treatment strategies represent the outcome of decades of research and clinical experience on how to best intervene in this critical social problem. The information accumulated over this time frame has pointed to several factors that must be taken into account, including the sex or gender of affected individuals. While *sex* is considered a biological construct used to classify individuals as "male" or "female" based on reproductive organs assigned by chromosomes, *gender* is a psychosocial construct used to classify individuals based on self-representations as "male" or "female." To maintain consistency with the use of the term *gender* in most of the research in this area, this entry uses the term *gender* to describe the assignment of male and female labels to humans. Before considering the unique issues facing men and women in substance abuse prevention and treatment, a brief review of recent historical advances provides a context for the current state of knowledge in this area.

Recent Historical Developments

When the National Institute on Drug Abuse (NIDA) was founded in 1974, there were notable gaps in the scientific and clinical literature on gender differences in substance abuse prevention and treatment. Indeed, most of the research at that time was devoted to the study of prevention and treatment efforts designed by and for men and neglected women as subjects in substance abuse research. Based on the dearth of much-needed research on gender differences in this area, from its onset NIDA was committed to supporting studies on the unique substance abuse issues facing women.

Early efforts by NIDA included funding for research on treatment for pregnant, drug-dependent women and the impact of prenatal exposure to substances on the health and well-being of the developing fetus and infants. The focus shifted from opioid-dependent women in the 1970s and early 1980s to cocaine-dependent women in the mid- to late 1980s. The impetus for this shift was a growing social concern about the influx of crack cocaine into inner cities, along with the harmful effects of exposure to the developing fetus. In addition to disquiet about the prevalence and consequences of crack use, health workers also became concerned about the link between drug use and an increased risk for HIV/AIDS among drug-dependent women. Considering the public health and social impact of the growing problems for drug-dependent women and their children during this time, NIDA increased its funding initiatives to facilitate the development of programs targeting drug-dependent pregnant and postpartum women.

In 1994, a landmark change occurred in the study of gender issues in substance abuse prevention and treatment. At this time, the National Institutes of Health (NIH) began requiring the inclusion of women in all human research and mandating analyses of gender differences in outcomes from clinical trials in order to secure NIH funding. In the same year, NIDA held a conference to review the progress made through funding initiatives targeting the understanding, prevention, and treatment of drug abuse by women. A notable outcome of this conference was the recognition that the study of women would benefit from an expansion to include male–female differences. The rationale behind this development included awareness that this more comprehensive approach can foster understanding of the unique issues facing both women and men as consumers of substance abuse programs. The effect of this convergence in 1994 was a dramatic increase in the study of gender issues in prevention and treatment.

Women's Issues

Similar to early substance use research, many current women-focused studies examine specialized female populations, specifically pregnant women, postpartum women with infants, and those in the criminal justice system. Since the NIH's 1994 published guidelines on the inclusion of women and minorities, the amount of general women-focused research has greatly increased. Several women-specific effects of substance use have been focused upon in research. Due to several factors, particularly gastric metabolism, body water, and body size, women have been found to be more medically and biologically vulnerable to the negative repercussions of substance use than men. Further, research findings suggest that women are at higher risk for contracting sexually transmitted diseases as a consequence of their substance use and that women with substance abuse problems may have greater social difficulties.

Women's age of onset for substance use and associated problems differs among different age cohorts, with the onset being closest for men and women in the youngest generations. The initiation of using

substances has progressively occurred among younger ages, likely in relation to recent changes in women's social roles, with substance use becoming more socially acceptable for women. A convergence hypothesis purported in alcohol research suggests that drinking patterns among men and women will eventually become equal. In support of this hypothesis, male-to-female ratios of adolescent alcohol use initiation were found to be 1.8:1 in the 1970s and 1:1 in the 1990s. For some substances, such as cocaine and crack, the prevalence of women's use can surpass that of men. Overall, American lifetime prevalence estimates have found that 5% to 8% of women have alcohol use disorders and 5% to 6% of women have drug use disorders.

Alcohol researchers have also found that women progress to alcohol dependence and treatment at a quicker rate than do men: a phenomenon deemed the telescoping effect. The telescoping effect has been thoroughly demonstrated using various time points. For example, the length of time for men versus women (a) between first treatment and first drink (31.1 versus 27.2 years, respectively), (b) between treatment onset and development of first alcohol-related problem (14.7 versus 10.4 years), and (c) between treatment onset and regular alcohol use (15.0 versus 11.6 years) all demonstrate a shorter progression to alcohol treatment for women than for men. Additional evidence of a telescoping effect comes from the consistent finding that despite having used substances for fewer years and having consumed smaller quantities than men, the severity of substance use symptomatology at the onset of treatment is generally equal among men and women. However, the telescoping effect and gender differences found with alcohol use are weaker among other drugs. Researchers emphasize that the telescoping effect of a quicker progression to treatment is not a reflection of earlier societal intervention for women but is instead due to women's quicker progression from first recognizing alcohol problems to first treatment. The telescoping effect has been hypothesized to result from women's greater biological vulnerability (body fat, water proportions, estrogen influence, and metabolism) to psychoactive substances. Further, some researchers have suggested that the telescoping effect may reflect women's greater willingness to seek help. Research findings of a telescoping effect in the nonchemical addiction of pathological gambling, though, suggest that psychosocial factors also likely influence women's quicker progression to dependence and treatment.

Women face complex social pressures related to substance use, prevention, and treatment. Society holds a double standard of substance use for women: While women's substance problems are viewed as being more deviant than men's, women receive less social support and greater opposition from spouses or partners to entering substance-related treatment. Research has shown that women are more likely to be involved in a relationship with a substance-abusing partner than are men and that their continued use of substances is often supported by those in their social network. Consequently, they are less likely to report interpersonal, spousal, or familial problems in relation to their substance use; the most frequently reported reason a woman reports for seeking services is because her "life is out of control."

The most common route for women's entry into substance abuse treatment is by referral from a medical provider or a social worker. Some reasons for this treatment entry point may include negative social appraisals of women who are identified as having substance-related issues, who lack of social support, and who are concerned that they may lose custody of their children, each of which may be a substantial barrier to seeking targeted substance abuse treatment. Pregnancy and parenting are significant issues related to substance abuse prevention and treatment for women. Treatment service providers working with pregnant women must be cognizant of the systemic physical effects of substance use, which can prompt special attention when considering the unique and complementary health needs of both mother and the developing fetus. Women with substance abuse problems may also decline or delay treatment out of concern that providers will report them as unfit to care for their children. Further, difficulties with finding and affording child care limit women's access to treatment. Considering that women with substance abuse issues often have low educational attainment and low income, affording child care while they attend treatment can be a legitimate concern.

Researchers have also suggested that the substance use treatment entry point via medical provider or social worker may be related to women identifying their substance abuse problems as secondary to other mental health concerns. Along these lines, women entering substance abuse treatment have greater psychiatric comorbidity and symptomatology than men. For example, co-occurring substance use and depression or anxiety disorders are common among women.

The presence of a comorbid psychiatric disorder is associated with poor treatment outcomes, a situation that can complicate substance abuse treatment. In addition, women with substance use disorders have higher rates of past trauma than men. Histories of physical or sexual trauma may make mixed gender treatment settings or certain treatment approaches (e.g., confrontation, which can enhance feelings of shame and perpetuate feelings of powerlessness) less advantageous.

Several studies have focused on the effects of various types of substance treatment programs for women. With the suggestion that traditional interaction styles and societal male dominance may negatively impact women in mixed-gender treatment, several studies have focused on the effects of gender-specific treatment for women. Women-only treatment programs may be beneficial for treating pregnant women or women with dependent children. These programs are likely to be sensitive to women's unique treatment issues, such as child care and pregnancy. Some benefits of this specialized approach can include an increased likelihood to continue care after completion of a women-only residential substance abuse program. In contrast to women-specific treatment, mixed-gender substance treatment programs may provide more of a real-world atmosphere by having men and women together in treatment, where they can interact with one other.

In sum, women face unique biological, societal, and psychological vulnerabilities and barriers for substance use prevention and treatment. These factors can help account for research showing that women are overall less likely than men to enter specialized substance abuse treatment over the course of a lifetime. Prevention and treatment strategies aiming to enhance outcomes for women with substance use problems may be augmented by considering these and related gender-specific barriers. Furthermore, the advantages and disadvantages of women-only versus mixed-gender treatment may be a relevant consideration when designing programs for women with these problems.

Men's Issues

The catalyst for attending to gender as a relevant consideration was to stimulate the inclusion of women in clinical studies, so that they may be adequately represented as consumers of substance abuse prevention and treatment efforts. While much work remains to be done toward that end, recent findings also suggest that men as a group have gender-specific issues impacting prevention and treatment. Along these lines, research and clinical literature in the past 2 decades show that, despite a historical bias toward the inclusion of men in these studies as targets of treatment efforts, men as a group still face substance abuse issues worthy of focused attention.

One of the most consistent findings across epidemiological and clinical studies is that men are significantly more likely to have a current or lifetime diagnosis of substance abuse or dependence. Estimates of the gender differences in prevalence suggest that men are 1.5 to 2 times more likely than women to meet diagnostic criteria for a substance-related disorder. These prevalence estimates vary according to the type of substance, however. Although research suggests that men have a higher prevalence of abuse across most substances, these gender differences may vanish when considering abuse of prescription drugs such as sedatives or tranquilizers. Alternatively, gender differences in prevalence may be magnified in the case of alcohol.

Experts have speculated that sociocultural practices and expectations for men's behavior may help explain the overall gender differences found in substance abuse prevalence. For example, research on drinking contexts has shown that alcohol use occurs across a broader range of activities for men when compared to women. Moreover, heavy drinking is often more socially acceptable for men. Cultural expectations for men's alcohol use are suggested by research showing that men are more often shown using alcohol in television and movies and that men are more frequently targeted through beer advertisements linking alcohol use to sports and positive appraisal from attractive women. Other researchers suggest that substance abuse among men may be linked to the risk taking and adventurousness prescribed by traditional male role norms. Overall, these differences in prevalence help explain why men outnumber women in substance abuse treatment admissions by a ratio of 2 to 1. Considering the prevalence of substance abuse among men and the rate of treatment admissions, it is imperative that those who work with individuals who have substance abuse problems develop awareness of male-specific issues in prevention and treatment.

An important issue that should be considered is the mechanisms through which men enter substance abuse treatment. In particular, men are most likely to enter substance abuse treatment when referred by the criminal justice system. As a consequence, men's participation in treatment is most often involuntary. Although motivation to resolve legal issues may increase men's readiness to enter treatment, being forced into treatment may also compromise internal motivation to change their behavior beyond meeting the ostensible demands of the treatment program. This lack of internal motivation may help explain why even though men enter treatment with fewer negative prognostic indicators than do women, men fail to have better relative outcomes. Another critical issue is that men are less likely than women to seek help for health-related issues overall, a factor that could explicate findings showing that treatment seeking for substance abuse problems is lower than for other health-related issues, such as depression and anxiety. Men are also likely to seek less help when they do pursue it. Some research suggests that cultural expectations for men prescribed by traditional male role norms (such as independence, strength, and self-sufficiency) may be incompatible with help seeking. Consequently, men who are not compelled to seek treatment involuntarily may have difficulty initiating therapy for substance abuse problems.

Based on these issues and the broader literature on treatments designed to foster positive outcomes in men, a few treatment recommendations can be suggested. Substance abuse programs working with male participants may benefit from a group therapy format aimed at developing new ways of expressing masculinity that do not include substance abuse. Some research also suggests that men fare better in mixed-sex treatment, as participation alongside women can facilitate emotional disclosure. Other general strategies may include a structured, problem-focused approach and efforts designed to enhance motivation to change when readiness to change may be compromised by referral from criminal justice settings. Finally, outreach efforts sensitive to cultural expectations for men to maintain independence and self-sufficiency should be considered when developing and implementing treatment programs. When considered together, the high prevalence of substance abuse problems and lower likelihood of help seeking without outside influence among men suggest that prevention and treatment strategies that take these factors into account may offer benefit to men in need of substance abuse treatment.

Conclusion

Taken together, current research and clinical literature suggests that gender has a relevant impact on issues related to substance abuse prevention and treatment. It is notable that seeking help for substance abuse problems is compromised across both genders, often for reasons connected to differential social expectations for men and women. These factors jointly contribute to overall low help-seeking rates for substance use issues, which can attenuate the effects of even the best treatments. Considering the personal and societal costs associated with a substance abuse problem, along with diminished rates of help seeking, prevention efforts may offer the most promising solutions. However, further study of how best to integrate knowledge of gender issues in substance abuse prevention and treatment is necessary. In particular, although some studies have shown that gender-specific issues can impact treatment entry and process, recent findings fail to show that gender is a specific predictor of treatment retention, completion, or outcome.

Joshua P. Smith, Abigail A. Goldsmith,
and Rachel D. Thompson

See also Client/Treatment Matching; Maternal Drug Use; Prevention Strategies; Special Populations; Treatment Access and Retention; Violence, Intimate Partner and Substance Abuse Treatment; Women for Sobriety

Further Readings

Claus, R. E., Orwin, R. G., Kissin, W., Krupski, A., Campbell, K., & Stark, K. (2007). Does gender-specific substance abuse treatment for women promote continuity of care? *Journal of Substance Abuse Treatment, 32,* 27–39.

Dawson, D. A. (1996). Gender differences in the probability of alcohol treatment. *Journal of Substance Abuse, 8,* 211–225.

Godfrey, J. R. (2007). Toward optimal health: Kathleen Brady, Ph.D., M.D., discusses challenges of substance abuse in women. *Journal of Women's Health, 16,* 163–167.

Grenfield, S. F., Brooks, A. J., Gordon, S. M., Green, C. A., Kropp, F., McHugh, R. K., et al. (2007). Substance abuse treatment entry, retention, and outcome in women: A review of the literature. *Drug and Alcohol Dependence, 86,* 1–21.

Lemle, R., & Mishkind, M. E. (1989). Alcohol and masculinity. *Journal of Substance Abuse Treatment, 6,* 213–222.

Thom, B. (1986). Sex differences in help-seeking for alcohol problems: 1. The barriers to help-seeking. *British Journal of Addiction, 81,* 777–788.

Walitzer, K. S., & Dearing, R. L. (2006). Gender differences in alcohol and substance use relapse. *Clinical Psychology Review, 26,* 128–148.

Wetherington, C. L. (2007). Sex-gender differences in drug abuse: A shift in the burden of proof? *Experimental and Clinical Psychopharmacology, 15,* 411–417.

Zilberman, M., Tavares, H., & el-Guebaly, N. (2003). Gender similarities and differences: The prevalence and course of alcohol- and other substance-related disorders. *Journal of Addictive Diseases, 22,* 61–74.

GENETIC ASPECTS OF ADDICTION

The risk for addictions (substance use disorders [SUDs]) differs from person to person. These differences may be due to various factors, which may ultimately be traced to hereditary (genetic) and environmental causes. Genetic research takes into account both genetic and environmental factors, because all individual characteristics develop according to a genetic program as it unfolds under the influence of environment. The genetic program consists of genes, which are parts of DNA molecules found in almost all cells of the organism in their nucleus, in the structures called chromosomes. Humans have 23 different pairs of chromosomes. Each chromosome of a pair may have a different or the same variant of a gene. These variants are called alleles. Because some of the alleles may cause differences in proteins and other molecules encoded by the genes, they may also be related to differences in life processes regulated by these molecules, including those related to the risk for drug and alcohol use disorders. The genes of the organism make up its genotype. Genetic studies of SUD are conducted to relate genetic variants and environmental factors to individual differences (variation) in the risk for this disorder. This entry discusses the main concepts, methods, and examples of results of human genetic studies in SUD.

Addiction: Traits and Phenotypes

Human genetics as science originally developed through the study of "simple" genetic disorders, the risk for which is caused by mutations (relatively rare alleles) in single genes, resulting in distinct disease phenotypes (observed characteristics), readily distinguishable from the normal phenotype. Genetic studies of SUDs are complicated by their multiple causes and symptoms (clinical signs). In addition, an addicted individual often combines use of different illicit (drugs) and licit (alcohol, tobacco) substances. This results in a large number of potential symptom and drug combinations. To deal with such complexity, researchers of human genetics can use the idea of liability to a disorder.

The liability concept was introduced to human genetics for traits that are not simply inherited (unlike single-gene disorders) but nevertheless run in families. Liability is a sum result of the whole combination of circumstances—genetic and nongenetic—that make a person more or less likely to develop the disease. This trait is quantitative, like weight or stature. Unlike these directly measurable traits, but similar to intelligence, liability is not directly observable. Persons who have values (phenotypes) of liability that are above a certain point, called the threshold, are more likely to be diagnosed with SUD than those who do not reach the threshold. Whereas clinical diagnosis of the disorder is needed for treatment and prevention, it is not an optimal research tool both because it is imprecise and because binary (yes/no) variables generally provide less information than do continuous ones.

The alleles of the genes influencing SUD liability in an individual genotype make up the person's genetic predisposition to the disorder. Different alleles of these genes cause differences in the structure or the levels of hormones, receptors, enzymes, or other proteins that participate in drug-related processes. Genetic investigations employ methods that analyze these processes from the molecular level (gene structure and function) to complex physiological reactions of the nervous system and the brain, to individual variation in personality and behavior, to family and social factors. Despite difficulties in modeling complex human behavior in laboratory animals, certain genetic problems in SUD research have been addressed in animal studies. This entry, however, focuses on human research.

The variety of genetic studies in SUD generally falls into two categories: behavior genetic and molecular genetic research. The former studies are conducted at the level of the phenotype in families, twins, and adopted children to estimate the proportions of variations in SUD risk that can be accounted for by genetic and nongenetic factors. Molecular genetic (linkage and association) studies attempt to find genes related to variation in liability, or they test the role of particular genes in individual phenotypic differences.

Behavior Genetics

Behavior genetic studies have demonstrated that phenotypic variation in the liability to SUDs (phenotypic variance) is caused by differences in individual genotypes as well as in environmental conditions. The two main methods used to estimate genetic (heritability) and environmental components of phenotypic variation are twin and adoption studies. It is important to know heritability of liability because it allows evaluation of chances to discover genes that explain the genetic causes of SUD risk variation.

The twin method is based on the fact that the members of a pair of identical (monozygotic [MZ]) twins, developing from the same fertilized egg, share all their genes in common, whereas fraternal (dizygotic [DZ]) twins on average share only half of their genes that have common origin. Therefore, for those genes that have different alleles, only 50% of these alleles are shared in common by both DZ twins, thus creating predictable genetic differences between them. The other sources of differences and similarities between DZ twins are usually assumed to be the same as in MZ twins. Therefore, differences within an MZ twin pair are due to environmental influences that are unique to each member of the pair (thus called nonshared environment), while their similarity is due to their identical genotypes and environmental factors that act on both twins the same way (called shared environment). In contrast, the differences between DZ twins are due to both genes and environment.

In behavior genetic studies, the known differences in the genetic similarity within the pairs of MZ and DZ twins are related to the MZ–DZ differences in the within-pair similarity for a trait, such as the risk for SUD. This allows estimation of genetic and both types of environmental contribution to phenotypic variation, using mathematic (statistical) methods. For instance, a 100% similarity for a trait in MZ pairs, but only 50% similarity within DZ pairs (the same as the genetic similarity within these twin groups), would mean that phenotypic variation is entirely due to individual genetic differences. Heritability in this case would be 1 (or 100%). It is virtually impossible to observe such heritability, particularly because phenotyping (e.g., SUD diagnosis, or measurement of SUD risk or a psychological trait) cannot be done without error. The absence of differences in such intrapair similarity between MZ and DZ twins would suggest that any phenotypic variation observed is caused by environmental factors only.

Adoption studies are based on the assumption that all similarities between adoptive parents and children are due to shared environment, whereas almost all similarity between biological parents and their adopted-away children is genetic.

Importantly, heritability estimates pertain to the population rather than the individual. Even a high heritability of liability does not necessarily mean that the disorder in an individual is not preventable or curable. A low heritability of a trait does not mean that genes have nothing to do with its development. Moreover, it may indicate that it is under a very strict genetic control, so that no genetic variation is allowed by natural selection. For instance, the number of hands in humans, which varies mainly due to trauma, is likely to have a very low heritability. Nobody, however, would have doubts about the defining role of genes in their development and number.

Heritability, varying for different substance use disorders, has been estimated as high as 0.8 in both males and females. An adoption study in females showed a pattern of relationships between biological family background and SUD outcome similar to that in males, with strong associations between SUD and antisocialism in biological parents and drug abuse in offspring. Parallel results from twin studies of alcoholism show heritability estimates reaching 0.7 in males and 0.6 in females. Genetic components of variation in liabilities to alcohol and drug use disorders, substance use and smoking, as well as nicotine and alcohol dependence have been shown to correlate, suggesting that alleles of the same genes contribute to variation in the risk for SUD in general (common SUD liability). A biological background of alcohol problems predicted increased drug abuse in adoptees. There was no relationship between the substances abused by the biological parent (alcohol, drugs, or both) and by the adoptee. Twin studies also showed that addictions related to abuse of, or dependence on, different illicit drugs share virtually all genetic variation in the risk. This supports the common liability concept. Notably, it is common liability, rather than drug- or "stage"-specific factors posited by the so-called gateway theory, which likely underlies transitions in drug abuse development.

Behavior genetic research (adoption studies) has identified several environmental factors, such as marital discord and psychiatric problems in the adoptive family, as associated with increased drug abuse in adoptees. Siblings have also been shown to influence adolescent alcohol use. Parental loss, another environmental factor, increases risk of alcoholism. Familial religiosity is another environmental variable affecting the risk for SUD. Environment may also interact with genetic factors, that is, influence the strength or direction of their relationship with SUD liability. Vice versa, certain relationships of environment with the risk for SUD may depend on the person's genotype, as discussed in the next section.

Molecular Genetic Studies

The significant heritability of SUD liability and associated traits suggest the existence of genetic polymorphisms (when a gene has several alleles in the population) contributing to variation. The two main general approaches applied in the search for these polymorphisms are linkage and association studies.

Linkage studies evaluate whether transmission of the risk in families is related to the inheritance of DNA markers (variable sites in the DNA molecule, whose position there is known). Association studies examine whether individual differences in the risk are related to particular genes or genetic markers. The genes are selected because of information, obtained in other fields of study, about their role in the nervous system and its response to drugs. The large number of markers that have now been characterized enable association and linkage studies that can cover the whole genome to detect locations (loci) linked to or associated with the risk for SUD.

Most of positive findings in SUD genetic research have been obtained using association methods. It is possible that some findings are positive by chance only. Nevertheless, because potentially many genes contribute to variation in the SUD risk and their effects are small, some of the failures may be due to samples being insufficiently large to replicate an association. The findings may also depend on the population, including differences in their genetic composition, environment, and interactions between them. For instance, the ALDH2 gene that encodes an enzyme involved in alcohol's fate in the organism contributes to variation in the risk for alcoholism in East Asians. A very low activity of this enzyme, caused by an allele of the ALDH2 gene, is common in East Asia. It is related to a lowered risk for alcoholism, causing a very unpleasant sensation related to drinking. Absent in other populations, this allele, however, does not influence alcoholism risk in them.

Genes related to the dopamine system, in contrast, may have a more universal significance. Dopamine is one of the primary chemicals, called neurotransmitters, used by the nervous system for transmitting signals between cells called neurons. The dopamine system includes many components. It plays a role in experiencing pleasure (reward), including that obtained with drugs. The reward pathways for different drugs, to a large degree, share the same structures of the brain. Some studies published to date find association between the genes involved in the dopamine system and SUD liability—for instance, DRD2, DRD4, DRD5, and MAOA genes—whereas other studies failed to demonstrate any association. The MAOA gene, encoding an enzyme involved in several neurotransmitters in addition to dopamine, in addition, has been shown to influence the relationship of environmental conditions, such as parenting style, with traits related to SUD liability (antisocialism, risk for childhood behavior disorders). In turn, a study showed that when parenting is taken into account, the relationship between the MAOA gene and the risk for SUD itself becomes detectable. Numerous other genes and their interactions are potential targets for association research.

It should be emphasized that no gene related to the risk for SUD can be called an "addiction gene." Even if there were a gene strongly related to SUD liability, it would unlikely be due to an allele strongly related to the risk; on the contrary, the risk-associated allele is likely to be common among nonabusers of drugs, as the data to date show. It is possible that a practical outcome of genetic studies of SUD will be identification of environmental factors that are capable of offsetting even a high individual genetic predisposition to the disorder, enabling science-based prevention of the disorder. As it is likely that these genes are not specific to SUD, such environmental factors may have wide implications for socially important behavior.

Conclusion

Both genetic and environmental individual differences have been shown to play a role in variation in the risk for addictions in the population. Most of the genetic factors involved are not specific to a drug or even a drug-related behavior. Variations at numerous genes, particularly those involved in the neurobiological systems, are being studied as potential candidates in association studies of substance abuse. Environment also may play an important role in the risk variation, both independently and in interaction with genetic factors.

Michael Vanyukov

See also Brain Chemistry and Addiction; Neurobiology of Addiction; Neurotransmitters

Further Readings

Tarter, R. E., & Vanyukov, M. (1994). Alcoholism: A developmental disorder. *Journal of Consulting and Clinical Psychology, 62,* 1096–1107.

Tarter, R. E., & Vanyukov, M. (1999). Re-visiting the validity of the construct of resilience. In M. D. Glantz & J. L. Johnson (Eds.), *Resilience and development: Positive life adaptations* (pp. 85–100). New York: Plenum Press.

Tarter, R., Vanyukov, M., Kirisci, L., Reynolds, M., & Clark, D. (2006). Predictors of marijuana use in adolescents before and after licit drug use: Examination of the gateway hypothesis. *American Journal of Psychiatry, 163,* 2134–2140.

Vanyukov, M. M. (2004). Evolution, genes, and the environment: Neurobiological outcomes. In D. H. Fishbein (Ed.), *The science, treatment, and prevention of antisocial behaviors: Application to the criminal justice system* (Vol. 2, pp. 1–29). Kingston, NJ: Civic Research Institute.

Vanyukov, M. M., & Tarter, R. E. (2000). Genetic studies of substance abuse. *Drug and Alcohol Dependence, 59,* 101–123.

Vanyukov, M. M., Tarter, R. E., Kirisci, L., Kirillova, G. P., Maher, B. S., & Clark, D. B. (2003). Liability to substance use disorders: 1. Common mechanisms and manifestations. *Neuroscience and Biobehavioral Reviews, 27,* 507–515.

GRIEF, LOSS, AND SUBSTANCE ABUSE

Any discussion of relationships between and among grief, loss, and substance abuse must first begin with an overview of loss and the resulting grief. While grief is most commonly defined as an emotional response to loss, there are more wide-reaching consequences in one's life. Beyond emotional responses, there are social, physical, psychological, cognitive, and spiritual dimensions to consider. Significant loss affects holistic health, including the ability to manage emotions, to function within the social environment, to make sound decisions, and to engage spiritually to uncover or find meaning in precipitating loss.

Many discussions of grief, loss, and substance abuse take place within the context of death. Although death may be the most commonly referenced event leading one to grief, most people's lives are affected by grief and loss from a multitude of sources. In addition to the loss suffered through death, there is a broad range of adverse circumstances, life events, and transitions that often result in grief. The source of loss ranges from loss of employment (either voluntary or involuntary), loss of friendships, loss of beloved pets, loss of socioeconomic state, and loss of socioeconomic status through financial hardship or social isolation or ostracism.

Individual responses to loss are varied and unpredictable, depending to a large extent on a person's support system, coping skills, and life situation. An individual's grieving process is equally complex, influenced by such factors as personality, family, culture, and spiritual and religious beliefs and practices. Each of these elements plays an important role in how someone responds to loss and the grief that frequently accompanies the loss. The relationship between job loss and individual, social, and psychological problems is well documented by counselors and researchers. The potential for loss of income, socioeconomic status, social network, and sense of purpose are numerous and potentially painful for many people. For people who lack resources and appropriate coping skills, the trauma of loss may lead to substance abuse.

In addition to personal loss, loss occurs on a larger, more public scale. Increased substance abuse sometimes results from the reaction of many people to disasters, armed conflicts, and other forms of mass violence. In a study following the September 11, 2001, attack on the World Trade Center, researchers estimated that within 5 to 8 weeks after 9/11, 265,000 people experienced increased use of alcohol and other drugs, with 226,000 consuming more alcohol and 29,000 abusing more marijuana.

Grief, Loss, and Substance Abuse

There are multifarious relationships among and between substance abuse and issues of loss and grief. One of the most common connections is grief and loss as the stimulus to substance abuse, or causing more severe substance abuse.

Substance abuse may either begin or become more severe due to the death of a loved one, the end of a relationship, or other traumatic life transitions and experiences. An older person who loses a life partner through either death or separation may begin to abuse alcohol in response to the loneliness and grief. Unresolved grief often leads to challenges in other, seemingly unrelated areas of life. People who have experienced loss but have not yet had the opportunity to reflect and process the occurrence may seek solace in other ways, with substance abuse being among the most common.

Parents who experience the death of a child often exhibit symptoms of trauma, including post-traumatic stress disorder and intense grief reactions that place them at high risk for complicated grief and mourning. This grief response, coupled with a lack of support, can increase the risk that a parent may cope with the loss through increased substance use or abuse. In addition to complicated grief responses, some parents may have other risk factors for substance abuse, such as family history of substance abuse, depression, anxiety, current use patterns, previous addiction history, or extreme isolation and lack of support. Any of these risk factors, coupled with the recent death of a child, may signal the need for additional support and possible treatment.

Another commonly referenced relationship between loss, grief, and substance abuse is substance abuse leading to loss and grief. Substance abuse causes grief, loss, or both, for addicts' loved ones or those with whom the addict has significant relationships. For example, many addicts witness the end of important relationships in their lives as a result of their behavior or loved ones' response to their behavior.

A slightly less common but valid causal relationship is the grief or loss as a result of recovery from substance abuse. People who are recovering from addiction must often terminate relationships with people, places, and behavior that have enabled their abuse; this situation can result in perceived isolation. A shared culture and substantive supportive systems may no longer be available, leading to grief and bereavement.

Treatment

Counselors and therapists encounter clients at all stages of grief and witness a vast range of responses to loss, either prior to, during, immediately following, or many years following the loss. In the period prior to loss and immediately following, the individual experiencing the loss is frequently given significant attention and support. As time passes, however, there is often a decline in the amount of formal and informal support available to the person who has experienced the loss. In American culture particularly, people are expected to carry on their routine lives and to recover quickly from the loss. On the contrary, many people who experience loss report their need for support increasing in the years following the loss, just as the support is receding.

Counselors, therapists, and other helping professionals who begin working with people who are grieving should acknowledge the loss and work with the client to discover the best possible sources of support. Grief counseling for the loss, even years following the experience, offers inestimable value to the client.

Clients may present to counselors and therapists with seemingly unrelated issues, including substance abuse, illustrating the need for a comprehensive loss history. Topics discussed in sessions may include the impact of the loss on the client's life and his or her relationships with others, as well as any unresolved issues associated with the loss. Such discussions may include a review of the client's relationship with a loved one who has died or terminated a relationship, an exploration of the circumstances surrounding the loss, and support for the associated issues or losses that have occurred as a result of the initial loss. Regardless of the client's presenting issue, the counselor should refer the client to treatment if the client is using or abusing substances.

Several approaches have been used successfully with clients experiencing substance abuse related in some way to loss and grief, including addiction counseling, cognitive behavioral therapy, motivational interviewing, and supportive psychotherapy. Addiction counseling, which concentrates on the symptoms of substance abuse and impaired functioning, emphasizes the building and strengthening of appropriate coping strategies and tools for recovery. The primary goals of addiction counseling are to help the client cease and abstain from the addictive behavior and to recover from the problems caused by the substance abuse. The client has an active role in his or her counseling, taking responsibility for his or her recovery.

Cognitive behavioral therapy is a short-term approach that has been extensively evaluated in clinical trials and has empirical support as an effective treatment. Cognitive behavioral therapy has also demonstrated enduring qualities as well as efficacy in cases of severe substance abuse. The approach is structured and goal oriented, but it is also flexible enough to be used with a diverse client population in various settings.

Motivational interviewing is a more recent approach that has proven effective in addressing grief among substance abusers. Motivational interviewing is a set of formalized, theory-based therapist responses to help clients identify and acknowledge substance abuse behaviors and work toward cessation of the behavior. The strength of motivational interviewing is that the counselor or therapist has an active role in contributing to the degree of clients' motivation to change. Through the use of eight interaction technique strategies, counselors and therapists are able to facilitate and support a client's efforts to change.

Finally, social support and connectedness are essential for people who are struggling with substance abuse related to loss and grief. Bereavement groups are often an effective means through which people can relate with others who have experienced loss, many of whom may also be struggling with substance abuse as a result or cause of the loss.

Peggy Dupey

See also Co-Occurring Disorders; Post-Traumatic Stress Disorder; Psychosocial History

Further Readings

Compton, P., Monahan, G., & Simons-Cody, H. (1999). Motivational interviewing: An effective grief intervention for alcohol and drug abuse patients. *Nurse Practitioner, 24,* 27–47.

National Institute on Drug Abuse. (2005). Trauma-related substance abuse persists after mental health symptoms abate. *NIDA Notes Bulletin Board, 20*(2). Retrieved October 3, 2007, from http://www.drugabuse.gov/NIDA_notes/NNvol20N2/BBoard.html

Silove, D., & Bryant, R. (2006). Rapid assessments of mental health needs after disasters. *JAMA, 296,* 576–578.

Williams, J. S. (2002, November). Depression, PTSD, substance abuse increase in wake of September 11 attacks. *NIDA Notes Research Findings, 17*(4). Retrieved October 3, 2007, from http://www.drugabuse.gov/NIDA_notes/NNVol17N4/Depression.html

GROUP THERAPY AND COUNSELING

Groups play a central role in the treatment of substance abuse. The Association for Specialists in Group Work has categorized the various kinds of groups into four categories. Psychoeducational groups provide information and limited practice in using new knowledge. They are short term and might include such groups as "driving under the influence" (DUI) classes or educational groups for addicts beginning treatment. Counseling groups address common problems and focus less on education than on members' interactions and mutual problem solving. These are generally short term and might include such groups as support groups for children of alcoholics. Psychotherapy groups aim to change people on a deeper level than do the other kinds of groups. They are typically longer lasting and ongoing. Recovering substance abusers are usually seen as candidates for psychotherapy groups. Finally, task or work groups are not considered therapeutic in that they are focused on getting specific tasks accomplished (e.g., committees and project teams). This entry focuses on counseling and psychotherapy groups.

Therapeutic Components of Groups

Although individual counseling is certainly useful in many ways, there are several therapeutic factors operating in well-conducted therapeutic groups that affirm their vital importance.

Research has shown that, in general, group and individual therapies have essentially equivalent efficacy. However, it is clear that different processes occur in group and individual treatments. That is, each type of treatment contains specific therapeutic components or factors. One widely accepted list of such components is that by Irvin D. Yalom. Yalom defined therapeutic factors as the actual mechanisms of effecting change in the patient. The 11 factors that he identified are instillation of hope, universality, imparting information, altruism, corrective recapitulation of the primary family group, development of socializing techniques, imitative behaviors, interpersonal learning, group cohesiveness, catharsis, and existential factors.

Dennis M. Kivlighan and his colleagues found overlap among many of these factors. Indeed, they found four components underlying this (and similar) lists. These components are (1) emotional awareness or insight (including strong affective experiences associated with gaining awareness or insight); (2) relationship climate (including formation and maintenance of relationships between either client and therapist or client and other group members); (3) other- versus self-focus (including clients' focus outside of themselves, especially the factor of altruism); and (4) problem definition and change (the problem-solving aspect of therapy experiences, including cognitive identification and understanding of a problem and behavioral changes that may follow).

The two components of relationship climate and other- versus self-focus tend to operate prominently in group psychotherapies, while emotional awareness or insight and problem definition and change are more prominent processes in individual therapies. The primacy of the first two components in groups is consistent with Yalom's theory that other group members are the main source of change in group therapy. In other words, group therapy is effective, in large measure, specifically because of the impact of interpersonal and relational factors (e. g., altruism, group cohesiveness).

Of course, not all factors are equally operative in all groups. Group cohesiveness, for example, seems to be a strong factor in homogeneous groups, such as those conducted in substance abuse treatment settings. Group members in homogeneous groups also tend to report greater satisfaction with their therapy experiences. In general, there is a consensus that the factors perceived by clients as being most helpful are group cohesiveness, catharsis, and interpersonal learning.

Finally, effectiveness of group counseling and therapy is related to certain dimensions of group leadership. Morton Lieberman and Mitch Golant have identified five empirically based leader functions. These are (1) evoking/stimulating emotions (the leader uses a tactic to engage members and elicit emotional responses), (2) supporting/caring (offers support, friendship, and affection), (3) facilitating meaning attributions (providing a meaning structure in the face of members' anxieties; i.e., labeling experiences as these occur, teaching how to change by utilizing in-group exercises, introducing schemes of making sense of a member's confusing "problem" experiences), (4) exerting an executive/management function (this includes setting rules and norms for the group, setting goals with the group, and blocking "toxic" interactions), and (5) using one's self (including disclosing the therapist's feelings in the here-and-now of the group).

Although all of these functions are important, the two most significant, in terms of client outcomes, seem to be meaning attribution and management. Thus, the more that a leader provides members with schemas to understand their problems and frameworks for change and explains, compares, summarizes, and invites members to seek feedback, the more a client is likely to benefit from the group experience. Likewise, managing time effectively, setting rules and norms, and blocking toxic interactions all have beneficial effects for clients.

Basic Processes

While much has been written about group process, it is important to recognize that group counseling and therapy are essentially an experiential form of therapy. As such, they attempt to expand individuals' awareness of themselves, their feelings, their interactions with others, and others' perceptions of them. This emphasis on a group member's coming to know oneself (i.e., one's impact on others as well as others' perceptions of oneself and their feedback) is central to a therapeutic group.

The process of how a person comes to know him- or herself has historically been dealt with as a matter of introspection. It has often been assumed that thinking about what kind of person one is will lead to insight and to self-definition. One significant exception to this perspective has been the "self-perception theory" of Daryl Bem. According to self-perception theory, everyone comes to know oneself in just the same way that we come to know others. We observe our own behaviors in a various situations, and then we make attributions about our behaviors.

This is especially true in group therapy. To the extent that a group is experiential, it allows a member to experience oneself in various interpersonal situations and to observe oneself.

Self-concepts do change. People change their self-beliefs, for instance, based on the self-presentations they make to others, and such changes affect their behaviors and their self-concepts. Anita Kelly proposed that self-presentation and impression management strategies by psychotherapy clients are crucial to successful psychotherapy. She proposed a four-step model of change in psychotherapy based on a self-presentation that involves (1) clients performing various favorable self-presentations (e.g., altruistic acts in a group), (2) therapists (and group members) giving feedback based on the client's self-presentations, (3) such feedback leading to clients' shifts in self-beliefs (e.g., "I *am* an altruistic, helpful person"), and (4) changes in self-beliefs leading to changes in clients' self-concepts.

This perspective is significant because it puts self-description and self-definition at the center of group therapy. There appear to be six steps in the self-definition process in group counseling and psychotherapy. In a therapeutic group experience, people learn about themselves by observing their own behaviors:

1. They pay attention to (i.e., observe) the things they say to others about themselves.

2. The group therapist and other members encourage new behaviors, including new recognitions of feelings, new experiences, and new cognitions.

3. Members then try out new behaviors in (and outside of) the group.

4. With the counselor's help, they reflect on these tried-out behaviors: What do these behaviors say about the kind of persons they are or can become?

5. They then redefine their selves according to their new behaviors and the feedback that other members give them.

6. Feedback from other members and from the therapist allows them to check on their changes.

When this sequence happens, therapists often notice that the therapy is "working." It is therefore part of the group therapist's role to facilitate each step of this process.

One crucial element in this process is feedback from group members. However, feedback is not always easy for members to give. A carefully done study by D. Keith Moran and colleagues pointed out that group members are happy to give positive feedback to other members but are very reluctant to provide corrective feedback. This appears to happen because most do not want to risk the loss of acceptance by the group. There seem to be at least three tactics that the group therapist should employ in order to overcome this hesitancy. First, as Yalom has suggested, it is important to remind the group that therapy is not like ordinary social intercourse. Members should be more honest as well as sensitive with the others in the group. Second, the therapist should model giving corrective feedback in such a way that is helpful and not damaging. Third, feedback should be labeled, by the therapist, as an altruistic act whenever it is given appropriately and sensitively.

Twelve-Step Groups

The role of groups such as Alcoholics Anonymous and Narcotics Anonymous in the treatment of substance-abusing individuals cannot be ignored. Although Twelve-Step meetings clearly do not fall in the Association for Specialists in Group Work classification of therapy groups, they do seem to occupy a space somewhere between psychoeducational and counseling groups. It has been found that mental health professionals tend to view support groups significantly less positively than professionally led groups. Nevertheless, approximately 18% of the population of the United States have participated in support groups at some time in their lives, and almost 7% have done so in the past year. Furthermore, 50% of Twelve-Step group participants also obtain professional services for their substance abuse problems.

What do Twelve-Step groups have to offer? To the recovering person, they can be a lifeline to overcoming addiction and maintaining recovery. These groups utilize at least eight of the therapeutic factors outlined earlier. Instillation of hope occurs when members realize that others have overcome their problems and so they can as well. Universality occurs when members recognize that they are not alone in feelings of isolation and hopelessness. Imparting information occurs regularly in such groups. Altruism is a part of every Twelve-Step group, and it is the heart of the twelfth step itself (i.e., helping other alcoholics or addicts). Imitative behaviors often occur when members see how others have dealt with similar issues. Some groups achieve group cohesiveness to the extent that individual members "carry the group around in their heads" and thus internalize and feel close to it. Catharsis occurs often as members become emotional in meetings. Finally, existential factors abound in Twelve-Step groups. Indeed, many meetings are not about the alcohol or substance of abuse but rather focus on the meaning of one's life. For example, it is not possible to go through the painful experiences of recovery without at least implicitly asking oneself the question: "Why am I struggling to overcome this?" The answer always has to do with the reasons for going on with life.

Conclusion

Counseling and psychotherapy groups play a major role in the treatment of substance abuse. Among the most significant therapeutic factors operating in such groups are emotional awareness, the relationships and climate of the group, other- versus self-focus, and problem definition and accompanying change. Leadership of groups has been found to be very important, especially the functions of providing members a meaning structure in the face of their addiction experiences and providing a safe and non-toxic environment for personal growth. The process of self-definition is basic to all successful therapeutic experiences in both professionally led and support groups.

Rostyslaw W. Robak

See also Counseling Approaches; Family Therapy; Support Groups; Treatment Approaches and Strategies

Further Readings

Bem, D. J. (1972). Self-perception theory. In L. Berkowitz (Ed.), *Advances in experimental social psychology* (Vol. 6, pp. 1–62). New York: Academic Press.

Kessler, R. C., Mickelson, K. D., & Zhao, S. (1997). Patterns and correlates of self-help group membership in the United States. *Social Policy, 27,* 27–46.

Lieberman, M. A., & Golant, M. (2002). Leader behavior as perceived by cancer patients in professionally directed support groups and outcomes. *Group Dynamics: Theory, Research, and Practice, 6,* 267–276.

Morran, D. K., Stockton, R., & Bond, L. (1991). Delivery of positive and corrective feedback in counseling groups. *Journal of Counseling Psychology, 38,* 410–414.

Perrone, P. B., & Sedlacek, W. E. (2000). A comparison of group cohesiveness and client satisfaction in homogeneous and heterogeneous groups. *Journal for Specialists in Group Work, 25,* 243–251.

Robak, R. W. (2001). Self-definition in psychotherapy: Is it time to revisit self-perception theory? *North American Journal of Psychology, 3,* 529–534.

Salzer, M. S., Rappaport, J., & Segre, L. (1999). Professional appraisal of professionally led and self-help groups. *American Journal of Orthopsychiatry, 69,* 536–540.

Yalom, I. D., & Leszcz, M. (2005). *The theory and practice of group psychotherapy* (5th ed.). New York: Basic Books.

H

HALLUCINOGENS

Hallucinogens are drugs that cause hallucinations or distortions in a person's perception of reality. Hallucinations are described as seeing images or hearing sounds that are not actually present and can result from medications, disease, mental illness, and even insomnia. This entry is concerned with the history, effects, and classification of hallucinogens that are discussed and/or used most frequently: lysergic acid diethylamide (LSD), phencyclidine (PCP), ketamine (known on the street as *Special K*), psilocybin (street name, *magic mushrooms*), mescaline (peyote), methylenedioxymethamphetamine (MDMA or *ecstasy*) and dimethyltryptamine (DMT). However, drugs that are not labeled hallucinogens, such as marijuana and cocaine, may cause hallucinations when taken in high doses or combined with other drugs.

Hallucinogens challenge what one knows and believes about human behavior and how the brain works. They have raised an abundant amount of controversy, and there are many different opinions regarding whether the effects of hallucinogens are positive or negative. Several researchers have labeled hallucinogens among the safest illicit drugs since they are not physically addictive. However, the heavy use of hallucinogens can result in a psychological dependence, and hallucinogen use disorders are included as diagnostic categories in the *Diagnostic and Statistical Manual of Mental Disorders*. There are no known physical withdrawal symptoms associated with hallucinogens, and overdosing is rare.

The federal government categorizes most hallucinogens as Schedule I drugs, the classification used for the most dangerous drugs in the United States. Schedule I drugs have high potential for abuse and have no known recognized medical use. With the exception of ketamine (used as an animal tranquilizer), hallucinogens have no recognized medical use in the United States and are illegal to possess.

History

Several different cultures have utilized hallucinogens for centuries. Hallucinogens have been used for social purposes, rituals, and ceremonies. Indigenous peoples discovered hallucinogens in plant form and integrated them into their religious belief patterns. Traditionally, it was believed that hallucinogens created an enlightened sense of spirituality, opened users to the gods, and provided them with greater spiritual insight. These beliefs still hold true in some North and South American countries, as well as some Asian countries such as Malaysia and Borneo.

Hallucinogens have been used in medicine and research. In the 1950s, PCP was developed for use as an anesthetic in medical procedures. The use of PCP was short-lived because the effects were extreme and dangerous. Instead, ketamine was designed as a safer replacement. Additionally, researchers wanted to identify how hallucinogens work in the brain, and this desire led to the widespread use of LSD and ecstasy by psychiatrists and researchers in the 1950s. LSD specifically was used for therapy in an attempt to aid individuals in exploring thoughts and in expressing feelings.

Hallucinogens are notorious for their seemingly mind-expanding effects. As a result, there have been documented increases in the use of hallucinogens for recreational purposes during certain periods of time. For example, LSD was discovered in 1938 by Dr. Albert Hofmann, but it was not until the 1960s' freedom movement that hallucinogens became popular for recreational use. During this time, hallucinogens were considered mind-enhancing psychedelics, and LSD became a widespread drug of choice for many people.

In the late 1990s, ketamine, magic mushrooms, and ecstasy became popular club drugs used by teenagers and college-age adults. Since then, there has been a decrease in the use of hallucinogens by young adults. In the 2007 Monitoring the Future's annual survey of drug use by young people, the use of hallucinogens in the last 30 days by 12th graders, college students, and young adults was less than half than the rate in 1995. In 2006, less than 2% of these age groups reported hallucinogen use in the previous month.

Physiological and Psychological Effects

With the exception of PCP, hallucinogens have similar physiologic effects, although differences exist between onset, duration, and intensity. Hallucinogens affect the body in numerous ways. Generally, hallucinogens can cause in increased heart rate and blood pressure, high body temperature, dilated pupils, dizziness, nausea, loss of appetite, dry mouth, sweating, numbness, and tremors. Taken in high doses, hallucinogens may result in sedation or a loss of consciousness.

The hallucinogenic effects of these drugs are sensory, emotional, and psychological. Hallucinogens affect emotional well-being and alter a person's thought processes and mood. They also affect how the brain interprets reality. Typically, hallucinogens cause an individual to experience a distorted perception of reality, affecting one's sense of time, space, and surrounding environment, as well as the way one hears, thinks, and sees.

An individual inebriated by a hallucinogenic drug might hear sounds and voices that do not exist. Individuals may see faces in clouds or visualize things that are not actually present. Another side effect, synaesthesia, can occur when the senses become crossed or mixed-up. This crossing of senses leads the individual to believe that he or she is feeling color, hearing sights, or seeing sounds.

The outcome and side effects of a hallucinogenic experience is unique to each individual. The experience is greatly influenced by several factors: the type and dose of drug, the user's state of mind before and during use, the environment in which the drug is taken, and the user's previous experience with drugs.

The use of hallucinogens is often described as a very intense experience. Some individuals become insightful or develop a sense of euphoria and increased enlightenment. They may be giddy and experience stimulating visuals with vivid, deep colors. Others might hear or see things that are frightening. They may become anxious or uneasy. This emotion can result in a panic reaction, which can lead to mood swings, paranoia, or depression. Therefore, hallucinogens have been known to result in either a good trip (enlightened experience) or a bad trip (aversive reaction). Although hallucinogens do not mimic mental illness or psychosis, in some cases they can trigger a psychotic experience.

Long-Term Effects

Hallucinogen persisting perception disorder, commonly known as flashback, is a possible long-term effect of using hallucinogens. Flashbacks are defined as experiencing spontaneous hallucinations or hallucinogenic effects after an individual is no longer taking the drug. Other common chronic effects of hallucinogens include but are not limited to persistent psychosis, anxiety, paranoia, depression, and a lack of motivation.

Classification of Hallucinogens

Hallucinogens are organic compounds. Many occur naturally in plant form or are derived from plants, while several others are synthetic. The incredible variation of hallucinogens leads to the diversity of their uses, thus making it nearly impossible to understand their complexity without looking at their chemical structure and individual characteristics. This section explains how the chemical structure of hallucinogens affects how they work in the brain and provides a brief introduction to common drugs in each group.

Serotonin-Like Group

Serotonin is a neurotransmitter important in regulating anger, body temperature, mood, sleep, nausea, and appetite. Chemically and structurally, there are several hallucinogens that mimic the neurotransmitter serotonin and use it as their chemical messenger. These drugs are LSD, psilocybin, peyote, and DMT. All of these drugs work the same way and produce similar effects. They prohibit the breakdown of serotonin by binding to serotonin receptors. The drugs compete for the receptors, ultimately blocking the serotonin from binding. This disruption in the normal functioning prevents the uptake of serotonin and allows hallucinogens to work in the brain.

LSD is a semisynthetic drug manufactured from lysergic acid, the ergot fungus that grows on rye and other grains. According to the National Institute on Drug Abuse, LSD is the best known and most widely used hallucinogenic drug. It is also one of the most potent and mind-altering drugs. LSD is usually clear or white and is taken orally in the form of paper, sugar cubes, or liquid drops. The effects can last from 6 to 12 hours.

Magic mushrooms are another frequently used hallucinogen in the United States. Psilocybin is an alkaloid that provides the hallucinogenic effect of mushrooms. Alkaloids are nitrogen containing compounds produced by plants or fungi; some are poisonous, while others are used as analgesics. Mushrooms are usually eaten or made into tea and drank. The effects can last from 4 to 6 hours.

In the United States, peyote is a rare drug. Mescaline is an alkaloid of the peyote cactus that causes a hallucinogenic effect. There are several species of the peyote cactus that produce mescaline. Mescaline has occurred randomly in nature for thousands of years and is typically found and used by native tribes in Mexico and the southwestern United States. The effects of a typical dose (half a gram) can last up to 12 hours and may initially cause nausea.

DMT is a chemical derived from plants, but it can also be synthesized in a laboratory. The DMT experience is typical of other hallucinogens. However, the effects have a very short duration, usually lasting about 45 minutes. As a result, DMT is commonly known as the *businessman's special*. DMT is usually snorted or smoked.

Substituted Phenethylamines

Substituted phenethylamines act as a substitute for the neurotransmitter norepinephrine. Norepinephrine, also known as adrenaline, is a stress hormone that affects parts of the brain responsible for attention, focus, and depression. The hallucinogenic drug ecstasy has a similar chemical makeup to that of norepinephrine. This similarity triggers the different sensations throughout the body, allowing the hallucinogens to work in the brain.

Ecstasy was used for hunger suppression in World War I. It is known for producing euphoric sensations. The effects of ecstasy closely resemble amphetamines, and ecstasy does not produce common hallucinogenic effects. Ecstasy is taken orally. The effects vary according to the dose, usually ranging from 4 to 6 hours.

Dissociative Anesthetics

Dissociative drugs alter the dispersal of glutamate, a nonessential amino acid throughout the brain. These drugs obstruct the functioning of neurotransmitters by preventing their binding to its receptors. Glutamate is associated with an individual's perception of pain, memory, and reactions to the environment. The obstruction of glutamate alone is enough to produce the majority of the effects of dissociative drugs.

PCP is a dissociative drug that distorts perceptions and causes dissociation from self and the environment. The effects of PCP are similar to those of alcohol, amphetamines, and hallucinogens combined. PCP in high doses can cause seizures, coma, or a psychosis-like state, often leading to medical emergencies or arrest by law enforcement officials. PCP is usually injected or taken orally; however, it can also be smoked. The effects associated with PCP use typically last several hours.

Ketamine is currently used for animal anesthesia and has recently become a regulated drug due to an outbreak in its recreational use. Ketamine was developed in 1963 as a replacement for PCP. The effects of ketamine are similar to those of PCP; however, it has a shorter duration and is much less potent. Ketamine is typically injected or evaporated and then snorted. Similar to the aversive effects of other hallucinogens, users of ketamine have described a near death experience with feelings of extreme sensory detachment known as a *K-hole*.

Conclusion

Hallucinogens are complicated drugs that generate a copious amount of controversy. Hallucinogens affect the brain and body, ultimately causing a distorted perception of reality. Their use is diverse, and the effects are unique to each individual. Throughout history, hallucinogens have been used for both religious and medicinal purposes. There are several types of hallucinogens, and their diverse chemical structures affect the brain in different ways.

Janita Jerup, Sabina Mutisya, and Thomas Harrison

See also Brain Chemistry and Addiction; Club Drugs; Drugs, Classification of; Ecstasy; Illicit and Illegal Drugs; Neurotransmitters

Further Readings

Gossop, M. (2000). *Living with drugs* (pp. 123–136). Brookfield, VT: Ashgate.

Johnston, L. D., O'Malley, P. M., Bachman, J. G., & Schulenberg, J. E. (2007, December 11). *Overall, illicit drug use by American teens continues gradual decline in 2007.* University of Michigan News Service. Available from http://www.monitoringthefuture.org

Kuhn, C., Swartzwelder, S., & Wilson, W. (2003). *Buzzed: The straight facts about the most used and abused drugs from alcohol to ecstasy* (pp. 83–109). New York: W. W. Norton.

Monitoring the Future: http://monitoringthefuture.org

Pellerin, C. (1998). *Trips: How hallucinogens work in your brain.* New York: A Seven Stories Press.

U.S. Department of Health and Human Services, National Institute of Health. (2001). *National Institute on Drug Abuse research report series: Hallucinogens and dissociative drugs* (NIH Publication No. 0-14209). Available from http://www.drugabuse.gov

U.S. Department of Health and Human Services, Substance Abuse and Mental Health Services Administration. (2004). *Truth about hallucinogens: Tips for teens.* Available from http://www.samhsa.gov

Weil, A. (2004). *From chocolate to morphine: Everything you need to know about mind-altering drugs* (pp. 110–134). Boston: Houghton Mifflin.

HARM REDUCTION, PUBLIC HEALTH

Harm reduction refers to strategies designed to minimize the negative consequences of drug use. There is an acknowledgement that both legal and illicit drug use is a reality and cannot be totally eliminated. Furthermore, harm reduction proponents believe that

there are differences in the level of safety among the various methods of using drugs, and they believe that drug users should be assisted to use drugs in the safest manner possible.

Rationale

Promoters of harm reduction strategies begin with the assumption that drug use can never be eliminated from any society. Consequently, it makes little sense to use the legal system to punish drug users because these sanctions do not produce the desired results and they cause harm in the process. Although many people would like to achieve a drug free society, this is not a realistic goal and should not guide public policy. If the premise is accepted that drug free is impossible to achieve, the issue becomes how the harm associated with drug use can be reduced and minimized. As a result, harm reduction advocates have proposed and in many cases, implemented a wide variety of strategies to minimize the problems associated with illicit drug use. Most harm reduction efforts are focused on illegal substances because there are already harm reduction methods in place for those using legal drugs. For example, the use of designated drivers is a harm reduction approach to reduce the possible damage caused by intoxicated drivers. The individual who chooses to drink is not discouraged from drinking to the point of intoxication, only from driving in that condition. It should be noted that people using legal drugs are typically left alone and not subjected to harassment, arrest, and serious punishment, even though they may be damaging their health and causing problems for friends, family members, and employers.

U.S. Public Policy

The position of the federal government toward harm reduction, as reflected in the National Drug Control Strategy formulated by the Office on National Drug Control Policy, is clearly negative. From both Democratic and Republican administrations, this position has been consistently maintained. This position is reflected in the following statement from the 1999 National Drug Control Strategy:

> Many harm reduction partisans consider drug use a part of the human condition that will always be with us. While we agree that crime can never be eliminated

entirely, no one is arguing that we legalize other harmful activities. At best, harm reduction is a half-way measure, a half-hearted approach that would accept defeat. Increasing help is better than decreasing harm. Pretending that harmful activity will be reduced if we condone it under the law is foolhardy and irresponsible. (pp. 52–53)

Strategies

Ironically, some harm reduction strategies are widely used in the United States and actively promoted in the National Drug Control Strategy. For example, heroin substitution therapy (e.g. methadone maintenance) has been used in the treatment of heroin addicts since the mid-1960s. Methadone is a synthetic opioid that eliminates the unpleasant withdrawal from heroin but does not produce heroin's euphoria, allowing the patient to maintain a relatively normal life. Although methadone has traditionally been administered in a limited number of specialized clinics, a revision of federal guidelines now allows qualified providers to be certified to administer methadone. The purpose of this change was to make methadone more accessible for heroin addicts, since in most cases, a daily dose of methadone is necessary. Since methadone is an addictive substance, the purpose of methadone maintenance therapy is to reduce the harm caused by injecting heroin. More recently, a new opioid, buprenorphine, has been approved as a treatment for heroin addiction. Buprenorphine is administered in pill form (methadone is a liquid) by qualified physicians. A daily dose does not seem to be necessary, and the withdrawal symptoms are relatively mild. Although methadone can be diverted and abused, the pill form of buprenorphine contains another drug that blocks the euphoric properties if the drug is injected. Federal agencies such as the Center for Substance Abuse Treatment and the National Institute on Drug Abuse have actively promoted buprenorphine. This is a harm reduction strategy to replace a harmful, addictive substance (heroin) with a less harmful, addictive substance (buprenorphine).

Drug courts, another harm reduction strategy in wide use in the United States, are specialized criminal courts that handle cases involving substance-abusing offenders. Supervision, drug testing, treatment services, sanctions, and incentives are used to divert these offenders from incarceration. In 1996, there were about 100 drug courts and nearly 1,800 by 2004. The need to reduce prison populations has been a strong motivator to increase the number of drug courts, and federal funding has regularly been increased to support these programs. With an emphasis on treatment rather than punishment (although punishment is implemented if offenders do not comply with treatment), drug courts are clearly among the harm reduction strategies. The goal is to reduce the harm that addicts cause society and themselves.

A harm reduction strategy that has been implemented in the United States and in many other countries but is opposed by the government is needle exchange programs. In these programs, intravenous drug users can exchange clean syringes for used ones. The purpose is to minimize the spread of HIV and hepatitis through infected needles. As of 1998, in the United States, there were 113 needle exchange programs in 80 cities in 38 states. In addition, these programs are common in many other countries. Many needle exchange programs include referrals for treatment and other support services as well as instruction for intravenous drug users on the proper procedures to clean their needles with bleach before use. The position of the opposition is that needle exchange programs imply that intravenous drug use is acceptable. Therefore, the federal government continues to ban federal funding for needle exchange programs in spite of evidence for their effectiveness in decreasing the transmission of HIV and lack of any evidence that these programs lead to increased drug use.

Heroin distribution programs, another harm reduction strategy, have been successfully operating in Switzerland. As the name implies, these programs involve providing heroin to addicts in controlled doses and in secure settings. In 1994 in Zurich, an experimental program was begun in which one group of addicts received heroin, one group got morphine, and a third group was administered methadone. The participants all had been using heroin for some time and had failed in earlier treatment. They were allowed to choose a dose level that would preclude drug seeking outside the clinic, where they were allowed to inject up to three times a day. They could not take drugs outside of the clinic and were offered support activities regarding employment, health, and family relationships. At the end of 3 years, the heroin group had improved health, employment, and social situations and had committed less crimes than before. Based on this evaluation, similar programs were opened in other parts of the country.

Drug consumption rooms are a controversial harm reduction strategy. These programs involve professionally supervised health care facilities where drug users can use illegal drugs in a safe, hygienic environment. The drug consumption room is part of a network of services for drug users and is separate from existing services for drug users or for the homeless. The goals of drug consumption rooms include making contact with drug users for the purpose of providing access to social, health, and treatment services; providing a safe, hygienic environment for drug use, particularly for intravenous drug use; reducing the harm of illegal drug use from overdose, the transmission of HIV and hepatitis, and bacterial infections; and minimizing public drug use and its associated problems. As of 2003, there were 72 drug consumption rooms in 39 cities in four European countries (Switzerland, the Netherlands, Germany, Spain). To participate, the clients must be dependent on heroin or cocaine. There is a registration process, personalized access cards, and limitations on numbers served. Consumption rooms do not advertise their services, and staff cannot help clients inject. However, staff can advise clients on safe injecting techniques. Obviously, drug dealing is not allowed. The staff ensures that hygienic and safety procedures are followed. Sterile equipment is provided, and the staff observes the administration of drugs.

In 2004, the European Monitoring Centre for Drugs and Drug Addiction reviewed the results of 15 research studies since 2000 on drug consumption rooms. In addition to the possible benefits of reduced high-risk drug use, increased access to treatment and support services, decreases in morbidity and mortality, and reductions in public drug use, the report also focused on the perceived risk of consumption rooms. These risks included increased drug use, initiation of new drug users, delaying treatment due to the perceived acceptance and comfort of drug use, and increases in public disorder by attracting drug users and drug dealers. The results of this review of studies found that consumption rooms do attract street users and older, long-term addicts who have never been in treatment. There was no evidence that consumption rooms recruit new users. Less risky drug use behavior was noted, with no increase in drug use. No conclusion about decreases in communicable diseases could be reached, but consumption rooms with adequate access did contribute to a reduction of drug-related deaths. The majority of clients accessed health care, social, and

treatment services, and there was no evidence that clients were more likely to delay treatment. The extent to which consumption rooms reduced public use and community problems was related to their accessibility, operating hours, and capacity. Consumption rooms located near illicit drug markets did not reduce this activity. The report concluded that consumption rooms were most effective when there was community acceptance of this program as part of a comprehensive strategy regarding drug-use problems.

With the rise in ecstasy use in the late 1990s, drug checking became a popular harm reduction strategy, particularly in Europe. As the name implies, drug checking involves testing a substance to determine its contents, with the intent to identify drugs with dangerous adulterants and to prevent the use of these substances. Drug checking has been used to test heroin but came into wider use as a harm reduction strategy when risky imitations of ecstasy came on the market and caused adverse reactions and even death among users. In European countries, warnings about dangerous ecstasy identified by drug checking have been communicated on the Internet. With on-site testing techniques, ecstasy tablets can be tested at raves or other party events with large numbers of young people, and the results immediately communicated to the participants. The drug checking service is combined with providing information and education about the risks of drug use and referrals for treatment or other services.

As with many harm reduction strategies, critics argue that drug checking encourages drug use and creates an environment that is accepting of drug use. Studies in Germany and in the Netherlands have not shown that drug checking encourages or increases drug use. These studies have found that unsafe pills were not taken, and users became cautious and critical of black market drugs.

Regulating the supply of a substance or access to it is another type of harm reduction strategy. Regulating is not the same as the supply reduction activities in the National Drug Control Strategy that involve interdiction of illegal drugs or destroying marijuana plants. For example, limitations on the location and density of retail alcohol outlets have been shown to be related to reductions in alcohol consumption, traffic accidents, and alcohol-related problems. With regard to marijuana, the Dutch try to control access by only allowing sales to adults and by limiting the number of licensed coffee houses. Supply is controlled by specifying the maximum amount of marijuana that can be sold to any customer and the amount of marijuana that can be kept on the premises. Some countries have made an attempt to control marijuana supplies by specifying the number of plants an individual can cultivate without a significant consequence. There are obvious problems with these supply control strategies because the supply of a drug is dependent upon the production and distribution of the substance. In other words, if a country wanted to control the supply of marijuana, it would have to control marijuana growing and/or importation as well as whatever distribution network exists.

Organizations

There are organizations in the United States devoted to harm reduction. For example, the Harm Reduction Coalition is a nonprofit organization committed to improving the health and well-being of drug users and communities affected by drug-related harm. The organization promotes effective harm reduction services and policies at the national, regional, and local levels through education and training, community organizing, policy advocacy, and publications.

Another organization involved in harm reduction, as well as legalization and decriminalization initiatives, is the Drug Policy Alliance. This organization is a merger of the Lindesmith Center and the Drug Policy Foundation. The goals of the Drug Policy Alliance are as follows:

- making marijuana legally available for medical purposes;
- curtailing drug testing not related to detecting impairment;
- ending asset forfeiture abuses and restoring constitutional protections against unreasonable searches and seizures;
- redirecting most government drug-control resources from criminal justice and interdiction to public health and education;
- supporting public health measures, notably syringe exchange and other harm-reduction programs, to reduce HIV/AIDS, hepatitis, and other infectious diseases;
- supporting effective, science-based drug education and ending support for ineffective programs;
- making methadone maintenance and other effective drug treatment more accessible and available;

- removing obstacles to proper use of opioid and other medications for treatment of pain and terminal disease;
- repealing mandatory minimum sentences for nonviolent drug offenses and ending incarceration for simple drug possession;
- ending criminal penalties for marijuana, except those involving distribution of drugs to children;
- ending invidious discrimination against people with past drug abuse problems or offenses; and
- ending racially discriminatory drug policies and enforcement measures.

The Drug Policy Alliance is involved in a variety of local, state, and national legislative and policy initiatives. For example, the organization has spearheaded a ballot measure in Oakland, California, to decriminalize marijuana, has funded legal actions involving medical marijuana patients, and has helped cities adopt needle exchange programs.

Conclusion

The premise behind harm reduction strategies is that illicit drug use can never be eliminated from society; therefore, it makes sense to do whatever is reasonable to reduce the harm caused by illicit drug use. Although the position of the U.S. government is opposed to harm reduction, the reality is that policymakers are only opposed to controversial, politically volatile strategies. Although the government will not fund needle exchange programs, it advocates heroin substitution therapies. Given the tremendous economic and human costs resulting from illicit drug use and the lack of progress in reducing these costs through the strategies that have been used for years, it would make sense to carefully examine harm reduction strategies that have been successfully implemented in other countries.

Gary L. Fisher

See also Decriminalization; Legalization of Drugs; National Drug Control Strategy; Needle Exchange Programs; Public Policy, Drugs; Public Policy, Treatment; War on Drugs

Further Readings

Bullington, B., Bollinger, L., & Shelley, T. (2004). Trends in European drug policies: A new beginning or more of the same? *Journal of Drug Issues, 34,* 481–490.

Drug Policy Alliance. (2007). *About the alliance.* Retrieved August 23, 2007, from http://www.drugpolicy.org/about

Fisher, G. L. (2006). *Rethinking our war on drugs: Candid talk about controversial issues.* Westport, CT: Praeger.

Harm Reduction Coalition. (2007). *About HRC.* Retrieved August 23, 2007, from http://www.harmreduction.org

HARM REDUCTION PSYCHOTHERAPY

Harm reduction is a movement that began in Europe in the 1970s as a public alternative to the moral and criminal models of addressing problematic substance use. The essence of this philosophy is to reduce the harmful consequences of substance use to both the individual and to society without requiring abstinence as a goal or precondition of treatment—a requirement that exists in many traditional mainstream treatment approaches to this day. Harm reduction has now spread throughout most of the world and is part of the national drug policy of most developed countries, except the United States.

Harm reduction psychotherapy (HRP) is a relatively recent and almost uniquely U.S. invention that reflects the encounter of psychotherapists who were working with psychodynamic and/or cognitive behavioral approaches to addiction treatment with the insights of the harm reduction movement. The aim of this entry is to present a distillation of the essence of HRP that draws on the work of such major innovators as Edith Springer, Alan Marlatt, Andrew Tatarsky, Patt Denning, Jeannie Little, and Frederick Rotgers.

Background

In the late 1980s, with the advent of the HIV/AIDS epidemic, harm reduction gained a foothold throughout the world. Once it became apparent that substance users, particularly intravenous injecting heroin-using individuals, were not only likely to get the disease, but also were at risk for transmitting it to others, the stage was set to shift the focus from drug-use cessation to stopping the spread of HIV. Needle exchanges and low-threshold, easily-accessible methadone programs became frontline actions in efforts to stop the spread of the disease. The focus was on strategies to help patients change their behavior in a positive direction to reduce the harmful consequences of their substance use. In short, as Earnest Drucker and colleagues have pointed out, AIDS took precedence over addiction.

Harm Reduction Philosophy

Out of the incorporation of this public health perspective, a new clinical philosophy emerged that Marlatt has called *compassionate pragmatism.* Tatarsky, in his book, has outlined six core ideas that characterize the harm reduction model:

1. *Meeting the client as an individual:* This idea reflects a belief that patients come with different internal worlds, strengths, needs, vulnerabilities, biologies, social backgrounds, and use histories; consequently, their patterns of use and the meanings that they hold will be unique for each user. For treatment to be successful, it must be tailored, as best as possible, to the patients' specific needs.

2. *Starting where the patient is:* This idea means accepting the patients with whatever goals and level of motivation for change that they come in with.

3. *Assuming the client has strengths that can be supported:* Patients are more than their problems. In many respects, to have survived in a world of active users and drug dealers speaks to deeper inner resources. The goal here would be to use these to help the patient move forward in a positive way.

4. *Accepting small incremental changes as steps in the right direction:* For most people, change will involve small steps, steps that may take time to integrate before the person can move on.

5. *Not holding abstinence (or any other preconceived notions) as a necessary precondition of the therapy before really getting to know the individual:* The belief is that the goals of the treatment will emerge out of the therapist–patient relationship and dialogue. This practice enables patients to begin where they are motivated to begin and have a therapy that is shaped to their needs.

6. *Developing a collaborative, empowering relationship with the client:* In line with psychotherapeutic traditions, there is an emphasis on egalitarianism, on a teamwork approach to clarifying issues, choosing goals, developing strategies, and implementing actions.

Understanding Drug Use

From an HRP perspective, people use substances to meet a variety of psychological, social, or biological needs. The psychological reasons incorporate the view that substance use can be adaptive, a view embodied in Edward Khantizian's self-medication hypothesis. For example, substances may be used to quell the pain of anxiety or depression, help block intrusive traumatic memories, overcome a sense of inner deadness, increase the ability of those with attention deficit hyperactivity disorder to focus, and reduce the symptoms of psychosis. Leon Wurmser, in turn, has looked at the role of the inner critic, or the harsh, punitive superego, in the use of substances. For many, alcohol or drugs serve as a kind of revolt against or escape from this experience of internal tyranny.

Tatarsky emphasizes that many of these adaptive uses of drugs also carry meaning that is related to difficult interpersonal histories. Given these histories, current relationships or internal relational schemas cause individuals pain and difficulty, and as a way of coping, substance users have found that the drug takes away the pain, at least temporarily. A drug may also be seen as a comforting and controllable stand-in for untrustworthy and unpredictable people.

A useful metaphor for integrating these ideas is to view people as being in relationships with the substances they use. These relationships fall along a continuum from healthy to unhealthy—just like relationships with people. Denning suggested that the terms *abuse* and *dependence* are ways of envisioning types of relationships to substances.

The social motivations for drug use are threefold. The first, as Denning and Springer have argued, is that many people suffer from their position or role in society due to poverty, unemployment, minority group membership, sexual orientation, or living in a high-crime environment and have, or believe they have, few possibilities for changing these difficult circumstances. Drug use becomes a method for coping with the pain associated with these difficult social realities.

The second, which overlaps with the first, is that substance use is a way to make social connections and to forge an identity. Tammy Anderson has made the case that for those who are having difficulty making successful claims to mainstream identities, the drug culture provides a rebel or outsider identity that is often fairly easy to gain access to. Scott Kellogg has noted that this social view incorporates a more complex view of substances as providers of reinforcement and meaning. For many individuals, not only does abstinence mean giving up a chemical, but also it means giving up a world and an identity in that world.

The third motivating force, which is interwoven with the other two, is the role of biology in reinforcing the use of substances. In the best of situations, people differ genetically in their responsiveness to different substances, and these differences render people more or less susceptible to finding drug use pleasurable. The scientific evidence is mounting that exposure to trauma—whether acute and dramatic or continuous—can lead to changes in brain chemistry and can leave the individual in chronic states of discomfort and/or make him or her more vulnerable to the effects of stress. It is also likely that the effects of poverty and other social ills can have a similar effect on the brain. These kinds of brain alterations can set the stage for the ability of a substance to, temporarily, bring the brain into an optimal state. This neurobiological model provides an organic understanding for the self-medication hypothesis and the trauma-oriented observations of those working in the psychological realm.

The end result is a situation in which drug use, abuse, and addiction can be understood as a complex biopsychosocial phenomena. Treatment conceptualizations and plans will need to be geared toward an understanding of the interplay of these forces.

Therapeutic Process

Therapeutic Alliance

Harm reduction therapists give the relationship with the patient, or the therapeutic alliance, central importance in their efforts. Without an alliance, there can be no work and no recovery. Making requirements about abstinence at the start of treatment for patients who are not prepared or willing to stop does not foster a good connection and is thus seen as being profoundly antitherapeutic and something to be avoided. Since many of these patients also have histories of problematic attachments, it is to be hoped that the therapy relationship will provide them with one that is attuned and affirming.

Assessment

Therapy begins with a period of assessment, and this assessment is done within a multiple-meaning framework. Not only are therapists interested in the amount, duration, and frequency of use, but also they want to know about how drug use is connected to different personal and social experiences in terms of their meaning and function.

The assessment process also serves as a vehicle for building the therapeutic alliance. As Denning put it, the goal will be the creation of an investigative team. Beyond that, assessment is viewed as an ongoing primary focus of therapy that is geared toward an ever-deepening clarification of the nature of problematic substance use and its relation to the larger context of the person.

Psychotherapeutic Goals

A treatment plan will be developed collaboratively based both on the therapist's assessment and what the patient wants from therapy. This plan will most likely include substance and non-substance-related situations. Goals for each of these problems will be chosen, and strategies for reaching each of them will be formulated. Marlatt and Rotgers each found that when patients were offered the option of pursuing either moderation or abstinence goals regarding their drinking that retention and positive outcomes significantly increased—regardless of the goal chosen.

In terms of substance use, the information from the assessment, combined with the motivational state of the patient, can be used to decide whether the goal will be to (a) continue with the current pattern but monitor it for problems, (b) make changes to reduce harm, (c) move toward a state of moderation, or (d) embrace abstinence as a goal.

Marlatt has suggested that substance use is best viewed as varying along a continuum of harmful consequences with chaotic use on one end and moderate, nonproblematic use and abstinence on the other. From this perspective, the goal of harm reduction interventions is to support the patient in making changes in substance use that move along the continuum in the direction of reduced harm. Thus, any step that reduces harm is defined as a success. Kellogg, taking a somewhat broader perspective on the role of goals in harm reduction interventions, has emphasized the importance of seeing abstinence or moderation as the ultimate,

if not the immediate, goal of the harm reduction enterprise. By keeping this endpoint in mind, the therapeutic encounter will, hopefully, contain a positive tension between the immediate or short-term goals of the patient and the long-term goals of abstinence or true moderation. This gradualist perspective on the interrelationship between goals and action can help increase the psychotherapeutic momentum.

For patients who are not seeking to achieve abstinence, Tatarsky has suggested that the ideal substance use plan be developed. This plan is worked out with the patient and is geared to maximize the positive benefits of drug use while minimizing the dangers to self and others. Developing this plan is an exercise designed to support the patient in assessing what is problematic about substance use and what are realistic goals for the him or her.

Difficulties in following through with the plan are examined in detail. Exploration of these failures can be a source of rich information about the patient's inner world. Actual techniques could include a retelling of the story with particular attention to the emotional valence of the situation, asking the patient to associate to the various details of the event, or as Jeffery Young does in his work, having the patient bring up images or memories from the past that connect to what has transpired.

Motivational Interventions

Harm reductionists have embraced the stages of change model that was developed by James Prochaska and Carlo DiClemente. In the precontemplation stage, the individual is not acknowledging that they have a problem with substances. The goal in this stage is to develop a positive therapeutic alliance that will promote the self-reflection and self-assessment that may lead patients to discover or identify the problematic consequences of their use.

In the second phase, contemplation, the patient is ambivalent about his or her drug use. Two interventions are commonly used here. Marlatt has emphasized the utility of using a decisional balance, a cognitive behavioral technique in which patients list the positives and negatives of both their current situation and of making a change. Motivational interviewing is a reflective psychotherapeutic approach developed by William Miller. In this approach, the therapist seeks to draw out and accentuate the inner conflict that the patient has about his or her drug use.

As the conflicting forces within become clearer and the cognitive dissonance more pronounced, the patient may be willing to consider resolving the conflict by changing his or her pattern of consumption.

The preparation stage follows. In this stage, the patient is moving from the abstract to the concrete. Long-term goals are selected, short-term strategies and objectives are devised to help reach those goals, barriers are acknowledged and plans to overcome them are made, and systems of support that could help in the process are identified.

The action stage has been the primary focus of mainstream treatment programs. In this stage, patients implement the planned actions—using clean needles more frequently, changing the method of taking their favored substances, eliminating specific drugs from their lives, or joining a methadone program.

The maintenance stage follows. As awareness has grown of the high rate of relapse following treatment, increasing attention has been paid to the importance of maintaining the gains the individual has achieved. Marlatt's classic work on this issue, *Relapse Prevention,* has outlined an approach for helping patients in this phase. This approach involves identifying the internal and external risk factors that could increase the likelihood that the patients would revert back to the earlier behavior. The plan is to teach patients new attitudes and new coping skills to help them successfully navigate these situations in ways that support their new choices.

Treatment Techniques

Given the comprehensive nature of HRP, psychotherapists will, ideally, be skilled in the psychodynamic, cognitive behavioral, and experiential techniques that are commonly used in integrative psychotherapies. A good place to begin is to help the patient become more aware of their drug-use process. This can be done by increasing their awareness though self-observation, which involves the cultivation of a stance of nonjudgmental, compassionate observation of the self. The benefit of this observing ego is that the person is no longer completely consumed by the addictive practice; instead, he or she is creating some inner space that provides him or her with the possibility of internal dialogue and change.

Denning and colleagues have been inspired by Norman Zinberg's work on drug, set, and setting. This view is based on the idea that the totality of the substance-induced experience develops out of the nexus of the neurotransmitter changes induced by the chemical (drug), the personality and cognitive attitude of the user (set), and the particular setting (i.e., with friends or alone, in a familiar or unfamiliar setting). Because these combinations will be different for each user, the resulting drug experiences will again be unique, and since each of these contribute to the outcome (although not necessarily in equal amounts), effective changes can be made through targeting one or more of these factors.

Pioneering work was done on changing drug-use patterns in this arena by Dan Bigg of the Chicago Recovery Alliance. Known as substance use management, the interventions focus on making alterations in the amount, type, and frequency of drug use and/or in the route of administration. Intervening with a person's set involves understanding that people may use the same substance in different ways or use different substances at different times depending on their emotional state. In terms of setting, the most straightforward is the question of whether people are using alone or with others. For those who go to bars and then repeatedly drive when they are too intoxicated to do so safely, it might be wise for them to drink at home. For those who tend to isolate and are using dangerously high levels of drugs, it might be best for them to try to use with others so that their use does not become fatal.

Drug Use During Treatment

As a core principle, it is to be expected that people will be using substances while in treatment. HRP aims to understand the specific meanings this use has to the patient and to respond accordingly. In terms of in-session intoxication, patients may be trying to express their ambivalence about changing their pattern of use. It may also be an attempt by the patients to share their experiences of being intoxicated directly with the therapist so that he or she will better understand them. Finally, patients also drink or get high to give them the courage to speak about things that are frightening or painful. Continued substance use outside of the session may reveal an issue about their level of motivation. Again, it may also reflect the possibility that the meanings that underlie their use have not been sufficiently addressed.

HRP is, at its core, about the reduction of harm and about bringing a better quality of life to the patient. At times, substance use is clearly self-destructive, life threatening, and potentially harmful to others; it may also reflect suicidal, self-harming, or homicidal wishes. In situations in which patients are putting themselves in immediate danger, the therapist will be required to take action. Harm reduction in these circumstances means not colluding with self- or other-destructiveness; it involves taking a position in favor of life and positive change, and it may look very much like a traditional limit-setting intervention. These responses can range from suggesting that evidence is mounting, that moderation or controlled use is clearly not working, that the patients may need to consider abstinence as a goal, and/or that they may need to enter more intensive, structured treatment.

Countertransference

Working with patients of any kind engenders feelings, and sometimes strong feelings, in the therapist. Substance users may be a particularly evocative group of patients in this regard. There are several reasons for response.

Given the ubiquitous nature of addictive behaviors, it is quite likely that psychotherapists have had unpleasant or even traumatic encounters with people who use alcohol and drugs in their personal lives. This personal experience, consciously or unconsciously, often contributes to therapists motivation to work with substance users. In these cases, it is likely that personal countertransference reactions based on this history will be evoked by experiences with the patient.

In mainstream addiction treatment settings, the clinical institution may be putting overt or covert pressure on the therapist to "get" their patients sober. This pressure may also be rooted in obligations to funding sources. This means that counselor's success may be based on patient abstinence. Understanding therapeutic success in this manner is likely to lead to feelings of frustration and dislike as the practitioner is trapped between the patient and the administration.

A related kind of countertransference can take place with practitioners who have successfully overcome their own addictions. Knowing that it can be done, it seems particularly frustrating to work with patients who appear to refuse to take the steps that would lead to their healing.

With addictions and drug use, countertransference also has societal roots. Kellogg and Elisa Triffleman have argued that addiction is unusual among the psychiatric disorders in that our society is torn between whether it envisions problematic drug and alcohol use as a disease to be healed or as a crime to be punished. This ambivalence permeates the treatment system as a whole, including the psyches of the treatment staff and the patients. Although harm reduction, at its best, represents the triumph of the medical over the criminal model, it does not mean that, even with the best of intentions, therapists do not carry punitive and stigmatizing voices within them. The solution is that therapists will need to engage in some form of self-examination and monitor their experience during and after their sessions to identify what has been triggered within them.

Horizontal and Vertical Interventions

Finally, it may be helpful to envision the challenge of HRP as the ability to work on two dimensions simultaneously. Traditional or mainstream treatment approaches have often focused on what might be called *horizontal* interventions or on therapeutic activities that are primarily focused on changing drug-using behavior. Earlier psychodynamic models tended to focus on what might be called *vertical* interventions; that is, they sought to understand the traumas, conflicts, and pain that were often at the root of the continued use. It now seems likely that each of these alone is an incomplete way to treat individuals who use substances in problematic ways and that harm reduction psychotherapists will need to be able to work skillfully in both dimensions.

Conclusion

Harm reduction psychotherapy is a new and exciting addition to the addiction treatment armamentarium that has great potential to make treatment more attractive to drug-using patients, to increase patient retention, and to improve successful outcomes. It is based on an expanded view of who can be treated and a corresponding emphasis of the need for treatment to be highly flexible and individualized to fit to the unique complexity of the individual. HRP aims to engage patients wherever they are interested in beginning treatment and support them in a process of positive change with abstinence as one possible goal among many. Thus, HRP builds upon abstinence-based treatment in its more ambitious goal of expanding the reach of traditional treatment.

Scott Kellogg and Andrew Tatarsky

See also Client Engagement; Harm Reduction, Public Health; Moderation Approaches to Alcohol Problems; Moderation in Use; Moderation Management; Needle Exchange Programs

Further Readings

Anderson, T. L. (1998). A cultural-identity theory of drug abuse. *Sociology of Crime, Law, and Deviance, 1,* 233–262.

Denning, P. (2000). *Practicing harm reduction psychotherapy.* New York: Guilford Press.

Denning, P., Little, J., & Glickman, A. (2004). *Over the influence: The harm reduction guide for managing drugs and alcohol.* New York: Guilford Press.

Drucker, E., Nadelmann, E., Newman, R. G., Wodak, A., McKneely, J., Malinowska-Semprucht, K., et al. (2004). Harm reduction: Pragmatic drug policies for public health and safety. In J. H. Lowinson, P. Ruiz, R. B. Millman, & J. G. Langrod (Eds.), *Substance abuse: A comprehensive textbook* (pp. 1229–1250). Baltimore: Williams & Wilkins.

Heather, N., Wodak, A., Nadelman, E., & O'Hare, P. (1993). *Psychoactive drugs and harm reduction: From faith to science.* London: Whurr.

Kellogg, S. H. (2003). On "gradualism" and the building of the harm reduction-abstinence continuum. *Journal of Substance Abuse Treatment, 25,* 241–247.

Kellogg, S. H., & Kreek, M. J. (2005). Gradualism, identity, reinforcements, and change. *International Journal of Drug Policy, 16,* 369–375.

Kellogg, S., & Triffleman, E. (1998). Treating substance-abuse patients with histories of violence: Reactions, perspectives, and interventions. *Psychotherapy: Research, Theory, Practice, Training, 35,* 405–414.

Marlatt, G. A. (1998). *Harm reduction: Pragmatic strategies for managing high risk behavior.* New York: Guilford Press.

Marlatt, G. A., & Donovan, D. (2005). *Relapse prevention* (2nd ed.). New York: Guilford Press.

Miller, W. R. (2000). *TIP 35: Enhancing motivation for change in substance abuse treatment* (Inventory No. BKD342). Rockville, MD: Center for Substance Abuse Treatment. Available from http://ncadistore.samhsa.gov

Prochaska, J. O, & DiClemente, C. C. (1982). Transtheoretical therapy: Towards a more integrative model of change. *Psychotherapy: Theory, Research, and Practice, 19,* 276–288.

Rotgers, F., Little, J., & Denning, P. (2005, July). Harm reduction and traditional treatment: Shared goals and values. *Addiction Professional,* pp. 20–26. Retrieved from http://findarticles.com/p/articles/mi_m0QTQ/is_4_3/ai_n25112626

Safran J. D., & Muran, J. C. (2000). *Negotiating the therapeutic alliance: A relational treatment guide.* New York: Guilford Press.

Tatarsky, A. (2002). *Harm reduction psychotherapy: A new treatment for drug and alcohol problems.* Northvale, NJ: Jason Aronson.

Tatarsky, A. (2003). Harm reduction psychotherapy: Extending the reach of traditional substance use treatment. *Journal of Substance Abuse Treatment, 25,* 249–256.

Wurmser, L. (1978). *The hidden dimension: Psychodynamics in compulsive drug use.* New York: Jason Aronson.

Young, J. E., Klosko, J. S., & Weishaar, M. E. (2003). *Schema therapy.* New York: Guilford Press.

Zinberg, N. E. (1984). *Drug, set, and setting: The basis for controlled intoxicant use.* New Haven, CT: Yale University Press.

HASHISH

See MARIJUANA

HEALTH CARE SYSTEM AND SUBSTANCE ABUSE

The relationship between substance use disorders and health is well documented according to the World Health Organization (WHO). Alcohol and drug abuse problems can be seen in schools, the workplace, primary care practices, mental health agencies, and within the criminal justice system. It is apparent that there are significant barriers to treatment including access to services, greater health care costs, rising insurance premiums, the increasing number of people who are uninsured, and the weak infrastructures of many treatment programs. This entry describes substance abuse prevalence rates, disease burden of alcohol and drug abuse, and barriers to effective substance abuse treatment. A recommendation to link primary health care and substance abuse treatment is also discussed.

Alcohol and Drug Prevalence Rates and Disease Burden

According to a 2005 to 2006 U.S. survey of states from the Substance Abuse and Mental Health

Services Administration, the rate of alcohol use during a 1-month period ranged from a low of 32.4% in Utah to a high of 63.1% in Wisconsin. These statistics were further broken down into rates of dependence or abuse, binge drinking, perception of risk of binge drinking, and underage drinking. The national rate of alcohol dependence or abuse for individuals 12 years and older was 9.2%. In the area of binge drinking, the rate for 12- to 17-year-olds was 10.1%, slightly lower than the 10.5% recorded the year before. The highest rates of binge drinking occurred in the 18- to 25-year-old age group with figures of 56.5% in North Dakota, about twice the rate for individuals ages 26 or older (Wisconsin at 27.4%) and almost 4 times the highest rate among youths ages 12 to 17 (Montana at 15.3%).

Alcohol consumption has health as well as social consequences due to intoxication, dependence, and other biochemical effects. Although evidence suggests that intoxication contributes to car crashes and domestic violence, it has also been shown to cause chronic health and social problems. According to the WHO, there are causal relationships between average amount of alcohol consumption and over 60 types of disease and injury. Most of these relationships are detrimental, although there are some beneficial relationships in terms of coronary heart disease, stroke, and diabetes mellitus if consumption is low to moderate and is combined with nonbinge patterns of drinking.

Alcohol use has major implications for disease burden and mortality rates. Worldwide, alcohol causes 3.2% of deaths (1.8 million) with 16% of the global burden occurring in the Americas, according to WHO. The proportion is much higher in males (5.6% of deaths) than females (0.6% of deaths). In addition, the proportion of disease burden within subregions of the world attributable to alcohol is greatest in the Americas and in Europe, where it ranges from 8% to 18% for males and 2% to 4% for females. Besides the direct effects of intoxication and addiction, alcohol is estimated to cause about 20% to 30% of each of the following worldwide: esophageal cancer, liver cancer, cirrhosis of the liver, homicide, epilepsy, and motor vehicle accidents.

The WHO believes that illicit drug use is on the rise worldwide, causing significant disease burden, even though there is a paucity of research quantifying the risks. Available prevalence rates for opioid use in the past year among people over the age of 15 vary from 0.02% to 0.04% in the Western Pacific region to 0.4% to 0.6% in the Eastern Mediterranean region. Cocaine use also varies in a similar way. The prevalence rate of amphetamine use is estimated to be 0.1% to 0.3% in most regions. Available data for stimulants and opioids, including cocaine and heroin, indicate that 0.4% of deaths (0.2 million) worldwide are caused by illicit drug use. There is higher risk among men than among women with the most at-risk patterns found among dependent users who frequently inject drugs and have done so over periods of years. Illicit drugs account for the highest percentage of disease burden among low mortality, industrialized countries in the Americas, Eastern Mediterranean, and European regions. Studies of treated injecting opioid users show this pattern is associated with increased overall mortality, including deaths caused by HIV/AIDS, overdose, suicide, and trauma. Several other adverse health and social effects that are more difficult to measure are important to note including other blood borne diseases such as hepatitis B and hepatitis C and criminal activity associated with drug abuse and addiction.

Barriers to Effective Substance Abuse Treatment

There are several major barriers to treating substance abuse. First is access to appropriate services. Treatment programs for substance use disorders are often lacking services that include primary medical care. This care is especially important since research indicates that those patients who receive primary care have reduced alcohol and drug severity. Treatment programs are faced with making referrals to other agencies for needed primary medical care or mental health services. Making referrals assumes that clients will actually follow through and access medical services.

Second, based on statistics from the National Coalition for Health Care and the Bureau of Labor Education, health care costs continue to rise at an alarming rate. The United States has the most expensive health care system in the world. National health care expenditures increased by 6.9% in the United

States in 2005. The total amount spent during this time was $2 trillion, which breaks down to about $6,700 a person and represents 16% of the gross domestic product (GDP). By 2015, these statistics are expected to rise to $4 trillion, translating to 20% of the GDP.

Third, complicating treatment even more is the fact that health insurance premiums in the United States have increased 7.7%, twice the rate of inflation. This increase averages to an annual health care premium of $11,500 for a family of four and $4,200 for individual coverage.

Another barrier impacting access to services is lack of health insurance. In the United States, there are over 47 million people without health insurance. The Kaiser Commission on Medicaid and the Uninsured Health believes that insurance is a critical component of the ability of people to access health care because those individuals with health insurance were more likely to link with a primary care provider. According to the WHO, the greatest threats to health are poverty, homelessness, lack of education, and low-level jobs.

A. Thomas McLellan and Kathleen Meyers identified several other barriers to addiction services in their evaluation of the status of the U.S. treatment system for adults through findings from a nationally representative survey of 175 specialty treatment programs. First, they found that staff working in addictions treatment programs had inadequate training. Historically, many addictions professionals have been individuals who are in recovery. In the last 8 years, there has been a paradigm shift in substance abuse education with an increased emphasis on upgrading the profession through advanced educational programs.

Problems in the structure of substance abuse programs were also identified as barriers to treatment. Many programs are dependent on local and state funding formulas that are not adequate to providing the best care available. The organizational, administrative, and personnel infrastructures of many treatment programs are fragile and unstable, making them unable to implement evidence-based care. High turnover and inadequate pay are among the contributing factors to the tenuous infrastructure found in many addictions programs. In addition, the lack of service linkages significantly impacts the provision of appropriate treatment.

Linking Primary Health Care to Addiction Treatment

There is growing evidence that linking substance abuse treatment with primary health care, including mental health services, is important and can positively impact treatment outcomes. Service linkages can occur in several ways. The first is an independent model where primary medical care is offsite. In the independent model, patients are referred to existing systems of primary medical care in the community. Several treatment models can be implemented within a primary care setting, including (a) a brief therapy model including psycho educational materials, (b) treatment from an on-site behavioral health professional, or (c) a referral-based system where patients are referred to a community-based substance abuse treatment program. The second type of service linkage is known as an integrated model where primary medical care is part of an addictions treatment program or is configured with addictions treatment as part of primary medical care services. For integrated models, primary medical care services may be provided on site at the substance abuse treatment facility or addictions treatment may be a part of primary care services. Both independent and integrated models appear to have a positive effect on addictions treatment outcomes.

Several studies reinforce the positive consequences of independent service linkages. One study by R. Saitz, N. J. Horton, and colleagues found that 63% of 400 people participating in a detoxification program linked with primary medical care when referred off-site for these services. In addition, those individuals with health insurance, support from family or friends, and other recent visits to a medical clinic or physician were much more liable to link with primary care. Another study by Saitz, M. J. Larson, and colleagues indicated that provision of primary care was associated with a lower chance of drug and alcohol severity for 391 participants. The researchers in this study purposely decided to implement a linkage model with primary care in the community since there had been little investigation in the area. Although the independent model has some support in the literature, the integrated model appears to be more effective for patients due to increased accessibility, ability to engage patients, and increased capacity to meet the needs of those with substance abuse-related medical conditions.

Other research studies show the positive impact of integrated models of primary medical care and substance abuse treatment. In one study by C. Weisner and colleagues, 592 men and women were randomly assigned to either an integrated model of treatment or an independent model. Results indicated that both groups demonstrated positive outcomes on all drug and alcohol measures including addiction severity, substance abuse-related medical conditions, medical status, health care utilization patterns, and treatment costs. Even though both groups displayed positive outcomes, patients in the integrated program had significantly higher abstinence rates, lower inpatient emergency department use, and decreased medical costs. Another study found that on-site delivery of primary care decreased emergency department visits and hospital stays for some methadone patients. Finally, a group of researchers found that a brief therapy model including psychoeducational materials within the primary care environment could significantly decrease stigma and reluctance to seek treatment. Their view was that this type of integrated model allowed for coordination between the primary care provider and substance abuse specialist.

Conclusion

People with substance use disorders have a disproportionately higher incident of medical problems compared to the general population due in part to the many barriers to primary health care. With access to care as a primary barrier, service linkages are an appropriate alternative to solving the problem. Although both independent and integrated models of service linkages have been found to be effective, it appears that an integrated model has the most potential for delivering positive outcomes over time. Improvements were seen in addiction severity, substance abuse–related medical conditions, medical status, health care utilization patterns, treatment costs, abstinence rates, inpatient emergency department use and hospital stays, and medical costs. In addition, several researchers found that a brief therapy model within the primary care environment could significantly decrease stigma and reluctance to seek treatment.

Although there is growing evidence that integrated models of service linkages are effective, more research is needed in this area. Specific areas of future inquiry might include an evaluation of treatment models, dual diagnosis programs, and the relationship between certain medical conditions and substance use disorders.

Patricia A. Markos

See also American Society of Addiction Medicine; Brief Interventions; Electronic Health Records; Health Insurance Portability and Accountability Act; Medical Consequences; Substance Use Disorders

Further Readings

Ernst, D., Miller, W. R., & Rollnick, S. (2007). Treating substance abuse in primary care: A demonstration project. *International Journal of Integrated Care, 7.* Retrieved from http://www.pubmedcentral.nih.gov/articlerender.fcgi?artid=2092396

Friedmann, P. D., Hendrickson, J., Gerstein, D., Zhang, Z., & Stein, M. D. (2006). Do mechanisms that link addiction treatment patients to primary care influence subsequent utilization of emergency and hospital care? *Med Care, 44*(1), 8–15.

The Henry J. Kaiser Family Foundation. (2008). *Medicaid benefits: Online database.* Retrieved from http://www.kff.org/medicaid/benefits/index.jsp

Hughes, A., Sathe, N., & Spagnola, K. (2008). *State estimates of substance use from the 2005–2006 national surveys on drug use and health* (DHHS Publication No. SMA 08-4311, NSDUH Series H-33). Rockville, MD: Substance Abuse and Mental Health Services Administration, Office of Applied Studies. Retrieved from http://oas.samhsa.gov/2k6state/2k6state.pdf

McLellan, A. T., & Meyers, K. (2004). Impact of substance abuse on the diagnosis, course, and treatment of mood disorders. *Biological Psychiatry, 56*(10), 764–770.

National Coalition for Health Care. (2008). *Health insurance cost.* Retrieved from http://www.nchc.org/facts/cost.shtml

Nilsen, P., Aalto, M., Nendtsen, P., & Seppa, K. (2006). Effectiveness of strategies to implement brief alcohol intervention in primary healthcare, *Scandinavian Journal of Primary Health Care, 24*(1), 5–15.

Saitz, R., Horton, N. J., Larson, M. J., Winter, M., & Samet, J. H. (2005). Primary medical care and reductions in addiction severity: A prospective cohort study. *Research Report, Addiction, 100*(1), 70–78.

Saitz, R., Larson, M. J., Horton, N. J., Winter, M., & Samet, J. H. (2004). Linkage with primary medical care in a prospective cohort of adults with addictions in inpatient detoxification: Room for improvement. *Health Services Research, 39*(3), 587–606.

Taleff, M. J. (2003). The state of addictions education programs: Results of a national cross-sectional survey. *Journal of Teaching in the Addictions, 2*(1), 59–66.

Weisner, C., Mertens, J., Parthasarathy, S., Moore, C., & Lu, W. (2001). Improved effectiveness from integrating primary medical care with addiction treatment. A randomized controlled trial. *JAMA, 286,* 1715–1723.

World Health Organization. (2007). *Global information system on alcohol and health.* Retrieved from http://www.who.int/substance_abuse/en

World Health Organization. (2008). *WHO expert committee on drug dependence.* Retrieved May 15, 2008, from http://www.who.int/substance_abuse/right_committee/en/index.html

World Health Organization. (2008). *WHO expert committee on problems related to alcohol consumption.* Retrieved May 15, 2008, from http://www.who.int/substance_abuse/expert_committee_alcohol/en/index.html

HEALTH INSURANCE PORTABILITY AND ACCOUNTABILITY ACT

The Health Insurance Portability and Accountability Act (HIPAA) of 1996, a federal act, included a number of provisions for simplifying the administration of health care. In an effort to maintain protection for the privacy of health care information, Congress incorporated into HIPAA the requirement to protect health care information. The Standards for Privacy of Individually Identifiable Health Information was passed in 2001 and became effective on April 14, 2003, for large organizations and in April 2004 for small organizations. These standards are commonly referred to as the Privacy Act. The Privacy Act is quite relevant to substance abuse treatment providers as it institutes a number of protections for individuals receiving health care services (regardless of what kind of health care) if the provider of the services utilizes electronic billing.

The Privacy Act standardized many common and good business practices for protecting the privacy of information. It also establishes a number of patient rights and provides patients with information about these rights by requiring distribution of the Notice of Privacy Practice. All providers are required to provide a copy of their Notice of Privacy Practice to recipients of services (although many health care recipients are called patients, some are called clients, consumers, or

other names; even if the provider uses a name other than patients, the Notice of Privacy Practice is likely applicable to these individuals).

The Privacy Act identifies the type of information that needs to be protected. This information is called protected health care information (PHI). PHI is any information that is created or obtained during the course of providing health care services. This information can be communicated orally or recorded through any form of media (e.g., on paper, videotape, electronically). The information may relate to current, past, or future health care services. Some common examples of protected health care information include the recipient's name, date of birth, social security number, address, telephone numbers (including cell phone), e-mail address, license plate number, dates of services, billing information, diagnosis, and clinical assessment information.

Protection of PHI is assured when the health care provider uses reasonable safeguards to avoid unauthorized disclosure. An unauthorized disclosure occurs when a person receives the recipient's information (either intentionally or unintentionally) without the recipient's expressed authorization to do so and without the disclosure being allowable or required by the Privacy Act. Commonplace reasonable safeguards include locking records in filing cabinets or locked rooms; restricting the access to records to only those needing to have the information for treatment, payment, or operations purposes; and ensuring that when information is disclosed, it has been authorized or allowable.

Disclosure of PHI is always allowable to the patient. According to HIPAA, it is also allowable when it is for treatment, payment, or operations purposes; when it has been authorized for disclosure; and when it is required to be disclosed. Disclosure of PHI can be required by law, including but not limited to, when required by court orders or subpoenas issued by a court or government entity. It is also required when requested by the recipient of health care services and required when the Secretary of the U.S. Department Health and Human Services requests the information for an investigation.

In addition to following HIPAA Privacy Act guidelines, substance abuse providers may also need to follow the rules of 42 CFR Part 2, Confidentiality of Alcohol and Drug Abuse Patient Records. The rule of thumb is that the more stringent rules apply. If the process set forth in this statute (42 CFR Part 2) is more stringent, as is the case with disclosure of information, then 42 CFR Part 2 must be followed. For example, even though HIPAA allows disclosure for payment purposes, 42 CFR Part 2 requires a signed authorization prior to disclosure.

When PHI is disclosed, the health care provider must ensure that only the minimum necessary amount of information sufficient for the purpose of the disclosure is disclosed. However, this requirement does not apply to disclosures made for treatment purposes, disclosures made to the recipient of the health care services, and disclosures made based on the authorization of the recipient or disclosures that are required.

Patients have additional rights, which include the right to request an accounting of disclosure of their protected health care information, the right to correct erroneous or incorrect information contained in the patient record, and the right to limit how and where confidential communications are conducted. Organizations establish procedures to abide by these rights.

In addition, the Privacy Act requires that all of an organization's workforce (employees, contractual employees, and volunteers) are trained on the organization's policies and procedures with respect to the Privacy Act and their responsibility for following the act. Organizations are also expected to assign a staff person as the privacy officer who acts as a contact point for patient complaints.

Compliance with the Privacy Act is legally bound, and there are financial and legal consequences for failure to follow the rule. Any individual with concerns about an organization's actions with regard to protecting the privacy of a patient is able to set forth a formal complaint to the organization's privacy officer or to the Department of Health and Human Services' Office of Civil Rights.

In conclusion, all individuals working in a substance abuse provider's agency should be well aware of the rules with regards to protecting the confidentiality of patient information through the Privacy Act and 42 CFR Part 2. Organizations should have in place solid policies and procedures that follow these statutes, provide for the rights of patients, and reduce the incidents of unauthorized disclosure of information.

Tory Lynch-Dahmm

See also Confidentiality; Electronic Health Records; Health Care System and Substance Abuse

Further Readings

U.S. Department of Health and Human Services. (2007). *Office of Civil Rights—HIPAA*. Retrieved November 1, 2007, from http://www.hhs.gov/ocr/hipaa

Hepatitis C

Worldwide, 170 million people are infected with the hepatitis C virus (HCV). HCV is the most prevalent bloodborne infection in the United States with an estimated 3.2 million to 3.5 million people chronically infected, and it is the most common cause of chronic liver disease, cirrhosis, and liver cancer in the United States. Although the natural history of chronic HCV infection varies greatly, it is estimated that 60% to 80% of people infected with HCV will develop chronic hepatitis. A majority will eventually develop symptoms or signs of liver damage after an average of 13 years. One third of these people will develop cirrhosis of the liver after an average of 20 years, and 20% to 40% of those who develop cirrhosis will develop liver failure or liver cancer on average 25 to 30 years after initial infection with HCV.

Most HCV infection appears to be transmitted through exposures to infected blood, such as blood transfusions, organ transplants, and injecting drug use. The incidence of HCV infection among blood transfusion recipients has fallen dramatically since 1990, when tests became available for screening blood donors for HCV antibodies. Injecting drug use is now the risk factor most commonly reported by hepatitis C patients and accounts for most HCV transmission in the United States.

Injecting Drug Users and HCV

Prevalence of HCV infection among injecting drug users (IDUs) ranges from 50% to 95%, according to the National Institutes of Health Consensus Development Program. HCV infection usually occurs relatively soon after initiation of injecting drug use with over 50% of IDUs infected in the first year, 75% within 2 years, and over 80% 3 or more years after. Although direct sharing of syringes (i.e., multiperson use of a syringe) is the most efficient method of HCV transmission, sharing of drug preparation equipment (e.g., spoons and cookers for mixing drugs, cotton filters, and water for dissolving drugs or rinsing syringes) may account for a sizable proportion of HCV incidence among IDUs.

Noninjecting Drug Users and HCV

Although the prevalence is much lower than among IDUs, illicit drug users that have never injected (non-IDUs) are also at increased risk for HCV infection. Estimates of HCV prevalence among non-IDUs range from 2% to 35%, according to R. Scheinmann and colleagues. Although there is debate about the mechanisms of HCV infection among non-IDUs, several mechanisms have been implicated, which include engaging in high-risk sexual practices, sharing of non-injection drug paraphernalia, and tattooing. Although HCV is not readily transmitted sexually, sexual transmission does occur. Elevated levels of HCV infection have been observed among patients seeking treatment for sexually transmitted infections (STIs), particularly those that involve genital ulcers such as syphilis, chancroid, and herpes simplex virus type 2. Stimulants such as crack cocaine, powder cocaine, and methamphetamine have been associated with increased frequency of sex, greater numbers of sexual partners, exchanges involving sex for drugs, higher rates of STIs, and extended duration during sexual encounters, all of which may increase the risk of HCV infection. HIV infection also increases the risk of contracting HCV sexually. Non-IDUs may also increase their risk for HCV infection by sharing of paraphernalia such as straws for snorting or inhaling powder cocaine and pipes for smoking crack cocaine, particularly if they contain small amounts of blood from sores inside the nose from irritations caused by the cocaine or from burns on the lips from crack pipes.

Alcohol and HCV

HCV prevalence is higher among alcoholics than among the general population, and alcohol is an aggravating factor for individuals with hepatitis C. Moderate alcohol use (e.g. one to two drinks per day) in hepatitis C patients has been associated with significantly increased serum HCV RNA levels and increased histological activity. Decreases in alcohol consumption have been associated with decreased viral load and histological activity. Consumption of greater than four alcoholic drinks per day in women and six drinks per day in men for a period of more than 5 years have been associated with increased progression to cirrhosis within 20 years of infection. The effect of alcohol consumption on the progression of hepatitis C liver disease appears to be additive for levels of alcohol consumption below five drinks per day and multiplicative for alcohol consumption above 12 drinks per day. Alcohol consumption has also been associated with increased risk of liver cancer and a reduction in the effectiveness of treatment for hepatitis C. Both the National Institute of Diabetes and Digestive and Kidney Diseases and the U.S. Centers for Disease Control and Prevention recommend abstinence from alcohol for people who test positive for HCV.

Illicit Drug Abusers and Alcohol

Illicit drug abuse among alcoholics and alcohol abuse among illicit drug users are common. Because alcohol accelerates the progression of chronic hepatitis C, it is particularly important that individuals with HCV infection know the risks of alcohol use.

Treatment for Hepatitis C

The currently recommended treatment for HCV infection is pegylated interferon alfa in combination with ribavirin. The recommended duration of treatment is 48 weeks for patients with HCV genotype 1 and 24 weeks for patients with genotype 2 or 3. Treatment is considered successful if it produces a sustained viral response, which is defined as no detectable virus 24 weeks after the end of treatment. Sustained viral response rates range from approximately 50% in patients with genotype 1 to 80% in patients with genotypes 2 and 3. Treatment can be difficult to tolerate though, and many people experience adverse side effects including fatigue, flulike symptoms, depression, fever, and anemia. These side effects cause some patients to discontinue treatment.

Prior to 2002, injecting drug use was an exclusionary criteria for HCV treatment due to concerns about difficulties adhering to treatment, psychiatric problems, and possible re-infection following successful treatment. Recommendations in the National Institutes on Health 2002 Consensus Statement on HCV revised this criteria, and current recommendations state that decisions to treat IDUs should be made on a case by case basis.

In conclusion, prevention of new HCV infections among IDUs who are not yet infected will require behavioral interventions that are sufficiently powerful to virtually eliminate injection-related risk behaviors. Non-IDUs are also at increased risk for HCV, but there is less certainty regarding the specific behaviors that lead to infection. Slowing the onset of serious liver disease among infected drug users, IDUs as well as non-IDUs that are already infected will require increased access to existing treatments for HCV infection and behavioral interventions to reduce factors, such as alcohol use, that increase the rate and probability of HCV progression.

William A. Zule

See also HIV/AIDS; Injection Drug Use; Medical Consequences; Needle Exchange Programs

Further Readings

National Institute of Diabetes and Digestive and Kidney Diseases, National Institutes of Health. (2006). *Chronic hepatitis C: Current disease management*. Retrieved September 25, 2007, from http://digestive.niddk.nih.gov/ddiseases/pubs/chronichepc/index.htm

National Institutes of Health Consensus Development Program. (2002, June 10–12). *Management of hepatitis C: 2002*. Retrieved September 25, 2007, from http://consensus.nih.gov/2002/2002Hepatitisc2002116html.htm

Scheinmann, R., Hagan, H., Lelutiu-Weinberger, C., Stern, R., Des Jarlais, D. C., Flom, P. L., et al. (2007). Non-injection drug use and hepatitis C virus: A systematic review. *Drug and Alcohol Dependence, 89,* 1–12.

World Health Organization. (2007). *Hepatitis C*. Retrieved September 25, 2007, from http://www.who.int/vaccine_research/diseases/viral_cancers/en/index2.html

HEROIN

Heroin, chemical formula $C_{21}H_{23}NO_5$, is a drug that is created from extracts of the opium poppy plant. An imitator of endorphins, heroin is known to create a sense of euphoria and well-being a short time after being introduced into the bloodstream. Heroin has an extremely high potential for addiction, and tolerance can occur quickly. Although illegal in the United States, heroin is a legal prescription in other countries under the name diamorphine. In its natural form, heroin usually exists as a brown or white powder. Popular street names for heroin include *H, brown sugar, horse, black tar, Harry, Bobby, smack, junk, dope, moop, sweet lady, Halloween, B, Ghetto D, honk, diesel, gear, skag, Jenny, brown, ice cube, jim nix, big time,* and *calipop.*

History

As long ago as 3400 BC, opium poppies were growing in Mesopotamia. The poppy plant is native to Asia and to the Middle East, is able to grow to 3 or 4 feet tall, and blooms with white, red, or purple flowers. When the poppies are blooming, the petals fall off, leaving behind a seedpod the size of an egg. When the seedpod is cut open, a milky white sap leaks out. Upon drying, the sap turns to a thick brown resin known as opium. A chemical analysis of opium reveals that two elements account for a majority of its action: codeine and morphine. C. R. Alder Wright, an English chemist, is credited with first creating heroin. In 1874 at St. Mary's Hospital Medical School in London, England, he had originally been researching the combination of morphine and a combination of acids. Boiling anhydrous morphine alkaloid and acetic anhydride for numerous hours created diacetylmorphine— a much more powerful form of morphine. Heroin did not become popular until 23 years after Wright's experiments when Felix Hoffman reproduced diacetylmorphine, instead of the codeine as he had intended. Bayer pharmaceuticals renamed the diacetylmorphine Hoffman created as heroin; this new product was actually close to twice the potency of morphine. Today's heroin is stronger than when first developed and can be 3 to 10 times the potency of morphine. Heroin has a greater potency than morphine because it is more lipid soluble than morphine. In addition, heroin travels to the brain faster and in higher amounts than morphine. The popularity of heroin spread rapidly and from 1898 to 1910. It was used as an ingredient in children's cough medicine, and ironically, as a cure for morphine addiction. Later, when Bayer Pharmaceuticals realized heroin actually converts to morphine after crossing the blood–brain barrier, its abuse potential was discovered, and its use in medicines was discontinued. Originally, when heroin was prescribed and sold for medical reasons, casual users could legally obtain heroin. In 1914, the Harrison Narcotic Act was passed as the first federal effort to regulate production, sales, and purchase of addictive substances. In 1924, the U.S. Congress passed additional laws that banned any contact with heroin, including the sale, import, or creation of the drug. The Controlled Substances Act of 1970 divided drugs into five schedules. They range from Schedule I with the highest abuse potential to Schedule V with a low potential for abuse. Heroin is classified as a Schedule I substance and has no current medical use. The only legal use for a Schedule I substance in the United States is for experimental or research purposes. The Drug Enforcement Agency is responsible for enforcement of these schedules and penalties. According to the Substance Abuse and Mental Health Services Administration, there were 338,000 current heroin users in 2006.

Usage and Effects

Heroin use is associated with intense and immediate euphoria. Next, the user feels a sense of gradual anesthetizing, drowsiness, lethargy, and sleepiness. Heroin can be administered several different ways: injection, smoking, or snorting. Heroin is ineffective if ingested. In terms of administration, intravenous injection is the quickest way to achieve a high (7–8 seconds). When heroin is injected, the initial rush of euphoria lasts less than a minute before relaxation and drowsiness takes over. An intramuscular injection produces a slower onset of euphoria (5–8 minutes), while snorting or smoking heroin delays effects even longer (10–15 minutes). Warm skin, dry mouth, and heavy extremities are effects often reported following the initial rush of euphoria.

Speedballing is another variation of heroin administration. Users combine cocaine and heroin before injecting the mixture intravenously. It may also be dissolved in water and snorted or smoked. The rush the user feels from speedballing is much more severe than with one of the drugs alone, but it is also more dangerous. The risk of death from overdosing is much higher because of the combination of a short-acting stimulant, cocaine, with a longer acting depressant, heroin. Smoking heroin requires users to heat heroin in its powder form and inhale the vapors, often referred to as *chasing the dragon*. Gravely serious health consequences

are associated with heroin use. Depending on the route of administration, severe conditions can arise just from the method of taking the drug. The most significant examples concern injection heroin users. Poor decision making while under the influence can lead to the contraction of numerous diseases. Whether it is unprotected sexual intercourse or the decision to use dirty syringes, HIV/AIDS, hepatitis, and other bloodborne diseases are very real consequences of heroin use. Collapsed veins and bloodstream infections are other possible consequences of injection use. In general, fatal overdose, spontaneous abortion, and decreased mental functioning can occur after use. Long-term effects appear after a user repeatedly takes the drug over an extended period. Heart lining and vein infections, liver disease, abscesses, and numerous pulmonary complications may arise. During pregnancy, heroin abuse is associated with low birth weight, irritability, shorter gestation, and general withdrawal symptoms once the infant is born. Large doses of heroin are often fatal. Heroin has been responsible for many suicides and murders. In addition, heroin that is cut with other powerful drugs makes overdoses more likely. Although heroin can be extremely addictive, not everyone who uses it automatically becomes addicted. A portion of heroin users, called *chippers*, take heroin only infrequently or on the weekends. Chippers use in a controlled manner and do not fit the mold of a opioid addict. Among other characteristics, they can have the drug around without having to use it; they rarely binge and do not use the drug as an escape from life's daily hassles.

Withdrawal

Symptoms of withdrawal from heroin occur 6 to 8 hours after the last dose. Withdrawal time frames may vary depending on how often and how much heroin is used and on the level of tolerance of the user. Symptoms of withdrawal include sweating, drug craving, muscle and bone pain, insomnia, cold sweats, nausea and vomiting, diarrhea, cramps, fever, cold flashes and goose bumps, restless leg syndrome, and abnormal genital sensitivity. In addition, users may experience uncontrollable kicking movements, which are referred to as *kicking the habit*. *Itchy blood* is a term users often apply to a painful condition during withdrawal. It refers to a compulsive and out-of-control scratching that can cause bleeding and scabs on the skin as well as bruises.

Occasionally, users will employ a cold turkey approach to heroin withdrawal. They will stop using without any assistance from symptom-aiding drugs, and their negative effects of withdrawal are severe.

Treatment of Addiction

The National Institutes of Health concluded in 1997 that drug addiction to opioids is a brain disease, and when treated as a medical disorder, it can be dealt with efficiently. There are two general approaches to aid in heroin withdrawal. The first involves using a long-acting or short-acting opioid in place of heroin and then weaning the user of all drugs. In the second approach, benzodiazepines are used to aid anxiety during withdrawal from heroin. Some long-acting or short-acting opioids that may be used in place of heroin include methadone, buprenorphine, naloxone, naltrexone, and nalmefene. Methadone is used most often as a substitute for heroin in treatment for addiction. Methadone is actually a synthetic opioid, and its duration of action is around 24 hours. It is considered a less harmful substitute for heroin because although it has a high potential for addiction itself, it avoids the rapid cycles of high and withdrawal due to the 24-hour action period. The danger with methadone is that users may become addicted to methadone itself, with a longer and more intense withdrawal period than the initial heroin withdrawal. It is possible that withdrawal symptoms from methadone can continue for over a month, which is why use is gradually tapered off. Methadone maintenance clinics have been established in some cities because methadone is not carried by regular pharmacies or easily prescribed by regular physicians. These clinics are a more accessible way to treat addiction for many users.

Buprenorphine is considered less risky than methadone in terms of addiction potential and is also more easily accessed. It is also associated with a lower level of physical dependence than other medications. Naloxone, nalmefene, and naltrexone are known for blocking the effects of all opioids, including heroin. Specifically, naltrexone has effects that last from 1 to 3 days, depending on the history of the user and the dose. Naltrexone works by preventing the user from feeling the pleasurable results of heroin use and is also useful in prevention of relapse. Naloxone is often used in cases where an overdose of heroin is suspected. It works by countering the effects of an overdose,

specifically the dangerous and severe depression of the central nervous system and respiratory system. Naloxone is fast-acting when injected and begins working approximately 2 minutes after an injection. Naloxone has actually been added as a component of emergency kits for heroin users in an attempt to decrease the amount of deadly overdoses.

The second approach for heroin treatment involves benzodiazepines to aid with the severe anxiety of withdrawal. The most popular benzodiazepine used is oxazepam (Serax). Just like the long and short-acting opioids, benzodiazepines must be used with caution because they also have an abuse potential. Opioid users may also frequently use other central nervous system depressants, which can unsafely react with benzodiazepines. Other less critical symptoms of withdrawal can be treated with pharmaceuticals. For example, clonidine (Catapres) is used to treat general aches and pains. The muscle relaxant baclofen can aid with the restless leg syndrome, and loperamide can assist in curbing diarrhea. The majority of professionals believe in a combination therapy approach to heroin treatment that includes both pharmacologic tools and behavioral therapies. Residential and outpatient therapies are used most often, but contingency management therapy and cognitive behavioral interventions are new treatments that show success. Contingency management therapy utilizes a system where patients receive points for every negative drug test they complete and then subsequently redeem those points for things that will assist them in their recovery. Cognitive behavioral interventions work with patients to adjust their stress reactions so that they are better able to cope with everyday life.

Harm Reduction

Harm reduction strategies play a major role in heroin addiction treatment. Believers in harm reduction aim to minimize harms that may develop as a result of heroin use. For instance, any other method of administration of the drug other than injection is considered safer because of the high potential for infections and overdose linked to injection drug use. Methadone treatments may be considered by some people to be a harm reduction strategy. Needle exchange programs (NEPs) are another strategy favored by harm reduction proponents. NEPs involve exchanging used, dirty needles for clean ones. Some NEPs also offer education on safer injecting techniques and safe disposal of used syringes as well as information on drug treatment resources.

Conclusion

Heroin is a dangerous drug that remains popular among different segments of the population. Because use is a serious problem in the United States, health professionals must be informed on heroin addiction and its consequences. If public officials, policymakers, and the public are made aware of the issues, it is possible to develop programs, create policies, and take action to ensure that feasible prevention and treatment options are available on the local and national level.

Maria Theresa Wessel, Jeanne Martino-McAllister, and Elizabeth C. Gallon

See also Buprenorphine; Methadone Maintenance Therapy; Morphine; Naloxone; Needle Exchange Programs; Opioids; Rapid Opioid Detoxification

Further Readings

Drug Enforcement Agency. (2005). *Drug scheduling.* Retrieved October 7, 2007, from http://www.usdoj.gov/ dea/pubs/scheduling.html

Goldberg, R. (2006). *Drugs across the spectrum* (5th ed.). Belmont, CA: Thomson/Wadsworth.

Hanson, G. R., Venturelli, P. J., & Fleckstein, A. E. (2006). Narcotics (opioids). In *Drugs and society* (9th ed., chap. 9). New York: Jones and Bartlett.

Levinthal, C. F. (2008). Narcotics, opium, heroin, and synthetic opioids. In *Drugs, behavior and modern society* (5th ed., chap. 5). Boston: Allyn & Bacon.

McKim, W. (2007). Opiates and opioids. In *Drugs and behavior: An introduction to behavioral pharmacology* (6th ed., chap. 12). Upper Saddle River, NJ: Prentice Hall.

National Institute on Drug Abuse. (2007). *NIDA infofacts: Heroin.* Retrieved September 20, 2007, from http://www.drugabuse.gov/infofacts/heroin.html

Spiess, M., & Fallows, D. (2006). *ONDCP drug policy information clearinghouse factsheet: Drug related crime.* Retrieved September 20, 2007, from http://www .whitehousedrugpolicy.gov/publications/factsht/crime/ index.html

Substance Abuse and Mental Health Services Administration. (2005, November 5). Youth drug use continues to decline. *SAMHSA Newsletter, 13*(5). Retrieved September 15, 2007, from http://www.samhsa.gov/SAMHSA_news/ VolumeXIII_5/article6.htm

Volkow, N. D. (2005). Heroin abuse and addiction. *National Institute on Drug Abuse Research Report Series.* Retrieved September 15, 2007, from http://www.nida.nih .gov/ResearchReports/Heroin/Heroin.html

HIGH-RISK BEHAVIORS

High-risk behaviors are those acts that place individuals at a greater disadvantage to abuse or depend on substances. These behaviors are often health compromising acts that are preexisting or comorbid with substance use. High-risk behaviors are risk factors that, according to the National Institute on Drug Abuse (NIDA), can be both additive and potent. As an additive effect, the more risk behaviors a person has, the more the chance for substance abuse. In terms of potency, the presence of some high-risk behaviors leads to a greater chance of substance abuse than does the presence of other high-risk behaviors. Identification of these behaviors is important to substance abuse prevention, treatment, and recovery because if not targeted for prevention or addressed in treatment, these behaviors can hinder efforts to address problematic substance use and interrupt the recovery process. The effectiveness of prevention and treatment models depends greatly on proper identification of high-risk behaviors, the proper development of treatment models, and the proper application of model components to address these behaviors.

Prevention of substance abuse begins with the identification of the behaviors that increase the likelihood that individuals will initiate the substance use process. Several high-risk behaviors become consequent to substance use and must be addressed in treatment, and individuals must understand the extent of their high-risk behaviors as they go through the process of recovery. As such, research efforts attempt to identify these behaviors within specified populations to provide evidence-based prevention, intervention, and treatment models to intercept and divert these behaviors when targeting substance abuse. High-risk behaviors can exist at the individual, family, peer, and community levels and tend to vary across youth and adult populations. It should be noted that individual level risk behaviors can be influenced by family, peer, and community high-risk behaviors and vice versa.

Individual-Level Behaviors

Individual-level high-risk behaviors include substance use–related behaviors and problem behaviors. Both types are often the focus of prevention and treatment programs, particularly when targeting youth. Prevention and treatment efforts seek to either reduce the identified behaviors or enhance protective factors to combat the risk. According to the Substance Abuse and Mental Health Services Administration (SAMHSA), conceptual models that focus on both risk and protective factors have been major developments in prevention theory and programming, and nearly all prevention programs begin with an understanding of factors that place individuals at risk for problem behaviors.

Substance Use–Related Behaviors

High-risk behaviors that are substance related include the early onset of substance use, underage and binge drinking, cigarette smoking, inhalant use, and the misuse of prescription drugs such as pain relievers, sedatives, and stimulants.

Early onset of substance use and underage drinking pose the greatest risks for later abuse or dependence on substances. Numerous studies indicate that many adults who abuse substances tended to begin their substance use prior to adulthood. According to the National Survey on Drug Use and Health (NSDUH), nearly 1 in 25 teens as young as ages 12 to 13 report past-month use of an illicit drug, and as the age increases, the rate is a high as one in five. Due to this rapid increase, many prevention programs are targeted to elementary- and middle school–age children.

The NSDUH provides estimates that there are 11 million current underage drinkers, and those who start drinking before the age of 15 are 5 times more likely to have alcohol-related problems in adulthood. Binge drinking is another dangerous high-risk behavior that is highly prevalent among youth as well as among adults. Binge drinking occurs in two out of five 18- to 25-year-olds. The prevalence and concern for underage drinking and binge drinking is so high that in 2006 the 109th Congress passed the Stop Underage Drinking Act, H.R. 864. The act authorizes the use of federal funds to identify the scope of the problem and to conduct research into the effects of underage drinking and binge drinking on brain development among students.

Cigarette smoking is considered a high-risk behavior in terms of substance abuse. According to SAMHSA, research studies indicate that substance use is more frequent in smokers than in nonsmokers. Because of this higher prevalence, cigarette smoking is often targeted in prevention models.

More recently, prescription drug misuse has become the focus of research studies on substance use. Not only is prescription misuse highly prevalent in the elderly, but it is a high-risk behavior among youth as well. The NSDUH survey also reveals that youth are almost half of the individuals who use prescription drugs for nonmedical reasons.

Inhalant use is high-risk behavior that is more prevalent in youth than in adults. The NSDUH reveals that the rate of inhalant use rises each year as youth tend to use inhalants because of the relative ease of access. Because of this ease of access, younger children are often experimenting with various inhalants. In fact, statistics indicate that roughly 3% of children within the United States have experimented with inhalants by the time they are in the fourth grade, and between the years of 2002 to 2003, approximately 8.6% of youth ages 12 to 13 had used inhalants in their lifetime. Of these 12- to 13-year-olds, 35% also had illicit drug use that is a fourfold increase over the percentage of illicit drug use in those who did not use inhalants. This finding is particularly salient for treatment and recovery processes as the use of inhalants to the point of abuse can become chronic and persist into adulthood.

Problem Behaviors

Problem behaviors such as fighting, aggression, gang involvement, and impulsive and sensation seeking behaviors are high-risk behaviors for substance abuse. Problem behavior theory posits that, particularly for youth, a series of behaviors often coexist or come into existence among individuals who display one behavior. Evidence from the NSDUH indicates that youth at the greatest risk are involved in a series of problem behaviors including poly substance use. Other high-risk individual behaviors include poor academic achievement and inappropriate social behavior. For adults, criminal behaviors are high-risk behaviors that are associated with substance abuse. According to results of the 2005 NSDUH, 26% of recent parolees were current illicit drug users, and 29% of those on probation were current drug users. These rates are substantially higher than rates within the general population.

Family-Level Behaviors

Family-level behaviors such as substance use by immediate family members increases the likelihood of use by individuals due to a modeling of substance use behaviors. For youth, this modeling of high-risk behaviors attributes to perceptions that substance use is an acceptable behavior. Familial substance use is a high-risk behavior that is salient to youth and adults. Parental substance use in particular has this distinction. The National Institute on Alcohol Abuse and Alcoholism cautions adults of alcoholic parents to maintain moderate drinking patterns if they choose to drink due to the heightened increase of vulnerability to alcoholism.

Abuse and maltreatment within the home are both behaviors at the family level that are high-risk for substance use because they lead members of the family to seek out alternatives ways to cope with the situation. NIDA reports that two thirds of patients in drug treatment report being the victim of child abuse. Whether for youth or adults, research indicates that behaviors of other family members can have a significant impact on whether or not others within the home will engage in the use of substances. There is some indication that these family-level high-risk behaviors, including familial substance use, create situations of high stress. To address the stress within the family, members may engage in substance use as a coping mechanism. The behaviors of the family are key targets in prevention research.

Peer-Level Behaviors

Peer-level high-risk behaviors include peer substance use, peer pressure, the desire for peer conformity, and the association with deviant peers. The theory of differential association explains how networks of peers influence behavior. It posits that the values of reference groups reinforce behaviors. Thus, if a person's reference group places a high value on substance use, the individual will be more likely to engage in such an act. Peer behaviors appear more relevant for youth populations than for adult populations. In the case of youth, attempts to separate from parents and to gain the acceptance of peers will heavily influence whether or not the youth will engage in the behaviors that are modeled by the peers. Substance use by youth is not performed because it is expected by peers, but because it becomes a natural part of the youth's

functioning if the peer group happens to place a high value on substance use.

Community-Level Behaviors

Community high-risk behaviors are more difficult to conceptualize, but they include tendencies within groups that demonstrate an acceptance and promotion of substance use among residents. These community factors place a significant amount of stress on residents within the community to conform. These practices include advertising practices that target low-income areas and behaviors associated with community disorganization including residential mobility. Communities with high levels of disorganization create environments of high tolerance for individual-risk behaviors. For instance, community disorganization can facilitate the availability of drugs. National surveys indicate that many youth in urban areas report relative ease in acquiring illicit drugs. Drug selling in neighborhoods makes it less likely that individuals will have to go outside of their community for their drug supply. In communities with high concentrations of poverty, community resources are sparse to combat the negative influx of the drug culture. High levels of residential mobility is another high-risk community-level behavior that can contribute to substance abuse as it contributes to community disorganization and family instability.

Conclusion

Identification of high-risk behaviors is a pivotal part of successful prevention, treatment, and recovery efforts. High-risk behaviors have to be targeted for prevention, but also they must be targeted in treatment efforts. Individuals must learn skills that help them cope with problem situations that enhance the likelihood of engaging in high-risk behaviors. The importance of understanding and identification of high-risk behaviors is further highlighted by the dedicated research centers that specifically focus on high-risk behaviors. One example is the Health and Human Development Program's development of the Center for Research on High Risk Behaviors that recognizes substance use as a risky behavior and seeks to identify why individuals become involved in the behavior and ways to reduce the behavior.

To facilitate efforts to address high-risk behaviors and prevent the initiation of substance use, NIDA published guidelines for prevention programs for youth that include specific principles for addressing high-risk behaviors. These principles include addressing all forms of drug use, including inhalants and prescription drugs, and targeting modifiable risk factors from an individual perspective. From a family perspective, principles for prevention include targeting parenting behaviors that lead to risk for drug abuse. These guidelines, though specific for youth, can also be applied to prevention programs with adults. As a general principle, NIDA suggests that prevention programs should attempt to target risks as they apply to specific populations.

Sharon D. Johnson

See also High-Risk Situations; Risk and Protective Factor Theory; Underage Drinking

Further Readings

Department of Health and Human Services. (2007). *The Surgeon General's call to action to prevent and reduce underage drinking*. Rockville, MD: Department of Health and Human Services, Office of the Surgeon General. Retrieved June 29, 2007, from http://www.surgeongeneral.gov/topics/underagedrinking

National Institute on Alcoholism and Alcohol Abuse. (2003). *A family history of alcoholism: Are you at risk?* (NIH Pub. No. 03-5340). Washington, DC: Author. Available from http://www.niaaa.nih.gov

National Institute on Drug Abuse. (2003). *Preventing drug use among children and adolescents: A research based guide for parents, educators and community leaders* (2nd ed.). Washington, DC: Author. Retrieved from http://www.drugabuse.gov/NIDAHome.html

National Institute on Drug Abuse. (2007). *Drugs, brains, and behavior: The science of addiction* (NIH Pub No. 07-5605). Washington, DC: Author. Retrieved from http://www.drugabuse.gov/NIDAHome.html

Schinke, S., Brounstein, P., & Gardner, S. (2002). *Science-Based Prevention Programs and Principles 2002: Effective substance abuse and mental health programs for every community* (DHHS Pub. No. SMA 03-3764). Rockville, MD: Center for Substance Abuse Prevention, Substance Abuse and Mental Health Services Administration. Available from http://ncadi.samhsa.gov

Substance Abuse and Mental Health Services Administration. (2006). *Results from the 2005 National Survey on Drug Use and Health: National findings* (DHHS Publication No. SMA 06-4194). Rockville, MD: Author. Retrieved from http://www.oas.samhsa.gov/NSDUH/2k5NSDUH/2k5Results.htm

HIGH-RISK SITUATIONS

High-risk situations refer to any condition that may increase the chance for engagement in any undesirable behavior. In the context of drug and alcohol treatment, a high-risk situation is any cognition, emotion, location, event, or experience that could escalate the potential to use or overuse a substance. This entry reviews both the original linear model and the later dynamic model of relapse as they relate to high-risk situations and reviews cognitive behavioral treatment options of identifying and preparing for high-risk situations.

Models of Relapse

Two primary models of relapse will be explained and examined below. The initial linear model of relapse views high-risk situations as an antecedent, resulting either in successful coping or relapse. The more recent dynamic model incorporates that theory with a dynamic perspective of interrelationships among different situations.

Linear Model

The linear model of relapse posits that following exposure to a high-risk situation, outcomes will progress in one of two linear frames. In the first instance, an effective coping response is elicited following a high-risk situation. As the response is effective, the individual will experience increased self-efficacy and therefore, a decreased probability of relapse. In the second occurrence, the high-risk situation fails to elicit an effective coping response, leading to decreased self-efficacy combined with positive outcome expectancies (or the belief that using will be reinforcing). This combination may lead to a lapse, or initial use of the substance, resulting in experiencing the effects of the substance. Depending on the individual's cognitions related to the lapse, two additional outcomes are possible. If the individual views the lapse as an unfortunate occurrence or as a learning opportunity, he or she may resume the prelapse goal of abstinence or moderation. Conversely, relapse or increased usage may follow if the individual experiences an abstinence violation effect (AVE). Common components of AVE include a feeling of loss of control over the ability to abstain from use and internal, stable, global attributions of the lapse.

A taxonomy of high-risk situations was developed to identify the precipitating events in relapse and is subdivided into eight categories: coping with negative emotional states, coping with negative physical-psychological states, enhancement of positive emotional states, testing personal control, giving in to temptations and urges, coping with interpersonal conflict, social pressure, and enhancement of positive emotional states. Each of the categories is briefly discussed.

Intrapersonal High-Risk Situations

Research studies indicate that negative emotional states are positively correlated with and predictive of relapse; however, many individual factors contribute to this risk. For example, different negative emotions (sadness, anger, grief) have different risks to different individuals. Similarly, negative physical and psychological states (such as chronic pain) may also pose a risk for relapse. As suggested by the categories, the risk may lie more in the individual's ability to cope with the emotions or sensations rather than the intensity or duration of the experience. A further emotional trigger may come from enhancing positive emotional states, rewards, or celebrations, but the research is mixed. Although some studies support this increased risk, others have determined that positive emotions may be more associated with less frequent and severe relapse.

Testing personal control may also increase the risk for lapse. In this instance, an individual may intentionally place himself or herself in a high-risk situation (returning to a bar where he or she habitually drank) as a test of willpower. In these circumstances, the risk may outweigh the preparation and coping strategies employed by the individual, leading to an increased risk of lapse. Finally, urges and temptations indicate an increased probability of relapse in specific circumstances and individuals, particularly when they do not subside and when they are present first thing in the morning. Again, the individual's

ability to cope with urges and temptations appears to be more predictive than just the experience of them.

Interpersonal High-Risk Situations

Interpersonal situations include coping with conflict, social pressure, and again enhancement of positive emotional states. The positive emotional states in this category refer more specifically to group celebrations and special occasions (going out after work on the weekend, a wedding) rather than based on internal mood and emotion. Social pressure can be present in many indirect forms (invitation to a barbeque) as well as overt encouragement or teasing and jeering. Finally, coping with conflict again illustrates the importance of positive coping strategies.

The linear model and hierarchy explains relapse by a series of if-then responses following exposure to a myriad of high-risk situations. In contrast, the dynamic model incorporates many of these situations with other potential contributors to clarify the interaction of these and other factors.

Dynamic Model

The dynamic model of relapse identifies two primary types of high-risk situations: static and dynamic. Static situations are rare and essentially are situations that are always (or by default, never) risky to the individual. More often than not, a combination of situations will produce different outcomes, even if one of the situations is identical. In the dynamic model, passing by the alleyway at night while feeling depressed may lead to a lapse, but passing by the alleyway in the morning while feeling happy may not increase risk.

The dynamic model posits two primary distinctions, though there is great overlap between them: tonic processes, or chronic vulnerabilities, and phasic responses, or transient states. Both of these processes occur within the general context of high-risk situations. Seven categories comprise tonic and phasic processes, with one category solely considered tonic, two categories solely considered phasic, and the remaining four categories having features of both.

Tonic Processes

Only distal risks, which include predispositions such as family history, social support, and dependence on the substance, are included solely in the tonic category. These risks are not actually included in high-risk situations, but rather interact with the other factors such as emotions and cognitions. These vulnerabilities are unique to the individual, and while history is not destiny, they may interact with other processes to increase risk of lapse.

Tonic and Phasic Processes

Four categories have features identified with both tonic and phasic processes: physical withdrawal, cognitive processes, affective state, and coping behaviors. Physical withdrawal will have a baseline or tonic level for the individual, though peaks could be associated with phasic responses.

Cognitive processes include categories such as self-efficacy, outcome expectancies, motivation, and craving. Self-efficacy is a predictor of lapse and relapse, both at baseline (tonic) and during fluctuations (phasic). Initial belief in the ability to manage one's substance use can be increased both through interventions and dynamically through successes, though day-to-day variations can occur. Outcome expectancies are related to relapse, with negative expectancies decreasing the risk and positive expectancies increasing the risk. Positive expectancies indicate the individual assumes use or overuse of a substance will be reinforcing, whether through positive reinforcement of achieving some desired effect or negative reinforcement whereby an unpleasant state (pain, anxiety) is removed. Negative expectancies refer to the belief that something unpleasant could occur, or simply that using will not achieve the desired effect. Expectancies can be both explicit and implicit, increasing the difficulty of identifying and if necessary challenging these positive expectancies.

Baseline motivation refers to individuals' internal and/or external drives to meet their goals concerning substance use. Under the phasic process, motivation may oscillate as it interacts with other processes such as self-efficacy within high-risk situations. Motivation to not drink at work, for example, may be much stronger than motivation to not drink while on vacation. Finally, baseline craving as a cognitive process is strongly related to outcome expectancies, while fluctuations in cravings may be a result of interaction with other high-risk situations such as affective state or physical withdrawal.

Affective state risk factors include both baseline levels of positive and negative emotions (anger, sadness, happiness) as described previously, as well as fluctuations that interact with other situations. For example, someone struggling with depression might be at a greater of risk of lapsing following an unusually bad day or an unusually good day, depending on the interaction with other factors such as expectancies and coping skills. Spikes in specific cognitive processes may also interact directly with emotions, whereby a decrease in self-efficacy may interact with negative emotions and increase the risk of lapse.

Finally, coping behaviors constitute the last category of tonic and phasic processes. Baseline coping mechanisms such as self-regulation play an important role in reducing risk, though phasic identification and implementation of specific strategies also predict positive outcomes. The dynamic nature of coping behaviors lies in their interaction with other processes. For example, a negative affective state such as anger may reduce the likelihood of using a coping strategy that may increase the likelihood of lapse, thereby reducing self-efficacy that may lead to further dismissal of strategies. Conversely, successful implementation of a coping strategy may help dissipate a phasic negative emotion, thereby creating a new positive expectancy related to self-control.

Phasic Responses

Two final categories comprise phasic responses: substance use behavior and perceived effects. The preceding paragraphs have incorporated both topics into the discussion and examples. Substance use behavior includes lapses if abstinence is a goal and includes quantity and frequency for moderation. Use is related to the perceived effects, through either positive or negative reinforcement or the abstinence violation effect. In the case of a goal of abstinence, a combination of low baseline motivation with high phasic negative emotion might result in use of the identified substance. If the negative emotion dissipates, the perceived effect may be that the drug was negatively reinforcing, increasing the risk of further use. Even if the drug is not reinforcing, the abstinence violation effect or belief that a lapse indicates failure and hopelessness may also increase risk. Conversely, if appropriate coping skills are used and the substance is not used, there may be an increase in self-efficacy that could also be positively reinforcing for emotions. There are an infinite number of interactions within the dynamic model.

Treatment Options

Given that high-risk situations potentially include baseline and variations in physical withdrawal, self-efficacy, outcome expectancies, motivation, craving, affective states, coping behaviors, self-regulation, substance use or misuse, and perceived effects, identification of a single situation and solution is impractical if not impossible. Standard relapse prevention treatment incorporates a number of these factors by first identifying high-risk situations that might be more salient for the client and then by developing clear alternatives to employ in risky situations. Great attention is paid to generalization due to the unlimited number of interactions the client may experience. Restructuring is often useful in treatment as well, as it directly interacts with cognitive processes that may increase risk of use. In addition, both mindfulness and acceptance approaches have been employed to counter effects of craving and urges, including the techniques of observation and urge surfing.

Conclusion

The definition of high-risk situations has evolved from a perception of greater risk at specific times of day and locations to include a dynamic model of interactions between myriad factors at both stationary and fluctuating levels. Distal risks, physical withdrawal, cognitive processes, affective state, coping behaviors, substance use behavior, and perceived effects all interact with each other, producing a unique situation for the individual. Cognitive behavioral treatments such as relapse prevention, acceptance, and mindfulness all play individual roles as well as interact to reduce the probability of lapse or relapse in high-risk situations.

Diane E. Logan and G. Alan Marlatt

See also Abstinence Violation Effect; Cognitive Behavioral Therapy; Craving; Expectancies; Relapse; Relapse Prevention

Further Readings

Carey, K. B. (1995). Alcohol-related expectancies predict quantity and frequency of heavy drinking among college students. *Psychology of Addictive Behaviors, 9*(4), 236–241.

Gwaltney, C. J., Shiffman, S., Balabanis, M. H., & Paty, J. A. (2005). Dynamic self-efficacy and outcome expectancies: Prediction of smoking lapse and relapse. *Journal of Consulting and Clinical Psychology, 62*(3), 611–619.

Larimer, M. E., Palmer, R. S., & Marlatt, G. A. (1999). Relapse prevention: An overview of Marlatt's cognitive-behavioral model. *Alcohol Research and Health, 23*(2), 151–160.

Marlatt, G. A. (1996). Taxonomy of high-risk situations for alcohol relapse: Evaluation and development of a cognitive-behavioral model [Supplement]. *Addiction, 91*, 37–49.

Marlatt, G. A., & Gordon, J. R. (Eds.). (1985). *Relapse prevention: Maintenance strategies in the treatment of addictive behaviors.* New York: Guilford Press.

Marlatt, G. A., & Ostafin, B. D. (2006). Being mindful of automaticity in addiction: A clinical perspective. In R. W. Wiers & A. W. Stacy (Eds.), *Handbook of implicit cognition and addiction* (pp. 489–495). Thousand Oaks, CA: Sage.

Witkiewitz, K., & Marlatt, G. A. (2004). Relapse prevention for alcohol and drug problems: That was Zen, this is Tao. *American Psychologist, 59*(4), 224–235.

Witkiewitz, K., & Marlatt, G. A. (Eds.). (2007). *Therapist's guide to evidence-based relapse prevention.* London: Academic Press.

Witkiewitz, K., Marlatt, G. A., & Walker, D. (2005). Mindfulness-based relapse prevention for alcohol and substance use disorders. *Journal of Cognitive Psychotherapy, 19*(3), 211–228.

HISPANICS/LATINOS, ISSUES IN PREVENTION AND TREATMENT

See RACIAL AND ETHNIC MINORITIES, ISSUES IN PREVENTION; RACIAL AND ETHNIC MINORITIES, ISSUES IN TREATMENT

HIV/AIDS

Since the first cases of human immunodeficiency virus (HIV) were reported in 1981, HIV has become a worldwide pandemic. HIV is a retrovirus that attacks and kills the body's critical immune cells known as helper-T and CD4 cells causing a gradual deterioration of the immune system. Once a person has been infected with HIV, or becomes HIV-positive, the virus replicates for years without symptoms. The point at which immune cells reach critically low levels and symptoms occur is denoted acquired immunodeficiency syndrome (AIDS). There is no cure for AIDS, and millions of people worldwide die from the disease every year.

Transmission

HIV is transmitted through the exchange of bodily fluids. Fluids such as blood, saliva, semen, vaginal and anal secretions, and breast milk may all contain the virus and are the most common vehicles for transmission. The transmission of HIV from one individual to another can occur in a number of ways. The most common form of transmission occurs through unprotected sexual activity, with anal sex representing the highest risk, followed by vaginal sex, and then oral sex. Although oral sex is a lower risk activity, the rates of transmission are potentially higher than originally thought. Blood-to-blood transmission is common through the sharing of needles and other surgical instruments. Intravenous drug use is implicated in transmission through needle sharing, but the sharing of knifes or scalpels in performing surgeries is a common practice in underdeveloped countries, and this transmission method has only recently been addressed. Transmission through breastfeeding can also occur, and this is the most common method of passage from an HIV-positive mother to an HIV-negative newborn. HIV can also be transmitted through blood transfusions, although blood screenings for HIV that have occurred after 1985 in the United States have virtually eliminated this method of transmission.

Interestingly, because HIV cannot survive in open air for more than a few minutes, transmission through household objects such as toothbrushes or razors is exceedingly rare. There are two or three case reports of HIV transmission through the sharing of a toothbrush or a razor, and in these cases the toothbrush or razor was used immediately after an infected person and probably contained some blood residue. Although HIV is present in saliva, the amounts of the virus in saliva are so low that a person would have to be exposed to relatively large amounts of infected saliva in order for transmission to occur, and there are no proven cases of HIV being transmitted solely from kissing. Also, HIV cannot be transmitted through a mosquito bite. Unlike malaria, HIV is not present in the anticoagulant saliva that a mosquito injects into its victim when it bites, so no HIV-infected blood can be passed from the mosquito to the person.

Replication

Once people are exposed to HIV-infected fluids and the virus enters their bloodstream, the virus is quickly attacked by antibodies known as CD4 cells or helper-T cells. The antibody binds to the protein coat of the virus, and then a conformational change in the binding protein allows the virus to fuse with the plasma membrane and enter the CD4 cell's cytoplasm, at which point the CD4 cell has become infected. The virus then excretes the genetic material from its core (i.e., RNA for retroviruses) into the cytoplasm of the CD4 cell, along with proteins such as reverse transcriptase, which allow transcription of a DNA strand from the viral RNA transcript. The viral DNA is then spliced into the genome of the CD4 cell with the help of a viral enzyme. This process effectively "hijacks" the cellular machinery so that instead of functioning normally, the CD4 cell begins to make viral RNA and viral proteins that congregate in the cytoplasm and are subsequently assembled into immature viruses. After assembly, the HIV particle separates from the host cell to form a plasma membrane coat, and the internal proteins and RNA are further spliced, creating a mature and infectious HIV particle.

HIV spreads rapidly throughout the body after initial infection, mostly congregating in the lymph tissue. Within the first 2 months, many people will develop the physical symptoms of a typical viral infection, such as fever. The body reacts as it would to the presence of any pathogen, with an immune response that will reduce but not eliminate the HIV levels in the body. After this initial reaction, an HIV-infected person will appear asymptomatic, usually for 2 to 10 years while the virus replicates and gradually degrades and destroys the body's immune cells, along with their ability to communicate and fight infections. This process is the transition from HIV to AIDS. Several years later, during the next stage in the cycle, the person develops general inflammation of the lymph areas. This symptom is the first physical manifestation of AIDS. Full-blown AIDS is the next stage, at which point antibody levels are so low that the person cannot fight what healthy people consider normal pathogenic infections. The individual may develop deterioration of neurological function, possibly developing AIDS dementia, and they will most likely succumb to an opportunistic infection such as pneumonia or tuberculosis.

Risk Factors

Throughout the world, 25 million people have died from HIV, with more than 500,000 deaths in the United States alone. In the 1980s, the majority of new cases in the United States were exposed through homosexual contact, which fed rumors that HIV was simply a "gay plague." However, the majority of cases worldwide result from heterosexual contact. This discrepancy begs the question: What factors put a person at risk for exposure to and thus contraction of, HIV? There are three recognized behaviors that have been associated with increased exposure to HIV, but there are also other high-risk groups to whom prevention efforts must be tailored. These behaviors are intravenous drug use or IDU, homosexual contact or men-having-sex-with-men, and unprotected heterosexual contact, often associated with substance abuse.

Critically, there are disproportionately high levels of infection among the Hispanic and African American populations, some of whom fall into the categories listed above. In fact, in 2003, an estimated 47% of the 1.2 million individuals infected with HIV living in the United States were non-Hispanic Blacks. Of the 40,000 new cases of HIV infection every year, 50% are African American, despite their accounting for only 13% of the general population. Similarly, 18% of new HIV-infection cases occur in Hispanic individuals, even though they make up only 13% of the general population. HIV is the number one cause of death for African American men ages 25 to 44 years old and for African American women ages 25 to 34. African Americans make up the highest percentage of new HIV cases in every age category. These statistics indicate that the spread of HIV infection among these groups must be specifically addressed in order to gain a better understanding of why the incidence of HIV among these groups is so high and to continue to develop prevention programs that target risk factors unique to these groups.

To date, many HIV-prevention interventions have targeted minority and inner-city women and adolescents. The goal of these programs is prevention through a focus on education and intervention-based treatments to reduce high-risk behaviors such as drug use and unprotected sex. Some programs have targeted adolescents for peer-education or for group education, while others target drug-abusing individuals through behavioral interventions. Results have shown that some behavioral intervention treatments have been successful in reducing high-risk behaviors among their target populations. However, many of these programs are client-specific, and more effort must be made to provide services to specific high-risk populations, such as substance abusing and dependent individuals.

Intravenous drug use has been a consistent method of HIV transmission. Among drug users, HIV can be transmitted through sharing needles and through the sharing of other drug paraphernalia such as cotton swabs, rinse water, and cookers. Professionals have sought to reduce HIV transmission by reducing the high-risk behaviors many IDUs engage in through intervention, often centering the programs in drug treatment centers. However, these programs may represent only those patients looking to reduce their drug use. Data collection has shown that HIV infection rates may be twice as high in community drug users as in those who initiated drug treatment. The intervention methods that have proven useful focus on education as well as on using behavioral intervention techniques to lower high-risk sexual behaviors and high-risk drug behaviors such as sharing needles, or association with "shooting galleries," where drug users congregate to share drugs and needles. As high-risk drug use and sexual behaviors are decreased, HIV seroincidence levels are, of course, likely to decrease. Needle exchange programs are designed to lower exposure to HIV by allowing IDUs the opportunity to exchange their used, and possibly infectious, needles for sterile ones, which are offered at private and public clinics. The practice remains controversial, with opponents arguing that the programs encourage drug use, and current laws prohibit the use of federal funding for needle exchange programs.

Substance Abuse

Substance abuse has a strong link to HIV in the United States. In addition to the risk of direct exposure to HIV by injecting drugs and needle sharing, research conducted by the National Institute on Drug Abuse and the National Institute on Alcohol Abuse and Alcoholism indicates that drug and alcohol consumption lead to an increase in other behaviors that put people at risk for HIV exposure. For example, drug and alcohol use can lead to such behaviors such as unprotected sex when intoxicated, exchanging sex for drugs, and overall poor decision-making ability and impulsiveness. All of these are considered high-risk behaviors or have been shown to lead to an increased risk of HIV exposure. As these and other risk behaviors are targeted by interventions, the incidence of HIV transmission is expected to decrease.

Unprotected sex while intoxicated is a common problem for adolescents as well as young adults and college students. Possibly seen as a harmless vice or less of a health risk than drug use, these individuals do not usually see themselves as engaging in high-risk behaviors. Individuals who engage in unprotected sex with multiple partners may justify their behaviors by downplaying the high-risk aspect of their encounters, or they may be more sensitized to their risk than those who engage with single partners. Oftentimes, individuals who are most at risk to be HIV-positive are least motivated to terminate high-risk behaviors that may increase the spread of HIV. Many of these individuals will avoid having an HIV test simply because they fear the results, which might cause them to appreciate that they are probably spreading the virus. Drug users have been found to avoid HIV testing due to inconvenience, distrust of clinical staff, and fears of blood-draws.

Prevention Measures

As mentioned previously, several intervention-based programs have been tailored toward drug treatment as an HIV prevention measure. Program staff in these facilities integrate behavioral interventions, education, and logistical procedures to help motivate drug users to lower their high-risk behaviors. Among IDUs in treatment, the chain of events seems to be simple: Individuals who enter drug treatment centers decrease their overall drug use, which leads to lower high-risk behaviors, leading to lower transmission risk for HIV, which leads to lower numbers of HIV-infected individuals in the community. A variety of prevention-based outcome studies specifically tailored to lower-income, high-risk groups or IDUs have been shown to be effective. Follow-up evaluations of programs targeting these groups have indicated lower high-risk sexual behaviors and increased condom use, while lowering drug use. Also, needle exchange programs are being implemented in major cities in the United States and have shown promising results in decreasing needle sharing. Similar prevention measures have recently been implemented targeting prevention of high-risk behaviors for HIV-positive individuals. Motivating seropositive individuals to lower drug use and other high-risk behaviors is important because they can maintain a low viral count and a high CD4 cell count through a combination of medical and lifestyle variables.

Antiretroviral Treatment

Several drugs have been designed to combat HIV infection. This combination has become known as *antiretroviral treatment* (ART) or *highly active antiretroviral treatment*. There are several different physiological pathways that these drugs target, but one underlying factor is that adherence to these drugs makes it possible to turn HIV and AIDS from a fatal disease to a syndrome that can be managed over the course of a lifetime.

Antiretroviral drugs are designed to affect the virus' ability to replicate once inside the cell. This effect is accomplished through the targeting of several biochemical pathways. One of these is a class of drugs called *protease inhibitors*, which target the splicing of the protein and viral RNA in the immature virus, thereby inhibiting its ability to become a mature and infectious virus. A second type of drug is known as nucleotide-nucleoside reverse transcriptase inhibitors, which target the function of the enzyme reverse transcriptase and its ability to produce a viable DNA strand from its viral RNA transcript. This drug provides the cell with faulty building blocks from which the enzyme will construct the viral DNA. If a faulty viral DNA is constructed, than proper viral proteins and RNA cannot be made from it, and the virus cannot be replicated. Another type is nonnucleotide-nucleoside reverse transcriptase inhibitors, which physically target the reverse transcriptase enzyme. The drug physically binds to the enzyme and prevents it from transcribing a viral DNA molecule from the RNA, thus prohibiting the first step in viral replication.

One of the newer mechanisms to be targeted by antiretroviral drugs is called an entry inhibitor, which targets the antibody's ability to bind the virus. If the antibody is unable to bind HIV, it cannot enter the cell, and thus, the person cannot become infected. This new classification of drugs is in its infancy, but the ability of HIV to become absorbed by the cells and the ability of CD4 cells to become infected looks to be at the forefront of new HIV-related research.

However, adherence to the antiretroviral medications is of the utmost importance. HIV replication enzymes do not have the proofreading mechanisms of prokaryotes and eukaryotes and therefore, cannot produce DNA and RNA with the same fidelity. As a result, the virus mutates at a surprising rate. Inconsistent adherence to the HIV medications has been shown to lead to the formation of resistant strains of the virus. This resistance is due to the virus' ability to evolve methods of replication in the presence of the drug at lower-than-optimal levels required to completely debilitate the virus' replication enzymes. Medication-resistant strains of HIV have been isolated from individuals, and these strains have a distinct advantage over medication-sensitive strains for replication and survival.

ART usually consists of a cocktail of medications that are administered on a daily basis. Patients have said that strict adherence may produce uncomfortable side effects, and many HIV-positive individuals are drug abusers who do not have the motivation to maintain the regimen over time. Inconsistencies in the adherence to the medication regimen are associated with lower levels of CD4 cells in the body, which correspond with higher levels of viral RNA, or viral load. These factors will lower the body's ability to fight the HIV infection and will increase the onset of AIDS. It also can produce a higher probability of medication-resistant strains of the virus, which may be transmitted to other individuals. For this reason, it is important to design antiretroviral regimens that stress strict adherence and underscore the reasons for this.

Further studies to examine the dynamics of ART adherence are urgently needed. Programs such as the KHARMA project have been tailored to increase medication adherence while also lowering high-risk behaviors for HIV-positive women. This ambitious project uses education about the importance of the ART adherence, as well as a motivational group intervention to reduce drug use and sexual activity. This encompasses several of the most important aspects of HIV prevention, such as educating a group of high-risk individuals, lowering high-risk drug and sexual behaviors, and adherence to ART. These issues must be confronted as higher rates of alcohol and substance use have been correlated with lower rates of adherence to ART. As substance use rates increase, adherence to ART decreases, which is coupled with higher rates of HIV viral load and with lower rates of CD4 cells. In short, if high-risk behaviors such as substance abuse interfere with ART adherence, these behaviors must be decreased if optimal treatment is to be followed.

Conclusion

Although major strides have been made in prevention measures for HIV and its links to substance abuse, much work remains to be done. Clearly this is a disease that must be brought to the forefront of worldwide research efforts. Intervention and prevention programs must be specifically tailored to high-risk groups to find what measures are successful and to determine how to bridge the gaps between research

findings and the clinical applications of those findings. Successful prevention techniques can be used in conjunction with biomolecular discoveries to allow clinicians and researchers a way to look at programs that can isolate the links between HIV and substance abuse, allowing for practical clinical execution.

*John Fordham, Bradley C. Donohue,
and Daniel N. Allen*

Authors' note: This entry was supported by a grant from the National Institute on Drug Abuse (NIDA 1R01DA020548-01A1).

See also Hepatitis C; Medical Consequences; Needle Exchange Programs; Sexually Transmitted Diseases

Further Readings

Centers for Disease Control. (2007). *HIV/AIDS surveillance report, 2005* (Vol. 17). Atlanta, GA: U.S. Department of Health and Human Services, Centers for Disease Control. Retrieved from http://www.cdc.gov/hiv/topics/surveillance/resources/reports

National Institute for Allergy and Infectious Diseases. (2004). *How HIV causes AIDS.* Bethesda, MD: U.S. Department of Health and Human Services. Retrieved from http://www.aegis.com/topics/basics/hivandaids.html

Roberts, K. J. (2002). Physician-patient relationships, patient satisfaction, and antiretroviral medication adherence among HIV-infected adults attending a public health clinic. *AIDS Patient Care and STDs, 16,* 43–50.

Sonnex, C., Petherick, A., Hart, G. J., & Adler, M. W. (1989). An appraisal of HIV antibody test counseling of injection drug users. *AIDS Care, 1,* 307–311.

HOMELESS, SUBSTANCE ABUSE AND TREATMENT

According to the Stewart B. McKinney Homeless Assistance Act of 1987, homelessness is defined as the lack of a regular and adequate nighttime residence including a nighttime residence that is either a supervised shelter, an institution that provides temporary assistance, or a public or private place not ordinarily used as sleeping accommodations for humans.

Homelessness in the United States is a significant social issue with as many as 3.5 million people estimated to be homeless during the course of a year and 700,000 to 800,000 people homeless on any given night. The U.S. idea of who is homeless has changed over the years. In the 1950s, the stereotype was an older, White, male alcoholic who lived on the streets in an urban slum; by the 1980s, the new generation of homeless also included minorities, drug users, women, families with children, senior adults, people who are mentally ill, and those who are unemployed. Compared to the 1960s and 1970s, more people now live on the streets or in shelters than ever before. For example, in the 2006 U.S. Mayors Conference survey assessing hunger and homelessness in the United States, requests for emergency food assistance increased by 7% on average, and requests for emergency shelter increased in 74% of the 23 cities surveyed. Members of families made up 48% of the people requesting emergency food assistance. Although it is true that many homeless people suffer situational hardships causing their homelessness, others experience substance use disorders, mental illness, physical disabilities, or mental incapacities. Today, considering the events of Hurricanes Katrina and Rita, these numbers have increased even more.

People who are homeless struggle for food, safety, shelter, and services. Some people actually choose to live on the street rather than in homeless shelters out of fear for their safety. Shelters are often dangerous and overcrowded with unmet nutritional needs, poor service delivery, severe emotional problems within families, and substandard living conditions.

Substance Abuse

It is often difficult to make precise estimates of prevalence of different problems within the homeless population. With this in mind, Robert Huebner and colleagues estimated that 45% of people who are homeless are alcohol abusive or dependent and an additional 30% are drug abusive. Often these individuals are polydrug users, using more than one drug at a time.

In addition, the National Coalition for the Homeless estimated that as many as 22% to 50% of the population of people who are homeless in the United States are mentally ill. Many individuals who are homeless are dually diagnosed; that is, they have been diagnosed as having a substance abuse disorder and a psychiatric disorder. Even more alarming are the high rates of people who are homeless and drug

abusers with HIV infection. Those people who are dually diagnosed and homeless face many obstacles to recovery, including increased risk for victimization and violence; frequent cycling between the streets, jails, emergency rooms, and hospitals; and rarely showing improvement in their symptoms or functioning. Also, many of the agencies working with substance abusers who are homeless will not take those with psychiatric problems, and many who work with individuals who are homeless and mentally ill will not accept those who are substance abusing.

Contributing Causal Factors

There are many theories of the etiology of homelessness. One of the primary causes of homelessness is poverty, and contributing to poverty is unemployment. This causal relationship has become especially evident after the events of September 11, 2001, and more recently, Hurricanes Katrina and Rita. Many companies have experienced severe cutbacks and layoffs. Many people are homeless or on the verge of homelessness as a result of these events. Low-paying jobs also contribute to poverty and homelessness. A report from the U.S. Council of Mayors suggested that having a job is no longer a guarantee against homelessness and in fact, approximately 27% of people who are homeless have jobs. In addition, many shelters cannot accommodate entire families due to lack of bed space and must turn people away and back onto the streets. In general, there is a lack of support for people who are homeless, leaving many to fend for themselves on the streets with issues in substance abuse and medical and mental health.

Prior to the events of September 11, 2001, and the more recent hurricanes, the United States was experiencing a booming economy that increased the cost of houses far beyond what minimum wage workers could afford. The same holds true now, with a weakened economy and the cost for houses high. This lack of affordable housing seems to be a major contributing factor for homelessness with the federal housing budget decreasing 30% while requests for subsidized housing significantly increased. It is no surprise then that people have found themselves without homes and are unable to locate affordable housing alternatives.

Substance use disorders and mental illness are other identified causes of homelessness. Research by

Nancy Jainchill and colleagues indicated that two thirds of the entire homeless population abuse alcohol, and 50% use drugs. It appears that the substance-abusing man is no longer the stereotypical homeless person. Women have surfaced as substance abusers in the homeless population research and on the streets. In women, substance use not only creates general life problems, but it also complicates issues surrounding homelessness. Substance use not only contributes to homelessness, but it also keeps women from being self-supportive. When combined with women experiencing mental illness, substance using and abusing women have little hope for a self-sufficient life. To exacerbate the problem, homeless pregnant mothers who drink while pregnant place their unborn fetus at risk for fetal alcohol effects. Treatment programs to deal with this issue have not been effective.

According to the National Homeless Coalition and other researchers, the incidence of psychiatric disorders, including substance use disorders, among people who are homeless ranges from 22% to 50%. Additional statistics over the years have varied, for example, the Governor's Advisory Board Report in Baltimore established that 70% of the homeless population experienced mental illness. In a New York City study, 61% of the homeless population interviewed was diagnosed as schizophrenic, 28% presented with schizoaffective disorder, 25% abused alcohol, and 17% abused illicit drugs. Of 246 patients in the study, 90% were labeled with a primary psychotic diagnosis. It is not unusual for people who experience homelessness and mental illness to have co-occurring substance abuse and mental health diagnoses.

Domestic violence, lack of affordable health care, and a disorder of academic functioning, specifically learning disabilities, have also been identified as causes of homelessness. In the 2006 Conference of Mayors, 46% of cities surveyed identified domestic violence as a primary cause of homelessness. The area of academic functioning is a relatively new area being explored as a cause of homelessness. There does appear to be a relationship between homelessness and learning disability because members of both groups face a number of similar life challenges including education, daily routines and life skills, self-esteem, and social interactions. It also appears that the majority of individuals in both groups is either unemployed or underemployed, and view getting a job that pays a living wage as their top priority.

Treatment Programs

Many problems confront those who work with clients who are homeless and have substance use disorders. Most people who are homeless do not have a support network such as family, relatives, or friends. They are usually surrounded by other homeless who are using drugs and/or alcohol, and life for these clients is usually more about survival than about personal growth, development, or changing life styles. It is not uncommon for someone who is homeless and a substance abuser to have other problems parallel with the dependency, such as mental disorders and physical disorders. Many of the available treatment programs have attempted to address some or all of these problems. There are several different theoretical models currently being used to treat substance abusers who are homeless. Most of these models were developed through a demonstration program of the United States National Institute on Alcohol Abuse and Alcoholism (NIAAA).

Treatment Models

Oxford Houses

Oxford Houses began as a grassroots, nonprofit corporation by a group of men living in Silver Springs, Maryland, in 1975. By 1988, the program had expanded to 13 Oxford Houses in the Washington, D.C., area and in Pennsylvania. At about the same time, the U.S. Anti-Drug Act of 1988 was enacted and created new revolving funds within each state to be used for self-run and self-supported recovery houses. The model required by this law was based on the experiences and replications of Oxford Houses. As of 1997, there were over 870 houses being operated under the nonprofit Oxford Houses umbrella.

There are four fundamental characteristics to both the Oxford Houses model and the requirements of the act of 1988: (1) no paid staff, (2) operate democratically, (3) expel residents who relapse into using alcohol or drugs, and (4) be financially self-supporting. There is a fifth tenet required by Oxford Houses, which is officers are to be elected by majority vote of the residents and are changed every 6 months.

Alcohol-Free Living Center

The Alcohol-Free Living Center (AFLC) was a relatively new concept similar to the Oxford Houses, but with some differences. Each AFLC unit essentially ran itself and tried to be self-supporting where the units were usually satellites of a parent treatment agency offering a comprehensive range of services. Each individual AFLC had a residential manager who is usually a recovering addict and a program manager who was employed by the parent agency. AFLCs varied in size from just a few people (six) living in a house to a large number (174) living in a renovated hotel. Like Oxford Houses, the goal of the AFLC was to combat the revolving door syndrome.

NIAAA Community Demonstration Projects

The first major comprehensive legislative response to the plight of the homeless was the 1987 passage of the Stewart B. McKinney Homeless Assistance Act. Section 613 of the McKinney Act provided funds for NIAAA to support a demonstration program for homeless individuals with alcohol and other drug abuse problems that would be innovative. Numerous problems were encountered in setting up these programs including the randomization of clients to different study groups. Counselors, caseworkers, and others wanted to assign clients according to a needs-based assessment. This technique made sense; however, for research purposes, the clients had to be randomly assigned to a treatment design. Examples of community demonstration programs include the Amity Settlement Services for Education and Transition in Tucson, Arizona, a therapeutic community model, rooted in Alcoholic's Anonymous (AA) Twelve Step model; the First Things First project that addressed the problems of residential instability and long-term substance treatment in Chicago for people who were homeless and substance abusers; and the New Orleans Homeless Substance Abusers Program, which supports permanent sobriety, residential stability, economic independence, and reduction in family estrangement.

Special Homeless Populations

Several specialized treatment program models for people who are homeless have emerged over the years. They included the Grant Street Partnership (GSP), a community demonstration project in New Haven,

Connecticut, that was unique compared to other NIAAA programs because it targeted people who were homeless and cocaine abusers. The goal of GSP was to provide short-term shelter and day treatment programs, one of the first of this type in the United States. In Seattle, Washington, the Systems Alliance and Support program targeted chronic public inebriates, and in Washington, D.C., the Dual Diagnosis Project was developed for people who were dually diagnosed and homeless.

Conclusion

Most of the programs operate on the philosophy that housing is the first problem that needed to be addressed. Before drug problems can be addressed, basic needs must be met. The AFLC model and the Oxford Houses are two types of treatment programs founded on these principles, as well as the therapeutic community approach.

All of the research based community demonstration projects used some form of case management in their designs. People who are homeless and substance abusers do not have "one-stop shopping" convenience available to them when trying to access services they may need within the community.

The AFLCs and the Oxford Houses would appear to be the most successful approaches to the problem and by far the most cost-effective. However, these approaches seem to be effective because the participants have already reached a point in their lives where they are ready to begin recovery from addiction. Most of the research projects were involved in a variety of attempts to create the process that brings or assists the client to the threshold of recovery. This process provided counseling, support, encouragement, education, goals, structure, and many other things necessary to achieving the threshold of recovery. It appears that those programs that incorporated a multidimensional approach were the most successful.

More research is needed in this area. Many of the demonstration projects described in this article are lacking outcome data. Some have preliminary data indicating positive results, although none of the studies include any longitudinal or generalization data. In addition, research results from most of the studies are at least 10 years old.

Patricia A. Markos

See also Co-Occurring Disorders; Special Populations

Further Readings

Drake, R. E., Osher, F. C., & Wallach, M. A. (1991). Homelessness and dual diagnosis. *American Psychologist, 46,* 1149–1169.

Huebner, R., Perl, H., Murray, P., Scott, J., & Tutunjian, B. (1993). The NIAAA cooperative agreement program for homeless persons with alcohol and other drug problems: An overview. *Alcoholism Treatment Quarterly, 10*(3/4), 5–20.

Jainchill, N., Hawke, I., & Yagelka, J. (2000). Gender, psychopathology, and patterns of homelessness among clients in shelter-based TCs. *American Journal of Drug and Alcohol Abuse, 26,* 553.

Korenbaum, S., & Burney, G. (1987). Program planning for alcohol-free living centers. *Alcohol, Health & Research World, 1*(3), 68–73.

Markos, P. A. (2004). Trauma, substance use disorders, and people who are homeless. *Guidance & Counselling, 20,* 31–36.

Molloy, J. (1993). *Self-run, self-supported houses for more effective recovery from alcohol and drug addiction* (DHHS Publication No. SMS 93-1678). Rockville, MD: U.S. Department of Health & Human Services.

National Coalition for the Homeless. (2005). *How many people experience homelessness?* Retrieved from http://www .nationalhomeless.org/publications/facts/How_Many.pdf

Russell, B. (1991). *Silent sisters: A study of homeless women.* New York: Hemisphere Publishing.

Silver, M. A., & McKinnon, K. (1993). Characteristics of homeless patients discharged from an intensive placement unit. *Hospital and Community Psychiatry, 44,* 576–578.

U.S. Conference of Mayors. (2006). *Hunger and homelessness survey.* Retrieved from http://usmayors.org/ uscm/hungersurvey/2006/report06.pdf

Wright, J., Devine, J., & Eddington, N. (1993). The New Orleans homeless substance abusers program. *Treatment Quarterly, 10*(3/4), 51–64.

I

ICE

See METHAMPHETAMINE

ILLICIT AND ILLEGAL DRUGS

Substance abuse is among the major public health concerns of the 20th century. However defined, excessive use of illegal drugs and prescribed medications is an all-too-common societal problem, not only in the United States, but across the globe. The negative effects of excessive substance use influence not only the individuals who use these substances but also their immediate and extended families and society in general. Moreover, illicit substance use is connected to many of the most pressing of our societal ills, including illness, crime, violence, and homelessness.

Scope of the Problem

For illicit psychoactive substances, the lifetime prevalence of drug abuse or dependence is roughly 6% in the United States, with lifetime cannabis abuse (i.e., 4.6%) being the most common. The World Health Organization estimates that 28 million people worldwide incur significant health risks by using psychoactive substances other than alcohol. Annually, heroin and cocaine use claims 10,000 lives. Moreover, the results of the 2006 National Survey on Drug Use and Health revealed the following staggering statistics:

(a) An estimated 20.4 million Americans, 12 or older, are current users of illegal drugs; (b) marijuana is the most commonly used drug, used by nearly 73% of current drug users; (c) of the 9.6 million current users of illegal drugs other than marijuana, 7 million are current users of psychotherapeutic drugs (e.g., tranquilizers, sedatives, and stimulants), and most of these users (5.2 million) use prescription pain medication for nonmedical purposes; (d) approximately 12.3 million Americans 12 or older have tried ecstasy at least once in their lifetime; (e) 338,000 Americans reported current heroin use; (f) 1 million Americans 12 or older are current users of hallucinogens; (g) 2.4 million Americans 12 or older are current users of cocaine and 702,000 use crack cocaine; and (h) 731,000 Americans reported current use of methamphetamine.

Estimates of the yearly economic social costs arising from illicit drug use are enormous. According to the Office of National Drug Control Policy, in the year 2000, Americans spent an estimated $36 billion on cocaine, $11 billion on marijuana, $10 billion on heroin, $5.4 billion on methamphetamine, and $2.4 billion on other illegal drugs. An estimated 260 tons of cocaine and 13.3 tons of heroin were used by Americans in 2000. Relatedly, individuals who abuse drugs consume a disproportionately large share of social resources (drug abuse treatment, treatment of secondary health effects, social welfare programs, and criminal justice system). In fact, estimates from the Office of National Drug Control Policy of the societal cost of drug abuse was over $180 billion for the year 2002, with an average annual rise in costs of 5.3% per year since 1992.

Common Drugs of Abuse

Most drugs are typically developed for medicinal purposes with the intention to be used to treat specific disorders (e.g., psychological, mental, physical) or to minimize pain (i.e., morphine). However, when these drugs are not taken as prescribed (e.g., taking more pills than necessary), there is a potential for abuse or dependence.

This section provides a general description of common drugs of abuse. The effects and symptoms listed for each drug have been adapted and modified from information collected from the National Institute on Drug Abuse (NIDA).

Hallucinogens

Hallucinogens are drugs that produce altered states of feeling and perception and sometimes cause flashbacks. Lysergic acid diethylamide (LSD) and phencyclidine (PCP) are the two most commonly abused hallucinogens. In fact, 1% of Americans 12 years and older report use.

PCP is a white powder that dissolves in liquid (e.g., water or alcohol). On the street, PCP is typically sold as a tablet, capsule, or colored powder. There are three primary ways of ingestion: (1) snorted, (2) smoked, or (3) swallowed. The primary effects associated with PCP use are a distortion of the senses, which produces feelings of detachment from the environment and self (i.e., "dissociation").

PCP abuse may result in memory loss, speech troubles, difficulty thinking, depression, and weight loss. Low or moderate doses of PCP may cause the user to experience an increase in breathing rate as well as a rise in blood pressure and pulse rate. When taken in high doses, PCP may cause a decrease in pulse rate and respiration. More specifically, the substance abuser may experience nausea, vomiting, blurred vision, drooling, loss of balance, and, in extreme cases, coma or death.

LSD creates distortions in the way a person perceives reality by disrupting the interaction of nerve cells and serotonin, which is involved in the control of behavioral, perceptual, and regulatory systems, and results in the person experiencing sounds and sensations that do not exist. The effects of LSD vary and depend on the characteristics of the user (e.g., mood, expectations, surroundings). Typically, the user will begin to feel the effects of the drug within 30 to 90 minutes after ingestion. Physical symptoms of LSD use include dilated pupils, increased body temperature, increased heart rate and blood pressure, and sweating. In addition, the changes in sensation and feeling are usually much more intense and may be characterized by a rapid cycling of emotions, which in severe cases, may cause panic, contribute to accidents, and possibly result in death.

Marijuana

Marijuana is the most widely used illegal drug in the United States. It is estimated that more than 40% of Americans 12 years and older have used marijuana in their lifetime. Derived from the plant *Cannabis sativa*, it is a mix of dry shredded flowers, stems, and seeds. Typically, marijuana is either smoked as a cigarette (i.e., "joint") or in a pipe (i.e., "bong"). In addition, marijuana may also take the form of hashish (which is a more concentrated, resinous form of marijuana) or a hashish oil, which is a black, sticky liquid. Common street names for marijuana include *pot, herb, weed, grass, ganja*, and *hash*. The primary chemical in marijuana is THC (delta-9-tetrahydrocannabinol), which binds to certain protein receptors in the brain and produces a sense of relaxation for the user.

Short-term effects of marijuana use can include memory and learning problems, distorted perceptions, thought difficulties, loss of coordination, paranoid thinking, increased high-risk behaviors, and heart rate. Long-term effects of chronic use may include changes in activity of the stress-response system and changes in the activity of dopamine nerve cells, which can help regulate motivation and reward impulses and result in panic attacks. Smoking marijuana can also cause burning and stinging sensations in the mouth and throat and is often accompanied by a heavy cough, which may contribute to respiratory infections.

Club Drugs

Club drugs are recreational drugs typically consumed at dance clubs, parties, or concerts (e.g., techno or punk rock). Methylenedioxymethamphetamine (MDMA), also known as ecstasy, is a synthetic, psychoactive drug. Besides *ecstasy*, common street names for MDMA include *Adam, hug, beans*, and *love drug*. MDMA has the qualities of both a stimulant and psychedelic and has an energizing effect, produces distortions in time, and causes hallucinations. From a biological perspective, MDMA primarily affects neurons in the brain that use serotonin, which produce changes in mood, aggression, sleeping patterns, and pain threshold.

Extensive use of MDMA can cause memory problems and may result in loss of consciousness. In addition, overuse of MDMA may also create problems with regulating body temperature, which may produce liver, kidney, and cardiovascular problems. Lastly, MDMA users may also experience psychological difficulties in the form of depression, drug craving, and anxiety.

Historically used at exclusive "rave" events, club drugs are now being found in more common places, such as bars and parties. Other examples of club drugs include ketamine, Rohypnol (i.e., *roofies*), gamma-hydroxybutyrate (GHB), and gamma-butyro-lactone (GBL).

Stimulants

NIDA defines stimulants as drugs that elevate mood, increase feelings of well-being, increase alertness, and stimulate energy. Common stimulants include methamphetamine and cocaine.

Methamphetamine

Because of its highly addictive nature, methamphetamine is classified as a Schedule II drug. On the street, methamphetamine is commonly referred to as *speed, crank, meth,* and *chalk.* Methamphetamine can be ingested in a variety of ways: swallowed, snorted, injected, or smoked. A derivative of methamphetamine, methamphetamine hydrochloride, is composed of clear, chunky crystals and is often called *ice, crystal,* or *glass* because of its physical appearance.

Methamphetamine use may cause significant changes in brain activity, resulting in reduced motor speed and impaired learning ability. More recently, researchers have found that methamphetamine use has damaged areas in the brain typically associated with emotion and memory. Other difficulties associated with methamphetamine use include decreased appetite, rapid heart rate, respiratory problems, irregular heart beat, increased blood pressure, and hypothermia.

Cocaine

Cocaine is typically ingested by snorting, although some users prefer to inject the drug in order to get a more concentrated and intense high. Common street names for cocaine include *coke, flake, snow,* and *blow.* Cocaine causes the body to feel as if there is an immediate danger, which causes the release of neurotransmitters. More specifically, while the body feels the chemistry of fright, tension, and anxiety, the brain is indicating things are fine. In essence, cocaine use heightens the body's sensitivity to stress, except the user does not realize this is occurring.

When cocaine is cooked with baking soda (i.e., sodium bicarbonate) and water, it hardens when heat dried; this form of cocaine is commonly referred to as *crack.* When smoked, the sodium bicarbonate produces a crackling sound; thus, the name crack. Crack is cut into bars or chips (i.e., "rocks") and smoked in a glass pipe. Crack became popular during the 1980s, in part because it was a cheap alternative to cocaine.

Opioids

Heroin

Processed from morphine, heroin is derived from the opium poppy plant, *Papaver somniferum.* Whereas pure heroin is in powder form, the street varieties may take many different forms (e.g., chunky, solid, coarse) but is usually sold in powder form. Heroin is a rapidly acting drug and is commonly referred to as *smack, H, skag,* or *junk*; it may be ingested by injecting, sniffing, or smoking it.

Heroin abuse is associated with myriad serious health problems, including overdose (lethal and nonlethal), spontaneous abortion, collapsed veins, HIV/AIDS, and hepatitis. The latter two problems result from contaminated needles. Heroin users typically report feeling a "rush" (i.e., sense of euphoria) and warm flushing of the skin, dry mouth, and a sense of heaviness in both the arms and legs. Subsequent to the initial feeling of euphoria, the user experiences alternating states of wakefulness and drowsiness (i.e., the "nod").

Conclusion

Illegal substance use is among the most pressing and intransigent health problems facing society today. Illicit drugs directly cause many medical problems. Substance abusers are at an increased risk for health problems such as cancer, cardiovascular disease, overdose (fatal and nonfatal), hepatitis, and HIV infection and AIDS. NIDA research has shown that almost every drug of abuse harms some tissue or organ. In addition, illegal substance use also tends to have important social implications and has been found to negatively impact employment, school achievement, socioeconomic status, and family functioning. Moreover, illegal substance use contributes to an increased possibility of arrest, conviction, and incarceration.

Keith Klostermann

See also Club Drugs; Cocaine and Crack; Drugs, Classification of; Ecstasy; Hallucinogens; Heroin; Marijuana; Methamphetamine

Further Readings

Johnston, L. D., O'Malley, P. M., Bachman, J. G., & Schulenberg, J. E. (2008). *Monitoring the Future national results on adolescent drug use: Overview of key findings, 2007* (NIH Publication No. 08-6418). Bethesda, MD: National Institute on Drug Abuse. Retrieved June 3, 2008, from http://www.monitoringthefuture.org/new.html

National Institute on Drug Abuse. (2007). *Drugs of abuse information*. Retrieved August 23, 2007, from http://www.nida.nih.gov/drugpages.html

Office of National Drug Control Policy (ONDCP). (2004). *The economic cost of drug abuse in the United States 1992–2002* (Publication No. 207303). Washington, DC: Executive Office of the President.

Substance Abuse and Mental Health Services Administration. (2007). *Results from the 2006 National Survey on Drug Use and Health: National findings* (Office of Applied Studies, NSDUH Series H-32, DHHS Publication No. SMA 07-4293). Rockville, MD. Retrieved June 3, 2008, from http://oas.samhsa.gov/NSDUH/2k6NSDUH/2k6results.cfm#Ch2

World Health Organization. (n.d.). *Management of substance abuse*. Retrieved September 11, 2007, from http://www.who.int/substance_abuse/en/

IMPAIRED PROFESSIONALS

Impairment of therapists, counselors, medical staff, and academicians plagues the helping professions.

Although these professionals may be considered experts in assessing and treating the clinical distress and impairment of the general population, there is reluctance in identifying their own impairments. This creates the potential for them to cause harm to themselves and to those that they serve. The credibility of the profession and its purposes may be questioned when helping professionals are unable to manage their own distress or impairment.

It is important to recognize that the interpretation of professional impairment is multifaceted. The variances in conceptualizations have resulted in a number of causal factors and types of impairment. The current research surrounding professional impairment has focused primarily on areas of substance abuse, sexual misconduct, and emotional and mental health issues. The majority of work, however, has focused on substance use and abuse among helping professionals, and this topic is therefore the focus of this entry.

Substance Use Disorders Among Helping Professionals

Collectively, substance use disorders (SUDs) are the most prevalent behavioral health problem in the United States. It is estimated that approximately 810,000 individuals are dependent on opioids, 2.5 million individuals are addicted to cocaine, and approximately 3 million people are thought to be addicted to marijuana. Alcohol, however, is the substance involved in the preponderance of the drug abuse and addiction problems in this country. Of the estimated 119 million Americans who use alcohol, 16.27 million are thought to be physically dependent on it. Consequently, it is estimated that alcoholism alone accounts for 85% of the drug addiction in the United States.

Contrary to stereotypical notions of addicts, such as drunks on skid row and drug users in jail, the majority of addicts are employed. It is estimated that fully 76% of illicit drug abusers in the United States are employed, as are 81% of the binge drinkers and 81% of the heavy drinkers. In light of these numbers, it therefore should come as little surprise that some of whom Robert Coombs calls "pedestal professionals"—physicians and other health care professionals, airline pilots, and attorneys—are also members of the addicted population.

Despite high levels of education and specialized training, professionals are not exempt from developing alcohol and other drug dependencies. In fact, research suggests that these widely admired professionals, especially health care professionals, are particularly vulnerable to drug abuse. Douglas Talbott, founder of the Talbott-Marsh Recovery Center in Atlanta, Georgia, has suggested that drug addiction can be a common occupational hazard of health care professionals.

Research has recently focused on examining potential SUD issues among health care professionals. In a survey of nearly 4,500 nursing professionals, 32% reported that they used alcohol, cocaine, prescription drugs, or marijuana on a regular basis. Among those surveyed, emergency room nurses were 3.5 times more likely to use cocaine or marijuana, and oncology nurses were more than twice as likely to binge drink. Interestingly, nicotine use was nearly 3 times more prevalent among psychiatric nurses. Among physicians, it has been estimated that 8% to 12% will develop a SUD and that emergency room physicians and anesthesiologists are most at risk. Counselors and psychologists—those generally on the frontline of SUD treatment—also have an elevated prevalence of SUDs. It has been estimated that around 10% of psychologists report current drinking problems. Another study of counseling psychologists indicated that approximately 6% used marijuana, 7% used tranquilizers, 1% used stimulants, and 3% used opioids at least occasionally. The most influential risk factor for developing SUDs among all of the professionals just described was job-related stress.

Education and Training and SUDs

Efficient, hard-working, and respected by both their colleagues and their communities, many addicted professionals tend to graduate in the top third of their classes. Ironically, however, the academic environment that provides them with the education and the opportunities to develop their professional skills may also be, for some, the same environment that enables the development of a future SUD. Many students attend colleges where recreational drug use, and in particular alcohol, is the social norm.

Even though the legal age to purchase alcohol is 21 in most states, more than 90% of college students view drinking as a central part of their social lives. Additionally, as a group, college students drink more heavily than their noncollege peers. Although binge drinking becomes less common for most individuals after the age of 23, approximately 5% to 19% of

those students surveyed continue to drink abusively over extended periods of time. Consequently, behavioral patterns of alcohol consumption acquired in college can, for some, continue into adult life and professional practice.

Professional training itself can also impede emotional development and consequently lead to an increased risk of developing SUDs. Although institutions providing professional training generally ensure that their graduates are intellectually and technically competent, many have a poor record of encouraging their up-and-coming professionals to develop emotionally. Emotional expressions generally incur a risk of appearing unprofessional. Therefore, in order to appear competent and strong, some individuals learn to rely on drugs to either suppress or alter their emotions. Additionally, the chronic overwork, fatigue, and sleep deprivation that accompany the rigors of specialized training can push trainees beyond their own stamina, which may result in intensified emotional problems and place them at further risk for burnout, depression, and substance abuse. Clearly these issues are most prevalent among nurses and physicians, who may not have learned appropriate ways to relieve stress and anxiety and hence turn to substance use to alleviate their burden. Most counseling and psychological professionals are taught ways to self-monitor throughout their training, but the risk for compassion fatigue and professional burnout remain elevated.

Owing to professional training and education, many helping professionals have the irrational belief that they can, solely through the use of their intellectual resources, solve all of their own personal problems. Furthermore, many professionals are committed to the belief that both high academic and professional achievement and competency will prevent the development of an SUD. The data, unfortunately, tell a much different story.

Denial and Underreporting of SUDs

Denial is a universal and profound defense mechanism. Denial has a healthy aspect in aiding the ability of patients to live with their illness(es) and in helping individuals deal with threatening situations. Individuals in the helping professions often learn the value of denying illness in themselves and also at times deny that they, too, can become ill or succumb to a SUD problem.

Professionals historically have been reluctant to report impaired colleagues because of a number of factors, including fear of retaliation or litigation from the accused practitioner. Instead, associates often help conceal the secret by ignoring, making excuses for, or otherwise covering up a colleague's addiction. However, enabling strategies that shield the addict from the legal, social, and work-related consequences of continued use further exacerbate the problem. Most professional associations have implemented ethical guidelines for their members that require them to report impaired colleagues. Unfortunately, however, research suggests that most professionals do not report incidences of SUDs among their colleagues.

Further compounding the problem is the impaired professional's own reluctance to admit to having an SUD. Many professionals view their professional status as an essential part of their identity. Anything that threatens their status and identity may leave them feel frightened, disgraced, and worthless. These unpleasant feelings may exacerbate the addictive behavior. Additionally, many helping professionals find it particularly difficult to move into the role of the patient. They verbalize fears of losing dignity; they experience injury to their sense of self, pride, and power; they believe themselves to be foolish; and they are disturbed by their loss of self-esteem. Their actions may be accompanied and complicated further by feelings of guilt or a sense of shame.

Signs of Impairment

Signs of impairment among professionals who suffer from SUDs manifest in several ways. The physical, mental, and behavioral symptoms mirror those that are stereotypically associated with addicts in the general population. Common symptoms include headaches, fatigue, inability to make important decisions, inability to focus, slurred or altered speech, and changes in normative behaviors. Obviously, professionals with these symptoms will find it difficult to appropriately handle the requirements of their jobs.

As is true for all addicts, difficulties and problems in family and social relationships as well as monetary and legal difficulties become manifest before difficulties in the work site are noticed. The most prominent sign of addictive illness is often a personality change. This change occurs sooner in the use of opioids and cocaine than with alcohol use and dependence, which most often develops slowly over many years.

Healthy and Unhealthy Motivations

The choice to become a helping professional often centers around the need for achievement, desire for admiration, personal growth, intellectual stimulation, and the desire to help those in need. Although these are admirable motivations to have as a helping professional, the pressure to fulfill these needs and motivations can sometimes lead to the overwhelming stress that leads to the development of SUDs.

Ultimately, it is up to the professional to differentiate between healthy and unhealthy motives. Entering the profession with healthy motives requires consciousness and thoughtfulness. Unhealthy motives usually involve an excessive need to satisfy unresolved childhood or adult difficulties or conflicts, potential earnings, advice giving, being in recovery from a prior addiction, or creating an identity for oneself. Those that enter the profession with unhealthy motives may have an increased risk of developing inappropriate coping mechanisms, such as drug or alcohol use.

Colleague Assistance Programs

In the 1980s, the field of psychology began to research the issue of impaired professionals and what effect it could have on both the profession and the public. The result was that much was learned about the prevalence of impaired professionals. Indeed, the work done by psychologists during this time provided the groundwork necessary to define what impairment among professionals meant, how to study impairment among professionals, and how to help colleagues find assistance when necessary.

The American Psychological Association (APA) spearheaded the early work on professional impairment. They formed the Advisory Committee on the Impaired Psychologist (ACIP), which produced an information manual widely circulated among the state associations. In 1986 the APA published the book *Professional in Distress: Issues, Syndromes, and Solutions in Psychology.* The APA Council of Representatives issued a resolution in 1988 outlining its intention to provide information and assistance to the states, and state psychological associations were encouraged to create and implement programs for impaired professionals. The subsequent growth of state association programs indicates efforts on behalf of the profession to deal with the effects of impairment on professional and ethical standards of practice.

Conclusion

Much work has been done examining the impact of trauma and stress on those in the helping professions. Physicians, nurse, counselors, and psychologists must always remain vigilant to self-monitor and to find appropriate means to deal with the inherent stressors of their jobs—stressors that can lead to an increased use of substances or to the development of SUDs. Of equal importance, too, is that professionals need to monitor one another as a service to their profession and to the people that they treat.

Larry Ashley, Chad L. Cross, and Peter Mansky

See also American Society of Addiction Medicine; Employee Assistance Program; Enabling; Workplace Drug Use

Further Readings

Angres, D. H., Talbott, G. D., & Bettinardi-Angres K. (1998). *Healing the healer, the addicted physician.* Madison, CT: Psychosocial Press.

Bissell, L. (1989). A historical review: Alcohol and drugs in the professions. In T. Hester (Ed.), *Professionals and their addictions* (pp. 3–23). Macon, GA: Charter Medical.

Coombs, R. (1997). *Drug-impaired professionals.* Cambridge, MA: Harvard University Press.

Crosby, L. R., & Bissell, L. (1989). *To care enough: Intervention with chemically dependent colleagues. A guide for healthcare and other professionals.* Minneapolis, MN: Johnson Institute.

Cross, C. L., & Ashley, L. (2007) Trauma and addiction: Implications for helping professionals. *Journal of Psychosocial Nursing, 45,* 24–31.

Mansky, P. A. (2004). Impaired physicians. In M. Galanter & H. Kleber (Eds.), *Textbook of substance abuse treatment third edition* (pp. 265–290). Washington, DC: American Psychiatric Press.

INDIAN HEALTH SERVICES

The Indian Health Service (IHS), an agency within the U.S. Department of Health and Human Services, provides federal health services to American Indians and Alaskan Natives (AI/AN). The AI/AN comprise 560 federally recognized tribes; tribal nations range from fewer than 100 enrolled members to more than 100,000. The majority of AI/AN live in metropolitan areas, with more than half living in six states: Oklahoma, California, Arizona, New Mexico, Alaska, and Washington. The IHS currently provides health services to approximately 1.8 million of the 3.3 million AI/AN, with an annual appropriation of $3 billion.

The first regular appropriations of funds for the relief of distress and conservation of health among AI/AN was due to the Snyder Act of 1921. In 1954, the U.S. government transferred the responsibility for provision of health care from the Bureau of Indian Affairs to the Department of Health, Education, and Welfare under the Transfer Act of 1954. As a result, the IHS was established to undertake wide-ranging responsibility for Indian health, including medical, dental, public health, and environmental health services. Health and medical care for AI/AN is currently available through IHS in the 35 states that contain Indian reservations or Alaska Native corporations. The IHS delivery system is divided into 12 administrative jurisdictions, called area offices, based on geographical boundaries. These 12 area offices are further subdivided into 127 service units, each of which may include several smaller satellite facilities and field health stations.

In the mid-1970s, two pieces of legislation were passed which had a great impact on the Native American population. The Indian Self-Determination and Education Assistance Act of 1975 provided the legal framework for individual tribes to create and operate their medical delivery systems to meet their self-defined needs. Federally recognized tribes were allowed to contract with the federal government to assume management of their health care programs. In 1976, the Indian Health Care Improvement Act specified a number of areas in which Indian people may manage contracts: training programs, specific health services, health facilities, waste disposal programs, and urban Indian clinics. Title V of that act provided support for urban health centers. Currently, there are 34 urban Indian programs receiving federal funding. Although 55% of the AI/AN population lives in urban areas, less than 1% of the IHS budget is dedicated to urban Indian health programs.

The mission of IHS is to raise the physical, mental, social, and spiritual health to the highest level among AI/AN. The IHS goal is to ensure that comprehensive, culturally acceptable personal and public health services are accessible and available to all AI/AN people. Federally recognized tribes enjoy a government-to-government relationship with the United States. To carry out its mission, the IHS assists tribes in developing health programs through technical assistance and management training; assists tribes in coordinating health planning and obtaining and using federal, state, and local resources; and provides comprehensive health care, including prevention programs and hospitalization.

American Indians suffer high mortality and morbidity rates. IHS has identified alcohol and other drug abuse as the most pressing health problem in American Indian communities. According to the National Center for Health Statistics, the overall mortality rate was 35% higher for American Indians than for all other ethnic groups in the United States, combined, and deaths from alcoholism were 7 times greater than deaths among other groups. Alcoholism deaths occur more commonly among Native men than women, with the highest rates occurring in the age group 45 to 54 years. It is estimated that 80% of suicides and 93% of homicides are associated with alcohol; 65% resulting from motor vehicle crashes and 25% from other unintentional injuries. The IHS is currently funding more than 200 substance abuse programs serving Indian reservations and urban communities. However, there is a shortage of funding—the current IHS budget allows health care funding for AI/AN at approximately 40% of the rate for the rest of the American population.

The IHS has several divisions to assist with health promotion and disease prevention. The Division of Behavioral Health (DBH) supports initiatives that strive to eliminate behavioral health diseases and conditions. Within this division, there are 16 primary prevention focus areas including diabetes, mental health, and substance abuse. Within the DBH primary prevention focus area of substance abuse is the Alcoholism and Substance Abuse Program (ASAP), which serves to reduce the prevalence and incidence of alcoholism and other drug dependencies. It provides support and resources for AI/AN communities to achieve excellence in holistic alcohol and other drug treatments, rehabilitation, and prevention services. Additionally, ASAP activities include development and management of a coordinated information management system measuring alcohol problems and substance abuse

among AI/AN, programmatic evaluation and research, national leadership focusing on at-risk youth, and developmentally disabled service provision (e.g., fetal alcohol syndrome, fetal alcohol effects). Currently, 97% of the ASAP budget is earmarked for contracted or compacted services, including approximately 300 AI/AN ASAPs that provide treatment and prevention services to both rural and urban communities.

Karen Kopera-Frye

See also Racial and Ethnic Minorities, Issues in Alcohol and Other Drug Use; Racial and Ethnic Minorities, Issues in Prevention; Racial and Ethnic Minorities, Issues in Treatment; Special Populations; Substance Abuse and Mental Health Services Administration

Further Readings

Indian Health Service. (2006). *Indian Health Service fact sheet.* Retrieved December 30, 2007, from http://www.ihs.gov/PublicInfo/PublicAffairs/Welcome_Info/ThisFacts.asp

Indian Health Service. (2007). *Behavioral health primary prevention focus areas: Substance abuse: Resources.* Retrieved February 5, 2008, from http://www.ihs.gov/NonMedicalPrograms/HPDP/index.cfm?module=focus&option=subs

U.S. Department of Health and Human Services. (2002). *Alcohol use among American Indians and Alaska Natives* (National Institute on Alcohol Abuse and Alcoholism Research Monograph No. 37; NIH Publication No. 02-4231). Bethesda, MD: National Institute on Alcohol Abuse and Alcoholism.

INFORMATION DISSEMINATION

Prevention is a process of influencing people to change their behavior by adopting positive behaviors or avoiding negative ones. The work of prevention is accomplished through a variety of strategies that differ in their form, intensity, and expected outcome. Information dissemination is one of six specific strategies identified by the U.S. national Center for Substance Abuse Prevention as essential to a comprehensive community approach to preventing substance abuse. Other prevention strategies include education, alternatives, problem identification and referral, community-based process, and environmental strategies.

Information dissemination is characterized by one-way communication from the source to the audience, with limited contact between the two. This strategy can involve a single message or multiple messages designed to be delivered on a repeated or sequential basis. Examples of information dissemination activities include the following:

- Clearinghouse or information resource center(s)
- Resource directories
- Media campaigns
- Brochures
- Radio and TV public service announcements
- Speaking engagements
- Health fairs and health promotion
- Telephone or electronic information lines

Whereas some of these activities involve the use of mass media, others, such as health fairs or information lines, may be single-contact situations between a sender and a receiver of the prevention messages.

Process of Development

Regardless of the particular form in which information is disseminated, the following description provides a capsule view of the process. First, the developer of the strategy analyzes the target audience to determine needs, cultural characteristics, and the most appropriate methodology for dissemination. Next, the program provides information about a particular problem, why it is important, and how the audience can act to prevent or mitigate it. The audience hears the message, gains knowledge, and changes its attitude about the problem and is motivated to act. The audience changes its behavior and adopts more effective or healthful practices and avoids negative behaviors. Finally, the changed behavior leads to improved social, health, or environmental outcomes for the audience members individually and, in the aggregate, for the population or system.

Target Populations

Information dissemination activities may be targeted at broad, general audiences or at very specific target populations. The target audience for information dissemination activities can be defined by using the classification system developed by the Institute of Medicine in 1994. This system categorizes audiences as universal, selective, or indicated. Universal prevention audiences are large populations such as the general community or all students within a school. These audiences are identified and targeted without regard to their comparative level of risk for substance abuse. The mission of prevention with universal audiences is to delay the onset of substance use or deter the occurrence of substance abuse by providing all individuals with the information and attitudes necessary to prevent the problem. Universal prevention approaches are based on the assumption that all members of the population share the same general risk for substance abuse, although the risk may vary greatly among individuals within that population. Information is disseminated to universal prevention audiences without any prior screening for substance abuse risk. The National Media Campaign, conducted by the Office of National Drug Control Policy, is probably the best-known information dissemination program targeted at a universal audience.

Selective prevention audiences are subgroups of the general population that are determined to be at risk for substance abuse based on their common biological, psychological, social, or environmental risk factors. Targeted subgroups may be defined by age, gender, family history, place of residence, victimization by physical or sexual abuse, or other risk factors. It is important to recognize that the focus on selective prevention audiences targets the entire subgroup regardless of the degree of risk for any individual within the group. The selective audience receives the prevention message because the subgroup, as a whole, is at higher risk for substance abuse than is the general population.

Indicated prevention audiences are individuals who may or may not already be using alcohol, tobacco, or other drugs but exhibit risk factors that increase their chances of developing a drug abuse problem. Strategies targeted at indicated audiences are designed to prevent the onset or progression of substance abuse in these individuals. For indicated prevention audiences, prevention activities address risk factors associated with the individual, such as conduct disorders and alienation from parents, school, and positive peer groups. Often, less emphasis is placed on assessing or addressing environmental influences, such as community values, when targeting indicated audiences.

Activities and Methods

Information dissemination activities utilize a combination of informative and persuasive communication techniques and a variety of methods to deliver prevention messages intended to instill knowledge, change attitudes, and increase awareness about alcohol and other drug use, abuse, and addiction. Messages may also focus on the effects of substances and substance abuse on individuals, families, and communities or inform the audience about available prevention and treatment programs and services. Even though knowledge alone is not necessarily sufficient to precipitate or sustain behavioral change, it is an essential first component in the process of such change.

Many factors contribute to effective information dissemination. Four major factors are (1) the message source, (2) believability of the message, (3) environmental factors, and (4) comprehension and retention of the message. For a persuasive message to have its intended impact, the message source must be seen as credible. Credibility involves recognized expertise, a desire to do what is right, and a perception that the sender of the message respects the individuals receiving the message. The perceived credibility of a prevention message is often proportional to the strength of the science on which it is based.

The believability of the message is very much related to the credibility of the message source. For a prevention message to be believable, it must be congruent with the audience's existing knowledge and belief systems. Environmental factors are the conditions under which the prevention information is received. This can include interruptions and distractions that can affect whether a message is heard and understood. In an environment that is not conducive to presenting a prevention message, the likelihood of message comprehension and retention decreases. Obviously, for a persuasive message to be effective it must be understood and recalled. Another key factor that affects comprehension of the message is the language level of the message. The prevention message must be conveyed in language that is understood by the receiver of the message.

Information dissemination may be the prevention strategy of choice when creating an initial exposure to prevention concepts. Messages that increase awareness and knowledge may be required to develop a readiness to adopt positive behaviors or avoid negative behaviors in the intended audience. Increased awareness and knowledge are often prerequisites to behavioral change.

Strengths and Limitations

One strength of information dissemination is the ability for messages to reach large numbers of people, often at a relatively low cost. Although mass media such as television advertisements can be fairly expensive, when the number of contacts is considered, the cost per individual is minimal. Some methods of information dissemination can be performed by persons without specialized training or experience, though others require specific skills or training. Using this strategy, information can be presented in stepped levels of complexity and variable dosages (levels of intensity or numbers of repetitions). Another strength of information dissemination is that is can be utilized with universal, selected, or indicated audiences. In addition, changes in awareness and knowledge can be relatively easy to measure in selected or indicated populations.

Limitations of information dissemination programs include the fact that awareness and knowledge alone may be insufficient to stimulate behavioral change or maintain long-term behavioral change. The dose or level of exposure in information dissemination strategies can be relatively low and may be insufficient to achieve the desired effect. Information dissemination that is targeted at universal audiences may not be particularly cost-effective, as it targets individuals who may not be at significant risk for substance abuse. The benefits of awareness and knowledge programs are highly dependent on the readiness of the audience to learn and on individual learning styles.

Research Results

The Center for Substance Abuse Prevention has summarized the available research in the area of information dissemination. Their most significant finding is that information dissemination campaigns should be viewed as complementary to more intensive and interactive prevention approaches. Effective use of the media is enhanced when the intervention is combined with other prevention strategies (e.g., education, enforcement of existing laws). While the dissemination of information regarding alcohol, tobacco, and other drugs can increase knowledge regarding the hazards of substance use and aid in the development of negative attitudes toward alcohol, tobacco, and other drug use, programs that involve booster sessions or multiple exposures over time can help move participants from awareness to action in changing their behavior as well as to help individuals maintain their changed behavior over longer periods.

Effective use of the mass media to change substance-related knowledge, behavior, and attitudes relies on creating messages that appeal to the audience's existing belief systems and address motives for using substances or perceptions of substance use. For example, when information dissemination results in a higher perception of the risk associated with a particular substance, individuals are more likely to avoid that substance. A key to success in the use of television and radio for information dissemination is selection of choice air times, that is, when the intended audience is more likely to be viewing or listening. Free public service announcements can enhance any media campaign but, by themselves, are unlikely to have an impact if they air at times when few members of the target population are likely to hear them. Information campaigns should allow for the specific media preferences of their target audience, utilizing broadcast, print, and electronic media appropriately. The images and sounds utilized in such campaigns should resonate with the target audience. Youth-oriented mass media campaigns have been found to be more effective if they avoid the use of authority figures and exhortations. Focus group research indicates that overbearing messages are likely to lose the target audience.

Information dissemination programs are not difficult to evaluate if the focus is primarily on process or formative evaluation. The number of contacts made or brochures distributed can be easily obtained. The number and frequency of media placements is also easy to track. When evaluation turns to outcome or summative evaluation, however, the process becomes more difficult, especially with universal prevention audiences. The process is slightly easier with selected audiences and more manageable with indicated prevention audiences, when specific individuals are targeted for receiving the information. Short-term outcomes for information dissemination are increases in knowledge and awareness and adoption or intensification of attitudes that deter individuals from using or abusing alcohol, tobacco, and other drugs. Intermediate outcomes include changes in behavior—either adoption of positive behaviors or avoidance of negative behaviors.

Long-term outcomes include maintenance of behavior change for individuals and population-level changes in substance use and abuse indicators. These effects are easiest to measure in indicated prevention audiences, where specific individuals have been identified for participation in the program. Even in the best evaluations of information dissemination projects, the data seldom go beyond short-term outcomes. The assumption seems to be that the short-term outcomes will lead to the intermediate outcomes, which in turn will lead to desirable long-term effects. However, there is no certainty that such links will actually occur; in fact, it is highly unlikely unless the information dissemination strategy is part of a long-term comprehensive prevention approach that utilizes multiple strategies in addition to information dissemination.

Gail D. Dixon

See also Center for Substance Abuse Prevention; Institute of Medicine Classification System; National Media Campaign; Office of National Drug Control Policy; Prevention Evaluation; Prevention Populations; Prevention Strategies

Further Readings

Gordon, R. (1983). An operational classification of disease prevention. *Public Health Reports, 98*, 107–109.

Gordon, R. (1987). An operational classification of disease prevention. In J. A. Steinberg & M. M. Silverman (Eds.), *Preventing mental disorders: A research perspective* (pp. 20–26). Rockville, MD: Department of Health and Human Services.

Mrazek, P. J., & Haggerty, R. J. (Eds.). (1994). *Reducing risks for mental disorders: Frontiers for preventive intervention research.* Washington, DC: National Academy Press.

Substance Abuse and Mental Health Services Administration, Center for Substance Abuse Prevention. (2002). *Science-based prevention programs and principles 2002: Effective substance abuse and mental health programs for every community* (DHHS Publication No. SMA 03-3764). Washington, DC: Government Printing Office.

INFORMED CONSENT

Informed consent is a foundation in the ethical practice of counseling. Not only does informed consent provide the groundwork for matters that affect the entire course and direction of the counseling relationship, it guides the practice of client autonomy. Informed consent refers to the freedom of choice a client has regarding whether or not to enter into a counseling relationship, the right to understand the nature of the counseling process, and relevant information concerning the counselor.

Due to the significant amount of information contained in the informed consent, both verbal communication and written communication are necessary. Any discussions of informed consent are to be documented by the counselor and, when appropriate, signed by the client. The informed consent process is used as a means to continuously monitor the goals and strategies of counseling. Rather than a onetime event at the onset of the counseling relationship, informed consent is an ongoing, collaborative process between the client and the counselor for the duration of the counseling process.

Underlying issues related to informed consent include the roles, rights, and responsibilities of the client and the counselor, as well as all parties involved. Topics that, at minimum, are included in the informed consent document are referenced in the Code of Ethics provided by the American Counseling Association (ACA), NAADAC (the Association for Addiction Professionals), as well as individual state certification or licensure boards. The following subject matter is typically included in this process, although this is not an all-inclusive list.

In clinical practice, the informed consent document includes a description of the client's right to confidentiality, program procedures that safeguard them, and exceptions imposed by federal, state, or agency regulations. An explanation of the counselor's background—that is, expertise, training, credentials, and theoretical orientation—is provided. Clients have a right to know which treatment modalities are to be employed and the expected benefits and potential risks of the services. Typical approaches to addiction counseling include individual, group, and couples and family therapy, in addition to medication management, support group attendance, and drug testing. Alternative approaches that might be available to the client should also be presented. Information about the anticipated duration of treatment and any situation potentially resulting in premature termination of treatment or circumstances in which a referral may be necessary are discussed. An explanation of client's rights in

regard to an organization's policy and procedures and means to resolve disputes are included. Financial responsibility, payment options, and any other monetary obligations of the counseling relationship need to be clearly explained.

Informed consent is also utilized in research initiatives. The investigator is responsible to ensure participants are informed of any associated risks and provide them with relevant information necessary to make decisions about participation in the research project. An institutional review board oversees the research process to ensure all necessary information is provided in an comprehensible manner to participants.

Ethical considerations for the informed consent process are particularly relevant to substance abuse counseling. Individuals enter treatment with varying levels of cognitive abilities, particularly if they have recently been under the influence of drugs, alcohol, or both. In the case of detoxification, clients may actually be under the influence of substances when they agree to engage in the process. Additional factors to consider are the client's motivation for entering treatment, medical and emotional condition, and legal constraints. Such factors can significantly impair the client's autonomy and ability to provide informed consent. Once clients have initially entered treatment and are stabilized, particularly if they have gone through detoxification, information pertaining to the counseling process outlined in the informed consent is again reviewed. Under all circumstances, counselors need to respect the client's autonomy and right to consent or withdraw, of their own accord, from treatment.

When a client's ability to provide a meaningful informed consent is questionable, a third party with appropriate qualifications may intervene. If an individual is unable to provide informed consent, a representative of the client may do so. However, agreement from the individual is still necessary. Working with adolescents poses an additional consideration in that consent is required from the parent or guardian, as well as the individual receiving services.

Clients seeking substance abuse treatment may be mandated through court order, probation or parole, or child protective services. In some cases, an intervention may have precipitated the person's entering into treatment. Employers may require an employee to seek treatment as a condition of continued employment. Individuals holding a specialized professional license may be required to undergo treatment as a condition of maintaining licensure. In all cases where treatment is coerced or mandated, conditions and circumstances under which information is reported back to referral sources should be clearly articulated in the informed consent document.

Unique to substance abuse counseling are additional legal considerations for treatment programs receiving federal funds either directly or indirectly. Under federal mandate, regulation 42 CFR Part 2, individuals seeking or receiving substance abuse treatment receive stringent confidentiality protection. Information about any client applying for or receiving services or referral for other treatment are protected under confidentiality laws and may be disseminated only with client consent. Details regarding a client's consent to release information and specific circumstances that permit disclosure should be explicit in the informed consent document.

Drug testing, such as urinalysis, is often used for the purpose of ongoing substance abuse treatment and is within the ethical standard practice of health care. Routine, random drug testing requires informed consent similar to that for other medical conditions. However, there are circumstances when explicit consent is not possible, such as in trauma or overdose. In these situations, informed consent is not required for clinical drug testing.

Jill Russett

See also Confidentiality; Ethical Standards for Addiction Professionals; Ethics; Health Insurance Portability and Accountability Act; NAADAC, the Association for Addiction Professionals

Further Readings

American Counseling Association. (2005). *Code of ethics.* Retrieved March 8, 2007, from http://www.counseling.org/Resources/CodeOfEthics/TP/Home/CT2.aspx

Cottone, R. R., & Robine, S. (1998). Addictions and ex-offender counseling. In R. R. Cottone & V. M. Tarvydas (Eds.), *Ethical and professional issues in counseling* (pp. 383–394). Columbus, OH: Merrill.

NAADAC, the Association for Addiction Professionals. (2004). *Code of ethics.* Retrieved March 8, 2007, from http://naadac.org/documents/index.php?CategoryID=23

Walker, R., Logan, T. K., Clark, J., & Leukefeld, C. (2005). Informed consent to undergo treatment for substance abuse: A recommended approach. *Journal of Substance Abuse Treatment, 29*(4), 241–251.

INHALANTS

The National Institute on Drug Abuse defines inhalants as volatile substances that produce chemical vapors that can be inhaled to induce a psychoactive (i.e., mind-altering) effect. While a multitude of other substances may be ingested, inhalants, as the name implies, are taken primarily through inhalation (i.e., either the nose or mouth). More specifically, inhalants can be abused by (a) sniffing or snorting sufficient concentrations of fumes from containers, (b) spraying aerosols into the nose or mouth, (c) sniffing fumes from substances sprayed or poured onto a rag and then placed into a bag (i.e., "bagging"), (d) heavily breathing into an inhalant soaked rag stuffed in the mouth (i.e., "huffing"), and (e) inhaling from nitrous oxide–filled balloons. Given their accessibility, inhalants are commonly the first drugs abused by young people.

A variety of common products contain substances that can be inhaled. Typically, inhalants are classified into four categories: (1) volatile solvents, (2) aerosols, (3) gases, and (4) nitrates. The information contained in this entry has been adapted and modified from the National Institute on Drug Abuse.

Volatile Solvents

Volatile solvents are liquids that vaporize at room temperatures, which are found in a variety of inexpensive, easily accessible, household products. Examples of volatile solvents include paint thinner and remover, dry-cleaning fluid, degreasers, gasoline, glue, nail polish remover, and felt tip markers.

Toluene (i.e., methyl benzene) is a common ingredient among most solvents. In an effort to prevent inhalant abuse, a number of industries have added mustard oil to products containing toluene because, upon inhalation, it causes nasal irritation. Hydrocarbon solvents, petroleum, and natural gas are the most commonly abused inhalants, with the exception of amyl nitrate and nitrous oxide.

Aerosols

Aerosols are sprays that contain propellants and solvents. Examples of aerosols include spray paints, deodorant, hair spray, and cooking oil sprays.

Gases

This category includes medical anesthetics (e.g., ether, chloroform, nitrous oxide [i.e., "laughing gas"]) as well as gases used in household products (e.g., butane lighters, propane tanks, whipped cream dispensers).

Nitrates

Although other inhalants are used to alter mood, nitrates are used primarily as a sexual enhancer. Whereas the use of other inhalants act directly on the central nervous system, nitrates serve as a muscle relaxant and act to dilate blood vessels. Examples of nitrates include cyclohexyl nitrate, isoamyl nitrite, and isobutyl nitrate, which are commonly referred to as "poppers" or "snappers." Although the Consumer Product Safety Commission has prohibited the use of nitrates, they can still be found in items such as video head cleaner, room deodorizer, or liquid aroma.

Trends in Inhalant Use

Because of their accessibility, inhalants are typically the first drugs used by young people. In particular, adolescents and preadolescents tend to be the group most associated with inhalant abuse, with the majority of inhalant abusers being under the age of 25. More specifically, according to the National Survey on Drug Use and Health and the Monitoring the Future (MTF) study, inhalant abuse is widespread among young people in the United States. In fact, approximately 3% of children have tried inhalants by the time they enter fourth grade. Along these lines, data from national surveys suggest that inhalant abuse reaches its peak between the seventh and ninth grades, with eight graders typically reporting the highest rates of abuse. In addition, according to the 2006 MTF data, 10.5% of eighth-grade females reported using inhalants in the previous year, compared to 7.8% of eighth-grade males. Moreover, among 12th-grade students, 3.9% of females and 5.1% of males reported using inhalants. While inhalant abuse is not location specific—in other words, people in rural, suburban, and urban areas abuse inhalants—other factors that have been associated with inhalant abuse include adverse socioeconomic conditions, a history of childhood abuse, poor grades, and dropping out of school.

Consequences of Inhalant Abuse

Since most inhalants produce a rapid high, similar to being drunk, the use of inhalants offers a more accessible and cheaper way for children and adolescents to achieve an alcohol-like high. As a result, many young people abuse inhalants hoping for a quick high, without being fully aware of the serious negative consequences associated with this behavior. Although most inhalants differ in their chemical compositions, they all produce effects similar to anesthetics and act to slow down the body's functions. Regular abuse of inhalants can cause serious physical complications (e.g., damage to the brain, heart, lungs, or kidneys). Even a single session of repeated inhalations can lead to heart failure by altering normal heart rhythms or preventing enough oxygen from reaching the lungs; in some cases, this can result in death (i.e., sudden sniffing death). The consequences of long-term inhalant abuse may include short-term memory loss, heart failure, hearing loss, numbness, central nervous system damage, blood oxygen depletion, and death. The abuse of inhalants may also result in both permanent and temporary physical problems. For example, permanent effects associated with inhalant abuse include hearing loss, peripheral neuropathies, brain damage, and bone marrow damage. Temporary effects of abuse may include liver and kidney damage and blood oxygen depletion. As noted by Susan Gray and Marilyn Zide, warning signs of inhalant abuse may include difficulties in school or work, a chemical odor to the breath, red eyes, confused appearance, and irritability.

Conclusion

Because of their relatively low cost and accessibility, inhalants are the drug of choice for many young people. Although some abusers may become dependent on inhalants, the probability of developing tolerance is small. In addition, it is also unlikely that the user will experience withdrawal when he or she stops using. However, inhalant abuse over a long period may result in physical and social problems.

Keith Klostermann

See also Amyl Nitrite; Drugs, Classification of; Monitoring the Future; School Drug Policies

Further Readings

Abadinsky, H. (2004). *Drugs: An introduction.* Belmont, CA: Thomson.

Gray, S. W., & Zide, M. R. (2006). *Psychopathology: A competency-based treatment model for social workers.* Belmont, CA: Thomson.

Hormes, J. T., Filley, C. M., & Rosenberg, N. L. (1986). Neurologic sequelae of chronic solvent vapor abuse. *Neurology, 36,* 698–702.

National Institute on Drug Abuse. (2004). *National survey results on drug use from the Monitoring the Future Study, 2004.* Available at http://www.monitoringthefuture.org

National Institute on Drug Abuse. (2004). *NIDA InfoFacts: Inhalants.* Retrieved April 28, 2008, from http://www.nida.nih.gov/Infofacts/Inhalants.html

Substance Abuse and Mental Health Services Administration. (2004). *Results from the 2003 National Survey on Drug Use and Health: National findings* (Office of Applied Studies, NSDUH Series H-25, DHHS Publication No. SMA 04-3964). Rockville, MD: Author.

INJECTION DRUG USE

In surveys such as the National Survey on Drug Use and Health, injection drug use is defined as the use of a needle to inject a drug that is not prescribed for the user or only for the feeling or experience that the drug causes. Injection drug use in a survey is assessed by asking the respondents whether they had injected heroin, cocaine, methamphetamines, or other stimulants during a specified time. Investigators, such as Vlahov and colleagues, have performed physical examinations to ascertain the presence of track marks and other physical evidence of injection drug use. Injection drug users are at high risk for human immunodeficiency virus (HIV), hepatitis C, and other bloodborne infections.

Prevalence

The National Survey on Drug Use and Health is an annual survey sponsored by the Substance Abuse and Mental Health Services Administration (SAMHSA). The survey collects data by administering questionnaires to a representative sample of the population age 12 or older through face-to-face interviews at their place of residence. According to the reports prepared by SAMHSA in 2003 and 2005, approximately 0.2% of Americans age 12 or older had injected heroin, cocaine, methamphetamines, or other stimulants during the past year. The prevalence of past-year injection drug use is higher among young adults ages 18 to 25 (0.3%) than among adolescents ages 12 to 17 (0.1%) and older adults age 50 or older (0.02%). There also are regional variations in injection drug use with a high prevalence among individuals residing in the western region of the United States (0.3%).

In 2007, Armstrong reported that an estimated 1.5% of noninstitutionalized Americans have ever injected drugs for nonmedical reasons. According to Wu and Howard, 0.3% of American adolescents ages 12 to 17 reported having ever injected drugs and nonstudents were more likely than students to report lifetime injection drug use (1.7 vs. 0.3%).

Needles

The National Survey on Drug Use and Health asked injection drug users how they obtained their needles the last time they injected drugs. According to the 2003 reports prepared by SAMHSA, close to one half (47%) of past-year injection drug users bought needles from a pharmacy, 9% bought them on the street, and 4% obtained them from needle exchange. Other less-common needle sources include drug dealers, a shooting gallery, and stealing from others. The 2005 report indicated that 17% of past-year injection drug users obtained their needles from needle exchange. Needle exchange is one of several interventions aimed at preventing the spread of HIV infection among injection drug users and their sexual partners.

Reasons for Use

In 2003, Calzavara and colleagues examined reasons for drug use among injection drug users. They found that, among those who injected drugs in the year prior to incarceration, reasons commonly given for drug use were "makes me feel good" (76%); "because I'm addicted" (69%); "a way to escape reality" (59%); "helps me deal with feelings of sadness" (51%); "helps me forget how much I miss those I care about (family, friends, etc.)" (50%); and "helps me deal with feelings of frustration" (50%).

Bloodborne Infections

Risky injection behaviors among recent injection drug users are not uncommon. The National Survey on

Drug Use and Health found that approximately 64% of past-year injection drug users did not clean their needle with bleach before the last time they had used one to inject a drug, and 51% reused a needle that they had used before. Approximately 13% used a needle that they knew or suspected someone else had used before them, and 18% used a needle that someone else used after them.

HIV infection is closely linked with injection drug use. In 2000, Chitwood and colleagues studied a sample of injection drug users recruited from the streets of Miami-Dade County, Florida. They found that new injectors had a lower HIV seroprevalence than long-term injectors (13.3 vs. 24.7%) and that both new and long-term drug injectors exhibited a high level of current HIV-related risk behaviors.

It appears that many young or recently initiated injection drug users have engaged in unsafe injection and/or sexual practices that place them at high risk for HIV and hepatitis viral infections. For example, Kral and colleagues found that young injectors (under 30 years) were more likely than old injectors (30 years or older) to share syringes in the past month, to report drug overdose in the past 15 months, and to report engaging in unprotected sex in the past 6 months.

According to U.S. investigators, rates of HIV and hepatitis virus infections rise within the first two years following initiation of injection drug use. For instance, Garfein and colleagues found high seroprevalence rates of hepatitis C virus (64.7%), hepatitis B virus (49.8%), and HIV (13.9%) among those who had injected for 1 year or less. Two sets of behaviors that increase injection drug users' risk of becoming HIV-infected are unsafe injection practices and high-risk sexual behaviors.

Populations at Risk

Research suggests that street youths, drug users, and those involved with the criminal justice system are at risk for initiating injection drug use. In a study of street-recruited youth ages 14 to 25 years in Montreal, Canada, Roy and colleagues found that more than one third of street youth reported having ever injected drugs: 14% and 26% were former and recent injectors, respectively. During a mean 6.9-month observation period, 7% of noninjectors initiated injection drug use (injecting cocaine or heroin), and 58% of new injectors reported borrowing used needles.

In 2003, Calzavara and colleagues reported that 68% of inmates used illicit drugs in the year prior to incarceration and 32% reported a history of injection drug use. More than one half (53%) of injection drug users injected a drug in the year prior to their current incarnation, and daily injection was common among those recent injectors (45%). Drugs most commonly injected were cocaine (67%), heroin (49%), other opioids (39%), and crack cocaine (26%).

In 2004, Wu and colleagues examined the prevalence of injection drug use in a representative sample of lifetime stimulant users age 12 or older. They found that approximately one in seven (15%) lifetime stimulant users had ever injected a drug for nonmedical reasons. About one tenth of stimulant users reported having ever injected a stimulant (11%) or cocaine (11%). Less than one tenth (8%) of stimulant users had ever injected heroin.

According to a 2001 report by U.S. Centers for Disease Control and Prevention, there is a high prevalence of injection drug use among drug users admitted to addiction treatment programs. Clients who were admitted to New Jersey addiction program centers were categorized into three groups: users of heroin and cocaine, users of heroin who did not use cocaine, and users of cocaine who did not use heroin. The 1999 data indicate that 45% of users of heroin and cocaine were injection drug users compared with 37% of users of heroin who did not use cocaine and 2% of users of cocaine who did not use heroin.

Risk Factors

Studies have identified several characteristics that are associated with injection drug use, such as childhood misbehaviors, inhalant use, marijuana use, dropping out of school, running away from home, early sex-trading, childhood sexual abuse, recent experience of violence victimization, and involvement with the criminal justice system.

Longitudinal Studies

Longitudinal patterns of injection drug use were examined among a cohort of 1,339 injection drug users recruited into the AIDS Link to Injection Experience (ALIVE) Study in Baltimore, Maryland, through community outreach efforts. This study was initiated in 1988, and follow-up continued through 2000. According to Galai and colleagues, over a

12-year study period, four patterns were noted: 29% of participants remained persistent drug injectors, 20% ceased injection, 14% relapsed once, and 37% had multiple transitions (i.e., multiple cessations and multiple relapses). The observed long-term injection patterns indicate that drug addiction is a chronic disease.

The long-term trend in HIV incidence and associated risk behaviors between 1988 and 1998 also were determined among the cohort of HIV-seronegative injection drug users in Baltimore, Maryland. According to Nelson and colleagues, 277 persons were found to be HIV-positive during 8,826.45 person-years of follow-up, an incidence of 3.14 per 100 person-years. HIV infections were associated with injection of cocaine, more frequent injection, needle sharing, and injection in a shooting gallery. Sexual behavior variables associated with HIV infections included a sexually transmitted infection, male homosexual behavior, and sex with another injector.

Public Health Implications

According to the 2006 reports by U.S. Centers for Disease Control and Prevention, since the HIV/AIDS epidemic began, injection drug use has directly and indirectly accounted for more than one third (36%) of AIDS cases in the United States. Of the 42,156 new cases of AIDS reported in 2000, 11,635 (28%) were related to injection drug use. Injection drug use contributes to the spread of HIV through sharing syringes and other equipment for drug injection, as well as through sexual transmission (e.g., having sex with an injector who is HIV-positive). Children born to mothers who contracted HIV through sharing needles or having sex with an injector also may become infected. The rate of mother-to-child transmission has decreased in the United States since treatment protocols for HIV-positive pregnant women became widely available in the mid- to late 1990s.

Conclusion

There is a continued need for innovative prevention programs that target subgroups at risk for injection drug use, such as young drug users, homeless people, and people who are involved with the criminal justice system. Additional efforts also are needed to engage drug users in drug treatment and HIV prevention in order to sustain cessation of drug use and to prevent adverse health and social outcomes among injectors.

Li-Tzy Wu and Daniel J. Pilowsky

See also Harm Reduction, Public Health; Medical Consequences; National Epidemiologic Survey on Alcohol and Related Conditions; Needle Exchange Programs; Office of National Drug Control Policy

Further Readings

Armstrong, G. L. (2007). Injection drug users in the United States, 1979–2002: An aging population. *Archives of Internal Medicine 167*(2), 166–173.

Calzavara, L. M., Burchell, A. N., Schlossberg, J., Myers, T., Escobar, M., Wallace, E., et al. (2003). Prior opiate injection and incarceration history predict injection drug use among inmates. *Addiction, 98*(9), 1257–1265.

Centers for Disease Control and Prevention. (2001). Trends in injection drug use among persons entering addiction treatment—New Jersey, 1992–1999. *Morbidity and Mortality Weekly Report, 50*(19), 378–381.

Centers for Disease Control and Prevention. (2006). Achievements in public health: Reduction in perinatal transmission of HIV infection—United States, 1985–2005. *Morbidity and Mortality Weekly Report, 55*(21), 592–597.

Centers for Disease Control and Prevention. (2006). *Drug-associated HIV transmission continues in the United States.* Retrieved June 1, 2008, from http://www.cdc.gov/hiv/resources/factsheets/PDF/idu.pdf

Chitwood, D. D., Sanchez, J., Comerford, M., Page, J. B., McBride, D. C., & Kitner, K. R. (2000). First injection and current risk factors for HIV among new and long-term injection drug users. *AIDS Care, 12*(3), 313–320.

Galai, N., Safaeian, M., Vlahov, D., Bolotin, A., & Celentano, D. D. (2003). ALIVE Study. Longitudinal patterns of drug injection behavior in the ALIVE Study cohort, 1988–2000: Description and determinants. *American Journal of Epidemiology 158*(7), 695–704.

Garfein, R. S., Vlahov, D., Galai, N., Doherty, M. C., & Nelson, K. E. (1996). Viral infections in short-term injection drug users: the prevalence of the hepatitis C, hepatitis B, human immunodeficiency, and human T-lymphotropic viruses. *American Journal of Public Health, 86*(5), 655–661.

Kral, A. H., Lorvick, J., & Edlin, B. R. (2000). Sex- and drug-related risk among populations of younger and older injection drug users in adjacent neighborhoods in San Francisco. *Journal of Acquired Immune Deficiency Syndromes, 24*(2), 162–167.

Nelson, K. E., Galai, N., Safaeian, M., Strathdee, S. A., Celentano, D. D., & Vlahov, D. (2002). Temporal trends in the incidence of human immunodeficiency virus infection and risk behavior among injection drug users in Baltimore, Maryland, 1988–1998. *American Journal of Epidemiology 156*(7), 641–653.

Roy, E., Lemire, N., Haley, N., Boivin, J. F., Frappier, J. Y., & Claessens, C. (1998). Injection drug use among street youth: A dynamic process. *Canadian Journal of Public Health, 89*(4), 239–240.

Substance Abuse and Mental Health Services Administration. (2003). *Injection drug use.* Rockville, MD: Author.

Substance Abuse and Mental Health Services Administration. (2005). *Injection drug use update 2002 and 2003.* Rockville, MD: Author.

Vlahov, D., Anthony, J. C., Munoz, A., Margolick, J., Nelson, K. E., Celentano, D. D., et al. (1991). The ALIVE study, a longitudinal study of HIV-1 infection in intravenous drug users: Description of methods and characteristics of participants. *NIDA Research Monograph, 109*, 75–100.

Wu, L. T., & Howard, M. O. (2007). Is inhalant use a risk factor for heroin and injection drug use among adolescents in the United States? *Addictive Behaviors, 32*(2), 265–281.

Wu, L. T., Pilowsky, D. J., Wechsberg, W. M., & Schlenger, W. E. (2004). Injection drug use among stimulant users in a national sample. *American Journal of Drug and Alcohol Abuse, 30*(1), 61–83.

INPATIENT TREATMENT

See RESIDENTIAL TREATMENT

INSTITUTE OF MEDICINE CLASSIFICATION SYSTEM

Classification systems are tools to help researchers, practitioners, and others think about large-scale problems. To avoid misuse of these tools, and to get the maximum benefit, a classification system's nature, strengths, and weaknesses must be understood. The Institute of Medicine's (IOM) classification of preventive interventions is important to the practice of substance abuse prevention.

Prior to 1994, substance abuse prevention used a public health classification system that designated "primary prevention" as stopping a problem before it starts, "secondary prevention" as stopping a problem early in its course, and "tertiary prevention" as minimizing further injury, disease, or disability among those with a problem. This system was originally designed to apply to physical illness. This system was helpful in some ways, but not easy to apply, especially to substance abuse prevention. For example, "tertiary prevention" fits into treatment systems but is not congruent with abstinence-based substance abuse prevention.

In 1994, the IOM issued a report called "Reducing Risks for Mental Disorders: Frontiers for Preventive Intervention Research." As part of its analysis, IOM proposed the use of a newer classification system, based on the work of R. Gordon. This new system divided mental disorder prevention into three categories: universal, selective, and indicated. The categories were based partly on the nature of the services provided rather than just the status of the service recipients.

Universal preventive interventions were defined as those for the general public or a population group (i.e., community, school, or neighborhood) with no screening to assess the risk for substance abuse of the participants. An example for substance abuse prevention would be a parenting program designed to be offered to all parents of teens in a community, irrespective of whether alcohol or other drug use by their teen had been an issue. The IOM made a cost–benefit argument for universal prevention because these interventions generally have a low cost per individual. If the interventions are perceived as effective and acceptable to the population and there is a low risk of undesirable unintended effects from the interventions, then universal prevention is worthwhile.

Selective preventive interventions are designed for groups with risk factors that indicate increased chance of developing a mental disorder. An example for substance abuse prevention would be a parenting program targeted toward parents of children experiencing academic failure. Because academic failure is a known risk factor for substance abuse (and vice versa), a prevention program that focused on this group might be appropriate, even if the cost per individual was higher than it would be for a universal population.

The IOM's report was created very specifically for the purpose of reviewing research about prevention of mental disorders, rather than substance abuse prevention. The IOM's definition of indicated preventive interventions was especially focused toward this purpose. The definition targeted people with signs of a mental disorder whose symptoms were not yet severe enough to allow the application of a diagnosis. As applied to substance abuse prevention, this has often been taken to mean youth who have "experimented" with some substance use but have not experienced sufficient problems to be diagnosed with a substance use disorder. A wide range of interpretations have been applied to the meaning of *indicated,* including use of the term whenever individual case management services are involved.

Substance abuse prevention professionals should be aware of three shortcomings in the use of the IOM system for substance abuse prevention. One is that the notion of "universal prevention interventions" heavily implies use of a "host" (i.e., person) strategy (in the public health host-agent-environment trilogy), and so may not fit well with the current trend toward more environmentally focused efforts. A working group in Illinois in 1998 proposed that "universal" be divided into "universal inoculation" and "social change." The former aims to reach and directly affect large numbers of persons (i.e., host strategies), while the latter aims to achieve widespread change by working with organizational entities (such as government, parent groups, or community-based organizations) that can profoundly affect communitywide risk and protective conditions (i.e., environmental strategies).

A second consideration in applying the IOM system to substance abuse prevention is that the IOM explicitly excluded health promotion from the classification system. This was done not out of doubt about the value of health promotion but simply to correspond to the mission of the group, which focused on the prevention of specific mental disorders. "Asset-based" prevention work that does not fall within the realm of the three IOM classifications may be considered to be in an additional category of "health promotion," if that is appropriate to the particular situation.

A third weakness of the IOM classification system is one that plagues all attempts to reduce complex reality to a typology: The definitions are heavily influenced by the context in which they are applied. As was acknowledged in the original IOM report, treatment of one problem could be considered prevention of another, so one must be very clear about the problem(s) one is preventing. For example, some prevention programs may talk about prevention of youth *use*

of substances, another may talk about prevention of substance *abuse,* and another may talk about prevention of *addiction.* Each goal may be appropriate, but preventing addiction among youth who are already regularly using alcohol or other drugs is a very different problem than prevention of any substance use among the general population of youth.

The IOM report made a point of placing the three-part classification within a larger typology that included two aspects of treatment (case identification and standard treatment) and two aspects of "maintenance" following initial treatment (compliance with treatment and after-care). This serves as a reminder that substance abuse services can be considered along an analogous continuum that includes prevention, treatment, and a growing variety of posttreatment programs for relapse prevention and ongoing recovery. In most cases, "substance abuse prevention" and relapse prevention are very different, but there can be some overlap. For example, when a prevention initiative raises community awareness of the role played by alcohol promotion in initiation of youth drinking and proposes local, state, or national policy changes to restrict such promotion, it may also be helping recovering individuals by decreasing cues toward their resumption of drinking. Preventionists who understand the IOM classification system can make use of it while not being restricted to the limits of the 1994 report.

Alan Markwood

See also Community-Based Processes; Environmental Approaches; Information Dissemination; Prevention Education

Further Readings

Mrazek, P. J., & Haggerty, R. J. (Eds.). (1994). *Reducing risks for mental disorders: Frontiers for preventive intervention research.* Washington, DC: National Academy of Sciences.

SAMHSA's Mental Health Information Center. (n.d.). *Clinical preventive services in substance abuse and mental health update: From science to services.* Retrieved March 28, 2007, from http://mentalhealth.samhsa.gov/publications/allpubs/SMA04-3906/ii.asp

Southwest Center for the Application of Prevention Technology. (n.d.). *IOMAFF response.* Retrieved March 28, 2007, from http://captus.samhsa.gov/southwest/documents/IOMAFFresponse.doc

INSURANCE PARITY

Insurance parity refers to equality in health insurance benefit coverage for treatment of substance use disorders as compared to benefits for treating other medical problems. Over the past 2 decades, policies to mandate equal benefit coverage for mental health and—to a lesser extent—substance use disorders in employer-sponsored health plans have been a topic of policy debate. Over time, this debate has increasingly been informed by research evaluating the impact of parity mandates that have already been adopted.

Parity in insurance coverage for mental and substance use disorders (often called "behavioral health" benefits) arose as a policy issue because health insurance plans offered by employers have historically covered other medical conditions more generously than they do mental health and substance abuse problems. By the mid-1990s, most employers offered insurance that provided a benefit for mental and substance use disorders, and therefore the vast majority of people with private insurance have some coverage. But these benefits are often more limited; they have lower annual or lifetime dollar limits; cover fewer outpatient visits, fewer hospital-days, or both; and require higher co-payments, higher deductibles, or both.

Parity Laws

In the past decade, the federal government and a growing number of states have enacted legislation mandating that employers offer parity in their health insurance coverage for behavioral health benefits. These laws vary with respect to the types of employers, behavioral health problems, and benefit limits that are encompassed in the parity mandates.

At the federal level, the Mental Health Parity Act (MHPA) was passed by Congress in 1996 and became effective in January 1998. Opponents of parity warned that it would greatly increase costs of insurance, and in light of these concerns, the MHPA was very limited in scope. The act requires that employers who offer health insurance with mental health benefits provide lifetime and annual dollar limits that are equal to those for other medical benefits. The parity provisions do not extend to substance use disorders. Even for mental disorders, there are no requirements for parity in limits on number of inpatient days, number of outpatient visits, or in dollar

amounts required for deductibles or co-payments. Furthermore, it applies only to employers with more than 50 employees. Although the MHPA represented an important legislative victory for mental health advocates, its limited scope resulted in limited impact. In 2007, Congress debated a bill to extend parity to substance use disorders and provide for equal benefits beyond dollar limits; at this writing the bill is still under consideration. Under President Clinton's directive, the health plans that provide benefits to all federal employees under the Federal Employee Health Benefits (FEHB) program were mandated to implement parity in benefits for mental and substance use disorders as of January 2001. The mandate called for equity across all benefit limits including dollar limits, limits on visits and inpatient days, and deductibles and co-payments. This was a far-reaching parity mandate, affecting about 8.5 million health plan enrollees.

Many states have also enacted parity legislation. Prior to the federal MHPA in 1996 only five states had adopted parity mandates, but the pace of state parity mandates quickly increased following the MHPA. Early legislation, however, was largely focused on equating particular benefits for specific mental health conditions; substance use disorders were generally excluded. Legislation including substance use disorders was slow to develop because of the absence of a well-organized advocacy community and lower public support for treatment of problems that are seen as self-incurred. In 2007, only 14 of the 36 states recognized by the National Alliance for Mental Illness as having enacted and implemented parity legislation include substance use disorders as a covered illness. Two of these states cover substance abuse services only for those with a diagnosed mental illness. Thus, benefit parity for substance abuse disorders still clearly lags behind that for mental health.

For a number of reasons, the state parity legislation that encompasses substance use disorders is likely to have little impact on insurance benefits. First, self-insured employers (including many large employers) are exempt from state insurance mandates by federal law. Second, many state laws have small firm exemptions, so that employers with 50 or fewer employees are not required to meet the parity requirements. Third, additional cost containment caps are included in many state provisions (e.g., Arkansas and Indiana), so that if offering these benefits could lead to an anticipated increase in health care costs above 4%, the firm or insurer is exempt. Fourth, some policies do not apply to all plans in the state. For example, North Carolina's policy applies only to state employees, and Minnesota's policy applies only to HMOs. Finally, these laws apply to specific types of benefits. For example, Massachusetts's legislation applies only to annual dollar limits and visit restrictions and not to cost-sharing requirements.

Arguments for Limited Benefits

The primary arguments for limiting coverage for these services are based on two economic considerations referred to as *moral hazard* and *adverse selection*. Moral hazard refers to the problem that individuals with insurance are inclined to use more medical services than they would if they had to pay the full cost of those services. Evidence supporting the moral hazard problem with mental health services comes from the RAND Health Insurance Experiment (conducted in the 1970s); however, this study did not examine substance abuse services. A strong response to the out-of-pocket price of treatment like that found in the Health Insurance Experiment for mental health services suggests that consumers are not valuing this kind of treatment as highly as other medical care. Benefit limits provide a mechanism for balancing the incentive to use services that are not highly valued.

Adverse selection refers to the problem that plans with more generous insurance coverage for mental health and addiction services could attract individuals who anticipate greater use of these types of medical services, generating higher costs for the insurer with more generous coverage. Health plans and employers can guard against this risk by limiting benefits.

Opponents to parity legislation argue that these laws increase the cost of insurance because of the presence of moral hazard and adverse selection in the health care market. Increased costs are ultimately transferred from insurance plans to employers and, in turn, increase the cost of doing business, increase costs of insurance for employees, or put people at greater risk of not having insurance coverage at all. Moreover, there is public skepticism about the effectiveness of treatment, fueling concerns that added costs are not justified by their health benefits.

Arguments for Parity

Advocates for broader parity mandates argue that social costs of substance abuse are extremely high and that treatment of individuals with these problems will result in social cost savings that more than offset the costs of treatment. The treatment research literature documents effectiveness of a variety of treatment practices in reducing substance use and associated social problems and thus supports this view. However, it is not known the extent to which usual services received for substance abuse problems by those with private health insurance are consistent with evidence-based practices.

Available research examining the impact of implementing parity also generally supports arguments for parity mandates by showing that fears of rising costs are largely unfounded. Contrary to predictions based on moral hazard and adverse selection, benefit parity does not appear to increase use of services, or if so, to result in small increases. Most research to date has focused on the impact of implementing parity in mental health benefits, but a few studies have addressed substance abuse treatment benefits. An evaluation of the comprehensive parity ruling implemented in the FEHB program found no significant increase in use of services attributable to parity for five of seven large plans studied, a decrease in use for one plan, and an increase in use in the remaining plan studied. These results can be explained by the fact that in recent years, utilization and costs of behavioral health services are, within most private insurance plans, contained by managed care organizations. In fact, the single FEHB plan that showed an increase in use attributable to parity was the only one that did not manage its behavioral health benefits through a contract with a managed behavioral health care organization. Other studies of substance abuse parity mandates (e.g., in Virginia and for state government employees in Ohio) also suggest minimal impact on utilization of services in the context of managed care.

Conclusion

Recent data reported by Jon Gabel and colleagues show little change in substance abuse treatment benefits since the mid-1990s. About 9 of 10 workers has some coverage for substance abuse treatment services, but most have more limited benefits and higher cost-sharing requirements for their substance abuse treatment benefits than for other medical benefits. Adjusted for inflation, total private insurance spending on substance abuse treatment has remained relatively steady over this time.

Given experience to date with implementation of parity policies, particularly the comprehensive parity mandate of the FEHB program, it is easy to wonder why benefit parity remains such a contentious policy issue and broader federal parity legislation has yet to be passed. Weak public advocacy and relatively limited research on substance abuse benefit parity undoubtedly play a role. And even though few commercial plan enrollees ever use substance abuse treatment services, high prevalence of substance use disorders in the population is well documented. It is perhaps not surprising that some remain politically opposed to parity legislation because they fear burdening employers and workers with escalating costs of insurance should the floodgates of all this pent-up need for services unexpectedly be opened.

In the debate surrounding parity, the full implications of having entered into an era of managed health care, particularly in behavioral health care, have been underappreciated. Projections of costs of parity have often assumed a world of health care like that of the 1970s Health Insurance Experiment, before managed care, when benefit limits were the only mechanism available for employers to control costs. Today, however, the great majority of privately insured people have behavioral health benefits under some form of managed care, where supply restrictions can be used in lieu of benefit design to influence utilization of services. Design of benefits with various limitations and cost-sharing is one way of controlling costs of health care; managed care is another. Benefit design controls costs through incentives that influence consumer "demand" for services, but it is a crude tool that eliminates not only low-value "discretionary" care but also appropriate care for those with severe disorders and highest need for services. Managed care controls costs by influencing "supply" of services, for example, through negotiated reductions in fees with a network of preferred providers and review of appropriateness of services to eliminate unnecessary use. Managed care is a more finely tuned and potentially appealing cost-containment strategy than benefit design, because it can offer a more flexible benefit with health services tailored to need by clinicians and case managers.

Under managed care, arguments against insurance benefit parity are greatly weakened. Even with benefit parity, concerns arise that managed care can discourage access to care and encourage skimping on the quality of care. These issues are likely to rise to the fore of substance abuse treatment advocacy when comprehensive parity is achieved.

M. Audrey Burnam and Rosalie Liccardo Pacula

See also Economic Costs of Alcohol and Drug Abuse; Evidence-Based Treatment; Health Care System and Substance Abuse; Public Policy, Treatment; Substance Use Disorders; Treatment Effectiveness

Further Readings

Burnam, M. A., & Escarce, J. J. (1999). Equity in managed care for mental disorders. *Health Affairs, 18*(5), 22–31.

Frank, R. G., & McGuire, T. G. (1998). Parity for mental health and substance abuse care under managed care. *Journal of Mental Health Policy and Economics, 1*(4), 153–159.

Gabel, J. R., Whitmore, H., Pickreign, J. D., Levit, K. R., Coffey, R. M., & Vandivort-Warren, R. (2007). Substance abuse benefits: Still limited after all these years, *Health Affairs, 26*(4), w474–w482.

Goldman, H. H., Frank, R. G., Burnam, M. A., et al. (2006). Behavioral health insurance parity for federal employees. *New England Journal of Medicine, 354*, 1378–1386.

National Alliance on Mental Illness. (n.d.). *State mental health parity laws 2007*. Retrieved June 1, 2008, from http://www.nami.org/Template.cfm?Section=Issue_Spotlights&template=/ContentManagement/ContentDisplay.cfm&ContentID=45351

Newhouse, J. P., and the Insurance Experiment Group. (1993). *Free for all? Lessons from the RAND Health Insurance Experiment.* Cambridge, MA: Harvard University Press.

Ridgely, M. S., Burnam, M. A., Barry, C. L., Goldman, H. H., & Hennessy, K. D. (2006). Health plans respond to parity: Managing behavioral health care in the Federal Employees Health Benefit Program. *Milbank Quarterly, 84*(1), 201–218.

INTERNATIONAL COALITION FOR ADDICTION STUDIES EDUCATION

Although addiction studies is a venerable field dating from the mid-20th century, there were a small number of curricula at colleges and universities until the late 1970s. At that time, state and national systems for credentialing of addiction counselors were established, and academic programs were put in place to offer the educational requirements for addiction counselor certification. In 1990, it became apparent that the complexion of addiction counseling was changing. This was manifested in an aging workforce, in advancements toward credentialing and licensure of addictions professionals, and in an increasingly complex body of addictions research that challenged current practitioners in the field. A group of addiction studies educators from around the United States formed a germinal organization to address this urgent workforce development need. Thus was born the International Coalition for Addiction Studies Education (INCASE).

As a relative newcomer to the many and varied addictions organizations around the country and around the world, INCASE initially struggled to find its niche and the audience with which to share its vision, mission, and goals. Addictions educators are found in many different academic departments and divisions: INCASE presidents have included a criminologist, a nurse educator, an anthropologist, human service educators and psychologists. With the publication of *Addiction Counseling Competencies: The Knowledge, Skills and Attitudes of Professional Practice* in 1997 (published by the Center for Substance Abuse Treatment [CSAT] in the Substance Abuse and Mental Health Services Administration), INCASE found both a purpose and a well-articulated role with direction. INCASE members served as field reviewers, consultants, and as members of the National Steering Committee on Addiction Counselor Competencies that voted to adopt the document as a statement from and for the field.

Initially, the multiple purposes of the organization included to disseminate professional knowledge and share ideas regarding addiction studies curricula; to conduct international seminars, workshops, and conferences in order to provide members with educational opportunities; to encourage and promote ongoing research and scholarship in the field of addictions studies; to develop standards for, and implementation of, an accreditation process for competent and comprehensive addiction studies education providers; to explore related funding sources and opportunities; to initiate discussions of reciprocity within and between nations, states, and provinces; and to develop liaisons with other organizations providing related educational services or who have related interests. Although originally broad in scope, these purposes evolved over time and are now a much more functional set of goals and objectives within the capabilities of a small but disciplined volunteer organization of educators.

Today, INCASE shares the characteristics of a traditional organization with both mission and vision statements. As a mission, INCASE has a succinct purpose: promoting new knowledge and advancing teaching and curriculum development as seminal to improving addiction professionals' education. As a vision, INCASE sees itself as important and contributory in workforce development; the education and clinical training of competent, well-informed practitioners; the production and dissemination of new knowledge; the development of products to advance the professional discipline; partnering with like-minded groups; and engaging in dialogue with allied or affiliated groups on issues of certification, licensure, supervision, and continuing education.

To meet these goals, INCASE has organized itself to be responsive to the rapidly changing environment of the addiction studies arena. As an organization, INCASE is interested in developing an identity as educators and as participants in the growth of this profession. To that end, INCASE members engage in conversations with other groups such as the Addiction Technology Transfer Centers, NAADAC (the Association for Addiction Professionals), the International Certification and Reciprocity Consortium, the Annapolis Coalition, the Association for Medical Education and Research in Substance Abuse, and many others. National conferences, held since 1994, have been cosponsored with state counselor bodies and Addiction Technology Transfer Centers, and have received support from the Center for Substance Abuse Treatment and the National Institute on Drug Abuse. As might be expected of academics who are traditionally employed and retained based on teaching, research, and service activities, INCASE characteristically focuses its efforts in three principal areas: curriculum development; program review and approval; and development, research, and planning.

Curriculum Development

The *Addiction Counseling Competencies* laid the platform for the construction of curricular experiences that would meet or exceed those minimum competencies of effective addictions practitioners. Included in this academic and educational format were the knowledge, skills, and attitudes one could expect of an individual in professional clinical practice. INCASE found itself at the heart of the matter at varied levels, from workshop presentations for continuing education to providing substantive academic programs for degree-seeking individuals at the associate, baccalaureate, master's, and doctoral levels. Today, emphasis in clinical preparation is not only founded on knowledge but also on the application of learning to achieve effective clinical outcomes; on an understanding of the history regarding what has worked but also on an appreciation for a projected future of improved practice; and on immersion into the research to improve both preparation and practice in place of running in fear from the science of addiction.

Program Review and Approval

In organizing a program approval process for higher education addictions curricula, INCASE hopes to further the goals of quality assurance and promulgation of program standards. It is of equal importance to educators to promote the development of articulation networks and transferability and portability of degrees; to provide a resource for the creation, expansion, and upgrading of addictions curricula; and to ensure that the classroom is a bridge from science to practice in the preparation of the addictions workforce. Self-governance within the addictions higher education field, helping addictions educators advocate for their existence and needs within their institutional environment, and aiding students in moving up educational and career ladders by providing legitimacy to the curricula and academic programs they have completed are core to the mission and vision of INCASE.

Development, Research, and Planning

INCASE produces its own journal, *The Journal of Teaching in the Addictions*, a forum for the presentation of manuscripts addressing new knowledge, strategies, teaching techniques, and enhancement of workforce development. It is engaged in the future, insistent on preparing practitioners for tomorrow's workplace. It provides a supportive environment for colleagues to share via a listserve, conferences, and a platform to discuss and review curriculum and teaching strategies. INCASE is pursuing grants to further its mission and vision of continued enhancement of the workforce in academic, personal, and professional dispositions. INCASE prides itself on staying at least abreast, if not ahead, of this ever-changing discipline.

The International Coalition of Addiction Studies Education, though relatively young, is emerging as a leader in the overall preparation of the next generation of addictions practitioners.

Michael D. Loos

See also Addiction Technology Transfer Centers; American Society of Addiction Medicine; Certification and Licensing; NAADAC, the Association for Addiction Professionals

Further Readings

Center for Substance Abuse Treatment. (2002). *Addiction counseling competencies: The knowledge, skills and attitudes of professional practice*. Retrieved May 30, 2007, from http://www.treatment.org/Taps/tap21/TAP21Toc.html
International Coalition for Addiction Studies Education: http://incase-edu.net/default.aspx

INTERNET ADDICTION

It is estimated that more than 210 million Americans access the Internet on a regular basis, making the United States by far the top World Wide Web user in the world. Specialists estimate that between 6% and 14% of Internet users in the United States have a destructive dependency on the Web and that the vast majority of these people do not realize they have a problem.

Internet addiction has been formally recognized as a disorder by the American Psychological Association, although it is not listed in the *Diagnostic and Statistical Manual of Mental Disorders, Fourth Edition, Text Revision* (*DSM-IV-TR*). The term *Internet addiction disorder* (IAD) first made headlines in 1995 when psychiatrist Ivan K. Goldberg posted a parody online spoofing the *DSM-IV* by using the criteria for pathological gambling and calling it "Internet Addiction Disorder." At the time, spending excessive time online was not considered a disorder, disease, or addiction, but soon Goldberg realized his joke was a lot more serious than originally planned, as he started receiving hundreds of requests for consultations.

Goldberg took his spoof even further, creating an Internet addiction support group online, something critics jokingly compared to holding an Alcoholics

Anonymous meeting at a cocktail party. Ironically, Goldberg is still one of those skeptics who refuse to recognize Internet addiction as a real addiction, calling it simply a symptom of other, existing disorders.

Many researchers agree with Goldberg. Sara Keisler, of Carnegie Mellon University, calls Internet addiction a "fad illness." Others argue that Internet addiction has as much medical merit as "telephone addiction" or "television addiction."

However, supporters of the diagnosis say that Internet addiction can have much more serious consequences than other destructive habits, because the Internet can lead obsessive users to other addictions like gambling or pornography. Just like pathological gambling, Internet addiction is considered a "pure" addiction or an impulse control disorder because it does not involve the use of intoxicating drugs.

Internet addiction typically starts with casual use of e-mail or other simple online applications, many times for work or school purposes. In a relatively short time, it progresses into an activity that results in major disruptions in life. Some mental health professionals compare Internet addiction to alcoholism or drug addiction, at least in the way it can destroy different aspects of a person's life.

As people begin to make the Internet an important part of their daily routine, they get channeled into different areas of the World Wide Web. Some of the most popular destinations for would be addicts include chat rooms, shopping sites, pornography, day trading, gambling, social networking sites like MySpace and Facebook, dating sites, downloading music and other digital files, instant messaging, blogging, or even reading news and sports.

Preliminary research shows that most Internet addicts are usually struggling with other issues such as depression and anxiety. For them, the Internet offers an escape from reality, and the fact that it is easily accessible, affordable, and anonymous makes them more susceptible to becoming addicted.

Kimberly S. Young, founder of the Center for Internet Addiction Recovery, developed one of the most efficient instruments for diagnosing Internet addiction, the Internet Addiction Test. This test is a 20-item questionnaire that measures mild, moderate, and severe levels of Internet addiction by quizzing the participants on things like the amount of time they spend online, the feelings and mood swings that people experience when they are on- or off-line, how

personal and professional relationships have been affected by the person's Internet usage, and the importance that the Internet has on a person's life overall.

According to Young, some of the symptoms associated with Internet addiction are preoccupation with the Internet, use of the Internet in increasing amounts of time in order to achieve satisfaction, unsuccessful efforts to cut back usage, a change in mood or feelings of depression when off-line, lying about the extent of the problem, using the Internet to escape other problems, and jeopardizing real-life relationships, career, or educational opportunities because of excessive use of the Internet.

The biggest problem with Internet addiction continues to be, and perhaps will always be, the effects that the addiction has on a person's off-line world. A married person may meet someone else through a chat room and cheat on his or her spouse. A high school or college student might drop in his or her grades, or even drop out of school altogether because of an Internet addiction. Personal finances can be greatly affected with shopping or even gambling sites. Using the Internet for non-work-related purposes has also been cited as being one of the top corporate time-wasting activities, costing corporations millions of dollars every year.

Even though Internet addiction is considered a relatively new illness, many mental health professionals are treating their patients with some of the same approaches used to treat chemical dependency, including Twelve-Step programs. As with some other behavioral addictions, treating Internet addiction usually does not require total abstinence, as the goal is to reduce the time a person spends online and getting them to take control of the areas of their life that have become unmanageable due to excessive Internet usage.

Some formal treatment programs for Internet addiction have been developed. For example, the Illinois Institute for Addiction Recovery has an inpatient program designed for computer addicts, located at Proctor Hospital campuses in Peoria, Bloomington, and Springfield. Doctors there say that they have seen some of the same withdrawal symptoms in excessive computer users as they see in alcoholics and drug addicts. Sierra Tucson Drug Treatment Center in Arizona also has a program to combat Internet addiction. Patients here are encouraged to attend Alcoholics Anonymous or Narcotics Anonymous meetings as part of their recovery.

Published studies on Internet addiction are still scarce compared to studies on addictions that have been around for decades, and some mental health professionals are still skeptical to call excessive use of the Internet an actual addiction because it lacks some of the characteristics and consequences of conventionally recognized addictions. However, few can deny that excessive Internet use is a growing problem among the general population, and it needs to be further researched as more people get access to, and spend more time on, computers and other devices connected to the Internet.

José Pacheco and Gary L. Fisher

See also Other Addictions; Sex Addiction; Shopping Addiction; Substitute Addictions

Further Readings

DeAngelis, T. (2000). Is Internet addiction real? *Monitor on Psychology, 31*(4). Retrieved February 12, 2008, from http://www.apa.org/monitor/apr00/addiction.html

Greenfield, D. N. (1999). *Virtual addiction: Help for netheads, cyberfreaks, and those who love them.* Oakland, CA: New Harbinger.

Grohol, J. M. (2005). *Internet addiction guide.* Retrieved February 12, 2008, from http://psychcentral.com/netaddiction/

Suler, J. (2004). Computer and cyberspace addiction. *International Journal of Applied Psychoanalytic Studies, 1,* 359–362. Retrieved February 12, 2008, from http://www-usr.rider.edu/~suler/psycyber/cybaddict.html

Young, K. S. (1998). *Caught in the net: How to recognize the signs of internet addiction—and a winning strategy for recovery.* New York: Wiley.

INTERVENTION

See JOHNSON MODEL INTERVENTION; MOTIVATIONAL INTERVIEWING

INTRAVENOUS DRUG USE

See INJECTION DRUG USE

INVENTORY OF DRINKING SITUATIONS

The Inventory of Drinking Situations (IDS) was developed by Helen Annis and colleagues at the Addiction Research Foundation in Toronto, Canada. The IDS draws its theoretical basis from Alan Marlatt's eight categories of high-risk drinking situations and is intended to provide an individualized profile of a problem drinker's particular high-risk situations that can then be used to structure and guide treatment.

The IDS is available in two forms. The original IDS consisted of 100 items representing particular situations in which people consume alcohol (e.g., "when I'm alone at home" or "when I've had a hard day at work"). Subsequent refinement of the instrument, including its revision to include drugs other than alcohol, has resulted in a final instrument that captures frequency of drinking in up to 50 different situations commonly reported by heavy drinkers as being ones in which they are most likely to drink. Factor analytic studies of the IDS have further grouped these eight situations into three factors: Negative Affective States, Positive Affective States, and Testing Personal Control. A short (42 items) form of the IDS was described by Carl Isenhart in 1993. The short form has been shown to have adequate reliability and validity compared to the long form, but it does not cover the full range of high-risk situations described by Marlatt, focusing on only five of the eight types of situations in Marlatt's typology.

In Marlatt's model, the key to understanding and preventing relapse is to understand the specific situations in which the individual was at high risk to use alcohol or other drugs. These high-risk situations are divided into eight categories of which include unpleasant emotions, physical discomfort, pleasant emotions, testing personal control, urges and temptations, social problems at work, social tension, and positive social situations. The respondent is asked to indicate on a Likert scale how often they consumed alcohol in the situations presented during the previous year. A summary "profile" of specific types of high-risk situations for the individual respondent is then generated and can be used to guide the teaching of relapse prevention strategies that target the situations in which the respondent was most likely to drink and therefore are considered most likely to trigger relapse.

For example, if a client reported her most frequent drinking in situations involving unpleasant emotions, the clinician might focus on teaching the client affect management strategies, such as cognitive restructuring or thought disputation, as coping strategies that could be implemented instead of drinking alcohol. The clinician and client can then use the IDS as a guide to efficiently structuring treatment for less frequently encountered high-risk situations, thus making the treatment process both more efficient and more effective.

The IDS has also lead to the development of another questionnaire, the Situational Confidence Questionnaire (SCQ) by Annis and colleagues. The SCQ uses the same situations as the IDS but asks the respondent to rate his or her confidence that he or she could encounter the situation without drinking. Taken together, the IDS and SCQ comprise a useful tandem of instruments for both treatment planning and treatment outcome assessment. Thus, following an initial assessment of high-risk situations with the IDS, and the teaching and implementation of coping strategies that do not involve drinking, the clinician can assess the extent to which the client is confident in his or her ability to encounter the high-risk situations identified by the IDS and cope without using alcohol. This assessment of confidence or self-efficacy is a critical one in helping to gauge both the likelihood of relapse and the ability to identify situations in which coping skills may fail. This then permits further anticipatory planning and coping skills training for the client.

In using the IDS to plan treatment interventions, the clinician may either complete the IDS with the client or have the client do so independently. Using the profile of high-risk situations generated, the clinician and client jointly identify those high-risk situations that are most likely to occur in the client's life and can then develop specific coping strategies the client can use in order to cope effectively without drinking.

Should the client subsequently relapse, the IDS can assist the clinician and the client in understanding that relapse and in planning subsequent relapse prevention treatment by indicating other situations that initially seemed less important but that may have played a role in the client's current relapse.

Later work by Annis and colleagues has extended the basic theory behind the IDS to the development of an Inventory of Drug-Taking Situations. Subsequent work has resulted in an instrument that combines assessment of high-risk situations for both alcohol and other drugs.

The IDS has been translated into a number of languages, including French, Spanish, German and Swedish, and has demonstrated adequate reliability and validity in all versions. The main disadvantage of the IDS comes with clients whose literacy level is below the eighth-grade level at which the items are written. However, the IDS can still be a useful tool with those clients if the items are read to the client by the clinician.

Frederick Rotgers

See also Assessment; Assessment Instruments; High-Risk Situations; Relapse; Relapse Prevention

Further Readings

Annis, H. M., & Graham, J. M. (1988). *Situational Confidence Questionnaire.* Toronto, ON, Canada: Addiction Research Foundation.

Annis, H. M., Graham, J. M., & Davis, C. S. (1987). *Inventory of Drinking Situations (IDS) user's guide.* Toronto, ON, Canada: Addiction Research Foundation.

Annis, H. M., Turner, N. E., & Sklar, S. M. (1997). *Inventory of Drug-Taking Situations.* Toronto, ON, Canada: Center for Addiction and Mental Health.

Cannon, D. S., Leeka, J. K., Patterson, E. T., & Baker, T. B. (1990). Principal components analysis of the inventory of drinking situations: Empirical categories of drinking by alcoholics. *Addictive Behaviors, 15,* 265–269.

Isenhart, C. E. (1991). Factor structure of the Inventory of Drinking Situations. *Journal of Substance Abuse, 3,* 59–71.

Isenhart, C. E. (1993). Psychometric evaluation of a short form of the Inventory of Drinking Situations. *Journal of Studies on Alcohol, 54,* 345–349.

Marlatt, G. A., & Donovan, D. M. (2005). *Relapse prevention: Maintenance strategies in the treatment of addictive behaviors* (2nd ed.). New York: Guilford Press.

Jellinek, E. M. (1890–1963)

Following repeal of the National Prohibition Act, the United States began the shift from a moral to a scientific approach to alcohol problems, emphasizing a disease concept of alcoholism and treatment for alcoholics. E. M. Jellinek was at the forefront of this change, helping to shape the policies and programs of the new alcoholism movement during the 1940s and 1950s. Through his work with the Research Council on Problems of Alcohol, the Yale Section of Alcohol Studies, and the World Health Organization (WHO), he influenced and helped disseminate the work of alcohol researchers and treatment professionals around the world.

Born in New York City, Jellinek was raised in Hungary and educated at the Universities of Berlin, Leipzig, and Grenoble. His studies ranged from philosophy and theology to language and linguistics, but his claims to various degrees from European and Latin American universities have been impossible to verify. Leaving Hungary in the 1920s, he spent several years in Sierra Leone before taking a job with the United Fruit Company in Honduras. In 1931, he returned to the United States to become Director of the Biometric Laboratory at the Memorial Foundation for Neuroendocrine Research in Worcester, Massachusetts, where he studied the neuroendocrine effects of schizophrenia.

Jellinek was nearly 50 years old when he accepted an offer in 1938 from the Research Council on Problems of Alcohol—an association of concerned researchers and physicians. He directed a major review of the existing research literature on the effects of alcohol on the individual. When the funding ended in 1941, Howard Haggard, Director of the Laboratory of Applied Physiology at Yale University, brought Jellinek and the project to Yale and made him Managing Editor of the *Quarterly Journal of Studies on Alcohol,* which Haggard had founded in 1940. Jellinek subsequently coauthored several review articles as well as two monographs, stemming from the literature review project.

At Yale, Jellinek quickly rose to a leadership position in the Laboratory of Applied Physiology. In 1943, with Haggard, he founded and directed the Yale School of Alcohol Studies, the first program to train alcoholism professionals. He also established the Yale Plan Clinics, the first outpatient alcoholism treatment programs. In 1944, with Marty Mann, the first woman to recover in Alcoholics Anonymous, he sponsored the creation of the National Committee for Education on Alcoholism. This program became a major tool for raising public awareness about the disease of alcoholism. When Haggard established a formal section of alcohol studies within the Yale laboratory in 1943, he named Jellinek as director.

During his career at Yale, Jellinek developed his own research interests, mainly in the area of epidemiology. He made various attempts to quantify the numbers of alcoholics, primarily based on liver cirrhosis deaths, which ultimately led to the Jellinek Estimation Formula, published by the WHO in 1951. He also assisted in a survey conducted by Alcoholics Anonymous to determine the course of alcoholism. His analysis, supplemented with subsequent survey data, led to his classic publication in 1952 describing the phases of alcohol addiction.

Jellinek left Yale in 1948 to set up a similar research institute at Texas Christian University. Without sufficient financial support, the venture failed in 1951. By that time, he had moved on to Geneva as consultant to the new Alcoholism Subcommittee of the WHO's Expert Committee on Mental Health. There he renewed his epidemiological work, using his estimation formula to help calculate alcoholism problems in various European and Latin American countries. He also convinced the WHO to disseminate abstracts from Yale's alcohol literature review project to research centers around the world.

Jellinek left the WHO in 1955 and spent 2 years with the short-lived International Institute for Research on Problems of Alcohol. In 1957, he accepted a grant from philanthropist R. Brinkley Smithers to return to the United States to prepare a national report on alcoholism. The final report, published in 1960 as *The Disease Concept of Alcoholism*, identified five distinct types of alcoholics: alpha (psychological dependence without loss of control), beta (physiological complications, such as cirrhosis, but no physical or psychological dependence), gamma (increased tolerance, withdrawal signs, loss of control), delta (increased tolerance and inability to abstain), and epsilon (heavy binge drinking).

While completing *The Disease Concept of Alcoholism,* Jellinek also served as a consultant to the Addiction Research Foundation of Toronto and the Alcoholism Foundation of Alberta in Canada. Then in 1961, he joined the staff of the Cooperative Commission on the Study of Alcohol Problems. The commission was a U.S.–Canadian effort to make policy recommendations on alcohol problems. While at the commission, Jellinek secured funding from the National Institute of Mental Health (NIMH) to compile an *Encyclopedia of Problems of Alcohol* to bring together the research knowledge on the subject. He died suddenly of a heart attack in 1963, leaving the work unfinished. The NIMH terminated the project, feeling that no one else was qualified to undertake it.

In just over 20 years, Jellinek helped establish a modern alcoholism field based on research, professional education, and public awareness. His own efforts to estimate the numbers of alcoholics, to delineate stages in the addiction process, and to identify different types of alcoholics provided important tools to build on this scientific approach to alcohol problems.

Penny Booth Page

See also Alcoholics Anonymous; Disease Concept; National Council on Alcoholism and Drug Dependence

Further Readings

Jellinek, E. M. (1951). Jellinek estimation formula. In World Health Organization, Expert Committee on Mental Health, *Report on the first session of the alcoholism subcommittee* (WHO Technical Report Series No. 42, Annex 2, pp. 21–24). Geneva: World Health Organization.

Jellinek, E. M. (1952). Phases of alcohol addiction. *Quarterly Journal of Studies on Alcohol, 13,* 673–684.

Jellinek, E. M. (1960). *The disease concept of alcoholism.* New Haven, CT: Hillhouse Press.

Page, P. B. (1988). The origins of alcohol studies: E. M. Jellinek and the documentation of the alcohol research literature. *British Journal of Addiction, 83,* 1095–1103.

Page, P. B. (1997). E. M. Jellinek and the evolution of alcohol studies: A critical essay. *Addiction, 92,* 1619–1637.

JOHNSON MODEL INTERVENTION

Vernon Johnson, the founder of the Johnson Institute associated with the Minnesota model of treatment, described the process of intervention that has been widely used in motivating alcoholics-addicts to seek treatment in his books *I'll Quit Tomorrow* and *Intervention: How to Help Someone Who Doesn't Want Help.* The Johnson intervention is based on the disease model of addiction. There is a need to forcefully motivate the alcoholic to enter treatment because the alternatives are dire. The Johnson intervention is seen as a dynamic, emotionally charged, confrontation by significant persons in the alcoholic's-addict's life.

The major reason for the need for forcefulness in the Johnson intervention model is the impenetrable denial systems developed by alcoholics-addicts. These denial systems are often used to explain the difficulty of motivating alcoholics-addicts to seek treatment. Therefore, this type of intervention is designed to counteract denial through dramatic means.

The rationale of the Johnson model of intervention is to break through the denial system of the alcoholic-addict by confronting the person with the crises that he or she caused. The confrontation is done by significant persons in the alcoholic's-addict's life. Through this confrontation, it is hoped that the intervention process will *raise the bottom.* The bottom may be extremely serious (e.g., injury, health problems, loss of family, death), and those who care about the alcoholic-addict would be anxious to avoid the bottom. The confrontational intervention would serve to precipitate a crisis in the life of the alcoholic-addict that is not life-threatening or otherwise damaging, but that would result in treatment. This is the concept of raising the bottom.

To raise the bottom, Johnson believed that the alcoholic-addict needed a clear view of reality as presented by the significant people in their life. Meeting this need means clearly stating specific facts about the person's behavior and the consequences of these behaviors in an objective, unequivocal, and caring manner.

In his books, Johnson outlined the specific procedures for conducting an intervention. Although Johnson wrote a book designed to enable a layperson to organize and implement an intervention, it is highly recommended that an intervention be facilitated by a trained mental health professional. These events can be volatile and emotionally charged.

First of all, there must be two or more people involved in the intervention who are close to the alcoholic-addict and who have witnessed his or her behavior while intoxicated. Having two or more people involved offers support for those confronting the alcoholic-addict, emphasizes the seriousness of the situation to the person, and helps to dispute attempts by the alcoholic-addict to dismiss or discount the events of any one person. Clearly, someone must determine the composition of the intervention team—usually, this is done by the person or people who have instigated the intervention. Participants may include spouses or lovers, children, parents, employers, teachers, or friends. Individuals who are seen as being influential in the life of the alcoholic-addicts would be valuable participants. It is sometimes the case that those people who are the most intimately involved with the alcoholic-addict are not helpful in the intervention because of their emotional closeness to the alcoholic-addict and consequent inability to refrain from nonproductive interactions during the intervention. In addition, Johnson suggested that each person on the intervention team be educated about the disease concept.

Each participant in the intervention develops a list of specific incidents of alcohol or other drug-related behavior and describes the effect that each incident had on the participant. Specificity is important to avoid generalized statements that can be disputed. Although it is important for participants to relate the effect of the alcohol and/or drug-related behavior on them, the tone

should be nonjudgmental. Because the intervention may become quite emotional, it is suggested that the participants write down the specific events so that they can remember them during the intervention.

Each participant must also decide what action he or she will be willing to take if the alcoholic-addict refuses treatment. The actions must be serious enough to have an impact, and the participant must be willing to follow through. Thus, spouses and lovers may decide to leave the relationship, employers to terminate, or friends to disengage. Obviously, if the intervention does not result in the person's seeking treatment and if participants do not follow through on their actions, it will be extremely difficult to intervene in the future.

Someone on the intervention team must do some homework and determine the treatment options available, the cost of treatment, availability of insurance, and other hurdles such as job and family responsibilities. All of these details must be cleared up before the intervention so that all the alcoholic-addict has to say is "yes" (i.e., agree to go to treatment).

Clearly, preparation for the intervention is essential. The intervention team must meet on several occasions to rehearse the intervention and to role-play possible scenarios. The order in which people will speak should be predetermined. Someone must be assigned the responsibility of getting the alcoholic-addict to the intervention and of getting the person there sober. Often, deception is used, since the alcoholic-addict would refuse to attend if the true purpose of the intervention were known. Participants need to be prepared for the emotional reaction of the alcoholic-addict. He or she may become angry when the purpose of the intervention is revealed. He or she may simply leave.

When the alcoholic-addict arrives at the intervention, the facilitator (who should be a mental health professional) tells the alcoholic-addict that the people in the room are there because they care and are concerned. The facilitator tells the alcoholic-addict that the people want to describe what they have been seeing. The alcoholic-addict is asked to listen to each person and will then be given an opportunity to talk. Each participant (in the predetermined order) expresses love, caring, and/or concern and describes the specific incidents he or she has prepared. The final participant, who should be the most influential, begins the discussion of what is being asked of the alcoholic-addict (i.e., treatment). The facilitator will usually need to contribute to the discussion of available treatment options, should intervene when the alcoholic-addict interrupts with arguments or rationalizations, and may need to remind the alcoholic-addict just to listen until everyone has finished. The facilitator should also intervene when nonproductive interactions occur between a participant and the alcoholic-addict.

Johnson model interventions were very popular 10 to 20 years ago. The development of motivational interviewing as an alternative has dramatically reduced the frequency of Johnson model interventions. Still, very traditional treatment programs that adhere to the Minnesota model of treatment may still conduct Johnson model interventions prior to treatment admission.

Gary L. Fisher

See also Client Engagement; Coercion and Treatment; Motivational Interviewing; Minnesota Model; Resistance in Treatment; Stages of Change Model

Further Readings

Johnson, V. E. (1973). *I'll quit tomorrow.* Toronto, ON, Canada: Harper & Row.

Johnson, V. E. (1986). *Intervention: How to help someone who doesn't want help. A step-by-step guide for families and friends of chemically dependent persons.* Minneapolis, MN: Johnson Institute Books.

JOIN TOGETHER

Illicit drugs and inappropriate alcohol use are national public health problems that are expressed differently in every community. Therefore, solutions to more effective prevention and treatment must occur through community-based strategies and action. In the late 1980s and early 1990s, the Robert Wood Johnson Foundation was looking for a way to attack drug and alcohol problems in communities. There were hundreds of community organizations eager to address the issue, but they were often run by volunteers who had few strategic planning skills, no access to current research, and very limited funds. They were often operating in isolation from similar groups and working in a policy environment that was hostile to effective prevention and treatment. Furthermore, the idea that alcohol and drug dependence was a disease with biologic, psychological, and behavioral components was not well established or accepted.

Join Together was launched at the Boston University School of Public Health in 1991 through an initial grant of $5 million from the Robert Wood Johnson Foundation with a mission to help leaders in communities address the leadership, strategy, funding, and policy challenges they faced. The group continues to operate as part of the Boston University School of Public Health with funding from Robert Wood Johnson and other foundations, corporations, and government agencies. Today, the program is one of the nation's largest providers of research information, planning assistance, and advocacy support for people who are working to improve strategies that prevent and treat alcohol and drug problems.

Join Together was the first group of its kind to make strategic use of Web technology, and currently, more than a million people consult its main Web site (www.jointogether.org) annually. More than 35,000 prevention and treatment professionals subscribe to one or more of its electronic newsletters. Join Together members include community leaders, public officials, doctors, nurses, and other treatment professionals, as well as parole officers, clergy, people from labor unions and employee assistance programs, and parents and families—anyone trying to help someone tackle a problem with addiction.

Although the Internet was only embryonic in the early 1990s, Join Together believed electronic communication could become a vehicle to connect people with others who were working on the same issue, disseminate accurate and timely information, and rally action on alcohol and drug policy issues. Its first program relied on a commercial time sharing system, but plans were developed that enabled the first version of Join Together Online to go live on the Internet within a month of the release of the first public browser in 1995.

One of Join Together's initial challenges was to identify, document, and gain access to the thousands of groups that existed throughout the country. Through lists collected from state agencies and other sources, mail surveys were conducted to gather information about what the groups were doing and what they needed. The answers formed the basis for technical assistance, leadership programs, and Web content development. Join Together continues to set its information and support agenda in response to regular surveys of community-level prevention and treatment leaders, but they are now done online.

Join Together's news and information services have evolved as technology caught up with its ambitions. Every week Join Together creates online summaries of approximately 100 new research reports, press stories, and program updates from all over the country. These are freely available on the main site, syndicated through an RSS feed to hundreds of other alcohol, drug, and tobacco Web sites, and repackaged into daily and weekly focused electronic newsletters distributed free to more than 35,000 subscribers.

Web technology also enables Join Together to initiate action campaigns on alcohol or drug issues at the national, individual state, or community level. For example, in 2006, Join Together led a national effort to get major chain stores to remove alcohol drinking games from their shelves and Web sites. It also used its Web technology to help a local group of activists launch a campaign against alcohol advertising on the regional public transit busses and subways.

From 1992 to 1999, Join Together ran a national leadership recognition program called the Join Together Fellows Program. Each competitively selected group represented all parts of the country and a mix of activists and professionals including coalition leaders, mayors, judges, police chiefs, business and union leaders, clergy, treatment and prevention counselors, and doctors and nurses. Many directors of state drug and alcohol programs were Join Together Fellows early in their careers. The mayor of San Francisco and a former head of the federal Department of Health and Human Services' Center for Substance Abuse Prevention as well as several judges have all been fellows.

Join Together is committed to using scientific evidence and demonstrated best practices as the basis for its information and technical assistance programs. The group believes it has demonstrated that strategies based on valid local data and relying on evidence-based solutions are more likely to be effective than efforts that rely on impressions and ideology. For example, communities that participated in the Fighting Back program, administered by Join Together, significantly reduced alcohol-related automobile deaths after they increased access to treatment and stepped up enforcement.

Creating sound and sane public policy on alcohol and drugs is another Join Together goal. From time to time, national policy panels are created to examine a particular issue and formulate recommendations for action. Members of panels include former and present elected officials, subject experts, and community activists. They gather information through background research and public hearings. Their findings and recommendations are published in print and online and are widely distributed to the targeted audiences throughout the country. A recent

panel chaired by the former Mayor of Baltimore and current Dean of the Howard University Law School Kurt Schmoke addressed issues of legal and social discrimination faced by people with alcohol and drug problems. The panel found that legally sanctioned discrimination often continues long after a person enters successful recovery and creates a lifetime of punishment. The panel recommended changes in federal and state laws and regulations to end these practices. In 2006, a panel chaired by former Governor of Massachusetts Michael Dukakis and Kansas State Representative Pat George focused on ways to improve state government organization of alcohol and drug services and strategies. The report called for new leadership from governors, legislatures, and courts and recommended organizational changes at the state level.

Although Join Together's primary mission has been to assist community leaders and strategies, its early internet capacity enabled it to pioneer applications aimed at helping individuals who smoke, drink too much, or use illicit drugs. In 1995, Nathan Cobb, then a Join Together staff member, created QuitNet as a free online program and community to help individuals quit smoking. Join Together sponsored the service, and it grew very rapidly. In 2000, in cooperation with Boston University, it was transformed to a private company and began providing services to state and private smoking cessation programs. QuitNet now operates as part of Healthways, Inc. and was used by more than one million people in 2007 in the United States and other countries.

Join Together also created and sponsors Web-based free screening programs to help individuals learn about the health related risks of their own drinking and/or drug taking. The Web site www.alcoholscreening.org was launched in 2002. In 2007, more than 15,000 individuals a month completed self-screens. The Web site www.drugscreening.org was launched in 2007 due to the rapid growth in use.

David Rosenbloom

See also Community-Based Processes; Prevention Strategies; Public Policy, Alcohol

Further Readings

Alcohol Screening: http://www.alcoholscreening.org
Drug Screening: http://www.drugscreening.org
Join Together: http://www.jointogether.org

L

LEGAL ACTION CENTER

The Legal Action Center is a nonprofit law and policy organization whose stated mission is to combat discrimination against individuals with a history of addiction, HIV/AIDS, or criminal records. The Legal Action Center helps individuals reclaim their lives, and it also advocates for reasonable public policies on issues related to addiction, AIDS, and/or criminal histories.

In 1973, the Vera Institute of Justice in New York City established the Legal Action Center to fight issues arising from the overlap of addiction and crime, particularly by assisting those most directly impacted. During the middle of the 1980s, AIDS was added to the mission of the Legal Action Center as it became evident that persons with alcohol and other drug problems and/or those with criminal records were at an increased risk for HIV/AIDS. The Legal Action Center is dedicated to fighting the prejudice and stigma that frequently keeps people with personal histories of addiction, crime, and/or HIV/AIDS from fully participating in mainstream society. Beginning with several class action suits and other cases in the 1970s and 1980s, the Legal Action Center has successfully challenged discrimination in granting government benefits, employment, and other areas with precedent setting litigation. For example, the Legal Action Center was instrumental in ensuring that the Americans with Disabilities Act (ADA) and the Fair Housing Act specifically forbid discrimination against those in recovery from alcohol and other drug use. One high profile case that the Legal Action Center litigated was *Traynor v. Turnage*, which they took successfully all the way to the U.S. Supreme Court and eventually got Congress to overturn the Veterans Administration ruling that classified alcoholism as willful misconduct instead of as a disease.

The Legal Action Center provides legal services to help fight discrimination, to protect privacy, and to assist with a wide range of legal issues. This legal assistance is provided nationally to help individuals in treatment, or otherwise in recovery, to deal with discriminations or privacy violations. Legal services are also available to individuals and agencies that assist individuals with criminal records or with HIV/AIDS. Assistance is intended to help eliminate legal barriers that could prevent people from gaining employment, housing, zoning, and other basic necessities. In addition to legal assistance, the Legal Action Center conducts many other programs and services.

The Legal Action Center engages in policy advocacy for the expansion of alcohol, drug, and HIV/AIDS treatment, prevention, and research. It also advocates for social welfare reform policies that will promote sobriety, increase employment, and reduce discrimination. The Legal Action Center conducts public policy research through the Arthur Liman Policy Research Institute in areas related to addiction, AIDS, and criminal justice.

The Legal Action Center is committed to helping bring about a fairer and more effective criminal justice system and strives to uphold the rights of those individuals with criminal justice records who seek to reenter society and to live crime free lives, as well as for those already rehabilitated. The Legal Action Center advocates for reform of sentencing laws and campaigns for greater funding of alternatives to incarceration and for community corrections. Attention is also paid to removing the potentially debilitating legal barriers that make it so difficult for individuals with criminal justice records to be successful in many important areas of life, not the least of which is employment and housing.

The Legal Action Center provides education, training, and technical assistance to individuals, service providers, and governmental agencies on issues such as confidentiality, discrimination, and managed care. The Legal Action Center also helps government agencies, community-based organizations, public advocates, and other interested individuals understand how and when varied mechanisms and systems of reimbursement interact with substance abuse treatment agencies. In addition, the Legal Action Center fights against discrimination and privacy violations for people with HIV/AIDS, providing training and technical assistance on issues such as HIV testing, partner notification, living will and health care proxies, syringe deregulation, permanency planning, and HIV/AIDS reporting.

The Legal Action Center produces a series of assorted publications and videos on topics such as the Federal Alcohol and Drug Confidentiality Regulations (42 CFR Part 2), drug testing, syringe exchange, the ADA, drug law reform, and criminal records expungement. Online confidentiality courses are also available from the Legal Action Center, such as the Introduction to Confidentiality and Advanced Confidentiality. Sample forms and other materials are available for use by substance abuse treatment agencies, such as how to comply with the Federal Alcohol and Drug Confidentiality Regulations (42 CFR Part 2) and with the Health Insurance Portability and Accountability Act requirements. Other initiatives include the National H.I.R.E. (helping individuals with criminal records reenter through employment) Network and the Women's Initiative to Stop HIV. The National H.I.R.E. Network has over 5,000 members and is dedicated to increasing the number and quantity of work opportunities available to individuals with criminal justice records.

The Legal Action Center maintains a useful Web site and provides news alerts and a newsletter, the *Washington Weekly Roundup*, free of charge. Many additional publications are available for purchase from the Legal Action Center (http://www.lac.org).

Victor B. Stolberg

See also Confidentiality; Criminal Justice Populations; Discrimination, Addicted and Recovering Individuals; HIV/AIDS; Informed Consent; Public Policy, Treatment

Further Readings

Galbraith, S., Bockvar, K., & Polnac, J. (1994). *Best practices: Models of care for pregnant alcoholic and drug dependent women and their children*. New York: Legal Action Center.

Goodman, R. (1995). *Employment discrimination and how to deal with it*. New York: Legal Action Center.

Legal Action Center. (2006). *Confidentiality and communication: A guide to the federal drug & alcohol confidentiality law and HIPAA*. New York: Author.

Rubinstein, G. (2001). *Getting to work: How TANF can support ex-offender parents in the transition to self-sufficiency*. New York: Legal Action Center.

Samuels, P., & Mukamal, D. (2004). *After prison: Roadblocks to reentry: A report on state legal barriers facing people with criminal records*. New York: Legal Action Center.

LEGALIZATION OF DRUGS

Public opinion about drug use and drug abuse is difficult to ascertain. It would be completely impossible to live in an entirely drug-free society in that drugs help alleviate pain and misery, correct organic and social dysfunction, and treat disease. And yet, drug use and abuse can serve to create some of the very conditions that drug therapy seeks to control. Drugs create disease, damage organs and tissue, engender social and psychological problems, and create physical and interpersonal pain. Furthermore, drug use and abuse creates, at the social level, crime and criminal activities that the non-drug-abusing members of society deem unacceptable. The use of many drugs represents a crime, irrespective of the individual or social harms done by the drug or by the person under the influence of the drug. So why then is there such considerable and constant interest in the idea of drug legalization?

Historically, the topic of drug criminalization and drug legalization has emerged several times. Usually, the discussion about criminalization occurs when there is something else happening in the society that is related to drug use and the public believes (perhaps wrongfully) that criminalization will solve the problem. Sometimes the criminalization helps, sometimes there is no noticeable or immediate effect, and sometimes the criminalization creates more problems; discussion then ensues regarding undoing the criminalization. Usually, this discussion centers either on a cost-benefit analysis of the laws or on the morality of drug use and the idea that it should remain illegal, regardless of the costs.

History

In 1914, the United States sought to control what was perceived as a growing threat to society by limiting access to cocaine, allowing it to only be obtained through a prescription offered by a health professional. In 1919, this act, known as the Harrison Act, was amended to make all distribution of cocaine illegal. In the same period, alcohol was outlawed through the Volstead Act, a prohibition that lasted until 1933.

Supporters of drug legalization cite multiple examples of miscarriages of justice and ask pointed questions in an attempt to show the illogical nature of drug laws and drug law enforcement. For instance, why was alcohol banned and not other addictive substances like tobacco? Why do similar substances, for example, powdered and crack cocaine, carry different punishments? These advocates of drug legalization are quick to point out that crime rates dropped dramatically after the approval of the 21st Amendment, which repealed the Volstead Act in 1933.

Current Issues

Even the most ardent supporters of drug legalization do not support the total and complete removal of all controls on drug use and possession. Juveniles and others who lack mature reasoning skills must be protected, but limited drug legalization could yield social and economic benefits far beyond the risks and costs to society. There is a great deal of drug use in society, and the majority of these users are adults who use these drugs for purely recreational purposes. This use does not generate thefts or robberies, it does not result in children being abused or neglected, and it rarely serves the interest of the justice system. In the 1970s, recreational drug use was treated with benign neglect by the justice system, and the majority of society had no problem with this unofficial policy.

Today, however, the mere use of drugs creates the threat of adjudication and incarceration even when there is no other harm associated with the behavior because drug use is illegal. If drug use was legal, the use would cease to be a social or legal problem.

Not all drug use is inconsequential. It would be unreasonable to assume that drug use does not generate crime beyond the simple purchase, possession, and use of the drug. Drug use does lead to crime in many cases. So how can the supporters of drug legalization advocate making them legal when the use of the drug is often either the cause or the result of crime? These advocates point out that drugs are a simple commodity, governed by the same market forces as legal commodities. It stands to reason, therefore, that the cost of the drug is a function of the availability, the demand, and the cost of production, which includes the growing or synthesizing of the substance, the processing and packaging of the drug into manageable and marketable units, and the distribution to the end user. All of these stages, due to the illegal nature of the substance, carry risk of detection and apprehension. This risk (and the associated losses caused by detection and apprehension) must be calculated into the cost of production, thereby increasing the cost of the product to the end consumer. As the risks of detection and apprehension increase, production and sales must increase to offset losses caused by confiscation, as will the legal costs associated with defense. In short, increases in enforcement lead to more production and to increased costs to end users. Since a certain proportion of the end users support their drug use through illegal activities, increases in enforcement that result in corresponding increases in both risk and price lead directly to increases in the numbers of crimes that are used to generate the money necessary to purchase the drugs. At the same time, these increases in enforcement add persons to the justice system who have been apprehended for the production, possession, use, and sales of the drug.

Arguments in Favor of Legalization

Legalization advocates argue that the legalization and control of select drugs would simultaneously drop the cost of the drugs to the end user while improving the quality and safety of the product. Add to this the reduced number of persons processed through the justice system and the diminished dollar value of drug-related crimes and you have an equation with few negatives and multiple advantages. The costs associated with policing, apprehending, adjudicating, and incarcerating drug and drug-related crime would greatly decrease, allowing increased spending in areas neglected since the onset of the War on Drugs.

Positions such as this argument are usually considered the domain of libertarians and those who oppose laws in many forms, not just those associated with drugs. It is, however, important to note that the position that supports limiting the laws that criminalize drug use and possession has proponents on both sides of the political spectrum. In 1999, then-governor of New Mexico, Gary Johnson (a Republican), argued that the War on Drugs had been a multibillion dollar failure and that he supported drug legalization for many reasons. In response to Johnson's statements, Barry McCaffrey, the director of the Office of National Drug Control Policy, called Governor Johnson's statements and his position on drug legalization irresponsible.

Arguments in favor of drug legalization have almost always focused on the potential financial savings to society, as well as on the increased funding available for other worthy programs if less money was being spent on a War on Drugs that cannot be won. Although some opponents of legalization acknowledge that there may be financial savings associated with legalization, the risk of increased social costs and the associated social disintegration make the option of legalization less socially and economically viable.

Arguments Against Legalization

In May 2003, the Drug Enforcement Administration (DEA) released a report titled *Speaking Out Against Drug Legalization*, which focused on the dangers of legalization. Rather than disputing the points made by the legalization advocates, the DEA argued that the legalization debate has become more intense due to drug legalization trends in Europe. The DEA contends, however, that the social situation in Europe is distinctly different from that of the United States, and policies that work there would likely be disastrous in the United States.

The DEA report contends that the War on Drugs is working. Drug use is decreasing and approximately 95% of all Americans do not use illegal drugs of any type. Treatment efforts and prevention are also working, and the progress made in the treatment and prevention areas would be undone by legalization. The justice

system is often the primary conduit that gets users into treatment programs. And, although not all treatment is successful the first time it is attempted, eventually many of these users stop using drugs due to aging and the cumulative effects of treatment programming. The leverage provided by a court order or referral would disappear if drugs were legalized, and a critical element of deterrence would also vanish, making increased use of now-illegal drugs a virtual certainty.

Those who support legalization cite how the cost of drug law enforcement would diminish substantially if the drug laws were repealed, but those who support the retention of these laws cite reports that indicate the small overall impact this would have on the national budget. The DEA report notes that the entire budget for drug control ($12.9 billion in 2008) only constitutes a minor portion of the U.S. budget, and the social and financial costs of drug use and addiction far outweigh the meager savings associated with the repeal of these laws. To support the idea that the legalization of drugs would lead to more addiction and increases in related social costs, the DEA provides the experience of Alaska as an example. In the 1970s, Alaska experimented with the legalization of marijuana, and within a short period of time, the youth in Alaska were using marijuana at twice the rate of youth in the lower 48 states. Alaskans decided in 1990 that the experiment had failed, and they subsequently voted to recriminalize marijuana in 1990. In the Netherlands, a similar situation occurred when heroin use and addiction tripled within a couple years of the legalization of marijuana. Although marijuana legalization may have kept some persons out of the justice system, the accessibility and lack of deterrence may have created more marijuana users and subsequently, more heroin users and addicts. By increasing access to a low-level drug, critics believe it may have sent a message to the citizens that drug use in general, regardless of the level, was acceptable.

Finally, those who support legalization often cite the medical uses of drugs such as marijuana. The criminalization of these drugs makes it much harder for persons with chronic health problems to get relief. Legal medications may not be as effective, and they may cost the consumer much more than illegal drugs would. According to the DEA, there are options for these persons, and these options are both safer than street-grade drugs and are legal. Marinol, which contains the active ingredient in marijuana (THC), is claimed to have the same effect as smoking marijuana, is legal, and does not cause the damage to the lungs that inhaling marijuana smoke can cause.

Conclusion

As stated earlier, discussing drug legalization places at odds the areas of morality and economic logic. The discussion is not a true debate because the sides rarely even consider the same issues to be central to the argument. Those in favor of legalization discuss the savings to the justice system and the economic costs of locking up relatively nondangerous offenders while opponents of legalization discuss the risk to society caused by relaxing drug laws and the possible negative consequences of the removal of legal constraints on drug use. The one area that the two sides can debate is on the War on Drugs. Each side, however, argues that the War on Drugs is the best reason to support their side. Those who support retaining the current drug laws believe that the War on Drugs is going well (as evidenced by the diminishing numbers of users), and without drug laws, many former drug users would have never received the help necessary to stop using. Opponents of drug laws maintain that the War on Drugs has been a monumental waste of time and money and repealing the laws would allow spending in areas that would yield much greater benefits to all of society. Even though the two sides are discussing the same basic issue, they each define success on the War on Drugs differently, and consequently, they disagree on the success of the war and the value of the laws that make the War on Drugs necessary. In short, there is no clear answer to the drug legalization question, but strong evidence exists in support of each side of the discussion.

Matthew Leone

See also Decriminalization; Harm Reduction Psychotherapy; Harm Reduction, Public Health; National Drug Control Strategy; Public Policy, Drugs

Further Readings

Balkin, K. F. (2005). *Drug legalization.* Farmington Hills, MI: Greenhaven Press.

Fish, J. M. (2006). *Drugs and society: U.S. public policy.* Lanham, MD: Rowman & Littlefield.

Leuw, E., & Marshall, I. H. (Eds.). (1996). *Between prohibition and legalization: The Dutch experiment in drug policy.* Amsterdam: Kugler.

Payne, B. K., & Gainey, R. R. (Eds.). (2005). *Drugs and policing: A scientific perspective.* Springfield, IL: Charles C Thomas.

Roleff, T. L. (Ed.). (2004). *The War on Drugs: Opposing viewpoints.* San Diego, CA: Greenhaven Press.

Timmons, M. (2007). *Disputed moral issues: A reader.* New York: Oxford University Press.

Vallance, T. R. (1993). *Prohibition's second failure: The quest for a rational and humane drug policy.* Westport, CT: Praeger.

Wodak, A., & Owens, R. (Eds.). (1996). *Drug prohibition: A call for change.* Portland, OR: International Specialized Books Services.

LEVO-ALPHA ACETYL METHADOL

There are currently three Food and Drug Administration (FDA)–approved opioid agonist treatments for opioid addiction, which include methadone hydrochloride, buprenorphine hydrochloride, and levo-alpha acetyl methadol (LAAM). All three of these drugs are long-acting opioids, which bind to opioid receptors and thus block opioids from binding to these receptors. LAAM, as well as the other opioid agonist treatments, are long-acting drugs that have minimal psychoactive effects. Use of LAAM thus permits opioid-addicted individuals to engage normally in daily routines while decreasing craving or drug-seeking behaviors.

LAAM may also be labeled as *levomethadyl acetate hydrochloride* or *levacetylmethadol*. LAAM was developed in the 1960s and was under investigation as a medication in the treatment of opioid dependence until the 1990s. In 1993, LAAM was approved by the FDA as a medication for opioid dependence. LAAM offers improvements over drugs like methadone because it has a significantly longer duration of action. However, despite the initial excitement over the introduction of LAAM for the treatment of opioid dependence, use of LAAM was found to be associated with adverse side effects, in particular, cardiac symptomatology. Such findings have since decreased the enthusiasm and thus have limited the demand for this drug.

Similar to methadone, LAAM is an oral medication. It is a synthetic opioid whose properties ameliorate symptoms for patients experiencing withdrawal from opioids. The mechanism of action for LAAM is to bind to pain receptors in the brain, and this binding action results in a decrease in patient cravings for heroin or other opioids and a decrease in withdrawal symptoms. More specifically, LAAM acts as a mu (μ) opioid receptor agonist. It has effects that are qualitatively similar to both morphine and methadone, but has the unique characteristic of a longer duration of action. LAAM provides opioid effects for 48 to 72 hours or longer depending on the dose. In contrast, methadone provides opioid effects for approximately 24 hours. This increase in the duration of action presents a significant improvement for patients being treated for opioid dependence. Although some studies indicate that LAAM is less potent than methadone, at least one study has demonstrated that under acute dosing conditions, LAAM may be significantly more potent relative to methadone. Despite its long duration of action, it should be noted that withdrawal from LAAM can be difficult.

Recommendations for Use

Because LAAM is less familiar to patients (e.g., relative to methadone) as an option for treatment of opioid addiction, patients may have reservations about using LAAM. Thus, for patients being prescribed LAAM, further counseling, support, and psychoeducation may be necessary. Those who may be more likely to benefit from LAAM, relative to other medications, are those who would prefer or require reduced frequency of clinic visits. For example, individuals whose employment would be interrupted by daily visits to receive methadone or who have difficulty obtaining daily transportation to a methadone clinic may be good candidates for use of LAAM. In addition, LAAM may be appropriate for individuals who worry about the stigma of methadone.

The FDA recently issued a warning about the use of LAAM following a small number of reports of a ventricular arrhythmia condition that were filed following the use of LAAM; this cardiac condition is called *torsade de pointes*. As a consequence of reports of torsade de pointes following use of LAAM, the FDA currently requires a warning to be included with packaging that LAAM should not be used as a first-line treatment of opioid addiction. Due to reports of cardiac problems associated with LAAM, use of LAAM has declined, and availability may eventually be discontinued. The manufacturer recommends that all patients who are prescribed LAAM receive an electrocardiogram before use of LAAM is initiated. In

addition, follow-up electrocardiograms after steady-state dosage has been achieved are also recommended to provide continued monitoring of cardiac health.

Patients can be transferred to LAAM not only from opioid use, but also from methadone use. Thus, if methadone was ineffective, LAAM can be presented as another drug to try. Of note, LAAM is available in approximately 10% of opioid agonist treatment centers. This relatively low availability is due in part to higher costs associated with monitoring via electrocardiograms and because the manufacturer began to limit production due to related concerns about cardiac health.

Properties of LAAM

Use of LAAM in place of opioids prevents withdrawal symptoms. In blocking withdrawal, LAAM does not produce a subjective high, but rather acts to block the effects of other opioids. Research has demonstrated that LAAM and methadone have similar efficacy levels, as well as similar outcome levels of heroin use. In addition, despite the small number of reported cases of torsade de pointes, studies also suggest similar safety levels for use of LAAM and methadone.

With respect to mechanisms of action, the primary difference between methadone and LAAM is that LAAM is the alpha-acetyl congener of methadone. LAAM is metabolized by the liver into four metabolites, including nor-levomethadyl and dinor-levomethadyl. Similar to methadone, LAAM is metabolized by the hepatic P450 isozyme CYP3A4. Methadone and LAAM have the same protein binding sights in plasma and thus, if taken together, have additive effects.

LAAM is commercially available in a liquid suspension form, and is taken orally. It is absorbed by the gastrointestinal tract, but has a slower onset of effect compared to methadone (90 minutes vs. 30 minutes) and is longer acting (48–72 hours vs. 24–36 hours). After the effect of LAAM has subsided, withdrawal symptoms are likely to be intense.

Conclusion

LAAM is a long-acting synthetic opioid used for the treatment of opioid dependence and has demonstrated similar efficacy rates for opioid dependence as compared to methadone treatment. Because LAAM is longer acting than methadone, it has benefits for individuals who are unable to schedule daily visits to a methadone clinic. However, due to cardiac problems that are associated with the use of LAAM, treatment requires consistent monitoring of cardiac health. Despite these limitations, LAAM may be a viable alternative to use of methadone in the treatment of opioid dependence.

Yael Chatav and Gregory L. Stuart

See also Buprenorphine; Heroin; Methadone; Methadone Maintenance Therapy; Opioids

Further Readings

Krantz, M. J., & Mehler, P. S. (2007). Treating opioid dependence. *Archives of Internal Medicine, 164,* 277–288.

M

Marijuana

Marijuana is the common way to refer to a class of drugs called *cannabinols*. The cannabinols include marijuana (*grass*, *pot*, *weed*, *joint*, *reefer*, *dube*), hashish, Charas, Bhang, ganja, and sinsemilla. The active ingredient is delta-9-tetrahydrocannabinol (THC). Hashish and Charas have a THC content of 7% to 14%; ganja and sinsemilla, 4% to 7%; and bhang and marijuana, 2% to 5%. However, modern growing techniques have increased the THC content of marijuana sold illicitly. For simplicity, the various forms of cannabinols will be referred to as *marijuana*.

The earliest references to the drug date back to 2700 BC. In the 1700s, the hemp plant (*cannabis sativa*) was grown in the colonies for its fiber, which was used in rope. Beginning in 1926, states began to outlaw the use of marijuana since it was claimed to cause criminal behavior and violence. Marijuana use became popular with mainstream young people in the 1960s. Some states have basically decriminalized possession of small amounts of marijuana, although according to the federal government, it remains a Schedule I drug, meaning that marijuana has no approved medical uses and has a high abuse potential.

Prevalence

Marijuana is the most widely used illegal drug. The result of the 2006 National Survey on Drug Use and Health showed that nearly 97.8 million Americans reported using marijuana sometime in their life, 25 million had used marijuana in the past year, and more than 14.8 million had used this drug in the past month. The number of past-month users is nearly 7 times the number of past-month users of cocaine, the next most widely used illegal drug and more than double the number of past-month nonmedical users of prescription drugs. Among young people, ages 12 to 17, 6.7% reported using marijuana in the past month, and 16% of young adults ages 18 to 25 used marijuana in the past month. Over 2 million people used marijuana for the first time in 2006.

Major Effects

Acute Physical and Psychological Effects

Marijuana is usually smoked in cigarette form or in pipes. It can also be ingested, normally by baking it in brownies or cookies. Marijuana users experience euphoria; enhancement of taste, touch, and smell; relaxation; increased appetite; altered time sense; and impaired immediate recall. An enhanced perception of the humor of situations or events may occur. The physiological effects of marijuana include increase in pulse rate and blood pressure, dilation of blood vessels in the cornea (which produces bloodshot eyes), and dry mouth. Motor skills and reaction time are slowed.

Marijuana intoxication has an adverse effect on attention span, short-term memory, and psychomotor performance. Anxiety and panic attacks can occur, primarily in new users who are not familiar with marijuana's effects. At very high doses, some people experience delusions and hallucinations. There are no cases of fatal marijuana poisoning, and humans are unlikely to be able to ingest a fatal dose. The effect of marijuana intoxication impairs motor and cognitive abilities necessary to safely drive a car or operate machinery. The extent to which marijuana is involved in auto accidents is unclear. Many motorists intoxicated with marijuana drive more slowly and carefully and take fewer risks. However, there is an increased risk of accidents after using marijuana, but marijuana alone does not appear to contribute a great deal to accidents. Marijuana in combination with alcohol does.

Physical Effects of Chronic Use

Marijuana smoke contains carcinogens. However, because of nondefinitive or conflicting results, additional research on the association between smoking marijuana and certain cancers should be conducted. There is no evidence that the rate of infectious diseases is increased among heavy marijuana users. However, with very high doses of marijuana, animal studies have shown immune system impairment, reduced resistance to infection, and compromises in the immune defense system in the lungs. Studies of HIV patients who use marijuana have not produced evidence of an accelerated progression to AIDS. The use of marijuana during pregnancy is associated with small birthweight but not with an increased risk of birth defects. Similar but smaller, behavioral, and developmental effects resulting from maternal tobacco use have been seen in studies of infants prenatally exposed to marijuana. Animal studies have demonstrated disruption in the reproduction system from chronic administration of THC. However, no definitive research has been conducted on the impact of heavy marijuana use on the reproductive systems of humans. The changes in heart rate and blood pressure from marijuana use are not likely to have an adverse impact on healthy adults but could be harmful to those with hypertension, at high risk for strokes, or with clogged heart arteries. Because marijuana smoke contains many of the same carcinogens found in tobacco smoke, it is likely that marijuana smoking increases the risk of respiratory cancers, especially if used in combination with tobacco. The regular use of smoked marijuana impairs the functioning of the airways and can cause chronic bronchitis. There is no evidence of any adverse effect of marijuana on the liver or gastrointestinal system.

Psychological Effects of Chronic Use

In the late 1960s, an amotivational syndrome was described in which young marijuana users were seen as apathetic, withdrawn, lethargic and unmotivated. However, there is no evidence of a unique syndrome with these symptoms that is attributable to marijuana use. These symptoms are more likely the result of marijuana dependence. Clearly, heavy marijuana use can lead to dependence on the drug characterized by a combination of social, legal, financial, family, educational, and occupational problems; withdrawal symptoms when drug use is discontinued; and difficulty in controlling the use of marijuana in spite of the intention to do so. The rate of abuse and dependence problems from marijuana is lower than that of alcohol, and more people with marijuana problems are able to discontinue their use without treatment than is found with other addicting substances. Daily long-term use of marijuana may adversely impact memory, attention, and the integration of complex information in subtle ways. However, there does not seem to be any severe impairment of cognitive functioning. There is still some uncertainty regarding whether all the impairments are reversible after a long period of abstinence.

Although there is a relationship between heavy marijuana use and mental health problems, the nature of this relationship is open to interpretation. Young people who use marijuana are at high risk for mental health problems. Some of this is explained by the fact that these young people were at high risk for mental health problems before they began to use marijuana. In addition, young people who begin using marijuana at a young age are more likely to affiliate with delinquent and/or drug-using peers, which increases their risk for a variety of problems. Finally, it should be noted that the early first use of tobacco and alcohol is also associated with later mental health problems. Therefore, the likely mediating variables that explain the association between marijuana and mental health problems involve the predisposing characteristics of the users and the lifestyle associated with illegal drug use.

There is evidence that marijuana can precipitate psychosis in people who are vulnerable to developing psychotic disorders. In other words, some people will develop schizophrenia or another psychotic disorder if the proper environmental conditions are present (e.g., trauma). The heavy use of marijuana may be one of those environmental factors. In spite of the implication that marijuana can cause schizophrenia, this does not seem likely. When marijuana use has increased among adults, the incidence of schizophrenia has been stable or decreased.

Similarly, there is an association between adolescent marijuana use and noncompletion of high school, involvement in drug-related crime, early pregnancy, and divorce. Again, the characteristics of the adolescent marijuana user seem to be the factors that explain these associations. However, there is little doubt that the early use of marijuana is among the risk factors that are associated with a variety of adolescent problems.

Medical Uses of Marijuana

In 1999, the Institute of Medicine (IOM) prepared a report at the request of the federal government on the scientific evidence regarding medical uses for marijuana. The conclusion was that there was scientific evidence for the potential therapeutic value of THC for pain relief, nausea and vomiting control, and appetite stimulation. However, the IOM report also indicated that smoking marijuana was an imprecise method to deliver THC and produced harmful substances through smoking. The report also discussed the psychological effects of marijuana, such as anxiety reduction, sedation, and euphoria. It was determined that these psychological effects can influence the therapeutic effects in potentially beneficial or harmful ways. For example, some older patients reported that the psychological effects were disturbing. For patients with AIDS wasting syndrome, the combination of appetite stimulation with the psychological effects of anxiety reduction, sedation, and euphoria could be beneficial.

The IOM report also examined the risks associated with the medical use of marijuana. With the exception of the harms associated with smoking, the detrimental effects of marijuana were seen as being within the range that is tolerated for other medications. The acute effects included diminished psychomotor performance, which could impact driving or the operation of dangerous equipment. A small number of marijuana users experienced unpleasant feelings from the drug. The acute effects on the immune system could not be firmly established but if such effects exist, were not severe enough to rule out the use of marijuana for medicinal purposes. With regard to chronic effects, the conclusion was that marijuana smoke is associated with increased risk of cancer, lung damage, and poor pregnancy outcomes. There was no convincing evidence that marijuana smoke does or does not cause respiratory cancer.

There are claims that marijuana is also beneficial in the control of muscle spasticity and in reducing intraocular pressure from glaucoma. The IOM report did not find compelling evidence to support or refute this claim with regard to muscle spasticity and concluded that marijuana was not effective treatment for glaucoma.

Treatment Admissions and Emergency Room Visits

According to information from the federal government, admissions to treatment in which the patient reported marijuana was the primary substance of abuse more than doubled from 1993 to 2003. In 1993, 7% of all admissions mentioned marijuana as the primary drug of choice, while 16% reported this in 2003. However, most of this increase was driven by referrals from the criminal justice system. In 1993, 48% of the marijuana treatment admissions were referred from the criminal justice system and 57% in 2003. Therefore, it is not possible to tell if the increase in treatment admissions is due to law enforcement changes (i.e., drug courts) or actual increases in marijuana dependence.

According to the Drug Abuse Warning Network, there were 627,923 emergency room visits related to drugs in the last half of 2003, and 12.7% of these visits included marijuana as a drug that either induced or related to the emergency room visit. In 4.5% of these cases, the emergency room visit involved a suicide attempt, 10.9% involved a desire for detoxification, and nearly all of the rest (84%) were categorized as *other*. In comparison, cocaine accounted for 20.1% of the drug-related emergency room visits, heroin was involved in 7.6%, and methamphetamine was mentioned in 4% of the cases. Therefore, marijuana was mentioned more often than any other illegal drug except cocaine.

Gateway Theory

Does marijuana use lead to other drug use? This idea is frequently referred to as the gateway theory. That is, the use of marijuana is a gateway to the use of other drugs. There is no evidence that there is something inherent in marijuana that causes a person to use other drugs. Although there is no disputing the fact that marijuana users are more likely than nonmarijuana users to use other drugs and that the earlier the age of first use of marijuana, the more likely the individual is to use other drugs, the relationship between these facts and the gateway theory is controversial. There is no evidence that marijuana has some pharmacological property that would cause a user to crave other drugs. The most likely explanations for the relationships between marijuana and other drug use involve the characteristics of marijuana users and peer and environmental influences. Those individuals who use marijuana at an early age and/or use marijuana heavily may have genetic, personality, and attitudinal characteristics that predispose them to use mind-altering substances. Since marijuana is the most widely available illegal drug and is perceived as the least harmful illegal drug, it makes sense that this drug would be used first. The fact that tobacco and alcohol use almost always precedes marijuana use is further evidence that the most widely available substance will be used first. Furthermore, those young people who use marijuana are affiliating with peers who also use marijuana, who are accepting of illegal drug use, who generally support the experimentation of other drugs, and who have some knowledge of how to secure illegal drugs. These generalizations do not always fit, since there are certainly peer groups who use marijuana but who disapprove of the use of other drugs and not all marijuana users progress to the use of other drugs. In fact, most do not. However, it is not difficult to conceptualize a 13-year-old who begins to use marijuana as associating with a peer group that is accepting of drug use in general, while an 18-year-old who first uses marijuana may be involved in a peer group whose illegal drug use is limited to marijuana. The 13-year-old initiate is much more likely to be rebellious, risk-taking, and unconventional than the 18-year-old initiate. This difference would explain the relationship between age of first use of marijuana and the use of other drugs.

Conclusion

Marijuana is the most widely used illegal drug. Although it is classified as a Schedule I drug by the federal government, marijuana is clearly not as dangerous acutely or chronically as drugs that have lower classifications. However, marijuana, like all mind-altering substances, is a drug that has damaging effects acutely and chronically and can result in dependence among heavy users. The available scientific evidence is that there is some likelihood that marijuana has medical uses, particularly in the alleviation of nausea, pain relief, and in appetite stimulation in people with serious, life-threatening medical conditions.

Gary L. Fisher

See also Amotivational Syndrome; Cannabis Youth Treatment Study; Decriminalization; Gateway Drugs Theory; Legalization of Drugs; Public Policy, Drugs

Further Readings

Fisher, G. L. (2006). Chapter 4: How dangerous is marijuana? In *Rethinking our war on drugs: Candid talk about controversial issues* (pp. 71–86). Westport, CT: Praeger.

Hall, W., & Liccardo-Pacula, R. (2003). *Cannabis use and dependence: Public health and public policy.* Cambridge, UK: Cambridge University Press.

Joy, J. E., Watson, S. J., & Benson J. A., Jr. (Eds.). (1999). *Marijuana and medicine: Assessing the science base.* Washington, DC: National Academy Press.

MATERNAL DRUG USE

Maternal substance abuse, as the term is used here, refers to any maternal substance use disorder ranging from substance abuse, in which the use of a substance continues despite negative consequences, to dependence, the salient feature of which is loss of control over the amount of or frequency with which the substance is consumed. Maternal substance abuse covers all of the illicit substances of abuse, as well as alcohol and tobacco. This section covers the stigma associated with and the complexity of the problem of maternal substance abuse and the effects of maternal substance abuse on embryos and fetuses, as well as on children and adolescents. Also discussed are effective treatment options and support for long-term recovery.

Stigma

The stigma of addiction is particularly severe for women who are mothers. Even within the substance abuse treatment field, pregnant women seeking treatment can be judged by those with an incomplete understanding of addiction, and in society at large, the criticism can range from harsh moral judgment to criminal sanctions for prenatal drug use. In the eyes of the public, the notion that addiction is a disease and not a crime often does not extend to mothers, and the illegal behavior that often provides a woman with her substances adds to the level of criticism and judgment she experiences.

A frequent criticism leveled at mothers with addictions is that if they really loved their children, they would not use substances. This common judgment connects two myths in one sentence: love for their children and motivation and ability to stop using substances. A mother's love is considered to be stronger than any other form of love—if it cannot force a woman to relinquish her hold on substances, then there must be something wrong with the mother, and she must not really love her children. Substance dependence and love for children are not connected, and addiction is not a disease that can be cured by intense desire alone.

American society has become accustomed to alleviating woes through use of substances. Even products completely unrelated to one's happiness are associated with good feelings through the advertising industry. It is no wonder that women succumb to the use of substances ostensibly to cure them of uncomfortable conditions (pregnancy is many things, but comfortable is not one of them!). If the relationship with the substance is of longer standing than the pregnancy (and it generally is), it is highly unlikely that the pregnant woman who has relied upon the substance to alleviate discomfort, loneliness, depression, despair, or anxiety will be able to simply stop using because she has found out she is pregnant.

Prenatal Substance Abuse

Knowledge of the risks of substance use during pregnancy is relatively new. Even now, marijuana is sometimes recommended to alleviate nausea and lack of appetite associated with early pregnancy. Women have used tobacco during pregnancy for as long as the use of tobacco by women has been considered socially acceptable (and before that, in secret), and use of tranquilizers, opioids, and plant-based stimulants to control or alter feelings or behavior by women has continued into pregnancy for those women already using substances. Among pregnant women and mothers who are active in their addictions, the use of stimulants such as cocaine or methamphetamine to trigger labor is well known and is used to relieve the discomfort of late pregnancy by inducing labor.

The teratogenic effects of alcohol on the fetus are quite well documented now, however. That portion of the fetus's body (and brain) that is being formed during the time of heavy prenatal alcohol exposure is damaged by the alcohol to which it is exposed. Being a teratogen, the alcohol causes the cells in this part of the body to divide in a different order than they should, and this sometimes leads to deformities in some facial features, as well as in those parts of the body being formed at the time the alcohol is used, and in the brain of the fetus. Even today, some well-meaning physicians tell their pregnant patients that it is okay to have a drink now and then in order to remain relaxed, thinking that the stress of attempting to remain abstinent from alcohol may be more damaging to the fetus than the alcohol would be. No safe level of alcohol use during pregnancy has been established, however, and mothers can discover through specialized evaluation later in their children's lives that the difficulties that they experience may be attributed to their alcohol use during pregnancy.

Newborns who have been prenatally exposed to substances are sometimes referred to in the media as *addicted infants* or as *the littlest addicts*. This terminology is misleading in that substance-exposed newborns may be physically dependent upon a substance (and may experience mild to severe withdrawal symptoms based on the nature of the drug, the level of exposure in utero, and the knowledge base of the neonatologist working with the mother–infant dyad), but they could not be properly labeled *addicted* or *dependent upon substances* because they do not display other symptoms of chemical dependency, such as lack of control over the use of the substance or time spent in seeking the substance.

Services are available for children who were exposed prenatally to drugs, tobacco, and alcohol, although nothing can cure prenatal substance exposure. Typically, the earlier in the child's life the exposure is identified, the better the long-term prognosis for the child's ability to function normally. Mothers tell of their guilt and shame at not having been able to stop using despite knowledge of the damage being done to their unborn children. Asking for professional help with their children's developmental and behavioral problems is particularly difficult when that request must be followed by a candid disclosure of the substance use and other behaviors in which the mother engaged during her pregnancy. Despite this difficulty, the ability to alter the child's environment in order to maximize chances of success and play to the child's strengths can make the difference between the perception of failure and hopefulness for the future for both parent and child.

Trauma

A basic understanding of trauma and the role it plays in the lives of many addicted women explains much to those seeking to provide help to mothers with substance use disorders. Estimates of the prevalence of trauma in the lives of women in treatment for substance use disorders average approximately 70% or more. Sometimes women turn to substance use to numb the painful feelings or symptoms caused by the trauma, and other times, the trauma is a result of events or circumstances connected with the addiction itself. Pregnancy and childbirth, as well as motherhood (all of which are associated with increased hormonal levels and significant levels of stress), can trigger symptoms associated with past trauma. The resulting pain, anxiety, guilt, and other negative feelings lead to a sometimes overwhelming desire to use, to increase use, or to give up on sobriety. For women with histories of sexual trauma, the experience of pregnancy and childbirth can be extremely triggering due to the loss of control she experiences over her own body during this time. As the mother of a growing child, a woman may find herself experiencing flashbacks to traumatic events that took place in her own childhood as her child enters the same stage of development at which these events took place for her. If her own past victimization has not been worked through (i.e., she has not acknowledged her experiences and feelings and has not gained an understanding of the effects of her abuse upon her current view of the world and of herself), she may leave her own child vulnerable to victimization. If her inability to protect her child results in the removal of that child from her care, her guilt and feelings of powerlessness increase, as well as her sense of failure as a mother.

For a mother whose infant tests positive for substances at birth and whose resources do not allow her to retain custody of that infant, the resulting loss can be devastating as the hormones released during birth become combined with the chemicals in her brain and body driving her addiction. If the same woman has had previous experiences with children being removed from her custody at birth, each subsequent loss and repeat of this experience compounds the trauma of the previous experiences. This cycle can lead to desires to replace the "lost" children with another child, resulting in numerous substance exposed births, unless this cycle is interrupted by treatment and recovery.

For many addicted mothers, their own childhood experiences leave them without a clear sense of the role of motherhood and how this can be carried out in a healthy, structured, and nurturing manner. Many grew up in homes in which one or both of their parents had substance use disorders that were active during the time their children were growing up. The unpredictability of the environments in which many of these women grew up led to incomplete lessons in problem solving—the lack of logical association between action and punishment leads to a lack of understanding of cause and effect. Substance use is often role modeled as the most common coping or problem-solving skill to the detriment of other more effective and well thought out methods. Mothers born into families in where there is parental substance abuse also are not protected as effectively by their parents as they might otherwise be. Because of this lack, they sometimes lack skills to provide effective protection to their own children, leaving them vulnerable to neglect by the mother and/or physical or sexual harm at the hands of their parents and others.

Relationships

Women's identities are formed to a large degree by the relationships in their lives, both during childhood and as adults. For a woman with a substance use disorder, these relationships are perceived through the lens presented by the substance, which can cause significant distortions in the interactions between people. One primitive example of this distortion is the new mother who has smoked marijuana throughout her pregnancy and who continues to use during the first year of her child's life. Major neural connections are made within the infant's brain during this first year, based primarily upon interactions with the environment and the people within it. If these interactions are primarily with the mother who uses marijuana regularly, then the mother's perceptions of the child may be such that she misses important opportunities to help the child's brain develop. For example, 1-month-old infants begin to focus their eyes upon faces for the first time, and very often this focus may be on the face of the mother. If the infant gives off a facial cue or message that he or she is seeing the mother's face and the mother misses the cue, the infant will present the cue for response only a limited number of times before that cue is extinguished and the baby seeks relational interaction elsewhere, or not at all. Although this miss may not be defined as abuse or neglect under current legal definitions, the problems it presents are clear.

Relationships with partners or significant others may be affected severely by substance use disorders by the woman and/or her partner. Women with substance use disorders may be impacted by their partners' expectations of their behavior. These expectations may be very punitive toward their substance use, they may reinforce the women's continued use if substance use is something the partners engage in together, or they may involve the women's substance use disorder in divorce and child custody proceedings. Each of these different scenarios plays out in a different way, but in each case, in order to support the woman's efforts at treatment, the relationship would need to be addressed.

Treatment

In response to the advent of public fear regarding the effects of children prenatally exposed to crack cocaine on society, treatment programs have been developed specifically for women and their children together. In these programs, treatment for the mother's substance use disorder takes place along side of the delivery of services to promote health and well-being in their children. Services offered in these facilities for women include psychoeducational groups covering topics such as substances of abuse, the effects of trauma on the lives of women and children, and parenting groups. They also include more traditional addiction treatment topics, such as relapse prevention and the development of nonusing support networks in their lives. Children receive primary health care, developmental assessments and services to address any needs defined through these assessments, and socialization and play opportunities with other children. In addition, child care is frequently provided on site if the women need to leave the facility for medical appointments, to take advantage of vocational services, or to complete other portions of their treatment off site.

As the threat of involvement with the child protection system is one of the biggest fears women have about entering treatment for substance use disorders, programs such as these can help alleviate that fear and promote participation in treatment. In a controlled environment, with many professionals monitoring the safety of and care for the children there, women find it easier to work on their addictions and parenting skills together. They are more likely to retain custody of their

children in these settings than they would be if they were participating in traditional outpatient or other residential treatment that did not make provisions for the participation of children and other family members. Conversely, as the desire to parent their children well is also one of the biggest motivators for women seeking treatment, these programs can offer the services to meet that need. This paradox, embodied in every effort to engage and retain mothers in addiction treatment, is rarely resolved completely. Treatment programs for mothers with their children together are now being expanded to include the entire family as a whole, recognizing the interwoven impact of maternal substance abuse upon all members of the family.

Support Groups

The relational nature of women's growth and development throughout the life span makes women's support groups a natural component of their recovery. Either during participation in formal treatment or following its completion, women can benefit greatly from participation in recovery support groups. Traditional Twelve-Step groups are widely available, and some gender-specific meetings offer childcare for parents who need it in order to attend. One criticism that has been leveled at Alcoholics Anonymous and its offspring models such as Cocaine Anonymous and Narcotics Anonymous is that the wording of the first step is inappropriate and may be harmful for women who have histories of trauma and oppression. An alternative and women-positive model is Women for Sobriety, founded by Jean Kirkpatrick. Information regarding times and locations of upcoming meetings is kept confidential but can be obtained through contacts available on its Web site, www.womenforsobriety.org.

Conclusion

Although maternal drug use and addiction creates and is created by many social conditions including oppression, discrimination, unequal access to resources, and weak societal structure, the good news is that the relational nature of women's development lends itself well to treatment and recovery when treatment is tailored to meet their needs. Increasing attention to the unique dynamics of maternal addiction in recent years has the potential to affect the safety and well-being of many generations to come.

Karen Mooney

See also Fetal Effects of Alcohol and Other Drugs; Children of Alcoholics; Gender Issues; Violence, Intimate Partner and Substance Abuse Treatment; Women for Sobriety

Further Readings

Besharov, D. J. (Ed.). (1994). *When drug addicts have children: Reorienting child welfare's response.* Washington, DC: The Child Welfare League of America, American Enterprise Institute.

Kandall, S. R. (1996). *Substance and shadow: Women and addiction in the United States.* Cambridge, MA: Harvard University Press.

Pagliaro, A. M., & Pagliaro, L. A. (2000). *Substance use among women.* Philadelphia: Taylor & Francis.

Straussner, S. L. A., & Brown, S. (2002). *The handbook of addiction treatment for women.* San Francisco: Jossey-Bass.

MATRIX MODEL

The Matrix Model is an intensive outpatient substance abuse treatment approach designed for treating individuals who abuse or who are dependent on stimulant drugs, such as cocaine or methamphetamine. This treatment model, developed in 1986 by the Matrix Institute of Los Angeles, California, came about out of a growing need for evidence-based practices in the treatment of stimulant disorders. The Matrix Institute is a nonprofit organization established in 1984. Its purpose is to disseminate empirically based information to treatment professionals in order to improve the quality of treatment for substance use disorders. Staff from the Matrix Institute developed the Matrix Model through the assimilation of numerous empirically tested treatment approaches. The Matrix Model includes elements of cognitive behavioral therapy, relapse prevention, psychoeducation, family therapy, and Twelve-Step group support. The goal of the Matrix Model is to provide stimulant users with the skills necessary to stop using, remain in treatment, and avoid relapse. Moreover, treatment clients not only receive direction and support for themselves from a counselor, their family members are included as an integral part of the client's continued recovery.

The Matrix Model is a form of long-term outpatient therapy lasting approximately 1 year. In this approach, treatment is divided into two parts: intensive treatment and continuing care. The intensive phase of treatment includes a combination of various group sessions, family education, and individual counseling. Upon successful completion of 16 weeks of intensive treatment, the clients enter the continuing care phase. During the continuing care phase, clients continue attending social support group sessions. During these sessions, clients learn how to socialize with other clients who are further along in the program. This is a mentoring approach that allows the clients who have been in recovery longer to act as role models for newer clients. The continuing care phase lasts for 36 weeks.

Sessions

During the first 16 weeks of treatment, the clients attend several outpatient sessions per week. These sessions include individual-conjoint family sessions, which include the client, the primary counselor, and possibly the client's family. In addition to individual sessions, clients are scheduled to attend several other group sessions including early recovery skills group sessions, relapse prevention group sessions, family education group sessions, and social support group sessions. Furthermore, clients are strongly encouraged to attend Twelve-Step or mutual-help groups such as Cocaine Anonymous.

Individual-Conjoint Sessions

A primary counselor is assigned to each client. The relationship between the counselor and the client is considered essential to the therapy. The primary counselor meets with each client individually or preferably conjointly with the client and his or her family for a total of three 50-minute sessions during the first 16 weeks of treatment. The first and the last of these sessions are intended to begin and end treatment in such a way that fosters treatment engagement and transition into continuing recovery. The middle session is used to provide an assessment of client progress and to coordinate services with other referral sources if needed.

The goals of individual-conjoint sessions include (a) to give clients and their families a chance to establish rapport with the counselor and the opportunity to learn about treatment, (b) to provide a safe environment where clients can discuss issues and work out solutions with family members under counselor supervision, (c) to set aside time for clients to openly discuss their addiction with a counselor, and (d) to allow clients opportunities to receive reinforcement and encouragement for positive change.

The Matrix Model supports the inclusion of family members or other significant others in the individual-conjoint sessions whenever possible. Clients most likely do not live secluded lives. Failure to include those with whom the client has primary relationships may impede treatment success and continued recovery. Counselors using the Matrix Model are encouraged to be conscious of how client recovery interacts with and is influenced by the family system.

Early Recovery Skills Group

Early Recovery Skills (ERS) groups typically involve up to 10 clients per session and are attended by clients twice per week during the first 4 weeks of treatment. ERS sessions are facilitated by the counselor and co-led by a client. Client co-leaders in ERS groups must have a minimum of 8 weeks of abstinence from drugs and alcohol, regular attendance in relapse prevention groups and individual-conjoint sessions, and must be willing to serve as a co-leaders for at least 3 months.

Clients in ERS are relatively new to treatment and may be feeling overwhelmed and out of control; therefore, it is necessary for these sessions to remain structured. This sense of structure can help ease any out-of-control feelings the client may be experiencing and also fosters a sense of confidence in the treatment process. The purpose of ERS sessions is twofold: first, to send a message to clients that behavior change is within their control and that ERS sessions can provide strategies for change and opportunities to practice new behaviors and, second, to communicate to clients that while professional treatment may aid in providing support and information, for optimal success a client should seek out additional mutual-help or Twelve-Step groups.

The goals of ERS sessions are (a) to introduce clients to basic recovery skills in structured groups, (b) to introduce clients to mutual-help or Twelve-Step programs, (c) to aid in client adjustment to participation in group sessions, (d) to provide an opportunity for the co-leader to model early recovery behavior, and (e) to provide the co-leader a chance to increase his or her own self-esteem and reinforcement of growth.

Relapse Prevention Group

Perhaps the most fundamental of the Matrix Model groups is the relapse prevention (RP) group. Clients attend RP a total of 32 times, two times per week during the first 16 weeks of treatment. Each of these sessions lasts approximately 90 minutes and concentrates on a specific topic. Examples of the sessions covered in RP group include (a) guilt and shame, (b) work and recovery, (c) truthfulness, (d) boredom, (e) motivation for recovery, (f) sex and recovery, (g) emotional triggers, and (h) acceptance. Client co-leaders in RP must have at least 1 year of abstinence from alcohol and drugs, have completed the entire Matrix Model treatment program, be actively participating in Twelve-Step or mutual-help groups, and be willing to be a co-leader for at least 6 months.

The principals behind the RP groups are that relapse is not a random event, and it follows a predictable pattern; furthermore, signs of impending relapse are identifiable by both client and counselor. Clients showing signs of heading toward relapse can be redirected with counselor support. Additionally, clients remaining steady in recovery are provided with encouragement to stay the course.

The goals of the RP group are as follows: (a) to encourage clients to interact with others in recovery, (b) to make clients aware of the difficulties of recovery and triggers of relapse, (c) to provide clients with strategies to use in maintaining their recovery, (d) to allow clients to benefit from the recovery experiences of the co-leader, (e) to give the counselor the chance to observe the interactions of clients, and (f) to give clients the opportunity to participate in a long-term group experience.

Family Education Group

Clients attend twelve 90-minute family education groups throughout the first 16 weeks of treatment. The primary counselor is responsible for inviting their clients' family members to these groups and educates and encourages participation by both the clients and their family members. The purpose of this group is to provide a safe environment for clients and their family to learn about and become comfortable with the recovery process. Information on stimulant dependence, other substance use, treatment, and recovery is presented during these sessions. Moreover, family members are taught ways in which they can support and aid their loved one's recovery.

Social Support Group

The last and longest phase of treatment includes 36 weeks of social support group or continuing care. Clients begin social support during their last month of primary treatment and continue attending these groups one time per week for the remainder of their treatment. The purpose of the social support sessions is to enable clients to learn socialization skills that will aid in their long-term recovery. These groups are typically facilitated by the counselor, but may be led by the co-leader. Social support groups provide an excellent opportunity for the co-leader to help other clients achieve continued recovery, while also strengthening their own recovery by becoming role models. Examples of topics discussed in social support sessions include anger, commitment, cravings, depression, friendship, honesty, and spirituality.

The goals of the social support group are to (a) allow clients a safe place to practice new social skills, (b) allow coleaders to serve as role models to other clients, (c) give clients an opportunity to increase their supportive social network, and (d) provide less structured meetings for clients in order to ease them into feeling comfortable in support groups without counselor assistance.

Role of Counselor

The Matrix Model should be implemented by counselors who have several years of experience. Although the materials provided by the Matrix Institute are well ordered and comprehensible, a counselor should have well-developed counseling skills and experience with both cognitive behavioral and motivational approaches in order to use this approach. The role of the primary counselor is to be familiar with materials from each group their client may be attending and to integrate all aspects of the Matrix Model with support groups and other services the client may be receiving. In addition to facilitating substance abuse treatment, primary counselors need to be able to coordinate and remain aware of other services that clients may be receiving, including mental health, psychiatric, and vocational services. Finally, it is imperative that counselors using the Matrix Model be culturally competent and sensitive to cultural differences within their client caseload.

Materials

In an effort to protect the integrity of the Matrix Model and to allow for extensive dissemination of the approach to treatment providers, the Matrix Institute has compiled a detailed manual of the approach. The manual includes instructions for use; a counselor's treatment manual and family education manual, including a CD-ROM with PowerPoint slides; and a client's handbook and treatment companion, including worksheets that accompany therapy sessions. The counselor's treatment manual includes all materials needed for a counselor to facilitate each group session and individual-conjoint session. The materials include a description of the topics to be discussed, goals for each session, a list of client handouts, homework assignments, and additional notes for the counselor to be aware of during the sessions. All of the Matrix Model materials are available through the U.S. Department of Health and Human Services, Substance Abuse and Mental Health Services Administration (SAMHSA), Center for Substance Abuse Treatment. Electronic copies can be obtained through SAMHSA's National Clearinghouse for Alcohol and Drug Information at www.ncadi.samhsa.gov.

D. Shane Koch and S. J. Davis

See also Cognitive Behavioral Therapy; Evidence-Based Treatment; Methamphetamine; Motivational Enhancement Therapy; Treatment Approaches and Strategies

Further Readings

Center for Substance Abuse Treatment. (2006). *Counselor's treatment manual: Matrix intensive outpatient treatment for people with stimulant use disorders* (SHHS Publication No. SMS 06-4152). Rockville, MD: Substance Abuse and Mental Health Services Administration. Available from http://ncadi.samhsa.gov

Obert, J., McCann, M. J., Marinelli-Casey, P., Weiner, A., Minsky, S., Brethen, P., et al. (2000). The Matrix Model of outpatient stimulant abuse treatment: History and description. *Journal of Psychiatric Drugs, 32*(2) 157–164.

Rawson, R. A., Shoptaw, S. J., Obert, J. L., McCann, M. J., Hasson, A. L., Marinelli-Casey, P. J., et al. (1995). An intensive outpatient approach for cocaine abuse treatment: The Matrix Model. *Journal of Substance Abuse Treatment, 12*(2), 117–127.

Shoptaw, S., Rawson, R. A., McCann, M. J., & Obert, J. L. (1994). The Matrix Model of outpatient stimulant abuse treatment: Evidence of efficacy. *Journal of Addictive Diseases, 13*(4), 129–141.

MEDIA CAMPAIGNS

See NATIONAL MEDIA CAMPAIGN

MEDICAL CONSEQUENCES

The National Survey on Drug Use and Health estimated that in 2006, 20.4 million Americans ages 12 years or older used an illicit drug in the month prior to the survey. About 7 million could be classified with a substance abuse or dependence disorder in the past year. Substance abuse can be defined as a harmful pattern of drug use that results in repeated adverse consequences, such as the failure to meet social obligations or encountering legal problems. The consequences of substance abuse can and often do lead to serious medical problems for not only the individual who uses drugs but also for the society at large. Some of the negative effects can occur after using a huge quantity of drugs or after using for an extended period; while in other cases, a negative effect may occur immediately after just one use. Nevertheless, research has shown that abusing drugs can cause damage to the brain and to all other organ systems as a result of changes brought about by the direct and indirect effects of drug use.

Neurological Effects

All drugs manipulate the brain in way that results in the excessive release of chemicals, such as dopamine and serotonin, which can produce a euphoric effect within the user. But as mentioned before, most of the effects of drug use are not positive. Over time, long-term substance abuse can change the brain structure in way that eventually leads to dependence or addiction. In most instances of substance dependence, the user needs to continue using a particular substance in order to avoid experiencing withdrawal symptoms. The symptoms of withdrawal depend on the substance but can include tachycardia (increased heart rate), hypertension (high blood pressure), nausea, sweating, tremors, seizures, and visual hallucinations. In rare instances involving certain types of substances, withdrawal can lead to death. Addiction is a brain disease characterized by uncontrollable, compulsive drug craving, seeking, and use, even in the face of negative health and social consequences. So individuals addicted to drugs are not only physically dependent but also psychologically dependent as well. Once addiction sets in, the likelihood of developing some kind of medical ailment is increased. In addition to the effects listed above, changes in the brain chemistry can lead to problems with memory, attention, and more serious psychological problems such as paranoia, depression, aggression, and hallucinations. The abuse of drugs can also cause widespread brain damage, seizures, and strokes.

Cardiovascular Effects

The abuse of drugs can have a damaging effect on the cardiovascular system. Some drugs, such as cocaine, cause an increase in blood pressure and heart rate, which increases the risk of cardiac arrest and heart failure. The use of drugs can also lead to disturbances in heart rhythm. The use of inhalants has been shown to induce irregular and rapid heart rhythms, which can lead to heart failure and death within minutes of sniffing. The chronic act of injecting heroin has been known to cause bacterial infections of the blood vessels and heart valves and can lead to scarred and/or collapsed veins.

Respiratory Effects

The lungs transport oxygen from the atmosphere into the bloodstream and carbon dioxide from the bloodstream into the atmosphere. The abuse of drugs can disrupt this process in many ways. Some drugs can cause an increase in breathing that makes the lungs work harder, while others can cause breathing to slow down or can reduce the capability of the lungs to absorb oxygen. Long-term use of some drugs can also have a corrosive effect on the lung tissue, which can lead to a variety of respiratory problems such as asthma, bronchitis, and emphysema.

Gastrointestinal Effects

Using drugs can have an adverse effect on the gastrointestinal system. Some of the short-term effects of drug use on the gastrointestinal system include nausea, vomiting, severe stomach cramps, and pains. Chronic abuse of certain drugs can lead to stomach ulcers and even cancers of the gastrointestinal system.

Kidney Damage

The kidneys are responsible for cleansing the blood by filtering it of waste and toxins. Drug abuse can often lead to high levels of toxins and waste being introduced into the bloodstream. This waste can cause the kidneys to become overworked and poisoned as these organs try to rid the bloodstream of these extreme amounts of toxins and waste. This along with increases in body temperature and muscle breakdown can cause kidney damage or even failure.

Liver Damage

The liver plays a huge role in just about every process that takes place in the body and is essential in keeping the body running properly. It removes or neutralizes poisons, germs, and bacteria from the blood. It also produces bile to help the body to absorb nutrients digested by the stomach. Chronic use of some drugs, such as inhalants and steroids, can cause severe damage to the liver, which can lead to the breakdown of normal bodily functions and complete liver failure.

Musculoskeletal Effects

The use of some drugs such as steroids can signal the body to stop growing or developing earlier then they would have. This can lead to stunted growth or permanent sexual immaturity. Other drugs can cause violent muscle spasms or muscle weakness. PCP is known to cause muscle contractions, which, when severe, can result in kidney damage or failure as a consequence of muscle cells breaking down.

Hormonal Effects

Drugs such as steroids are known to have a damaging effect on normal hormone levels, causing both reversible and irreversible changes. In men, these changes can include breast formation, testicular atrophy, infertility, and male-patterned baldness. In women the abuse of steroids causes masculinization. So, females may experience a deepening of the voice, facial hair growth, a decrease in breast size and body fat, enlargement of the clitoris, and male-pattern baldness.

Indirect Effects

As shown in the previous sections, drugs of abuse can directly cause many medical problems. They can also indirectly impact the health of the user as result of the circumstances and behaviors associated with drug abuse. Different routes of administration can produce different adverse effects on the body. For instance, snorting cocaine can lead to nosebleeds, problems with swallowing, hoarseness, and an overall irritation of the nasal septum, which can lead to a chronically inflamed, runny nose.

Injecting drugs can cause blood clots, scarred and/or collapsed veins, and severe skin infections. In addition to these effects, the sharing of injection equipment or fluids increases the risk of the user acquiring some kind of infectious disease such as hepatitis (HCV) and HIV. In fact, research has shown that injection drug users (IDU) represent the highest risk group for acquiring HCV infection. It is estimated that almost 80% of new HCV infections occurring in the United States are among IDUs.

The abuse of some drugs can repress inhibitions and lead people to take risks while under the influence, such as engaging in impulsive sexual activity. This activity of course, increases the risk of contracting HIV or some other sexually transmitted disease. Drugs can also lead people to engage in other unsafe behaviors such as driving under influence or getting into a fight, which can result in injuries that require medical care.

Drug abuse can complicate the treatment of other illnesses or injuries. Research has shown that a large proportion of chronic drug abusers do not comply with their medication regimens and many do not seek proper medical care. Also, some illicit drugs are known to negatively interact with medications used for treating diseases. So, if a user continues to use an illicit drug while taking medication for a medical condition, this can cause the medication to become less effective as well as cause other adverse effects.

Societal Effects

Many of the consequences of drug abuse can have a negative impact on the health of the non-drug-abusing public. Not only are drug abusers more likely to contract HIV and other sexually transmitted diseases due to engaging in high-risk behaviors such as having unprotected sex, they also risk passing these diseases onto their sexual partners. In addition to this, many drug abusers are at greater risk for contracting other diseases such as tuberculosis (TB) if their immune system has been compromised due to various factors such as long-term drug use, inadequate nutrition, or HIV/AIDS. Furthermore, even if they do seek medical attention, many are not compliant with their treatment regimes and continue to compromise their health by using alcohol and other drugs. This has led to the development of a multidrug resistant strain (MDR) of TB that does not respond to the usual medication. Since TB is an airborne disease, the spread of TB and MDR can be rapid in crowded situations and public institutions such as hospitals or prisons, which potentially places millions of nonaddicted individuals at risk for a serious and possibly deadly disease.

Prenatal Effects

According to the National Institute on Drug Abuse, more than 5% of the 4 million women who gave birth in the United States in 1992 used illegal drugs while they were pregnant. Abusing drugs while pregnant not only harms the body of the user but also the developing fetus. The full extent of prenatal exposure to drugs is unknown because there are many factors (such as the amount and number of drugs abused, extent of prenatal care, socioeconomic conditions, maternal nutrition, and other health conditions) that can make it difficult to determine the direct impact of a particular drug on fetal and child outcomes. But it is known that abusing drugs increases the risk of miscarriage and other developmental abnormalities. Premature birth can also occur. Studies on babies born to mothers who use cocaine have shown that they are often delivered prematurely and have low birthweights. Using drugs while pregnant can also the increase the chances of the infant becoming dependent on the substance that is being abuse, which can result in the infant experiencing withdrawal symptoms after birth.

Conclusion

Substance abuse is a major problem in society today. Studies have shown that drug users have a greater risk of developing health problems than nonusers as a result of the negative effects that various drugs have on the body and other factors associated with the drug-using lifestyle. In addition, substance abuse can lead to the premature death of the user due to overdoses and drug-related accidents, homicides, and diseases. Based on estimates from a study conducted by The Lewin Group, drug abuse is one of the most costly health problems in the United States due to direct costs (health care costs associated with treating drug-related illnesses)

and indirect costs (loss of potential productivity from crime-related costs, illness, disability, or death). In 2002 alone, the overall economic cost came to about $180.9 billion, with $15.8 billion of that amount attributed to health care costs and $128.6 billion to productivity costs. Given that substance abuse is a complex and pervasive health issue, education, prevention, and treatment efforts must encompass a public-health approach in order to effectively combat this costly disease.

Stacy B. Calhoun

See also Brain Chemistry and Addiction; Fetal Effects of Alcohol and Other Drugs; Hepatitis C; High-Risk Behaviors; HIV/AIDS; Sexually Transmitted Diseases; Tuberculosis

Further Readings

Brick, J. (Ed.). (2004). *Handbook of the medical consequences of alcohol and drug abuse.* Binghamton, NY: Haworth Press.

Edlin, B. R., Kresina, T. F., Raymond, D. B., Carden, M. R., Gourevitch, M. N., Rich, J. D., et al. (2005). Overcoming barriers to prevention, care, and treatment of hepatitis C in illicit drug users. *Clinical Infectious Diseases, 40,* S276–S285.

Greenwell, L., & Brecht, M. (2003). Self-reported health status among treated methamphetamine users. *The American Journal of Drug and Alcohol Abuse, 29,* 75–104.

Khalsa, J., Francis, H., & Mazin, R. (2003). Bloodborne and sexually transmitted infections in drug abusers in the United States, Latin America, the Caribbean, and Spain. *Clinical Infectious Diseases, 37,* S331–S337.

Mertens, J. R., Lu, Y. W., Parthasarathy, S., Moore, C., & Weisner, C. (2003). Medical and psychiatric conditions of alcohol and drug treatment patients in an HMO. *Archives of Internal Medicine, 163,* 2511–2517.

Smeriglio, V. L., & Wilcox, H. C. (1999). Prenatal drug exposure and child outcome. Past, present, future. *Clinics in Perinatology, 26,* 1–16.

MEDICAL USE OF MARIJUANA

Medical marijuana (*cannabis sativa*) refers to the medically controlled use of marijuana or tetrahydrocannabinol (THC, the main psychoactive ingredient in marijuana) by patients seeking a means to address medical problems including nausea, vomiting, weight loss, multiple sclerosis, asthma, inflammation, glaucoma, poor appetite, spasticity, chronic pain, and acute pain. There is a consensus that marijuana's medical use developed first in China, spreading to India, Rome, and Greece by the 1st century and eventually reaching Europe and Africa. The use of marijuana as medicine finally spread to the European colonies in North America sometime in the 18th century.

Thus, the use of medically controlled marijuana in the United States predates the 1937 Marihuana Tax Act, which rendered cannabis illegal even with a physician's prescription. Moral crusades condemning the use of marijuana for any purpose prior to the 1937 Marihuana Tax Act and widespread illegal use of marijuana since the passage of that law contributes to the contemporary controversy over developing clinical studies to assess the efficacy of medical treatments using marijuana. Although a few states did enact legislation (primarily in the 1970s and 1980s) that allows physicians to prescribe marijuana, federal law prohibiting this practice prevents physicians from prescribing marijuana as medication. Currently, the federal government of the United States does not recognize marijuana as serving any legitimate medical function. However, some synthetic cannabinoids, for example, dronabinol, fall into the Schedule III drug category. These synthetic cannabinoids mimic some of marijuana's medical effects while costing considerably more. However, because they have a standardized dosage, regulators consider these to have a low potential for abuse.

The contemporary debate over medical marijuana consists of two opposing arguments. One side of the debate suggests that medical marijuana is unnecessary because existing drugs address all conditions that medical marijuana may ameliorate. Opponents suggest that medical marijuana is more effective and less expensive than existing legal drugs. Although in the United States medical marijuana legislation is limited to compassionate use laws in approximately 13 states, global legislation (and attitudes) toward both marijuana and medical marijuana vary greatly, and there is a social movement industry centered around marijuana use, particularly decriminalizing-legalizing the medical use of marijuana.

Contemporary Debate

Many studies conducted in the 1970s, some of which resulted in follow-up studies in the 1980s and 1990s, confirm that cannabinoid drugs are effective in treating appetite loss, glaucoma, nausea and vomiting,

pain, spasticity, and weight loss. Opponents of decriminalizing-legalizing marijuana for medical use contend that legal drugs, such as dronabinol, alleviate medical conditions as efficiently as marijuana. To this argument, supporters of medical marijuana reply that the presence of an existing treatment does not preclude developing and approving alternative treatments. For example, there is more than one drug therapy approved for the treatment of depression and more than one kind of pain medication. In addition, the legal cannabinoid drug dronabinol, which mimics the effect of marijuana, has more side effects than inhaled marijuana, costs more, takes longer for a patient to experience the beneficial effects, and presents ingestion difficulty for both vomiting patients and patients whose symptoms include throat swelling. It is also far easier for patients to control their dosage of inhaled marijuana because they can monitor their body's reactions and cease inhaling when undesirable side effects present themselves, an advantage that cannot be obtained with a dosage-standardized pill.

Almost 40 years ago, tests demonstrated that inhaled marijuana was effective in treating glaucoma by lowering pressure within the eye, thus protecting the patient from damage to the optic nerve. However, alternative treatments developed in the late 1990s are equally efficacious in safeguarding the optic nerve. Additionally, The American Academy of Ophthalmology does not promote marijuana as a safe or effective treatment for glaucoma because while marijuana may reduce intraocular pressure, at the high dosage required to treat glaucoma (8–10 per day) undesirable side effects appear.

Further research on using medical marijuana to treat glaucoma is unlikely. Though studies show that it is an effective means of reducing intraocular pressure, existing treatments protect the optic nerve as effectively without the numerous side effects of a therapeutic dosage of marijuana. However, professional organizations such as The American Academy of Ophthalmology and The National Eye Institute, while not currently endorsing medical marijuana as a glaucoma treatment, state their willingness to reconsider this position following further research.

Although case studies testing the effectiveness of inhaled marijuana on both specific and general pain, including pain induced by surgical intervention, headache, and chronic illness do exist, it is difficult to separate the actual effect of inhaled or ingested marijuana on physical pain from the expectation that inhaled marijuana produces a pain-relieving effect (the placebo effect).

Conclusions drawn from large-scale studies assessing the effectiveness of marijuana on acute pain are mixed. In one 1977 study, most respondents preferred a presurgical intervention of diazepam (antianxiety medication) or a placebo to intravenous THC prior to tooth extraction. However, at least one controlled experiment conducted in 1974 using more reliable measures of pain tolerance indicate that higher doses of THC may reduce acute pain.

One 1975 study regarding the efficacy of marijuana for treating chronic pain resulting from cancer demonstrated that chronic pain caused by cancer responds to high doses of oral THC (20 mg) and high doses of codeine (120 mg) comparably. However, researchers also concluded that the negative side effects of high-dosage oral THC were more negative than that of high-dosage codeine, including anxiety, paranoia, dizziness, and depression. However, this study utilized oral, rather than inhaled doses, which affects several factors related to the efficacy of treatment, including strength and absorption of the drug. Although it is true that the use of marijuana induces side effects, not all patients experience these effects, and indeed, some patients may prefer the side effects of marijuana use to the pain cancer causes.

In addition to treating chronic pain resulting from cancer, numerous studies demonstrate that both orally ingested and inhaled marijuana is effective in treating nausea and vomiting related to cancer treatments. Studies also demonstrated that the synthetic cannabinoids nabilone and levonantradol reduced nausea and vomiting when taken prior to treatment. The differing anti-emetic effects of inhaled marijuana, ingested marijuana, and synthetic cannabinoids warrants further research because inhaled marijuana is more cost-effective, offers patients more control overdosage, and serves as an additional drug with which to rotate patients developing tolerance to existing anti-emetics. Additionally, because medicines vary in their impact on the individual, some patients may find inhaled marijuana more effective than standard antinausea drugs. Although it is true that medically controlled marijuana does present side effects, patients may prefer these side effects to chemotherapy-induced nausea.

U.S. Legislation

The 1970 Comprehensive Drug Abuse Prevention and Control Act divided substances into categories based on their medical use and potential for addiction.

Marijuana, along with heroin, mescaline, and lysergic acid diethylamide (LSD), is a Schedule I drug, meaning that the Drug Enforcement Administration legally classifies marijuana and cannabis as (a) carrying a high potential for abuse, (b) without currently accepted medical use in the United States, and/or (c) lacking accepted safe use even with medical supervision. Even with this classification, for a brief period, the federal government allowed citizens to apply for relief from this law as part of a compassionate use program. A compassionate use exception would allow collection of data regarding the efficacy of medical marijuana; however, the federal government discontinued compassionate use exceptions in 1992 despite the increasing number of people who applied for it every year.

Since marijuana is a Schedule I drug, physicians cannot legally prescribe it, and possession of the drug can lead to large fines and/or jail time. However, the use of medical marijuana outside the United States, state legislation related to medical marijuana developed over the past 10 years, and contemporary efforts to reschedule marijuana to allow medical use provides evidence for the conflicting attitudes that characterize the current climate toward medical marijuana.

California's 1996 Compassionate Use Act (Proposition 215) states that a seriously ill Californian may use marijuana with a physician's recommendation that the patient might benefit from its use. Since 2000, legislators in Hawaii, Vermont, and Rhode Island have passed bills protecting seriously ill patients from prosecution for using marijuana as medicine. In 2007, New Mexico's legislators passed a law giving the state Department of Health a mandate to develop rules for the use and distribution of medical marijuana to patients authorized by the state. These are only some of the examples of state laws regarding medical marijuana.

A ruling in *Conant v. Walters* in 2002 found that federal authorities could not legally sanction physicians for frankly discussing medical marijuana with patients. Although the holding did not affect physicians' inability to prescribe medical marijuana, it did affirm that physicians could legally endorse or recommend the use of marijuana to patients.

Social Movements, Global Attitudes

National and international social movement organizations supporting the decriminalization or legalization of marijuana, particularly medical marijuana, continue to thrive. These social movement organizations include the Drug Policy Foundation and the Drug Policy Alliance operating in the United States, The National Organization for the Reform of Marijuana Laws operating in the United Kingdom and the United States, the European Movement for the Normalization of Drug Policy, and the International Anti-Prohibition League.

Drug laws in Western Europe vary widely from country to country. Today, in some European countries, it is a criminal offense to use medical marijuana; in some, it is a civil matter; and in a few, marijuana is completely decriminalized. Most recent legislation demonstrates a trend of moving away from harsh penalties for marijuana use and toward a harm reduction model that would allow more patients to access marijuana for medical use. In 2003, the Netherlands, continuing its trend of liberal drug policy and legislation, became the first country to enact federal regulations that allowed pharmacies to distribute medical cannabis.

In recent years, the United Kingdom moved toward harm reduction policies in its drug laws. Marijuana is decriminalized and simple possession does not result in arrest. However, in the United Kingdom, medical marijuana is not legal. This policy means that even patients using marijuana to address medical conditions are subject to verbal warnings and the confiscation of the drug. In Canada, patients may use medical marijuana if (a) they suffer from serious illness, (b) existing treatments do not provide relief for either the illness or symptoms related to treatment of the illness, and (c) the benefits offered to the patients outweigh the risks posed by use of marijuana. Mexico's drug laws are similar to the United States, and Mexico does not currently have any laws decriminalizing or legalizing medical marijuana.

Conclusion

Proponents of medical marijuana focus on the benefit of inhaling smoke rather than on ingesting pills when treating patients with nausea, as well as on the importance of developing medical alternatives for patients who fail to respond to conventional drug therapy. Current federal legislation in the United States creates difficulty for large-scale assessment of medical marijuana's effectiveness as a treatment, though older studies (primarily from the 1970s) confirm the efficacy of cannabinoids for treating a variety of maladies. Contemporaneously, following California's 1996

Proposition 215, several states enacted compassionate use laws that allow patients to use marijuana with a physician's recommendation without legal penalty. Opponents of legalizing and/or decriminalizing marijuana for medical purposes aver that existing drugs offer sufficient treatment for all medical conditions that may respond to marijuana, as well as argue that marijuana causes harmful physiological effects. Both the potential medical benefits and negative side effects created by medically controlled marijuana warrant further research.

Heather M. Griffiths

See also Cannabis Youth Treatment Study; Decriminalization; Harm Reduction, Public Health; Marijuana; War on Drugs

Further Readings

Bock, A. W. (2000). *Waiting to inhale: The politics of medical marijuana.* Santa Ana, CA: Seven Locks Press.
Earlywine, M. (2002). *Understanding marijuana: A new look at the scientific evidence.* New York: Oxford University Press.
Fisher, G. L. (2006). *Rethinking our war on drugs: Candid talk about controversial issues.* Westport, CT: Praeger.
Huggins, L. E. (Ed.). (2005). *Drug war deadlock: The policy battle continues.* Stanford, CA: Hoover Institution Press.
Joy, J. E. (1999). *Marijuana and medicine: Assessing the science base.* Washington, DC: The National Academies Press.

MENTORING

In the larger context of health and social service provision, formal treatment for substance abuse is a relative newcomer to the field, emerging only in the last several decades. Substance abuse treatment originated primarily from grassroots effort, first through churches and the temperance movement and later from the Twelve-Step movement whose genesis began with Alcoholics Anonymous in 1939. Although the first federal monies for substance abuse treatment also emerged in the 1930s in the form of funding for a program in Lexington, Kentucky, in 1935, and for a smaller program in Fort Worth, Texas, in 1938, it was not until the passage of the Narcotic Addict and Rehabilitation Act of 1966 and the Comprehensive Alcoholism Prevention and Treatment Act (Hughes Act) of 1970 that a national infrastructure began to develop to systematically address both the prevention of, and treatment for, substance dependence and alcoholism. As is often the case with grassroots origins, early leaders in substance abuse treatment were often those who had successfully overcome their own addictions. Following Twelve-Step principles of giving back to the community, treatment program graduates were often subsequently employed as substance abuse counselors and continued their career development paths upward toward senior management positions. Thus, a legacy of peer leadership and mentorship in substance abuse was born.

Changes in the Field

However, as the field of substance abuse has developed into a mainstream public health concern with regular budget allocations from the federal, state, and county governments, concomitant requirements for treatment service elements have increasingly begun to shape, monitor, and circumscribe the demands of substance abuse treatment provision. In addition, the rise of substance abuse research and clinical outcome trials in the quest for evidence-based treatment practices has also intensified the regulations placed on treatment providers in order to obtain funding from governmental block grants.

As a result of these new external demands, the specificity and nature of skills needed for successful leadership in substance abuse treatment in the 21st century is radically different from what was necessary a few short decades earlier. Not only must newly emerging substance abuse leaders be well versed in the diagnosis and treatment of addiction, but also stakeholders need to understand the interaction effects of addiction as it relates to trauma, mental illness, criminal justice, and child welfare domains. In addition, as substance abuse treatment has increasingly become corporate big business, leaders increasingly need to develop specific management skills, including but not limited to contract management; development of financial revenue from multiple and divergent funding streams; data collection, outcome monitoring, and participation in research; large property acquisition and buildings management; public policy development; and political advocacy efforts with various governmental agencies. As the culture of substance abuse codevelops from the avenues of recovery as well as from research, clinical service, and corporate business expertise, the development of new leaders via specific mentoring opportunities is crucial.

This need for mentorship is necessary not only to develop effective leaders for single-agency substance abuse prevention and treatment providers but also to mentor and grow key public health, public policy, and state and national leadership positions. Furthermore, it is essential that current field leaders, particularly those in national stakeholder positions, recognize that emergent trailblazers will be developing new models for prevention and treatment and will need to provide and allow opportunities for these new leaders to succeed.

Workforce Concerns

The need for mentoring and cultivating new leaders in substance abuse has reached a critical juncture in the last decade. Demographic data for the substance abuse workforce indicates two significant trends: first, that the average age of an employee in this field is higher than for other professions, with the mean age hovering between 45 and 50 years, and, second, that there is an excessive rate of workforce turnover, with up to 33% of employees vacating substance abuse positions annually, a rate three times higher than the national average workforce turnover of 11% across all employment fields. This workforce turnover negatively impact frontline staff positions but also key leadership roles. It has been estimated that for the 50 state directors who are responsible for all substance abuse treatment and prevention efforts for the constituents within their geographic boundaries, there is 30% turnover in these key positions every 2 years. Further complicating workforce development concerns, demographic data indicates that the ethnic distribution of substance abuse staff is not diversely represented, with a range of 70% to 90% of employees being non-Hispanic Caucasians. Another significant workforce concern is the paucity of remuneration in substance abuse, whereby compensation for work is consistently less than equivalent jobs in other social services provision, both for frontline service and senior administrative positions.

Mentorship Initiatives

Recognizing that single-agency leaders were struggling to consistently generate and cultivate the resources and structure for successful workforce development on their own, in 1993, the Addiction Technology Transfer Center (ATTC) network was created to aid in these efforts. Under the auspices of the Substance Abuse and Mental Health Services

Administration (SAMHSA), 14 regional ATTCs across the nation were developed to provide linkage to local and national resources, to facilitate collaboration between agencies, and to conduct technical assistance trainings and subsequently promote the dissemination of substance abuse prevention and treatment best practices.

Although the ATTCs demonstrated continued success in increasing the skill set of substance abuse practitioners, it became evident that in order to nurture and grow the nation's next generation of leaders would require more than informal mentoring. To achieve more effective succession planning, in October 2003, the Southern Coast ATTC implemented a pilot Leadership Institute program, which was designed to provide a more structured approach to the mentoring process.

In collaboration with the Graduate School of the U.S. Department of Agriculture, the Leadership Institute inducts mentorship protégés in a 6-month program comprising four core elements: (1) evaluation of leadership gaps and potential candidates' management interests and abilities; (2) a thorough 360-degree evaluation of strengths and weaknesses by the protégés supervisors, peers, and supervisees, resulting in developmental suggestions and an action plan; (3) participation in an intensive 5-day immersion course with a subsequent pair-matching of protégé and mentor; and (4) 6 months of ongoing experiential mentoring between protégé–mentor pairs, for a recommended minimum of 1 to 4 hours per week, culminating in the completion of a specific project designed to fulfill one of the protégé's leadership development goals.

Based on the success of this pilot project, SAMHSA's Center for Substance Abuse Treatment created the Partners for Recovery (PFR) initiative with the other ATTCs, and utilizing this model has subsequently implemented regional Leadership Institutes across the country. As of mid-2007, 354 protégés have graduated from the PFR Leadership Institutes.

Conclusion

In addition to the benefits of structured mentorship models, it is equally important to recognize and incorporate the values and successes of the field's self-help and recovery origins. Substance abuse treatment has a long history of nonhierarchical, democratic leadership from within its own. Communication in substance abuse is omnidirectional, with feedback provided not only leader to leader and leader to client but also client to client and client to leader. Despite the increasing skill set required for effective leadership, it is important to embed the strengths of historical peer leadership and recovery values within newly emergent business demands and continually developing governmental oversight. Toward that end, a culture of mentorship both within and without organizations may provide the optimal path for balancing the historical values of substance abuse treatment with the contiguous need for more business, research, and co-occurring clinical service skills.

Elke Rechberger

See also Addiction Technology Transfer Centers; Business Improvement Practices; Center for Substance Abuse Treatment; Clinical Supervision of Addiction Counselors; Substance Abuse and Mental Health Services Administration

Further Readings

Addiction Technology Transfer Center National Office, PFR/ATTC Leadership Institute: http://www.nattc .org/leaderInst/index.htm

Daigle, J. (2002). *Leadership in substance abuse treatment and recovery.* Retrieved September 8, 2007, from http://www.pfr.samhsa.gov/docs/Daigle_Leadership_ Paper_4-14-2005.pdf

Graduate School, U.S. Department of Agriculture, Leadership Development Programs: http://grad.usda.gov/index.php? option=com_content&task=view&id=188&Itemid=200

McCarty, D., & Goldman, H. H. (2005). Treatment for alcohol and drug dependence: History, workforce, organization, financing, and emerging policies. In J. H. Lowinson, P. Ruiz, R. B. Millman, & J. G. Langrod (Eds.), *Substance abuse: A comprehensive textbook* (4th ed., pp. 1346–1360). Philadelphia: Lippincott, Williams & Wilkins.

Substance Abuse and Mental Health Services Administration, Partners for Recovery. (n.d.). *Partners for recovery leadership institutes prepare future leaders in the addiction treatment field.* Retrieved September 9, 2007, from http://pfr.samhsa.gov/leadership_ institutes.html

TASC, Inc. (2004). *Leadership development in substance abuse treatment and recovery: Lessons learned and future directions.* Retrieved September 8, 2007, from http:// www.pfr.samhsa.gov/docs/Leadership_paper_TASC_4-14- 2005.pdf

METHADONE

With hundreds of thousands of people abusing heroin and other opioids such as oxycodone and hydrocodone, methadone treatment clinics are found worldwide. These clinics are intended to assist injection drug users and prescription opioid abusers from the numerous physical and mental health problems that go hand in hand with substance abuse and dependence. Although methadone has been found to be beneficial in treating heroin dependence, methadone itself has a potentially problematic addiction potential of its own. Other alternatives such as buprenorphine (Suboxone) have been developed in order to prevent such abuse from developing.

Methadone is used medicinally with management of cancer pain and other chronic pain. Indeed, physicians outside of addiction treatment facilities have very limited prescription privileges for methadone, and are generally limited to prescribing it for pain management. It is a synthetic opioid (derived from morphine) and has analgesic effects that help reduce pain. Methadone-related deaths have seen a drastic increase throughout the world since it was first developed. It is of particular note that of those who die from methadone related overdoses, the majority are prescribed methadone for pain.

Methadone is most often used in treating those with opioid addiction through licensed methadone maintenance programs. It is generally given only to a patient in a clinical setting, but on rare occasions, it will be sent home with a patient. Not only does methadone help substance abusers avoid cravings for opioids, but it also blocks the euphoric effects commonly associated with abuse and the many unwanted withdrawal symptoms associated with opioids. Although it is a highly regulated drug, it is still found sold on the streets illegally, which is one of the reasons that it is usually dispensed at a clinic and not sent home with a patient. Once sold, substance abusers will mix methadone with other drugs such as Xanax in order to get the same effect as heroin.

Methadone's effects are not as intense as that of heroin, yet they can be just as addicting. Methadone maintenance has been used for heroin addicts for years; however, the abuse of this drug has lead to increases in addiction, abuse, overdose, and death. In this instance, methadone may simply be providing substitute addiction among drug users. It is for this reason that alternative medications have been developed in order to prevent such addiction. The abuse of methadone is most likely due to concomitant increases in heroin and prescription opioid use. Also, substance abusers are turning to methadone when they cannot obtain other drugs such as heroin.

Studies indicate that the average patient in methadone maintenance can be described as a Caucasian female in her mid-30s who lives in a county with a population of over a million. Although heroin abuse is commonly found in people who enroll in methadone maintenance programs, it is also common to see prescription opioid abuse reported in these enrollees. Not only is the abuse potential high in those treated with methadone, but since it is usually given under supervision, the cost of this treatment is relatively high. This cost may deter substance abusers from entering and remaining in treatment; however, government subsidies to some facilities do allow treatment for individuals who are underinsured, uninsured, or otherwise unable to afford treatment.

Prescription drugs can sometimes be viewed as legal and more socially acceptable. Access to drugs such as methadone is relatively easy, and it is not uncommon to see it sold in much safer locations than illicit drugs such as heroin or cocaine. Prescription opioids such as methadone are sold at higher costs than heroin, and their abuse potential is most commonly found in suburban areas where access to money is not as limited as it may be in inner cities or rural areas.

Methadone Alternatives

Buprenorphine

Since the abuse potential and death rates of prescription opioid analgesics have seen an unwanted increase over the years, alternatives such as buprenorphine have been prescribed in place of methadone.

Buprenorphine was approved by the Food and Drug Administration (FDA) after numerous years of testing. The mu opioid receptors that mediate analgesia (relief from pain) are partially displaced by buprenorphine, and it has its own characteristics that are unique and set it apart from heroin and methadone. Like methadone, buprenorphine is used as an alternative in detoxification of opioid substance abusers. Although more expensive than methadone, buprenorphine has a lower rate of illicit use and has also been found to be a safer medication. Unlike heroin and methadone, once buprenorphine is discontinued, withdrawal symptoms are relatively mild and overdose risk is lower. One of buprenorphine's beneficial characteristics involves the fact that it has a high affinity for the mu receptor and helps in preventing other opioids (e.g., heroin) from binding to the receptors. Thus, if it is given to an individual who has already taken an opioid such as heroin, buprenorphine will take the place of heroin and help with symptoms of withdrawal.

Suboxone

Although buprenorphine has been found to be an effective drug in treatment for opioid addiction, there is still abuse potential, especially when buprenorphine is crushed and injected intravenously. Thus, an alternative mixture of buprenorphine and naloxone (Suboxone) has been developed in order to deter intravenous use. This buprenorphine-naloxone mixture is usually found in a 4:1 ratio and is suitable for unsupervised administration unlike methadone and buprenorphine. Overdose due to respiratory depression is less likely with Suboxone, and withdrawal symptoms are also much lower than with methadone use.

Conclusion

Although methadone is a common and widely used prescription drug in the treatment of opioid addiction, there are also many unwanted and deleterious effects associated with its use. Thus, drugs such as buprenorphine have been developed in order to help avoid the potential risks involved with opioid maintenance. Careful consideration must be taken when determining what drug is administered in opioid treatment in order to help reduce abuse and death rates due to prescription opioid addiction.

Melanie L. Gulmatico-Mullin and Chad L. Cross

See also Buprenorphine; Heroin; Methadone Maintenance Treatment; Opioids; OxyContin; Pain Management; Prescription Drugs

Further Readings

Bell, J., Byron, G., Gibon, A., & Morris, A. (2004). A pilot study of buprenorphine-naloxone combination tablet (Suboxone®) in treatment of opioid dependence. *Drug and Alcohol Review, 23*, 311–317.

Inaba, D., & Cohen, W. E. (2004). *Uppers, downers all arounders.* Ashland, OR: CNS Publications.

Jones, H. E. (2004). Practical consideration for the clinical use of buprenorphine. *Science & Practice Perspectives, 2*, 2–43.

Rosenblum, A., Parrino, M., Schnoll, S. H., Fong, C., Maxwell, C., Cleland, C. M., et al. (2007). Prescription opioid abuse among enrollees into methadone maintenance treatment. *Drug and Alcohol Dependence, 20*, 64–71.

METHADONE MAINTENANCE TREATMENT

Methadone maintenance treatment (MMT) has been the primary form of treatment for heroin addiction for many years and has been recognized as the most effective treatment for this condition by the Institute of Medicine and the National Institutes of Health. As a treatment for opioid dependence, MMT involves the daily administration of the oral opioid agonist methadone, a long-acting, orally administered drug, to replace the shorter acting heroin that is usually injected. As a maintenance medication, methadone has distinct advantages. When administered in adequate oral doses, a single dose lasts between 24 and 36 hours. Methadone is dispensed orally in different forms, which include tablets (also called diskettes), powder, and liquid. Most importantly, methadone relieves the persistent narcotic craving or hunger that is believed to be the major reason for relapse to heroin. MMT involves providing drug abusers with methadone in a clinical setting, a methadone maintenance treatment program (MMTP). In the United States alone, there are more than 1,200 MMTPs, with an estimated staff of 20,000 serving more than 220,000 patients annually. MMT is intended to do three things for patients who participate: (1) keep the patient from going into withdrawal, (2) keep the patient comfortable and free from craving street opioids, and (3) block the effects of street opioids.

The operations of a MMTP are regulated by federal and state regulations. MMTPs are staffed by physicians, physician assistants, nurses, social workers, addiction counselors, case managers, vocational counselors, HIV counselors, and administrative supervisors. The methadone dose is determined by the physician, who adjusts it according to the patient's need, withdrawal, and craving symptoms. Daily dispensing and observation of methadone, supervised urine drug screens, and other medical treatments (i.e., HIV/AIDS and hepatitis screening) are provided by nurses and physicians assistants. Clinical staff members provide individual and group counseling, case management, cognitive and behavioral treatments, and psychotherapy. The ability to provide all of these treatments in one location has made MMT the most effective treatment for opiate dependence to date.

Effectiveness

For over 30 years, methadone maintenance has been the most extensively researched form of maintenance treatment for opioid dependence in the United States. Methadone has been demonstrated repeatedly to be a safe and effective treatment with minimal side effects when used with appropriate safeguards and psychosocial services. Randomized trials have shown that methadone treatment, even with minimal counseling, is far superior to no treatment. Studies have shown that heroin users in MMT show marked reductions in illicit drug use and criminal activity and improvements in employment rates and psychological status.

Research has shown that program characteristics are critical factors in successful outcomes. The major factors in treatment retention are methadone dosage and length of time in treatment. Patients maintained on a daily dose of 60 milligrams (mg) or more had longer retention in treatment, less use of heroin and other drugs (including cocaine), and a lower incidence of HIV infection and AIDS. Other studies demonstrate the effectiveness of methadone was even greater for patients on a 70-mg dose and more pronounced for patients on 80 mg a day or more (further-reduced intravenous heroin). Studies also show that doses in excess of 100 mg a day are safe and necessary to eliminate opioid abuse and, in some cases, reduce abuse of alcohol and other drugs.

Many studies have documented a substantial reduction in criminal behavior from pretreatment behavior. Like most other factors, reduction in criminal behavior increases with length of time in treatment. This trend has been consistent throughout the almost 4 decades of methadone treatment in a variety of settings. Drug-offense arrests decline because MMT patients reduce or stop buying and using illegal drugs. Arrests decline because MMT patients no longer need to finance a costly heroin addiction and because treatment allows many patients to stabilize their lives and obtain legitimate employment. Other factors that influence retention in treatment are well-trained staff, trusting and confidential relationships between patients and program staff, clear policies and procedures, low staff turnover, high patient morale, and flexible policies for take-home methadone.

MMT is also an important point of contact with service providers and supplies an opportunity to teach drug users harm reduction techniques such as how to prevent HIV/AIDS, hepatitis, and other health problems that endanger drug users. Studies have confirmed that methadone maintenance treatment plays a crucial role in the prevention of transmission of HIV infection among injectors of heroin, reducing the risk four- to sixfold. MMT reduces the frequency of injecting and of needle sharing.

The success of methadone in reducing crime, death, disease, and drug use is well documented. Compared to the other major drug treatment modalities—inpatient detoxification, drug-free residential and outpatient treatment, and therapeutic communities—methadone is the most rigorously studied and has yielded the best results.

Special Issues of Women

Women's health care needs necessitate a better integration of medical care and addiction treatment. Most methadone clinics are unable to adequately coordinate specialty care for pregnancy, sexually transmitted diseases, and menopause, and few have reproductive health care available to women on site. As a result, most women will seek care from a prenatal care provider with limited experience caring for women on methadone, and the patient may be reluctant to disclose that she is on methadone due to negative attitudes and stigma. Nonetheless, many women view methadone treatment as the only means to obtain medical care and as a defense against losing their children to child welfare authorities. In addition, due to the aging of this population, menopause affects many women in methadone treatment. Menopausal symptoms mimic some of the effects of narcotic withdrawal and are easily confused (by both patients and practitioners) with symptoms related to improper methadone dosage. Yet little attention is currently paid to menopausal care with methadone treatment.

Additional Approaches

The system of methadone treatment in the United States has changed very little since its inception more than 30 years ago. Methadone treatment in this country remains almost exclusively based in specialized methadone treatment clinics—the only model permitted under a set of federal and state regulations in place for over 30 years. But this single model of care varies greatly in its quality and generally employs large clinics (averaging 300 patients) that, due to their large size and visibility, are often unpopular with the communities they serve. Because of the limitations of this single model and the strong local resistance to opening any new methadone clinics, fewer than 15% of opioid addicts are in MMT in the United States. Despite the increased urgency of AIDS and years of serious efforts to address opioid addiction through expanded methadone treatment, the number of enrollment slots (about 220,000 nationally) has increased very little since the 1970s.

These considerations led to renewed efforts on the part of medical and public health authorities to reform and expand methadone treatment in the United States. In 1996, the Institute of Medicine issued a series of studies and a report calling for the expansion and modification of methadone treatment, and in 1997, a National Institute of Health Consensus Conference reasserted the conceptualization of opioid addiction as a medical disorder. It called for "effective medical treatment of opiate addiction" through the reduction of misperceptions and stigma, improved medical training, assurance of greater access to methadone, and the reduction of unnecessary regulations which restrict the availability and quality of methadone treatment. The Center for Substance Abuse Treatment and the American Society of Addiction Medicine, working with the American Methadone Treatment Association, convened a task force to revise the regulations and support innovation in practice to increase treatment availability.

Medical Maintenance

The only alternative model of care that has been used in the United States is medical maintenance (MM), available to about 5,000 very-long-term patients since the 1960s. MM provides services to a highly select group, that is, private patients who are employed with several years of abstinence from illicit drugs—criteria currently met by approximately 5% to 10% of all current patients in MMTPs. In this model, physicians provide take-home methadone directly from their offices.

There have been several small demonstration projects limited to a few programs in New York, Chicago, and Baltimore in the 1980s. These produced positive results for their patients. The strict criteria for acceptance includes 5 or more years in continuous treatment, stable and verifiable employment, financial self sufficiency (all pay private fees for their treatment), and no criminal involvement or use of illegal drugs or alcohol abuse within 3 or more years. These patients are considered to be socially rehabilitated and are dispensed their medication at monthly visits to the doctor who also supplies them with 30 days of medication. Results of this approach have been excellent for these patients—with over 85% retention, little or no evidence of concurrent illicit drug use, continued employment, and good social adjustment. These outcomes are comparable or superior to those seen in usual care in methadone clinics.

In Connecticut, six community practitioners prescribed methadone to 46 patients using a MM model with monthly visits and weekly pickup from the practitioners' offices. There were a low percentage of patients who became clinically unstable during the 6-month period of the program. Patient satisfaction with the medical maintenance was very high, and the majority expressed that, if given the option, they would prefer to receive methadone maintenance in their physicians' offices.

Another model in Washington transferred 31 stable methadone patients to a unit of the outpatient medical clinic that provides their primary medical care. In this medical model, methadone is distributed through a pharmacy unit with weekly and biweekly pickup, which keeps separate records for methadone patients. Patients had the option of continuing with psychosocial services at MMTPs. The goal of the program was to implement MM outside of the experimental context that prevented previous medical maintenance programs from being replicated widely. Overall, the patients felt that they were leading a more productive life outside of treatment with some requesting decreases in their levels of methadone, but most patients requested increases (>100 mg) in order to reduce the frequency of their office visits. Clinicians learned about treating this population with a noticeable decrease in stigma. However, even with a 1-year criterion of stability, only 10% of potential patients qualified for MM with pharmacy dispensing.

Office-Based Opioid Treatment

Office-based opioid treatment (OBOT) provides medically supervised maintenance treatment for opioid dependent individuals through primary care physician practices in conjunction with community pharmacies dispensing. This model is a well-established clinical practice throughout the world with hundreds of thousands of patients in care in dozens of countries, but not in the United States. Office-based care in conjunction with community pharmacy dispensing can clearly increase access as current methadone maintenance delivery in specially licensed, centralized programs reaches only an estimated 15% of patients with opioid dependence because of limited treatment slots and geographical constraints. Greater access is needed to cope with the upsurge in heroin use and in the increasing proportion of HIV transmission resulting from injecting-drug use. This model holds appeal because it would expand methadone treatment options to rural and underserved communities, embed treatment in an environment that is less stigmatized, and integrate treatment with other health management in the United States.

A 1-year pilot demonstration study was implemented with the aim of assessing the safety, feasibility, and efficacy of a primary care; community pharmacy; and social work model for methadone maintenance treatment in an urban New Mexican community. Five medical practitioners provided continuous and comprehensive care for 12 stable (minimum 6 months of no illicit drug use) female patients. Patients met monthly with the prescribing physician for clinical review and urine toxicology. Five community pharmacists supervised the self-administration and dispensing of take-home methadone. As in MMTP, doses administered at the pharmacy were observed, but unlike most MMTPs, dosing took place in a private consultation area. A master's-level social worker coordinated all patient care and provided all psychosocial treatment and documentation according to federal and state regulations. The results suggested that properly selected, trained, and supervised medical providers and pharmacists can safely and effectively manage and dispense methadone for maintenance. This pilot supports the practice and implementation of

physicians, pharmacists, and social workers to provide community-based treatment to expand the options available for MMT in the United States.

In another pilot study, a primary care physician prescribed and a community pharmacist observed and dispensed take-home methadone to 10 stable MMTP patients in Lancaster, Pennsylvania, which, at the time of the pilot, had hundreds of heroin users but no methadone clinic. Patients met monthly with the prescribing physician (a general internist) in the office for clinical review, urine toxicology, and individual counseling. Methadone dispensing with an observed dose at each visit occurred at a family-owned, community pharmacy. Patients were followed for 24 months. This model of OBOT (one doctor, one pharmacy, and a small group of patients) allowed stable MMTP patients to be in methadone treatment in a community setting and produced clinical results equal or superior to the MMTP, at lower cost and with greater patient satisfaction.

The introduction of buprenorphine (another opioid maintenance medication similar in its action to methadone) and its FDA approval in the United States may allow this drug to be routinely employed in an OBOT model (i.e., with medications prescribed by a general or primary care physician and dispensed by community pharmacists).

Conclusion

MMT has been recognized as the most effective treatment for opioid addiction for many years. Although the benefits of MMT in reducing illicit drug use, criminal behavior, and the transmission of HIV and other communicable diseases is unquestioned, access to MMT has been limited due to stringent federal and state regulations on the dispensing of methadone. Stigma toward opioid addicts and misconceptions about MMT has contributed to the problems in changing regulations. The result has been that many communities, particularly in rural areas, have limited access to MMT, and inconvenience may prevent some opioid addicts from accessing this treatment. Recently, models of dispensing methadone through primary care settings and community-based pharmacies have yielded promising results, and a widespread application of these models would solve many of the problems of the current system of MMT.

Ellen Tuchman

See also Buprenorphine; Harm Reduction, Public Health; Heroin; Levo-Alpha Acetyl Methadol; Methadone; Needle Exchange Programs; Pharmacological Approaches to Treatment

Further Readings

Ball, J. C., & Ross, A. (1991). *The effectiveness of methadone maintenance treatment.* New York: Springer-Verlag.

D'Aunno, T., & Vaughn, T. E. (1992). Variations in methadone treatment practices: Results from a national study. *JAMA, 267,* 253–258.

Drucker, E., Rice, S., Ganse, G., Bonuck, K., & Tuchman, E. (2007). The Lancaster office based opiate treatment program: A case study and prototype for community physicians and pharmacists providing methadone maintenance treatment in the US. *Addictive Disorders and Their Treatment, 6,* 121–135.

Fiellin, D. A., O'Connor, P. A., Chawarski, M., Pakes, J. P., Pantalon, M. V., & Schottenfeld, R. S. (2001). Methadone maintenance in primary care: A randomized controlled trial. *JAMA, 286,* 1724–1731.

Joseph, H., Stancliff, S., & Langrod, J. (2000). Methadone maintenance treatment (MMT): A review of historical and clinical issues. *The Mount Sinai Journal of Medicine, 67,* 347–364.

Salsitz, E. A., Joseph, H., Frank, B., Perez, J., Richman, B. L., Salomon, N., et al. (2000). Methadone medical maintenance (MMM): Treating chronic opioid dependence in private medical practice—A summary report (1983–1998). *The Mount Sinai Journal of Medicine, 67,* 388–397.

Tuchman, E. (2003). Methadone and menopause: The aging population of women in drug treatment. *Journal of Social Work Practice in the Addictions, 3,* 14–26.

Tuchman, E., Gregory, C., Simson, J., & Drucker, E. (2006). Safety, efficacy, and feasibility of office based prescribing and community pharmacy dispensing of methadone: Results of a pilot study in New Mexico. *Journal of Addictive Disorders and Their Treatment, 5,* 43–51.

METHAMPHETAMINE

Methamphetamine production, use, and abuse are becoming widespread, affecting many Americans. Most methamphetamine production is occurring within the U.S. borders. This drug not only ruins the user's life but also has negative consequences on families, friends, communities, the environment, the government, and law enforcement agencies. Millions of tax dollars and countless man-hours must be spent each year to address control, prevention, and intervention of this devastating drug.

Methamphetamine (chemical formula $C_{10}H_{15}N$) is a synthetic central nervous system stimulant and an incredibly potent and dangerous drug. Methamphetamine is noted for its extreme toxicity and severely addictive properties. Central nervous system stimulants work by speeding up mental and physical processes within the body. Many stimulants closely resemble the chemical structure of hormones that direct the brain into an artificial fight-or-flight state. By introducing methamphetamine into the body, the user can experience a high commonly referred to as euphoria. In a methamphetamine-induced euphoric state, the user will experience elevated alertness and attention, an increase in energy, raised blood pressure, elevated heart rate, and increased respiration. Other effects may include restlessness, an irregular heart rhythm, psychotic episodes, tremors, headaches, increased impulsiveness, and aggression. When a user takes methamphetamine, it quickly enters the brain causing a rush of the neurotransmitters norepinephrine, dopamine and serotonin. Norepinephrine affects alertness and arousal. Serotonin in the brain helps control aggression and anger, sleep, appetite, and sexuality. Dopamine levels control behavior, movement, the ability to experience pleasure and pain, and the brain's motivation and reward center. The elevated level of these neurotransmitters is followed by a cascading effect as the amount released slowly diminishes.

Methamphetamine generally comes in three forms: powder, a larger crystal form, or a pill, usually by prescription. Common street names for methamphetamine include *meth, speed, crystal meth, crank, glass, shard, tweak, chalk,* and *ice.*

Methamphetamine was first synthesized in 1919 by A. Ogata, a Japanese chemist. During World War II, methamphetamine was distributed in bulk as a performance enhancer for soldiers. The overuse of methamphetamine during the war led to widespread addiction issues throughout Japan post–World War II. In the 1940s, methamphetamine was sold under the trade name Methadrine as an antidepressant and also an appetite suppressant for obesity.

Manufacturing

Some methamphetamine is produced legally according to the rules and regulations of the federal government and distributed through a prescription for certain medical conditions such as narcolepsy (frequent and uncontrollable episodes of sleep). Illegal methamphetamine, however, is produced in clandestine or *tabletop* laboratories. These labs are referred to as tabletop due to their easy portability. Lab portability is a major factor for the producers of methamphetamine, as they tend to travel frequently to avoid law enforcement and to supply their product to a large number of dealers and users.

Large-scale illegal methamphetamine labs, or superlabs, outside of the United States produce a large portion of the methamphetamine that enters the United States. Although a significant proportion of the drug is imported, the ease in obtaining the necessary components to manufacture methamphetamine is the principal reason why small-scale methamphetamine production has increased exponentially over the last several years. Methamphetamine can be produced using pseudoephedrine from cold and allergy medications as well as from other ingredients from household products such as white gasoline, muriatic acid, acetone, denatured alcohol, drain cleaner, and battery acid. Individually, each of the ingredients is legal and has a specific purpose, but when all are combined, the results are dangerous and sometimes deadly to the manufacturer, the user, and often the innocent bystander.

Although production of methamphetamine is relatively simple, the use of highly volatile and flammable chemicals makes the production of methamphetamine extremely dangerous with serious and sometimes deadly consequences. The mixture of such volatile chemicals often results in explosions of the labs and causes chemical burns to the manufacturers and those in close proximity. It is estimated that for every pound of methamphetamine produced, there may be up to 5 pounds of toxic waste that needs to be disposed. These toxic by-products of methamphetamine production are frequently dumped into freshwater ecosystems, as well as in fields, forests, and sewage systems. This influx of toxic waste has a tremendous negative effect on wildlife and water quality in the area surrounding the dump site. The toxic gases that result from methamphetamine production adhere to many surfaces inside of the lab area including carpets and walls. These tainted facilities are extremely expensive to correctly clean. Until these facilities have been cleaned, they are uninhabitable.

Routes of Administration

Methamphetamine can be introduced into the body in many ways. The principal route of administration for medical use of methamphetamine is oral intake, by swallowing a prescribed pill. In recreational methamphetamine use, however, the drug is usually smoked, snorted, injected intravenously (after being dissolved in water), or inserted into the anal cavity or urethra to be absorbed by the mucous membranes.

When smoking the drug, the methamphetamine is vaporized, or heated until the fumes are able to be inhaled. Generally speaking, inhalation is the fastest mechanism for introducing a drug to the brain, even more so than intravenous use. As with all modes of administration, injecting the methamphetamine is inherently dangerous. Injection can carry serious consequences due to the risk of disease transmission through the use and reuse of syringes. Injection is also dangerous due to the difficulty in gauging a proper dose for beginning users (see Overdosing section). What may be the proper dose for one user to achieve a desired high may not be the proper dose for another user. Dissolving the methamphetamine in water or alcohol and inserting it into the anus or urethra is said to intensify sexual pleasure, but little research has been done to investigate the validity of this method.

Short-Term Effects

There are many signs and symptoms of methamphetamine use that will be present in users. Although these effects are common, not all users will exhibit the same signs and symptoms. Methamphetamine users may experience euphoria followed by depression, paranoia, and nervousness; decreased appetite; rapid eye movement; dilated pupils; fever; excessive sweating; hallucinations; aggression; impaired speech; increased heart rate; and convulsions.

Long-Term Effects

Many of the short-term effects of methamphetamine use will continue to be present in long-term users, but chronic users tend to have more severe effects including kidney and lung disorders, brain damage, liver damage, extreme weight loss, nose bleeds, constant scratching or picking of the skin, damaged blood vessels, discolored teeth or tooth loss, paranoia, chronic hallucinations, insomnia, malnutrition, increased susceptibility to illness, stroke, and repetitive motor activity, referred to as behavioral stereotypy. Long-term use can also cause cardiovascular problems such as elevated blood pressure, rapid heart rate, and circulatory complications leading to stroke(s). Although these are some of the most common signs of long-term methamphetamine use, signs and symptoms are certainly not limited to the aforementioned.

With long-term use of methamphetamine, dependence will develop. Most addicts will develop a tolerance for the drug as well. This tolerance forces the user to increase the dosage or to change the route of administration of the drug in order to achieve the desired effects. In many cases with long-term use, the drug user will pass up food and sleep in what is known as a *binge* in order to maximize the use and effects of methamphetamine. Some users may binge for several days and go without sleep during that time.

Overdosing

Because illegal methamphetamine is produced in homemade labs and can be manufactured using different components and amounts of ingredients, the potency of methamphetamine can vary greatly from one batch to another. This inconsistency in the potency of illegal methamphetamine makes it nearly impossible to predict what will be an appropriate dose for a methamphetamine user. If users introduce more methamphetamine into their bodies than can be processed, the result is what is known as an overdose. The symptoms of a methamphetamine overdose can include sudden spike in blood pressure, abrupt rise in body temperature (externally visible through excessive sweating), convulsions, dilated pupils, rapid respiration, and collapse.

As the methamphetamine takes effect on the user's body, norepinephrine is released in the brain. Norepinephrine stimulates the heart, causing acceleration in heart rate. As the heart beats faster, the body temperature rises. The body compensates for the increase in temperature by sweating since the evaporation of sweat on the skin cools the body. After an extended period of sweating, the body lacks the fluids to produce any more sweat and becomes dehydrated. As the heart rate continues to increase, blood vessels constrict, causing limited flow of oxygenated blood throughout the body. Without proper oxygen, kidney tissue starts to deteriorate and can no longer filter the methamphetamine toxins out of the body. With the sharp increase in body temperature (hyperthermia) and a lack of circulating oxygen, muscle tissue starts to breakdown. As the muscles break down they produce proteins that are normally absorbed by the kidneys. When there is a large influx of these proteins, the kidneys cannot compensate and begin to shut down as the overdosed user goes into renal (kidney) failure.

Use During Pregnancy

The medical community believes that the use of methamphetamine by a pregnant mother places the unborn fetus at serious risk for abnormalities and developmental issues. Although it is not conclusive, research suggests that methamphetamine use during pregnancy is linked to issues in the child such as heart and circulatory problems, central nervous system abnormalities, urinary and reproductive system complications, and deformed extremities. Many studies suggest that babies exposed to methamphetamine in utero have a tendency to be asocial and have problems with motor skill development, have short attention spans, and are extremely irritable, causing them to cry more frequently and for longer periods. Methamphetamine use during pregnancy puts the mother at a higher risk for spontaneous abortions or miscarriage. Research has shown that children born to parents who use methamphetamine are at an increased risk for neglect and child abuse, in addition to an increased risk of burns and deaths from accidents and explosions in methamphetamine labs in the homes.

Legislation in the United States

Recent increases in methamphetamine production, sale, use, and arrests have led to the creation and enforcement of many new laws. Under the U.S. Controlled Substances Act, methamphetamine is listed as a Schedule II drug due to its high potential for abuse, which may lead to severe psychological or physical dependence. However, it does have some medical uses, which are limited to narcolepsy and short-term weight reduction programs. As a Schedule II drug, methamphetamine manufactured for medical use is subject to production quotas set by the U.S. Drug Enforcement Agency.

The Federal Combat Methamphetamine Epidemic Act, signed into law in March 2006, placed restrictions on the sale of over-the-counter medications containing primary ingredients used to manufacture methamphetamine such as pseudoephedrine, ephedrine, and phenylpropanolamine products. Purchasers of such products must sign in and are restricted to the purchase of no more than 9 grams of these products in any given 30-day period. In addition, under this act penalties were increased for people manufacturing methamphetamine in residences where children live.

Conclusion

With more information about the use of methamphetamine, federal government, health agencies, and community-based prevention efforts including law enforcement, social services, and educational institutions must plan effective prevention, intervention, and treatment programs to curtail this devastating problem and save lives.

Maria Theresa Wessel, Jeanne Martino-McAllister, and Bryan J. Wedel

See also Amphetamines; Central Nervous System Stimulants; Cocaine and Crack; Drugs, Classification of; Matrix Model; Public Policy, Drugs

Further Readings

Centers for Disease Control and Prevention. (2007, January). *CDC HIV/AIDS fact sheet: Methamphetamine use and risk for HIV/AIDS.* Retrieved July 12, 2007, from http://www.cdc.gov/hiv/resources/factsheets/meth.htm

National Institute on Drug Abuse. (n.d.). *Research report series: Methamphetamine abuse and addiction.* Retrieved August 3, 2007, from http://www.drugabuse.gov/ResearchReports/methamph/methamph3.html

Office of National Drug Control Policy. (2007). *Drug facts: Methamphetamine.* Retrieved July 11, 2007, from http://www.whitehousedrugpolicy.gov/drugfact/methamphetamine/index.html

Prairie View Prevention Services. (2000). *Meth use signs and symptoms. METH Awareness and Prevention Project of South Dakota.* Retrieved June 13, 2007, from http://www.mappsd.org/Signs%20&%20Symptoms.htm

U.S. Drug Enforcement Administration. (n.d.). *Methamphetamine.* Retrieved July 18, 2007, from http://www.usdoj.gov/dea/concern/meth.html

METHODS OF DRUG ADMINISTRATION

Drugs can enter the body in numerous ways. Whether a particular substance is taken for strictly medicinal purposes or for recreational purposes, no effect(s) will occur in the body unless absorption of the substance takes place. In the case of drugs of abuse (i.e., psychoactive drugs), the central nervous system will be activated in some way in order to cause the desired, and often times undesired, effect(s).

Absorption of substances can occur through either an enteral route or a parenteral route. Enteral routes include those methods that require absorption through the gastrointestinal tract (e.g., oral ingestion or rectal absorption). Enteral routes are generally safer in that the active substance may get diluted or broken down prior to reaching the bloodstream; this safety is also a disadvantage in that metabolism of the drug may result in irregular absorption, gastrointestinal discomfort, and/or dangerous metabolic breakdown products. Parenteral routes include all other forms of absorption (e.g., injection, pulmonary, or topical absorption). Parenteral routes are more rapid and eliminate gastrointestinal breakdown; unfortunately, however, the potential for overdose and infection is greatly increased.

In more general terms, there are five common ways in which chemical substances (including illicit substances) enter the body. These include inhalation of volatilized vapors, injection into the skin or bloodstream, absorption by contact with a mucous membrane, ingestion through the alimentary tract, and absorption through the dermis.

Inhalation

The most rapid and arguably the most common method of absorption of psychoactive drugs occurs via inhalation. This method can be used with any substance that can be volatilized and inhaled. Most often a substance is heated or burned until vapors are released, and then these vapors are taken into the lungs. However, vapors need not come from heated substances. Liquids can also be inhaled into the lungs using nebulizers, and any substance that can be turned into tiny droplets can be inhaled in this way. Owing to the large surface area of the alveoli of the lungs and the millions of tiny capillaries that line these alveoli, drugs that are inhaled can reach the brain in less than 10 seconds.

Medically, inhalation of drugs saves lives because the effect is so fast (e.g., *inhalers* or *puffers* used to counteract acute asthma symptoms). Alternatively, substance abusers find reprieve from withdrawal symptoms quite quickly and reach a rapid and desired high by volatilizing common substances (e.g., methamphetamine and cocaine) that have been buffered into altered compounds (e.g., *crystal meth* or *ice* and *crack cocaine*). The most commonly inhaled psychoactive substance is nicotine. An obvious negative effect of this method of use is irritation of the epithelial lining of the trachea and lungs and the potential development of cancerous lesions.

Because the effects of substances can be felt so quickly using this method, substance users often claim that they can self-regulate their intake until a desired effect is achieved. This ability is easily illustrated by a marijuana smoker who inhales one-to-two puffs or by a cigarette smoker who smokes only part of a cigarette. It should be noted, however, that self-regulation is not an exact science, and substance abusers can easily overdose via inhalation. Indeed, self-regulation via inhalation would require that the user know precisely the concentration of the active substance in the drug of choice, and it is widely known that street-grade drugs vary quite drastically in their concentration.

Injection

This parenteral route of administration is also quite rapid. For illicit drugs, a substance is injected directly into the body in one of three ways, as described below. Note, however, that in addition to those discussed, medically there are four additional injection routes generally not used by illicit drug users:

1. intrathecal—into a cavity or space,

2. intraperitoneal—into the peritoneum or visceral lining,

3. intracerebral—into the brain, and

4. intra-arterial—direct injection into the arteries.

For illicit drug users, the most rapid and most dangerous method of injection is intravenous injection (referred to as *IV* or *slamming*), wherein a user directly injects a substance into the bloodstream and feels the effect(s) in less than 30 seconds. Because a large amount of a substance enters the body at one time, a rapid and intense rush results. If a user inadvertently injects too much or obtains a substance that is of a higher quality (i.e., concentration) than normal, overdose is often a result. In fact, many substance abusers have been found deceased with a syringe still in their arm. Another route of injection is intramuscular injection (referred to as *IM* or *muscling*), wherein a user injects a substance into the muscle tissue (e.g., steroids). Since the substance must first be absorbed into muscle tissue and then into the bloodstream, effects generally are not felt for 3 to 5 minutes after injection; the large range of time here is because absorption via the muscle depends on the amount of blood flow to the region. The last route of injection is infradermal or subcutaneous injection (referred to as *ID* or *sub-Q* or *skin popping*), wherein a substance in injected just under the surface of the skin (i.e., infradermally) or just under the skin layers (i.e., subcutaneously). As with intramuscular injection, substances taken in this way must first be absorbed through tissue before entering into the bloodstream making the effects less intense and delaying the response by 3 to 5 minutes. Also, this is the leading cause of tissue necrosis in injection drug users, causing ulceration and sloughing of tissue around the injection site. Any of these routes of injection are particularly dangerous since users must use needles, greatly increasing the risk of exposure to a number of bloodborne infections (e.g., HIV, hepatitis) and dangerous adulterants and impurities.

Mucous Membranes

Absorption through the mucosal membranes is another method of drug administration. For certain substances of abuse, insufflation (referred to as *snorting*) provides a common route of exposure that results in the desired effect in 3 to 5 minutes. Insufflation allows drugs to make contact with the lining of the nasal passages, which are heavily lined by blood vessels. Consistent and persistent insufflation can permanently damage tissue and lessen the rate of absorption of psychoactive substances. In addition, the high acidic content of some substances (e.g., cocaine hydrochloride) can permanently damage and/or alter tissues.

Mucosal absorption can also be accomplished by placing a substance under the tongue (referred to as *sublingual* absorption), between the cheek and gum (referred to as *buccal* absorption), or by use of suppositories. Because mucous membranes are found throughout the body, reports of unusual drug abuse are sometimes noted (e.g., vaginal absorption). Another interesting, and very dangerous, twist to mucosal absorption gained popularity in England and involved *snorting* alcohol. Alcohol absorbed in this way can be particularly dangerous in that this toxin enters the bloodstream rapidly and undiluted since it does not first enter the alimentary system and hence avoids first-pass hepatic metabolism. In addition to snorting alcohol directly, some have experimented with vaporizing alcohol and then inhaling it into the lung tissue (as described for nebulized drugs above). Although proponents claim that the amount of alcohol consumed in this way is small, scientists and physicians warn that there is an increased risk of brain damage.

Digestion

Absorption via the alimentary tract is one of the oldest and most widely used routes of drug administration. Historically and presently, many herbal remedies are taken by drinking various steeped concoctions, and the most commonly employed way to take medications is by ingesting liquids and pills. Certainly, drugs of abuse are often taken by mouth, and alcohol, the most widely used and abused of the psychoactive substances, is primarily taken by ingestion. Most substances, with the exception of limited amounts of alcohol and barbiturates, are not absorbed directly by the stomach. Rather, most absorption takes place in the small intestines. In general, weak acids generally are absorbed more readily from the stomach and weak bases from the intestines.

Ingestion of foods and liquids can reduce and/or slow absorption in the alimentary tract. Further, the liver metabolizes ingested substances prior to their distribution to the body, and this reduces the overall effect of many substances. However, it should be noted that some substances, for example, some benzodiazepines, are metabolized into highly active metabolites by the liver. Owing to liver metabolism and relatively slow rate of digestion, absorption by the alimentary tract is upwards of 20 to 30 minutes.

Contact Absorption

The final route of absorption of psychoactive substances is by contact absorption. Many ophthalmologic drugs are administered by using eye drops because of the relatively large number of ocular capillaries. Interestingly, LSD and other illicit substances have

also been taken in this way. Another common way to absorb drugs is by direct contact with the skin (referred to as *transdermal* absorption). Commonly, medication patches (e.g., fentanyl) and nicotine patches are used to administer low-levels of substances over a long time. Because the low number of capillaries under the skin and the difficulty of getting substances through the dermis, absorption of drugs using this route can take several hours to several days. Absorption can be aided and quickened by the use of certain solvents that are readily absorbed by the skin (e.g., dimethyl sulfoxide).

Research and Summary

The National Institute on Drug Abuse provides educational materials on all drugs of abuse. As can be seen in the adapted illustration (Table 1), many drugs enter the body through multiple routes.

Other than anecdotal reporting of administrative routes of exposure that are commonly part of surveys conducted by researchers and clinicians, few studies are designed with the specific intent of providing drug use methods as reported by the substance-using population. One such study, however, does provide an interesting account of drug use. A study conducted by Carl Latkin, Amy Knowlton, and Susan Sherman consisted of interviews of nearly 1,800 individual drug users in the Baltimore area; about half of the participants were chosen to participate in the study because they reported using opioids and/or cocaine. Of the participants, 63 different patterns of use of heroin and/or cocaine were identified (e.g., heroin insufflation only, smoking crack and heroin). Indeed, simply assessing methods of drug administration can be a complex task, particularly since those who abuse or are dependent on drugs are generally associated with using multiple substances.

Conclusion

Drugs can enter the body in any number of ways. Administration of medically necessary drugs has been extensively studied over the last several centuries to find the most appropriate way to treat particular ailments. In addition, modern chemistry has resulted in more complex administration possibilities (e.g., enteric coating to reduce gastrointestinal breakdown or buffering to reduce stomach upset). Unfortunately, modern street chemistry has also kept pace with medical developments, and hence illicit

Table 1   Drugs of Abuse and Common Administrative Routes

Drug Category	Examples	Inhalation	Injection	Mucosal Absorption	Alimentary Absorption	Dermal Absorption
Cannabinoids	THC, Hashish	X			X	
Depressants	Barbiturates					
	Benzodiazepines		X	X	X	
	GHB					
Dissociative	Ketamine	X	X	X	X	
Anesthetics	Phencyclidine					
Hallucinogens	LSD, Mescaline, Psilocybin	X		X	X	
Opiates &	Morphine, Opium,	X	X	X	X	X
Opioids	Codeine, Fentanyl, Oxycodone					
Stimulants	Methamphetamine, Cocaine, MDMA, Nicotine	X	X	X	X	
Others	Steroids, Inhalants	X	X	X	X	X

Source: Adapted from National Institute on Drug Abuse. (2003). *Commonly abused drugs.* Retrieved from http://www.drugabuse.gov/DrugPages/DrugsofAbuse.html

drugs are often designed to be taken in alternative ways to increase the active dose of the drug or to decrease the absorption time into the bloodstream (e.g., smoking crack cocaine as opposed to insufflation of powder cocaine). Other unfortunate side effects of using medical routes of administration for illicit drugs include the potential of developing dangerous infections, accidental overdose because of exposure to high drug concentrations, and the spread of communicable diseases.

Chad L. Cross

See also Hepatitis C; HIV/AIDS; Intravenous Drug Use

Further Readings

Inaba, D. S., & Cohen, W. E. (2004). *Uppers, downers, all arounders: Physical and mental effects of psychoactive drugs* (5th ed.). Ashland, OR: CNS Publications.

Latkin, C. A., Knowlton, A. R., & Sherman, S. (2001). Routes of drug administration, differential affiliation, and lifestyle stability among cocaine and opiate users: Implications to HIV prevention. *Journal of Substance Abuse, 13,* 89–102.

National Institute on Drug Abuse. (2003). *Commonly abused drugs.* Retrieved from http://www.drugabuse.gov/DrugPages/DrugsofAbuse.html

MICHIGAN ALCOHOL SCREENING TEST

The Michigan Alcohol Screening Test (MAST) is a patient self-report alcoholism screening measure. The items ask individuals about a range of alcohol-related problems (e.g., Item 10: Have you gotten into fights when drinking?), the extent to which they have had diminished control over drinking (e.g., Item 4: Can you stop drinking without a struggle after one or two drinks?), and symptoms of alcohol tolerance and withdrawal (e.g., Item 19: Have you ever had delirium tremens [DTs], severe shaking, heard voices, or seen things that weren't there after heavy drinking?). Consistently, the MAST has been shown to perform well in identifying individuals who have abused alcohol or been dependent on it.

The MAST contains 25 yes or no questions that are differentially weighted. Individuals complete the MAST individually as a questionnaire or in an interview format. The measure yields an overall score ranging from 0 to 53 by summing individual items as follows: no answers get a score of 0, and yes answers get a score of 1, 2, or 5 depending on the inherent severity of the symptom covered in the item. The recommended interpretation of the total score is for 0 to 4 to indicate absence of alcoholism, 5 to 6 to suggest possible alcoholism, and 7 or more to indicate probable alcoholism. Symptoms included in the MAST are not explicitly linked to any standard diagnostic criteria for alcohol use disorders.

It takes approximately 5 minutes to administer the MAST and 2 minutes to score it. It can be scored by the administrator or by computer. No special training is required for administration. Several briefer versions of the MAST also are available. These tests include the 13-item Short MAST (SMAST), the 10-item Brief MAST, and a geriatric version called the MAST-G. All of these instruments are in the public domain and do not require permission for use.

The MAST scores have been shown to be consistent when re-administered to the same individuals over brief periods (1-day to 1-week intervals) and several months, demonstrating that the scale is reliable. The MAST also has been shown to accurately detect alcohol use disorders when checked against clinician-interview diagnoses. Different cutoff scores have been examined to yield the best combination of correctly distinguishing individuals with true alcohol use disorders from those persons who do not have drinking problems. Cutoff scores between 5 and 15 have been recommended. The MAST scores also have been shown to correspond with other measures of alcohol use severity. Notably, the originator of the MAST, Melvin Selzer, found that the 13-item SMAST was as effective as the MAST in screening for alcoholism. SMAST scores of 0 to 1 suggest no problems with alcoholism. SMAST scores of 2 point to possible alcohol use problems. SMAST scores of 3 or higher are likely to meet criteria for alcohol abuse or dependence. Selzer concluded that when time is limited, the SMAST may be substituted for the MAST.

The strengths of the MAST include that it can be administered reliably in a variety of clinical and non-clinical settings, including when used in psychiatric settings. It also provides a gross, general measure of lifetime problem severity that can be used for choosing treatment intensity and guiding further inquiry into alcohol-related problems. Because the items do not specify a time frame, however, the scale does not distinguish between current and past alcohol problems and, therefore, is not useful as a change measure. It also does not assess drinking frequency and quantity. Furthermore, because the focus is typically on late-stage symptoms of alcoholism, it may miss less severe use or patterns of use that occur earlier in the course of the illness and thus not perform as well as a screening

measure in populations where drinking patterns may vary more widely (e.g., college students). Finally, because the intent of the MAST questions is straightforward, individuals may easily disguise actual problems related to their lifetime history of drinking.

Steve Martino

See also Alcohol Use Disorders Identification Test; Inventory of Drinking Situations; Screening; Screening Instruments

Further Readings

Clements, S. (1998). A critical evaluation of several alcohol screening instruments using the CIDI-SAM as a criterion measure. *Alcoholism: Clinical and Experimental Research, 22,* 985–993.

Pokorny, A. D., Miller, B. A., & Kaplan, H. B. (1972). The brief MAST: A shortened version of the Michigan Alcoholism Screening Test. *American Journal of Psychiatry, 129,* 342–345.

Ross, H. E., Gavin, D. R., & Skinner, H. A. (1990). Diagnostic validity of the MAST and the Alcohol Dependence Scale in the assessment of DSM-III alcohol disorders. *Journal of Studies on Alcohol, 51,* 506–513.

Selzer, M. L. (1971). The Michigan Alcoholism Screening Test: The quest for a new diagnostic instrument. *American Journal of Psychiatry, 127,* 1653–1658.

Selzer, M. L., Vinokur, A., & van Roojen, L. (1975). A self-administered Michigan Alcoholism Screening Test (SMAST). *Journal of Studies on Alcohol, 36,* 117–126.

Zung, B. J. (1979). Psychometric properties of the MAST and two briefer versions. *Journal of Studies on Alcohol, 40,* 845–859.

Zung, B. J. (1982). Evaluation of the Michigan Alcoholism Screening Test (MAST) in assessing lifetime and recent problems. *Journal of Clinical Psychology, 38,* 425–439.

MINNESOTA MODEL

The Minnesota model refers to a structured treatment model for alcoholism that began in the late 1940s and early 1950s in the state of Minnesota. Today, it is the leading model for addiction treatment for many alcohol and other drug treatment centers in the United States and worldwide.

The development of the Minnesota model of treatment for alcoholism and other drug addiction arose from the confluence of a series of historical events.

This history is recounted in 1993 by Jerry Spicer, who was at the time president of the Hazelden Foundation. Three important events took place involving a small number of recovering individuals and health professionals strongly influenced by Alcoholics Anonymous (AA). These three events reflect an evolution from informal and basic Twelve-Step programs to a more formal, multidisciplinary treatment program.

The first event was the development of what would become known as Pioneer House in Minneapolis, Minnesota. Originating as a treatment center based on the Twelve-Step model and receiving its first support from the city Relief Department in 1948, this recovery program came about through the efforts of Patrick Cronin, the first documented person to recover through AA in Minnesota. He and several other persons in recovery first began an AA club that allowed people to stay over night and that subsequently developed into a treatment center. This first AA-based treatment center was eventually housed in an old stone building that had been a potato warehouse. The program was christened Pioneer House and is now owned by Hazelden and has been renamed the Hazelden Center for Youth and Families, which offers services for addicted adolescents.

Another event important to the establishment of the Minnesota model was the development of Hazelden, a private treatment program for alcoholics first funded in 1949 by a group of Minnesota businessmen on land made available by Richard Lilly who was a local entrepreneur and philanthropist. Lilly was inspired to stop drinking and to help other alcoholics when he fortuitously landed unhurt on a barge full of sand in the Mississippi River after he drove off the side of a bridge while returning home drunk. The Hazelden program in the early 1950s was organized using the principles of the AA program of recovery within a therapeutic community located in a peaceful rural setting.

The third and most important historical event was the establishment of the original philosophy and initial treatment program that would become known as the Minnesota model by two professionals at the Wilmar State Hospital. Wilmar was the only state hospital in Minnesota that was required to accept alcoholics and addicts. Nelson Bradley met Daniel Anderson at a state hospital in Hastings, Minnesota, where Bradley was staff physician and Anderson was an attendant. Later, in 1950, when Dr. Bradley was named superintendent of Wilmar State Hospital, he hired Anderson as a key staff person. At that time, the hospital housed about 1,800 mentally ill patients, including approximately 100 *inebriates* (a term that was used at the time to refer to persons whose use of alcohol or other drugs caused serious harm). These inebriates were mostly legally committed chronic, desocialized, and homeless alcoholics. Bradley and Anderson recognized that alcoholics and addicts needed a specialized program at the hospital, separate from the mentally ill patients. The first major step was hiring alcoholics as counselors who were in recovery through the Twelve-Step program for the chemically dependent clients at the hospital. This resulted in a 28-day inpatient treatment program with participation in AA and family involvement. A multidisciplinary team was put in place that included physicians, psychologists, social workers, and clergy. Anderson was later hired as director of Hazelden in 1961 and brought with him the key components of the model.

The Minnesota model, developed at Wilmar in the early 1950s, provides the perspective that alcoholism is an illness in its own right, that it is a chronic and primary disease and is in no way due to choice or volition of the afflicted individual. Analysis of the data on early program effectiveness resulted in an important assumption of the model that initial motivation for treatment is not related to outcome. Recovery rates were similar for individuals who voluntarily came for treatment and for those who entered the program as a result of court action or family pressure.

The core of the program has remained stable since its initial development. However, programs, both nationally and internationally, that adopt the Minnesota model as their central organizing structure supplement the basic model with a broad range of other compatible techniques, procedures, and services derived from contemporary clinical practice and empirically based research. Currently, numerous clinically and empirically supported approaches, such as cognitive behavioral therapy, motivational interviewing, and mindfulness meditation, are used to enhance ongoing recovery. Cognitive behavioral therapy is included to address issues such as anger, anxiety, self-pity, and other emotions that put the recovering person at risk of relapse. For example, a series of booklets for both counselors and clients, published by the Hazelden Foundation, focuses on rational-emotive behavior therapy techniques aimed at changing irrational thoughts and behaviors that are associated with increased relapse potential. Motivational interviewing and mindfulness meditation are used as means to develop meaning and significance for living beyond self-centered interests.

Programs may also provide the opportunity to use cutting-edge medications to reduce cravings or act as antagonists to the physiological effects of various chemicals. Services for coexisting psychiatric disturbances are an important recent component of many programs and are often available through coordination with mental health agencies.

The orientation remains a caring versus curing mode with emphasis on managing the illness rather than on ameliorating it. The Twelve-Step program of recovery provides the essential elements of the treatment process and allows for continuity of support following treatment through AA meetings. The major therapeutic modality of the model is group participation. Groups include a variety of educational lectures and discussions related to the disease of addiction as well as effective strategies for maintaining sobriety. Peer groups are also an important part of the program where individuals in recovery help themselves by helping others. Psychoeducational groups provide knowledge and skills applicable to addiction-related issues, such as anger, blame, resentment, anxiety, grandiosity, self-pity, or procrastination. Finally, groups for family members are important as a means to both educate significant others related to characteristics of addiction, to develop effective roles of family members to foster the recovery process, and to directly help family members whose lives have been negatively impacted by the addicted person.

Evaluation of the effectiveness of Minnesota model of treatment has been an ongoing effort since the late 1950s. In a review of research studies from 1957 through mid 1980s, Christopher Cook concluded that the model has an established research base supporting its effectiveness with the majority of clients who are treated with this model. More recent research completed by Randy Stichfield and Patricia Owens at Hazelden found that 53% of adult clients treated with this model reported abstinence at a 1-year follow-up with an additional 35% reporting reduced alcohol and other drug use. Similar findings have been published regarding the use of the model with adolescents, with 53% of teens who completed treatment reporting abstinence with minor slips over a 12-month period compared to 15% to 28% abstinence of teens who

failed to complete the program or who were on a waiting list control group. In a recent study comparing the Minnesota day clinic treatment program with traditional public psychosocial treatment, researchers in Denmark found that through a 12-month follow-up period, 35% of Minnesota day clinic patients abstained while only 20% of patients treated in the public outpatient clinic did.

Today, the Minnesota model is also known as the Hazelden model due to the Hazelden treatment center continuing the legacy of the original model through ongoing evaluation of research and the enhancement of the model with newer and more effective techniques. Scientific studies of addiction treatment conducted by The Butler Center for Research at Hazelden are made available to addiction professionals and researchers worldwide through educational programs and publications.

Clayton Shorkey and Michael Uebel

See also Alcoholics Anonymous; Evidence-Based Treatment; Recovery; Treatment of Alcohol and Drug Use Disorders; Treatment Strategies and Approaches; Twelve-Step Recovery Programs

Further Readings

Anderson, D. J. (1981). *Perspectives on treatment: The Minnesota experience.* Center City, MN: Hazelden Foundation.

Anderson, D. J., McGovern, J. P., & DuPont, R. L. (1999). The origins of the Minnesota model of addiction treatment—A first person account. *Journal of Addictive Diseases, 18,* 107–114.

Cook, C. C. H. (1988). The Minnesota model in the management of drug and alcohol dependency: Miracle, method or myth? Part II. Evidence and conclusions. *British Journal of Addiction, 83,* 735–748.

Grønbæk, M., & Nielsen, B. (2007). A randomized controlled trial of Minnesota day clinic treatment of alcoholics. *Addiction, 102,* 381–388.

Spicer, J. (1993). *The Minnesota model: The evolution of the multidisciplinary approach to addiction recovery.* Center City, MN: Hazelden Foundation.

Stinchfield, R., & Owen, P. (1998). Hazelden's model of treatment and its outcome. *Addictive Behaviors, 23,* 669–683.

Winters, K. C., Stinchfield, R. D., Opland, E., Weller, C., & Latimer, W. W. (2000). The effectiveness of the Minnesota model approach in the treatment of adolescent drug abusers. *Addiction, 95,* 601–612.

MODERATION APPROACHES TO ALCOHOL PROBLEMS

Moderation training and the concept of moderation of drinking at safe levels as a resolution of problem drinking have a long history. Although still somewhat controversial in the United States, moderation training and moderation as a goal of treatment for problem drinkers have wide acceptance in most Western European countries, as well as in Canada and Australia. Historian of addictions treatment William White has identified self-help groups whose aim was promoting moderate drinking rather than abstinence as long ago as the 1880s in the United States. These groups, however, were overwhelmed by the political power of the American Temperance Movement, which focused on abstinence as the only acceptable goal for problem drinkers, and the notion of moderation as a resolution of drinking problems did not surface systematically again in the United States and in Europe until the second half of the 20th century. In 1962, D. L. Davies reported on a series of alcohol dependent individuals who seemed to have achieved moderate drinking after years of problem drinking.

Since Davies's first report, and with the advent of behavioral and cognitive behavioral approaches to treating problem drinking, moderation training has gradually become a mainstream approach outside the United States, although still controversial among U.S. clinicians who espouse Twelve-Step approaches. Nonetheless, because research has supported their effectiveness, moderation approaches have garnered significantly more research attention and significantly more research support than virtually any other treatment approach for alcohol problems. In a 2000 paper in the *Journal of Studies on Alcohol,* Nick Heather and colleagues described behavioral self-control training (BSCT), one form of moderation-focused treatment, as perhaps the most researched single treatment modality in the alcohol problems field and as supported by the second largest number of positive studies of any treatment modality in the literature. Despite having been developed and extensively studied by William Miller and colleagues at the University of New Mexico in the United States, BSCT has been largely ignored by mainstream alcohol treatment providers. Researcher Harold Rosenberg, who has reviewed both predictive factors associated with successful moderation and the acceptance of moderation approaches by clinicians, has documented that outside the United States, moderation-focused treatments are much more widely accepted and used.

Philosophy

Moderation training approaches fall within a category of interventions that focus on harm reduction rather than on eliminating the use of the substance altogether. Harm reduction approaches, while sometimes incorporating abstinence as a goal of intervention, typically focus on other factors associated with substance use, specifically the negative consequences associated with use. In drinkers whose use of alcohol has created problems, harm reduction approaches, exemplified by moderation training, focus on helping individuals restructure their use of alcohol in ways that will minimize negative consequences associated with drinking rather than on eliminating drinking altogether. Thus, although some individuals who undergo moderation training eventually may elect to abstain from alcohol either permanently or temporarily, most enter moderation training with the goal of reducing their drinking to levels of alcohol consumption that are pleasant and create minimal negative consequences for the individual.

Approaches

Although a number of moderation training approaches have been developed over the years, only a few have been adequately tested for effectiveness. With the exception of the Behavioral Alcohol Screening and Intervention for College Students (B.A.S.I.C.S.) developed by Alan Marlatt and colleagues at the Alcohol Skills Training Program in the late 1980s, all of the most studied and validated moderation approaches were developed in the late 1970s and early 1980s. Three approaches represent the most efficacious approaches to moderation: *Drinkwise* developed at the Addiction Research Foundation in Toronto, Canada, by Martha Sanchez-Craig and colleagues; BSCT, developed by Miller and colleagues at the University of New Mexico; and Guided-Self Change developed by Linda Sobell and Mark Sobell at the Addiction Research Foundation and Nova Southeastern University. At least two other moderation focused treatments have been reported in the literature: a cue exposure program developed and studied by Heather in the United Kingdom, and the use of naltrexone as a moderation tool reported by Henry Kranzler and colleagues in the United States. Moderation-focused general treatments (which essentially are standard treatments in which the client is allowed to choose moderation instead of abstinence as their treatment goal) have been reported and studied in Sweden, Norway, Australia, New Zealand, Spain, and Canada.

Defining Moderation

One of the critical aspects of moderation training is the definition of moderation that is used in determining when and whether a client has achieved moderate drinking. There are a number of different definitions of moderation that have appeared over the decades since moderation approaches were first developed. Each approach to moderation varies slightly from the others, but all tend to focus around three characteristics: (1) a specific limit to the number of standard drinks per day that a person may consume, (2) a specific limit to the number of standard drinks a person may consume over the course of a typical week, and (3) a specific limit to the number of days in a typical week that the person may consume alcohol. Guidelines also specify different limits for men and women based on research showing distinct differences between men and women with respect to how alcohol is metabolized.

One typical definition of moderate drinking that has been adopted by the support group Moderation Management (MM) is one derived from empirical studies of the relationship between drinking and negative consequences associated with drinking by researchers at the Addiction Research Foundation in Canada and at the National Institute on Alcohol Abuse and Alcoholism. This set of guidelines specifies that for the average man, moderate drinking consists of consuming no more than four standard drinks per drinking day with no more than 4 drinking days per week and a total of no more than 16 standard drinks per week. For women, the guidelines specify no more than three drinks per drinking day with no more than 3 drinking days for a total of no more than nine drinks per week.

Another approach to defining moderate drinking is to use peak blood alcohol concentration (BAC) as the guide. Unlike the specific number of drinks limits described above, peak BAC definitions are fixed. To use the example of MM again, MM specifies a peak

BAC level of .05% as a maximum BAC that the individual may achieve and still be considered to be drinking moderately. Practically, peak BAC guidelines permit much more flexibility than do number of drinks guidelines in that the peak BAC that a specific person will achieve with a specific number of drinks varies by sex, weight, and the duration of the drinking episode. For example, for a 100-pound woman, the number of drinks she may consume and not exceed a peak BAC of .05% in a drinking episode of 4 hours is dramatically less than the number of drinks a 200-pound man may consume in the same 4 hours and not exceed a peak BAC level of .05%. The 100-pound woman may only be able to consume one or two drinks in 4 hours and remain below .05%, while the 200-pound man may be able to consume five or six drinks in the same time period and not exceed .05%.

When comparing number of drinks guidelines with peak BAC guidelines, it is clear that there is great variability in the extent to which the two sets of guidelines coordinate with each other. For a particularly heavy woman, for example, three drinks (the number of drinks considered moderate by MM for women over one drinking episode) will result in dramatically different peak BACs depending on the length of the drinking episode than the same number of drinks will for a petite woman. For this reason, most moderation training programs suggest that clients choose a metric to guide drinking and to develop a personalized set of limits that keeps both number of drinks and peak BAC within safe limits.

Clients

A recurrent question among clinicians has been to ask for which clients a moderation approach is appropriate. Concerned with both ethical and safe practice and in the context of the idea that some clients simply cannot moderate their drinking consistently over time, clinicians are frequently concerned about doing moderation training with their clients.

Research on this question has been somewhat mixed, but generally studies of the efficacy of moderation training approaches have suggested that those clients with lower levels of alcohol dependence are more likely to be able to successfully moderate their drinking over time. Nonetheless, there have been both anecdotal reports and research reports over the past decade that suggest that for more seriously dependent clients who are highly committed to moderating their drinking, moderation training may be effective. In one study by Heather, in fact, more severely dependent drinkers actually showed greater improvements on a variety of measures of drinking than did drinkers who were less alcohol dependent.

A large body of research on client choice of drinking goals in treatment (moderation or abstinence or a combination) has suggested that when clients are permitted to choose the goal of treatment, they do better regardless of whether the chosen goal is moderation or abstinence. This same body of research has also suggested that working with clients who choose moderation may in fact facilitate a shift in client goal to abstinence among clients who do not, after assessment, appear likely to become successful moderators.

At present, what can be said in response to this question is that clinicians should explain the risks of moderation approaches as well as the potential benefits but then rely upon client preference in guiding treatment in the early stages. Given that many of the skills necessary to successfully moderate one's drinking are also applicable to the maintenance of abstinence, it is likely that actively working toward moderation with virtually all clients who choose that goal will produce positive benefits (either in terms of success at moderating or the provision of strong experiential data supporting goal shift to abstinence) regardless of whether the client achieves successful moderation.

Basics of Moderation Training

The same basic principles are used throughout the various moderation training approaches. The approaches differ from each other along only two dimensions: (1) the extent to which training is coupled with ancillary social skills over and above those detailed below and (2) the extent to which training is therapist delivered versus delivered through bibliotherapy and/or a computer program.

Principles and Variations

Five basic principles are used in all moderation training approaches. These approaches are strongly client centered in the sense that client autonomy and ability to make personal decisions about drinking is recognized and reinforced. The decisions about whether or not to follow particular aspects of the training explicitly rest with the client, as does the choice of

drinking goal. Clients are assumed to be capable of making effective decisions about drinking, and the desire to moderate is not viewed as a symptom of denial or other failure of problem recognition.

Moderation approaches emphasize goal setting and commitment on the part of the client. This emphasis is consistent with research indicating that when clients are strongly committed to specific behavioral goals, they are much more likely to achieve those goals. The key conditions for eliciting commitment revolve around the clinician's respect for and reinforcement of client autonomy and decision-making capacity noted above.

Moderation approaches focus on helping clients understand and adhere to specific guidelines for how many drinks to consume on a given occasion and for how many drinking occasions are safe during a given week. Although the guidelines are specific, as discussed previously, they may be tailored to specific client goals and preferences, all with the aim of helping the client establish a safe relationship with alcohol.

Self-monitoring of either drinking behavior or urges to drink (if the client has decided to abstain in preparation for an attempt at moderation, see below) is a central component of all moderation training approaches with the exception of cue exposure and medication. Clients are taught techniques to assist them in keeping track of drinks within and across drinking episodes. It is usually suggested that clients track number of drinks per drinking day during and after the period of training and to use instances in which moderate limits were exceeded as learning situations to refine their skills at accomplishing moderation.

Even clients who are highly committed to moderation may have days that their drinking exceeds moderate limits (whether general or self-imposed). Contingency planning and tailored skills training is used to help clients cope with these instances and to use them to develop new skills. For example, a client may find that at a birthday party for an old school friend she or he drank more than the drink limit she or he had set. After examining what happened in the situation, the client concludes that she or he was more ready to accede to the urgings of the host to have another one than she or he really wanted to be. In this circumstance, training in saying no thanks gracefully and assertively might be called for to assist this client in coping with similar high-risk situations in the future. Skills training is tailored to specific client self-analyses of drinking episodes in which moderate guidelines are exceeded.

Role of Abstinence in Moderation

Some moderation training approaches suggest that a useful way for clients to begin the process of learning to moderate is to initiate a short period of abstinence, typically 30 days. During that time, several things are accomplished. First, heavy drinking clients essentially detox from alcohol and begin to experience enhanced physical well-being as a result (frequently increased energy, sounder sleep, and a general feeling of better health). Second, the client who begins self-monitoring during this abstinent period will begin to understand more clearly the conditions under which he or she used alcohol to cope rather than as a pleasurable accompaniment to meals or social gatherings. Finally, an abstinence period of 30 days reduces the individual's tolerance to alcohol. For clients who drink largely for the psychoactive effect of alcohol (the "buzz"), this may result in a greater psychoactive effect with less alcohol, thus facilitating the client's efforts to keep within moderate limits.

Personalized and Normative Feedback About Drinking

All moderation approaches make use of some form of personalized normative feedback about how the individual's drinking compares to some general standard (e.g., drinking limits or population consumption levels). One approach, Marlatt's B.A.S.I.C.S., makes use of annual brief sessions with a counselor in which the student is provided with both normative information about how much people in his or her age group actually drink (as opposed to what the individual might perceive based on observations of heavy drinking peers alone) and brief feedback about the individual's own self-reported drinking over time. Combined with minimal social skills training, this approach has been highly effective in randomized controlled trials at reducing alcohol-related harm among college student heavy episodic drinkers.

Variations in Delivery of Moderation Training

As noted above, moderation training has been delivered through several mechanisms. Which of these mechanisms is used depends largely on client preference. Many clients want to have regular face to face contact with a therapist, and moderation training may be delivered in that way. However, moderation training has also been shown to be effective with less direct therapist involvement. For example, Sobell and Sobell's guided self-change program is essentially a self-help bibliotherapy process in which written assignments are given to clients who then carry them out and check in only periodically with a therapist. Reid Hester has designed a computer administered version of behavioral self-control training, Behavioral Self-Control Training for Windows, that has been shown in a randomized controlled trial to be as effective as a therapist-delivered version of behavioral self-control training. Hester has also designed and tested an Internet-delivered version of Miller's Drinkers Checkup that has also been shown in a randomized controlled trial to be as effective as a therapist delivered version.

Conclusion

Despite their somewhat controversial nature among traditional abstinence-focused treatment providers, moderation approaches are among the demonstrably most effective approaches to helping drinkers reduce drinking-related harm that are currently available. As such, they deserve wider incorporation into treatment programs in the United States than they now enjoy. Outside the United States, where the abstinence-only, temperance-driven ideology that dominates much of alcohol treatment in the United States is less hegemonic, moderation approaches have wide acceptance among treatment providers. Moderation approaches rely on established cognitive behavioral and motivational interventions and form a group of interventions that would likely be much more acceptable to problem drinkers with milder levels of dependence than are current abstinence-focused approaches.

Frederick Rotgers

See also Blood Alcohol Concentration; Cognitive Behavioral Therapy; College Students, Alcohol Use and Abuse; Evidence-Based Treatment; Harm Reduction Psychotherapy; Moderation in Use; Moderation Management

Further Readings

Dimeff, L. A., Baer, J. S., Kivlahan, D. R., & Marlatt, G. A. (1999). *Brief alcohol screening and intervention for college students (B.A.S.I.C.S.): A harm reduction approach.* New York: Guilford Press.

Heather, N., Brodie, J., Wale, S., Wilkinson, G., Luce, A.,Webb, E., et al. (2000). A randomized controlled trial of moderation-oriented cue exposure. *Journal of Studies on Alcohol, 61,* 561–570.

Miller, W. R., & Munoz, R. F. (2004). *Controlling your drinking: Tools to make moderation work for you.* New York: Guilford Press.

Rotgers, F., Kern, M. F., & Hoeltzel, R. (2002). *Responsible drinking: A MODERATION MANAGEMENT® approach for problem drinkers.* Oakland, CA: New Harbinger.

Sanchez-Craig, M. (1996). *DrinkWise: How to quit drinking or cut down.* Toronto, ON, Canada: Addiction Research Foundation.

Sobell, M. B., & Sobell, L. C. (1987). *Moderation as a goal or outcome of treatment for alcohol problems: A dialogue.* New York: Haworth Press.

Sobell, M. B., & Sobell, L. C. (1993). *Problem drinkers: Guided self-change treatment.* New York: Guilford Press.

Sobell, M. B., & Sobell, L. C. (2005). Guided self-change model of treatment for substance use disorders. *Journal of Cognitive Psychotherapy, 19,* 199–210.

Walters, G. D. (2000). Behavioral self-control training for problem drinkers: A meta-analysis of randomized controlled studies. *Behavior Therapy, 31,* 135–149.

MODERATION IN USE

Moderation in the use of intoxicating substances generally refers to a level of use that is not accompanied by detrimental health or lifestyle outcomes. Although moderate substance use has long held a privileged position in Western society, in the past century, emphasis on moderation has decreased in favor of abstinence. Indeed, proposals that moderate use represents an appropriate, generally harmless, lifestyle choice remain controversial, especially in the United States. However, in the last 3 decades, the scientific community has come to increasingly recognize moderation as a legitimate treatment goal for some individuals with substance use related problems, particularly for those whose difficulties involve the excessive use of alcohol.

Moderation as a Lifestyle Choice

The principle of moderation in the use of intoxicating substances has been recognized since the dawn of Western civilization. The ancient Greeks listed temperance among the four central virtues, and the Old Testament counseled against drunkenness but also described alcohol as emanating from divine provenance. Indeed, an emphasis on moderation characterized Christian doctrine for several centuries, and this orientation remained largely unchallenged until the middle of the 19th century. Early critics of moderation argued that abstinence was a more exemplary stance toward alcohol use, as it presented a more robust defense against moral turpitude than did moderation. Antimoderation sentiment gained popularity throughout the latter half of the 19th and early part of the 20th century in the United States and reached its pinnacle in the ill-fated prohibition movement of the 1920s. Since the repeal of prohibition in the United States in 1933, the moderate use of alcohol has regained widespread acceptance. Indeed, the majority of adults in the United States and other Western nations enjoy alcohol in moderation.

Although moderation is a generally accepted principle in alcohol use, attitudes toward the use of other intoxicating substances continue to emphasize abstinence. The use of cannabis, which is the most widely used intoxicant after alcohol, is prohibited in most Western nations. According to the National Survey on Drug Use and Health, more than 10% or over 25 million adults in the United States report having used cannabis in the past year. These rates of use are comparable to those reported for other Western nations, and in consideration of this widespread cannabis use, several nations have reduced legal sanctions and enforcement of laws related to cannabis. The reduction of these sanctions might allow for a reevaluation of the consequences of moderate cannabis use, and for a more comprehensive determination of the feasibility of moderation with regard to this widely used intoxicant. In contrast to the increasing social leniency toward cannabis, the use of other substances such as cocaine and opioids is associated with severe sanctions in virtually all Western societies. Currently, highly punitive sociolegal attitudes toward these substances prohibit an investigation of whether these drugs may be used in moderation, since their use is inherently criminal and associated with negative consequences.

Moderation as a Treatment Goal

A proportion of individuals who use intoxicating substances experience significant deleterious outcomes and seek professional assistance in resolving their substance use problems. Trends in the treatment of substance use such as Alcoholics Anonymous and related Twelve-Step recovery programs have emphasized abstinence as a preferred goal of treatment. However, in the past several decades increasing attention has been devoted to treatments including behavioral self-control training and Moderation Management that recognize goals other than abstinence, such as controlled use and harm reduction. Importantly, these programs do not conceptualize moderation as necessarily preferable to abstinence but instead recognize that the adoption of less harmful patterns of use is a viable alternative for many individuals who seek to reduce the negative consequences associated with substance use.

There is substantial empirical support for the efficacy of moderation-based treatments for alcohol use among individuals who have not been severely dependent on alcohol. However, the extent to which moderate use is endorsed as an acceptable treatment goal varies considerably across Western nations. Surveys of Western European nations suggest that moderate drinking outcomes are endorsed by approximately 75% of treatment facilities. In contrast, moderate use goals are endorsed by slightly more than 50% of treatment providers in Canada and by fewer than 30% of providers in the United States. These differences are largely reflective of differences in the treatment cultures of the respective nations. Specifically, the prevalence of the disease model of alcoholism in North America and its reliance on former treatment recipients as treatment providers have resulted in a distrust of alternatives to abstinence. Indeed, powerlessness against alcohol is a central tenet of the disease model and provides an emotionally compelling premise for rejecting moderate use as a valid treatment aim.

Given resistance to the recognition of moderation as a valid aim of alcohol treatment in the United States, it is not surprising that treatments aimed at moderation in the use of other substances has received little support. Nonetheless, the emergence of less punitive attitudes toward substance use in Canada and Europe may be conducive to the development of moderation-based treatments for substances other than alcohol. Such treatments may provide valuable assistance to individuals who struggle with problems related to the excessive use of these substances, but the viability of moderation of use of these substances is an empirical question.

Zach Walsh and Gregory Stuart

See also Cultural Aspects; Decriminalization; Harm Reduction, Public Health; Moderation Approaches to Alcohol Problems; Moderation Management; Social Drinking

Further Readings

Iversen, L. (2005). Long-term effects of exposure to cannabis. *Current Opinion in Pharmacology, 5,* 69–72.

Saladin, M. E., & Santa Ana, E. J. (2004). Controlled drinking: More than just a controversy. *Current Opinion in Psychiatry, 17,* 175–187.

Schippers, G. M., & Nelissen, H. (2006). Working with controlled use as a goal in regular substance use outpatient treatment in Amsterdam. *Addiction Research and Theory, 14,* 51–58.

West, J. (2003). *Drinking with Calvin and Luther: A history of alcohol in the church.* Lincoln, CA: Oakdown.

MODERATION MANAGEMENT

Moderation Management (MM) is a harm reduction–focused self-help support group for problem drinkers who want to reduce or stop drinking. MM was founded in 1994 by Audrey Kishline, a housewife from Ann Arbor, Michigan, and incorporated in 1995. Relying on a strong basis in research supporting the effectiveness of moderation training approaches with problem drinkers, MM provides support in several different forms for people attempting to change their drinking habits. MM sponsors face to face meetings around the United States and maintains a number of e-mail list-serves and a variety of international online chat rooms devoted to providing support for MM members in their efforts to reduce drinking to healthy, nonharmful levels. MM also sponsors an online drinking self-monitoring program called Abstar (Abstar and other information about MM can be found on the MM Web site at www.moderation.org). MM has members in the United States, South America, and Europe.

The basic program of MM is based on cognitive behavioral moderation training approaches including William Miller and Ricardo Munoz's behavioral self-control training, and Martha Sanchez-Craig's *DrinkWise*. Drawing on these two well-researched treatments, MM holds a number of assumptions about problem drinkers and behavior change that are consistent with research in these areas. These assumptions, as listed on the MM Web site, are as follows:

- Problem drinkers should be offered a choice of behavioral change goals.
- Harmful drinking habits should be addressed at a very early stage, before problems become severe.
- Problem drinkers can make informed choices about moderation or abstinence goals based upon educational information and the experiences shared at self-help groups.
- Harm reduction is a worthwhile goal, especially when the total elimination of harm or risk is not a realistic option.
- People should not be forced to change in ways they do not choose willingly.
- Moderation is a natural part of the process from harmful drinking, whether moderation or abstinence becomes the final goal. Most individuals who are able to maintain total abstinence first attempted to reduce their drinking, unsuccessfully. Moderation programs shorten the process of discovering if moderation is a workable solution by providing concrete guidelines about the limits of moderate alcohol consumption.

MM's assumptions are further guided in their implementation by a clearly stated set of values with respect to helping people resolve problems associated with drinking. These values are also stated on the MM Web site:

- Members take personal responsibility for their own recovery from a drinking problem.
- People helping people is the strength of the organization.
- People who help others to recover also help themselves.
- Self-esteem and self-management are essential to recovery.
- Members treat each other with respect and dignity.

Two important components of the MM program are the use of empirically derived drinking limits that assist members in determining what level of drinking is likely to be safe for them, and a recommendation that members begin the process of moderating their drinking by abstaining from alcohol for up to 30 days.

MM's drinking limits are an amalgam of empirically derived drinking guidelines that have been generated over the years by researchers in both the United States and other countries. The limits, which are considered to be the maximum safe amount an individual may drink during one drinking episode, are no more than four drinks per day for males, with no more than 14 drinks in a given week, and 3 drinks per day for females, with no more than 9 drinks in given week. Members are also provided with blood alcohol concentration (BAC) charts to assist them in calculating their own level of intoxication and helping ensure that even if limits are exceeded on a given day, the member will not exceed a BAC that is safe (generally .05%).

At the beginning of moderation efforts, MM members are encouraged to abstain from all alcohol use for a period of 30 days, although shorter or longer periods are also considered helpful. There are three reasons for this recommendation, which is not a binding one or a prescription but rather a suggestion to members: (1) 30 days of abstinence help lower tolerance so when the member resumes drinking, he or she will experience greater subjective effects with fewer drinks; (2) having a period of 30 days without drinking frequently has significant benefits to the individual's health and sense of well-being with improved sleep and more energy often noted by MM members during periods of abstinence; and (3) eliminating alcohol from the member's life for a short period highlights both situations in which the member is strongly tempted to drink and helps to bring out and clarify ways in which alcohol served as a coping tool for that individual.

MM is the only self-help support group for people who want to resolve problems with alcohol that accepts any healthy change (not solely abstinence) in drinking as a positive outcome. Relying on its values and assumptions, MM promotes members' self-examination and self-regulation in ways that the member chooses and is willing to commit to pursuing. MM is a program of personal empowerment and self-efficacy that rejects the idea that alcohol problems are universally manifestations of a biologically based disease. Although MM specifically supports member efforts of moderation, studies of MM members have shown that as many as 30% pursue abstinence as their primary goal.

Research on MM conducted by Keith Humphreys and colleagues of Stanford University and Ana Kosok of Columbia University has also shown that MM attracts a disproportionately large (compared to other alcohol support groups) proportion of women, that members tend to have less severe drinking problems than people who opt for support from Alcoholics Anonymous (AA), and that MM members tend to be better educated and more affluent than the average AA member. MM members frequently state that they would never have pursued an abstinence-only program, but nonetheless, many MM members ultimately choose abstinence from alcohol as their goal. These data suggest that MM is the first large-scale personal harm reduction program to reach predominantly middle-class problem drinkers, most of whom are not alcohol dependent and for whom abstinence-only support and change programs are not only unlikely to be acceptable but avoided as well. As such, MM fills a major gap in services for problem drinkers that has been largely unaddressed in the United States.

Controversy and MM

Despite its strong empirical basis and scientific support, MM has not met with a ready reception among treatment providers in the United States. Few programs or practitioners, if any, include MM among the support groups to which their clients are referred. This reflects a continued belief in the United States that abstinence is the only acceptable resolution for alcohol-related problems and that persons seeking help for such problems must be actively induced to pursue abstinence as their goal.

This skepticism with regard to moderate drinking goals and outcomes has persisted and has been a focus of controversy surrounding MM when the group's founder, Kishline, was involved in a drunk-driving accident that resulted in two deaths in the late 1990s. Opponents of moderation approaches generally and MM in particular pointed to the program of MM as being responsible for Kishline's difficulties, despite the fact that Kishline had recognized that she was unable to moderate her drinking successfully and was attending AA meetings for several months prior to the accident. This suggestion that the attempt at moderation was responsible for Kishline's difficulties is an example of the passionate opposition to MM and moderation approaches by many within the abstinence-only community. Despite such opposition, MM has continued to grow, particularly in its Internet-based formats, and is increasingly attracting members from among people who would not seek other abstinence-only support to overcome problem drinking.

Frederick Rotgers

See also Harm Reduction Psychotherapy; Moderation Approaches to Alcohol Problems; Moderation in Use; Natural Recovery; Peer Recovery Support Services

Further Readings

Kishline, A. (1994). *Moderate drinking: The Moderation Management™ guide for people who want to reduce their drinking.* New York: Crown Trade Paperbacks.

Miller, W. R., & Munoz, R. (2006). *Controlling your drinking.* New York: Guilford Press.

Moderation Management. (2007). *What is Moderation Management?* Retrieved April 5, 2007 from http://www.moderation.org/whatisMM.shtml

Rotgers, F., Kern, M. F., & Hoeltzel, R. (2002). *Responsible drinking: A MODERATION MANAGEMENT™ approach for problem drinkers.* Oakland, CA: New Harbinger.

MONITORING THE FUTURE

Monitoring the Future (MTF), started in 1975, is a large-scale, long-term study of American youths, college students, and adults through age 45. The study grew out of an increasing concern regarding the health risks of both legal and illegal substance use during adolescence. Illegal drugs emerged from specific youth subcultures to the general adolescent population in the 1960s and have remained a national concern ever since. In order to adequately understand and respond to adolescent substance use, it became obvious that reliable and valid data were needed. For more than 30 years now, the MTF has gathered data that assesses the prevalence and trends of adolescent substance use and has impacted many policy and intervention efforts to curb adolescent substance use.

Since the study's inception, significant changes have occurred regarding the use of and attitudes toward most of the licit and illicit substances investigated in the survey. Among those changes, for example, is the almost incessant emergence of new drugs and alterations of known substances. Thanks to the continuous collection and reporting of self-report data, the MTF has successfully mapped the changing landscape of substance use and its contributing factors among American adolescents and young adults.

The study is conducted by the University of Michigan's Institute for Social Research and has been funded continuously by a number of investigator-initiated research grants from the National Institute on Drug Abuse. Principal Investigators are Lloyd D. Johnston, Jerald G. Bachman (both are Research Professors and Distinguished Research Scientists at the University of Michigan's Institute for Social Research), Patrick M. O'Malley (Research Professor at the University of Michigan's Institute for Social Research), John E. Schulenberg (Research Professor at the University of Michigan's Institute for Social Research and Center for Human Growth and Development and Professor of Developmental Psychology in the Department of Psychology), and John M. Wallace, Jr. (Associate Professor at the University of Pittsburgh's School of Social Work, Visiting Associate Professor at the University of Michigan's School of Social Work, and a Faculty Associate at the Institute for Social Research).

Study Design and Methods

Goals and Purposes

The underlying rationale for undertaking the MTF study was the belief that the hidden behavior at issue was in need of systematic research and reporting. During the 1960s, adolescent substance use had become more widespread with no indication that use would disappear in the future. The original survey included only self-reports from high school seniors. The age range was subsequently increased to include younger students to account for the fact that the onset of substance use typically takes place during early adolescence. In addition, the researchers argued it was important to survey those adolescents who drop out of school before graduation.

The MTF has 11 key objectives. At the top of the list is the assessment of prevalence and trends in substance use as well as the determination of causal factors contributing to adolescents' use of licit and illicit substances. Furthermore, among other goals, the study seeks to (a) determine risk factors for various patterns of drug use, (b) gain insight into the lifestyles and values inherent in different substance use patterns, (c) examine differences and similarities between different subgroups of adolescent users and nonusers, (d) analyze which social environmental factors contribute to or protect adolescents from substance use, (e) assess the impact of major life transitions (e.g., college, employment, marriage,

pregnancy) on substance use patterns, (f) determine and evaluate age and cohort effects, (g) examine potential consequences of substance use, and (h) investigate trends in multiple substance use.

Sampling and Field Procedures

To achieve the study's objectives, a team of researchers collect extensive data from nationally representative samples of 8th, 10th, and 12th graders. In addition, yearly follow-up surveys are carried out with representative samples of high school seniors until they reach age 30. After that, additional data from those young adults is collected every 5 years. The 2007 wave was the 33rd survey of high school seniors, the 28th of college students, and the 17th survey of 8th and 10th graders in the series.

To date, the study includes between 44,000 and 50,000 secondary school students. About 420 public and private high schools and middle schools participate in the project. For each of the targeted grade levels, data are collected for about 15,000 to 17,000 students. The follow-up surveys include about 8,000 college students and young adults between 19 and 30 years of age.

Data collection takes place during the springtime. A multistage random sampling design is used where geographic areas are selected first, followed by the determination of schools in each selected area, and finally, individual classes in each of the schools. Any resulting unequal probabilities of selection are corrected with sampling weights procedures during the analysis stage.

Parental consent is mandatory for participation in the study. Prior to data collection, parents receive information about the study along with a consent form. However, even with parental consent, participation in the study is voluntary. The survey instrument is administered during a regular class in the students' classroom. Self-report are anonymous for the two lower grade levels, and confidential for high school seniors. Respondents are randomly assigned to fill out one of six questionnaires. Each version of the questionnaire contains a set of core questions about the respondent's background and substance use, as well as different subsets of various categories of questions. In total, there are approximately 1,400 to 1,500 variables across the various survey instruments. Surveys for 8th and 10th graders contain fewer questions.

Key Measures

The core questions of the study relate to substance use. The following drugs are included in the questionnaire: alcohol, tobacco, marijuana-hashish, inhalants, nitrites, hallucinogens (LSD separately), PCP, MDMA (i.e., *ecstasy*), cocaine, crack, heroin, OxyContin, Vicodin, amphetamines, Ritalin (methylphenidate), methamphetamine, crystal methamphetamine (i.e., *ice*), sedatives (barbiturates), Quaaludes (methaqualone), tranquilizers, Rohypnol, GHB (gamma hydroxybutyrate), ketamine, and steroids.

With the exception of tobacco, a set of questions about the frequency of use is asked to determine past-month, past-year, and lifetime usage levels for the various drugs. For cigarettes, questions cover only past-month use. In addition to the regular alcohol use measure, students are asked about the frequency of getting drunk and about drinking five or more drinks in a row (binge drinking). Information on substance use is augmented by questions about age of onset, likelihood of future use, perceived availability of drugs, exposure to drugs, experience of feeling high, perception of the harmfulness of drugs, disapproval of drug use, and attitudes about legalization of drugs. Besides reporting their personal attitudes, students are asked how they think their parents and peers feel about drug use.

A second set of key measures includes questions about respondents' background and demographics (e.g., respondents' sex, race-ethnicity, college plans, residential information, and parental education). Information about the respondents' family situation is collected as well. The survey further covers questions about a series of deviant and delinquent behaviors (e.g., theft, vandalism, drunk driving, and carrying weapons to school), incidents of victimization, deviance proneness (e.g., self-esteem, self-control, and risk-taking tendency), and attitudes toward various issues (e.g., religion, sex roles, ecology, and major social institutions).

Long-Term Trends and Recent Findings

According to reports from the MTF study, the 1990s marked some important changes in the drug-using behavior of adolescents. As risk perceptions and disapproval decreased, the use of illicit substances increased significantly for all three grade levels in the first half of the decade.

In 1997 through 1998, use began to decline for the first time in 6 years. Although numbers dropped significantly for 8th graders during the following years, use among 10th and 12th graders seemed to just level off. In 2002 and 2003, overall use of illicit substances finally dropped significantly among the older age cohorts. Unfortunately, the most recent waves of data indicate that the long-term decline may be coming to an end.

Marijuana

Marijuana, the most commonly used illicit drug among adolescents and young adults, experienced a surge in the early 1990s until 1997 for middle and high school students. More specifically, annual prevalence rates for 8th graders jumped from 6% to 18%, while those for 10th graders more than doubled (from 15% to 35%). Use among high school seniors also rose significantly (from 22% to 39%), albeit not as extremely as in the younger cohorts. Interestingly, rates for college students and young adults were fairly stable during that period. Because of this discrepancy, researchers argue that the changes in consumption behavior witnessed during the 1990s reflect cohort effects rather than broad secular trends. Beginning in 1997, annual prevalence began to slowly decline for 8th graders and modest declines for 10th and 12th grades started 1 year later. The downward trend is still ongoing, though not statistically significant.

A reliable indicator for changes in use has been the measure of perceived risk. Parallel to increases in use, perceived risk of marijuana fell during the late 1970s and again in the 1990s. Disapproval of marijuana use dropped significantly in the 1990s, but has increased some in recent years.

Tobacco

Similar to the overall rate of illicit substance use mentioned above, rates of current cigarette smoking among 8th- and 10th-grade students increased by approximately 50% during the early 1990s. The upward trend halted in 1996 and declined in the following years, but recently the rate held steady, indicating a halt to the long-term decline in current smoking among these adolescents. Long-term trends for current smoking among high school seniors nearly parallel those of the younger cohorts, albeit with a 1-year time lag. Data from college students and young adults did not evidence declines in the smoking rate until after 1999 and 2004, respectively. Data indicate a clear cohort effect for cigarette use.

According to most recent data, 3% of 8th graders, 7% of 10th graders, 12% of high school seniors, 9% of college students, and 19% of young adults qualify as current smokers. Adolescents most commonly pick up smoking between sixth and ninth grade.

Risk perceptions of smoking decreased between 1993 and 1995, followed by a significant increase until 2000. Since then, data shows a leveling off in perceived risk associated with a pack-a-day smoking. Disapproval of smoking declined in the first half of the 1990s until 1996, when it began to steadily increase.

Alcohol

The majority of survey respondents report experience with alcohol. Approximately 39% of eighth-grade students reported having tried alcohol, compared with 62% of 10th graders. By the time students graduate from high school, 72% have used alcohol. Finally, 85% of college students had had at least one drink in their lifetime. Long-term trends in alcohol use indicate slight declines in drinking among all three grade levels between 1991 and 1995, followed by an upward shift until 1996 to 1997 that corresponds to the trend of increased use of illicit substances during that same period. Since then, more downward drifts materialized, with a significant decrease in drinking after 2002.

More concerning than simply trying alcohol, however, are figures on occasional heavy drinking episodes (five or more drinks in a row at least once in the prior 2 weeks). After gradual increases for all grades in the early 1990s, rates began to decline in the second half of the decade. In 2007, 10% of 8th graders, 22% of 10th graders, and 26% of 12th graders reported heavy drinking. Heavy drinking typically peaks in the early 20s, as evidenced by the 40% of college students who reported engaging in such drinking behavior. Self-reports of having been drunk in the past month have followed a very comparable pattern for all three grades.

Long-term data from the MTF thus evidences that trends and patterns of alcohol use show more similarities with illicit drug use than differences.

Gender Differences

Overall, males are more likely to use both licit and illicit substances than females. Gender differences are rare and fairly insignificant among the youngest age cohorts. Younger females show slightly higher rates of use only for inhalants and amphetamines. Although males of all ages drink more and drink more often, the gender gap has been decreasing, as is the case for gender differences in use of other substances.

Tanja C. Link

See also Adolescents, Substance Abuse and Treatment; Behavioral Risk Factor Surveillance System; College Students, Drug Use and Abuse; National Epidemiologic Survey on Alcohol and Related Conditions; National Survey on Drug Use and Health; National Institute on Drug Abuse; Underage Drinking

Further Readings

Bachman, J. G., Johnston, L. D., O'Malley, P. M., & Schulenberg, J. E. (2006). *The Monitoring the Future project after thirty-two years: Design and procedures* (Monitoring the Future Occasional Paper No. 64) [Electronic version]. Ann Arbor, MI: Institute for Social Research. Available at http://monitoringthefuture.org

Johnston, L. D., O'Malley, P. M., Bachman, J. G., & Schulenberg, J. E. (2006). *The aims and objectives of the Monitoring the Future study and progress toward fulfilling them as of 2006.* (Monitoring the Future Occasional Paper No. 65) [Electronic version]. Ann Arbor, MI: Institute for Social Research. Available from http://monitoringthefuture.org

Johnston, L. D., O'Malley, P. M., Bachman, J. G., & Schulenberg, J. E. (2007). *Demographic subgroup trends for various licit and illicit drugs, 1975–2008.* (Monitoring the Future Occasional Paper No. 67) [Electronic version]. Ann Arbor, MI: Institute for Social Research. Available from http://monitoringthefuture.org

Johnston, L. D., O'Malley, P. M., Bachman, J. G., & Schulenberg, J. E. (2007). *Monitoring the Future national survey results on drug use, 1975–2006: Vol. 1. Secondary school students* (NIH Publication No. 07-6205). Bethesda, MD: National Institute on Drug Abuse. Available from http://monitoringthefuture.org

MORAL MODEL

For several hundred years, conceptions of tobacco, alcohol, and drug dependence have been based on incongruent beliefs involving moral judgments and medical considerations. To this day, neither set of beliefs has supplanted the other. As a result, in the general population there is much disagreement and confusion about the nature of addiction and how to best address problems involving substance abuse. These conflicting views are at the center of the ongoing debate about public policies on tobacco, alcohol, and other drug abuse prevention and treatment. The moral model can be considered the philosophical foundation of much of the U.S. federal drug control policy and the so-called War on Drugs.

Features of the Model

In the moral model, addiction represents a refusal to abide by some ethical or moral code of conduct. Excessive drinking or drug use is considered freely chosen behavior that is at best irresponsible and at worst evil. This conception of addiction does not require one to equate addiction with the sinfulness of committing rape, larceny, or murder. Nevertheless, in this view addiction is seen as misbehavior because substance use is thought to be freely chosen conduct. Persons who are dependent upon a substance are not considered to have experienced a loss of control. Instead, they are seen as selfish and hedonistic and personally responsible for creating suffering for themselves and others. Therefore, they are blameworthy and the justified targets of punishment and are thought to deserve the health and medical problems, employment problems, and legal sanctions that they encounter. Furthermore, punishment is perceived to be a viable and credible means of deterring further involvement in substance use and abuse. Relapse is generally considered evidence of lingering evil that needs to be suppressed with the threat of further sanctions.

In American culture, the moral model of addiction has long been the guiding conceptual framework of politically conservative groups, law enforcement organizations, and some zealous religious communities. Also, U.S. politicians have been known to appeal to this sentiment by proposing tougher legal penalties for possession and distribution of illicit drugs, underage drinking, and for alcohol-impaired driving. Unfortunately, U.S. history is marked by failed government efforts to eliminate addiction via criminal legislation and law enforcement actions. The crackdown on Chinese opium smokers in the 1800s and the enactment of Prohibition in the early 20th century stand as two noteworthy examples.

Disease Models

To fully understand the conceptual underpinnings of the moral model, it is necessary to contrast them with those of the disease models of addiction. In the latter view, substance use and abuse is seen through a different lens—it is considered to be a disease process. Persons who are dependent upon a drug are thought to be suffering from an underlying disease process that causes compulsive use. In other words, the high rate and volume of use are merely the manifest symptoms of a latent or less apparent illness. The exact nature of the illness is not fully understood at this point, but many proponents of the disease models believe that it has genetic origins. For these reasons, it is hypothesized that individuals cannot smoke, drink, or drug themselves into addiction. If the disease (possibly arising from a genetic vulnerability) is not present, then a dependency will not usually develop.

The addiction-as-a-disease conception maintains that the alcoholic and addict are victims of an illness. The afflicted individual is not evil or irresponsible, just sick. Thus, it is believed that substance abuse is not freely chosen; rather, the excessive smoking, drinking, or drugging is seen to be beyond the control of the sufferer. In fact, a common feature of the disease conceptions is believed to be the loss of control over substance use. It is hypothesized that once an addict has consumed a small amount of a drug, intense cravings are triggered via physiological mechanisms, and these cravings lead to compulsive overuse. This mechanism is beyond the personal control of the addict.

Since drug-dependent persons are seen as suffering from an illness, the logical conclusion is that they deserve compassionate care, help, and treatment. Because the condition is considered a disease, medically supervised treatment is thought to be legitimate. Clearly, the acceptance and rise of the disease model of addiction over the past 50 years or so has been responsible for the allocation of resources to help individuals with substance abuse problems. Without the advent of the disease models, it is likely that there would be little, if any, assistance available to substance abusers in the United States today.

There are also a number of disadvantages to the disease models. Several of the key concepts of these models have not held up under scientific scrutiny. For example, the loss-of-control hypothesis, the supposedly progressive course of alcoholism, and the belief that a return to controlled drinking is impossible are all propositions that have been seriously challenged by scientific investigations.

Supreme Court Decision of 1988

In 1988, the U.S. Supreme Court weighed in on the controversy surrounding the two competing definitions of alcoholism. In a 4-to-3 ruling on a narrow issue, the court concluded that the Veterans Administration had the authority to define some types of alcoholism as a willful misconduct rather than as a disease in determining eligibility for specific veteran benefits. Writing for the majority, Justice Byron R. White indicated that the court was not deciding whether alcoholism was a disease, but instead was upholding the authority of the Veteran's Administration to make decisions about the treatment of a disorder that, according to medical research, is not fully understood. The majority opinion stated that under these circumstances, it was reasonable for the Veteran's Administration to identify alcoholism as willful misconduct.

Behavioral Science Theories

In addition to the moral model and the disease models, there are number of other conceptual frameworks that arise out the social and behavioral sciences that provide a distinct perspective on the nature of addiction and how to address these problems. The position of some in the social and behavioral sciences is that addiction is a learned pattern of behavior shaped by the same laws that shape all human behavior. Essentially, then, addiction is learned. It is neither sinful (as the moral model purports) nor out of control (as the disease models purport). Instead, it is seen as a problem behavior that is clearly under the control of environmental, family, social, and/or even cognitive contingencies. As in the disease models, the person with an addiction problem is seen as a victim—not a victim of a disease, but a victim of destructive learning conditions. For the most part, addictive behavior is not freely chosen, although some behavioral science theories (e.g., social learning theory) do assert that addicts retain some degree of control over their drinking or drug use.

It is important to understand the value placed upon objectivity in the behavioral sciences. When alcoholism (or addiction) is described as a maladaptive behavior, this description is very different from describing the condition as misbehavior (the moral model). Behavioral scientists avoid passing judgment on the rightness or wrongness of substance abuse. By maladaptive, the behavioral scientist means that the behavior pattern has destructive consequences for addicts and/or their families (and possibly society). It does not imply that the addicts are bad or irresponsible.

In this behavioral science view, the most appropriate interventions are based on learning principles and definitely not on punishment as advocated by the moral model. Typically, clients are taught skills to prevent relapse. The medical aspects of treatment are attended to when necessary, but they are generally deemphasized. Interventions based on behavioral science theory are labor intensive and evaluation focused. Though these characteristics are consistent with today's emphases on efficiency and accountability, many prevention and treatment programs are slow to adopt this kind of empirical approach because of inadequate resources and training opportunities.

Conclusion

The moral model will not fade in importance because it has several advantages over those perspectives that embrace disease conceptions or other theories. One advantage of the moral model is that it is straightforward and clear. There is little ambiguity or murkiness associated with this viewpoint. Furthermore, it is absolute; there is no need for theorizing or philosophizing about the nature of addiction. Addiction is thought to simply be wrong behavior that needs to be confronted and addressed with punishment. Scientific investigation of the problem is believed to be unnecessary because that which must be done to correct it (i.e., provision of punishment) is already well understood. In this view, our society's inability to adequately address substance abuse problems reflects a widespread moral decay and the decline of conservative, family-based values.

Nevertheless, the moral model also has several weaknesses. First, science suggests that tobacco, alcohol, and other drug dependencies are anything but a simple phenomena. They appear to be multifactorial in origin, stemming from pharmacological, biological, psychological, and social factors. The apparent complexity of addiction is underscored by the variety of diverse theories seeking to explain it. Moreover, as science has begun to shed light on various aspects of compulsive substance use and abuse, it has become clearer that much still remains to be learned. The genetic vulnerability hypothesis, alcohol expectancy theory, and the purported stabilizing effects of alcoholism on family structure are all cases in point.

Another disadvantage with the moral point of view is that it is not at all clear that these dependencies are freely chosen. The various disease models of addiction maintain that exactly the opposite is the case. That is, excessive drinking or drugging represents a loss of control that is considered a chief symptom of an underlying disease process. A further point of departure is offered by the behavioral sciences, where, at least in several theoretical perspectives, a high rate of drug self-administration is understood to be under the control of social or environmental contingencies. These contingencies are usually external to alcoholics or addicts and are not under their personal control. Thus, both the disease models and the behavioral sciences challenge the notion that addiction is willful misconduct.

A third disadvantage with the addiction-as-sin position is that history suggests that punishment is an ineffective means of reducing the prevalence of addictive problems in the population. Aside from the possibility of inhumane sanctions, a reasonably strong case can be made, based upon historical precedents, that striking back at substance abusers via governmental authority simply does not work over an extended period of time. Law enforcement crackdowns often have the unintended effects of being an impetus for strengthening organized crime networks, creating underground markets, bolstering disrespect for the law, clogging court dockets, and overloading prison systems with inmates convicted of drug crimes.

Dennis L. Thombs

See also Coercion and Treatment; Crime and Substance Abuse; Disease Concept; Decriminalization; Legalization of Drugs; Psychological Model of Addiction; Social Learning Model of Addiction Behaviors; Sociocultural Models of Addiction; War on Drugs

Further Readings

Conrad, P. (1992). Medicalization and social control. *Annual Review of Sociology, 18,* 209–232.

Conrad, P., & Schneider, J. W. (1992). *Deviance and medicalization: From badness to sickness.* Philadelphia: Temple University Press.

Cox, W. M. (1985). Personality correlates of substance abuse. In M. Galizio & S. A. Maisto (Eds.), *Determinants of substance abuse: Biological, psychological, environmental factors* (chap. 7). New York: Plenum Press.

Des Jarlais, D. C. (2000). Prospects for a public health perspective on psychoactive drug use. *American Journal of Public Health, 90*(3), 335–337.

Peele, S. (1985). *The meaning of addiction: Compulsive experience and its interpretation.* Lexington, MA: D.C. Heath.

Thombs, D. L. (2006). *Introduction to addictive behaviors* (3rd ed.). New York: Guilford Press.

Torres, S. (1997). An effective supervision strategy for substance-abusing offenders. *Federal Probation, 61*(2), 38–44.

Yalisove, D. (1998). The origins and evolution of the disease concept of treatment. *Journal of Studies on Alcohol, 59,* 469–476.

MORPHINE

Morphine is an opioid that acts directly on the central nervous system to relieve pain. Morphine, in effect, mimics our endogenous opioids. Morphine also produces sleepiness, mood alteration (euphoria or dysphoria), reduced gastrointestinal motility, diminished respiration, peripheral vasodilatation, and pupil contraction. Morphine can be administered through injection, orally, by inhalation, through rectal suppositories, and is available in capsules and in extended-release tablets. Some chronic pain patients have an implanted morphine pump. Morphine is also used for epidural injections. Morphine is the only opioid that has been approved by the Food and Drug Administration for intrathecal administration. Morphine crosses the placenta and has been found in breast milk. Morphine is contraindicated for use in patients with acute alcoholism, delirium tremens, convulsive disorders, acute pancreatitis, renal failure, bronchial asthma, and head injury.

Morphine is a derivative of the juice of the opium poppy, *Papaver somniferum.* By weight, morphine constitutes about 10% of opium, the coagulated juice of the poppy plant. Since pure morphine is not very water soluble, morphine is generally produced as a morphine sulfate, an odorless white crystalline powder that darkens with exposure to light.

In about 1805, Friedrich Wilhelm Serturner, a German pharmacist, was the first to isolate and identify the organic alkaloid compound, morphine, from the gum resin excreted from the opium poppy. Serturner used hot water to extract the opium and then used ammonia to precipitate out the bitter crystalline morphine. This research set the stage for the identification of other alkaloids, such as strychnine in 1818, caffeine in 1821, and nicotine in 1828. Serturner named his new substance morphium after the Greek god of dreams, Morpheus. By the 1820s, morphine was available from pharmaceutical companies and other sources across Western Europe. By the 1850s, the development of hypodermic syringes with hollow pointed needles by Francis Rynd and Charles Pravaz permitted the widespread administration of morphine. Morphine was initially used as a cure for opium addiction, as well as for its analgesic and antitussive effects. Like many other drugs, morphine became hailed as a panacea soon after its introduction. The regular use of morphine by soldiers during and after the U.S. Civil War, as well as the subsequent Franco-Prussian War in Europe, led to morphine addiction being known as the *soldier's disease*. During the 19th century, morphine was commonly used in remedies for assorted conditions, including headaches, diarrhea, menstrual pains, and colic. Morphine was thought to be a useful cure for alcoholism, even though it was known to be addictive. Physicians and others considered alcoholism to be worse than morphine addiction. It was regularly included in an array of patent medicines and could also be ordered by mail. Growing public concern with this accessibility led to the passage of the Pure Food and Drug Act in 1906 and then to the Harrison Narcotic Act in 1914. An unintended effect of the Harrison Narcotic Act was the closure of the few drug treatment programs then available. Ironically, heroin was introduced to treat morphine addiction. Heroin is metabolized into morphine by the removal of the acetyl groups.

Morphine is a highly effective painkiller. It is commonly prescribed for the relief of severe pain, such as that associated with surgery or cancer. Side effects of morphine include nausea, vomiting, constipation, blurred vision, lethargy, and respiratory suppression. The effects of morphine are generally potentiated by alkaline substance and antagonized by acidic substances. The analgesic effects are potentiated by melatonin, methocarbamol, and chlorpromazine.

Morphine is a highly addictive substance, with tolerance and dependence developing rapidly. The direct analgesic effect of morphine appears to become attenuated over the history of use. Successive administration of the drug appears to elicit a compensatory learned hyperalgesic response leading to tolerance. This process seems to be a combination of the conditioned association to the rituals accompanying use as well as to the systemic effects of the substance. Overdose is possible, resulting in depressed respiration, constriction of the pupils, cold and clammy skin, stupor or coma, sometimes accompanied by drop in a blood pressure and slowed heart rate. The effects of morphine can be countered by the use of opioid antagonists, such as naltrexone or naloxone. Methadone and buprenorphine have been used to treat morphine addiction. Clonidine (Catapres) can be used for relief of withdrawal symptoms. Rapid detoxification has been attempted through joint administration of clonidine and naloxone. Levo-alpha acetyl mehadol (i.e., LAAM) and naltrexone, a longer acting opioid antagonist, can be given to prevent relapse. The half-life of morphine is between 1.5 and 4.5 hours. Morphine is eliminated primarily through renal excretion.

Physical dependence to morphine results in moderate to severe withdrawal symptoms in those who suddenly stop using the drug. Signs of withdrawal can include restlessness, drippy nose, teary eyes, sweating, yawning, gooseflesh, and sleep disturbance during the first 24 hours, with other symptoms becoming more severe over the next 72 hours including extreme irritability; anxiety; nausea; spasms and twitching of muscles; abdominal, leg, and back pains; hot and cold flashes; diarrhea; vomiting; and insomnia. Although extremely uncomfortable, the symptoms of withdrawal are not physically dangerous in otherwise healthy individuals. However, it is important to maintain appropriate fluid and electrolyte balance during the abstinence syndrome. Withdrawal treatment is primarily supportive and concerned with symptom relief.

Morphine sulfate is marketed under names such as MS-Contin, Infumorph, Roxanol, Duramorph, Oramorph, and MSIR. In the United States, morphine is classified legally under the Controlled Substances Act (21 U.S.C. 801–886) of the Comprehensive Drug Abuse and Prevention Act 1970 as a Schedule II drug by the Drug Enforcement Agency (DEA Number 9300). Schedule II drugs have a high potential for severe dependence but can be medically useful, such is clearly the case with morphine. Internationally, morphine is listed as a Schedule I drug under the Single Convention on Narcotic Drugs.

Victor B. Stolberg

See also Buprenorphine; Heroin; Methadone; Naloxone; Naltrexone; Opioids; Pain Management

Further Readings

Hamilton, G. R., & Baskett, T. F. (2000). In the arms of Morpheus, the development of morphine for postoperartive pain relief. *Canadian Journal of Anaesthesia, 47,* 367–374.

Schmitz, R. (1985). Friedrich Wilhelm Serturner and the discovery of morphine. *Pharmacy in History, 27,* 61–74.

Siegel, S. (1977). Morphine tolerance acquisition as an associative process. *Journal of Experimental Psychology: Animal Behavior Process, 3,* 1–13.

Motivational Enhancement Therapy

Motivational Enhancement Therapy (MET) is a counseling approach that combines motivational interviewing (MI) and personalized feedback of assessment results. This intervention can be applied to a wide variety of behavioral domains but originated in the area of addictions and has been most widely applied to individuals with alcoholism and substance use disorders. MET was developed and tested empirically in a format that involved an assessment of factors related to the early effects of alcohol and a 1-hour review of results in a MI consistent style. Although the term *Motivational Enhancement Therapy* was first used to describe the treatment approach used in Project MATCH (described further in this entry), it has broadened to signify the combination of MI and feedback within any clinical or research context. In fact, the first application of MET occurred before its implementation in Project MATCH, and many trials since Project MATCH have used the approach. Since its inception, MET has been tested in a variety of clinical trials and among populations with varying substance abuse issues. The intervention is generally effective, although there is high variability in its effect.

Motivational Interviewing

MI is therapeutic approach that aids individuals in exploring and resolving ambivalence about change. The approach is consistent with client-centered treatment approaches, as it relies heavily on the expression of empathy through reflective listening. However, MI is also directive in its use of techniques to facilitate the exploration of ambivalence and draw out client arguments for change.

MI operates under the assumption that motivation to change should be elicited from the client, instead of imposed from without. In MI, the interventionist resists taking on the expert role and instead seeks to join patients as a nonjudgmental companion in their exploration of ambivalence. MI is intended to facilitate change by aiding patients in identifying and mobilizing their own intrinsic values, helping them to develop discrepancies between these values and their current behavior, and encouraging and supporting commitment to change. The developers point out that, while specific learnable skills are an important part of the intervention, if it is seen simply as a collection of techniques, its spirit and likely effectiveness will be lost.

MI was first described by William Miller as an extension of his intuitive clinical perspectives on the nature of change. The intervention was further described and elaborated by Miller and Stephen Rollnick in the book *Motivational Interviewing: Preparing People for Change,* which is now in its second edition. The first empirical tests of MI were actually tests of MET, as they combined the intervention with reporting of personalized assessment results.

Early Applications

The first empirical tests of MET were conducted by Miller, the codeveloper of MI, in the late 1980s. In multiple clinical trials, MET was tested as part of an intervention labeled the Drinkers Check-up, in which individuals were given a 2-hour battery of assessment instruments that are sensitive to the early effects of alcohol. Assessment instruments included behavioral measures, such as quantity and frequency of alcohol use, neuropsychological measures, such as executive functioning and attention tasks, and biomedical indexes, such as serum samples to be assayed for liver function. Following assessment, Drinker's Check-up participants received personalized objective feedback in which their assessment scores were compared to normative samples or other objective criteria. Participants were given a written personalized feedback report, which was reviewed by a clinician who helped the participant to understand and interpret the feedback relative to normative samples. Consistent with MI, feedback was given in a client-centered, empathic style, and labeling and confrontation were avoided.

Early applications of the Drinker's Check-up found that self-referred problem drinkers who received the intervention experienced significant reductions in drinking. A follow-up study compared feedback styles, randomizing participants to an MI-consistent or confrontational style. No significant differences in outcome were found between the two groups, but variability in therapist style led the researchers to conduct post hoc analyses in which they determined that confrontational therapist behavior was highly correlated with poor drinking outcome.

Several other early investigations tested the efficacy of the intervention as a prelude to treatment entry. In the first randomized study on the topic, outpatient substance abuse patients either received MI-consistent feedback of assessment results or an attention-placebo intervention at intake to treatment. Results demonstrated that MI patients had improved outcomes and were more likely to attend their first outpatient treatment session. Follow-up investigations replicated the findings with different populations and settings. MET was found to enhance treatment engagement when added to the intake session of residential alcohol treatment participants. In addition, MET was found to be an effective prelude to treatment for polysubstance-using outpatient adolescents.

Large Multisite Trials

Following the promising early findings of MET, the intervention has been tested more extensively in large, multisite clinical trials. Three of those trials, including Project MATCH, the Cannabis Youth Treatment project, and the Clinical Trials Network community-based studies, are discussed.

Project MATCH

The Drinker's Check-up was expanded to a four-session intervention, and a manual was created for Project MATCH. Project MATCH was a large, multisite

clinical research trial, designed to test whether specific patient characteristics interacted with treatment modality to predict outcome. Alcohol outpatients and aftercare patients were given an extensive assessment battery and randomized to one of three treatment conditions, including 12 sessions of cognitive behavioral therapy, 12 sessions of Twelve-Step Facilitation therapy, or 4 sessions of MET. Few specific patient–treatment matching results were found in the trial, and few differences in outcome were noted between treatment condition. However, all interventions resulted in significant improvements among participants, including the shorter duration MET intervention.

The MET intervention tested within Project MATCH was composed of four treatment sessions spread out across 12 weeks. The first two treatment sessions focused on feedback of assessment results, exploration of motivation to change, and discussion of future plans. The last two sessions took place at 6 weeks and 12 weeks and were designed to further explore change and reinforce progress. The Project MATCH intervention manual describes the basic principles of MI, including expressing empathy, developing a discrepancy, avoiding argumentation, rolling with resistance, and supporting self-efficacy. The intervention is described in two phases. In phase one, the therapist builds motivation for change by presenting feedback and eliciting self-motivating statements through the use of reflective listening and other important strategies. In phase two, the therapist is encouraged to recognize readiness for change and strengthen commitment through information, advice, and the development of a change plan. The intervention also allowed for the inclusion of a significant other.

Cannabis Youth Treatment Project (CYT)

As part of the CYT project randomized, multisite clinical trial, MET was combined with cognitive behavioral therapy (CBT) to form a five session intervention for outpatient youth with cannabis use disorders. The intervention combined two sessions of individual MET with three group session of CBT. CYT was designed to test the efficacy of this intervention compared to other interventions, including 12 sessions of adolescent Community Reinforcement Approach, 12 sessions of multidimensional family therapy, and two interventions that added additional sessions to the MET-CBT combination. In the trial, all interventions were found to improve participant substance use across time, and no differences between interventions were found. However, the MET-CBT combination was more cost-effective.

The MET-CBT intervention has a corresponding manual, which describes the intervention protocol for the two sessions of MET. During the first session, therapists are encouraged to build rapport and increase motivation for change by helping youth explore and resolve ambivalence about change. In addition, the feedback report is reviewed. During the second session, goals are identified and participants are prepared for CBT group sessions. CBT sessions focused on developing skills for living a drug-free life, but therapists were encouraged to rely on their MI skills throughout the intervention.

Clinical Trials Network Studies

Two multisite investigations of MET have been conducted within community-based treatment programs that are part of the National Institute on Drug Abuse's Clinical Trials Network. In the first study, investigators compared outcomes for outpatient substance users who received a standard intake-evaluation with those who received an intake-evaluation with components of MET. Consistent with the goals of the Clinical Trials Network, the study was done using community-based treatment programs and therapists. MET participants were found to have increased treatment retention; however, differences in substance use were not observed. The MET intervention is described in a manual that is based on adaptations of other manuals, including Project MATCH. The intervention involved providing feedback in an empathic style and eliciting change talk using directive MI techniques.

In another Clinical Trials Network multisite trial, outpatient substance users were randomly assigned to three sessions of MET or three session of standard treatment. The intervention embodied the spirit of MI, using client-centered and directive strategies to elicit change talk and motivation to change. No differences in treatment retention or short-term substance use outcomes were observed between the two groups. However, long-term substance use outcomes were superior for MET participants. Follow-up analyses revealed a variety of factors that interacted with treatment condition, including differential effects across sites. An intervention manual was created and that was based largely on the Project MATCH manual.

Other Outcome Studies

Given the early promising findings MET, the intervention has been widely studied in a variety of alcohol and substance use settings. In fact, the majority of clinical trials that have been conducted on the efficacy of MI in addictions use a MET intervention format. Clinical trials have expanded in breadth from early alcohol studies to include investigations targeting opioid, cocaine, marijuana, and dually diagnosed patients. Recent meta-analytic findings suggest that MET generally has a positive impact on patients, with moderate effect sizes observed when comparing it to other treatment approaches. However, results vary widely across studies, with some investigations finding highly positive findings when comparing MET to other evidence-based interventions and other investigations failing to find positive effects when comparing MET to standard care. This variability in findings can also be found within multisite clinical trials, where the effects of MET have been found to vary significantly by site. Several factors have been hypothesized to influence this variability in outcomes. For example, MET may show diminished effectiveness when applied to substance users with multiple psychosocial risk factors. In addition, MET interventions which are limited to one treatment session may be less promising. Finally, differences in therapist training vary widely across and within studies, likely contributing to variability in outcome.

Conclusion

MET is a widely utilized treatment approach that combines MI and the reporting of personalized feedback results. MET was first tested empirically with patients with alcohol problems as part of the Drinker's Checkup. Further studies tested MET as a prelude to treatment or as a part of the treatment intake process. The promising early findings of MET led to several randomized, multisite clinical trials and other investigations that have had generally favorable, but variable results.

Jennifer E. Hettema

See also Brief Interventions; Cannabis Youth Treatment Study; Cognitive Behavioral Therapy; Evidence-Based Treatment; Motivational Interviewing; Project MATCH

Further Readings

Ball, S. A., Martino, S., Charla, N., Frankforter, T. L., Van Horn, D., Crits-Christoph, P., et al. (2007). Site matters:

Multisite randomized trial of Motivational Enhancement Therapy in community drug clinics. *Journal of Consulting and Clinical Psychology, 75,* 556–567.

Miller, W. R., Benefield, R. G., & Tonigan, J. S. (1993). Enhancing motivation for change in problem drinking: A controlled comparison of two therapist styles. *Journal of Consulting and Clinical Psychology, 61,* 455–461.

Miller, W. R., & Rollnick, S. (2002). *Motivational interviewing: Preparing people for change.* New York: Guilford Press.

Miller, W. R., & Sovereign, R. G. (1989). The check-up: A model for early intervention in addictive behaviors. In T. Loberg, W. R. Miller, P. E. Nathan, & G. A. Marlatt (Eds.), *Addictive behaviors: Prevention and early intervention* (pp. 219–231). Amsterdam: Swets & Zeitlinger.

Miller, W. R., Zweben, A., DiClemente, C. C., & Rychtarik, R. G. (1992). *Motivational Enhancement Therapy manual: A clinical research guide for therapists treating individuals with alcohol abuse and dependence.* Rockville, MD: National Institute on Alcohol Abuse and Alcoholism.

Sampl, S., & Kadden, R. (2001). *Motivational Enhancement Therapy and cognitive behavioral therapy for adolescent cannabis users: 5 sessions, cannabis youth treatment (CYT) series* (vol. 1). Rockville, MD: Center for Substance Abuse Treatment, Substance Abuse and Mental Health Services Administration.

Motivational Interviewing

Motivational interviewing (MI) is a client-centered, directive therapy for helping individuals to explore and resolve ambivalence about change. Although MI has been applied to a wide variety of behavioral domains, it arose as a treatment for substance abuse and has been most widely tested and applied in this area.

Overview

MI is a therapeutic approach designed to help individuals explore and resolve ambivalence about change. The approach is both client-centered and directive in its use of techniques to facilitate the exploration of ambivalence and draw out client utterances regarding change. MI can be implemented in a variety of formats and by a range of interventionists. However, it is typically applied as a brief intervention of one to two sessions. Thus, its duration is often much shorter than most other evidence-based substance abuse treatments. MI can be administered as a stand-alone treatment, as a prelude to other treatment approaches, or in combination with other interventions. It is also commonly combined with objective feedback. Treatment agents also vary greatly, ranging from physicians to community layperson volunteers. The flexibility of MI makes it applicable to a wide variety of settings, but this diversity in applications can present some challenges to researchers who wish to draw generalized conclusions regarding its effect.

Brief History

MI was originally conceptualized by William Miller, who was influenced by clinical experience, previous psychotherapy traditions, and empirical findings in cognitive psychology. Miller credits the formal conceptualization of MI with a sabbatical experience in Norway during which he was encouraged by trainees to explain and verbalize decision rules for his clinical approach. This process motivated him to describe the rationale for his approach in writing. After publishing his first description of MI in 1983, Miller joined with Stephen Rollnick to further develop the intervention and to create the first edition of the book *Motivational Interviewing* in 1991. The book is now in its second edition.

MI has its roots in client-centered, Rogerian therapy, which holds that all individuals house within them the potential to change and that unconditional positive regard by therapists can help germinate positive change. Both techniques rely on the use of reflective listening to communicate empathy and facilitate exploration of change. However, although traditional client-centered therapy is nondirective in its use of reflective listening, MI uses reflective techniques strategically to encourage the exploration of ambivalence and elicit change talk.

Several cognitive psychology principles also influenced the development of MI. Cognitive dissonance theory argues that perceived discrepancies between beliefs and behavior are uncomfortable for individuals and can motivate them to reduce dissonance by changing their behavior. MI relies on this principle in its attempts to help clients identify important goals or values and then develop a discrepancy between these goals and values and their current behavior. In addition, Daryl Bem's self-perception theory holds that individuals' beliefs can be influenced in part by their own verbal behavior. Consequently, MI aims to facilitate change talk and commitment language on the part of the client.

Spirit

The developers of MI point out that, while specific learnable skills are an important part of the intervention, if it is seen simply as a collection of techniques, its spirit and likely effectiveness will be lost. MI is intended to facilitate change by aiding clients in identifying and mobilizing their own intrinsic values, helping them to develop discrepancies between these values and their current behavior, and encouraging and supporting commitment to change. To achieve these goals, the therapist operates within the spirit of MI, relying on certain assumptions regarding the nature of human change. Three important constructs help describe the spirit of MI: collaboration, evocation, and autonomy.

Collaboration

The relationship between client and therapist is seen as an important aspect of MI. Instead of the expert–recipient dynamic that dominates many psychotherapeutic interventions, the client and therapist are seen more as partners or companions. The role of the therapist is to join with the client and be supportive through the exploration of ambivalence. In this role, the therapist is encouraged to be aware of his or her own aspirations and avoid direct persuasion, as this is seen as an ineffective means of promoting behavior change. As the developers point out, because of this, the intervention can often been perceived as quiet and eliciting when compared to more directive or skills-based approaches.

Evocation

Within MI, motivation to change is not imposed from without, but elicited from the client. Interventionists often see themselves as being uniquely situated to see the potential dangers of clients' behaviors and hold a great deal of information regarding corrective courses of action. This position can lead to temptation to use direct persuasion as a means to change

behavior, despite evidence that suggests that this approach is not effective. In MI, instead of the therapist generating reasons and contingencies to stimulate behavior change, interventionists are encouraged to identify and mobilize the client's own intrinsic motivation. MI operates under the assumption that clients have important goals and values that, if drawn out, can promote healthy behavior change.

Autonomy

Within MI, responsibility for change lies with client, and it is the therapist's job to communicate and respects the client's freedom of choice. Here, it is the client's responsibility to articulate and resolve his or her own ambivalence. The therapist can support this process by affirming that the client has the ability and right to make decisions about change that are in line with his or her goals and values.

The Four Principles

Several basic principles are key to the successful implementation of MI, including expressing empathy, developing a discrepancy, supporting self-efficacy, and rolling with resistance.

Expressing Empathy

Within MI, empathy is largely operationalized as the skillful application of reflective listening, or accurate empathy. This therapist behavior is thought to communicate to the client that he or she is accepted and understood, as it provides a safe atmosphere for the client to explore ambivalence and decisions about change. MI operates under the seemingly paradoxical principle that respectfully accepting clients' ambivalence toward change, including positive feelings about maladaptive behaviors, is the most effective means of motivating positive behavior change.

Developing a Discrepancy

In addition to communicating an acceptance and understanding of the client, MI techniques can be used in a strategic manner to help clients resolve ambivalence in the direction of positive behavior change. One such technique involves helping clients to consider important goals and values in the context of their current behavior. When a discrepancy exists between these constructs, the client may then be motivated to reduce dissonance. In seeking to develop a discrepancy, although the MI therapist may encourage the client to identify and articulate what is important to him or her, consider values in the context of current behavior, or imagine the future having and not having made changes, it is the client who must ultimately determine whether a discrepancy exists and whether that discrepancy is sufficient reason to change.

Support Self-Efficacy

In MI, it is acknowledged that a desire to change may not be sufficient to motivate change, if the individual does not believe that he or she is capable. Clients' beliefs about their chances of success can often influence behavior in a way that makes them self-fulfilling. Consequently, another goal of MI is to increase the client's confidence regarding his or her chances of success. To accomplish this, MI utilizes techniques that affirm strengths and past successes and emphasize personal responsibility for change.

Roll with Resistance

MI views resistance as a byproduct of the interaction between client and therapist. Consequently, a strong emphasis is placed on the importance of therapist behavior in response to such resistance. Therapists are encouraged to respond to resistance with acceptance and empathy, versus confrontation, counter-arguments, or therapist generated reasons to change. MI also normalizes resistance, by seeing it as normal aspect of ambivalence and representative of the clients underlying struggle to find resolution.

The Core Skills: OARS

Four basic skills can be used to help accomplish the goals of MI.

Open-Ended Questions

Open-ended questions are inquiries that cannot be answered with a simple yes or no response and instead encourage the client to speak in more depth about a particular issue. This technique is often used to provoke client talk (e.g., "What brings you in today?") or steer the conversation in specific directions

(e.g., "What have your friends and family said about your substance use?). Open-ended questions can also be used to help clients explore their ambivalence (e.g., "What are some things you like and don't like about your substance use?") or can be strategically placed to encourage clients to think about their behavior in different ways (e.g., "If you continued using substances in this way, what do you think your life might be like 5 years from now?). Open-ended questions can be used in a directive fashion to accomplish the goals of MI; however, interactions that take the form of question-answer-question-answer may reduce collaborative spirit and restrict exploration on the part of the client.

Affirmations

Affirmations are statements that reinforce client strengths, efforts, progress, or accomplishments. Affirmations can take many forms, including compliments (e.g., "You have accomplished a lot since our last meeting.") and expressions appreciation (e.g., "I appreciate you taking the time think about these difficult issues with me."). Affirmations serve to reinforce positive client behaviors, increase rapport between client and therapist, and build confidence or self-efficacy.

Reflections

Reflections are the most commonly utilized skill within MI. Therapists implementing MI actively listen to clients using reflective listening techniques, with the intention of helping clients to feel heard, valued, and understood. Within MI, reflections are conceptualized as hypotheses or guesses about the meaning of what a client has said. Reflections can vary in depth, ranging from simple repetitions of what the client has said, to paraphrases that have increased depth or add meaning. Reflections can also vary in focus, being strategically used to highlight the emotional content or ambivalence in client utterances. Structurally, reflections are formed as statements that inflect down at the end. Using reflective listening helps ensure that the therapist is accurately understanding the meaning of what the client has said and communicates to the client that the therapist is interested and invested in understanding. Reflective listening allows the client to openly explore ambivalence in an environment that is nonjudgmental and free from unsolicited advice.

Summaries

Summaries are a special form of reflection in which the therapist reflects back a larger sample of a client's thoughts or feelings. Summaries are commonly used to highlight ambivalence, reflecting two or more ways that a client feels about a situation. In addition, they can be used to highlight discrepancies in a client's behavior, by reflecting what is important to the client and his or her current high-risk behaviors. Finally, reflections can be used to transition for one topic to another or at the end of a session to integrate the information that has been shared by the client.

Empirical Evidence

Many clinical trials of MI have been conducted in the area of substance abuse. One early clinical trial of MI that helped to establish it as a valid treatment approach was Project MATCH, a randomized, multisite clinical trial comparing Twelve-Step Facilitation therapy, cognitive behavioral therapy, and an adaptation of MI, Motivational Enhancement Therapy. All three interventions in the clinical trial were found to perform equally well in the treatment of alcohol-dependent clients. Despite this finding, other studies have generally found positive findings with small to moderate between-group effect sizes in the areas of alcoholism, substance abuse, and treatment engagement. Results to date appear less promising in the area of smoking cessation, with MI not appearing to consistently add any benefit to other commonly utilized treatment approaches. MI has also been shown to improve client behavior in areas related to substance abuse, such as high-risk sexual behavior and medication compliance.

Drawing generalized conclusions regarding the efficacy of MI has been challenging to researchers since it has been applied and tested in a variety of formats. In addition, clinical trials vary in their comparative method, with some studies comparing control groups or comparison interventions with pure MI and others combining or adding MI to another form of treatment. Early evidence seems to suggest that MI often performs equally as well or superior to other established treatments and that any superior effects of MI tend to be prolonged when MI is added as a prelude or adjunct to another treatment. In addition, preliminary research seems to suggest that MI may work better with Latino and African American populations.

In addition to outcome research, some process research has been conducted on MI. The role of language has been identified as a particularly salient factor. MI consistent therapist techniques have been found to increase client change talk, or expression of the desire, ability, reasons, need, and commitment to change. In turn, the presence and strength of this language within sessions has been found to predict client outcome, leading to an increased emphasis on encouraging therapist behaviors that lead to an increase in client change talk.

Another challenge involved in empirically studying MI is the inconsistency observed in the training of MI therapists. Teaching MI varies widely in both clinical and research settings, ranging from short didactic sessions to multiple day interactive trainings. This issue has been addressed in part by the Motivational Interviewing Network of Trainers, which provides standardized training for MI trainers themselves and has provided guidelines for different types and functions of training. Several treatment fidelity measures have also been developed to measure adherence to the treatment model. Early application of these instruments suggests that ongoing support through feedback, coaching, and supervision is necessary to maintain skillfulness in MI following training.

Conclusion

MI is a clinical approach to the treatment of substance abuse that is unique in its efforts to increase motivation by collaborating with clients and helping them to identify their own personal reasons for change. The spirit of MI is complimented by specific principles and clinical skills that communicate acceptance and confidence in helping clients to explore and identify reasons for change. MI has been tested empirically with generally positive findings, particularly when added as a prelude to another treatment approach or used with minority samples. Finally, early work suggests that clinicians wishing to utilize MI trainings should receive ongoing support following training.

Jennifer E. Hettema

See also Brief Interventions; Cannabis Youth Treatment Study; Counseling Approaches; Motivational Enhancement Therapy; Project MATCH

Further Readings

Amrhein, P. C. (2004). How does motivational interviewing work? What client talk reveals. *Motivational Interviewing:*

Theory, Research, and Practice [Special issue]. *Journal of Cognitive Psychotherapy* , *18*, 323–336.

Hettema, J. E., Steele, J., & Miller, W. R. (2005). Motivational interviewing. *Annual Review of Clinical Psychology, 1,* 91–111.

Miller, W. R., & Rollnick, S. (2002). *Motivational interviewing: Preparing people to change.* New York: Guilford Press.

Miller, W. R., Yahne, C. E., Moyers, T. B., Martinez, J., & Pirritano, M. (2004). A randomized trial of methods to help clinicians learn motivational interviewing. *Journal of Consulting and Clinical Psychology, 72,* 1050–1062.

Moyers, T. B. (2004). History and happenstance: How motivational interviewing got its start. *Journal of Cognitive Psychotherapy: An International Quar*terly, 18, 291–298.

Moyers, T. B., & Martin, T. (2006). Therapist influence on client language during motivational interviewing sessions. *Journal of Substance Abuse Treatment, 30,* 245–251.

Moyers, T. B., Martin, T., Manuel, J. K., Hendrickson, S. M. L., & Miller, W. R. (2005). Assessing competence in the use of motivational interviewing. *Journal of Substance Abuse Treatment, 28,* 19–26.

Rollnick S., & Miller, W. R. (1995). What is motivational interviewing? *Behavioural and Cognitive Psychotherapy, 23,* 325–334.

MULTICULTURALISM

Longevity, mobility, and other issues make our population demographics increasingly dynamic. Multiculturalism represents acknowledgement that assumptions, experiences, and meanings are not universal; that the worldviews they give rise to are not identical between or among individuals or groups; and that these numerous perspectives are all valid (even if seemingly undesirable or unjust). In health, mental health, and substance abuse treatment, cultural competency (the ability to work effectively with varied cultures and with that of the current client in particular) is positively correlated with clients' treatment entry, engagement, and favorable outcomes. In the last decade, cultural competency and culturally relevant interventions have been of increasing concern and interest among clinicians; researchers in psychology, social work, and public health; and policymakers as health disparities between non-Hispanic Whites and ethnic minorities persist—at least in part due to lack of cultural competency. The body of this entry defines and discusses relevant terms, articulates elements of culturally competent practice including skills required of practitioners for cultural competence, discusses current substance use epidemiological data for specific minority groups, and makes suggestions for development and evaluation of substance use intervention programs in light of multiculturalism.

Terms and Concepts

Several concepts and terms are central to the discussion of multiculturalism. *Culture* encompasses the socially constructed patterns, practices, and norms of behavior that guide our daily lives. Explanatory systems, meanings, values, expectations, and boundaries of acceptable or unacceptable behavior are all part of culture. Culture is distinct from one's physical appearance and demographic census category. Culture is socialized and transmitted through interactions with influences around us including interpersonal (e.g., family members, friends, acquaintances), communal (e.g., schools, religious organizations, worksites), and national (e.g., economic systems, mass media, Internet). Daily, people are socialized by others while simultaneously being a socializing agent for others. Each person may simultaneously be part of several cultures: in one's home, work or school, peer group, and community lives. The culture(s) people most identify with become their personal reference framework and have the greatest influence on their beliefs and behaviors.

Further, this framework stems from their personal history and also from the norms, roles, behaviors, expectations, and experiences currently and historically experienced by the cultural groups to which they belong. As culture becomes internalized, each person carries ideas about what is right and acceptable or wrong and unacceptable for others and for themselves. A *worldview* is based on these personal and collective experiences and the collective and individual meanings attached to them. Race and ethnicity are complex constructs that, while often considered to have universal definitions, are in fact the topic of much debate and inconsistent interpretation in the field. *Race* generally encompasses biologically heritable traits that may or may not influence aspects of groups' experiences. Historical and structural factors also play a large part in the conceptualization of race. *Ethnicity* connotes a shared identity among a group of people, which may stem from cultural (e.g., religious, linguistic), racial, or geographic (regional or national) attributes represented in the group. With both race and ethnicity, it is important to acknowledge that racial identity and ethnic identity are separate constructs and often the more useful constructs to consider when discussing multiculturalism. An important consideration for substance use assessment and intervention planning is that some racial and ethnic groups have histories of horrific injustices and chronic discrimination, sanctioned and maintained by government institutions and the majority population. Consequently, group members may be justifiably dubious of programs and aid offered by government, institutions, or those seemingly different from themselves.

Disability status may be another factor in cultural identification for some individuals. Further, as some believe alcoholism and substance abuse are diseases, clients may link illness and disability status with acknowledgement of their use. Consideration of this and general physical, mental, and emotional disabilities are important aspects of multiculturally competent care. Social class is not yet universally addressed within current literature discussing multiculturalism, cultural competency, and substance use treatment, but social classes have different cultures (e.g., consider role expectations, priorities, alternatives, explanatory styles, and other values) and should be considered in light of appropriate multicultural care.

It is important to recognize that while all culture-based worldviews are valid, they are not all treated equally. We may be exposed to varied influences and cultures, but there exists a dominant culture that is a common barometer for standards and normality. In the United States and in many Western countries, this dominant culture represents a non-Hispanic White, middle-class, Christian, male worldview—complete with values, expectations, rules of behavior, roles, priorities, and morals. Even if this is not one's own worldview, it is known to us because it is represented as normal in the media and codified in our social institutions (such as medicine and substance use interventions) and practices (such as medication researched on men being transferred for use with women without evaluation for sex differences in reaction or dosing). The more one identifies with the dominant culture, the harder it will be to see implicit assumptions, or how common knowledge or imperatives are only common to those within one's culture. Cultural competence in the rapidly changing and multicultural environment requires a rigorous and critical evaluation of the worldview and culture that people, as interventionists, hold. Unexamined, their internalized cultural ideas are blindly applied in their dealings with others (termed *ethnocentrism*).

Culturally Competent Interventions

As interventionists, unchecked cultural biases lead to ethnocentricity in the assumptions, framing, planning, and delivery of interventions to the frequent detriment of those with different worldviews. Cultural competency requires that one's interventions be acceptable, accessible, meaningful, and helpful to one's client or target populations. Several things are required to address those requirements: (a) the interventionist's awareness of his or her own culturally driven assumptions; (b) general epidemiological-type knowledge of cultural specifics of ethnic groups with which the client might identify; (c) collaboration with the client to understand his or her particular worldview and culture, which may or may not be what we expect or what is representative for people with his or her perceived characteristics; (d) flexibility to adjust elements of the intervention to bring it in line with the client so that it is acceptable, accessible, meaningful, and helpful to him or her; and (e) willingness and commitment to a process that, by design and nature, may challenge the status quo and the interventionist's personally held beliefs.

A tension between evidence-based substance use intervention and required fluidity in intervention planning for culturally competent care does exist. One of the difficulties with both epidemiological data and large, positivistic scientific methodological research studies is that the nuances of particular individual(s) get lost. That is to say, a particular assessment tool or intervention program may work with the "average" person, but it may systematically fail with specific individuals or populations because of cultural characteristics. Finding and addressing these instances is the thrust of culturally competent care. Qualitative research methods and population-specific randomized trials are ways of evaluating the specific needs and efficacy of programs within a given cultural population. However, the blending and changing nature of the multicultural population and the importance of the clients' most salient, particular cultural identity mean individualized assessment and intervention tailoring are the cornerstone of truly multiculturally competent care.

Multicultural substance use assessment and treatment starts from a multicultural framework with critical awareness of ones own cultural worldview and should generally include exploration of the following:

- The client's thoughts about problematic substance use—what are the boundaries, occasions, levels, and consequences of substance use in his or her cultural group? Do certain substances have different significance or meaning to the client? How would one know when substance use is a problem?

- What causes substance use problems? What would it mean to the client and his or her family if the client has a problem with substances? What are the consequences of having a substance use problem (social sanctions)? How would one behave if they have a problem?

- What assistance would be useful for a person with a substance use problem (sanctions, prayer, will power, is help possible)? Who controls this help and where could the client get help? Will the client be expected to discuss his or her substance use treatment with elders, extended family, or community members, and how might they help the client?

- What is an acceptable substance use treatment goal (abstinence, moderation with use at specific occasions, abstinence save for certain substances with cultural meaning)?

- What language does the client speak at home? Is the client conversant in English (as spoken, as written)? If the client has immigrated, what circumstances prompted the immigration? How long has the client been here? What is the client's legal status? How much has the client adapted to American life (*enculturation*)? What family or supports do they have here and who was left behind?

- Is the client religious or spiritual? Even if not now, what faiths or practices currently or previously surround the client?

- What concerns does the client have about working with a therapist or exploring substance use treatment in general? What personal or cultural knowledge does the client hold about programs such as this treatment and about health and health care in general? Are there specific fears or requirements that need to be considered in treatment planning? Physical requirements might include location, language, time, day care, wait room for escorts, or ability to pay co-pays or treatment fees. Philosophical requirements might include same sex interventionist or group members,

no mention of God or faith as part of treatment, or adequate privacy protections.

- Broadly consider general epidemiological information known about the client and consider or directly explore with the client what is acceptable, accessible, meaningful, and helpful to him or her (or target population) based on age, sex, sexual identity, racial identity, ethnic identity, religious identity, disability status, social class, language, living situation, and degree of national acculturation.

- Finally, consider how what is learned about the client's culture and worldview may aid the client in realizing mutual goals regarding the client's improved health and quality of life.

Epidemiological Data for Minority Groups

National studies conducted by government organizations such as the Substance Abuse and Mental Health Services Administration (SAMHSA), the National Institute on Alcohol Abuse and Alcoholism (NIAAA), and the Centers for Disease Control and Prevention (CDC) have identified many unique trends in alcohol and drug use among different populations. Unfortunately, these organizations typically do not use the same categorization systems, making comparisons and generalization problematic. In addition, by grouping together many different ethnicities into one race, many within-group differences are lost. The purpose of the following review is to introduce the reader to current epidemiological data, highlight the need for treatment options, and emphasize the inherent difficulties in a one-size-fits-all conceptualization of alcohol and drug use.

In reviewing SAMHSA studies on alcohol use, results show similar past-year use among Native Americans (63.7%), Mexican Americans (63.7%), and non-Hispanic Whites (58.7%). However, when considering only heavy drinking statistics, Mexican Americans have a disproportionate representation (6.9%, compared to 5.3% of non-Hispanic Whites and 4.6% of Native Americans). When comparing alcohol dependence trends reported by SAMHSA and NIAAA, Native Americans have the largest representation among individuals identified as alcohol dependent (ranging from 5.6% to 6.4%, compared with 4.0% of Hispanics and 5.6% of Mexican Americans, and 3.4%–3.8% of non-Hispanic Whites).

Substance use related health concerns are also variable and not necessarily proportional to drinking prevalence. For example, although African Americans reported less alcohol use in the past year (55.4%), less heavy alcohol use (4.7%), and a lower alcohol dependence rate (3.4%–3.6%), the percent of males with alcohol-related liver disease identified by NIAAA is almost double that for non-Hispanic Whites (8.3% compared to 5.3%). Hispanic males exceeded both groups with 12.7% diagnosed with alcohol-related liver disease. SAMHSA also identified substantial differences in need for drug treatment, ranging from 2.5% of non-Hispanic Whites to 3.6% of Mexican Americans to 3.9% of African Americans to 7.8% of Native Americans.

Prevalence of and patterns of alcohol use vary as well. The CDC found that alcohol use varied from 55.2% of non-Hispanic Whites to 52.4% of Hispanics to 48.8% of Native Americans to 46.6% of African Americans. In these findings, more non-Hispanic Whites reportedly consumed alcohol and were more likely to identify as a current drinker (63.6%, compared to 49.6% of Hispanics, 48.8% of Native Americans, and 46.6% of African Americans). In spite of these differences, heavy drinking rates, defined as consuming five or more drinks in one occasion, were very similar among Native Americans (33.2%), Hispanics (31.8%), and non-Hispanic Whites (32.5%). These findings indicate that although non-Hispanic Whites were more likely to use alcohol and identify as current drinkers, the risk of heavy drinking and associated consequences was disproportionately greater for Hispanics and Native Americans.

Many studies indicate alcohol and drug use rates among Asian Americans are lower than population norms, including the CDC's findings of 3.1% drug use, 37.4% alcohol use, and 12.4% binge alcohol use. However, this CDC study excluded Pacific Islanders due to a small sample size and did not distinguish between Asian American subgroups. Other studies suggest Pacific Islanders and Filipino Americans report much higher alcohol and drug use than Japanese and Chinese Americans subgroups, for instance. In addition, Asian American college student drinking is similar to and sometimes greater than the general population, indicating that the national surveys may be failing to detect some of the variance inherent in this population.

Again, the use of different categorical groupings among studies means both variance and similarity found among populations may be attributable to the consolidation of disparate groups that masks true differences. Further, apparent differences may also be attributable to treatment accessibility, problematic programming, or in the diagnostic system itself. Some ethnic groups have been thus far neglected in the literature, such as Arab Americans. Another significant limitation of recent studies is the limited categorization of biracial or multiracial individuals. In much of the current literature, study participants are limited to identifying as one race or on rare occasion, as two or more races, which equally loses the specific and complex nuance of multiracial, multiethnic individuals. With these limitations in mind, it is apparent that there is substantial variability in alcohol and substance use and impact among different cultural groups which is important to consider and incorporate into one's multicultural framework.

Development and Evaluation of Intervention Programs

When considering multiculturalism in the development and evaluation of substance use intervention programs, one must consider both content and processes. Focusing on principles known to be broadly efficacious across cultures in designing and evaluating interventions provides a concrete foundation to a complicated and multifaceted issue. Three such principles emerging from recent literature are discussed below.

One principle of multiculturally appropriate substance use intervention programs is that the environment and process of the delivery of treatment should be culturally sensitive and culturally relevant to clients. This principle often requires organizational, programmatic, and staff self-assessment of current (or planned) formal, informal, and physical infrastructures. Changes may be necessary to ensure cultural sensitivity and cultural relevance, including multicultural congruency between the physical environment, staff, and treatment delivery. This self-assessment should include considerations of process variables such as the following:

1. Are the cultural and linguistic competencies of individuals implementing the interventions appropriate for the clients being served? Will clients likely assess practitioners to be culturally competent to work with them?

2. Are assessment and intervention frameworks based on theory and tools that are sensitive to issues of oppression, discrimination, and racism?

3. Will clients be comfortable with the objects, symbols, and seating, and so on within waiting and meeting rooms and in written material?

4. Are the interventionists committed to a common goal of improving health and are willing and able to adapt to the cultural context of the clients served?

5. Are values and principles promoting diversity and commitment to effective treatment for all clients broadly and constantly reflected in the organization's formal and informal policies and procedures (including client outreach, assessment, treatment planning, billing, scheduling, and all personnel policies)?

A second principle shown to be effective with diverse cultural groups is meeting the client where he or she is. This principle is widely found in the substance use literature as a whole, but examining it with a focus on multiculturalism emphasizes some specific approaches and captures the content and parameters for multicultural substance use treatment.

Outreach is critical. This includes not only basic approaches such as physically entering the community, but also intentionally building rapport by gaining community buy-in, trust, and respect (e.g., conduct focus groups, consult with community leaders); work with the community to reach an understanding of what, when, and how substance use is normal or problematic to individual community members and the community as a whole; communicate and collaborate directly with the target community (e.g., build partnerships with existing community organizations, community leaders, and current programs within the community that may serve as referrals, treatment collaborators, or cultural consultants in the efforts); and clearly outline the incentives to participation in treatment (e.g., vouchers, input in treatment development).

In addition to the use of culturally sensitive and relevant outreach to inform the content aspect of appropriate multicultural care, it is imperative that each client be approached via a culturally integrated assessment. This assessment should culminate in a culturally sensitive diagnosis and lead to development of a culturally relevant treatment plan. There are real and valid differences in how an individual's cultural group

conceptualizes substance use and when it is a problem. The majority of assessment measures have not been adequately normed on diverse cultural groups and thus may generate under or overestimations of use, distress, consequences, and dependence. Suggested elements of culturally integrated assessment and culturally relevant treatment planning were bulleted for reference above.

Recognition of not only stressors related to minority status (racism, prejudice, discrimination) but also of group strengths (social support, values, traditions) should not be overlooked. Incorporating these and other cultural protective factors into substance use assessment and treatment or health behavior promotion planning is critical. This is a third principle of multicultural practice, the strengths perspective. Look for and therapeutically utilize sources of strength, support, tradition, expectations, meaning, and values with all clients, but particularly when working with clients with cultures and worldviews different from the therapist's, as their strengths may be found in unexpected places or easily overlooked.

An important part of competent multicultural case conceptualization is recognition of the injustices that can be and have been perpetuated by the mental health system both historically and presently (e.g., minority individuals are more likely to receive restrictive services than nonminority individuals despite the same diagnosis). This is important to recognize both to validate the client's concerns and to avoid perpetuating further injustices. It is easy to lose sight of the fact that personal interactions occur in larger contexts. Current context occurs amid racial and culturally based health disparities. Lack of attention to culturally specific factors, and their importance, as well as misinformation about group dynamics, statistics, and conditions can contribute to clients' problem behaviors and be inadvertently included in interventions intended to help the client.

Conclusion

In a pluralist society, multiculturalism accepts that varied personal and group histories give rise to numerous worldviews. Culturally competent care (known to relate to treatment entry, engagement, and better outcomes) must accommodate these worldviews and stems from adaptability of the interventionist and the intervention to provide substance use assessment and treatment that is acceptable, accessible, meaningful, and helpful to the client. Teasing out the boundaries of what is typical and expected within a different culture from what is atypical and problematic is a necessary component of culturally competent care.

This entry has been written in consideration of primary, direct intervention care efforts; public health level efforts have similar premises, but may also include identification of culturally sanctioned behavior that is problematic (both within dominant American society and also within the specific cultural community) that can be targeted for public education and group attitude and behavior change efforts (i.e., current trends in smoking behavior or binge drinking). This level of interventive agenda is beyond the scope of this entry, but should necessarily be approached in collaboration and partnership with targeted community group leaders to assure the community's interests are represented and honored and to avoid further oppression of marginalized or minority groups.

In general, both content and process are of concern for competent multicultural care and three principles of development and evaluation of intervention programs can guide direct-level program planning: (1) the environment and process of the delivery of treatment should be culturally sensitive and culturally relevant to clients, (2) meet the client where the client is, and (3) draw upon cultural strengths. Collaborating with cultural leaders of targeted service populations can help illuminate places where interventions or interventive organizations may need to adjust their assumptions or interventive or organizational protocols. Commitment, personal insight, and willingness are among five elements identified as required of interventionists to provide competent multicultural care. Programs in which the organization, the intervention, and the interventionist are all aligned in support of multiculturalism are preferable as each of these levels contributes to the context, content, and delivery of care to clients. Ultimately, culturally competent assessments and culturally relevant treatment plans stem from understanding the individual client within his or her own group context. Several bulleted suggestions that facilitate doing this have been offered.

Evidence-based programs normed on the general population offer tools shown to be efficacious. However, while being generally helpful, they may be systematically unhelpful to specific individuals or populations. The hope is that the discussion in this article will help the reader discern when standardized protocols may need to be adapted or created afresh to suit the needs and worldviews of specific target populations. The goal, after all, is helping people. Services offered need to be acceptable, accessible, meaningful, and helpful to the client. If clients fail to present or adhere to treatment, then the therapists have failed as well.

Michelle D. Garner, Diane E. Logan,
and Briana A. Woods

See also Assessment; Cultural Aspects; Racial and Ethnic Minorities, Issues in Alcohol and Other Drug Use; Special Populations; Treatment Access and Retention

Further Readings

Grant, B. F., Dawson, D. A., Stinson, F. S., Chou, S. P., Dufour, M. C., & Pickering, R. P. (2004). The 12-month prevalence and trends in DSM-IV alcohol abuse and dependence: United States, 1991–1992 and 2001–2002. *Drug Alcohol Depend, 74*(3), 223–234.

Hays, P. A. (2001). *Addressing cultural complexities in practice: A framework for clinicians and counselors.* Washington, DC: American Psychological Association.

National Institute on Alcohol Abuse and Alcoholism. (2006). *NIAAA: Social work education for the prevention and treatment of alcohol use disorders, Module 10H: Ethnicity, culture and alcohol.* Retrieved September 9, 2007, from http://pubs.niaaa.nih.gov/publications/Social/Module10HEthnicity&Culture/Module10H.html

National Institute on Alcohol Abuse and Alcoholism, Division of Clinical and Prevention Research Treatment Research Branch. (2003). National Institute on Alcohol Abuse and Alcoholism workshop on treatment research priorities and health disparities, Bethesda, MD, September 23–24, 2002. *Alcoholism: Clinical and Experimental Research, 27*(8), 1318–1388.

Office of Applied Studies. (1998). *Prevalence of substance use among racial and ethnic subgroups in the United States, 1991–1993* (DHHS Publication No. SMA 98-3202, NHSDA Series A-6). Retrieved September 10, 2007, from http://www.oas.samhsa.gov/NHSDA/Ethnic/toc.htm

Saadatmand, F., Stinson, F. S., Grant, B. F., & DuFour, M. C. (1999). *Liver cirrhosis mortality in the United States, 1970–96* (National Institute on Alcohol and Alcoholism Surveillance Report No. 52). Bethesda, MD: U.S. Department of Health and Human Services.

U.S. Department of Health and Human Services, National Center for Health Statistics. (2004). *National Health Interview Survey* (No. ICPSR04349-v2). Hyattsville, MD: U.S. Department of Health and Human Services, National

Center for Health Statistics. Retrieved September 10, 2007, from ftp://ftp.cdc.gov/pub/Health_Statistics/ NCHS/Publications/Health_US/hus06tables

U.S. Department of Health & Human Services Office of Minority Health. (2007). *What is cultural competency?* Retrieved December 18, 2006, from http://www.omhrc .gov/templates/browse.aspx?lvl=2&lvlID=11

U.S. Department of Health and Human Services Office of the Surgeon General-SAMHSA. (1999). *Mental health: Culture, race, and ethnicity supplemental to mental health: A report of the Surgeon General.* Retrieved December 18, 2006, from http://mentalhealth.samhsa .gov/cre/default.asp

Multidimensional Family Therapy

Multidimensional family therapy (MDFT), created by Howard A. Liddle, is a family-based treatment that was developed for adolescents with drug and behavior problems and for substance abuse prevention with early adolescents. MDFT as a community and home therapy works in a variety of environmental domains such as the self, family, school, peers, and neighborhood in an effort to eliminate or significantly reduce drug use, as well as providing alternatives to a drug-using lifestyle. It is a multiple systems-oriented and developmentally focused therapy that can be utilized to target the known areas of risk associated with adolescent drug abuse and delinquency. MDFT also focuses on enhancing those protective factors and processes that are understood to promote successful teen and family development.

Theoretical Basis

MDFT was developed in part from the social ecology theory, which suggests that children develop within several interconnected subsystems, such as schools, peer groups, neighborhoods, and families. By understanding and working with the influence of the subsystems that surround the troubled adolescents, lasting behavior changes are thought to be possible.

Research in adolescent developmental psychology and psychopathology has shown that the family is the main context of healthy identity formation, that peer influence operates in relation to the buffering effect of the family against a possibly deviant peer subculture, and that adolescents require the development of an interdependent (as opposed to emotionally separated) relationship with their parents. MDFT was created to allow for symptom reduction and the enhancement of prosocial and normative developmental functions by targeting the family as the basis for the intervention while at the same time allowing for curative processes to develop in several domains of functioning and across multiple systemic levels.

Structure

MDFT is recognized internationally as among the most effective treatments for adolescent substance misuse and has been developed and tested in different forms, increasing the flexibility of the program. This flexibility allows the format and components of MDFT to be modified to specifically meet the needs of different clinical populations. Sessions may occur multiple times during the week and can be tailored to take place in a variety of contexts such as in the home, in the MDFT clinic, in community settings, or by phone. The program is designed to produce behavioral changes in 3 to 6 months using 12 to 25 therapy sessions.

Session content may vary according to the stage of treatment; however, four assessment and intervention modules structure the approach within three stages. Stage one includes a comprehensive assessment covering the problems areas as well as areas of strength that the adolescent may possess and that may not be currently utilized. Assessment in MDFT is important in directing therapists as to where intervention is needed among the myriad of domains within an adolescent's life.

Stage two is the working phase of the treatment during which the therapist attempts to help the patient make significant changes within and across individual, family, peer, school, and other subsystems. The focus during this stage of treatment is on the facilitation of developmentally appropriate competence across a multitude of areas of the patient's life while teaching individualized communication and problem-solving skills. During this stage, parents are helped to examine their relationship with their child, as well as the strategies they use to influence their child. The therapists work to change negative family interaction patterns in order to change the family's everyday environment and to coach parents on innovative ways of reaching out to their children.

The third stage of treatment helps the family to cement the changes that have been made while preparing the adolescent and the family for their next stage of development. In this stage, progress and changes that have been made are acknowledged and any remaining issues that may need to be addressed are refined by the therapist. The main focuses during this stage are on having the family work to maintain the progress that has been made, to encourage the family to work on its own, and to help the family understand the ability to generalize and expand upon its new ideas and behaviors in current and future situations. These new skills, ideas, and behaviors are applied in treatment to new real-world situations to illustrate appropriate usage.

The four assessment and intervention modules within these stages are the adolescent module, the parent module, the family module, and the extrafamilial module. The adolescent module helps address developmental issues including peer relations, identity formation, prosocial involvement, and drug use and its consequences. The parent module helps the parents enhance parenting skills in areas such as monitoring and limit-setting, teaches them how to participate in their child's life outside of the family, and helps them learn how to rebuild emotional bonds with their adolescent. The family module works with the entire family to help them develop the motivation and skills to interact in more adaptive ways and rejuvenate their familial attachments. Finally, the extrafamilial module attempts to establish collaborative relationships among the various social systems with which the adolescent interacts. The core focus of each of the therapy sessions within these modules may cover a variety of subjects, such as the adolescent's developmental tasks and concerns, peer relations, involvement in legal and juvenile justice systems, and drug use as a way of coping with circumstances or psychological status.

MDFT is implemented by a clinical team that is comprised of one clinical supervisor for two to four therapists and may also include one to two case manager therapist assistants. The treatment length can vary, with one example of an intensive outpatient version of MDFT ranging between 16 and 25 sessions over 4 to 6 months, and another example of a less intensive version with twelve sessions over 3 months. MDFT has been implemented in over 16 sites throughout the United States, with clinical groups that have been comprised of ethnically and linguistically diverse adolescents at risk for abuse and/or abusing substances and their families, with ethnicities represented from White, African American, and Hispanic backgrounds. The parents of the adolescents who have been targeted in MDFT randomized controlled studies have had a range of economic and educational levels; however, the majority of families treated have been from disadvantaged inner-city communities. Adolescents treated in MDFT trials have ranged from high-risk early adolescents to multi-problem, juvenile justice-involved, dually diagnosed female and male adolescent substance abusers.

There are 10 clinical operating principles that create a framework for multidimensional family therapists to work from. These principles help guide the therapist as to what is prescribed and proscribed during the treatment process:

Principle 1: Adolescent drug abuse is a multidimensional phenomenon. This allows for MDFT clinical work to be guided by ecological and developmental research and perspectives.

Principle 2: Problem situations provide information and opportunity. Symptoms and problem situations provide assessment information and intervention opportunities to the therapists working on the case.

Principle 3: Change is multidetermined and multifaceted. Change comes from the effects of interaction among different systems, people, time periods, domains of functioning, and intra- and interpersonal processes, allowing a clinician to access multiple methods and paths to produce change.

Principle 4: Motivation is malleable. Not all of those who enter treatment are motivated to change and resistance to change may need to be understood as part of the therapy process.

Principle 5: Working relationships are critical. This points to the importance of making treatment possible through supportive and outcome-focused working relationships with familial and extrafamilial support systems while also working through relationship and life themes through therapeutic interactions.

Principle 6: Interventions are individualized. It is important for interventions to be customized according to each family seeking treatment in the program.

Principle 7: Planning and flexibility are two sides of the same therapeutic coin. This indicates the need for continuing evaluation on the part of the therapist as the intervention progresses to allow for changes to be made to the intervention plan if and when necessary.

Principle 8: Treatment and its multiple components are phasic. This explains the reason that the overall therapy process is organized and executed in stages, with progress in each area setting up the therapy for the next stage while still allowing for flexibility within the program.

Principle 9: Participation and motivation of those involved in therapy is a responsibility that belongs in large part to the therapist. It is the therapist's responsibility to provide, evaluate, and change the treatment as needed to prompt behavior change.

Principle 10: Therapist attitude and behavior are fundamental to success. Therapists should advocate for both the adolescent and the parent while understanding and using the therapists' own abilities to remain positive, creative, energetic, and committed despite whatever challenges may arise during therapy.

Through the process of understanding these 10 principles, therapists are able to be guided through the training and practice of MDFT.

Efficacy

MDFT has been tested in federally funded research projects since 1985, and this research has been able to provide evidence for the efficacy and effectiveness of MDFT for working with adolescent substance abuse. The studies have been conducted at several sites across the United States among adolescents ranging in ages from 11 to 18 across urban, suburban, and rural settings. MDFT studies include adolescent research participants who meet diagnostic criteria for substance use disorders, which are often comorbid with other problems such as delinquency and depression. MDFT has demonstrated superior outcomes relative to several other interventions such as cognitive behavioral therapy, family group therapy, peer group treatment, and comprehensive residential treatment when tested in six randomized controlled trials.

Five of the controlled clinical trials showed that substance use was reduced in MDFT to a significantly greater extent than all comparison treatments, with substance use decreasing 41% to 82% from intake to discharge. Also, both during the treatment and 12-month follow-up, youth taking part in MDFT showed higher rates of abstinence from substance use than those taking part in comparable treatments, with 56% showing abstinence from all substances and 64% showing either complete abstinence or substance use only once per month. At the 12-month follow-up, youth receiving MDFT showed a 58% reduction in marijuana use.

In addition to significantly reducing substance use, substance-related problems such as antisocial, delinquent, and externalizing behaviors were also significantly reduced. Among those treated with MDFT, school functioning was also seen to improve at higher rates than among those treated with other therapies. MDFT clients returned to school and earned passing grades 43% of the time as opposed to 17% of those treated with family therapy and 7% of those treated with peer group therapy. Family functioning and interaction has also been shown to improve at higher rates in MDFT when compared to family group or peer group therapy, and this improvement was maintained at 12-month follow-up.

MDFT has also been shown to work effectively as a community-based drug prevention program. In addition to the previously mentioned improvements, MDFT has demonstrated high effectiveness when used to treat youths with comorbid diagnoses and multiple impairments. MDFT is associated with decreased delinquent behavior and involvement with delinquent peers and reduced the likelihood of being arrested or placed on probation.

The average weekly cost of treatment with MDFT is significantly less than both community-based outpatient treatments and residential treatments. Training and treatment in MDFT is available in various locations throughout the United States, with research projects also currently taking place in Europe.

Nicole A. Kahhan, Katherine W. Follansbee,
and Gregory L. Stuart

See also Adolescents, Substance Abuse and Treatment; Brief Strategic Family Therapy; Cannabis Youth Treatment Study; Evidence-Based Treatment; Family Behavior Therapy; Family Therapy

Further Readings

Center for Treatment Research on Adolescent Drug Abuse. (2007). *Overview of multidimensional family therapy.* Retrieved December 20, 2007, from http://www.med .miami.edu/ctrada/x14.xml

Liddle, H. A. (2002). *Multidimensional family therapy.* Retrieved December 6, 2007, from http://www

.strengtheningfamilies.org/html/programs_1999/
10_MDFT.html

Liddle, H. A., Rodriguez, R. A., & Marvel, F. A. (2006). *Multidimensional family therapy* (MDFT): An effective treatment for adolescent substance abuse. Miami, FL: Center for Treatment Research on Adolescent Drug Abuse, University of Miami Miller School of Medicine.

SAMHSA model programs: Multidimensional family therapy. (2007). Retrieved December 6, 2007, from http://www .modelprograms.samhsa.gov/pdfs/model/multi.pdf